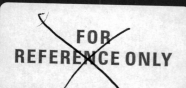

Thieme

Withdrawn

Ultrasound in Obstetrics and Gynecology

Volume 1: Obstetrics

WITHDRAWN

Eberhard Merz, M.D.
Professor and Director
Dept. of Obstetrics and Gynecology
Hospital Nordwest
Frankfurt/Main, Germany

Contributors

F. Bahlmann
G. Bernaschek
R. Bollmann
R. Chaoui
J. Deutinger
K.-H. Eichhorn
A.K. Ertan
F. Flock
D. Grab
J. Hartung
H.J. Hendrik
K. Kalache
S. Kupesic
A. Kurjak

E. Merz
H. Müntefering
I.J.M. Nijhuis
J.G. Nijhuis
H.-D. Rott
W. Schmidt
R. Terinde
U. Theile
B. Ulm
G. Weber
C. Welter
J. Wisser
H.-B. Wuermeling

1536 illustrations, most in color
213 tables

Second edition, fully revised

Thieme
Stuttgart · New York

Library of Congress Cataloging-in-Publication Data
is available from the publisher

1st German edition 1988
1st English edition 1991
1st Italian edition 1993
1st Spanish edition 1994

This book is an authorized and revised translation of Volume 2 of the 2nd German edition puplished and copyrighted 2002 by Georg Thieme Verlag, Stuttgart, Germany.
Titel of the German edition:
Sonographische Diagnostik in Gynäkologie und Geburtshilfe. Lehrbuch und Atlas in 2 Bänden. Band 2 Geburtshilfe.

Translator: Terry Telger, Waco, Texas, USA

Illustrators: Adrian Cornford, Reinheim-Zeilhard, Germany; Katharina Schumacher, Munich, Germany

© 2005 Georg Thieme Verlag
Rüdigerstraße 14, 70469 Stuttgart,
Germany
http://www.thieme.de
Thieme New York, 333 Seventh Avenue,
New York, NY 10001 USA
http://www.thieme.com

Typesetting: OADF Electronic Publishing, D-71155 Altdorf
Printed in Germany by Grammlich, Pliezhausen
ISBN 3-13-131882-1 (GTV)
ISBN 1-58890-147-5 (TNY)   1 2 3 4 5

Humanity owes its progress to the
dissatisfied.

— *Aldous Huxley*

For Christine, Beatrice and Véronique

WITHDRAWN

Contributors

Franz Bahlmann, MD
Priv. Doz.
Bürger Hospital
Dept. of Obstetrics and Gynecology
Frankfurt/Main, Germany

Gerhard Bernaschek, MD
Professor
General Hospital
University of Vienna
Dept. of Prenatal Diagnosis and Treatment
Vienna, Austria

Rainer Bollmann, MD
Professor
Humboldt University of Berlin
Campus Charité Mitte
Dept. of Prenatal Medicine
Berlin, Germany

Rabih Chaoui, MD
Professor
Humboldt University of Berlin
Campus Charité Mitte
Dept. of Prenatal Medicine
Berlin, Germany

Josef Deutinger, MD
Professor
General Hospital
University of Vienna
Dept. of Prenatal Diagnosis and Treatment
Vienna, Austria

Karl-Heinz Eichhorn, MD
Associate Professor
Weimar, Germany

A. Kubilay Ertan, MD
University of Homburg/S
Dept. of Obstetrics and Gynecology
Homburg/Saar, Germany

Felix Flock, MD
University of Ulm
Dept. of Obstetrics and Gynecology
Ulm, Germany

Dieter Grab, MD
Professor
Städtisches KH, München-Harlaching
Dept. of Obstetrics and Gynecology
Munich, Germany

John-Peter Hartung, MD
Prenatal Medicine and Ultrasound Practice
Berlin, Germany

Hans-Joachim Hendrik, MD
University of Homburg/S
Dept. of Obstetrics and Gynecology
Homburg/Saar, Germany

Karim Kalache, MD
Priv. Doz.
Humboldt University of Berlin
Campus Charité Mitte
Dept. of Prenatal Medicine
Berlin, Germany

Sanja Kupesic
Professor
Sveti Duh Hospital
Dept. of Obstetrics
University Medical School
Zagreb, Croatia

Asim Kurjak, MD
Professor
Sveti Duh Hospital
Dept. of Obstetrics
University Medical School
Zagreb, Croatia

Eberhard Merz, MD
Professor
Hospital Nordwest
Dept. of Obstetrics and Gynecology
Frankfurt/Main, Germany

Horst Müntefering, MD
Professor
University of Mainz
Dept. of Pediatric Pathology
Mainz, Germany

Ilse J. M. Nijhuis, MD
Professor
Medisch Spectrum Twente
Dept. of Pediatrics
Enschede, Netherlands

Jan G. Nijhuis, MD
Professor
Academic Hospital Maastricht
Dept. of Obstetrics and Gynecology
Maastricht, Netherlands

Hans-Dieter Rott, MD
Professor
Institute for Human Genetics
University of Erlangen-Nuremberg
Erlangen, Germany

Werner Schmidt, MD
Professor
University of Homburg/S
Dept. of Obstetrics and Gynecology
Homburg/Saar, Germany

Rainer Terinde, MD
Professor
University of Ulm
Dept. of Obstetrics and Gynecology
Ulm, Germany

Ursel Theile, MD
Professor
Institute for Human Genetics
Genetic Counseling Center
Johannes Gutenberg University Mainz
Mainz, Germany

Barbara Ulm, MD
Professor
General Hospital
University of Vienna
Dept. of Prenatal Diagnosis and Treatment
Vienna, Austria

Gerald Weber, MD
Prenatal Medicine and Ultrasound Practice
Mannheim, Germany

Christoph Welter, MD
Hospital Nordwest
Dept. of Gynecology
Frankfurt/Main, Germany

Josef Wisser, MD
Associate Professor
University of Zurich
Dept. of Obstetrics
Zurich, Switzerland

Hans-Bernhard Wuermeling, MD
Professor
Institute for Medical Law
University of Erlangen-Nuremberg
Erlangen, Germany

Preface to the Second Edition

When I. Donald, J. MacVicar, and T. G. Brown published the first obstetric ultrasound images in *Lancet* in 1958, they could not have envisioned the tremendous advances and extensive use that diagnostic ultrasound would achieve in prenatal diagnosis during subsequent decades. The basic evolution of diagnostic ultrasound has been from A-mode to B-mode scanning, then to real-time 2-D imaging and color Doppler sonography, and finally to real-time 3-D ultrasound technology. This progress has included many smaller but no less important evolutionary steps, such as advances in transducer designs and innovations in computer hardware and software. Today we have at our disposal a sophisticated sonographic technology that not only provides an increasingly detailed look at embryonic and fetal development and physiology but also permits the early detection of numerous pathologic conditions. As a result, the ultrasound examination has become an indispensable part of prenatal diagnosis and treatment.

Given the broad range of developments in ultrasound technology, it is not surprising that the number of publications dealing with ultrasonography have reached startling proportions. This has made it difficult even for specialists in obstetric ultrasound to keep abreast of the latest developments.

This second edition of *Ultrasound in Gynecology and Obstetrics* is designed to provide the prenatal diagnostician with a comprehensive, up-to-date review of transvaginal and abdominal sonography as they are applied to obstetrics. Besides offering copious information and illustrations, each chapter concludes with an extensive list of bibliographic references. As in the gynecologic volume, sonographic images in this volume are matched with clinical photographs so that the observer can gain a clearer appreciation of pathologic findings. This edition also gives special attention to biometry, providing growth charts and an appendix with tables listing the normal values that are most relevant to prenatal diagnosis.

The combined efforts of 26 contributors have resulted in a textbook and atlas that will familiarize hospital and office practitioners with the current applications of the various ultrasound techniques used in prenatal diagnosis and treatment while also guiding physicians in the sound and discriminating clinical use of these techniques.

I express thanks to all of my coauthors, who have contributed decisively to the success of this book. I also thank Dr. J. Bohl (Dept. of Neuropathology, University of Mainz) for preparing the pathoanatomic brain sections, Prof. H. Müntefering (head of the Dept. of Pediatric Pathology, University of Mainz) for providing various images of pathologic conditions, Prof. J. W. Spranger (executive director of the Mainz University Pediatric Hospital) for his help in reviewing the nomenclature for fetal limb anomalies, and Prof. S. Wellek (director of Mannheim Central Institute, Dept. of Biostatistics) for his extensive help in constructing growth charts and tables.

I am grateful to my secretary, Mrs. I. Künstler, for her help in the preparation of this book.

Finally, I am honored to thank Mr. Albrecht Hauff, the president of Thieme Medical Publishers, for the splendid production work that has gone into this book. I am also indebted to the staff at Thieme. Dr. Markus Becker (program planning), Dr. Antje Schönpflug (editorial), and Mr. Rolf-Dieter Zeller (production) worked with great understanding of my concepts and wishes in bringing this second edition to a successful completion.

Mainz, Summer, 2004

E. Merz

Abbreviations

AAPSS	= American Academy of Pediatrics Surgical Survey		**D-TGA**	= dextro-transposition of the great arteries
ABCD	= airway, breathing, circulation, differential diagnosis		**ECG**	= electrocardiography, electrocardiogram
AC	= abdominal circumference		**ECHO**	= enteric cytopathic human orphan
AChE	= acetylcholinesterase		**EUROCAT**	= European Union Registry of Congenital Anomalies and Twins
ACOG	= American College of Obstetricians and Gynecologists		**FHR**	= fetal heart rate
ADAM	= amniotic deformity, adhesions, mutilations		**FHRP**	= fetal heart rate pattern
ADPKD	= autosomal-dominant polycystic kidney disease		**FL**	= femur length
AEDF	= absent end-diastolic flow		**FISH**	= fluorescence in-situ hybridization
AFI	= amniotic fluid index		**FI**	= fibula
AFP	= alpha-fetoprotein		**FTA-ABS**	= fluorescence treponemal antibody absorption (test)
AGS	= adrenogenital syndrome		**GEPH**	= gestational edema, proteinuria, and hypertension
AMC	= arthrogryposis multiplex congenita		**GIFT**	= gamete intrafallopian transfer
ANF	= atrial natriuretic factor		**HC**	= head circumference
Ao	= Aorta		**hCG**	= human chorionic gonadotropin
AP	= anteroposterior		**β-hCG**	= β-human chorionic gonadotropin
ARPKD	= autosomal-recessive polycystic kidney disease		**Hct**	= hematocrit
ASD	= abdominal sagittal diameter; atrial septal defect		**HELLP**	= hemolysis, elevated liver enzymes, and low platelet count (syndrome)
AT	= acceleration time		**HIV**	= human immunodeficiency virus
ATD	= abdominal transverse diameter		**HLA**	= human leukocyte antigen
AV	= atrioventricular		**HLHS**	= hypoplastic left heart syndrome
AVP	= arginine vasopressin		**HSV**	= herpes simplex virus
AVSD	= atrioventricular septal defect		**ICSI**	= intracytoplasmic sperm injection
BPD	= biparietal diameter		**ICU**	= intensive-care unit
BTC	= bony thoracic circumference		**IFMSS**	= International Fetal Medicine and Surgery Society
BTSD	= bony thoracic sagittal diameter		**IPIR**	= intercostal-to-phrenic inhibitory reflex
BTTD	= bony thoracic transverse diameter		**IPKD**	= infantile polycystic kidney disease
BV	= bladder volume		I_{spta}	= spatial peak temporal average intensity
CATCH 22	= cardiac defects, abnormal facies, thymic hypoplasia, cleft palate, hypocalcemia (caused by defects in chromosome 22)		**IUD**	= intrauterine device
			IUFD	= intrauterine fetal death
CAVSD	= complete atrioventricular septal defect		**IUGR**	= intrauterine growth retardation
CCAM	= congenital cystic adenomatoid malformation		**i.v.**	= intravenous
CCHB	= complete congenital heart block		**IVC**	= inferior vena cava
CHAOS	= congenital high airway obstruction syndrome		**IVF**	= in-vitro fertilization
CMV	= cytomegalovirus		**IVF/ET**	= in-vitro fertilization/embryo transfer
CNS	= central nervous system		**IVS**	= interventricular septum
COFS	= cerebro-oculofacioskeletal syndrome		**LCM**	= lymphocytic choriomeningitis
CPM	= confined placental mosaicism		**LD**	= lung diameter
CRL	= crown-rump length		**LD/BTC**	= ratio of lung diameter and bony thoracic circumference
CRP	= C-reactive protein		**LGA**	= large for gestational age
CSF	= cerebrospinal fluid		**LSVC**	= left superior vena cava
CT	= computed tomography		**L-TGA**	= levo-transposition of the great arteries
CT ratio	= ratio of cardiac and thoracic diameters		**LV**	= left ventricle
CTA ratio	= ratio of cardiac and thoracic areas		**MCV**	= mean corpuscular volume
CTG	= cardiotocography, cardiotocogram		**MI**	= mechanical index
CVS	= chorionic villus sampling		**MIS**	= minimally invasive surgery
CW	= continuous wave		**MRI**	= magnetic resonance imaging
DA	= ductus arteriosus		**MSAFP**	= maternal serum alpha-fetoprotein
DEGUM	= Deutsche Gesellschaft für Ultraschall in der Medizin (German Society for Ultrasound in Medicine)		**MTX**	= methotrexate
			Nd:YAG	= neodymium-yttrium aluminum garnet
DOLV	= double-outlet left ventricle		**NIHF**	= nonimmune hydrops fetalis
DORV	= double-outlet right ventricle		**NSE**	= neuron-specific enolase

NT	=	nuchal translucency
ODS	=	Online Display Standard
OEIS	=	omphalocele, exstrophy, imperforate anus, spinal defects
OFD	=	occipitofrontal diameter
PA	=	pulmonary atresia
PA/IVS	=	pulmonary atresia with an intact ventricular septum
PAPP-A	=	pregnancy-associated plasma protein-A
PAPVR	=	partial anomalous pulmonary venous return
PCD	=	power color Doppler
PCR	=	polymerase chain reaction
PGE$_2$	=	prostaglandin E$_2$
PGI$_2$	=	prostaglandin I$_2$ (prostacyclin)
PI	=	pulsatility index
PIH	=	pregnancy-induced hypertension
PLA$_1$	=	phospholipase A$_1$
PLSVC	=	persistent left superior vena cava
PND	=	prenatal diagnosis
PRF	=	pulse repetition frequency
PSVT	=	paroxysmal supraventricular tachycardia
PT	=	pulmonary trunk
Ra	=	radius
RA	=	Right atrium
RADIUS	=	Routine Antenatal Diagnostic Imaging Ultrasound Study
REM	=	rapid eye movement
RF	=	reverse flow
RI	=	resistance index
ROI	=	region of interest
RV	=	right ventricle
SCID	=	severe combined immunodeficiency
SD	=	standard deviation
SGA	=	small for gestational age
SLE	=	systemic lupus erythematosus
SPTA	=	spatial peak temporal average
STIC	=	spatial-temporal image correlation
T$_3$	=	triiodothyronine
T$_4$	=	thyroxine
TA	=	tricuspid atresia
TAC	=	truncus arteriosus communis
TAPVD	=	total anomalous pulmonary venous drainage
TAPVR	=	total anomalous pulmonary venous return
TBII	=	thyrotropin-binding inhibitory immunoglobulin
TC	=	thoracic circumference
TCD	=	transverse cerebellar diameter
TDE	=	tissue Doppler echocardiography
TGA	=	transposition of the great arteries
Ti	=	tibia
TI	=	thermal index
TIB	=	thermal index for bone
TIC	=	thermal index for cranium
TIS	=	thermal index for soft tissues
TOF	=	tetralogy of Fallot
TORCH	=	toxoplasmosis, other infections, rubella, cytomegalovirus infections and herpes simplex virus
TP-ELISA	=	Treponema pallidum enzyme-linked immunosorbent assay
TPHA	=	Treponema pallidum hemagglutination (test)
TR	=	trachea
TRAP	=	twin reversed arterial perfusion
TSD	=	thoracic sagittal diameter

TSH	=	thyroid-stimulating hormone
TSI	=	thyroid-stimulating immunoglobulin
TTD	=	thoracic transverse diameter
TV	=	transfusion volume
TXA$_2$	=	thromboxane A$_2$
UI	=	ulna
V/H ratio	=	ventricular-hemispheric ratio
VACTERL	=	vertebral defects, anal atresia, cardiac anomalies, tracheoesophageal fistula with esophageal atresia, renal dysplasia, and limb anomalies
VATER	=	vertebral defects, imperforate anus, tracheoesophageal fistula, and radial and renal dysplasia
V$_{mean}$	=	mean flow velocity
VSD	=	ventricular septal defect

WITHDRAWN

Contents

Ultrasound in Obstetrics ... 1

1 Ultrasound Applications and Examination Techniques in Obstetrics ... 2
E. Merz

Minimum Equipment Requirements ... 2
Transvaginal Ultrasound ... 2
Abdominal Ultrasound ... 3

2 Ultrasound Screening ... 8
E. Merz und K.-H. Eichhorn

Prenatal Care ... 8
Ultrasound Screening ... 9
Targeted Imaging in High-Risk Pregnancies ... 14

3 Normal Early Pregnancy (First Trimester) ... 17
J. Wisser

Pregnancy Dating ... 17
Technique of Transvaginal Ultrasound ... 17
Ultrasound Embryology ... 17

4 Transvaginal Biometry and Gestational Age Assignment in the First Trimester ... 26
F. Bahlmann und E. Merz

Biometry ... 26
Gestational Age Assignment ... 28

5 Abnormalities of Early Pregnancy ... 32
E. Merz

Diagnostic Approach ... 32
Spontaneous Abortion ... 32
Molar Pregnancy and Choriocarcinoma ... 36
Ectopic Pregnancy ... 36
Less Common Forms of Ectopic Pregnancy ... 38

6 Transvaginal Detection of Fetal Anomalies ... 45
E. Merz

Detection of Fetal Anomalies in the First Trimester ... 45
Detection of Fetal Anomalies in the Second and Third Trimesters ... 46

7 Transvaginal Ultrasound of Maternal Disorders ... 49
E. Merz und G. Weber

Transvaginal Diagnosis of Uterine and Adnexal Masses in Pregnancy ... 49
Cervical Incompetence ... 49
Placental Localization in Placenta Previa ... 50
Evaluating the Postpartum Uterus ... 50

8 Pelvimetry with Transvaginal Ultrasound ... 55
J. Deutinger

Cephalopelvic Disproportion ... 55
X-Ray Pelvimetry ... 55
Ultrasound Pelvimetry ... 55

Abdominal Ultrasound ... 59

9 Normal Early Pregnancy, Biometry, and Gestational Age Assignment in the First Trimester ... 60
E. Merz

Basic Principles of Embryology ... 60
Pregnancy Detection by Abdominal Ultrasound ... 60
Development in the First Trimester ... 61
Biometry and Gestational Age Assignment in the First Trimester ... 61
Summary of Key Parameters ... 62

10 Abnormalities in the First Trimester ... 67
E. Merz

Spontaneous Abortion ... 67
Early Pregnancy with an IUD in Place ... 68
Molar Pregnancy ... 68
Choriocarcinoma ... 68
Ectopic Pregnancy ... 73
Early Detection of Fetal Anomalies in the First Trimester ... 78
Adnexal Masses and Uterine Fibroids in Early Pregnancy ... 78

11 Normal Ultrasound Anatomy of the Fetus in the Second and Third Trimesters ... 81
E. Merz

Head ... 81
Spinal Column ... 90
Neck Region K. Kalache und R. Bollmann ... 93
Thorax ... 97
Circulatory System (Fetal Circulation) ... 100
Heart R. Chaoui ... 106
Abdomen ... 122
Urinary Tract, Adrenal Glands, and Pelvis ... 126
Genitalia ... 129
Limbs ... 132

12 Fetal Biometry in the Second and Third Trimesters ... 139
E. Merz

Prerequisites ... 139
Basic Biometry ... 140
Extended Biometry (Organ Biometry) ... 142

13 Gestational Age Assignment in the Second and Third Trimesters ... *161*

E. Merz

Importance of Estimating Gestational Age ... *161*
Curves for Estimating Gestational Age ... *161*

14 Fetal Weight Estimation ... *163*

E. Merz

Importance of Fetal Weight Estimation ... *163*
Normal Curves and Definitions ... *163*
Ultrasound Estimation of Fetal Weight ... *163*

15 Fetal Behavior ... *168*

J.G. Nijhuis and I.J.M. Nijhuis

Fetal Behavioral Patterns and States in Detail ... *168*
Clinical Applications ... *171*
Fetal Neurology ... *171*
Conclusion ... *171*

16 Fetal Growth Disturbances in the Second and Third Trimesters ... *175*

E. Merz

Error in Dates ... *175*
Intrauterine Growth Retardation ... *175*
Macrosomia, Macrocephaly ... *177*

17 Immune Fetal Hydrops Due to Rhesus Incompatibility ... *184*

B. Ulm and G. Bernaschek

Occurrence, Pathogenesis, and Ultrasound Features ... *184*
Diagnosis ... *185*
Prognosis and Treatment ... *186*

18 Nonimmune Hydrops Fetalis (NIHF) ... *188*

J. Hartung and R. Bollmann

Occurrence, Pathogenesis, and Ultrasound Features ... *188*
Diseases Associated with NIHF ... *189*
Diagnosis ... *193*
Prognosis and Treatment ... *193*
Fetal Ascites ... *194*

19 Intrauterine Fetal Death ... *200*

E. Merz

Ultrasound Detection ... *200*
Intrauterine Fetal Death in Multiple Pregnancy ... *202*
Obstetric Management and Subsequent Pregnancy ... *202*

Ultrasound Examination of Fetal Anomalies ... *203*

20 General Detection of Fetal Anomalies ... *204*

H. Müntefering and E. Merz

Basic Principles ... *204*
General Ultrasound Diagnosis of Fetal Anomalies ... *207*
Implications of Suggestive Signs or a Detected Fetal Anomaly ... *208*

21 Anomalies of the Head ... *212*

E. Merz

Neural Tube Defects ... *212*
CNS Anomalies ... *217*
Facial Anomalies ... *234*

22 Anomalies of the Neck ... *246*

K. Kalache and R. Bollmann

Neoplasms ... *246*
Functional Impairment ... *248*
Conclusion ... *249*

23 Spina Bifida ... *253*

E. Merz

Occurrence, Pathogenesis, and Ultrasound Features ... *253*
Ultrasound Forms ... *254*
Diagnosis ... *255*
Prognosis and Prenatal Management ... *255*

24 Thoracic Anomalies ... *261*

E. Merz

Pulmonary Hypoplasia ... *261*
Hydrothorax, Chylothorax ... *261*
CCAM ... *262*
Bronchogenic Cysts ... *262*
Pulmonary Sequestration ... *263*
Diaphragmatic Hernia ... *263*
Pentalogy of Cantrell ... *264*

25 Anomalies and Diseases of the Fetal Heart ... *270*

R. Chaoui

Epidemiology and Indications for Fetal Echocardiography ... *270*
Prognosis of Cardiac Anomalies ... *271*
From Symptom to Diagnosis ... *271*
Specific Cardiac Anomalies and Diseases ... *273*
Fetal Arrhythmias ... *290*

26 Anomalies of the Gastrointestinal Tract and Anterior Abdominal Wall ... *297*

E. Merz

Atresias ... *297*
Meconium-Related Diseases ... *300*
Situs Inversus ... *301*
Ventral Abdominal Wall Defects ... *301*
Ultrasound Abnormalities of the Liver, Gallbladder, and Spleen ... *307*

27 Anomalies and Diseases of the Kidneys and Urinary Tract ... 312

R. Terinde and F. Flock

Embryology of the Kidneys ... 312
Incidence of Anomalies and Associated Anomalies ... 312
Ultrasound Survey ... 312
Diseases of the Kidneys ... 314

28 Genital Anomalies ... 329

E. Merz

Genital Anomalies in the Male Fetus ... 329
Hermaphroditism ... 329
Genital Anomalies in the Female Fetus ... 330

29 Sacrococcygeal Teratoma ... 333

G. Weber and E. Merz

30 Anomalies of the Extremities ... 336

E. Merz

Osteochondrodysplasias (Skeletal Dysplasias) ... 337
Fatal Skeletal Dysplasias ... 337
Nonfatal Skeletal Dysplasias ... 344
Limb Defects ... 349
Positional Abnormalities or Restricted Motion of
Fetal Limbs ... 353

31 Disorders and Anomalies of the Skin ... 359

E. Merz

Cutaneous Edema ... 359
Cutaneous Tumors ... 359
Hyperechoic Focal Skin Changes ... 360
Bullous Skin Changes ... 360
Hyperkeratotic Skin Disorders ... 360

32 General and Specific Ultrasound Suggestive Signs of Fetal Chromosome Abnormalities ... 363

B. Ulm and G. Bernaschek

General Suggestive Ultrasound Signs of Chromosomal
Abnormalities ... 363
Specific Ultrasound Suggestive Signs of Chromosomal
Abnormalities ... 370
Phenotypic Expression of Common Chromosomal
Abnormalities ... 371

33 Ultrasound Features of Infectious Diseases in Pregnancy ... 375

D. Grab and R. Terinde

The Most Common Infectious Diseases ... 376
Differential Diagnosis of the Most Common Ultrasound Features
of Infectious Diseases ... 381

Ultrasound of the Placenta, Umbilical Cord, and Amniotic Fluid ... 387

34 Placenta ... 388

E. Merz and G. Weber

Normal Placenta ... 388
Placental Abnormalities ... 393

35 Umbilical Cord ... 404

G. Weber and E. Merz

Normal Umbilical Cord ... 404
Abnormalities of the Umbilical Cord ... 404

36 Amniotic Fluid ... 409

G. Weber and E. Merz

Physiology and Pathophysiology ... 409
Ultrasound Assessment of Amniotic Fluid Volume ... 409

Ultrasound in Multiple Pregnancy ... 415

37 Multiple Pregnancies ... 416

E. Merz and C. Welter

Special Features of Multiple Pregnancies ... 416
Ultrasound of Multiple Pregnancy in the First Trimester ... 418
Ultrasound of Multiple Pregnancy in the Second and
Third Trimesters ... 423
Summary of the Management of Multiple Pregnancies ... 432

Maternal Ultrasound ... 437

38 Diagnosis of Maternal Disorders by Abdominal Ultrasound ... 438

E. Merz

Cervical Incompetence ... 438
Uterine Leiomyomas during Pregnancy ... 438
Pain during Pregnancy ... 438
Ultrasound Diagnosis of Symphyseal Distension during
Pregnancy ... 439

39 Abdominal Ultrasound in the Puerperium ... 443

E. Merz and G. Weber

Uterine Involution ... 443
Complications in the Puerperium ... 443
Follow-Up of Cesarean Section ... 443
Trauma to the Pelvic Floor ... 443

Doppler Ultrasound ... 447

40 Basic Principles of Doppler Ultrasound ... 448
F. Bahlmann

Historical Development ... 448
Basic Concepts ... 448
Doppler Techniques ... 449
Equipment-Related Factors that Affect the
Doppler Spectrum ... 449
Effects of Examination Technique on the
Doppler Spectrum ... 454
Newer Methods of Color Imaging ... 455

41 Hemodynamic Evaluation of Early Pregnancy ... 458
A. Kurjak and S. Kupesic

Normal Early Pregnancy ... 458
Early Pregnancy Loss ... 464

42 Uteroplacental Circulation ... 469
F. Bahlmann

Development of the Uteroplacental Vascular System ... 469
Doppler Ultrasound of the Uteroplacental Vessels ... 469
Clinical Significance of Uterine Doppler Ultrasound ... 471

43 Fetal Circulation ... 481
F. Bahlmann

Aspects of Fetal Physiology ... 481
Doppler Ultrasound of the Arterial System ... 481
Indications for Doppler Ultrasound ... 497

44 Perinatal Abnormalities and Fetal Outcome in Cases with Severely Abnormal Doppler-Flow Findings in the Umbilical Artery and Fetal Aorta ... 507
A.K. Ertan, H.J. Hendrik and W. Schmidt

High-Risk Pregnancies ... 507
Absent End-Diastolic Flow and Reverse Flow ... 507
Pathoanatomic Changes and Technical Issues ... 507
Clinical Results of AEDF and RF in the Umbilical Artery and/or Fetal Aorta ... 508
Summary ... 511

3-D Ultrasound ... 515

45 3-D Ultrasound in Prenatal Diagnosis ... 516
E. Merz

Capabilities of 3-D Ultrasound ... 516
Technique of Transvaginal and Abdominal 3-D Ultrasound ... 516
Problems with 3-D Ultrasound ... 519
Critical Appraisal and Outlook ... 520

Invasive Diagnosis and Treatment in Pregnancy ... 529

46 Invasive Prenatal Diagnosis ... 530
E. Merz

Amniocentesis ... 530
Chorionic Villus Sampling ... 533
Placental Biopsy in the Second and Third Trimesters ... 534
Cordocentesis ... 536
Percutaneous Procedures in the Fetus ... 539
Fetoscopy ... 539
Amnioinfusion ... 541

47 Fetal Therapy and Treatment of Abnormal Amniotic Fluid Volume ... 544
E. Merz

Fetal Therapy ... 544
Treatment of Abnormal Amniotic Fluid Volume ... 555

Safety and Genetic and Ethical Aspects of Prenatal Ultrasound Diagnosis ... 559

48 Safety Aspects of Diagnostic Ultrasound in Pregnancy ... 560
H.-D. Rott

Historical Development ... 560
Risk Assessment for Various Ultrasound Procedures ... 560
Safety Indices ... 561
Conclusions and Recommendations ... 563

49 Genetic Counseling for a Fetal Anomaly ... 564
U. Theile

Aims of Genetic Counseling ... 564
Counseling in Various Disorders ... 565
Conclusions ... 568

50 Ethical Considerations in Obstetric Ultrasound ... 572
H.-B. Wuermeling

Value System ... 572
Principles ... 572
Prenatal Diagnosis ... 575
Prenatal Therapy and Medical Experimentation ... 575

Appendix ... 577

51 Biometry Curves and Tables ... 578
E. Merz

Index ... 617

WITHDRAWN

Ultrasound in Obstetrics

WITHDRAWN

Ultrasound in Obstetrics

1 Ultrasound Applications and Examination Techniques in Obstetrics

Withdrawn

Noninvasive and without radiation risk, ultrasound is an ideal imaging modality in pregnancy. Owing to the tremendous evolution of ultrasound technology in recent years, we now have at our disposal a range of sophisticated techniques. The use of a particular technique will depend on the age of the pregnancy and the nature of the investigation. The available options include abdominal and transvaginal 2-D imaging, M-mode studies, Doppler and color Doppler, power color Doppler, and 3-D ultrasound.

Minimum Equipment Requirements

Real-time scanner. Modern ultrasound examinations in pregnancy require at least a real-time scanner with an abdominal transducer operating in the frequency range of 3–5 MHz and calibrated to a sound velocity of 1540 m/s. The transducer should provide an image width of 9.5 cm at a depth of 6 cm, and the system should provide at least 16 levels of gray (International Electrotechnical Commission [IEC] standard 1157). Documentation equipment should consist of a Polaroid or 35-mm camera, a video printer, or a video cassette recorder.

Vaginal transducer. A vaginal transducer is recommended for examinations in early pregnancy, although it is not essential. All ultrasound systems currently marketed for use in obstetrics and gynecology come equipped with an endovaginal transducer.

Transvaginal Ultrasound

▬ *Applications*

First trimester. Transvaginal ultrasound is used predominantly in the first trimester of pregnancy (1, 4, 8, 9, 14, 15, 16, 18, 20, 22, 24, 26, 28, 30). It can be used at this stage for the early detection of an intact or abnormal intrauterine pregnancy (especially in a retroflexed uterus whose cavity is more distant from the abdominal wall), the early diagnosis of multiple gestation, ectopic pregnancy (7, 23, 29), and fetal anomalies (25). Early transvaginal scanning is also used for the investigation of uterine anomalies (25) and uterine or adnexal masses (Table 1.1).

Late pregnancy. Transvaginal ultrasound is used much less often in late pregnancy, but it still has selected applications. These include the investigation of deeply situated fetal structures that are not accessible to abdominal scans (e.g., head and brain structures) (2), transvaginal Doppler ultrasound of the uterine artery (11), pelvimetry (10), the evaluation of cervical insufficiency (6, 12, 21, 27), precise evaluation of the internal cervical os to exclude placenta previa (13, 17), and the investigation of uterine bleeding or a mass in the cul-de-sac (Table 1.1).

Advantages. One advantage of transvaginal ultrasound is that it does not require a full bladder for examinations during early pregnancy. It also provides higher image resolution than abdominal ultrasound, as the structures of interest are always scanned within the focal zone of

Table 1.1 Applications of transvaginal ultrasound in early and late pregnancy

Early pregnancy
Detection of intact early pregnancy, especially in a retroflexed uterus
Early diagnosis of multiple pregnancy
Investigation of abnormal early pregnancy
Detection or exclusion of ectopic pregnancy
Early detection of fetal anomalies
Detection of uterine anomalies
Investigation of a pelvic mass

Late pregnancy
Fetal structures not accessible to abdominal scan
Late detection of fetal anomalies
Investigation of oligohydramnios
Pelvimetry
Diagnosis of cervical insufficiency in the second or third trimester
Investigation of placenta previa or low-lying placenta
Investigation of uterine bleeding
Investigation of a pelvic mass
Doppler ultrasound of the uterine artery

Table 1.2 Advantages and disadvantages of transvaginal ultrasound in relation to transabdominal ultrasound (adapted from 18)

Advantages
➢ The examination is performed with an empty bladder, offering several advantages: • Patient can be examined at any time • No waits or delays • Permits optimum comparison with palpable findings • Examination time is not limited by painful bladder distension • Examination can be done in patients who cannot fill their bladder completely
➢ Sharper image resolution than abdominal scans, since the pelvic organs are always within the focal zone of the transducer (especially with a retroflexed uterus)
➢ Image quality not compromised by bowel loops, obesity, or abdominal wall scars
➢ Panoramic scan gives a wide-angle view of the lower pelvis.

Disadvantages
➢ Unaccustomed viewing angle requires reorientation when imaging pelvic organs.
➢ The mid- and upper abdomen cannot be scanned transvaginally, so the method (aside from special detail studies) is not useful for the routine monitoring of fetal growth and anatomy in the second and third trimesters.
➢ High-sited ovarian tumors are not accessible to transvaginal scans in late pregnancy.

the transducer (3, 18) (Table 1.2). This is particularly advantageous in patients with a retroflexed uterus.

Disadvantages. Disadvantages of transvaginal ultrasound are that it displays the pelvic organs from a different perspective than abdominal ultrasound, and it has a limited scanning range in the cephalad direction. This may preclude the use of transvaginal scanning after the uterus has reached a certain size or may limit its use to specialized studies (Table 1.2).

Vaginal Transducers

Ultrasound transducers with various frequencies, scanning angles, and fields of view are available for transvaginal use (Fig. 1.**1**). Probes with a larger field of view provide a broader display of the internal genitalia. Most vaginal probes in current use operate at a frequency of 5–7.5 MHz and have a 120° field of view. A mechanical panoramic end-fire transducer offers the largest viewing angle of 240°. While this probe affords a wide-angle survey of the internal genitalia, it does not permit color Doppler imaging, which requires an electronic transducer.

Transvaginal Examination

Condom. Prior to the examination, the vaginal probe is sheathed with a condom that contains some coupling gel. The condom should be of the non-reservoir type, since air bubbles could collect in the reservoir and interfere with imaging. The outside of the condom is wetted with ultrasound gel or NaCl to lubricate the probe and improve acoustic coupling.

Patient position. As in gynecology, transvaginal ultrasound in obstetrics can be performed either in a gynecologic examination chair or on an ordinary examination table with the patient supine (Fig. 1.**2**). With the patient's legs flexed and slightly abducted, the probe is carefully inserted into the vagina and advanced just to the cervix.

Scanning sequence. The examination starts with a longitudinal midsagittal scan to establish orientation (Fig. 1.**3**). By raising and lowering the probe (Fig. 1.**4**) and angling it from side to side (Fig. 1.**3**), the examiner can explore the entire lower pelvis in various planes of section.

Image Orientation in Transvaginal Ultrasound

As in gynecology, the transvaginal image in obstetric patients should be displayed such that:
- a transvaginal image is clearly distinguishable from a transabdominal image, and
- a standard orientation system is used for superior/inferior, anterior/posterior, and left/right (5, 19).

The more superior structures should be displayed at the top of the transvaginal image in both sagittal and coronal scans (Table 1.**3**, Figs. 1.**5**, 1.**6**). In longitudinal scans, posterior structures should appear on the left side of the image and anterior structures on the right side (Table 1.**3**, Fig. 1.**5**).

Coronal scans should be anatomically oriented—i.e., structures on the anatomical right side of the lower pelvis should appear on the left side of the image, and structures on the left side should appear on the right (Table 1.**3**, Fig. 1.**6**).

Abdominal Ultrasound

Abdominal Examination

Full bladder. For abdominal ultrasound in early pregnancy, the maternal bladder should be well distended to displace bowel loops out of the lower pelvis and create an acoustic window for scanning the uterus and conceptus. By the end of the first trimester, the enlarging uterus has displaced the bowel so far cephalad that scanning can be performed with a full or empty bladder.

Abdominal ultrasound is performed routinely at the start of the second trimester. Vaginal ultrasound would be used in exceptional cases such as oligohydramnios, which can compromise abdominal scans, and for visualizing low fetal structures that are not accessible to transabdominal imaging (2).

Patient position. Normally the patient is positioned supine (Fig. 1.**7**). The lateral decubitus position may be preferable in late pregnancy to avoid a vena cava occlusion syndrome.

Scanning sequence. A routine abdominal examination starts with a longitudinal scan at the center of the lower abdomen (Fig. 1.**8**). This is followed by additional longitudinal, transverse (Fig. 1.**9**) and oblique scans (Figs. 1.**10**, 1.**11**) to obtain detailed views of the fetus (see Chapter 2 for further information).

Abdominal Transducers

Linear-array, curved-array or sector transducers can be used in obstetric abdominal ultrasound (Fig. 1.**12**). Less experienced examiners should use linear- or curved-array transducers. They are easier to manipulate, and it is easier to locate the desired scan plane than with a sector probe. At the same time, a sector probe require less manipulation to change from one scan plane to another, and the lateral pelvic regions are easier to examine with a sector probe. The standard frequency range of abdominal transducers is 3.5 to 5 MHz. In obese patients, initial scanning should be done with a 3.5-MHz probe for better penetration.

Image Orientation in Abdominal Ultrasound

As in gynecologic ultrasound, image orientation is an important consideration in obstetric abdominal ultrasound examinations (19).

Longitudinal scan. To ensure uniform orientation, the transducer should be positioned so that the superior portion of the uterus always appears on the left side of the longitudinal scan while the inferior portion is on the right side (Table 1.**4**). Thus, the fetal head always appears to the right of the trunk when the fetus is in a cephalic presentation (Fig. 1.**13**) and to the left of the trunk when the fetus is in a breech

Table 1.3   Image orientation in transvaginal ultrasound

Transvaginal sagittal scan	
Top of image	= superior (cranial)
Bottom of image	= inferior (caudal)
Right side of image	= anterior (ventral)
Left side of image	= posterior (dorsal)
Transvaginal coronal scan	
Top of image	= superior (cranial)
Bottom of image	= inferior (caudal)
Right side of image	= left
Left side of image	= right

Table 1.4   Image orientation in abdominal ultrasound

Abdominal sagittal scan	
Top of image	= anterior (ventral)
Bottom of image	= posterior (dorsal)
Right side of image	= inferior (caudal)
Left side of image	= superior (cranial)
Abdominal transverse scan	
Top of image	= anterior (ventral)
Bottom of image	= posterior (dorsal)
Right side of image	= left
Left side of image	= right

presentation (Fig. 1.**14**). In a dorsosuperior transverse lie, the fetal spine appears on the left side of the image (Fig. 1.**15**). In a dorsoinferior transverse lie, the spine appears on the right side.

Transverse scans. Transverse scans should have an anatomic orientation with the right side of the maternal abdomen appearing on the left side of the monitor and the maternal left side appearing on the right (Fig. 1.**16**). If the transducer placement is unclear, it can be checked by slipping a finger beneath the side of the probe and seeing if the finger appears on the correct side of the monitor. If not, the transducer should be rotated 180°.

Fetal position. For examinations in the second or third trimester, it is important to have a clear mental picture of the topographic position of the fetus, depending on whether the fetus is in a cephalic or breech presentation or transverse lie. This is necessary in order to detect abnormal positions of the fetal organs. In transverse scans, the spinal column of a vertex- or breech-presenting fetus will appear on the right side of the image in the first position and on the left side of the image in the second position.

Principal scan planes in the fetus. Three principal planes of section are distinguished in the fetus itself: sagittal, coronal, and transverse (axial) (Fig. 1.**17**). The scan planes necessary for evaluating the fetus are shown in Fig. 1.**18**.

Separate chapters are devoted to more specialized ultrasound techniques, including the various Doppler techniques and 3-D ultrasound.

References

1. Achiron, R., Achiron, A.: Transvaginal ultrasonic assessment of the early fetal brain. Ultrasound Obstet. Gynecol. 1 (1991) 336–344
2. Benacerraf, B., Estroff, J.A.: Transvaginal sonographic imaging of the low fetal head in the second trimester. J. Ultrasound Med. 8 (1989) 325–328
3. Bernaschek, G.: Vorteile der endosonographischen Diagnostik in Gynäkologie und Geburtshilfe. Geburtsh. u. Frauenheilk. 47 (1987) 471–475
4. Bernaschek, G., Deutinger, J., Kratochwil, A.: Endosonography in Obstetrics and Gynecology. Springer, Berlin 1989
5. Bernaschek, G., Deutinger, J.: Endosonography in obstetrics and gynecology: the importance of standardized image display. Obstet. Gynecol. 74 (1989) 817–820
6. Böhmer S., Degenhardt, F., Gerlach, C., Jagla, K., Schneider, J.: Vaginalsonographie versus vaginaler Tastbefund: Erste Erfahrungen bei 120 schwangeren Frauen mit Verdacht auf Zervixinsuffizienz. Z. Geburtsh. u. Perinat. 193 (1989) 115–123
7. Cacciatore, B., Stenman, U.H., Ylostalo, P.: Diagnosis of ectopic pregnancy by vaginal ultrasonography in combination with a discriminatory serum HCG level of 1000 IU/I (IRP). Brit. J. Obstet. Gynaecol. 7 (1990) 904–908
8. De Crespigny, L.C.: Early diagnosis of pregnancy failure with vaginal ultrasound. Amer. J. Obstet. Gynecol. 159 (1988) 408–409
9. Degenhardt, F.: Atlas der vaginalen Ultraschalldiagnostik. Edition Gynäkologie und Geburtsmedizin. Hrsg.: J. Schneider, H. Weitzel. Wissenschaftliche Verlagsgesellschaft, Stuttgart 1990
10. Deutinger J., Bernaschek, G.: Die vaginalsonographische Pelvimetrie als neue Methode zur sonographischen Bestimmung der inneren Beckenmaße. Geburtsh. u. Frauenheilk. 46 (1986) 345–347
11. Deutinger J., Rudelstorfer, R., Bernaschek, G.: Vaginosonographic velocimetry of both main uterine arteries by visual vessel recognition and pulsed Doppler method during pregnancy. Amer. J. Obstet. Gynecol. 159 (1988) 1072–1076
12. Eppel, W., Schurz, B., Frigo, P., Reinold, E.: Vaginosonographische Beobachtung des zervikalen Verschlußapparates unter besonderer Berücksichtigung der Parität. Geburtsh. u. Frauenheilk. 52 (1992) 148–151
13. Farine, D., Fox, H., Jakobson, S., Timor-Tritsch, I.E.: Vaginal ultrasound for diagnosis of placenta praevia. Amer. J. Obstet. Gynecol. 159 (1988) 566–569
14. Holzgreve, W., Westendorp, J., Tercanli, S., Schneider, H.P.G.: Ultraschalluntersuchungen in der Frühschwangerschaft. Ultraschall in Med. 12 (1991) 99–110
15. Krone, S., Wisser, J., Strowitzki, Th.: Anatomie des menschlichen Embryos im vaginalsonographischen Bild. Ultraschall Klin. Prax. 4 (1989) 205–209
16. Levi, C.S., Lyons, E.A., Linsay, D.J.: Early diagnosis of nonviable pregnancy with endovaginal US. Radiology 167 (1988) 383–385
17. Lim, B.H., Tan, C.E., Smith, A.P.M., Smith, N.C.: Transvaginal ultrasonography for diagnosis of placenta praevia. Lancet 1 (1989) 444
18. Merz, E.: Transvaginale oder transabdominale Ultraschalldiagnostik? Ein Vergleich zweier Methoden in Gynäkologie und Geburtshilfe. Ultraschall Klin. Prax. 2 (1987) 87–94
19. Merz, E.: Standardisierung der Bilddarstellung bei der transvaginalen Sonographie. Gynäkologie und Geburtshilfe 1 (1991) 37–38
20. Merz, E.: Aktueller Stand der Vaginosonographie. Teil II: Geburtshilfliche Diagnostik, neue Aspekte und Zukunftsaussichten. Ultraschall in Med. 15 (1994) 52–59
21. Raga, F., Simon, C., Strasser, J., Bonilla-Musoles, F.: Abdominale, perineale und vaginale sonographische Diagnose der Zervikalinsuffizienz. Ultraschall in Med. 13 (1992) 24–27
22. Rempen, A.: Vaginale Sonographie der intakten Gravidität im ersten Trimenon. Geburtsh. u. Frauenheilk. 47 (1987) 477–482
23. Rempen, A.: Vaginal sonography in ectopic pregnancy. A prospective evaluation. J. Ultrasound Med. 7 (1988) 381–387
24. Rempen, A.: Vaginale Sonographie im ersten Trimenon. 1. Qualitative Parameter. Z. Geburtsh. u. Perinat. 195 (1991) 114–122
25. Rottem, S., Bronshtein, M.: Transvaginal sonographic diagnosis of congenital anomalies between 9 weeks and 16 weeks' menstrual age. J. clin. Ultrasound 18 (1990) 307–314
26. Schurz, B., Wenzel, R., Eppel, W., Schon, H.J., Reinold, E.: Die Bedeutung der Vaginosonographie in der Frühschwangerschaft. Geburtsh. Frauenheilk. 50 (1990) 848–849
27. Stolz, W., Balde, M.D., Unteregger, B., Wallwiener, D., Bastert, G.: Die Beurteilung der Zervix in der Schwangerschaft mit Hilfe der Vaginalsonographie. Untersuchungen zur Zervixinsuffizienz. Geburtsh. u. Frauenheilk. 49 (1989) 1063–1066
28. Timor-Tritsch, I.E., Farine, D., Rosen, M.G.: A close look at early embryonic development with the high-frequency transvaginal transducer. Am. J. Obstet. Gynecol. 159 (1988) 676–681
29. Timor-Tritsch, I.E., Yeh, M.N., Peisner, D.B., Lesser, K.B., Slavik, T.A.: The use of transvaginal ultrasonography in the diagnosis of ectopic pregnancy. Am. J. Obstet. Gynecol. 161 (1989) 157–161
30. Voigt, H.J., Faschingbauer, C.: Pränatale Diagnostik mit Hilfe der Vaginalsonographie. Ultraschall Klin. Prax. 4 (1989) 199–204

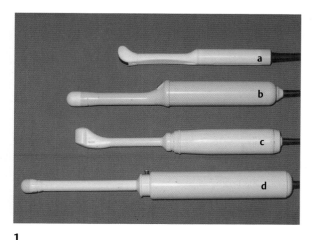

1

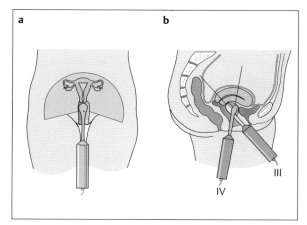

3

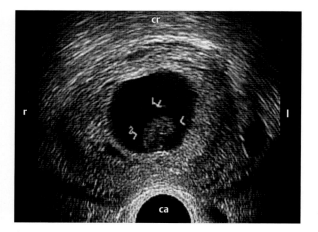

4

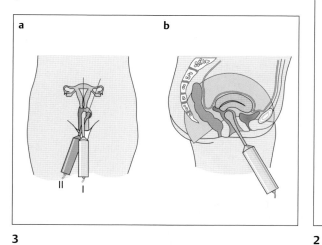

2

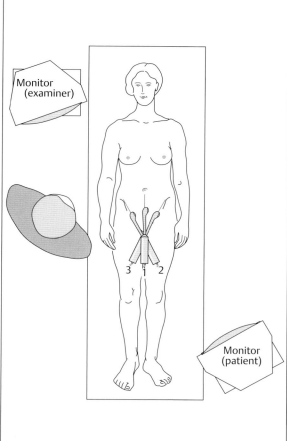

5

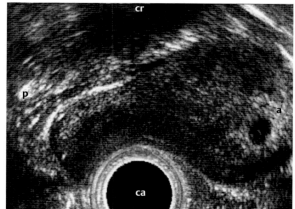

6

Transvaginal ultrasound

Fig. 1.**1**   Ultrasound probes for transvaginal use.
a , b Electronic end-fire probes.
c Mechanical panoramic end-fire probe.
d Mechanical side-fire probe (chiefly for endorectal use).

Fig. 1.**2**   Setup for transvaginal ultrasound on an examination table. The examiner sits to the left of the patient. Separate monitors are provided for the examiner and patient.
1 = Midsagittal scan,
2, 3 = Oblique scans through the lower pelvis.

Fig. 1.**3**   Schematic representation of longitudinal scan planes in transvaginal ultrasound with a 240° end-fire probe.
a AP view (I = longitudinal midline scan, II = oblique longitudinal scan).
b Lateral view of a longitudinal midline scan.

Fig. 1.**4**   Schematic representation of coronal scan planes in transvaginal ultrasound with a 240° end-fire probe.
a AP view. For clarity, the uterus is shown in a straightened position.
b Lateral view (III = transverse scan through the cervix, IV = transverse scan through the uterine corpus).

Fig. 1.**5**   Longitudinal scan through a gravid anteflexed uterus at 5 weeks, 5 days. The probe is in the anterior fornix.
cr = superior, ca = inferior,
p = posterior, a = anterior

Fig. 1.**6**   Transvaginal coronal scan shows a cross-sectional view of the uterine cavity at 8 weeks, 1 day. The markers indicate the size of the amniotic cavity. A section of the corpus luteum appears on the patient's left side.
cr = superior, ca = inferior,
r = right, l = left

Abdominal ultrasound

Fig. 1.**7**   Setup for abdominal ultrasound. The examiner sits to the left of the patient. Separate monitors are provided for the examiner and patient. I = Midsagittal scan, II = lateral sagittal scan, III–VIII = suprasymphyseal transverse scans, IX and X = oblique scans.

Fig. 1.**8**   Transducer placement for a midsagittal scan.

Fig. 1.**9**   Transducer placement for a suprasymphyseal transverse scan.

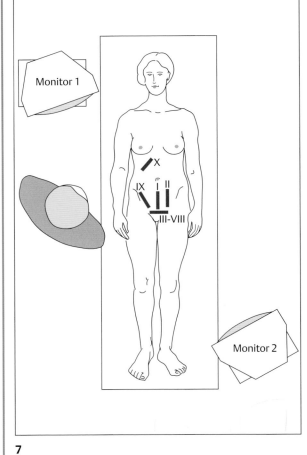

7

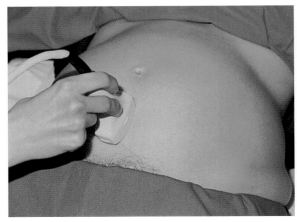

8

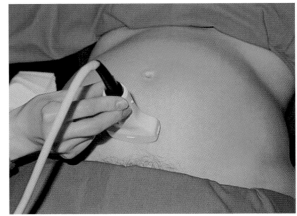

9

Fig. 1.**10**   Transducer placement for an oblique scan through the right abdomen.

Fig. 1.**11**   Transducer placement for an oblique scan through the right upper abdomen.

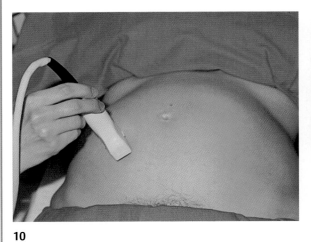

10

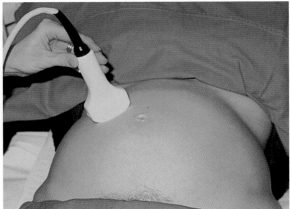

11

Fig. 1.**12**   Transducers for abdominal obstetric ultrasound.
a Linear transducer.
b Curved array transducer.
c Sector transducer.

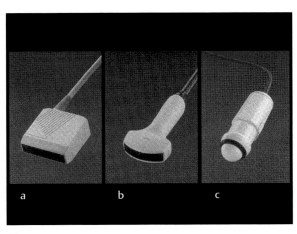

12

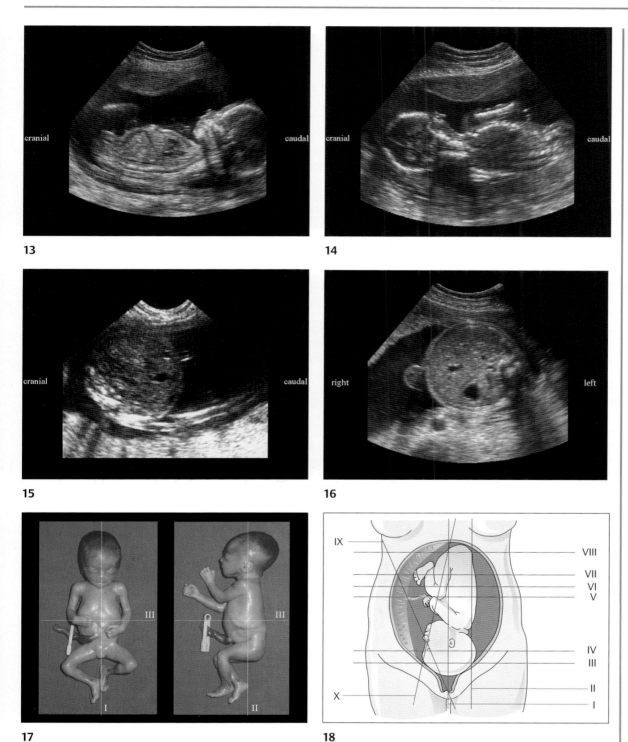

13

14

15

16

17   18

Image orientation

Fig. 1.**13**   Image orientation in a longitudinal scan of a vertex-presenting fetus. With correct transducer placement, the fetal head appears on the right side of the image and the fetal trunk on the left side.

Fig. 1.**14**   Image orientation in a longitudinal scan of a breech-presenting fetus. With correct transducer placement, the fetal head appears on the left side of the image and the fetal trunk on the right side.

Fig. 1.**15**   Image orientation in a midlongitudinal scan of a fetus in a dorsosuperior transverse lie. The fetal spine appears on the left side of the image. With a dorsoinferior transverse lie, the fetal spine would appear on the right side of the image.

Fig. 1.**16**   Image orientation in a transverse scan of a vertex-presenting fetus in the first position. With correct transducer placement, the anatomical left side of the patient should appear on the right side of the image, and the anatomical right side should appear on the left side of the image.

Fig. 1.**17**   Planes of section in the fetus. I = Sagittal plane, II = coronal plane, III = transverse (axial) plane.

Fig. 1.**18**   Diagram of scan planes for evaluating the biometric parameters and organs of a fetus in the cephalic presentation with the spine to the left (first position). I = midsagittal plane for general evaluation, II = plane for defining the spinal column, III = cerebral lateral ventricles, IV = cephalometry, V = thoracometry, VI = abdominometry, VII = kidneys, VIII = fetal urinary bladder, IX = placental cord insertion with a right sidewall placenta, X = femur

2 Ultrasound Screening

Prenatal Care

Goals. Screening examinations during pregnancy are an essential part of prenatal care. Among the various screening tests that are now offered to pregnant women, ultrasound has the broadest diagnostic spectrum. There is no modality that can detect as many abnormalities throughout pregnancy as ultrasound. Another important advantage of ultrasound is its low cost. Besides the early detection of a nonviable pregnancy (missed abortion, blighted ovum) or ectopic pregnancy, ultrasound at the end of the first trimester can detect gross fetal anomalies or at least show initial signs that are suggestive of anomalies. In the second and third trimesters, the primary emphasis is on the detection of fetal anomalies and growth disturbances as well as the diagnosis of placental, umbilical cord and amniotic fluid abnormalities.

First and second screening examinations. As early as 1979, the Federal Republic of Germany became the first country in the world to institute two ultrasound screening examinations as a routine part of prenatal care (33). The goal of the first ultrasound examination, scheduled between weeks 16 and 20, was to determine gestational age, assign a delivery date, detect multiple gestation, and check for fetal anomalies. The goal of the second examination, scheduled between weeks 32 and 36, was to evaluate fetal growth and detect any late-onset fetal anomalies or placental and amniotic fluid problems.

Screening at 10, 20, and 30 weeks' gestation. German prenatal care guidelines were revised on April 1, 1995, adding a third ultrasound examination to the prenatal program and setting a new schedule for the individual examinations. The goal of this "10–20–30" screening program is to create a framework for the earlier and more selective detection of abnormalities so that further diagnostic procedures can be instituted as required.

Examiner proficiency. Besides accurate dates, the detection of intrauterine abnormalities depends critically on the examination conditions, the equipment used, and especially on the experience and proficiency of the examiner. In Germany as in most European countries, the ultrasound examination is considered a physician-supplied service and is not delegated to ultrasound technicians (as in the U.S., for example).

Major anomalies. A priority goal in screening is the early detection of major fetal anomalies. Major anomalies are defined as malformations that affect fetal viability and/or quality of life and necessitate intervention (as defined by the European Union Registry of Congenital Anomalies and Twins, EUROCAT) (12, 13).

Incidence. Incidence data on major congenital anomalies vary considerably depending on the type of detection system used. With passive detection systems, major anomalies are found in approximately 2–3% of all newborns (14, 21, 24). With active detection systems (27, 40) in which newborns are systematically examined by specially trained physicians following a standard, uniform protocol, significantly higher values are found (7.3% of all newborns) (40). This means that of the approximately 800,000 babies that are delivered in Germany each year, some 50,000 to 60,000 will be born with major anomalies. In the U.S., 100,000 to 150,000 babies are born annually with severe malformations (51).

While these figures are relatively high, it should be considered from a diagnostic standpoint that a practicing gynecologist will encounter only a small number of fetal anomalies in any given year. Moreover, different anomalies show extreme variations in their incidence rates (from one in 200 to one in 250,000). An incidence of one in 1000 births (e.g., spina bifida) means that, statistically, it will take 10 years for a gynecologist who treats 100 pregnant women a year to see one such anomaly. With much rarer anomalies such as thanatophoric dysplasia (incidence of one in 100,000 births), the same gynecologist would have to practice for 1000 years before encountering a single case.

Three-level concept. Given the statistical hurdles, the effective detection of fetal anomalies can be achieved only by referring selected cases to properly equipped prenatal centers. As early as 1981, Hansmann (16) proposed a three-level concept requiring three different levels of examiner proficiency. In recent years this concept has been adopted and put into practice by the German Society for Ultrasound in Medicine (DEGUM).

- **Level I.** Level I screening examinations are conducted primarily by qualified office gynecologists who have a good working knowledge of normal fetal ultrasound anatomy and can perform accurate, basic biometry of fetal parts (crown–rump length [CRL], biparietal diameter [BPD], abdominal transverse diameter [ATD]). The examiner should also know the suggestive signs of a fetal anomaly.
- **Level II.** Level II examinations place greater demands on the examiner and equipment and are performed in a specialized office or hospital setting. The examiner should have several years' experience with ultrasound as well as specialized knowledge in the detection of fetal anomalies.
- **Level III.** Level III examinations are reserved for specialists who practice at prenatal centers, act as problem solvers for equivocal cases, and are active in scientific research.

This three-tiered concept is similar to the three screening levels recognized by the American College of Obstetricians and Gynecologists (ACOG): basic, limited, and comprehensive (1).

Ultimately, ultrasound screening can be effective only if abnormalities are successfully detected at the level I stage so that the patient can be referred to an appropriate center.

Table 2.1 Detection of anomalies in pregnancy (adapted from Garmel and D'Alton [15])

Authors	Patients (n)	Period of study	Sensitivity	Specificity
Lys et al. (28)	8316	1986	14%	98%
Li et al. (25)	678	1980–1981	38%	98%
Levi et al. (22)	13 309	1986–1987	34–55%	> 99%
Rosendahl et al. (44)	9012	1980–1988	58%	> 99%
Shirley et al. (52)	6183	1989–1990	67%	> 99%
Chitty et al. (7)	8785	1988–1989	74%	> 99%
Luck (26)	8523	1988–1991	85%	> 99%
RADIUS study (14)	15 151	1987–1991	35%	–
Levi et al. (24)	25 046	1984–1992	44,5%	99.93%
Quiesser-Luft et al. (40)	20 248	1990–1994	30.3%	–

Table 2.**2**   Detection of anomalies before 24 weeks (after Chitty [8])

Authors	Period	Number	Weeks gestation	Prevalence of abnormality in %	Sensitivity in %	Specificity in %	TOP* in %	Examiner
Rosendahl and Kivinen (44)	1980–1988	9012	18	1.03	39–40	99.9	0.16	Physician, midwife
Saari-Kempainen et al. (45)	1986–1987	4691	16–20	0.43	36–76.9	99.8	(20) 0.23	?
Chitty et al. (7)	1988–1989	8785	18–20	1.5	74.4	99.98	0.6	Radiographer, physician, technician
Levi et al. (23)	1984–1989	15654	16–20	2.3	21	100	?	Sonographer
Shirley et al. (52)	1989–1990	6412	19	1.4	60.7	99.98	0.45	Radiographer
Luck (26)	1988–1991	8844	19	1.9	85	99.9	0.28	Radiographer
Ewigman et al. (14)	1987–1991	7617	15–22	2.46	16.6		0.11	Technician, physician
Levi et al. (24)	1990–1992	9392	16–20	2.45	41	99.9	?	Physician, technician, sonographer

*TOP = termination of pregnancy.

Overall detection rates. Various studies in low-risk populations have shown that the overall detection rates for fetal anomalies vary over a wide range from 14% to 85% (Table 2.**1**). Average detection rates prior to 24 weeks' gestation are even lower (Table 2.**2**).

RADIUS study. The frequent low detection rates for fetal anomalies have often led critics to question the value of screening examinations. Serious doubts were raised by the Routine Antenatal Diagnostic Imaging Ultrasound Study (RADIUS) (14). This 1993 study involved a total of 15,151 cases, which were randomly divided into two groups. Group I received routine ultrasound screening at 15–22 weeks and 31–35 weeks, while group II received selective screening only when indicated. Analysis showed that only 16.6% of the anomalies in group I were detected prior to 24 weeks. The total anomaly detection rate in this group was 34.8%. The study also showed that the detection of an anomaly had no effect on perinatal outcome.

Helsinki Study and Belgian Multicenter Study. In contrast to the RADIUS study, which has been criticized for errors in methodology (7, 17), the Helsinki Study (34) and Belgian Multicenter Study (24) yielded markedly better results: ultrasound screening before 24 weeks detected 44.5% and 41% of congenital anomalies, respectively.

The importance of examiner experience was documented in the Belgian Multicenter Study (24). While the detection rate for fetal anomalies before 24 weeks was 40.4% during the period from 1984 to 1989, it rose significantly to 51.1% during the subsequent period from 1990 to 1992.

Other data. This euphoria has been dampened by recent data from German authors on the active detection of fetal anomalies. In a study of 20,248 newborn fetuses and infants, Queisser-Luft et al. (40) reported a total detection rate of only 30.3% for major anomalies.

Conclusion. These figures clearly demonstrate that screening for anomalies in a low-risk population is worthwhile only if the examiners are adequately qualified and patients with suspicious findings are selected for referral to appropriate centers. Repeated lower-level examinations with equivocal results tend only to subject worried parents to further anxiety. On the other hand, targeted imaging and the exclusion of a fetal anomaly can be an important source of reassurance for the parents.

Ultrasound Screening

Prenatal care guidelines issued in Germany on April 1, 1995 (20) have established the foundation for ultrasound screening in pregnancy. The guidelines call for a total of three ultrasound examinations scheduled at 8–12 weeks, 18–22 weeks, and 28–32 weeks (20) (Table 2.**3**).

First Ultrasound Screening (8–12 weeks)

Goals. The first ultrasound screening examination in the first trimester is generally transvaginal (5–7.5 MHz), but abdominal scanning is also acceptable. The goals of this initial screening examination are to detect an intact intrauterine pregnancy, determine gestational age, check for multiple pregnancy, and detect any abnormalities of embryonic development (Table 2.**4**).

Determining Gestational Age

An accurate ultrasound assignment of gestational age is possible only in the first trimester, since the range of variation of measurable parameters is smallest at that time.

Crown–rump length and biparietal diameter. The crown–rump length (CRL) is the most accurate parameter for determining gestational age. In principle, the gestational sac diameter can also be used to assess gestational age, but this parameter gives a less precise estimate due to its greater range of variance. Toward the end of the first trimester, the biparietal diameter (BPD) of the fetal head can be used as an alternative or adjunct in assigning gestational age. Within the first trimester, the confidence interval is ± 10 days for the chorionic sac diameter, ± 6 days for the crown–rump length, and ± 8 days for the biparietal diameter (43).

The various biometric parameters become increasingly variable as gestation progresses, and the range of variation by the third trimester is approximately ± 2 weeks.

Table 2.**3**   Ultrasound screening in pregnancy

First examination	8–12 weeks (= from start of 9th week to end of 12th week)
Second examination	18–22 weeks (= from start of 19th week to end of 22nd week)
Third examination	28–32 weeks (= from start of 29th week to end of 32nd week)

Table 2.**4**   Goals of the first screening examination (8–12 weeks)

➢ Detect an intact intrauterine pregnancy
➢ Check gestational age (CRL, BPD)
➢ Detect multiple gestation
➢ Detect embryonic developmental abnormalities and defects
➢ Check for suggestive signs of a fetal anomaly

Importance of accurate pregnancy dating. An accurate knowledge of gestational age is clinically important for several reasons:

- The accuracy of many tests used in prenatal medicine (AFP assay in maternal serum or amniotic fluid, triple test) depends on knowing the correct gestational age.
- Intrauterine growth retardation can be confidently diagnosed only if the gestational age has been verified at an early stage.
- Only an early confirmation of gestational age can avoid unnecessary induction of labor due to an erroneous belief that the pregnancy has been carried past term.

Another source of confusion is the fact that pregnancy is sometimes dated in completed weeks and sometimes in the current week. To eliminate this problem, gestational age should be stated in completed weeks whenever possible. Table 2.**5** shows the relationship between conceptual age and the current and completed menstrual age.

Detection of Twin Pregnancy

The ultrasound detection of twin pregnancy is based on the number of amniotic cavities and the type of placentation. Monoamniotic and monochorionic–diamniotic twins are at significantly higher risk for fetofetal transfusion syndrome and nutritive placental insufficiency than dichorionic–diamniotic twins.

Lambda sign. The lambda sign (49, 50) can be used in ultrasound to differentiate between a monochorionic and dichorionic placenta (Fig. 2.**1**). The sign refers to a chorionic tissue projection seen at the membrane–placental junction between the twins. This sign can be detected between 10 and 24 weeks when a dichorionic placenta is present. Absence of the lambda sign indicates a monochorionic–diamniotic placenta.

Developmental Disturbances and Anomalies

Abnormal early pregnancy. The monitoring of fetal biometric parameters and heart rate can provide early indications of an abnormal pregnancy. The findings listed in Table 2.**6** are considered unfavorable prognostic signs.

Fetal anomalies. Major anomalies such as anencephaly and large abdominal wall defects can be detected sonographically by the end of the first trimester. A detailed knowledge of the sonomorphologic development of the embryo is the key to avoiding the misinterpretation of normal changes, such as the physiologic umbilical hernia.

Nuchal Translucency

Detection of nuchal translucency. In recent years, the ultrasound detection of nuchal translucency (38) at the end of the first trimester has been recognized as an important suggestive sign in the diagnosis of chromosomal abnormalities, especially trisomy 21 (36,53,54). It is a transient sign, usually visible only between 11 ± 0 and 13 ± 6 weeks' gestation. Both abdominal and transvaginal scanning can demonstrate the sign in a midsagittal section of the embryo or fetus (Fig. 2.**2**). The thickness of the nuchal translucency is measured from the inner margin of the skin to the nuchal soft tissue (Fig. 2.**2**). A thickness above the 95th percentile is considered abnormal (Fig. 2.**3**). Measurements of 3 mm or greater are generally considered abnormal. An amniotic membrane that is not yet in full contact with the chorionic membrane can occasionally mimic nuchal translucency.

Table 2.**7** gives an overview on all the parameters that are important for nuchal translucency measurements.

Nuchal translucency thickness and chromosomal abnormalities. There is considerable variation in published reports on the sensitivity of nuchal translucency thickness as a marker of fetal chromosomal abnormalities. For example, one review of 1593 cases found sensitivities ranging from 0% to 100% with a mean incidence of 29% (53). In the study by Pandya et al. (39) in 1015 cases, a chromosomal defect was present in 19% of fetuses that showed ≥ 3 mm of nuchal translucency thickness.

The risk of a chromosomal defect increases markedly with nuchal translucency thickness (Table 2.**8**) (39, 53). Thus, whenever nuchal translucency thickness is 3 mm or more, karyotyping should be done by means of chorionic villus sampling or early amniocentesis. Younger women (< 35 years of age) who are not considered at high risk for chromosomal abnormalities can profit from this noninvasive ultrasound screening procedure. If increased nuchal translucency thickness is detected, these women can be selectively referred for an invasive diagnostic test.

Table 2.**5**   Correlation between conceptual age, current menstrual age, and completed menstrual age

Current conceptual age	Current week of menstrual age	Completed week of menstrual age
Day 41 conceptual age = day 6 of the 6th embryonic week	Day 55 menstrual age = day 6 of the 8th week (8/6 week)	55 days menstrual age = 7 completed weeks plus 6 days (7 weeks, 6 days)
Day 56 conceptual age = day 7 of the 8th embryonic week	Day 70 menstrual age = day 7 of the 10th week (10 weeks, 7 days)	Exactly 10 completed weeks = 70 days menstrual age (10 weeks, 0 days)

Table 2.**6**   Unfavorable prognostic signs in early pregnancy

> Gestational sac too small for the duration of amenorrhea
> Deformity of the gestational sac
> Nonvisualization of the embryo at 6 or more weeks' gestation
> No sign of heart activity at 7 or more weeks' gestation
> Mean diameter of gestational sac ≥ 3 cm with no detectable embryo
> No significant increase in mean gestational sac diameter during one week

Table 2.**7**   Important parameters for nuchal translucency (NT) measurement

> Gestation 11 + 0 until 13 + 6 weeks
> CRL 45–84 mm
> Midsagittal view of the fetus
> Fetal size > 75% of the image
> Neutral position of the fetus
> NT away from amnion
> Maximum translucency
> Calipers on-to-on

Table 2.**8**   Relationship between fetal nuchal translucency thickness and the frequency of chromosomal abnormalities (after Snijders et al. 53)

Nuchal translucency thickness			Chromosomal abnormalities					
			Trisomies			Sex-linked		Others*
	n	Total	21	18	13	45,X	47,XXY/ XXY	
3 mm	696	7%	24	8	2	1	4	11
4 mm	139	27%	26	5	3	-	-	4
5 mm	66	53%	24	8	2	-	-	1
6 mm	39	49%	6	9	1	3	-	-
7 mm	24	83%	6	10	1	3	-	-
8 mm	23	70%	6	6	3	1	-	-
9 mm	28	78%	8	5	1	6	-	-
Total	1015	19%	101	51	13	14	4	16

* Triploidies (n = 10); 47,XY+fr; 47,XX+22; 46,XX-4p; 46xym16; 47,XY+20; 47,X+22

The risk of a chromosomal defect increases markedly with nuchal translucency thickness (Table 2.**8**) and maternal age (Fig. 2.**4**).

The most effective method of screening for chromosomal defects is by a combination of maternal age, fetal nuchal translucency thickness and maternal serum free β-human chorionic gonadotropin (b-hCG) and pregnancy-associated plasma protein-A (PAPP-A) at 11–14 weeks of gestation (56, 57, 60). The detection rate is about 90% for a screen-positive rate of 5% (37).

Increased nuchal translucency thickness and structural defects. Structural defects (mainly heart defects, diaphragmatic defects, renal anomalies, and abdominal wall defects) are detected in 4% of cases where karyotyping indicates a normal chromosome set (39). Fetal echocardiography should be performed in such cases to detect or exclude a cardiac anomaly.

Second Ultrasound Screening (18–22 weeks)

Goals. The main goals of the second screening examination are to assess fetal development, search for fetal anomalies, estimate amniotic fluid volume, and evaluate the structure and location of the placenta (Table 2.**9**)

Biometry. Four of the quantitative parameters listed in Table 2.**10** can be used as basic biometric parameters. When the head and abdominal circumference are determined, it does not matter whether they are measured by tracing around them on the correct scan plane or by calculating the circumference from the transverse and sagittal diameters.

Anomalies

Recognition of suggestive signs. The primary goal of the second screening examination is to detect or exclude fetal anomalies. The basic screening program in Germany does not mandate a detailed search for fetal anomalies at this stage, other than the detection of anencephaly. It does require recognizing the suggestive signs for a fetal anomaly (Table 2.**11**) and, when such signs are found, referring the patient to a qualified center.

Further studies. If it is determined that the patient needs a more specialized ultrasound examination, it should be asked whether the examiner has the proficiency and equipment necessary to perform the examination. If this is not the case and if the patient is not referred elsewhere, the examining physician may be open to litigation. Also, an

Table 2.9   Goals of the second screening examination (18–22 weeks' gestation)

> ➤ Check for singleton or multiple pregnancy
> ➤ Confirm viability (heart action, motion)
> ➤ Evaluate amniotic fluid volume
> ➤ Evaluate placental location and structure
> ➤ Check growth parameters (biometry)
> ➤ Demonstrate accessible fetal structures

Table 2.10   Biometric parameters for the second and third screening examinations

> ➤ Biparietal head diameter (BPD)
> ➤ Fronto-occipital head diameter (FOD)
> ➤ Head circumference (HC)
> ➤ Abdominal transverse diameter (ATD)
> ➤ Abdominal sagittal diameter (ASD)
> ➤ Abdominal circumference (AC)
> ➤ Femur length (FL)
> ➤ Humerus length (HL)

Table 2.11   Ultrasound signs that suggest the presence of a fetal anomaly

> ➤ Abnormal amniotic fluid volume (poly- or oligohydramnios, anhydramnios)
> ➤ Fetal growth disturbance (early retardation, macrosomia)
> ➤ Disproportion between fetal parts (between head and trunk or head and extremities)
> ➤ Body surface abnormality (defect, protrusion, abnormal head shape [lemon sign])
> ➤ Internal abnormalities (fluid, cavity, atypical four-chamber view, banana sign)
> ➤ Cardiac arrhythmias
> ➤ Increased or decreased fetal movements
> ➤ Absence of an umbilical artery
> ➤ Abnormal placental structure (vacuolated placenta)

Table 2.12   Fetal anomalies that are associated with amniotic fluid abnormalities

Amniotic fluid abnormality	Fetal anomaly or disease
Hydramnios	➤ Impaired amniotic fluid absorption • Cleft lip and palate • Esophageal stenosis or atresia • Duodenal stenosis or atresia • Bowel obstruction ➤ Infection ➤ Increased urine production ➤ Anencephaly ➤ Diabetes, gestational diabetes ➤ Blood group incompatibility ➤ NIHF (nonimmune hydrops fetalis)
Oligohydramnios, anhydramnios	➤ Intrauterine growth retardation (IUGR) ➤ Potter's sequence • Renal agenesis • Sponge kidney • Multicystic kidneys • Impaired urinary transport ➤ Decreased urine production • IUGR with centralization of the fetal circulation • Genetic disease ➤ Premature rupture of membranes!
Combined hydramnios and oligohydramnios in twins	➤ Fetofetal transfusion syndrome ("stuck twin")

examiner who misses a fetal anomaly will be held to the quality standard of a specialized ultrasound expert (23).

Amniotic Fluid Volume

Polyhydramnios and oligohydramnios. Among the suggestive signs listed in Table 2.**11**, an abnormal amniotic fluid volume is the most important. Both polyhydramnios and oligohydramnios have a high association with fetal anomalies. The reported incidence of anomalies ranges from 7.9% (62) to 18% (18) in polyhydramnios and from 7% (31) to 13% (3, 41) in oligohydramnios.

Polyhydramnios is most commonly associated with malformations of the neural tube (anencephaly, spina bifida) and digestive tract (esophageal atresia, duodenal atresia) (Table 2.**12**). Oligohydramnios is usually associated with a renal anomaly or urinary tract obstruction. If amniotic fluid is absent (anhydramnios) and rupture of the fetal membranes is ruled out, the cause may be original Potter syndrome (bilateral renal agenesis), and further tests should be performed (Table 2.**12**).

Abnormal Fetal Growth

Proportional growth retardation. Proportional (symmetric) growth retardation of the fetus affecting both the head and trunk is suggestive of a fetal chromosomal abnormality (especially triploidy or trisomy 13, 18, and 21).

Disproportional growth. Isolated growth retardation affecting individual body parts may also signify a fetal anomaly. Disproportional growth can be detected only by measuring several growth parameters when the gestational age is precisely known.

Abnormal Fetal Structures

General fetal survey. Attention is given both to the fetal body surface and to internal structures.

Surface abnormalities. Fetal surface abnormalities include defects, such as anencephaly or rachischisis, as well as protrusions such as cervical hygroma, omphalocele, or myelomeningocele.

Abnormal head shape. An abnormal head shape (lemon sign, Fig. 2.**5**) (48, 61) is a reliable indicator of myelomeningocele. An abnormal structure within the fetal head, such as bowing of the cerebellum (banana sign, Fig. 2.**5**) (61), is another marker of myelomeningocele.

Intrafetal cystic masses (Table 2.**14**). Depending on their location, these internal masses may signify hydrocephalus or a stenotic lesion of the urinary or gastrointestinal tract. Fluid collections within the abdominal cavity or pericardium are found with severe fetal anemia (nonimmune or immune hydrops) or fetal heart failure.

Fetal Heart and Movement

Fetal heart. The first step in evaluating the fetal heart is to check its location. Displacement of the cardiac axis or the entire heart to the contralateral side is always suspicious for a diaphragmatic hernia. If a well-defined four-chamber view cannot be obtained, it should be assumed that a cardiac anomaly is present. Reports on the sensitivity of the four-chamber view in detecting a cardiac anomaly range from detection rates of 39% (59) to 92% (9). Gestational age is a significant factor. A sensitivity of approximately 50% is reported between 18 and 24 weeks' gestation (58).

Fetal movement. Fetal movement patterns can also provide important evidence of a fetal anomaly. Hectic, irregular movements suggest anomalous development of the central nervous system (e.g., anencephaly), while a paucity of fetal movement may signify a motor disturbance (e.g., high spina bifida or arthrogryposis multiplex congenita) (Table 2.**15**).

Umbilical Cord and Placenta

Evaluation of the umbilical cord. This requires defining the umbilical vein and both umbilical arteries. The absence of one umbilical artery (singular umbilical artery) is associated with a fetal anomaly in 7% (10) to 50% (6) of cases.

Abnormal placental structure. An abnormal placental structure is another important sign of fetal pathology. In particular, a large, vacuolated placenta is suspicious for chromosomal triploidy (5, 11).

Table 2.**13**   Association between fetal growth abnormalities and anomalies

Head size	Trunk size	Femur, humerus	Fetal anomalies and diseases
>	=	=	➢ **Macrocephaly** • Hydrocephalus • Familial large head (check parental head size)
<	=	=	➢ **Microcephaly** • Spina bifida • Fetal infection • Familial small head (check parental head size)
=	>	=	➢ **Early signs of hydrops fetalis** • Blood group incompatibility • NIHF (heart defect) • Fetal infection ➢ **Intra-abdominal mass** • Ascites • Bowel obstruction • Cystic kidneys • Impaired urinary transport • Intra-abdominal cysts
=	<	=	➢ **Early asymmetric IUGR** • Gastroschisis • Omphalocele
>	>	>	➢ **Hyperplastic growth** • Gestational diabetes • Familial large child (check parental body size)
<	<	<	➢ **Hypoplastic growth** • Genetic disease (triploidy, trisomy 13, 18, 21) • Familial small child (check parental body size)
=	=	<	➢ **Dwarfism** • Thanatophoric dysplasia • Chondrodysplasia ➢ **Bone mineralization disorders** • Osteogenesis imperfecta

Key to symbols:
= normal-for-date development; > too large for date; < too small for date

Table 2.**14**   Hypoechoic (liquid) mass within the fetus

Head	➢ Ventriculomegaly, hydrocephalus ➢ Choroid plexus cysts ➢ Holoprosencephaly ➢ Dandy-Walker syndrome ➢ Porencephaly
Thorax	➢ Pleural effusion ➢ Pericardial effusion ➢ Diaphragmatic hernia (stomach, bowel loops) ➢ Cysts (lung, bronchial tract)
Abdomen, retroperitoneum	➢ Ascites ➢ Double bubble (duodenal atresia) ➢ Bowel obstruction ➢ Renal pelvic congestion, hydronephrosis ➢ Multicystic kidneys ➢ Megalocystis ➢ Ovarian cyst ➢ Mesenteric cyst

Table 2.**15**   Fetal anomalies and disorders associated with abnormal fetal movement patterns

Hectic movements	Anencephaly
Weak movements	Hypoxia, sleep, drugs
No movements	Arthrogryposis multiplex congenita

Placental location. Placental location is important in the second trimester only if an invasive test is proposed (chorionic villus sampling, amniocentesis) or in patients with a central placenta previa (one entirely covering the internal os). Unlike a central placenta previa, a low-lying placenta or even a marginal placenta previa may still move cephalad as uterine growth progresses. The definitive evaluation of placental location in such cases should be postponed until the third trimester.

■ Third Ultrasound Screening (28–32 weeks)

Goals. The third ultrasound screening examination covers fetal position in addition to all of the points covered in the second examination (Table 2.**16**). The main priorities of the third screening examination are to evaluate fetal growth and detect any additional fetal abnormalities.

Biometry. The correct interpretation of biometric ultrasound parameters requires an accurate knowledge of gestational age, accurate visualization of the reference planes, and identifying the correct points for taking fetal measurements (see Chapter 12). The parameters that are measured in the third screening examination are the same as those checked in the second trimester (Table 2.**10**).

Evaluation of Fetal Growth

Intrauterine growth retardation and macrosomia. Both the detection of intrauterine growth retardation due to chronic placental insufficiency and the development of fetal macrosomia are of key importance in terms of further clinical management. Both growth abnormalities are diagnosed by ultrasound fetal biometry. Growth retardation is assumed to be present when ultrasound abdominal dimensions remain below the 5th percentile of the growth chart in serial examinations, and macrosomia is assumed to be present when abdominal dimensions are above the 95th percentile.

Growth charts. Growth charts have proven useful for the early detection of fetal growth abnormalities. In Germany, biometric data are entered on standard charts printed in the prenatal exam record that is issued to every pregnant woman. In this way the obstetrician can tell at a glance how fetal growth is progressing and whether there is any indication of proportional or disproportional growth retardation.

Body parameters. With the elongated (dolichocephalic) head shape that is often seen in breech-presenting fetuses, it is misleading to use BPD as the only growth parameter, since the narrow head leads to a small BPD measurement that can mimic growth retardation. If comparison of the biparietal diameter and transverse abdominal diameter indicates a growth discrepancy, additional body parameters such as head circumference (HC), abdominal circumference (AC), and the long limb bones should be included in the evaluation (see Chapter 12).

Serial biometric examinations. Serial biometry should be scheduled at intervals of no less than one week. Otherwise the measurement errors could be larger than the growth that has occurred since the last examination. It is also advisable to have one person perform all the examinations to avoid interpersonal measurement errors.

Doppler ultrasound. Whenever a fetal growth abnormality is detected in the third trimester, a Doppler examination (30, 47) should be performed to evaluate fetomaternal hemodynamics. Abnormal waveforms in the maternal circulation (uterine artery) and fetal circulation (umbilical artery, descending aorta, middle cerebral artery, ductus venosus) can be noted at an early stage, permitting the early detection of fetal compromise. Particularly in a high-risk population like that with seri-ous growth retardation, Doppler monitoring leads to a significant decline in fetal morbidity and mortality (2). Doppler ultrasound has not proved to be an effective screening method for low-risk populations, however.

Abnormalities of Late Onset

The prenatal detection of late-onset fetal abnormalities (e.g., growth discrepancy in twins, hydrocephalus, omphalocele, hydronephrosis) can be a critical factor in successful obstetric management. On the one hand, the location, timing, and mode of the delivery can be discussed with the parents once the late-onset condition has been diagnosed. Additionally, plans can be made to provide optimum neonatologic care for the newborn infant.

Fetal Position

Breech presentation. The detection of a breech presentation is extremely important in terms of obstetric management. Because a breech presentation in primiparae is now considered an indication for primary cesarean section and is unlikely to resolve spontaneously after 36 weeks' gestation, the patient can be referred for a planned cesarean delivery without delay.

Placenta and Amniotic Fluid

Besides the evaluation of fetal development and position, greater importance is being placed on the evaluation of placental location, placental structure, and amniotic fluid volume in the third trimester.

Placental location. In contrast to the first half of pregnancy, in which placental location is usually a minor concern, a low-lying placenta or placenta previa in the third trimester is important in terms of potential complications. If the lower margin of the placenta cannot be accurately defined by abdominal ultrasound, it can be clearly delineated from the internal os by transvaginal ultrasound.

Abnormal placental thickness. An abnormal placental thickness can be an important sign of possible complications. Placental thickness greater than 5 cm (placental hydrops) is a suggestive signs of incipient fetal hydrops (19). An extremely thin or markedly small placenta may signify placental insufficiency.

Structural changes. Structural changes in the placenta do not accurately reflect the functional competence of the organ. A circumscribed hyperechoic zone within the placenta may result from a placental infarction, which would lead to compromise of placental function. Local hypoechoic or anechoic areas in the placenta, on the other hand, often represent physiologic lacunae.

Abnormal amniotic fluid volume. It is not uncommon for an abnormal amniotic fluid volume to affect the course of the pregnancy in the third trimester. While polyhydramnios is associated with premature labor and potential preterm delivery, significant oligohydramnios may be an early sign of placental insufficiency.

Table 2.**16** Goals of the third screening examination (28–32 weeks)

> Check for singleton or multiple pregnancy
> Check viability (heart activity, movements)
> Evaluate amniotic fluid volume
> Evaluate placental location and structure
> Check growth parameters (biometry)
> Demonstrate accessible fetal structures
> Determine fetal lie

Uterus

Cervical incompetence. The transvaginal measurement of cervical length, with concurrent evaluation of the internal os, is essential for detecting cervical incompetence in a patient with premature uterine contractions or a palpable cervical abnormality. If the cervix is shortened to less than 30 mm or if there is appreciable opening of the internal os, the risk of preterm delivery is substantially increased.

Targeted Imaging in High-Risk Pregnancies

While routine screening has not yielded the desired results in nonselected populations, it has been shown that targeted ultrasound imaging by experienced examiners in high-risk pregnancies can achieve markedly higher anomaly detection rates in excess of 85% (Table 2.**17**).

Fetal Echocardiography

This particularly applies to the prenatal detection of heart defects. Heart defects are among the anomalies that are most frequently missed at screening, with detection rates ranging from 18% (59) to 39% (59). By contrast, detection rates as high as 92% (9) are achieved at prenatal centers that deal intensively with fetal echocardiography when the study includes a four-chamber view, the aortic and pulmonary outflow tracts, and color Doppler imaging.

Fetal Anomalies

The detection and assessment of fetal anomalies, as well as their definite exclusion, require an examiner who is very well versed in the physiology and pathophysiology of fetal development.

Chromosomal abnormalities. Various fetal abnormalities are not separate disease entities but are part of a syndrome or chromosomal abnormality and therefore warrant a targeted search for other associated anomalies. Thus, the selective sonomorphologic evaluation of all fetal body regions is essential for the comprehensive diagnosis of fetal anomalies. This is particularly evident with chromosomal abnormalities, which often are associated with subtle sonomorphologic changes (35) (Table 2.**18**). If we further consider that targeted imaging examinations are time-consuming and may take two hours or more to complete, it becomes clear that this type of examination can be accomplished only in highly specialized office or hospital settings that have the appropriate staff and equipment. Particularly when it comes to the fetal cardiovascular system, a competent examination requires a proficient examiner using state-of-the-art equipment (color Doppler).

First and second trimesters. An experienced sonographer can detect a variety of fetal malformations and even smaller defects in the second trimester when imaging conditions are good and the fetus is in a favorable position. With transvaginal ultrasound, various large defects (anencephaly, encephalocele, omphalocele) can be recognized as early as the first trimester.

Invasive techniques. Besides noninvasive ultrasound, the detailed investigation of a fetal anomaly usually requires an invasive diagnostic procedure. The principal options are chorionic villus sampling, amniocentesis, placentocentesis, cordocentesis, and fetoscopy. If the amniotic fluid volume is deficient (oligohydramnios, anhydramnios), amnioinfusion with physiologic NaCl solution can improve vision by creating a fluid pool around the fetus.

Table 2.**17**   Detection rates in targeted imaging (adapted from Garmel and D'Alton [15])

Authors	Patients (n)	Period	Sensitivity	Specificity
Sollie et al. (55)	481	1980–1985	86%	100%
Sabbagha et al. (46)	596	1980–1983	95%	99%
Campbell et al. (4)	2372	1978–1983	95%	> 99%
Manchester et al. (29)	257	1983–1995	99%	91%

Table 2.**18**   Various ultrasound markers that suggest a chromosomal abnormality

Brachycephaly	Trisomy 13, 18, 21; triploidy; XO
Microcephaly	Trisomy 13, 18; XO
Ventriculomegaly	Trisomy 13, 18, 21; triploidy; XO
Choroid plexus cysts	Trisomy 13, 18, 21
Enlarged cisterna magna	Trisomy 13, 18, 21
Cleft lip and palate	Trisomy 13, 18
Micrognathia	Trisomy 13, 18; triploidy
Nuchal translucency ≥ 3 mm (10–14 weeks)	Trisomy 13, 18, 21; triploidy
Nuchal fold > 5 mm (16–22 weeks)	Trisomy 21
Cervical hygroma	Trisomy 18, 21; XO
Heart defect	Trisomy 13, 18, 21; triploidy; XO
Omphalocele	Trisomy 13, 18; triploidy
Double bubble	Trisomy 13, 21
Slight bilateral dilation of renal pelvis	Trisomy 13, 18, 21; triploidy; XO
Hydrops	Trisomy 13, 18, 21; triploidy; XO
Retardation	Trisomy 13, 18, 21; triploidy; XO
Short femoral shaft	Trisomy 13, 18, 21; triploidy; XO

Three-dimensional ultrasound. Modern 3-D ultrasound permits a detailed tomographic evaluation of fetal anomalies. Besides providing an accurate sectional image analysis, this technique can also generate surface-rendered images and transparent views (32). In this way 3-D ultrasound can help parents appreciate the severity of a fetal defect, and in negative cases it can provide the parents with a photograph-like image of the normal fetus that is far more reassuring than a conventional 2-D ultrasonogram.

Patient information. Although rapid advances in ultrasound technology have enabled the increasingly detailed visualization of individual embryonic and fetal structures, it must be emphasized that ultrasound experts cannot successfully detect all malformations prenatally or define their specific features. Given the generally high expectations of patients who undergo targeted imaging for fetal anomalies, the patients should always be informed of this limitation verbally or on a consent form (42).

References

1. ACOG: Ultrasonography in Pregnancy. Washington DC, ACOG Technical Bulletin, Publication No. 187 (1993)
2. Alfirevic, Z., Neilson, J.P.: Doppler ultrasonography in high-risk pregnancies: systematic review with meta-analysis. Am. J. Obstet. Gynecol. 172 (1995) 1379–1387
3. Bastide, A., Manning, F., Harman, C., Lange, I., Morrison, I.: Ultrasound evaluation of amniotic fluid: Outcome of pregnancies with severe oligohydramnios. Am. J. Obstet. Gynecol. 154 (1986) 895–900
4. Campbell, S., Pearce, J.M.: The prenatal diagnosis of fetal structural anomalies by ultrasound. Clin. Obstet. Gynaecol. 10 (1983) 475–506
5. Casper, F.W., Merz, E., Seufert, R., Hoffmann, G.: Sonographische Diagnostik der fetalen Triploidie. Ultraschall 10 (1990) 311–313
6. Catanzarite, V.A., Hendricks, S.K., Maida, C., Westbrook, C., Cousins, L., Schrimmer, D.: Prenatal diagnosis of the two-vessel cord: implications for patient counseling and obstetric management. Ultrasound Obstet. Gynecol. 5 (1995) 98–105
7. Chitty, L.S., Hunt, G.H., Moore, J., Lobb, M.O.: Effectiveness of routine ultrasonography in detecting fetal structural abnormalities in a low risk population. Br. Med. J. 303 (1991) 1165–1169
8. Chitty, L.S.: Ultrasound screening for fetal abnormalities. Prenatal Diagnosis 15 (1995) 1241–1257
9. Copel, J.A., Pilu, G., Green, J., Hobbins, J.C., Kleinman, C.S.: Fetal echocardiographic screening for congenital heart disease: the importance of the four-chamber view. Am. J. Obstet. Gynecol. 157 (1987) 648–655
10. Csecsi, K., Kovacs, T., Hinchliffe, S.A., Papp, Z.: Incidence and associations of single umbilical artery in prenatally diagnosed malformed. midtrimester fetuses: a review of 62 cases. Am. J. Med. Genet., 43 (1992) 524–530
11. Donnenfeld, A.E., Mennuti, M.T.: Sonographic findings in fetuses with common chromosomal abnormalities. Clin. Obstet. Gynecol. 31 (1988) 80–96
12. EUROCAT report: Surveillance of Congenital Anomalies 1980–1988. Eurocat Central Registry, Department of Epidemiology, Catholic University of Louvain, Brussels (1991)
13. EUROCAT report 6: Surveillance of Congenital Anomalies in Europe 1980–1992, Brussels: EUROCAT Central Registry, Institute of Hygiene and Epidemiology (1995)
14. Ewigman, B.G., Crane, J.P., Frigoletto, F.D., LeFevre, M.L., Bain, R.P., McNellis, D. and the RADIUS Study Group: Effect of prenatal ultrasound screening of perinatal outcome. N. Engl. J. Med. 329 (1993) 821–827
15. Garmel, S.H., D'Alton, M.E.: Diagnostic Ultrasound in Pregnancy: An Overview. Semin. Perinat. 18 (1994) 117–132
16. Hansmann, M.: Nachweis und Ausschluss fetaler Entwicklungsstörungen mittels Ultraschallscreening und gezielter Untersuchung—ein Mehrstufenkonzept. Ultraschall 2 (1981) 206–220
17. Hansmann, M., Hackelöer, B.J.: Stellungnahme der Gesellschaft für Pränatal- und Geburtsmedizin sowie der Deutschen Gesellschaft für Ultraschall in der Medizin: "Ultraschalluntersuchungen in der Schwangerschaft". Der Frauenarzt 35 (1994) 505–506
18. Hobbins, J.C., Grannum, P.A.T., Berkowitz, R.L., Silverman, R., Mahoney, M.J.: Ultrasound in the diagnosis of congenital anomalies. Am. J. Obstet. Gynecol. 134 (1979) 331–345
19. Holländer, H.J.: Die Ultraschalldiagnostik während der Schwangerschaft. Urban & Schwarzenberg, Munich 1975
20. Hutzler, D.: Mitteilungen der kassenärztlichen Bundesvereinigung. Überarbeitete Neuauflage des Mutterpasses 1996. Deutsches Ärzteblatt 93, Heft 30 (1996) B-1556–B-1562
21. Kalter, H., Warkany, J.: Congenital malformations. Etiologic factors and their role in prevention. N. Engl. J. Med. 308 (1983) 424–431
22. Levi, S., Crouzet, P., Schaaps, J.P., Defoort, P., Coulon, R.; Buekens, P., de Brier, M..: Ultrasound screening for fetal malformations. Lancet I (1989) 678
23. Levi, S., Hyjazi, Y., Schaaps, J.P., Defoort, P., Coulon, R., Buekens, P.: Sensitivity and specificity of routine antenatal screening for congenital anomalies by ultrasound: the Belgian multicentric study. Ultrasound Obstet. Gynecol. 1 (1991) 102–110
24. Levi, S., Schaaps J.P., De Havay, P., Coulon, R., Defoort, P.: End-result of routine ultrasound screening for congenital anomalies: The Belgian Multicentric Study 1984–92. Ultrasound Obstet. Gynecol. 5 (1995) 366–371
25. Li, T.M., Greenes, R.A., Weisburg, M. et al.: Data assessing the usefulness of screening obstetrical ultrasonography for detecting fetal and placental abnormalities in uncomplicated pregnancy. Effects of screening a low-risk population. Med. Decis. Making 8 (1988) 48–54
26. Luck, C.: Value of routine ultrasound scanning at 19 weeks: a four year study of 8849 deliveries. Br. Med. J. 304 (1992) 1474–1478
27. Lynberg, M.C., Edmonds, L.D.: In: Halperin, W., Baker, E.L., Monson, R.R. (eds) Public Health Surveillance. Surveillance of Birth Defects, New York: Van Nostrand Reinhold (1992) 157–177
28. Lys, F., DeWals, P., Borlee-Grimee, I., Billiet, A., Vincotte-Mols, M., Levi, S.: Evaluation of routine ultrasound examination for the prenatal diagnosis of malformations. Europ. J. Obstet. Gyencol. Reprod. Biol. 30 (1989) 101–109
29. Manchester, D.K., Pretorius, D.H., Avery, C. et al.: Accuracy of ultrasound diagnoses in pregnancies complicated by suspected fetal anomalies. Prenat. Diagn. 8 (1988) 109–117
30. Marsal, K.: Rational use of Doppler ultrasound in perinatal medicine. J. Perinat. Med. 22 (1994) 463–474
31. Mercer, L.J., Brown, L.G., Petres, R.E., Messer, R.H.: A survey of pregnancies complicated by decreased amniotic fluid. Am. J. Obstet. Gynecol. 149 (1984) 355–361
32. Merz, E., Bahlmann, F., Weber, G.: Volume (3-D) scanning in the evaluation of fetal malformations .Ultrasound Obstet. Gynecol. 4 (1994) 339–345
33. Mutterschaftsrichtlinien vom 31.10.1979. Beilage 4/80 des Bundesanzeigers Nr. 22a vom 1.2.80
34. Newnham, J.P., Evans S.F., Michael, C.A., Stanley, F.J., Landau, L.I.: Effects of frequent ultrasound during pregnancy: A randomised controlled trial. Lancet 342 (1993) 887–891
35. Nicolaides, K., Shawwa, L., Brizot, M. Snijders, R.: Ultrasonographically detectable markers of fetal chromosomal defects. Ultrasound Obstet. Gynecol. 3 (1993) 56–69
36. Nicolaides, K.H., Sebire, N.J., Snijders, R.J.M.: Nuchal translucency and chromosomal defects. In Nicolaides, K.H. (ed.). The 11–14-week scan: The diagnosis of fetal abnormalities. Carnforth, UK, Parthenon Publishing (1999) 3–65
37. Nicolaides, K.H., Cicero, S., Liao, A.W.: One-stop clinic for assessment of risk of chromosomal defects at 12 weeks of gestation. Prenat. Neonat. Med. 5 (2000) 145–154
38. Pandya, P.P., Snijders, R.J.M., Johnson S.P., Brizot, M., Nicolaides, K.H.: Screening for fetal trisomies by maternal age and fetal nuchal translucency thickness at 10 to 14 weeks of gestation. Br. J. Obstet. Gynaecol. 102 (1995) 957–962
39. Pandya, P.P., Kondylios, A., Hilbert, L., Snijders, R.J.M., Nicolaides, K.H.: Chromosomal defects and outcome in 1015 fetuses with increased nuchal translucency. Ultrasound Obstet. Gynecol. 5 (1995) 15–19
40. Queisser-Luft, A., Stopfkuchen, H., Stolz, G., Schlaefer, K., Merz, E.: Prenatal diagnosis of major malformations: Quality control of routine ultrasound examinations based on a five-year study of 20 248 newborn fetuses and infants. Prenat. Diagn. 18 (1998) 567–576
41. Rabe, D, Leucht, W., Hendrik, H.J., Boos, R., Schmidt, W.: Sonographische Beurteilung der Fruchtwassermenge. II. Oligohydramnion—Bedeutung für den Schwangerschafts- u. Geburtsverlauf. Geburtsh. u. Frauenheilk. 46 (1986) 422–426
42. Ratzel, R.: Auswirkungen der Effizienzbewertung der Untersuchungen in der Schwanger-schaft auf die Aufklärung. Gynäkologe 29 (1996) 590–593
43. Rempen, A.: Vaginale Sonographie im ersten Trimenon. II. Quantitative Parameter. Z. Geburtsh. u. Perinat. 195 (1991)163–171
44. Rosendahl, H., Kivinen, S.: Antenatal detection of congenital malformations by routine ultrasonography. Obstet. Gynecol. 73 (1989) 947–951
45. Saari-Kemppainen, A., Karjalainen, O., Ylöstalo, P., Heinonen, O.P.: Ultrasound screening and perinatal mortality: controlled trial of systematic one-stage screening in pregnancy. Lancet 336 (1990) 387–391
46. Sabbagha, R.E., Sheikh, Z. Tamura, R.K.: Predictive value, sensitivity, and specificity of ultrasonic targeted imaging for fetal anomalies in gravid women at high risk for birth defects. Am. J. Obstet. Gynecol. 152 (1985) 822–827
47. Schneider, K.T.M.: Standards in der Perinatalmedizin—Dopplersonographie in der Schwangerschaft. Geburtsh. u. Frauenheilk. 56 (1996) M69–M73
48. Sebire, N.J., Noble, P.L., Thorpe-Beeston, J.G., Snijders, R.J., Nicolaides, K.H.: Presence of the "lemon" sign in fetuses with spina bifida at the 10–14-week scan. Ultrasound. Obstet. Gynecol. 10 (1997) 403–405
49. Sepulveda, W., Sebire, N.J., Hughes, K., Odibo, A., Nicolaides, K.H.: The lambda sign at 10–14 weeks of gestation as a predictor of chorionicity in twin pregnancies. Ultrasound Obstet. Gynecol. 7 (1996) 421–423
50. Sepulveda, W., Sebire, N.J., Hughes, K., Kalogeropoulos, A., Nicolaides, K.H.: Evolution of the lambda or twin-chorionic peak sign in dichorionic twin pregnancies. Obstet. Gynecol. 89 (1997) 439–441
51. Sever, L., Lynberg, M.C., Edmonds, L.D.: The impact of congenital malformations on public health. Teratology 48 (1993) 547–549
52. Shirley, I.M., Bottomley, F., Robinson, V.P.: Routine radiographer screening for fetal abnormalities by ultrasound in an unselected low risk population. Br. J. Radiol. 65 (1992) 565–569
53. Snijders, R.J.M., Pandya, P., Brizot, M.L., Nicolaides, K.H.: First trimester fetal nuchal translucency. In: Ultrasound Markers For Fetal Chromosomal defects. R.J.M. Snijders and K.H. Nicolaides (eds.). Carnforth, UK, Parthenon Publishing (1996) 121–156
54. Snijders, R.J.M., Noble, P., Sebire, N., Souka, A., Nicolaides, K.H.: UK multicentre project on assessment of risk of trisomy 21 by maternal age and fetal nuchal translucency thickness at 10–14 weeks of gestation. Lancet 351 (1998) 343–346
55. Sollie, J.E., Van Geijn, H.P., Arts, N.F.T.: Validity of a selective policy for ultrasound examination of fetal congenital anomalies. Europ. J. Obstet. Gynecol. Reprod. Biol. 27 (1988) 125–132
56. Spencer, K., Souter, V., Tul, N., Snijders, R., Nicolaides, K.H.: A screening program for trisomy 21 at 10–14 weeks using fetal nuchal translucency, maternal serum free b-human chorionic gonadotropin and pregnancy-associated plasma protein-A. Ultrasound Obstet. Gynecol. 13 (1999) 231–237
57. Spencer, K., Liao, A.W., Skentou, H., Cicero, S., Nicolaides, K.H.: Screening for triploidy by fetal nuchal translucency and maternal serum free b-HCG and PAPP-A at 10–14 weeks of gestation. Prenat. Diagn. 20 (2000) 495–499
58. Stümpflen, I., Stümpflen, A., Wimmer, M., Bernascheck, G.: Effect of detailed fetal echo-cardio-graphy as part of routine prenatal ultrasonographic screening on detection of congenital heart disease. Lancet 348 (1996) 854–857
59. Tegnander, E., Sik-Nes, S.H., Johansen, O.J., Linker, D.T.: Prenatal detection of heart defects at the routine fetal examination at 18 weeks in a non-selected population. Ultrasound Obstet. Gynecol. 5 (1995) 372–380
60. Tul, N., Spencer, K., Noble, P., Chan, C., Nicolaides, K.H.: Screening for trisomy 18 by fetal nuchal translucency and maternal serum free beta hCG and PAPP-A at 10–14 weeks of gestation. Prenat. Diagn. 19 (1999) 1035–1042
61. Van den Hof, M.C., Nicolaides, K.H., Campbell, J., Campbell, S.: Evaluation of the lemon and banana signs in one hundred thirty fetuses with open spina bifida. Am. J. Obstet. Gynecol. 162 (1990) 322–327
62. Zamah, N.M., Gillieson, M.S., Walters, J.H., Hall, P.F.: Sonographic detection of polyhydramnios: A five-year experience. Am. J. Obstet. Gynecol. 143 (1982) 523–227

First screening examination

Fig. 2.**1** Lambda sign in a dichorionic, diamniotic twin pregnancy at 11 weeks, 4 days.

Fig. 2.**2** Left: nuchal translucency of 8 mm thickness in a fetus with trisomy 21. Right: Only the maximum width of the hypoechoic area (blue crosses) is measured. The red crosses show various possible sites for an incorrect measurement.

Fig. 2.**3** Fetal nuchal translucency. Normal range as a function of CRL (in mm). The 5th, 50th, and 95th percentiles are shown (adapted from [36]).

Fig. 2.**4** Maternal age-related risk for trisomy 21 at 12 weeks of gestation and the effect of fetal nuchal translucency (NT) thickness (adapted from [37]).

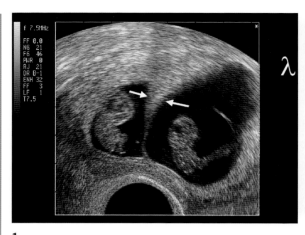

1

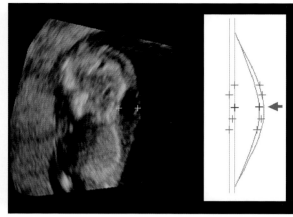

2

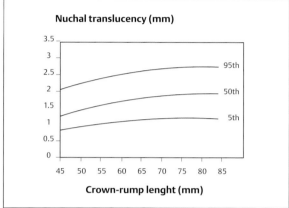

3

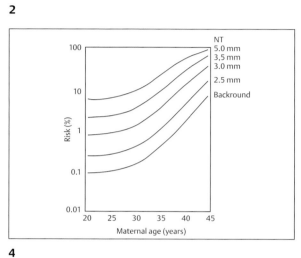

4

Second screening examination

Fig. 2.**5** Fetus with myelomeningocele at 27 weeks. Left: banana-shaped bowing of the cerebellum (banana sign). Right: concavities in the frontal part of the cranium (lemon sign).

5

3 Normal Early Pregnancy (First Trimester)

Pregnancy Dating

Menstrual age and conceptual age. Because the date of conception is not precisely known, it is customary in obstetrics to date a pregnancy in terms of menstrual age, which is counted from the first day of the last menstrual period. This is commonly referred to as the gestational age. In embryology, the conceptual age is used to designate the true age of the embryo counted from the date of conception (i.e., days postconception). Since the advent of reproductive medicine in the early 1980s, we are able to examine embryos of which the date of conception is precisely known.

Carnegie classification. For the first time, high-resolution transvaginal real-time ultrasound has been used to examine dated human embryos without disturbing their physical integrity or development. The Carnegie classification of the developmental stages in human embryos (5) is based on the parameters of maximum body length, external body shape, and the degree of development of the internal organs. Today this staging system can be correlated with the sonomorphologic findings of body length and body shape in living human embryos. The accurate dating of embryos examined in vivo enables us to check the gestational age figures in the Carnegie classification.

The normal development of the living human embryo will be reviewed in this chapter. Gestational age figures are based on conceptual age, but 14 days are added to obtain the menstrual age that is customarily used in obstetrics. Embryonic morphogenesis through 10 weeks' postmenstrual age is summarized in Table 3.**1**.

Table 3.1 Synopsis of human embryonic development (10)

Menstrual age	Carnegie stages	Ultrasound embryonic characteristics
Fifth week	6, 7	Implantation
Sixth week	8, 9, 10	Start of fetal circulation
Seventh week	11, 12, 13, 14	Separation from the yolk sac
Eighth week	15, 16, 17, 18	Dominance of brain development
Ninth week	19, 20	Completion of cardiogenesis and limb differentiation
Tenth week	21, 22, 23	Completion of organogenesis

Technique of Transvaginal Ultrasound

Modern ultrasound technology, including the use of high-resolution vaginal transducers, makes it possible to study ultrasound embryology in vivo. Several conditions must be satisfied, however, in order to accomplish this:

- The maternal bladder should be empty. A full bladder would lift the pregnant uterus out of the lower pelvis, and this would require applying an uncomfortable degree of pressure to obtain acceptable images.
- The patient is placed in a lithotomy position or supine with the buttocks elevated on a cushion. This increases the mobility of the vaginal probe in situ.

- Variable-frequency transducers should be set to the highest possible frequency, since higher frequencies correlate with higher image resolution.
- Ultrasound scanners for use in embryology should have a zoom feature that magnifies the image with minimal degradation.
- The examination should be done within the focal zone of the transducer to ensure that very small embryonic structures can be resolved. External pressure may have to be applied in some cases to move the uterus into the focal zone.

In principle, these conditions apply to all applications of transvaginal ultrasound. They are reviewed here because they are of fundamental importance in ultrasound embryology.

Ultrasound Embryology

Embryonic Development in the 5th Week of Menstrual Age (Day 15–21 Postconception)

Today the earliest phase of human development from conception to the initial cell divisions can be observed under the microscope within the framework of reproductive medical procedures (in-vitro fertilization/embryo transfer, IVF/ET; intracytoplasmic sperm injection, ICSI). When natural conception has occurred in the fallopian tube, we cannot directly observe the earliest stages of human embryonic development (Carnegie stages 1–5), and the conceptus can be visualized only after it has implanted in the uterine mucosa.

Chorionic sac. The earliest that we have been able to detect an implanted chorionic sac was on day 16 postconception. The sac diameter at that time was 2 mm (Figs. 3.**1**, 3.**2**). Two days later, the chorionic sac had doubled in size and already contained a recognizable yolk sac. The chorion appears as a circular echogenic structure bordering directly on the decidua. High-resolution color Doppler imaging can define maternal blood vessels between the decidua and chorion (Figs. 3.**3**, 3.**4**). By establishing this connection with the maternal circulation, the embryo secures the nutritional supply that is necessary for its further development.

Chorion frondosum. A hypoechoic structure in the uterine cavity can be identified as a chorionic sac only if it is surrounded by hyperplastic endometrium and displays an echogenic border, the chorion frondosum. If these signs are disregarded, a fluid collection in the uterine cavity (= pseudogestational sac) in an ectopic pregnancy may be misinterpreted as an intrauterine pregnancy.

Embryonic Development in the 6th Week of Menstrual Age (Day 22–28 Postconception)

Fetal pole. A fetal pole can usually be seen adjacent to the yolk sac at the start of the 6th week of menstrual age. Starting on day 23 postconception, we are consistently able to define a fetal pole in a normal pregnancy (10). It is still broadly adherent to the yolk sac at this time, initially appearing only as an echogenic structure about 1 mm long on the surface of the yolk sac.

Notochord. In subsequent days the early embryo appears pear-shaped in coronal section and contains a central notochord (Fig. 3.**5**). The neural tube begins to close from the rostral direction. This process concludes on day 38 of menstrual age with closure of the inferior neuropore.

Heart activity. Embryonic heart beats may be detected as early as the 23rd day postconception and are consistently detected by the 26th day (Fig. 3.**6**). The development of the cardiac pump and the parallel development of the vascular system provide a mechanism for distributing nutrients throughout the body of the embryo, enabling its further development during subsequent weeks.

Embryonic Development in the 7th Week of Menstrual Age (Day 29–35 Postconception)

Separation from the yolk sac. At the start of week 7 menstrual age, the embryo measures approximately 4 mm in length and its rostral pole begins to fold away from the yolk sac. The increasing longitudinal development of the embryo, made possible by acquiring a nutrient supply from the mother and distributing it via the cardiovascular system, leads to an increasing separation of the embryo from the yolk sac. At first this involves only a curling of the embryo, which is still broadly adherent to the yolk sac (Figs. 3.**7**, 3.**8**). But as the connecting stalk develops, the embryo increasingly separates from the yolk sac. Meanwhile the yolk sac is extruded into the extra-amniotic coelom, with only the vitelline duct connecting it to the embryonic vascular system (Figs. 3.**10**, 3.**11**).

C-shaped embryo. The embryo appears as a C-shaped figure at the end of 7 weeks' menstrual age (Figs. 3.**8**, 3.**9**). The amniotic membrane is still closely attached to the embryo, which consists of a dominant rostral pole and a smaller inferior pole (Fig. 3.**12**). Viewed in coronal section, limb buds can be distinguished on the lateral aspects of the body at the end of 7 weeks' menstrual age (Fig. 3.**13**).

Embryonic Development in the 8th Week of Menstrual Age (Day 36–42 Postconception)

Brain. The external shape of the head changes rapidly during this period, accompanied by rapid development of the embryonic brain. The maximum body length of the embryo is approximately 9 mm. M-mode scanning can already define two cardiac chambers separated by a distinct interventricular septum (Fig. 3.**14**). As early as day 36 postconception, we have been able to detect body movements reflecting the function of the embryonic central nervous system (10). Brain development proceeds rapidly during this period. By the end of the 8th postmenstrual week, the brain comprises approximately 50% of the total body length. The axis of the head is roughly perpendicular to the axis of the trunk (Figs. 3.**15**, 3.**16**). The telencephalon can always be identified by day 40 postconception. It first appears as a rostral, symmetrical outpouching from the prosencephalon and later envelops the diencephalon. Ultrasound confirms the development of the telencephalon by demonstrating the choroid plexus, which appears as a symmetrical, echogenic feature (Fig. 3.**17**). The rhombencephalon can be identified in the occipital head region (Fig. 3.**18**). The brain, then, is the first fetal organ system to undergo extensive structural differentiation, consistent with its central regulatory function.

Limbs. Brain development is paralleled by an initial segmental development of the embryo, which shows a marked increase in trunk width. Concomitant with this development of the mesoderm, the limbs begin to unfold and can be clearly identified with ultrasound (Fig. 3.**19**).

Amniotic membrane. The amniotic membrane also becomes clearly visible at this stage. It appears as an oval-shaped membrane outlining the body and limb contours of the embryo and marking the boundary between the amniotic and chorionic cavities. The vitelline duct and yolk sac are located in the extra-amniotic coelom (Fig. 3.**20**).

Embryonic Development in the 9th Week of Menstrual Age (Day 43–49 Postconception)

Limb differentiation. The embryo measures approximately 16 mm at the start of the 9th postmenstrual week. This stage is marked by changes in external body shape, characterized by longitudinal growth and differentiation of the limbs (Fig. 3.**21**). Differentiation of the upper limbs precedes that of the lower limbs by several days. But in all cases the upper limbs are clearly subdivided into an upper arm, forearm, and hand, and the lower limbs into a thigh, lower leg, and foot.

Physiologic umbilical hernia. A sagittal scan through the umbilical cord insertion at the end of this developmental stage demonstrates the physiologic umbilical hernia, which appears as a hyperechoic structure located in front of the embryonic abdominal wall (Figs. 3.**22**–3.**24**).

Heart. Also at this time, the embryonic heart completes its complex structural development (1). The ostium primum regresses during the 9th postmenstrual week, and the membranous interventricular septum closes (8), completely separating the systemic circulation from the pulmonary circulation. Further development is manifested by an increase in the epimyocardial mantle. Cardiogenesis is accompanied by a steady rise in the embryonic heart rate, culminating in a maximum rate that is about twice that of the maternal heart rate (Fig. 3.**25**).

Brain. During this stage the embryonic trunk straightens and the head begins to assume a more upright position. The midbrain flexure and dominant rhombencephalic fossa are clearly visible in a midsagittal scan (Fig. 3.**26**). Also, the contours of the telencephalon becomes increasingly distinct. A coronal scan from the posterior side demonstrates the structures of the axial skeleton (Fig. 3.**27**). The rhomboid fossa can be defined rostrally by tilting the coronal scan into the transverse plane.

Embryonic Development in the 10th Week of Menstrual Age (Day 50–56 Postconception)

Completion of organogenesis. Organogenesis is completed during the 10th week of menstrual age, and the major embryonic vessels can be defined with power color Doppler (Fig. 3.**28**). The embryo has a maximum body length of 23–31 mm.

Limbs. The limbs, which can be brought together only at the fingers and toes in the 9th postmenstrual week, lengthen and flex at the elbows and knees and can now reach across the fetal midline (Fig. 3.**29**). Details of the fingers and toes can be appreciated (Fig. 3.**30**). Isolated arm and leg movements can also be seen and are no longer attributable to spinal reflex actions (11).

Head. It is possible to discern the maxilla and mandible, which form the basic framework for the embryonic facial skeleton (Fig. 3.**31**). Development of the telencephalon becomes increasingly distinct, and the two hemispheres are separated by the falx cerebri (Fig. 3.**32**).

Trunk. A transverse Doppler scan through the embryonic trunk below the liver can clearly demonstrate the umbilical vessels and the adjacent bowel loops that have herniated into the umbilical cord insertion

(Fig. 3.**33**). The initially oblong amniotic cavity has expanded to a circular-shaped structure (Fig. 3.**33**), with a corresponding reduction in the size of the extra-amniotic coelom. The yolk sac is still clearly visible in the extra-amniotic coelom.

Fetal Development in the 11th Week of Menstrual Age (Day 57–63 Postconception)

Body shape. The organs that develop during organogenesis become sonographically visible during the coming weeks of fetal development. The maximum body length measures between 31 and 40 mm, and the BPD ranges from 14 to 18 mm (10) (Fig. 3.**34**). The contours of the facial profile become more distinct, although the frontal prominence of the calvaria is still the dominant feature (Fig. 3.**35**).

Trunk. The fetal urinary bladder can be seen in the lower part of the trunk (Fig. 3.**36**), at this stage consisting only of connective tissue and epithelial cells with no contractile elements (4). The amniotic cavity has expanded markedly, compressing the yolk sac in the extra-amniotic coelom (Fig. 3.**37**).

Fetal Development in the 12th Week of Menstrual Age (Day 64–70 Postconception

The maximum body length in this week is 41–53 mm, and the BPD increases from 18 to 21 mm. The stomach and bladder can be identified within the fetal abdomen (Fig. 3.**38**), and both kidneys can be seen in the retroperitoneum (Fig. 3.**39**). Thoracic scans can demonstrate the heart with its two chambers, which can be clearly visualized with color Doppler (Fig. 3.**40**). In a coronal scan of the face, both eyes can be identified (Fig. 3.**41**).

Fetal Development in the 13th Week of Menstrual Age (Day 71–77 Postconception)

Face. The fetus at the end of the first trimester has a maximum length of 71 mm and a BPD of 24 mm. The facial physiognomy is clearly discerned on a midsagittal scan through the head owing to the development of the facial skeleton and soft tissues (Fig. 3.**42**).

Abdomen and pelvis. The physiologic umbilical hernia can no longer be seen (Fig. 3.**43**). Discontinuities in the abdominal wall must now be classified as fetal pathology (6). Color Doppler imaging can define the principal blood vessels (Fig. 3.**44**). Smooth-muscle cells can be detected in the wall of the urinary bladder, but they still lack an autonomous nerve supply (3). The external genitalia are grossly visible at the end of 13 weeks (9).

Clinical Importance of Ultrasound Embryology

Diagnostic ultrasound in the first trimester gives doctors and parents a detailed look at early human development and provides impressive documentation of this period. A knowledge of the normal development of the human embryo on ultrasound images forms the basis for the early detection of embryofetal pathology.

Because the morphogenesis of the embryo proceeds at a rapid pace, it is very useful for the dating of embryos. This requires a very high degree of morphologic expertise, however, and so the age of a pregnancy in routine settings is determined by measuring the greatest embryonic length and the BPD. The essential aspects of morphologic development are reviewed in Table 3.**2**.

Table 3.2 Developmental milestones in the first trimester (adapted from 7, 9, and 10)

Ultrasound finding	Earliest visualization (menstrual age)	Definite visualization (menstrual age)
Chorionic cavity	Day 30	Day 32
Yolk sac	Day 32	Day 34
Fetal pole	Day 35	Day 37
Heart activity	Day 37	Day 40
Limbs	Day 47	Day 53
Telencephalon	Day 50	Day 54
Movements	Day 50	Day 56
Stomach	Week 10	Week 11
Urinary bladder	Week 11	Week 12
Genitalia	Week 12	Week 14

References

1. Cooper, M.H., O'Rahilly, R.: The human heart at seven postovulatory weeks. Acta Anat Basel 79 (1971) 280–299
2. Drews, M.: Taschenatlas der Embryologie. Stuttgart: Thieme (1994)
3. Gilpin, S.A., Gosling, J.A.: Smooth muscle in the wall of the developing human urinary bladder and urethra. J. Anat. 137 (1983) 503–512
4. Newman, J., Antonakopoulos, G.N.: The fine structure of the human fetal urinary bladder. Development and maturation. A light, transmission and scanning electron microscopic study. J. Anat. 166 (1989) 135–150
5. O'Rahilly, R., Müller, F.: Developmental stages in human embryos. Washington: Carnegie Inst. Wash. Publ. (1987) vol 637
6. Schmidt, W., Yarkoni, S., Crelin, E.S., Hobbins, J.C.: Sonographic visualization of anterior abdominal wall hernia in the first trimester. Obstet. Gynecol. 69 (1987) 911–915
7. Takeuchi, H.: Sonoembryology. In: Kurjak, A. (ed.): An Atlas of Ultrasonography in Obstetrics and Gynecology. Casterton: Parthenon Publishing Group (1992)
8. Teal, S.I., Moore, G.W., Hutchins, G.: Development of aortic and mitral valve continuity in the human embryonic heart. Am. J. Anat. 176 (1986) 447–460
9. Timor-Tritsch, I.E., Blumenfeld, Z., Rottem, S.: Sonoembryology. In: Timor-Tritsch, I.E., Rottem, S. (eds.): Transvaginal Sonography. Amsterdam: Elsevier (1991)
10. Wisser, J.: Vaginalsonographie im ersten Schwangerschaftsdrittel. Berlin: Springer (1995)
11. Wisser, J., Dudel, C.: Evaluation of human embryonic brain morphology and development of movement by transvaginal real-time sonography. In: Siegenthaler, W., Haas, R., (ed.): The decade of the brain. Stuttgart: Thieme (1995) 20–22

Week 5 of menstrual age

Fig. 3.**1** Transvaginal sonogram of an embryo that implanted in the decidua of the posterior uterine wall on the 17th day after conception (from 10, with permission of Springer Verlag, Heidelberg).

Fig. 3.**2** Embryo prior to reorganization (after 2).

Fig. 3.**3** Two days later, the embryo from Fig. 3.1 shows the development of a yolk sac. The implantation vessel is also definable by color Doppler imaging (from 10, with permission of Springer Verlag, Heidelberg).

Fig. 3.**4** Embryo after reorganization (after 2).

Week 6 of menstrual age

Fig. 3.**5** Embryo implanted in the uterus on postmenstrual day 40. The pear-shaped fetal pole is visible on the yolk sac.

Fig. 3.**6** Embryo implanted in the uterus on postmenstrual day 40. The M-mode trace indicates an embryonic heart rate of 105 bpm.

Week 7 of menstrual age

Fig. 3.**7** Embryo on postmenstrual day 43. The body is still broadly apposed to the yolk sac and exhibits lordosis.

Fig. 3.**8** By postmenstrual day 47, the embryo has separated from the yolk sac and shows a C-shape curvature.

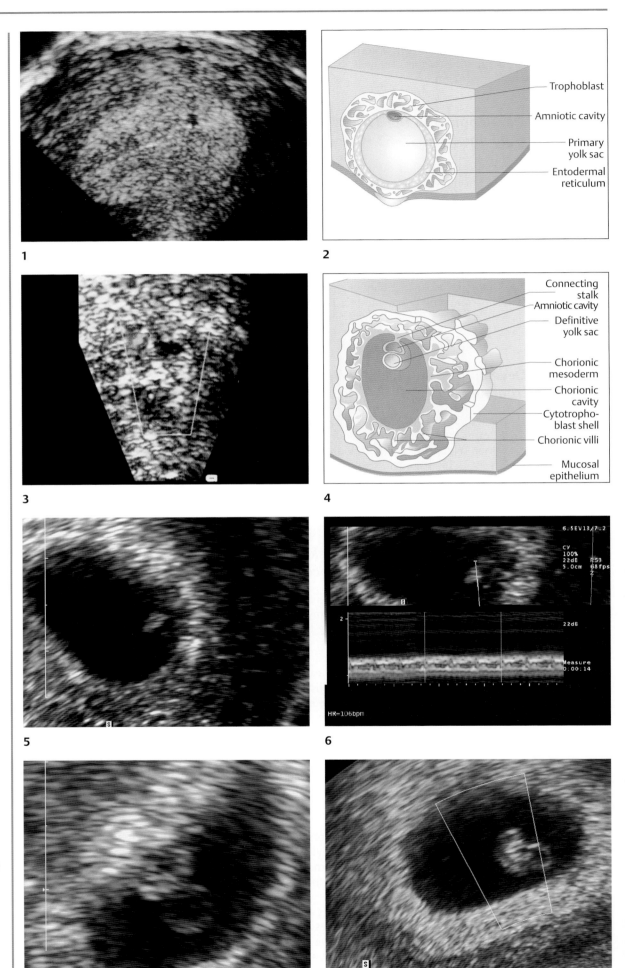

1

2
- Trophoblast
- Amniotic cavity
- Primary yolk sac
- Entodermal reticulum

3

4
- Connecting stalk
- Amniotic cavity
- Definitive yolk sac
- Chorionic mesoderm
- Chorionic cavity
- Cytotrophoblast shell
- Chorionic villi
- Mucosal epithelium

5

6

7

8

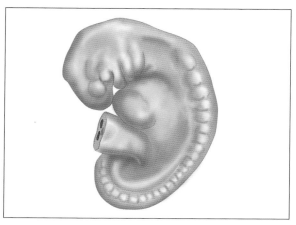

9

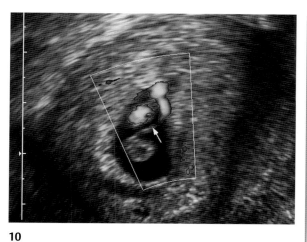

10

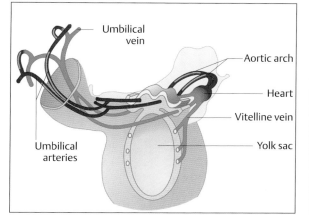

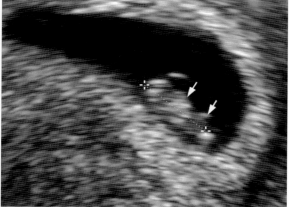

Umbilical
vein

Aortic arch

Heart

Vitelline vein

Umbilical
arteries

Yolk sac

11

12

13

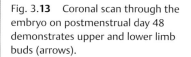

14

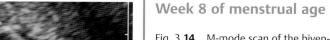

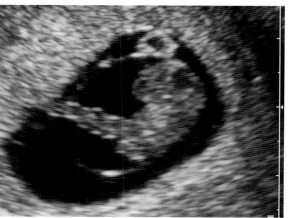

15

Fig. 3.**9** Development of the umbilical cord, viewed from the left side (after [2]).

Fig. 3.**10** On postmenstrual day 48 the yolk sac is in the extra-amniotic coelom and is linked to the embryo by the vitelline duct (arrow).

Fig. 3.**11** Course of the vitelline vein and umbilical vein (after [2]).

Fig. 3.**12** The embryo is closely enveloped by the amniotic membrane (arrow) on postmenstrual day 48.

Fig. 3.**13** Coronal scan through the embryo on postmenstrual day 48 demonstrates upper and lower limb buds (arrows).

Week 8 of menstrual age

Fig. 3.**14** M-mode scan of the biventricular embryonic heart on postmenstrual day 55. The cardiac diameter is 1.8 mm.

Fig. 3.**15** Midsagittal scan through the embryo on postmenstrual day 53 shows the dominance of brain development.

Fig. 3.**16**   Embryo 9.6 mm long, viewed from the right side (after [2]).

Fig. 3.**17**   Coronal scan on postmenstrual day 53 shows the telencephalon with symmetrical development of the cortical anlage. Arrows indicate the choroid plexus on each side.

Fig. 3.**18**   Coronal scan through the posterior superior fossa on postmenstrual day 55 demonstrates the rhombencephalon.

Fig. 3.**19**   The limbs are clearly identified on postmenstrual day 56 (short arrows: arms; long arrows: legs).

Fig. 3.**20**   On postmenstrual day 56, the embryo is surrounded by the amniotic membrane (arrows). The vitelline duct and yolk sac have been displaced into the chorionic cavity.

Week 9 of menstrual age

Fig. 3.**21**   On postmenstrual day 60, the upper limb of the embryo is seen to consist of three segments.

Fig. 3.**22**   Transverse scan through the abdomen of the embryo on postmenstrual day 60 shows an echogenic bulge in the umbilical area (arrow).

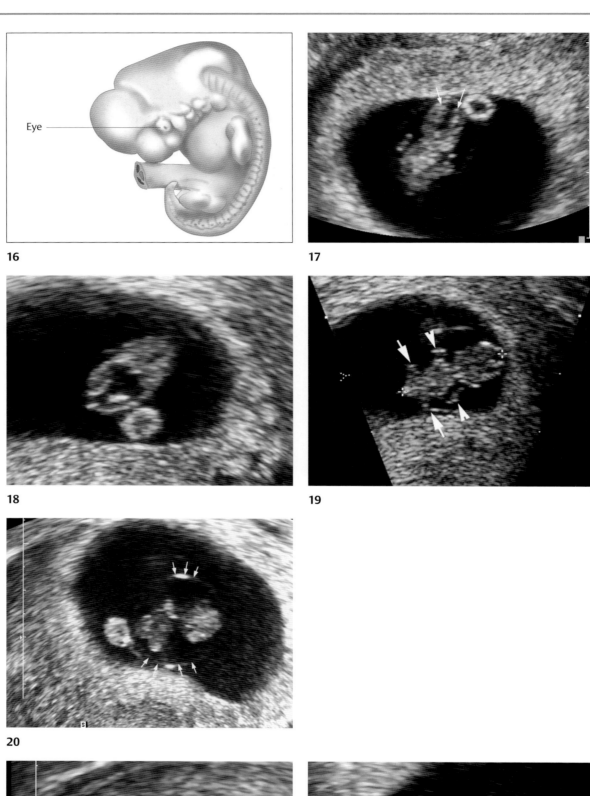

16

17

18

19

20

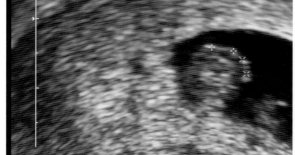

21

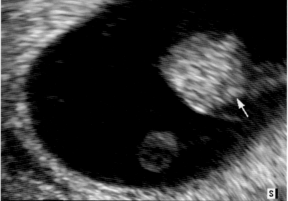

22

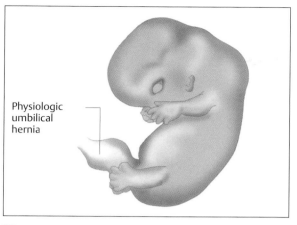

Physiologic umbilical hernia

23

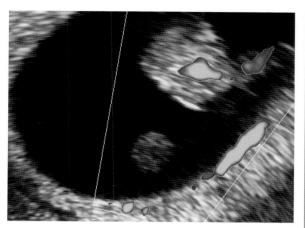

24

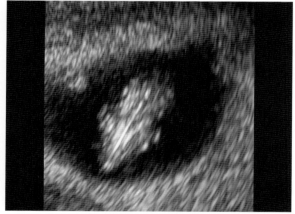

n = 348

Embryonic heart rate (BPM) vs. Menstrual age of embryo

25

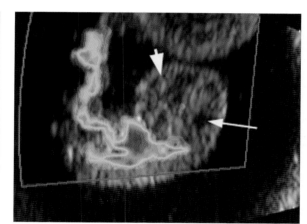

26

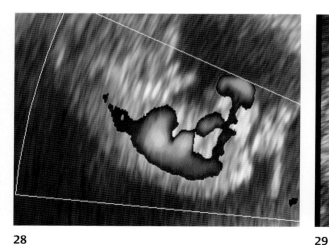

27

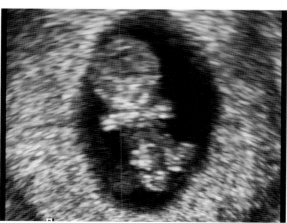

28   **29**

Fig. 3.**23**   Embryo 24 mm long on postmenstrual day 65. The physiologic umbilical hernia at this stage has expanded the fetal end of the cord.

Fig. 3.**24**   Power Doppler at the umbilical ring defines the embryonic vascular system and the physiologic umbilical hernia.

Fig. 3.**25**   Embryonic heart rate as a function of menstrual age (from [10], with permission of Springer Verlag, Heidelberg).

Fig. 3.**26**   Sagittal scan through the embryo on postmenstrual day 61 demonstrates the rhombencephalon (long arrow) and telencephalon (short arrow).

Fig. 3.**27**   Axial skeleton of the embryo on postmenstrual day 60.

Week 10 of menstrual age

Fig. 3.**28**   Power Doppler on postmenstrual day 66 demonstrates the embryonic vascular system with the heart, aorta, umbilical artery, umbilical vein, and carotid artery.

Fig. 3.**29**   In a coronal scan on postmenstrual day 66, the arms and legs have grown so long that they can reach across to the contralateral side.

Fig. 3.**30**   Four fingers (arrows) can be seen on postmenstrual day 66.

Fig. 3.**31**   Sagittal scan through the embryonic face on postmenstrual day 66 defines the basic structures of the facial skeleton with the mandible and maxilla.

Fig. 3.**32**   By day 67 the telencephalon has increased markedly in size and is beginning to enclose the diencephalon. Both hemispheres are clearly separated by the falx cerebri.

Fig. 3.**33**   The amniotic membrane envelops the embryo on postmenstrual day 66, appearing nearly circular (arrows). The extra-amniotic coelom is considerably more echogenic than the amniotic cavity. The cord insertion is thickened and shows the physiologic umbilical hernia.

Week 11 of menstrual age

Fig. 3.**34**   Transverse scan through the head of the embryo on postmenstrual day 72 for measuring the biparietal diameter. Both halves of the brain are clearly separated, and the cavum septi pellucidi is defined.

Fig. 3.**35**   Facial profile of an embryo on postmenstrual day 73.

Fig. 3.**36**   Coronal scan of the embryo on postmenstrual day 72. The urinary bladder appears as a hypoechoic structure in the lower pelvis (arrow).

Fig. 3.**37**   On postmenstrual day 72 the yolk sac (arrow) is compressed between the amniotic and chorionic membranes and is undergoing regression.

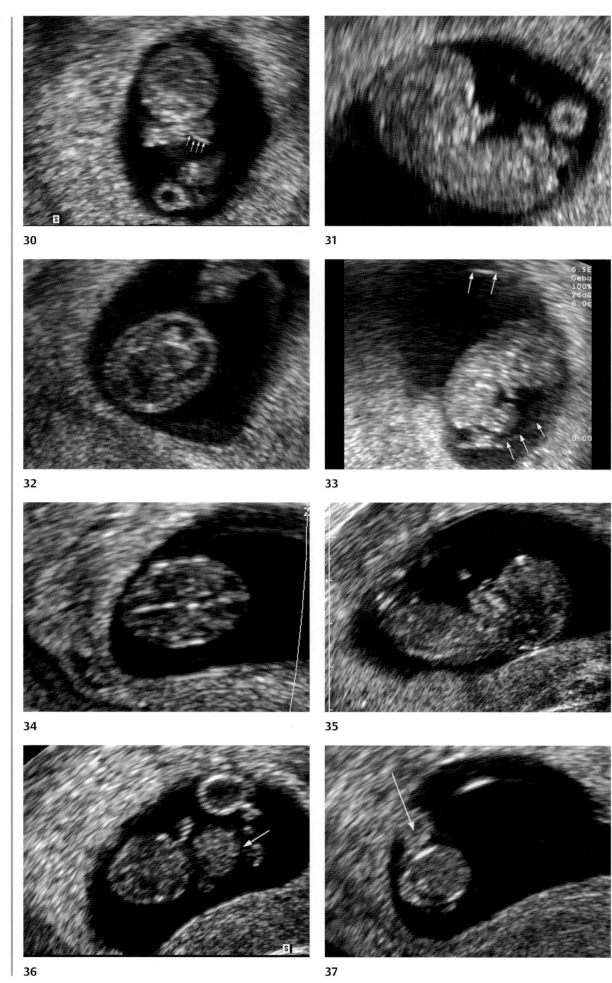

30

31

32

33

34

35

36

37

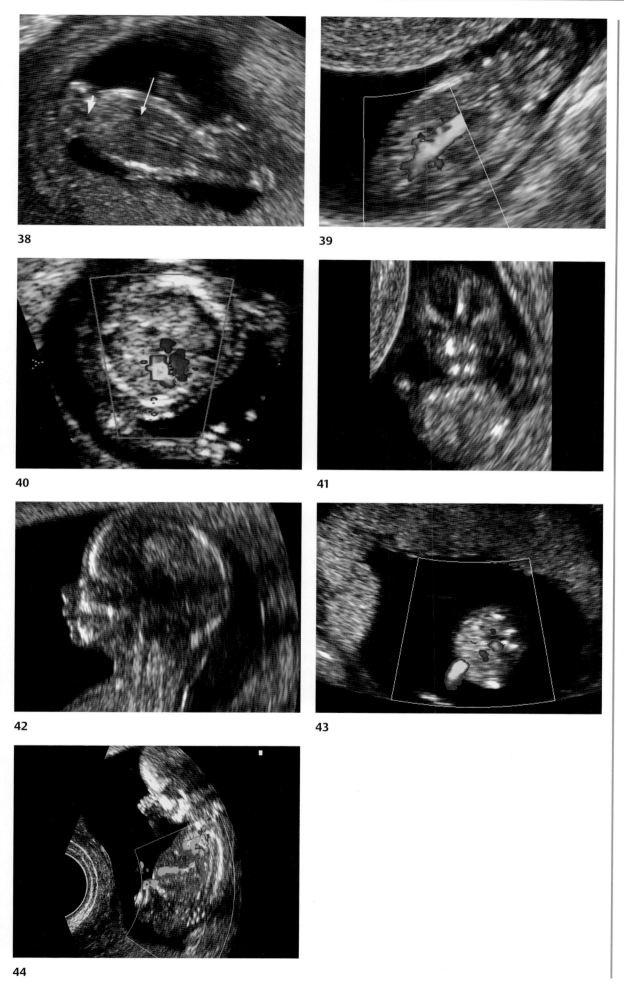

38

39

40

41

42

43

44

Week 12 of menstrual age

Fig. 3.**38** Coronal scan through the embryonic abdomen on postmenstrual day 81. The gastric bubble (long arrow) is visible in the left upper abdomen and the urinary bladder (short arrow) in the lower abdomen.

Fig. 3.**39** Coronal power Doppler scan through the retroperitoneum on postmenstrual day 81 demonstrates the aorta, the aortic bifurcation, and both renal arteries. The kidneys are hyperechoic.

Fig. 3.**40** Intrathoracic color Doppler scan on postmenstrual day 82 demonstrates the heart with its separate ventricular systems.

Fig. 3.**41** Coronal facial scan on postmenstrual day 81 demonstrates both eyes.

Week 13 of menstrual age

Fig. 3.**42** Facial profile on postmenstrual day 91.

Fig. 3.**43** Umbilical cord insertion on postmenstrual day 88. The abdominal wall is closed.

Fig. 3.**44** Thoracoabdominal vessels of a fetus on postmenstrual day 91.

4 Transvaginal Biometry and Gestational Age Assignment in the First Trimester

Biometry

Biometric data provide a tool for checking the progress of a pregnancy with regard to gestational age. Standardized image planes are of key importance in measuring biometric parameters. When small fetal dimensions are measured, precision biometry requires the use of a high-resolution vaginal probe (5–7.5 MHz) and zooming to obtain a magnified view of critical structures.

When the gestational age is known, a comparison of biometric parameters with reference charts permits the selective monitoring of embryofetal growth even during the first trimester.

Chorionic Sac

Detection. Transvaginal visualization of the chorionic sac at the earliest possible stage is important in confirming the presence of an intrauterine pregnancy and excluding ectopic gestation. The chorionic sac is the first pregnancy-specific structure that can be defined with ultrasound, and it can be detected just a few days after the missed period by transvaginal scanning (3, 9, 11, 41). It can be difficult to detect a chorionic sac at this early stage, however, particularly in a fibroid uterus. When the chorionic sac has reached 2–4 mm in diameter, it appears as an echogenic ring-like structure with a hypoechoic center embedded in the secretory endometrium.

Mean diameter of chorionic sac. The mean diameter of the gestational sac correlates closely with the rise in maternal serum hCG levels (Table 4.1). The mean diameter of the chorionic sac is defined as the arith-

metic mean of its greatest sagittal, transverse, and coronal diameters. The mutually perpendicular measurements are "inner-to-inner" dimensions—i.e., they are measured between the inner margins of the chorionic cavity (Fig. 4.1).

Growth rate. The chorionic sac shows an approximately linear growth rate during the first 10 weeks of menstrual age in both abdominal and transvaginal scans (Fig. 4.7a). It is circular during the initial weeks and becomes more elliptical toward the end of the first trimester. The sac has a reported mean growth rate of 1.13 mm/day between 5 and 11 weeks (34). Less than 0.6 mm/day of sac growth suggests that spontaneous abortion will probably occur (34). The mean sac diameter is approximately 5 mm at 5 weeks and approximately 50 mm at 11 weeks.

Abortion risk. When the chorionic sac has reached more than 8 mm in diameter, it should be possible to detect the yolk sac (26). A chorionic sac that is small in relation to the crown–rump length appears to be associated with a greater than 90% rate of spontaneous abortion (5). Other authors could predict abortion in 71% of cases when both the mean sac size and the crown–rump length were below one standard deviation (33).

Amniotic epithelium. Starting at the end of 7 weeks, the amniotic epithelium can be identified as a fine, echogenic membrane within the chorionic sac (2, 18, 38). During subsequent weeks the amniotic epithelium increasingly separates from the embryo, becoming adherent to the chorionic epithelium at 12–13 weeks.

Yolk Sac

First embryonic structure. The secondary yolk sac can be seen toward the end of the 5th week, appearing as a sharply circumscribed, echogenic ring-like structure within the chorionic cavity (41). It is the first embryonic structure that is detectable in the extraembryonic coelom between the amnion and chorion. It is connected to the embryo by the omphaloenteric (vitelline) duct. Given its embryonic origin, the ultrasound detection of a yolk sac rules out a blighted ovum and an ectopic pregnancy even before the embryo itself can be identified (35).

Detection. The yolk sac can be detected between 5 and 10 weeks' gestation in 80–90% of cases (17, 38). Its diameter is measured from outer-to-outer margin (Fig. 4.2) (42). Care is taken not to confuse the yolk sac with the embryonic head.

Growth pattern. The yolk sac exhibits a biphasic growth pattern. Its growth is almost linear between 5 and 8 weeks' gestation and then plateaus until the end of the first trimester (Fig. 4.7b). The size of the yolk sac is approximately 2 mm at 6 weeks and 6 mm at 11 weeks and correlates closely with embryonic development and crown–rump length (2, 18). It should be noted, however, that the growth patterns in both normal and abnormal early pregnancies show considerable variation (17, 37, 51).

Size and shape discrepancies. There is disagreement over the clinical relevance of a yolk sac size that is outside normal limits. While some authors have found a link between an enlarged yolk sac and an increased rate of spontaneous abortions and chromosomal abnormalities

Table 4.1 hCG levels (IU/L) correlated with mean gestational sac diameter (7)

Gestational sac diameter (mm)	Serum hCG level (mean) (IU/L)	95% confidence interval (IU/L)
3	710	1050–2800
4	2320	1440–3760
5	3100	1940–4980
6	4090	2580–6530
7	5340	3400–8450
8	6880	4420–10810
9	8770	5680–13660
10	11040	7220–17050
11	13730	9050–21040
12	16870	11230–25640
13	20480	13750–30880
14	24560	16650–36750
15	29110	19910–43220
16	34100	25530–50210
17	39460	27470–57640
18	45120	31700–65380
19	50970	36130–73280
20	56900	40700–81150
21	62760	45300–88790
22	68390	49810–95990
23	73640	54120–102540
24	78350	58100–108230
25	82370	61640–112870
26	85560	64600–116310
27	87820	66900–118420
28	89050	68460–119130
29	89230	69220–118420
30	88340	69150–116310

(19, 29, 39), other authors have found no relationship to pregnancy outcome (17, 26, 37). The absence of a yolk sac or a markedly smaller-than-normal yolk sac is considered a poor prognostic sign (6, 19, 39). A yolk sac with ill-defined margins or a distorted shape also seems to imply an unfavorable outcome (29). By 13 weeks' gestation, the yolk sac can no longer be seen due to fusion of the amniotic and chorionic epithelia.

Amniotic Cavity

Detection. Between 7 and 10 weeks' gestation, the amniotic cavity can be distinguished from the chorionic cavity by its different echogenicity. Whereas fine, homogeneous internal echoes can be seen within the chorionic cavity, the amniotic cavity is echo-free. The amniotic epithelium appears as a round, thin, echogenic membrane surrounding the embryo, first enveloping it closely and than separating from it after 7 weeks' gestation (2, 18, 41).

Mean diameter. As with the chorionic sac, the mean diameter of the amniotic cavity is defined as the arithmetic mean of its greatest sagittal, transverse, and coronal diameters (Fig. 4.3). The mutually perpendicular measurements are taken between the inner margins of the amniotic cavity.

Growth pattern. The amniotic cavity increasingly expands during subsequent weeks. Because the amniotic sac grows much faster than the chorionic sac (53), the amniotic epithelium becomes applied to the chorionic epithelium toward the end of the first trimester. By that stage only the amniotic cavity can be seen. As with the chorionic sac, the growth of the amniotic cavity follows a linear pattern (Fig. 4.7c). Its diameter is approximately 10 mm at 7 weeks and 50 mm at 12 weeks (2). A large amniotic cavity in relation to the crown–rump length appears to be associated with an increased rate of early embryonic death (24).

Crown–Rump Length

Maximum embryonic length. Transvaginal ultrasound can usually demonstrate the embryo by 6 weeks' gestation, located in close proximity to the yolk sac (33, 41, 49). The sonographically measured crown–rump length (CRL) is not the true CRL due to the curled position of the trunk and the flexed head. It is actually the maximum embryonic length (32), but the term "CRL" is used for simplicity. The CRL is measured from the superior to the inferior pole, preferably with the embryo in an extended position (Fig. 4.4).

Measurement errors. CRL measurements have a reported intra- and interobserver variability of 6.6% and 8.4%, respectively (46). The most common errors in CRL determinations are caused by measuring the embryo in a flexed position and by including the yolk sac in the measurement. The CRL grows in a nonlinear, exponential pattern with an increasing scatter of values toward the end of the first trimester (Fig. 4.7d).

Abdominal and vaginal ultrasound measurements. A comparison of the growth charts constructed with abdominal and transvaginal ultrasound shows no significant differences between the two methods (2, 10, 16, 21, 23, 27, 30, 31, 36, 42, 43, 44, 46, 48). However, the embryo can be detected approximately one week earlier by transvaginal scanning. Good agreement also exists with growth charts for embryos of precisely known conceptual age in the setting of IVF therapy (8, 52).

Singleton pregnancies. In singleton pregnancies of confirmed gestational age, a CRL below the 5th percentile is associated with an increased rate of trisomy 18 (25). All other chromosomal abnormalities

show no such relationship to CRL, however (25, 50). From 7 to 13 weeks' gestation, the CRL increases 15-fold from approximately 4 mm to approximately 58 mm (2). Figure 4.11a shows the estimated gestational age as a function of CRL (42).

Multiple pregnancies. No differences in CRL have been found between singleton pregnancies and higher-order multifetal pregnancies (45). But if multiple fetuses show a discordant CRL of 3 mm or more, the rate of embryonic loss under 9 weeks (= 63 days menstrual age) is approximately 50% (12). There are also reports that a below-normal CRL is associated with an increased rate of spontaneous abortion (33), congenital anomalies (51), and chromosomal abnormalities (13, 14, 15).

Biparietal Diameter

The biparietal diameter (BPD) can be measured at the end of 7 weeks' gestation (1, 4, 28). The measurement is taken from the outer-to-outer aspects of the skull at the level of the occipitofrontal plane (Figs. 4.5, 4.6). The BPD growth curve shows a linear increase during the first trimester (Fig. 4.7e) (2, 4, 28, 42). The BPD measures approximately 7 mm at 8 weeks and approximately 24 mm at 13 weeks (2, 42). The relationship between crown–rump length and biparietal diameter is shown in Table 4.2.

Abdomen

Growth pattern. The embryonic abdomen shows a linear growth pattern during the first trimester (4, 22, 27, 28, 42). The stomach and intrahepatic veins often cannot be visualized at this early stage. The level of the umbilical cord insertion, therefore, is used as the reference plane for abdominal biometry in the embryo (Fig. 4.8) (27). The embryonic abdomen can be successfully measured at the end of 8 weeks. The mean transverse abdominal diameter is approximately 6 mm, and the abdominal circumference is approximately 20 mm at 8 weeks (4, 27, 42) (Fig. 4.10a). Multiple regression analysis has shown that the abdominal dimensions correlate better with CRL than with gestational age (22, 27). The relationship between crown–rump length and abdominal circumference is shown in Table 4.2.

Physiologic umbilical hernia. The physiologic umbilical hernia can be detected with ultrasound between 10 and 12 weeks' gestation. It should not be included in abdominal measurements.

Femur

Definite limb buds can be recognized at 9 weeks' gestation (22, 27, 42). The most important biometric limb parameter at this stage is femur length, which is an outer-to-outer measurement of the ossified femoral shaft (Fig. 4.9). Abnormal measurements toward the end of the first trimester can already provide initial evidence for the presence of skele-

Table 4.2 Mean values and 95% confidence intervals (in mm) of biparietal diameter (BPD), abdominal circumference (AC), and femur length in relation to crown–rump length (CRL) (27)

CRL	BPD			AC			Femur length		
mm	2.5%	50%	97.5%	2.5%	50%	97.5%	2.5%	50%	97.5
5	1.9	4.8	7.7	1.6	10.9	20.1		0.2	3.4
15	4.7	7.6	10.4	10.9	20.1	29.2		1.9	5.0
25	7.6	10.5	13.4	20.1	29.2	38.3	0.5	3.6	6.6
35	10.5	13.4	16.2	29.3	38.3	47.3	2.2	5.2	8.2
45	13.4	16.2	19.1	38.5	47.5	56.6	4.0	6.9	9.9
55	16.2	19.1	22.0	47.6	56.7	65.7	5.6	8.5	11.5
65	19.1	22.0	24.8	56.7	65.8	75.0	7.2	10.2	13.2
75	21.9	24.8	27.7	65.8	75.0	84.2	8.8	11.9	15.0
85	24.7	27.7	30.6	74.8	84.1	93.5	10.5	13.5	16.7

tal dysplasia. Femur length is approximately 5 mm at 10 weeks (Fig. 4.**10b**) (27, 42). Table 4.**2** shows the relationship between crown–rump length and femur length.

Gestational Age Assignment

Crown–rump length. Reliable ultrasound determination of gestational age is possible only during the first trimester. The standard parameter for this assessment is the crown–rump length (CRL), as it shows the least variation compared with other biometric parameters. This was demonstrated during the 1970s by Robinson and Fleming (44) and Hansmann et al. (23) and confirmed in the early 1980s by Schmidt et al. (47). Robinson and Fleming (44) could estimate gestational age to an accuracy of ± 4.7 days (95% confidence interval) based on a single CRL measurement taken between 7 and 14 weeks. Hansmann et al. (23) achieved an accuracy of ± 7 days (2 SD) in the 7th week and ± 11 days (2 SD) at the end of the first half of pregnancy. Schmidt et al. (47) achieved an accuracy of ± 7 days to ± 10 days for the same period.

Recent data have been published on the dating accuracy of transvaginal ultrasound measurements obtained during the first trimester (40, 42, 52). Rempen (42) determined confidence intervals for gestational age at the 95th and 5th percentiles of ± 6 days for crown–rump length, ± 8 days for biparietal diameter and transverse abdominal diameter, and ± 9 days for mean chorionic sac diameter. Figure 4.**11a** shows estimated gestational age as a function of CRL (42).

Mean chorionic sac diameter. The mean chorionic sac diameter is useful for pregnancy dating only during the initial weeks of gestation (42). This parameter becomes much more variable toward the end of the first trimester and is less accurate than the CRL for gestational age assignment.

Biparietal diameter. The biparietal diameter becomes increasingly important for gestational age assignment toward the end of the first trimester (21) (Fig. 4.**11b**).

References

1. Bahlmann, F., Merz, E.: Sonomorphologie der normalen und gestörten Frühgravidität. Gynäkol. Prax. 19 (1995) 5–21
2. Bahlmann, F., Merz, E., Weber, G., Wellek, S., Engelhardt, O.: Transvaginale Ultraschallbiometrie in der Frühgravididtät – Ein Wachstumsmodell. Ultraschall in Med. 18 (1997) 196–204
3. Bernaschek, G., Rudelstorfer, R., Csaicsich, P.: Vaginal sonography versus serum human chorionic gonadotropin in early detection of pregnancy. Am. J. Obstet. Gynecol. 158 (1988) 608–612
4. Blaas, H.G., Eik-Nes, H., Bremnes, J.B.: The growth of the human embryo. A longitudinal biometric assessment from 7 to 12 weeks of gestation. Ultrasound Obstet. Gynecol. 12 (1998) 346–354
5. Bromley, B., Harlow, B.L., Laboda, L.A., Benacerraf, B.B.: Small sac size in the first trimester: A predictor of poor fetal outcome. Radiology 178 (1991) 375–377
6. Crooji, M.J., Westhuis, M., Schoemaker, J., Exalto, N.: Ultrasonographic measurement of the yolk sac. Brit. J. Obstet. Gynaecol. 89 (1982) 931–933
7. Daya, S., Woods, S., Ward, S., Lappalainen, R., Caco, C.: Transvaginal ultrasound scanning in early pregnancy and correlation with human chorionic gonadotropin levels. J. Clin. Ultrasound 19 (1991) 139–142
8. Daya, S.: Accuracy of gestational age estimation by means of fetal crown-rump length measurement. Obstet. Gynecol. 168 (1993) 903–908
9. De Crespigny, L.C., Cooper, D., McKenna, M.: Early detection of intrauterine pregnancy with ultrasound. J. Ultrasound Med. 7 (1988) 7–10
10. Degenhardt, F., Böhmer, S., Behrens, O., Mühlhaus, K.: Transvaginale Ultraschallbiometrie der Scheitel-Steiß-Länge im ersten Trimenon. Z. Geburtsh. u. Perinat. 192 (1988) 249–252
11. Degenhardt, F., Böhmer, S., Laabs, A.: Vaginalsonographische Ermittlung des Fruchtsackquerschnittes in der Frühschwangerschaft. Z. Geburtsh. u. Perinat. 193 (1989) 68–71
12. Dickey, R.P., Olar, T.T., Taylor, S.N. et al.: Incidence and significance of unequal gestational sac diameter or embryo crown-rump length in twin pregnancy. Hum. Reprod. 7 (1992) 1170–1172
13. Dickey, R.P., Olar, T.T., Taylor, S.N., Curole, D.N., Matulich, E.M.: Relationship of small gestational sac-crown-rump length differences to abortion and abortus karyotypes. Obstet. Gynecol. 79 (1992) 554–557
14. Dickey, R.P., Gasser, R.F., Olar, T.T. et al.: The relationship of initial embryo crown-rump length to pregnancy outcome and abnormal karyotype based on new growth curves for the 2–31mm embryo. Hum. Reprod. 9 (1994) 366–373
15. Drugan, A., Johnson, M.P., Isada, N.B. et al.: The smaller than expected first-trimester fetus is at increased risk for chromosome anomalies. Am. J. Obstet. Gynecol. 167 (1992) 1525–1528
16. Drumm, J.E., Clinch, J., MacKenzie, G.: The ultrasonic measurement of fetal crown-rump length as a method af assessing gestational age. Brit. J. Obstet. Gynaecol. 83 (1976) 417–421
17. Ferrazzi, E., Brambati, B., Lanzani, A. et al.: The yolk sac in early pregnancy failure. Am. J. Obstet. Gynecol. 158 (1988) 137–142
18. Funk, A., Fendel, H.: Ultraschallechographische Darstellbarkeit und Messung der Amnionhöhle und des Dottersacks in der frühen Schwangerschaft: Vergleichende Untersuchung von intakten und gestörten Schwangerschaften. Z. Geburtsh. u. Perinat. 192 (1988) 59–66
19. Funk, A., Eichenberg, S., Sohn, C.: Transvaginale Sonographie: Die differentialdiagnostische Bedeutung des sekundären Dottersackes in der Frühschwangerschaft. Z. Geburtsh. u. Perinat. 193 (1989)178–182
20. Goldstein, S.R., Snyder, J.R., Watson, C., Danon, M.: Very early pregnancy detection with endovaginal ultrasound. Obstet. Gynecol. 72 (1988) 200–204
21. Goldstein, S.R.: Embryonic ultrasonographic measurements: Crown-rump length revisited. Am. J. Obstet. Gynecol. 165 (1991) 497–501
22. Green, J.J., Hobbins, J.C.: Abdominal ultrasound examination of the first trimester fetus. Am. J. Obstet. Gynecol. 159 (1988) 165–175
23. Hansmann, M., Schuhmacher, H., Foebus, J., Voigt, U.: Ultraschallbiometrie der fetalen Scheitelsteißlänge in der ersten Schwangerschaftshälfte. Geburtsh. u. Frauenheilk. 39 (1979) 656–666
24. Horrow, M.M.: Enlarged amniotic cavity: A new sonographic sign of early embryonic death. AJR 158 (1992) 359–362
25. Kuhn, P., Brizot, M.L., Pandya, P.P., Snijders, R.J., Nicolaides, K.H.: Crown-rump length in chromosomally abnormal fetuses at 10 to 13 weeks' gestation. Am. J. Obstet. Gynecol. 172 (1995) 32–35
26. Kurtz, A.B., Needleman, L., Pennel, R.G., Baltarowich, O., Vilaro, M., Goldberg, B.B.: Can detection of the yolk sac in the first trimester be used to predict the outcome of pregnancy? A prospective sonographic study. AJR 158 (1992) 843–847
27. Kustermann, A., Zorzoli, A., Spagnolo, D., Nicolini, U.: Transvaginal sonography for fetal measurement in early pregnancy. Brit. J. Obstet. Gynecol. 99 (1992) 38–42
28. Lasser, D.M., Peisner, D.B., Vollebergh, J., Timor-Tritsch, I.: First-trimester fetal biometry using transvaginal sonsography. Ultrasound Obstet. Gynecol. 3 (1993) 104–108
29. Lindsay, D.J., Lovett, I.S., Lyons, E.A. et al.: Yolk sac diameter and shape at endovaginal US: Predictors of pregnancy outcome in the first trimester. Radiology 183 (1992) 115–118
30. Mac Gregor, S., Tamura, R., Sabbagha, E., Minogue, J., Gibson, M., Hoffmann, D.: Underestimation of gestational age by conventional crown-rump length dating curves. Obstet. Gynecol. 70 (1987) 344–348
31. Merz, E.: Vaginosonographie. Enke 1992
32. Merz, E.: Aktueller Stand der Vaginosonographie. Teil II. Geburtshilfliche Diagnostik, neue Aspekte und Zukunftsaussichten. Ultraschall in Med. 15 (1994) 52–59
33. Nazari, A., Check, J.H., Epstein, R.H., Dietterich, C., Farzanfar, S.: Relationship of small for dates sac size to crown-rump length and spontaneous abortion in patients with a known date of ovulation. Obstet. Gynecol. 78 (1991) 369–373

34. Nyberg, D.A., Mack, L.A., Laing, F.C., Patten, R.M.: Distinguishing normal from abnormal gestational sac drowth in early pregnancy. J. Ultrasound Med. 6 (1987) 23–27
35. Nyberg, D.A., Mack, L., Harvey, D., Wang, K.: Value of the yolk sac in evaluating early pregnancies. J. Ultrasound Med. 7 (1988) 129–135
36. Pennell, R.G., Needleman, L., Pajak, T. et al.: Prospective comparison of vaginal and abdominal sonography in normal early pregnancy. J. Ultrasound Med. 10 (1991) 63–67
37. Reece, E.A., Scioscia, A.L., Pinter, E. et al.: Prognostic significance of the human yolk sac assessment by ultrasonography. Am. J. Obstet. Gynecol. 159 (1988) 1191–1194
38. Rempen, A.: Vaginale Sonographie der intakten Gravidität im ersten Trimenon. Geburtsh. u. Frauenheilk. 47 (1987) 477–482
39. Rempen, A.: Der embryonale Dottersack bei gestörter Frühschwangerschaft. Geburtsh. u. Frauenheilk. 48 (1988) 804–808
40. Rempen, A.: Biometrie in der Frühgravidität (I.Trimenon). Gynäkologie u. Geburtshilfe 1 (1991) 23–28
41. Rempen, A.: Vaginale Sonographie im ersten Trimenon. I.Qualitative Parameter. Z. Geburtsh. u. Perinat. 195 (1991) 114–122
42. Rempen, A.: Vaginale Sonographie im ersten Trimenon. II.Quantitative Parameter. Z. Geburtsh. u. Perinat. 195 (1991) 163–171
43. Robinson, H.P.: Sonar measurements of the fetal crown-rump length as a means of assessing maturity in the first trimester of pregnancy. Brit. Med. J. 4 (1973) 28–31
44. Robinson, H.P., Fleming, J.E.E.: A critical evaluation of sonar crown-rump length measurements. Brit. J. Obstet. Gynaecol. 82 (1975) 702–710
45. Saade, G.R., Gray, G., Belfort, M.A., Carpenter, R.J., Moise, K.J.: Ultrasonographic measurement of crown-rump length in high-order multifetal pregnancies. Ultrasound Obstet. Gynecol. 11 (1998) 438–444
46. Schats, R., Van Os, H.C., Jansen, C.A., Wladimiroff, J.W.: The crown-rump length in early human pregnancy: a reappraisal. Brit. J. Obstet. Gynaecol. 98 (1991) 460–462
47. Schmidt, W., Hendrik, H.J., Kubli, F.: Ultraschallfetometrie – die Scheitel-Steißlänge in der ersten Schwangerschaftshälfte. Z. Geburtsh. Perinat. 185 (1981) 327–335
48. Silva, P.D., Mahairas, G., Schaper, A.M., Schauberger, C.W.: Early crown-rump length. A good predictor of gestational age. J. Reprod. Med. 35 (1990) 641–644
49. Timor-Tritsch, I.E., Farine, D., Rosen, M.G.: A close look at early embryonic development with the high-frequency transvaginal transducer. Am. J. Obstet. Gynecol. 159 (1988) 676–681
50. Wald, N.J., Smith, D., Kennard, A. et al.: Biparietal diameter and crown-rump length in fetuses with Down's syndrome: implications for antenatal serum screening for Down's syndrome. Brit. J. Obstet. Gynaecol. 100 (1993) 430–435
51. Weissman, A., Achiron, R., Lipitz, S., Blickstein, I., Mashiach, S.: The first-trimester growth-discordant twin: an omnious prenatal finding. Obstet. Gynecol. 84 (1994) 110–114
52. Wisser, J., Dirschedl, P., Krone, S.: Estimation of gestational age by transvaginal sonographic measurement of greatest embryonic length in dated human embryos. Ultrasound Obstet. Gynecol. 4 (1994) 457–462
53. Zimmer, E.Z., Chao, C.R., Santos, R.: Amniotic sac, fetal heart area, fetal curvature, and other morphometrics using first trimester vaginal ultrasonography and color doppler imaging. J. Ultrasound Med. 13 (1994) 685–690

Withdrawn

Biometry

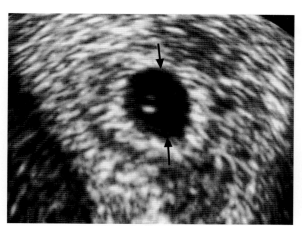

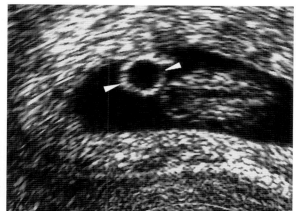

1

2

Fig. 4.**1** Transvaginal scan of the chorionic sac at 5 weeks, 4 days. Measurement are taken between the inner margins of the chorionic cavity (arrows).

Fig. 4.**2** Transvaginal scan of yolk sac at 7 weeks, 2 days. The outer-to-outer dimension is measured (arrows). The embryo appears as an oblong structure next to the yolk sac.

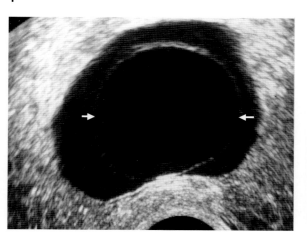

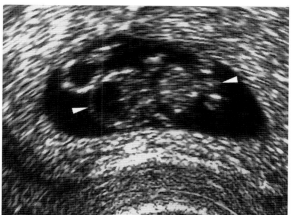

3

4

Fig. 4.**3** Transvaginal scan of the chorionic and amniotic cavities at 10 weeks. Measurement are taken between the inner margins of the amniotic cavity (arrows).

Fig. 4.**4** Transvaginal ultrasound measurement of crown–rump length at 8 weeks, 4 days (arrows). The hypoechoic structure within the embryonic head is normal and represents the rhombencephalon. The yolk sac can be seen to the left of the rhombencephalon.

Fig. 4.5 Transvaginal ultrasound measurement of biparietal diameter in an embryo at 8 weeks, 4 days. Outer-to-outer measurement (arrows).

Fig. 4.6 Transvaginal ultrasound measurement of biparietal diameter at 11 weeks, 1 day. The outer-to-outer BPD is measured at the level of the oc-cipitofrontal plane (arrows).

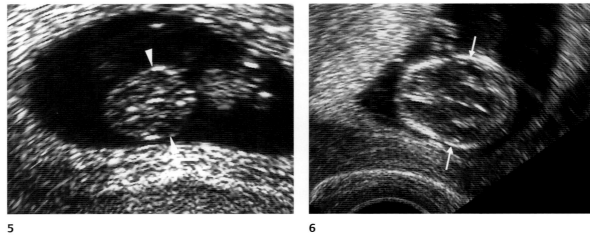

5

6

Fig. 4.7 Standard growth curves (5th, 50th, 95th percentiles) relating various parameters to menstrual age (2).
a Growth curve for chorionic sac diameter.
b Growth curve for yolk sac diameter.
c Growth curve for amniotic cavity diameter.
d Growth curve for crown–rump length.
e Growth curve for biparietal diameter.

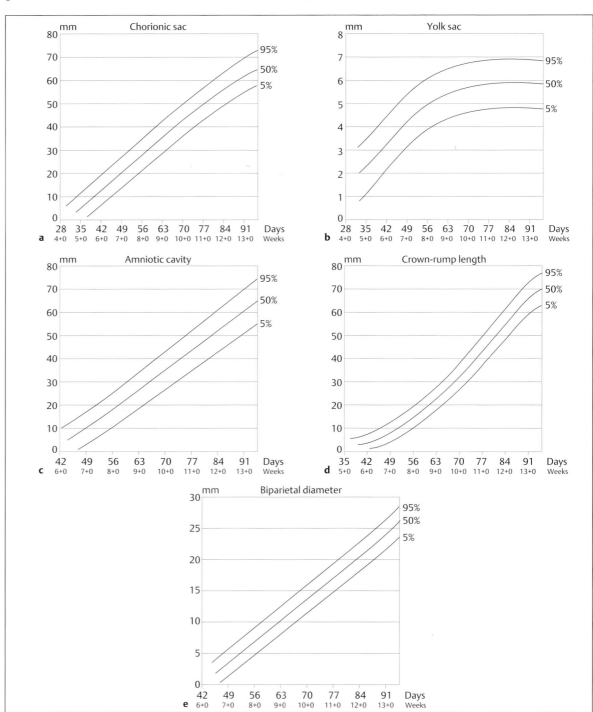

7

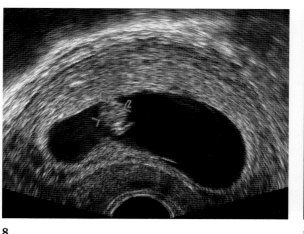

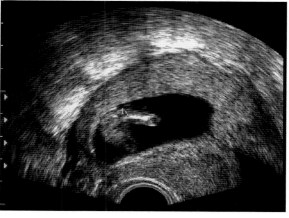

8   **9**

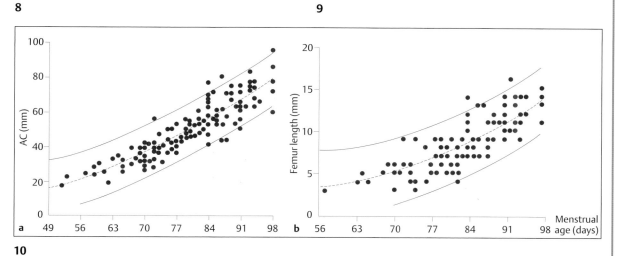

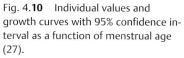

a 49 56 63 70 77 84 91 98   **b** 56 63 70 77 84 91 98 age (days)

10

Fig. 4.**8** Measurement of the embryonic abdomen at the level of the umbilical cord insertion (arrows). ATD 10 mm, ASD 10 mm (9 weeks, 2 days).

Fig. 4.**9** Transvaginal measurement of femur length (outer-to-outer, arrows) at 12 weeks, 4 days.

Fig. 4.**10** Individual values and growth curves with 95% confidence interval as a function of menstrual age (27).
a Abdominal circumference.
b Femur length.

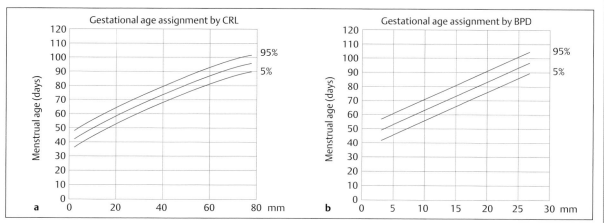

a 0 20 40 60 80 mm   **b** 0 5 10 15 20 25 30 mm

11

Gestational age assignment

Fig. 4.**11** Standard growth curves (5%, 50%, 95%) for gestational age assignment (based on data from Rempen [40]).
a Dating by crown–rump length (CRL).
b Dating by biparietal diameter (BPD).

5 Abnormalities of Early Pregnancy

Diagnostic Approach

Advantages of vaginal ultrasound. Transvaginal ultrasound has become an indispensable tool for the investigation of abnormal pregnancies. While abdominal ultrasound has made an essential contribution to the evaluation of abnormal early pregnancy (43), transvaginal ultrasound has further enhanced the capabilities of antenatal ultrasound (9, 23, 94).

The ultrasound examination may immediately follow the clinical examination. This is particularly important in an acute emergency situation such as a ruptured ectopic pregnancy. Factors that limit the usefulness of abdominal ultrasound (retroflexed uterus, marked obesity, bowel gas) have virtually no effect on transvaginal ultrasound.

Since vaginal ultrasound can directly detect signs of a live embryo or fetus, it can also distinguish an intact early pregnancy from a nonviable one (26, 40, 62, 93) more quickly and reliably than abdominal ultrasound or biochemical tests (99).

Detection of heart activity. In an intact pregnancy, cardiac pulsations should always be detectable in an embryo whose menstrual age is 46 days or more. The β-hCG level should be 47,171 mIU/mL or more (First International Reference Preparation). The mean chorionic sac diameter should be at least 18.3 mm, or the trophoblast thickness should be at least 5 mm (78). If these parameters are within normal limits for an early pregnancy but there is no detectable heart activity, the pregnancy is definitely nonviable. In most cases the patient can be given a definitive result immediately after the examination; there is no need for serial examinations like those that are often necessary in abdominal ultrasound. However, this applies only to cases in which the dates are known. If the last menstrual period is uncertain and a definite embryo or heart activity cannot be detected, the transvaginal scan should be repeated one week later before the pregnancy is declared to be nonviable. If the diagnosis is clear-cut based on ultrasound findings, unnecessary hormone assays can be omitted and the patient referred for immediate uterine evacuation. When embryonic heart activity is detected, the risk of pregnancy loss during the first 15 weeks is 8.6% (79).

Ultrasound criteria. Table 5.1 lists the ultrasound parameters that are important in the evaluation of abnormal early pregnancy. In doubtful cases, the ultrasound findings should always be compared with the serum hCG or β-hCG. Table 5.2 lists the ultrasound criteria that suggest an abnormal early intrauterine pregnancy.

Spontaneous Abortion

Incidence. Abortion is the most frequent complication of all clinically confirmed pregnancies. The incidence of spontaneous abortion is 2.1% up to maternal age 35 and rises thereafter to 16.1% (87).

Causes. Approximately 50–60% of spontaneous abortions in the first trimester are the result of a chromosomal abnormality (13). Most of these cases involve numerical aberrations caused by a failure of chromosome separation ("nondisjunction") during the first meiotic division of the gametes (14). While most of these chromosome errors are random events, a small percentage (approximately 2%) are based on structural chromosomal abnormalities in a phenotypically normal parent with balanced gametes (14). Thus, the diagnostic workup of abortion should include a chromosome analysis of the abortion products and also of the parents, especially in cases of recurrent miscarriage.

Spontaneous abortions may also be caused by abnormal placentation and by a failure of conversion of the spiral arteries into uteroplacental vessels (50, 68, 82).

Vaginal bleeding. The cardinal symptom of an abnormal early pregnancy in most cases is vaginal bleeding. First trimester bleeding occurs in approximately 25% of all pregnancies, and over half of these cases end in miscarriage. In a study of 550 pregnancies, Everett (32) found that vaginal bleeding occurred before 20 weeks in a total of 117 (21%), and that 67 (12%) of those pregnancies ended in miscarriage.

Because vaginal bleeding is a nonspecific symptom and cannot be interpreted on the basis of clinical or biochemical studies, it is left to ultrasound to establish the cause of the bleeding (Table 5.3).

Table 5.1 Parameters that are important in the ultrasound investigation of an abnormal early pregnancy

If an intrauterine gestational sac can be identified:
1. Detection of an intrauterine chorionic cavity
2. Detection of a yolk sac
3. Detection of an embryo
4. Detection of heart activity
5. Placental structure

If an intrauterine gestational sac cannot be identified:
1. Endometrial cavity
2. Detection of ectopic gestational sac
3. Detection of free fluid in the cul-de-sac
4. Detection of an adnexal mass

Table 5.2 Transvaginal ultrasound criteria for an abnormal early intrauterine pregnancy

1. Gestational sac > 12 mm with no visible yolk sac
2. Abnormal-appearing yolk sac (> 6 mm, abnormal structure)
3. Embryo > 5 mm with no heart activity
4. Indistinct embryonic structure
5. Distorted shape of gestational sac
6. Bradycardia < 85 bpm (between 5 and 8 weeks)
7. Detection of a subchorionic or retroplacental hematoma
8. Vacuolated placental structure
9. Separation of amniotic membrane > 14 weeks

■ *Threatened Abortion*

Clinical diagnosis. Threatened abortion is a clinical diagnosis that is made whenever pain and/or bleeding of unknown cause occur in early pregnancy. Due to the uncertainty that came with a threatened abortion, it was once common to recommend prolonged hospitalization. Today, however, transvaginal ultrasound makes it possible to detect early ultrasound changes and offer a prognosis based on the extent of the changes that are found.

Table 5.**3**   Causes of bleeding in early pregnancy

Pregnancy-related vaginal bleeding in early pregnancy	Pregnancy-unrelated vaginal bleeding in early pregnancy
Subchorionic hematoma	Colpitis
Retroplacental hematoma	Vulnerable cervical ectopia
Hydatidiform mole	Cervical polyp
Ectopic pregnancy	Pregnancy + IUD
Complete placenta previa	Cervical carcinoma

Hematoma. Ultrasound reveals an intrauterine pregnancy with definite fetal heart motion and an accompanying subchorionic, marginal-sinus or retroplacental hematoma. Small marginal-sinus hematomas are a relatively common finding at the inferior end of the gestational sac (Fig. 5.**1**). Larger subchorionic hematomas appear as a hypoechoic zone between the uterine wall and chorion, which has separated from the decidua (Fig. 5.**2**). A relatively fresh hematoma the same size as the gestational sac can mimic a multiple gestation. Retroplacental hematomas appear as hypoechoic zones located between the uterine wall and placenta (Fig. 5.**3**).

Prognostic factors. The prognosis depends on the extent of the hematoma, the age of the mother, and the age of the pregnancy. Bennett et al. (6) found an overall spontaneous abortion rate of 9.3% in 516 patients with first trimester bleeding. The rate was 7.7% in patients with small hematomas and 9.2% in patients with moderate hematomas. Large subchorionic hematomas were associated with a spontaneous abortion rate of 18.8%. The rate was 13.7% in women aged 35 years or older, versus 7.3% in younger women. With regard to gestational age, the authors found that bleeding up to 8 weeks' gestation was associated with a lower risk of spontaneous abortion (5.9%) than bleeding after 8 weeks (13.7%).

Kurjak et al. (56) conclude that the site of the hematoma, not its size, is the critical factor in pregnancy outcome. Most of the hematomas leading to abortion were found in the corpus or fundus of the uterus, not in the supracervical region.

Serial scans. Serial ultrasound scans of hematomas reveal various changes. Besides an increase or decrease in size, structural changes (increased echogenicity) may be noted as the hematoma becomes more organized. In some cases an organized hematoma can be difficult to distinguish from the placenta (Fig. 5.**4**).

Serial examinations have shown that patients with a hematoma are much more likely than normal controls to experience premature uterine contractions at some time during their pregnancy (34.5% versus 12.7%), resulting in a significantly higher rate of preterm delivery (21.9% versus 12.9%) (98).

Other signs. Comparing the development of the embryo with the development of the gestational sac and finding a marked growth discrepancy for gestational age is an early sign of an abnormal pregnancy. According to Laboda et al. (57), fetal bradycardia with a heart rate less than 85 bpm between 5 and 8 weeks' gestation is also a sign of impending abortion.

Various authors (38, 41, 45, 77) have shown that an abnormal yolk sac can be another sign of impending abortion. The yolk sac may be small and distorted or calcified (Fig. 5.**5**), or it may be abnormally large (>6 mm) (Fig. 5.**6**). An enlarged yolk sac is a nonspecific finding that does not correlate with a normal or abnormal karyotype (41).

Inevitable Abortion

With inevitable abortion, the miscarriage is already underway and the pregnancy can no longer be saved. Sonographically, the cervix is dilated and the gestational sac is markedly deformed and has entered the lower uterine segment (Fig. 5.**7**).

Complete Abortion

A complete abortion generally occurs only within the first 8 weeks of pregnancy. On ultrasound examination of the uterus, an embryo or gestational sac cannot be identified. Instead, a prominent decidual reaction is observed within the uterine cavity (Fig. 5.**8**). A pregnancy test administered at this stage is still positive, and color Doppler still shows an increase in uterine blood flow (Fig. 5.**9**). If transvaginal ultrasound shows no retained products of conception, usually there is no need to proceed with curettage (19, 64).

Incomplete Abortion

In contrast to a complete abortion, ultrasound after an incomplete abortion shows irregular intrauterine structures of varying echogenicity (2, 81). These echogenic areas correspond to retained products of conception, while hypoechoic areas represent small collections of blood (Fig. 5.**10**). Older, organized coagula are difficult to distinguish from retained products. If subsequent scans show markedly fewer echogenic structures within the uterine cavity after the administration of contrast medium, it may be assumed that the material was clotted intrauterine blood rather than retained products. In some incomplete abortions, residual products may be found only in the region of the cervix (Fig. 5.**11**), requiring differentiation from an abnormal cervical pregnancy.

Blighted Ovum

Empty gestational sac. A blighted ovum is defined as an anembryonic pregnancy in which the embryo and yolk sac are absent. Approximately one-third of spontaneous abortions are found to have an empty gestational sac (22). The incidence of chromosomal abnormalities is high (67%) but not significantly higher than in aborted embryonic pregnancies, in which 53% of cases are found to have an abnormal karyotype (69). The incidence of trisomies, however, is considerably higher in anembryonic abortions (74%) than in aborted embryonic pregnancies (35%). Ultrasound reveals an empty gestational sac, whose size is usually normal for date during the initial weeks (Fig. 5.**12**).

Differential diagnosis. If the gestational age is uncertain and the gestational sac is small, an error in dates by one week should be considered in the differential diagnosis. Transvaginal ultrasound should be repeated at one week to positively exclude a normal early pregnancy. If the second examination again shows no embryo or yolk sac, a blighted ovum may be diagnosed.

Missed Abortion

The incidence of missed abortion in singleton pregnancies between 10 and 14 weeks' gestation is approximately 2%. The incidence is twice as high in twin pregnancies (85).

Ultrasound findings. Ultrasound in missed abortion shows an embryo that is too small for gestational age (Fig. 5.**13**). The crown–rump length is below the 5th percentile in more than 90% of cases (3) (Fig. 5.**14**). The yolk sac is absent or rudimentary (37, 38). There is no sign of embryonic heart activity or body movements. If imaging conditions are unfavorable, however, pulsations transmitted from maternal vessels

Spontaneous abortion

Fig. 5.**1**   Small marginal-sinus hematoma at the inferior end of the gestational sac (arrow), 6 weeks, 5 days.

Fig. 5.**2**   Subchorionic hematoma (2.5 x 1.4 x 2.7 cm), 10 weeks.

Fig. 5.**3**   Retroplacental hematoma (2.4 x 0.9 cm) at 8 weeks, 5 days.

Fig. 5.**4**   Organized hematoma with thin internal echoes at the lower pole of the gestational sac (3.2 x 1.8 cm) at 7 weeks, 2 days. Corpus luteum cyst in the cul-de-sac (∗).

Fig. 5.**5**   Calcified yolk sac in a missed abortion at 9 weeks, 1 day.

Fig. 5.**6**   Abnormally large yolk sac (8 mm) in a missed abortion, 11 weeks.

Fig. 5.**7**   Inevitable abortion with a low gestational sac and contractile wave at 10 weeks, 6 days.

Fig. 5.**8**   Complete abortion with an empty uterine cavity.

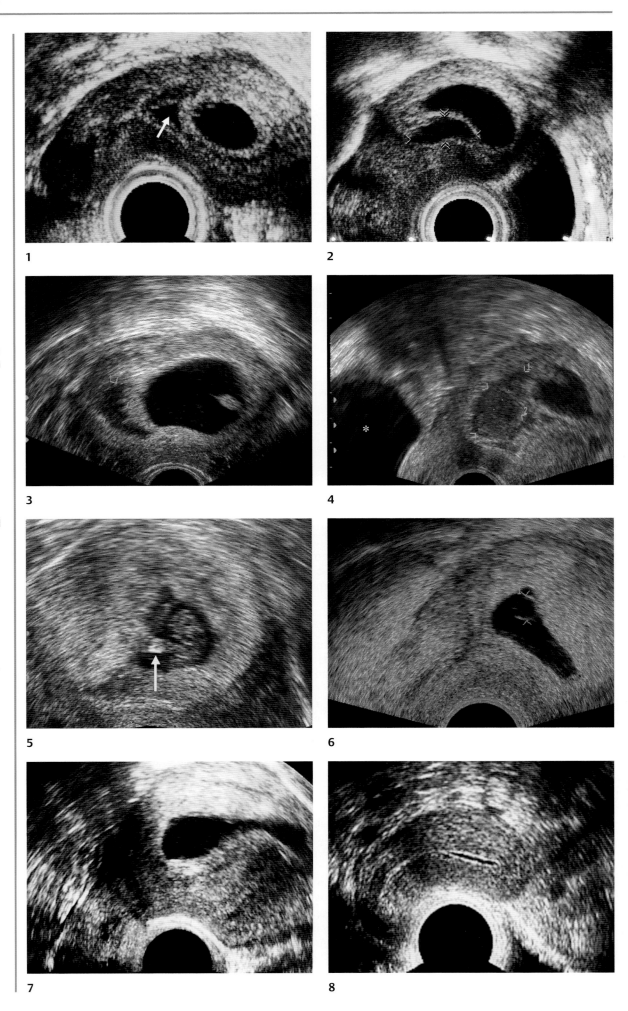

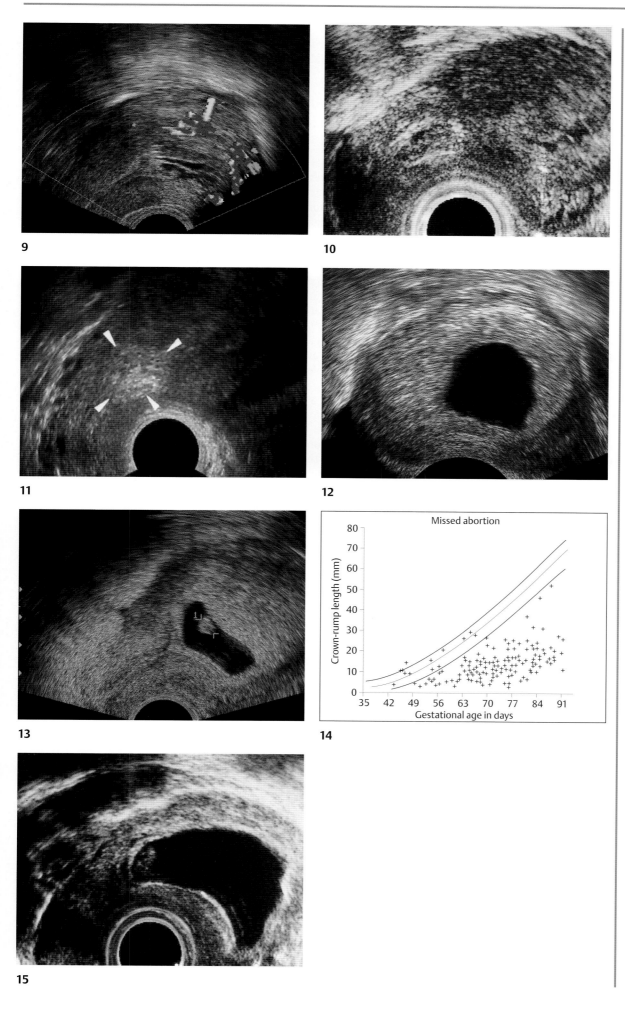

9

10

11

12

13

Missed abortion

14

15

Fig. 5.**9**   Complete abortion at 9 weeks, 5 days. Only a faint fluid crescent is visible in the uterine cavity. Color Doppler still demonstrates increased uterine blood flow.

Fig. 5.**10**   Incomplete abortion at 11 weeks, 5 days. Products of conception are still visible within the uterine cavity and at the level of the uterine isthmus.

Fig. 5.**11**   Incomplete abortion at 6 weeks, 5 days. Echogenic abortion remnants can be seen in the area of the uterine isthmus (arrows). Longitudinal scan of the uterus.

Fig. 5.**12**   Blighted ovum at 9 weeks, 1 day. Transverse scan shows an empty gestational sac.

Fig. 5.**13**   Missed abortion at 11 weeks. Longitudinal scan of the uterus shows an abnormally small crown–rump length of 7 mm.

Fig. 5.**14**   Crown–rump length in 146 cases of missed abortion (after Bahlmann et al. [3]).

Fig. 5.**15**   Missed abortion, 15 weeks. Note the marked discrepancy between the gestational sac and the small fetus.

can mimic embryonic movements or even heart activity. In doubtful cases, the uterus can be tapped briefly with the vaginal probe. This will elicit only a passive swaying of the dead conceptus rather than active embryonic movements.

Serial scans. Serial scans show no further increase in crown–rump length or amniotic sac size, whereas the chorionic sac may continue to develop as in a viable pregnancy. This leads to a marked discrepancy between the small embryo and the relatively large chorionic cavity. The amniotic fluid volume may become quite large (12) (Fig. 5.**15**).

Table 5.**4** reviews the ultrasound abnormalities that are seen in the various forms of spontaneous abortion.

■ *Pregnancy with an IUD in Place*

If a patient with an intrauterine device (IUD) in place for contraception becomes pregnant, ultrasound should be used as an initial study to determine whether the IUD is still inside the uterus. If the device has been expelled, the pregnancy can be continued without further risk. But if the IUD is still in utero, it must be decided whether extraction of the device is an option. This depends on the location of the IUD and the gestational age. Sonographically, the device appears as an echogenic structure of variable shape located below, next to, or above the gestational sac (Figs. 5.**16**, 5.**17**).

Removing the IUD. If the IUD is below or adjacent to the gestational sac, usually it can be safely extracted under ultrasound or hysteroscopic guidance if the precervical end of the thread is still visible. Even with occult IUDs, Sviggum et al. (91) could successfully retrieve the device in 8 of 9 women under ultrasound guidance.

Leaving the IUD in place. If the IUD is above the gestational sac, it should be left alone due to the increased risk of injury and abortion. The same applies to more advanced pregnancy (>12 weeks), in which even hysteroscopic retrieval can be problematic or impossible.

High-risk pregnancy. If the IUD is left in the uterus, the pregnancy is placed in the high-risk category due to the increased incidence of abortion (92) and other complications (infection, perforation, premature labor) (72). Accordingly, additional ultrasound follow-ups should be scheduled for these cases. Since an IUD in a gravid uterus is not known to increase the risk of fetal anomalies (8), there is no indication for pregnancy termination.

Ectopic pregnancy. If a gestational sac is not detected in a woman with a positive pregnancy test and an IUD in place, the adnexal region should be carefully explored to detect or exclude an ectopic pregnancy.

Molar Pregnancy and Choriocarcinoma

The transvaginal ultrasound appearance of a hydatidiform mole depends on the gestational age and whether the mole is partial or complete. The classic snowstorm pattern described by Donald (28) on abdominal ultrasonograms is not seen with transvaginal ultrasound owing to its higher resolution. Instead, vaginal scans show a variable degree of placental thickening with small, hypoechoic vacuoles, depending on the week of gestation (16, 52, 53).

Partial and complete mole. Normally a gestational sac and embryo are seen only with a partial mole (5) (Fig. 5.**18**). Because a partial mole has a high association with chromosomal polyploidy and especially triploidy (18, 39, 51), the ultrasound detection of an abnormal early pregnancy with a vacuolated placental structure should always prompt a chromosome analysis of the abortion products. Unlike a partial mole, a complete mole is not associated with a detectable gestational sac (Fig. 5.**19**).

It is rare for a molar pregnancy to be carried to term, but sporadic cases have been reported (20, 90).

β-hCG levels. Some moles are associated with the formation of thecalutein cysts on the ovaries. These lesions are attributed to the high urinary and serum levels of β-hCG that are typically present in molar pregnancies.

Invasive mole. An invasive mole is characterized by the aggressive growth of trophoblastic tissue into the myometrium (Fig. 5.**20**). Vaginal scanning demonstrates an irregular, hyperechoic myometrial structure with ill-defined hypoechoic areas representing sites of hemorrhagic necrosis. Color Doppler imaging demonstrates very high blood flow (Fig. 5.**21**). Ultrasound cannot distinguish an invasive mole from choriocarcinoma, which is characterized by a very nonhomogeneous, partly hypoechoic and partly hyperechoic structure (Figs. 5.**22**, 5.**23**). Scott et al. (84) described the occurrence of choriocarcinoma following in vitro fertilization.

Ectopic Pregnancy

Incidence and causes. Reports in recent years document a rise in the worldwide incidence of ectopic pregnancies from approximately 1% to 2.5% (61, 63). This rise has been attributed to an increased prevalence of pelvic infections, IUD use, and fertility treatments. More than 90% of ectopic pregnancies are tubal. Other sites are much less common (15) (Fig. 5.**24**).

Diagnosis. Today, most ectopic pregnancies are diagnosed by transvaginal ultrasound. Its high resolution makes it superior to transabdominal ultrasound for imaging the lower pelvis (17, 36, 67, 76, 95). Transvaginal ultrasound is particularly advantageous in acute diagnostic settings such as a suspected tubal rupture, as it can be performed at any time without the need for retrograde bladder distension as in abdominal ultrasound.

Detection rates. Ectopic pregnancy detection rates in excess of 90% can be achieved with transvaginal ultrasound (31, 47, 67, 76, 95). But the

Table 5.**4**   Ultrasound abnormalities in the various forms of abortion

Form of abortion	Ultrasound findings
Threatened abortion	➢ Detectable embryo and heart activity ➢ Detectable subchorionic or retroplacental hematoma
Inevitable abortion	➢ Distorted shape of gestational sac ➢ Embryo with or without heart activity ➢ Cervical dilation
Complete abortion	➢ Empty uterine cavity with decidual endometrial border
Incomplete abortion	➢ Uterus enlarged ➢ Echogenic structures visible within the uterine cavity
Blighted ovum	➢ Empty gestational sac with no sign of an embryo or yolk sac
Missed abortion	➢ No embryonic heart activity ➢ Small CRL

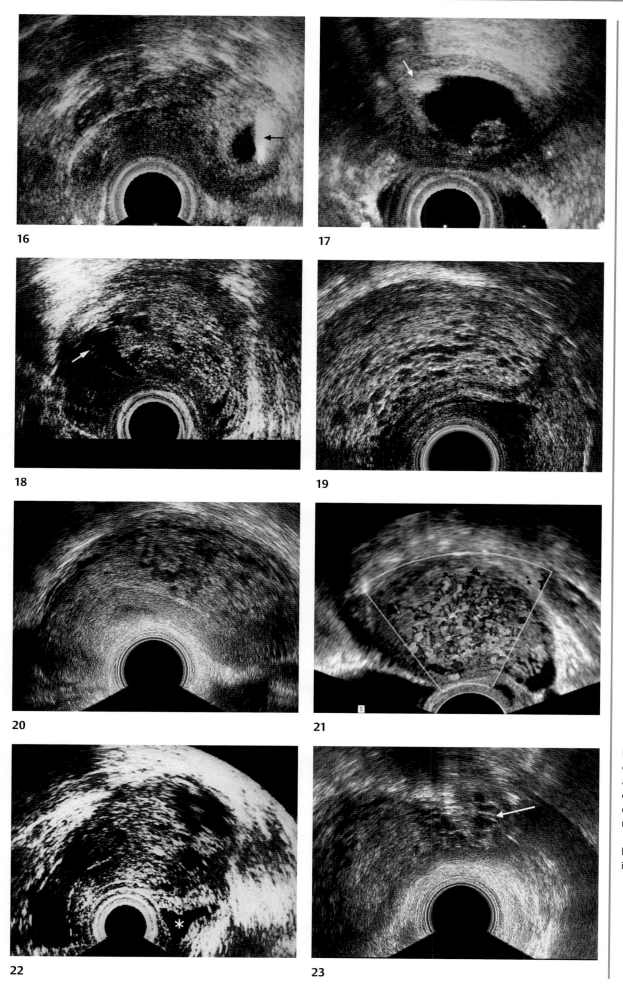

16

17

18

19

20

21

22

23

Pregnancy with an IUD in place

Fig. 5.**16** Early pregnancy (8 weeks, 3 days) with an IUD in the uterine fundus (arrow). Longitudinal scan of the uterus.

Fig. 5.**17** Early pregnancy (9 weeks, 5 days). Transverse scan of the uterus with an IUD on the right uterine wall (arrow).

Molar pregnancy and choriocarcinoma

Fig. 5.**18** Partial mole at 15 weeks. Longitudinal scan. The gestational sac is almost completely occupied by a greatly enlarged, vacuolated placenta. The isthmic area contains a crescent-shaped residual sac with a dead fetus (arrow).

Fig. 5.**19** Complete mole in a retroflexed uterus at 16 weeks. Longitudinal scan of the uterus shows extensive vacuolation of the placenta. A gestational sac cannot be identified.

Fig. 5.**20** Invasive mole infiltrating the myometrium in the posterior wall of an anteflexed uterus.

Fig. 5.**21** Color Doppler demonstrates hypervascularity in an invasive mole. Transverse scan of the uterus.

Fig. 5.**22** Choriocarcinoma, longitudinal scan. The fundus is occupied by an irregular mass of echogenic tissue containing some ill-defined, hypoechoic cystic areas (intratumoral hemorrhage). Urinary bladder (*).

Fig. 5.**23** Choriocarcinoma infiltrating the left ovary, transverse scan.

confident detection of ectopic pregnancy depends critically on the experience of the examiner. Also, an ectopic pregnancy is not always diagnosed at initial examination, and a second or third examination may be needed. Ectopic pregnancy should be suspected in all cases where the serum β-hCG level is higher than 300 mIU/mL (Second International Standard) and an intrauterine gestational sac is not found (10). Bateman et al. (4) state that in women with a normal singleton pregnancy, intrauterine sacs were consistently detected by ultrasound when the hCG level was 2004 mIU/mL or higher (First International Reference Preparation).

Therapeutic implications. The early detection of an ectopic pregnancy not only lowers the maternal risk but also increases the chance for successful conservative treatment. This is particularly true with tubal pregnancies. The earlier the ectopic pregnancy is detected in the fallopian tube, the greater the chance that the tubal wall is not yet irreversibly damaged, making it possible to preserve the tube. The goal of diagnosis, then, is to detect an ectopic pregnancy at the earliest possible stage.

Ultrasound Detection

Direct signs. The definitive sign of ectopic pregnancy is the ultrasound detection of an extrauterine trophoblastic ring with a central hypoechoic cavity and an embryo. This can be accomplished in only 53% of cases, however (66). A yolk sac can be identified in 30% of cases (Fig. 5.**25**). An embryo with heart activity can be detected in just 24% (76) or 27% (66) of cases (Figs. 5.**26**, 5.**27**).

Indirect signs. If a hyperechoic trophoblastic ring with a gestational sac cannot be found either inside or outside the uterus in a patient with a positive pregnancy test, the examiner should look for indirect signs of ectopic pregnancy such as an enlarged uterus with a thickened endometrium (Fig. 5.**28**), a central pseudogestational sac (Figs. 5.**29**, 5.**30**), free fluid in the cul-de-sac (Fig. 5.**28**), or an adnexal mass (Table 5.**5**). The pseudogestational sac is a small hemorrhagic area that is always located at the center of the uterine cavity (Figs. 5.**29**, 5.**30**). A true gestational sac, by contrast, always occupies an eccentric location. This is most clearly appreciated in a transverse scan of the uterus (Fig. 5.**30**). A true gestational sac is also distinguished by the fact that it contains either a visible yolk sac or an embryo (Fig. 5.**29**).

The detection of an early intrauterine pregnancy virtually excludes an ectopic pregnancy, because coexisting intrauterine and extrauterine gestations occur in just one of 30,000 pregnancies (7, 75).

Figure 5.**31** shows the diagnostic algorithm that should be followed for a suspected ectopic pregnancy.

Tubal Pregnancy

The ultrasound features of a tubal pregnancy vary according to whether it is an intact tubal pregnancy, a tubal abortion, or a tubal rupture.

Small, Intact Tubal Pregnancy

A small, intact tubal pregnancy may be found at various sites along the fallopian tube (Fig. 5.**32**). If implantation occurs in the proximal tubal segment, the pregnancy will be found close to the uterus. The more distal the tubal pregnancy is located, the more variable the site at which it may be detected with ultrasound. It may be close to the ovary or even within the cul-de-sac. In some cases vaginal ultrasound can detect the ectopic pregnancy at a very early stage, even before laparoscopy shows evidence of tubal expansion.

A corpus luteum occasionally mimics an ectopic pregnancy (Fig. 5.**33**). It appears as a hyperechoic ring-like structure that is

Table 5.5   Ultrasound parameters for the detection of ectopic pregnancy

Direct sign
➢ Detection of an echogenic trophoblastic ring with a gestational sac or yolk sac and/or an embryo (with or without heart activity)

Indirect signs
➢ Enlarged uterus with thickened endometrium and no evidence of an intrauterine gestational sac
➢ Small, centrally located pseudogestational sac
➢ Free fluid in the cul-de-sac (retrouterine hematocele)
➢ Adnexal mass with irregular margins (peritubal hematoma)

markedly smaller than a true ectopic pregnancy and can always be localized to the ovary.

Tubal Abortion

It is difficult to detect an echogenic trophoblastic ring in tubal abortion, especially in cases where a large peritubal hematoma has formed (Fig. 5.**34**). A suspected peritubal hematoma requires differentiation from a corpus luteum cyst, an endometriotic cyst, a distended bowel loop, and in rare cases from an abscess.

Tubal Rupture

A tubal rupture presents clinically with acute pain and a large amount of free fluid in the cul-de-sac. With fresh bleeding, a hypoechoic area is noted behind the uterus. This area may contain fine, punctate internal echoes (Fig. 5.**35**). If the rupture occurred some time ago and the hematoma is partially organized, it will appear as a streaky or hyperechoic structure.

If there is a significant collection of intra-abdominal blood, transvaginal ultrasound should be supplemented by transabdominal scans to check for blood in the mid- to upper abdomen (see Chapter 10).

Less Common Forms of Ectopic Pregnancy

Interstitial Pregnancy

Interstitial pregnancy results from implantation in the intramural portion of the fallopian tube (Fig. 5.**24**). Sonographically, the ectopic sac cannot be definitely localized to the uterine cavity or fallopian tube, as it is located within the myometrium (Fig. 5.**36**). Chen et al. (21) reported on the ultrasound detection of six cases.

Differential diagnosis. Interstitial pregnancy can be difficult to distinguish from a far lateral intrauterine pregnancy and from a pregnancy in one horn of a bicornuate uterus (Fig. 5.**37**).

Complications. The principal risk from an interstitial pregnancy is uterine rupture with life-threatening intra-abdominal hemorrhage.

Treatment. An unruptured interstitial pregnancy can be successfully managed by the systemic or local administration of methotrexate (25, 42).

Cervical Pregnancy

Cervical pregnancies account for less than 1% of ectopic pregnancies (1). They are easily recognized sonographically by their cervical location below a normal-size uterus with a thickened endometrium. The trophoblast quickly gains attachment to the uterine artery circulation,

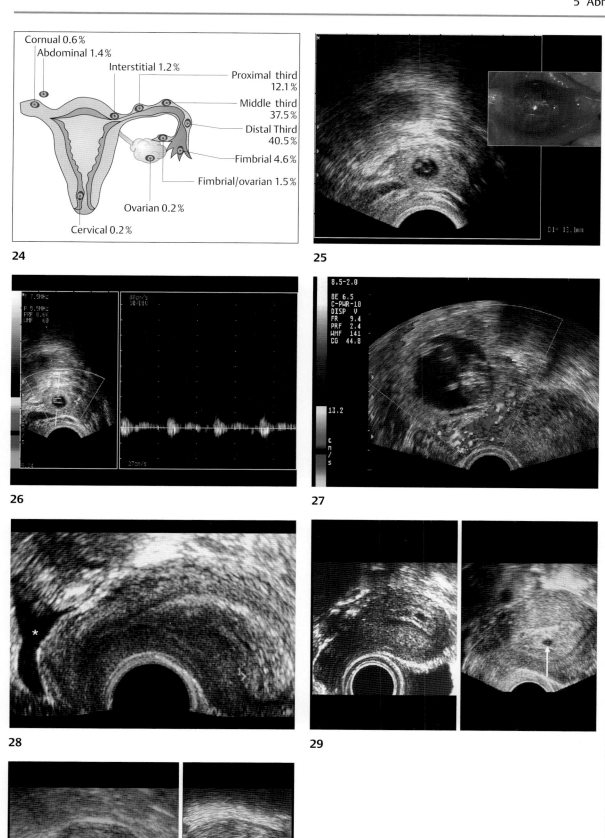

24

25

26

27

28

29

30

Ectopic pregnancy

Fig. 5.**24** Frequency of implantation sites in ectopic pregnancy (modified from Breen [15]).

Fig. 5.**25** Left-sided tubal pregnancy (5 weeks, 4 days) with a definable embryo (3 mm) and yolk sac (3 mm). The inset shows an intraoperative view of the expanded tube.

Fig. 5.**26** Intact left-sided ectopic pregnancy (6 weeks) with a Doppler display of embryonic heart activity.

Fig. 5.**27** Large, intact right-sided tubal pregnancy (10 weeks). Color Doppler shows a ring-like perfusion pattern. Transverse scan.

Fig. 5.**28** Ectopic pregnancy (7 weeks, 6 days) with thickened endometrium (1.6 cm diameter) and no sign of an intrauterine sac. Free fluid in the cul-de-sac appears as a hypoechoic area (∗).

Fig. 5.**29** Longitudinal scans of the uterus. Left: pseudogestational sac of ectopic pregnancy appears as a central, hypoechoic zone. Right: true gestational sac at a relatively central location. In contrast to the pseudogestational sac, a small yolk sac can be identified within the uterine cavity (arrow).

Fig. 5.**30** Transverse scan of the uterus. Left: centrally located pseudo-gestational sac of ectopic pregnancy. Right: normal early pregnancy with an eccentric gestational sac.

Fig. 5.**31** Diagnostic management of suspected ectopic pregnancy.
TVS = transvaginal sonography
MIS = minimally invasive surgery
MTX = methotrexate

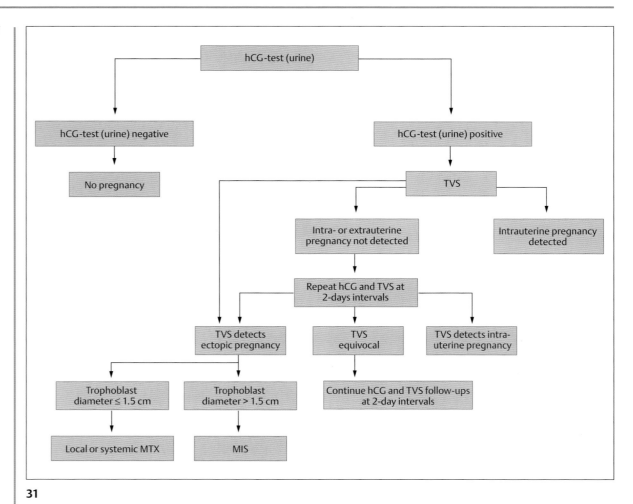

31

Fig. 5.**32** Left-sided tubal pregnancy at 6 weeks, 3 days. Small gestational sac with no sign of an embryo.

Fig. 5.**33** Left corpus luteum appears as a thin, echogenic ring-like structure with a hypoechoic center, 9 weeks.

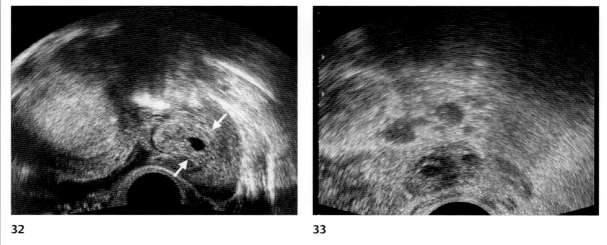

32   **33**

Fig. 5.**34** Left-sided tubal abortion with a peritubal hematoma (arrows). The hypoechoic corpus luteum of pregnancy can be seen medial to the tubal abortion.

Fig. 5.**35** Left-sided tubal rupture with a large amount of free fluid anterior and posterior to the retroflexed uterus. Longitudinal scan.

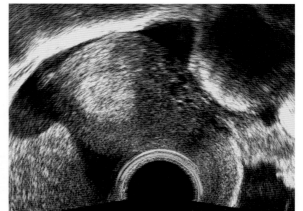

34   **35**

with color Doppler showing a distinctive ring-like pattern of blood flow to the ectopic sac (Fig. 5.**38**).

Treatment. Because surgical removal of the cervical pregnancy by curettage is associated with an extremely high risk of massive or intractable bleeding due to the rich cervical blood supply (74, 97), more and more cases are now being managed with methotrexate therapy (48, 49, 73, 96).

There are rare reports of cervical pregnancy culminating in a live birth (70).

Ovarian Pregnancy

Ovarian pregnancy has an estimated incidence of one in 7000 pregnancies and 1–6% of all ectopic pregnancies (80). It results either from the fertilization of a nonovulated ovum or from secondary implantation near the ovulation site. The clinical manifestations are similar to those of tubal pregnancy. Ovarian pregnancy can be reliably detected with ultrasound (46, 65, 80) only by demonstrating a hyperechoic ring-like structure in the ovarian region and identifying an embryo or yolk sac within the ectopic sac (Fig. 5.**39**).

Differential diagnosis. Differentiation is required from a fresh corpus luteum, which presents a similar echogenic ring-like structure (Fig. 5.**33**).

Abdominal Pregnancy

Owing to the high invasive potential of trophoblastic tissue, an ectopic pregnancy can implant anywhere in the abdominal cavity. Implantations have been described in the liver, diaphragm, spleen, and even in the mesentery (29) and anterior abdominal wall (100). Peritoneal implantation in the pelvic region is more common, however, occurring predominantly near the uterus (29).

Diagnosis. Abdominal pregnancy is difficult to diagnose by transvaginal ultrasound. It can be diagnosed only if the pregnancy is located within the pelvis, there is an "empty" uterus with a thickened endometrium and normal-appearing adnexal region, and an echogenic trophoblastic ring is found above, beside, or behind the uterus or in the area of the pelvic wall (Figs. 5.**40**, 5.**41**).

Differential diagnosis. There have been isolated reports of abdominal pregnancies reaching the third trimester or being carried to term (11, 29, 33). Advanced abdominal pregnancies are very difficult to distinguish from intrauterine pregnancies, but an extremely thin "uterine wall," especially in the area of the placenta, is a conspicuous finding on abdominal scans (see Chapter 10). If transvaginal ultrasound is then used to evaluate the uterus itself, it will show an unenlarged uterus within the lower pelvis.

Conservative Treatment of Ectopic Pregnancy by the Transvaginal Instillation of Methotrexate (MTX)

In recent years the medical treatment of unruptured ectopic pregnancies has evolved into a successful procedure that effectively supplements invasive and conservative surgical treatment options.

Agents used. Various agents have been used in the medical treatment of ectopic pregnancy, most notably methotrexate (24, 34, 35, 71, 89, 101), prostaglandins (27, 30, 59, 60), hyperosmolar glucose solution (58), potassium chloride (86), and mifepristone (RU-486) (54). Most clinical experience to date has been with the folic acid antagonist methotrexate. Prostaglandins have also been the subject of recent large studies, however (30).

Methotrexate. The goal of any medical treatment is the rapid devitalization of the hCG-producing trophoblast without harming the fallopian tube. Unlike prostaglandins, which damage the trophoblast through a vasoconstriction-induced ischemia while stimulating tubal peristalsis (44), methotrexate inhibits trophoblastic metabolism (83) without causing morphologic damage to the tube (55).

Local instillation. The local, transvaginal instillation of methotrexate into the ectopic sac is advantageous over systemic administration in that it requires a substantially smaller dose (10 mg) (66). This treatment is feasible, however, only if the ectopic sac can be positively identified (Fig. 5.**42**). Using low-dose MTX therapy, Merz et al. (66) successfully treated all cases in which the trophoblast diameter did not exceed 1.5 cm, regardless of the hCG level or the detection of embryonic heart activity.

Local MTX therapy in cervical pregnancy can reduce the trophoblast and cervical blood flow to a degree that permits secondary evacuation by curettage without risk of severe bleeding (Figs. 5.**43**–5.**45**).

References

1. Acosta, D.A.: Cervical pregnancy – a forgotten entitiy in family practice. J. Am. Board Fam. Pract. 10 (1997) 290–295
2. Alcazar, J.L., Balsonado, C., Laparte, C.: The reliability of transvaginal ultrasonography to detect retained tissue after spontaneous first-trimester abortion, clinically thought to be complete. Ultrasound Obstet. Gynecol. 6 (1995) 126–129
3. Bahlmann, F., Brockerhoff, P., Merz, E., Beckmann, K.: Transvaginale sonographische Diagnostik im Notfall. Notfälle und Notsituationen in der Frühgravidität. Notfallmedizin 22 (1996) 212–218
4. Bateman, B.G., Nunley, W.C. Jr., Kolp, L.A., Kitchin, J.D. III, Felder, R.: Vaginal sonography of early intrauterine and tubal pregnanecies. Obstet. Gynecol. 75 (1990) 421–427
5. Beinder, E., Voigt, H.J., Jäger, W., Wildt, L.: Partielle Blasenmole bei zytogenetisch unauffälligem Fetus. Geburtshilfe u. Frauenheilk. 55 (1995) 351–353
6. Bennett, G.L., Spernol, R., Beck, A.: Subchorionic hemorrhage in first-trimester pregnancies: prediction of pregnancy outcome with sonography. Radiology 200 (1996) 803–806
7. Berger, M.J., Taymor, M.L.: Simultaneous intrauterine and tubal pregnancies following ovulation induction. Am. J. Obstet. Gynec. 113 (1972) 812–813
8. Bernaschek, G., Spernol, R., Beck, A.: IUD-Lage bei intrauterinen Schwangerschaften. Geburtsh. u. Frauenheilk. 41 (1981) 645–647
9. Bernaschek, G.: Vorteile der endosonographischen Diagnostik in Gynäkologie und Geburtshilfe. Geburtsh. u. Frauenheilk. 47 (1987) 471–476
10. Bernaschek, G., Rudelstorfer, R., Csaicsich, P.: Vaginal sonography versus serum human chorionic gonadotropin in early detection of pregnancy. Am. J. Obstet. Gynecol. 158 (1988) 608–612
11. Binder, R.E.: Eine ausgetragene Bauchhöhlenschwangerschaft. Geburtsh. Frauenheilkd. 54 (1994) 587–588
12. Birnholz, J.C., Madanes, A.E.: Amniotic fluid accumulation in the first trimester. J. Ultrasound Med. 14 (1995) 597–602
13. Boue, J., Bou, A., Lazar, P.: Retrospective and prospective epidemiological studies of 1500 karyotyped spontaneous abortions. Teratology 12 (1975) 11–26
14. Brackertz, M., Schindler, D.: Indikationstellung zur Chromosomenanalyse bei der diagnostischen Abklärung wiederholter Aborte. Z. Geburtsh. u. Perinat. 189 (1985) 249–254
15. Breen, J. L.: A 21 year survey of 654 ectopic pregnancies. Am. J. Obstet. Gynecol. 106 (1970) 1004–1016
16. Burmeister, R., Tucker, R.: Ultrasonographic diagnosis of first trimester hydatidiform mole. J. Clin. Ultrasound 25 (1997) 36–38
17. Cacciatore, B., Stenman, U.H., Ylostalo, P.: Comparison of abdominal and vaginal sonography in suspected ectopic pregnancy. Obstet. Gynecol. 73 (1989) 770–774
18. Casper, F.W., Merz, E., Seufert, R., Hofmann, G.: Sonographische Diagnostik der fetalen Triploidie. Ultraschall Med. 11 (1990) 311–313
19. Cetin, A., Cetin, M.: Diagnostic and therapeutic decision-making with transvaginal sonography for first trimester spontaneous abortion, clinically thought to be incomplete or complete. Contraception 57 (1998) 393–397
20. Chen, F.P.: Molar pregnancy and living normal fetus coexisting until term: prenatal biochemical and sonographic diagnosis. Hum. Reprod. 12 (1997) 853–856
21. Chen, G.D., Lin, M.T., Lee, M.S.: Diagnosis of interstitial pregnancy with sonography. J. Clin. Ultrasound 22 (1994) 439–442
22. Coulam, C.B., Goodman, C., Dormann, A.: Comparison of ultrasonographic findings in spontaneous abortions with normal and abnormal karyotypes. Hum. Reprod. 12 (1997) 823–826
23. Cullen, M.T., Green, J.J., Reece, A., Hobbins, J.C.: A comparison of transvaginal and abdominal ultrasound in visualizing the first trimester conceptus. J. Ultasound Med. 8 (1989) 565–569
24. Darai, E., Benifla, J.L., Naouri, M. et al.: Transvaginal intratubal methotrexate treatment of ectopic pregnancy. Report of 100 cases. Hum. Reprod. 11 (1996) 420–424
25. De Bruyne, F., Tutschek, B., Hucke, J., Crombach, G.: Interstitial pregnancy treated with local and systemic methotrexate. Gynecol. Obstet. Invest. 46 (1998) 133–138

Less common forms of ectopic pregnancy

Fig. 5.**36**   Interstitial pregnancy in the cornual region of the left uterine tube at 5 weeks, 3 days. Transverse scan of the uterus.

Fig. 5.**37**   Intact early pregnancy in a bicornuate uterus at 8 weeks. The left uterine cornu contains a normal-size gestational sac with a normal embryo (arrow). The right cornu contains only a pseudogestational sac surrounded by thickened endometrium. Transverse scan of the uterus.

Fig. 5.**38**   Cervical pregnancy at 7 weeks, 2 days. Longitudinal scan of the uterus shows marked expansion of the cervix with minimal enlargement of the uterine corpus.

Fig. 5.**39**   Left image: right-sided ovarian pregnancy (6 weeks). An embryo is visible in the ectopic sac within the right ovary (arrow). Right image: left ovary for comparison.

Fig. 5.**40**   Abdominal pregnancy adjacent to the uterine fundus with rupture of the ectopic sac. Longitudinal scan of the uterus.

Fig. 5.**41**   Corresponding intraoperative view. The fetus has ruptured into the free abdominal cavity.

Conservative treatment of ectopic pregnancy

Fig. 5.**42**   Local methotrexate instillation for a left-sided ectopic pregnancy. A needle is passed transvaginally into the ectopic pregnancy (needle tip at the center of the ectopic sac). The fluid is aspirated, and methotrexate is instilled.

Fig. 5.**43**   Local MTX therapy for a cervical pregnancy (9 weeks). Appearance before MTX instillation.

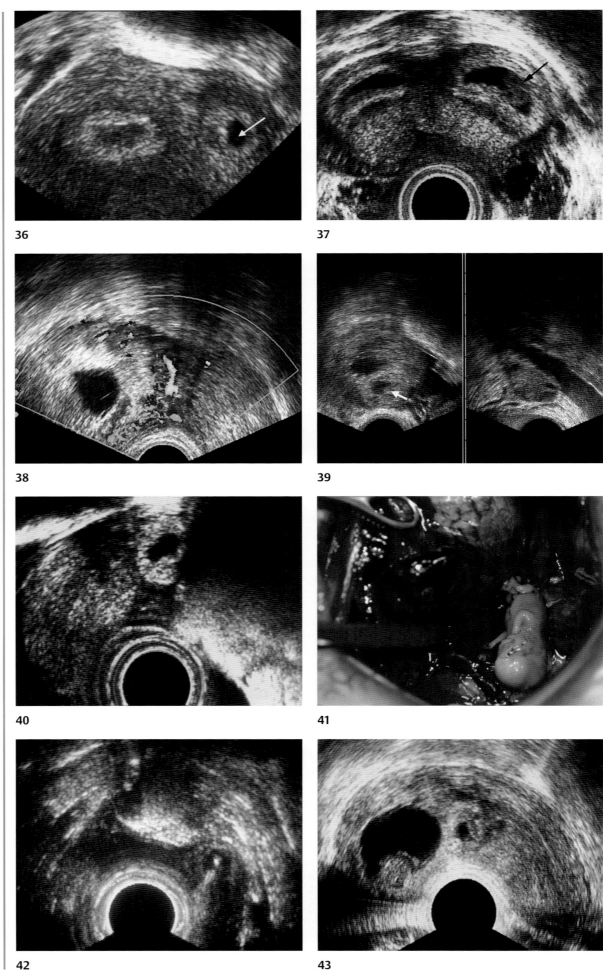

36

37

38

39

40

41

42

43

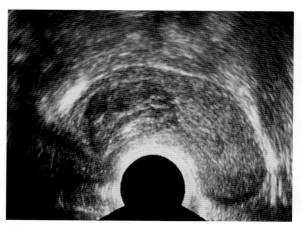

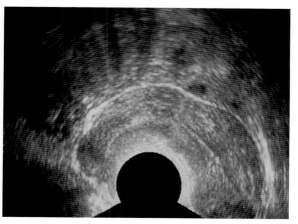

44

45

Fig. 5.**44** Same case as in Fig. 5.**43**, 16 days after MTX instillation. An organized hematoma can be seen within the cervix.

Fig. 5.**45** Same case as in Fig. 5.**43** and 5.**44**. 46 days after MTX instillation and instrumental evacuation of the hematoma in the interval.

26. De Crespigny, L.C.: Early diagnosis of pregnancy failure with transvaginal ultrasound. Am. J. Obstet. Gynecol. 159 (1988) 408–409
27. Degenhardt, F., Ebeling, B., Meier, B., Schlösser, H.W., Schneider, J.: Behandlung von Eileiterschwangerschaften mit Prostaglandinen. Geburtsh. u. Frauenheilk. 51 (1991) 649–652
28. Donald, I.: Ultrasonic echo sounding in obstetrical and gynecological diagnosis. Am. J. Obstet. Gynecol. 93 (1965) 935–941
29. Dubinsky, T.J., Guerra, F., Gormaz, G., Maklad, N.: Fetal survival in abdominal pregnancy: a review of 11 cases. J. Clin. Ultrasound 24 (1996) 513–517
30. Egarter, Ch., Fitz, R., Spona, J. et al.: Behandlung der Eileiterschwangerschaft mit Prostaglandinen: Eine Multicenterstudie. Geburtsh. Frauenheilkd. 49 (1989) 808–812
31. Enk, L., Wikland, M., Hammarberg, K., Lindblom, B.: The value of endovaginal sonography and urinary human chorionic gonadotropin tests for differentiation between intrauterine and ectopic pregnancy. J. Clin. Ultrasound 18 (1990) 73–78
32. Ewerett,C.: Incidence and outcome of bleeding before the 20th week of pregnancy: prospective study from general practice. BMJ 315 (1997) 32–34
33. Faustin, D., Halio, D., Shiffman, R., Flaxman, L., Castro, J.: Preoperative diagnosis of third trimester abdominal pregnancy by transvaginal ultrasound. J. Diagn. Med. Sonography 8 (1992) 89–90
34. Feichtinger, W., Kemeter, P.: Conservative treatment of ectopic pregnancy by transvaginal aspiration under sonographic control and methotrexate injection. Lancet I (1987) 381–382
35. Fernandez, H., Baton, C., Lelaidier, C., Frydman, R.: Conservative management of ectopic pregnancy: Prospective randomized clinical trial of methotrexate versus prostaglandin sulprostone by combined transvaginal and systemic administration. Fertil. Steril. 55 (1991) 746–750
36. Funk, A., Fendel, H.: Verbesserte Diagnostik der Extrauteringravidität durch die Endosonographie. Z. Geburtsh. u. Perinat. 192 (1988) 49–53
37. Funk, A., Fendel, H.: Ultraschallechographische Darstellbarkeit und Messung der Amnionhöhle und des Dottersacks in der frühen Schwangerschaft: Vergleichende Untersuchung von intakten und gestörten Schwangerschaften. Z. Geburtsh. u. Perinat. 192 (1988) 59–66
38. Funk, A., Eichenberg, S., Sohn, C.: Transvaginale Sonographie: Die differentialdiagnostische Bedeutung des sekundären Dottersackes in der Frühschwangerschaft. Z. Geburtsh. u. Perinat. 193 (1989) 178–182
39. Goldstein, D.P., Berkowitz, R.S.: Current management of complete and partial molar pregnancy. J. Reprod. Med. 39 (1994) 139–146
40. Goldstein, S. R.: Sonography in early pregnancy failure. Clin. Obstet. Gynecol. 37 (1994), 681–692
41. Goldstein, S.R, Kerenyi, T., Scher, J., Papp, C.: Correlation between karyotype and ultrasound findings in patients with failed early pregnancy. Ultrasound Obstet. Gynecol. 8 (1996) 314–317
42. Gucer, F., Hönigl, W.: Interstitielle Schwangerschaft und Management mit systemischer einmaliger Gabe von Methotrexat. Zentralbl. Gynäkol. 120 (1998) 306–308
43. Hackelöer, B.J., Hansmann, M.: Ultraschalldiagnostik in der Frühschwangerschaft. Gynäkologe 9 (1976) 108–122
44. Hahlin, M., Bokström, H., Lindblom, B.: Ectopic pregnancy: in vitro effects of prostaglandins on the oviduct and corpus luteum. Fertil. Steril. 47 (1987) 935–940
45. Harris, R.D., Vincent, L.M., Askin, F.B.: Yolk sac calcification: A sonographic finding associated with intrauterine embryonic demise in the first trimester. Radiology 166 (1988) 109–110
46. Hönigl, W., Reich, O.: Vaginosonographie bei ovarieller Gravidität. Ultraschall Med. 18 (1997) 233–236
47. Hopp, H., Schaar, P., Entezami, M. et al.: Diagnostische Sicherheit der Vaginalsonographie bei ektoper Gravidität. Geburtsh. Frauenheilkd. 55 (1995) 666–670
48. Hung, T.H., Jeng, C.J., Yang, Y.C., Wang, K.G., Lan, C.C.: Treatment of cervical pregnancy with methotrexate. Int. J. Gynaecol. Obstet. 53 (1996) 243–247
49. Hung, T.H., Chiu, T.H., Hsu, J.J., Chen, K.C., Hsieh, C.C., Hsieh, T.T.: Sonographic evolution of a living cervical pregnancy treated with intraamniotic instillation of methotrexate. J. Ultrasound Med.16 (1997) 843–847
50. Hustin, J. Schaaps, J.P., Jauniaux, E.: Histological study of the materno-embryonic interface in sponataneous abortion. Placenta 11 (1990) 477–486
51. Jauniaux, E., Kadri, R., Hustin,J.: Partial mole and triploidy: screening patients with first-trimester spontaneous abortion. Obstet. Gynecol. 88 (1996) 661–619

52. Jauniaux, E, Nicolaides, K.H.: Early ultrasound diagnosis and follow-up of molar pregnancies. Ultrasound Obstet. Gynecol. 9 (1997) 17–21
53. Jauniaux, E: Ultrasound diagnosis and follow-up of gestational trophoblastic disease. Ultrasound Obstet. Gynecol. 11 (1998) 367–377
54. Kenigsberg, D., Porte, J., Hull, M., Spitz, I.M.: Medical treatment of residual ectopic pregnancy: RU 486 and methotrexate. Fertil. Steril. 47 (1987) 702–703
55. Kooi, S., van Etten, F.H.P.M., Kock, H.C.L.V.: Histopathology of five tubes after treatment with methotrexate for a tubal pregnancy. Fertil. Steril. 57 (1992) 341–345
56. Kurjak, A., Schulman, H., Zudenigo, D., Kupesic, S., Kos, M., Goldenberg, M.: Subchorionic hematomas in early pregnancy: clinical outcome and blood flow patterns. J. Matern. Fetal Med. 5 (1996) 41–44
57. Laboda, L.A., Estroff, J.A., Benacerraf, B.R.: First trimester bradycardia. A sign of impending fetal loss. J. Ultrasound Med. 8 (1989) 561–563
58. Lang, P., Weiss, P.A.M., Mayer, H.O.: Local application of hyperosmolar glucose solution in tubal pregnancy. Lancet II (1989) 922–923
59. Lindblom, B., Källfelt, B., Hahlin, M., Hamberger, L.: Local Prostaglandin F2α injection for termination of ectopic pregnancy. Lancet I (1987) 776–777
60. Lindblom, B., Hahlin, M., Lundorff, P., Thornburn, J.: Treatment of tubal pregnancy by laparoscopic-guided injection of prostaglandin F2α. Fertil. Steril. 54 (1990) 404–408
61. Lübke, F., Focke, E., Torabi-Tillig, E.-H.: Wandel in der Diagnostik und Therapie der Extrauteringravididtät. Geburtsh. u. Frauenheilk. 49 (1989) 172–178
62. Macchiella, D., Merz, E.: Diagnostik der gestörten Frühgravidität. In: Merz, E. (Hrsg.): Vaginosonographie. Stuttgart: Enke 1992; S. 73–78
63. Mäkinen, J.I., Erkkola, R.U., Laippala, P. J.: Causes of the increase in the incidence of ectopic pregnancy. A study on 1017 patients from 1966 to 1985 in Turku, Finland. Am. J. Obstet. Gynecol. 160 (1989) 642–646
64. Mansur, M.M.: Ultrasound diagnosis of complete abortion can reduce need for curettage. Eur. J. Obstet. Gynecol. Reprod. Biol. 44 (1992) 65–69
65. Marcus, S.F., Brinsden, P.R.: Primary ovarian pregnancy after in vitro fertilization and embryo transfer: a report of seven cases. Fertil. Steril. 60 (1993) 167–169
66. Merz, E., Bahlmann, F., Weber, G. et al.: Unruptured tubal pregnancy: Local low-dose therapy with methotrexate under transvaginal ultrasonographic guidance. Gynecol. Obstet. Invest. 41 (1996) 76–81
67. Mesrogli, M., Degenhardt, F., Maas, D.H.A., Klaus, I., Busche, M., Schneider, J.: Tubargraviditäten: early pregnancy factor, Progesteron, beta-HCG und Vaginalsonographie als differentialdiagnostische Parameter. Z. Geburtsh. u. Perinat. 192 (1988) 130–132
68. Michel, M.Z., Khong, T.Y., Clark, D.A. et al.: A morphological and immunological study of human placental bed biopsies in miscarriage. Brit. J. Obstet. Gynaecol. 97 (1990) 984–988
69. Minelli, E., Buchi, C., Granata, P. et al.: Cytogenetic findings in sonographically defined blighted ovum abortions. Ann. Genet. 36 (1993) 107–110
70. Mitrani, L.: Cervical pregnancy ending in a live birth. J. Obst. Gynaecol. Brit. Commonwealth 80 (1973) 761–763
71. Ory, S.J., Villamiera, A.Z., Sand, P.K., Tamura, R.K.: Conservative treatment of ectopic pregnancy with methotrexate. Am. J. Obstet. Gynecol. 154 (1986) 1299–1306
72. Os, W.A.A. van: Komplikationen bei Intrauterinpessaranwendung und ihre Behandlung. In: Beller, F.K., Schweppe, K.W., Wagner, H.: Intrauterinpessare. Edition Medizin, VCH, Weinheim 1984
73. Pastorelli, G., Steiner, R., Haller, U.: Die Zervikalschwangerschaft. Eine gynäkologisch-geburtshilfliche Notfallsituation. Gynäkol. Geburtsh. Rundschau 37 (1997) 209–211
74. Pretzsch, G., Einenkel, J.D., Horn, L.C., Alexander, H.: Zervikale Gravidität: Kasuistik und Literaturübersicht. Zentrbl. Gynäkol. 119 (1997) 25–34
75. Reece, E.A., Petrie, R.H., Sirmans, M.F., Finster, M., Todd, W.D.: Combined intrauterine and extrauterine gestations: A review. Am. J. Obstet. Gynec. 146 (1983) 323–330
76. Rempen, A.: Vaginal sonography in ectopic pregnancy. A prospective evaluation. J. Ultrasound Med. 7 (1988) 381–387
77. Rempen, A.: Der embryonale Dottersack bei gestörter Frühschwangerschaft. Geburtsh. Frauenheilk. 48 (1988) 804–808
78. Rempen, A.: Diagnosis of viability in early pregnancy with vaginal sonography. J. Ultrasound Med. 9 (1990) 711–716
79. Rempen, A.: Die Aborthäufigkeit vitaler Schwangerschaften im ersten Trimenon. Zentralbl. Gynäkol. 115 (1993) 249–257

80. Riethmüller, D., Sautiere, J.L., Benoit, S., Roth, P., Schaal, J.P., Maillet, R.: Diagnostic echographique et traitement laparoscopique d'une grossesse avarienne d'un cas et revue de la literature. J. Gynecol. Obstet. Biol. Reprod. Paris. 25 (1996) 378–383

81. Rulin, M.C., Bornstein, S.G., Campbell, J. D.: The reliability of ultrasonography in the management of spontaneous abortion, clinically to be thought to be complete: a prospective study. Am. J. Obstet. Gynecol. 168 (1993) 12–15

82. Rushton, D.I.: Placental pathology in spontaneous miscarriage. In: Beard, R.W., Sharp, F. (eds.): Early Pregnancy Loss: Mechanisms and Treatment. London: Springer (1988) 149–157

83. Sand, P.K., Stubblefield, P.A., Ory, S.J.: Methotrexate inhibition of normal trophoblasts in vitro. Am. J. Obstet. Gynecol. 155 (1986) 324–329

84. Scott, P., Schupfer, G.K., Bruhwiler, H.: Chorionkarzinom nach In-vitro-Fertilisation. Geburtshilfe Frauenheilk. 55 (1995) 285–286

85. Sebire, N.J., Thomton, S., Hughes, K., Snijders, R.J., Nicolaides, K.H.: The prevalence and consequences of missed abortion in twin pregnancies at 10 to 14 weeks of gestation. Br. J. Obstet. Gynaecol. 104 (1997) 847–848

86. Shalev, E., Zalel, Y., Bustan, M., Weiner, E.: Ectopic pregnancy: sonographically-guided transvaginal reduction. Ultrasound Obstet. Gynecol. 1 (1991) 127–131

87. Smith, K.E., Buyalos, R.P.: The profound impact of patient age on pregnancy outcome after early detection of fetal cardiac activity. Fertil. Steril. 65 (1996) 35–40

88. Stabile, I., Campbell, S., Grudzinskas, J.G.: Ultrasound and circulating placental protein measurements in complications of early pregnancy. Br. J. Obstet. Gynecol. 96 (1989) 1182–1191

89. Stovall, T.G., Ling, F.W., Gray, L.A., Carson, S.A., Buster, J.E.: Methotrexate treatment of unruptured ectopic pregnancy: A report of 100 cases. Obstet. Gynecol. 77 (1991) 749–753

90. Suvanto-Luukkonen, E., Sundstrom, H., Penttinen, J., Jouppila, P.: Hydatidiform mole co-existent with a live fetus. Acta Obstet. Gynecol. Scand. 76 (1997) 380–381

91. Sviggum, O, Skjeldestad, F.E., Tuveng, J.M.: Ultrasonically guided retrieval of occult IUD in early pregnancy. Acta Obstet. Gynecol. Scand. 70 (1991) 355–357

92. Tatum, H.J., Schmidt, F.H., Jain, A.K.: Management and outcome of pregnancies associated with the Cooper T intrauterine contraceptive device. Amer. J. Obstet. Gynec. 126 (1976) 869–879

93. Terinde, R., Kozlowski, P.: Ultraschalldiagnostik der gestörten Frühgravidität. Gynäkologe 21 (1988) 210–219

94. Timor-Tritsch, I.E., Farine, D., Rosen, M.G.: A close look at early embryonic development with the high-frequency transvaginal transducer. Am. J. Obstet. Gynecol. 159 (1988) 676–681

95. Timor-Tritsch, I.E., Ming, N.Y., Peisner, D.B., Lesser, K.B., Slavik, T.A.: The use of transvaginal ultrasonography in the diagnosis of ectopic pregnancy. Am. J. Obstet. Gynecol. 161 (1989) 157–161

96. Timor-Tritsch, I.E., Monteagudo, A., Mandeville, E.O., Peisner, D.B., Anaya, G.P, Pirrone, E.C.: Successful treatment of viable cervical pregnancy by local injection of methotrexate guided by transvaginale ultrasonography. Am. J. Obstet. Gynecol. 170 (1994) 737–739

97. Ushakov, F.B., Elchalal, U., Aceman, P.J., Schenker, J.G.: Cervical pregnancy: past and future. Obstet. Gynecol. Surv. 52 (1997) 45–59

98. Weigel, M., Friese, K., Schmitt, W., Inthraphuvasak, J., Melchert, F.: Die prognostische Bedeutung intrauteriner Hämatome des I. und II.Trimenons für den Schwangerschafts- und Geburtsverlauf. Geburtsh. u. Frauenheilk. 51 (1991) 876–881

99. Wiedemann, R., Strowitzki, T., Sandner, R., Luppa, P., Hepp, H.: Wertigkeit hormoneller und sonographischer Parameter bei der Diagnostik der gestörten bzw. ungestörten Frühgravidität. Geburtsh. u. Frauenheilk. 49 (1989) 237–242

100. Zaki, Z.M.: An unusual presentation of ectopic pregnancy. Ultrasound Obstet. Gynecol. 11 (1998) 456–458

101. Zakut, H., Sadan, O., Katz, A., Dreval, D., Bernstein, D.: Management of tubal pregnancy with methotrexate. Brit. J. Obstet. Gynaecol. 96 (1989) 725–728

6 Transvaginal Detection of Fetal Anomalies

Detection of Fetal Anomalies in the First Trimester

By permitting the early, detailed visualization of normal embryonic structures, transvaginal ultrasound can be used to screen for serious fetal anomalies during the first trimester (1, 10, 12, 18, 20, 21, 22, 24).

Advantages. The early detection of fetal anomalies offers several advantages:
- Positive cases can be referred early for a chromosome analysis.
- If ultrasound detects a serious anomaly or if an abnormal karyotype is found, the pregnancy can be terminated at an early stage.
- If pregnancy termination is deemed necessary, it is less risky and more easily tolerated than termination at a later stage.

Another consideration is that some findings such as the physiologic umbilical hernia (27) or nuchal translucency (19, 25, 26, 28) can be detected only within a designated time window of approximately 4 weeks and cannot be seen thereafter. If the ultrasound examination is performed after that period, the changes can no longer be detected.

Supplement to pathologic findings. The ultrasound detection and careful documentation of a fetal anomaly are also important for the pediatric pathologist. Following a spontaneous abortion and D&C, or several days following intrauterine fetal death, the retrieved tissue is often so damaged and macerated that scant information can be gained from a gross and microscopic evaluation of the malformed embryo or fetus. In these cases the ultrasound images obtained before D&C can provide supplemental information that is valuable in making a specific diagnosis.

Prerequisite. In order to detect an early fetal anomaly, the examiner must be familiar with normal embryonic development. Otherwise a normal change, such as the physiologic umbilical hernia, might be mistaken for a malformation.

Detectable findings. Under optimal conditions, initial changes such as an umbilical cord cyst (Fig. 6.**1**) can be detected as early as 8 weeks' gestation. During the next 4–6 weeks, assuming the embryo is in a favorable position, vaginal ultrasound can detect various anomalies such as anencephaly (13, 21, 29), hydranencephaly (29), holoprosencephaly (9), encephalocele (8), nuchal cystic hygroma (5, 21, 29), cardiac anomalies (7, 11), omphalocele or renal abnormalities (6), and conjoined twins (14, 16).

Anencephaly

Anencephaly can be detected as early as 10 weeks' gestation (13). Absence of the superior vault is associated with an abnormal head/trunk ratio and abnormally large orbits (Fig. 6.**2**). The crown–rump length, however, is normal in most anencephalic fetuses (13).

Nuchal Translucency

Chromosomal abnormality. Some fetuses between 11 and 14 weeks' gestation display an unusual hypoechoic area in the nuchal region (Fig. 6.**3**). This condition, called nuchal edema or nuchal translucency, is a suggestive sign of a chromosomal anomaly (usually trisomy 21) (see Chapter 2). A nuchal translucency thickness ≥ 3 mm is associated with an increased risk of a chromosomal anomaly. The greater the measured diameter of the translucent area, the greater the risk of a chromosomal abnormality (trisomy 13, 18, 21; triploidy) (19, 25). When serum assays are combined with maternal age and nuchal translucency, a detection rate of 87% can be achieved for Down syndrome, with a false-positive rate of 5% (18).

Structural abnormalities. If karyotyping shows no chromosomal abnormalities, increased nuchal translucency thickness is found to correlate with various structural abnormalities and genetic syndromes (18, 26, 28). Souka et al. (26) published a review of the anomalies found in 15 studies. Conversely, when nuchal translucency thickness is less than 4.5 mm in a chromosomally normal pregnancy, the outcome in approximately 90% of cases is a healthy live birth (26).

Differential diagnosis. Amniotic membrane in contact with the fetal neck should be excluded, as it can mimic nuchal translucency (Fig. 6.**4**).

Cystic Hygroma

When cystic hygroma is present (Fig. 6.**5**), there is an approximately 75% chance that the fetus has Turner syndrome (45,XO). If chorionic villus sampling shows no chromosomal abnormalities, the outlook is less certain since the hygroma may resolve completely as the pregnancy progresses (15). A nonseptated cystic hygroma (5) appears to have a particularly favorable prognosis in this regard. It should be noted that a contiguous amniotic membrane can mimic a cystic hygroma.

Omphalocele

One should also be cautious in interpreting abdominal wall defects. The definitive diagnosis of an omphalocele (Fig. 6.**6**) should not be made until 12 weeks' gestation, since the physiologic umbilical hernia is still present from 8 to 11 weeks (27).

Conjoined Twins

There is always a risk of conjoined twins (e.g., thoracopagus, Fig. 6.**7**) in any monochorionic, monoamniotic multiple pregnancy. Under favorable examination conditions, transvaginal scanning can detect this type of anomaly prior to 10 weeks' gestation.

Equivocal Findings

Although transvaginal ultrasound can detect various anomalies during the first trimester, there are findings that cannot be confidently interpreted or assessed as to their prognostic significance. Examples include slight expansion of the renal pelves, which may be detected as early as 12 weeks' gestation (Fig. 6.**8**) and then disappear during the later course of the pregnancy. In most cases, the accurate interpretation of these equivocal findings requires one or more follow-up ultrasound examinations.

New ultrasound techniques. Newer ultrasound techniques such as 3-D transvaginal ultrasound (4, 17) can be used as adjuncts in the early diagnosis of embryofetal anomalies. Surface-rendered images in particular offer new display options and new tools for excluding anomalies in cases where there is a known risk of recurrence (see Chapter 44).

Detection of Fetal Anomalies in the Second and Third Trimesters

Transvaginal ultrasound can also be used in selected cases to detect anomalies at a later stage of pregnancy (2, 29). This particularly applies to cases in which the fetal head is so low in the lower pelvis that it cannot be completely evaluated by abdominal ultrasound, or the fetus is poorly visualized because of scant amniotic fluid (Fig. 6.**9**). Transvaginal ultrasound is often better in these cases for detecting or excluding a fetal anomaly (Fig. 6.**10**). It is also better for areas that are not clearly demonstrated by abdominal scanning (Fig. 6.**11**). Transvaginal ultrasound can also be used for cephalic biometry in cases where the fetal head is at a very low level.

References

1 . Achiron, R., Taadmor, O.: Screening for fetal anomalies during the first trimester of pregnancy: transvaginal versus transabdominal sonography. Ultrasound Obstet. Gynecol. 1 (1991) 186–191
2. Benacerraf, B.R., Estroff, J.A.: Transvaginal sonographic imaging of the low fetal head in the second trimester. J. Ultrasound Med. 8 (1989) 325–328
3. Bilardo, C.M., Pajkrt, E., de Graaf, I., Mol, B.W., Bleker, O.P.: Outcome of fetuses with enlarged nuchal translucency and normal karyotype. Ultrasound Obstet. Gynecol. 11 (1998) 401–406
4. Bonilla-Musoles, F,. Raga, F., Osborne, N., Blanes, J.: The use of three-dimensional (3D) ultrasound for the study of normal and pathological morphology of the human embryo and fetus: preliminary report. J. Ultrasound. Med. 14 (1995) 757–765
5. Bronshtein, M., Rottem, S., Yoffe, N., Blumenfeld, Z.: First-trimester and early second-trimester diagnosis of nuchal cystic hygroma by transvaginal sonography: Diverse prognosis of the septated from the nonseptated lesion. Am. J. Obstet. Gynecol. 161 (1989) 78–82
6. Bronshtein, M., Yoffe, N., Brandes, J.M., Blumenfeld, Z.: First-trimester and early second-trimester diagnosis of fetal urinary tract anomalies using transvaginal sonography. Prenatal Diagn. 10 (1990) 653–666
7. Bronshtein, M., Zimmer, E.Z., Milo, S., Ho, S.Y., Lorber, A., Gerlis, L.M.: Fetal cardiac abnormalities detected by transvaginal sonography at 12–16 weeks' gestation. Obstet. Gynecol. 78 (1991) 374–378
8. Bronshtein, M., Zimmer, E.Z.: Transvaginal sonographic follow-up on the formation of fetal cephalocele at 13–19 weeks' gestation. Obstet. Gynecol. 78 (1991) 528–530
9. Bronshtein, M., Wiener, Z.: Early transvaginal sonographic diagnosis of alobar holoprosencephaly. Prenatal Diagn. 11 (1991) 459–462
10. Cullen, M.T., Green, J.J., Scioscia, A.L., Gabrielli, S., Sanchez-Ramos, L., Hobbins, J.C.: Ultrasonography in the detection of aneuploidy in the first trimester. J. Ultrasound Med. 14 (1995) 559–563
11. Gembruch, U., Knöpfle, G., Chatterjee, M., Bald, R., Hansmann, M.: First-trimester diagnosis of fetal congenital heart disease by transvaginal two-dimensional and Doppler echocardiography. Obstet. Gynecol. 75 (1990) 496–498
12. Hernadi, L., Torocsik, M.: Screening for fetal anomalies in the 12th week of pregnancy by transvaginal sonography in an unselected population. Prenat. Diagn. 17 (1997) 753–759
13. Johnson, S.P., Sebire, N.J., Snijders, R.J.M., Tunkel, S, Nicolaides, K.H.: Ultrasound screening for anencephaly at 10–14 weeks of gestation. Ultrasound Obstet. Gynecol. 9 (1997) 14–16
14. Lam, Y.H., Sin, S.Y., Lam, C., Lee, C.P., Tang, M.H.Y., Tse, H.Y.: Prenatal sonographic diagnosis of conjoined twins in the first trimester: two case reports. Ultrasound Obstet. Gynecol. 11 (1998) 289–291
15. Macken, M.B., Grantmyre, E.B., Vincer, M.J.: Regression of nuchal cystic hygroma in utero. J. Ultrasound Med. 8 (1989) 101–103
16. Maymon, R., Halperin, R., Weinraub, Z., Herman, A., Schneider, D.: Three-dimensional transvaginal sonography of conjoined twins at 10 weeks: a case report. Ultrasound Obstet. Gynecol. 11 (1998) 292–294
17. Merz, E., Bahlmann, F., Welter, C., Miric-Tesanic, D.: Transvaginale 3D-Sonographie in der Frühgravidität. Gynäkologe 32 (1999) 213–219
18. Orlandi, F., Darmiani, G., Hallahan, T.W., Krantz, D.A., Marcri, J.N.: First trimester screening for fetal aneuploidy: biochemistry and nuchal translucency. Ultrasound Obstet. Gynecol 10 (1997) 381–386
19. Pandya, P.P., Kondylios, A., Hilbert, L., Snijders, R.J.M., Nicolaides, K.H.: Chromosomal defects and outcome in 1015 fetuses with increased nuchal translucency. Ultrasound Obstet. Gynecol. 5 (1995) 15–19
20. Quashie, C., Weiner, S., Bolognese, R.: Efficacy of first trimester transvaginal sonography in detecting normal fetal development. Am. J. Perinatol. 9 (1992) 209–213
21. Rottem, S., Bronshtein, M., Thaler, I., Brandes, J.M.: First trimester transvaginal sonographic diagnosis of fetal anomalies. Lancet I (1989) 444–445
22. Rottem, S., Bronshtein, M.: Transvaginal sonographic diagnosis of congenital anomalies between 9 weeks and 16 weeks. J. Clin. Ultrasound 18 (1990) 307–314
23. Rottem, S.: IRONFAN – a sonographic window into the natural history of fetal anomalies. International Registry of the Onset of Fetal Anomalies [editorial]. Ultrasound Obstet. Gynecol. 5 (1995) 361–363
24. Rottem, S.: Early detection of structural anomalies and markers of chromosomal aberrations by transvaginal ultrasonography. Curr. Opin. Obstet. Gynecol. 7 (1995) 122–125
25. Snijders, R.J.M., Pandya, P., Brizot, M.L., Nicolaides, K.H.: First trimester fetal nuchal translucency. In: Snijders, R.J.M., Nicolaides, K.H. (eds.): Ultrasound Markers For Fetal Chromosomal defects. The Parthenon Publishing Group 1996; S. 121–156
26. Souka, A.P., Snijders, R.J.M., Novakov, A., Soares, W., Nicolaides, K.H.: Defects and syndromes in chromosomally normal fetuses with increased nuchal translucency thickness at 10–14 weeks of gestation. Ultrasound Obstet. Gynecol. 11 (1998) 391–400
27. Timor-Tritsch, I.E., Warren, W.B., Peisner, D.B., Pirrone, E.: First-trimester midgut herniation: high-frequency transvaginal sonographic study. Am. J. Obstet. Gynecol. 161 (1989) 831–833
28. Van Vugt, J.M.G., Tinnmans, B.W.S., Van Zalen-Sprock, R.M.: Outcome and early childhood follow-up of chromosomally normal fetuses with increased nuchal translucency at 10–14 weeks' gestation. Ultrasound Obstet. Gynecol. 11 (1998) 407–409
29. Voigt, H.J., Faschingbauer, C.: Pränatale Diagnostik mit Hilfe der Vaginalsonographie. Ultraschall Klin. Prax. 4 (1989) 199–204

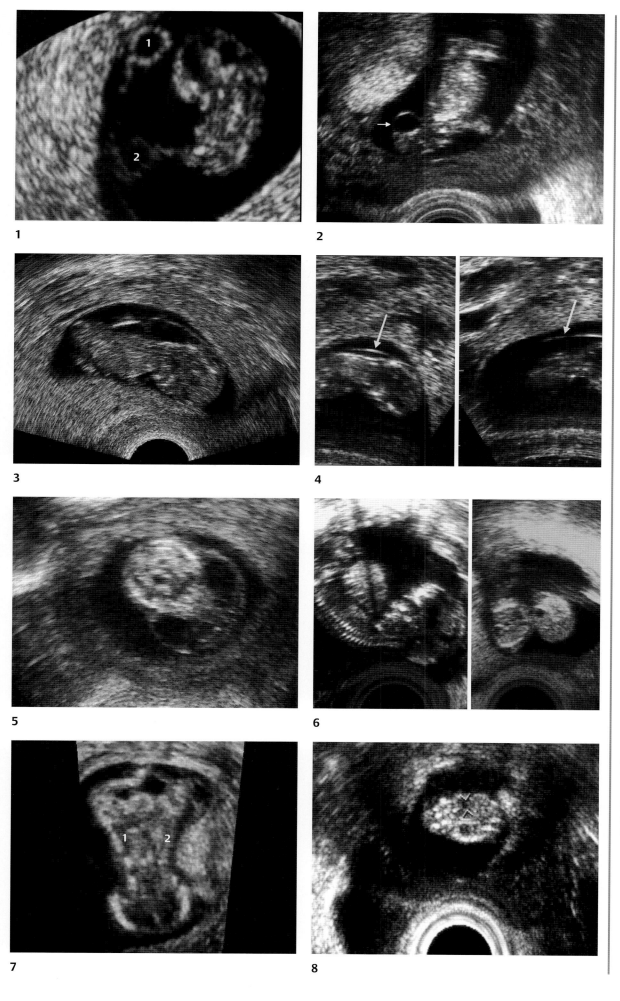

Fig. 6.**1**   Scan in early pregnancy (8 weeks) demonstrates two cystic structures in the amniotic epithelium. 1 = Yolk sac, 2 = umbilical cord cyst.

Fig. 6.**2**   Anencephaly (10 weeks) with absence of the superior vault and abnormally large orbits (arrow).

Fig. 6.**3**   Nuchal translucency thickness of 8 mm (11 weeks, 2 days). Karyotype: trisomy 21.

Fig. 6.**4**   Left: amniotic membrane behind the fetal head mimics nuchal translucency (12 weeks). Right: after fetal movement, the amniotic membrane is clearly seen as being separate from the fetus.

Fig. 6.**5**   Cystic hygroma (13 weeks).

Fig. 6.**6**   Large omphalocele (12 weeks, 5 days). Left: longitudinal scan. Right: transverse scan.

Fig. 6.**7**   Thoracopagus (13 weeks) with two spinal columns (1, 2) and one head.

Fig. 6.**8**   Subtle, bilateral renal pelvic dilatation. Pelvic width on the left side is 3 mm (arrows) (12 weeks).

Second and third trimesters

Fig. 6.9   Transabdominal sonogram of a fetal head in severe oligohydramnios (19 weeks). The fetal head is very difficult to evaluate in the transabdominal scan.

Fig. 6.10   Transvaginal scan of the same fetus clearly defines the head despite oligohydramnios. Small pools of amniotic fluid are visible on each side of the head.

Fig. 6.11   Small bilateral neck cysts (arrows) in a 14-week fetus. Left: longitudinal scan. Right: transverse scan showing both anterolateral neck cysts.

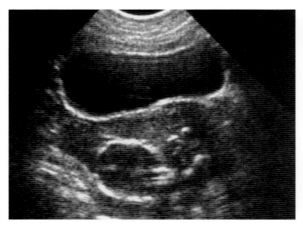

9

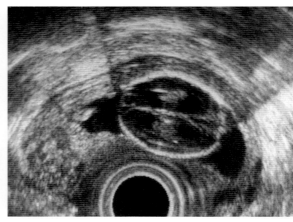

10

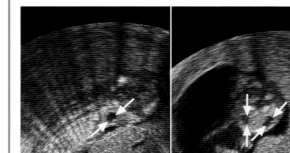

11

withdrawn

7 Transvaginal Ultrasound of Maternal Disorders

withdrawn

Transvaginal Diagnosis of Uterine and Adnexal Masses in Pregnancy

Uterine and adnexal abnormalities during pregnancy can be detected with transvaginal ultrasound only if they are still within the lower pelvis. This usually limits their detection to the first trimester and the start of the second trimester. Subsequent rapid enlargement of the uterus displaces the uterine corpus and adnexa superiorly, making them inaccessible to transvaginal scanning. Abdominal ultrasound must then be used to resolve equivocal findings (see Chapter 38).

Uterine Masses

Fibroids

The most common uterine tumors, fibroids (leiomyomas), can be detected and measured by transvaginal ultrasound in early pregnancy. They may complicate the pregnancy in varying degrees, depending on their size and location (20, 27) (Figs. 7.1, 7.**2**). While a pedunculated, subserosal fibroid of the uterine fundus will rarely jeopardize the fetus, an intramural or submucosal fibroid will increase the risk of preterm labor and spontaneous abortion. Nevertheless, three-fourths of these patients carry their pregnancy to term without serious problems (20). The most frequent complication is aseptic necrosis (25% of cases), but usually it is of a moderate degree (20). Because of their rich blood supply, fibroids in a pregnant uterus appear mostly hypoechoic. Fibroids can be measured and their growth monitored with serial scans, initially using transvaginal ultrasound and then changing to abdominal ultrasound later in the pregnancy.

Malignant Uterine Tumors

Malignant uterine tumors in pregnancy are somewhat rare compared with benign uterine masses. Cervical carcinoma should be suspected if the tumor has caused a barrel-like distension of the cervix and has a nonhomogeneous structure (Fig. 7.**3**).

Adnexal Masses

Both physiologic and pathologic adnexal findings are easily visualized with transvaginal ultrasound, especially in early pregnancy.

Benign Adnexal Masses

The most common adnexal mass is the physiologic corpus luteum of pregnancy. It appears sonographically as a sharply circumscribed, echo-free cyst adjacent to the uterus (Fig. 7.**4**). While the corpus luteum cyst subsequent regresses and can no longer be detected with ultrasound, true cystic ovarian masses remain visible as gestation progresses (Fig. 7.**5**). Also, serial transvaginal scans can detect any changes in the size of the mass as well as structural changes, like those seen in a hemorrhagic ovarian cyst. If the mass is too high in the abdomen for transvaginal evaluation, abnormal ultrasound should be performed.

One study found that adnexal masses can be detected sonographically in 4.1% of second- and third-trimester pregnancies, and that 81.6% of the masses are ovarian cysts with a mean diameter < 3.0 cm (16).

The need for surgical intervention depends on the sonomorphologic changes that are noted in serial examinations. The second trimester is the most favorable time for action in cases where surgery is required (28).

Malignant Adnexal Tumors

Malignant adnexal tumors are rare in pregnancy. Estimates range from one in 25,000 (5) to one in 18,000 pregnancies (21). Suspicious ultrasound changes are usually sites of mural papillomatous proliferation in cystic tumors, with color Doppler showing pronounced tumor angiogenesis and low Doppler indices. Grendys and Barnes (13) report a 2–5% risk of malignancy for ovarian masses that persist into the third trimester. Occasionally, manual examination will disclose an enlarged uterus with a solid adnexal mass that is identified by transvaginal scanning as a pelvic kidney (Fig. 7.**6**).

Cervical Incompetence

Characteristics

Definition and Incidence

Cervical incompetence refers to a weakness of the cervix and lower uterine segment. It is associated with painless, premature shortening of the cervix accompanied by dilatation and opening of the cervical os during pregnancy. In most cases this premature opening of the os occurs in the second trimester, usually between the 18th and 26th weeks (7). The incidence of cervical incompetence stated in the literature ranges from 0.2% to 2% (8, 19). Cervical incompetence is a frequent cause of late pregnancy failure and preterm delivery, although premature opening of the cervix does not always imply the start of parturition.

Anatomy and Physiology of the Cervix

The three main components of the cervix are smooth muscle, collagen fibers, and connective-tissue matrix. Unlike the myometrium, 65–70% of which consists of smooth muscle, the cervix contains only 25% smooth muscle in its upper portion, 16% in its central portion, and 6% in its lower portion.

When ripening of the cervix occurs during late pregnancy, the proportion of cervical connective tissue increases while the collagen fibrils are reduced (4, 12). Also, qualitative changes take place in the connective-tissue matrix, increasing the distensibility of the cervical tissue. Errors in the timing of these processes may have a role in the pathogenesis of cervical incompetence.

Diagnosis of Cervical Incompetence

For many years, manual and speculum examination were the only tools available for diagnosing cervical incompetence, and only the ectocervix could be evaluated. With the advent of obstetric ultrasound and especially transvaginal ultrasound, it became possible to measure the total length of the cervix objectively and noninvasively.

The history is of major importance in patients with cervical incompetence. Predisposing factors are a prior history of second trimester abortion, cervical trauma such as curettage or conization and cervical lacerations after childbirth, induced abortions, and infections (9, 18).

Palpation of the Cervix

Cervical palpation is done to assess cervical length and consistency, the position of the cervix in the pelvic canal, the width of the cervical os, and the level of the presenting part. Bishop (3) was the first to use a "pelvic score" to try and objectify cervical findings. But the value of the Bishop score is limited by the subjective evaluation of the parameters tested. Other limitations of the manual cervical examination are an inability to access the portion of the cervix located deep in the fornices and inability to evaluate the internal os when the external os is closed. The manual examination is useful, however, for evaluating the surface and consistency of the cervix and is an important guide in many situations (2, 29).

Ultrasound of the Cervix

The cervix in pregnancy can be scanned abdominally using the full-bladder technique. But for reasons of better reproducibility and image quality, transvaginal ultrasound measurement of the cervix is recommended. Several authors have emphasized the importance of vaginal ultrasound in examining the cervix and evaluating its competence (6, 11, 14, 17, 26).

Examination technique. The bladder should contain very little fluid (100 mL or less) for a vaginal ultrasound examination. A distended bladder can alter the shape of the cervix and compress the cervical canal, in some cases preventing the detection of cervical incompetence (22). The vaginal probe should be placed in the posterior third of the vagina without pressure (Fig. 7.**7**). If the probe is pressed too hard against the cervix, it can obscure cervical incompetence (Fig. 7.**8**). Initial orientation is established by locating the longitudinal axis of the cervix. The cervical canal should appear as a hypoechoic groove. The junction between the amniotic fluid and cervical canal is designated as the internal os. The external os is located at the lower end of the cervix and touches the posterior vaginal wall in the upper third of the vagina. Cervical length is defined as the distance between the internal os and external os. Cervical thickness at the center of the cervix is measured perpendicular to the cervical canal (10) (Fig. 7.**9**).

Normal values. The cervix in a normal pregnancy shows an individual pattern in which the relationship among various parameters such as cervical length and thickness and the width of the internal os remain constant. Normally the cervical length is always greater than the cervical thickness, and the internal os is closed. Shortly before term, the relationship changes in favor of cervical thickness. Cervical length during pregnancy can range from 30 to 70 mm (Figs. 7.**7**, 7.**9**), and the ultrasound width of the cervical canal ranges from 2 to 4 mm. Cervical thickness is in the range of 25–35 mm. Sonographically, no differences are observed between the cervix of a primipara and that of a multipara. The cervix in multiple pregnancies is significantly longer and thicker than in singleton pregnancies (7).

Table 7.1   Ultrasound changes that suggest cervical incompetence (after Varma [29])

➤ Cervical length < 1.5 cm
➤ Cervical width > 3 cm
➤ Expanded cervical canal > 8 mm
➤ Prolapsed membranes in cervical canal, especially with fetal parts

Cervical opening. Cervical opening is a dynamic process that begins sonographically with dilatation of the internal os (Fig. 7.**10**). This is followed by a shortening of the cervix and progressive widening of the internal os, which is continuous distally with the cervical canal. Sonographically, the cervical canal assumes the appearance of a hypoechoic V- or U-shaped funnel (Figs. 7.**10**–7.**13**). In transverse section, the widened cervical canal appears as a round or elliptical area of low echogenicity (Fig. 7.**14**). As widening of the cervical canal progresses, it leads ultimately to prolapse of the fetal membranes (Fig. 7.**15**).

Serial scans. Serial scans make it possible to diagnose progressive cervical shortening and also detect initial incompetence of the internal os at a time when the external os is still closed. According to Varma (29), the ultrasound changes listed in Table 7.**1** are suspicious for cervical incompetence.

Therapeutic implications. The ultrasound surveillance of cervical length can not only help in the early detection of cervical incompetence but in some cases can help to avoid cervical cerclage by showing a lack of further shortening on serial scans despite a clinical decrease in cervical length. On the other hand, if ultrasound shows cervical shortening to < 1.5 cm at 23 weeks, a cerclage procedure can significantly reduce the risk of preterm delivery (15). Following the placement of cerclage, the efficacy of the procedure can be checked by the ultrasound assessment of cervical length.

Conclusion. On the whole, ultrasound evaluation of the cervix during pregnancy is an essential tool in the diagnosis of cervical incompetence. The history, clinical examination, and palpable findings aid in the correct interpretation of cervical ultrasound findings.

Placental Localization in Placenta Previa

Although the incidence of placenta previa is just 0.5% during the second half of pregnancy, it is nevertheless associated with high perinatal morbidity and mortality (23).

Differentiation. Abdominal ultrasound in the second and third trimesters cannot always distinguish a true placenta previa from a low-lying placenta, making it necessary for many women to undergo prolonged hospitalization. Transvaginal ultrasound can help in differentiating these conditions (Figs. 7.**16**, 7.**17**).

Bleeding risk. The fear that using a vaginal probe in placenta previa might provoke heavy bleeding has not been confirmed (24). This is understandable when we consider that the probe need be inserted only a few centimeters into the vagina to define the lower uterine segment. Care should always be taken, however, to avoid compressing the cervix with the probe.

Evaluating the Postpartum Uterus

Transvaginal ultrasound can be used in the puerperium to investigate bleeding, involutional problems, or pain. This is possible only if there has been sufficient uterine involution for the vaginal scan to define the uterus in its full size. Because transvaginal ultrasound can define the uterine cavity as well as the lower uterine segment in patients who have had a cesarean section, it can easily detect intrauterine placental residues, membranes, and a hematoma in the area of the abdominal scar. Residual placenta and membranes usually appear as hyperechoic structures within the uterine cavity (25) (Figs. 7.**18**–7.**20**). The same applies to placental polyps (Fig. 7.**21**). A hematoma in the area of the abdominal scar appears hypoechoic.

References

1. Alcazar, J.L., Balsonado, C., Laparte, C.: The reliability of transvaginal ultrasonography to detect retained tissue after spontaneous first-trimester abortion, clinically thought to be complete. Ultrasound Obstet. Gynecol. 6 (1995) 126–129
2. Bader, W., Böhmer, S., Degenhardt, F., Schneider, J.: Vergleichende Betrachtungen der Cervix uteri in graviditate mittels Palpation und Vaginosonographie. Ultraschall Med. 13 (1992) 18–23
3. Bishop, E.M.: Pelvic scoring for elective induction. Obstet. Gynecol. 24 (1964) 264
4. Buchanan, D., Macer, J., Yonekura, M.L.: Cervical ripening with prostaglandin E2 vaginal suppositories. Obstet. Gynecol. 63 (1984) 659–664
5. Chung, A., Birnbaum, S.J.: Ovarian cancer associated with pregnancy. Obstet. Gynecol. 41 (1973) 211–216
6. Cook, C.M., Ellwood, D.A.: A longitudinal study of the cervix in pregnancy using transvaginal ultrasound. Brit. J. Obstet. Gynaecol. 103 (1996) 16–18
7. Eppel, W.: Die isthmozervikale Insuffizienz. Gynäkologe 28 (1995) 175–180
8. Eppel, W., Frigo, P., Schurz, B., Reinold, E.: Vaginosonographische Studie bei normaler und inkompetenter Zervix: Versuch einer mathematischen Beurteilung. Ultraschall Med. 11 (1990) 183–187
9. Eppel, W., Schurz, B., Frigo, P., Reinold, E.: Vaginosonographic surveillance of cervix after conization. Acta Obstet. Gynecol. Scand. 68 (1989) 89–91
10. Eppel, W., Schurz, B., Frigo, P., Reinold, E.: Die Zervix am Termin – eine sonographische Studie. Z. Geburtshilfe Perinatol. 195 (1991) 250–253
11. Eppel, W., Schurz, B., Frigo, P., Reinold, E.: Vaginosonographische Beobachtung des zervikalen Verschlußapparates unter besonderer Berücksichtigung der Parität. Geburtsh. Frauenheilk. 52 (1992) 148–151
12. Granström, L., Ekman, G., Ulmsten, U., Malmström, A.: Changes of the connective tissue in corpus and cervix uteri during ripening and labour in term pregnancy. Brit. J. Obstet. Gynaecol. 96 (1989) 1198–1202
13. Grendys, E.C.Jr., Barnes, W.A.: Ovarian cancer in pregnancy. Surg. Clin. North. Am. 75 (1995) 1–14
14. Guzman, E.R., Rosenberg, J.C., Houlihan, C., Ivan, J., Waldron, R., Knuppel, R.: A new method using vaginal ultrasound and transfundal pressure to evaluate the asymptomatic incompetent cervix. Obstet. Gynecol. 83 (1994) 248–252
15. Heath, V.C., Souka, A.P., Erasmus, I., Gibb, D.M., Nicolaides, K.H.: Cervical length at 23 weeks of gestation: the value of Shirodkar suture for the short cervix. Ultrasound Obstet. Gynecol. 12 (1998) 318–322
16. Hill, L.M., Connors-Beatty, D.J., Nowak, A., Tush, B.: The role of ultrasonography in the detection and management of adnexal masses during the second and third trimesters of pregnancy. Am. J. Obstet. Gynecol. 179 (1998) 703–707
17. Iams, J.D., Johnson, F.F., Sonek, J., Sachs, L., Gebauer, C., Samuels, P.: Cervical incompetence as a continuum: a study of ultrasonographic cervical length and obstetric performance. Am. J. Obstet. Gynecol. 172 (1995) 1097–1103
18. McDonald, H.M., O'Laughlin, J.A., Jolley, P., Vigneswaran, R., McDonald, P.J.: Vaginal infection and preterm labour. Brit. J. Obstet. Gynaecol. 98 (1991) 427–438
19. Michaels, W.H., Montgomery, C., Karu, J.: Ultrasound differentiation of the competent from the incompetent cervix: prevention of preterm delivery. Am. J. Obstet. Gynecol. 154 (1986) 537–546
20. Monnier, J.C., Bernardi, C., Lanciaux, B., Vinatier, D., Lefebvre, C.: L'association fibrome et grossese. A propos de 51 observations relevees d'avril 1976 a decembre 1984. Rev. Fr. Gynecol. Obstet. 81 (1986) 99–104
21. Munnell, E.W.: Primary ovarian tumours in pregnancy. Clin. Obstet. Gynecol. 6 (1963) 983
22. Pfersmann, C., Deutinger, J., Bernaschek, G.: Die Cervixlänge gegen Ende der Schwangerschaft – eine sonographische Studie. Geburtsh. Frauenheilk. 46 (1986) 213–214
23. Powell, M.C., Buckley, J., Price, H., Worthington, B.S., Symonds, E.M.: Magnetic resonance imaging and placenta praevia. Am. J. Obstet. Gynecol. 154 (1986) 565–569
24. Rotten, S., Bronshtein, M., Thaler, I., Brandes, J.: Transvaginal ultrasonography for diagnosis of placenta praevia. Lancet I (1989) 444–445
25. Rulin, M.C., Bornstein, S.G., Campbell, J. D.: The reliability of ultrasonography in the management of spontaneous abortion, clinically to be thought to be complete: a prospective study. Am. J. Obstet. Gynecol. 168 (1993) 12–15
26. Smith, C.V., Anderson, J.C., Matamoros, A., Rayburn, W.F.: Transvaginal sonography of cervical width and length during pregnancy. J. Ultrasound Med. 11 (1992) 465–467
27. Struzziero, E., Corbo, M.: Attualita sui fibromi in gravidanza. Minerva-Ginecol. 48 (1996) 15–16
28. Tanos, V., Schenker, J.G.: Ovarian cysts: a clinical dilemma. Gynecol. Endocrinol. 8 (1994) 59–67
29. Varma, T.R., Patel, R.H., Pillai, U.: Ultrasonic assessment of cervix in "at risk" patients. Int. J. Gynecol. Obstet. 25 (1987) 25–34

Uterine and adnexal masses

Fig. 7.**1**   Large, hypoechoic, subserosal anterior-wall fibroid (5 · 4.2 cm) in early pregnancy (7 weeks). Transvaginal coronal scan through the lower pelvis.

Fig. 7.**2**   Intramural posterior-wall fibroid, 4.3 cm in diameter, at 14 weeks.

Fig. 7.**3**   Cervical carcinoma (barrel-shaped tumor) with a mixed hyperechoic/hypoechoic structure (arrows), 32 weeks. Fetal head (*).

Fig. 7.**4**   Hypoechoic 5-cm corpus luteum cyst in the cul-de-sac in early pregnancy (5 weeks, 3 days).

Fig. 7.**5**   Dermoid cyst to the left of the uterus (arrows) at 8 weeks. Urinary bladder (1), gestational sac with embryo (2).

Fig. 7.**6**   Left pelvic kidney (arrows) in early pregnancy (6 weeks, 2 days). Oblique longitudinal scan through the lower pelvis.

Cervical incompetence

Fig. 7.**7**   Normal cervical length (55 mm) at 28 weeks (arrows). The vaginal probe has been positioned directly in front of the cervix without compressing it. Medial longitudinal scan.

Fig. 7.**8**   Cervical incompetence at 31 weeks. Cervical compression by the vaginal probe creates the appearance of an intact cervix 36 mm in length (arrows).

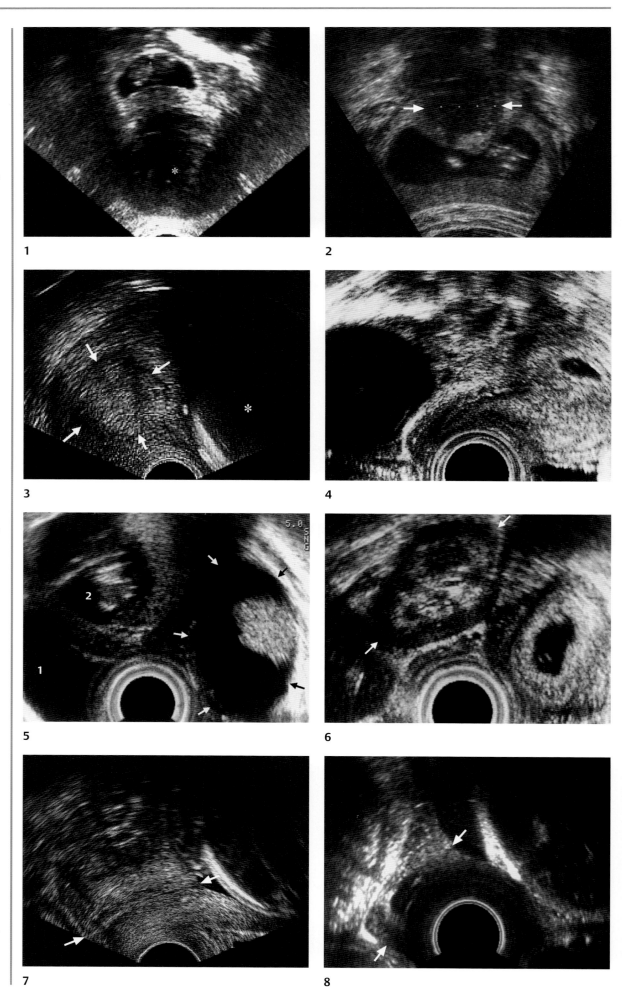

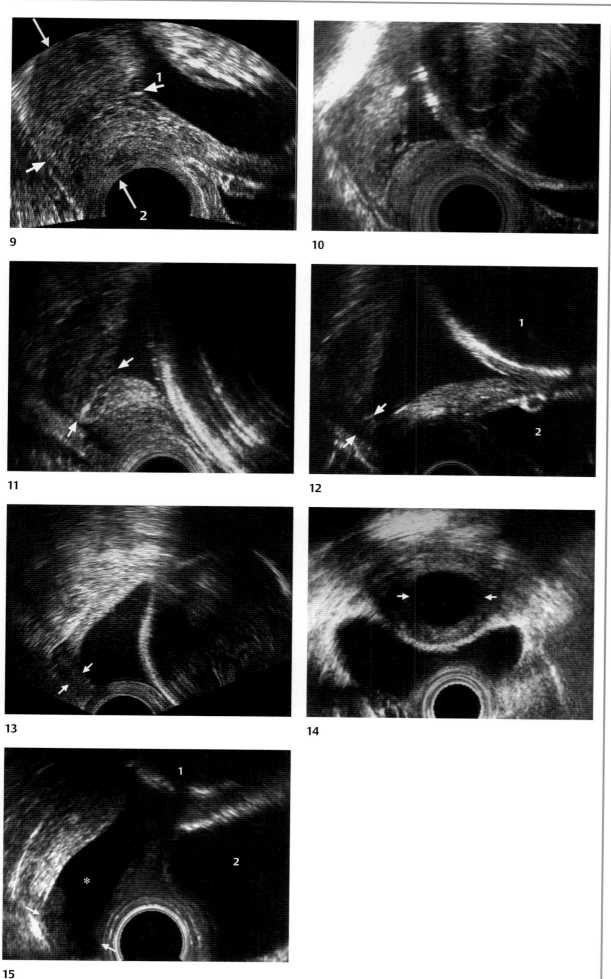

9

10

11

12

13

14

15

Fig. 7.**9**   Normal cervical length (34 mm) at 18 weeks (arrows 1). Medial longitudinal scan. Cervical thickness is measured across the center of the cervix (arrows 2).

Fig. 7.**10**   Incipient cervical incompetence, 30 weeks. Note the slight V-shaped dilatation of the internal os. Longitudinal scan.

Fig. 7.**11**   Progressive cervical incompetence, 33 weeks. V-shaped dilatation of the internal os is accompanied by marked shortening of the cervix to 22 mm (arrows). Longitudinal scan.

Fig. 7.**12**   Marked cervical incompetence with funnel-shaped expansion of the cervical canal from the inside. Residual cervix 9 mm. 31 weeks. Longitudinal scan. Fetal head (1), maternal bladder (2).

Fig. 7.**13**   Marked cervical incompetence with U-shaped expansion of the cervical canal by herniated membranes. The external os is still closed (arrows). 20 weeks. Longitudinal scan.

Fig. 7.**14**   Marked cervical incompetence in a transverse scan of the cervix, 30 weeks. Note the elliptical expansion of the cervical canal by the herniated amniotic sac (arrows).

Fig. 7.**15**   Complete membrane prolapse (∗) at 20 weeks. Longitudinal scan. The arrows mark the external os. Fetal head (1), maternal bladder (2).

Placenta previa

Fig. 7.**16** Partial placenta previa on the posterior uterine wall (arrows). Longitudinal scan. Cervix (1), posterior wall placenta (2), fetal head (3), maternal bladder (4).

Fig. 7.**17** Marginal placenta previa with a small hematoma at the inferior edge of the placenta (arrows). Longitudinal scan. Cervix (1), posterior wall placenta (2), fetal head (3), maternal bladder (4).

Postpartum uterus

Fig. 7.**18** Echogenic placental remnants in the uterine cavity 2 weeks postpartum. Longitudinal scan of the uterus.

Fig. 7.**19** Echogenic abortion products in the uterine cavity following pregnancy termination. Longitudinal scan of the uterus.

Fig. 7.**20** Specimen photograph corresponding to Fig. 7.**19**.

Fig. 7.**21** Echogenic placental polyp (arrow) 7 weeks after delivery. Longitudinal scan of the uterus.

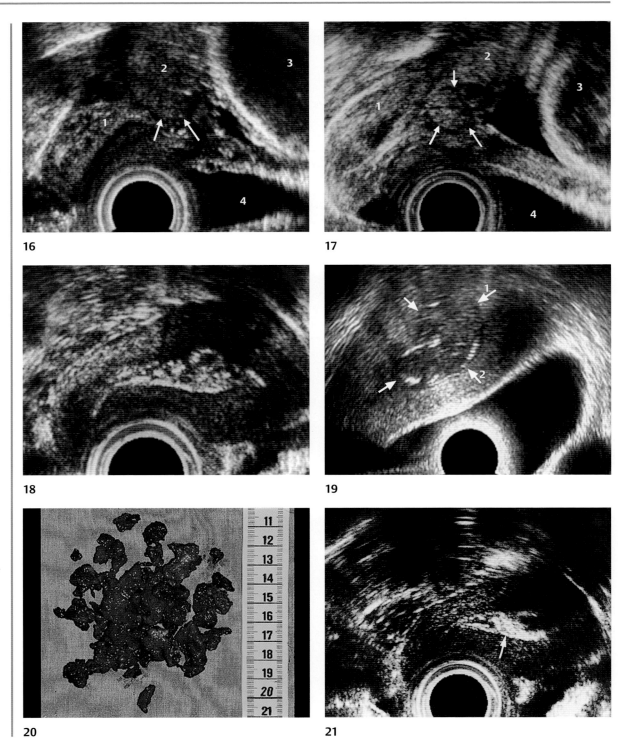

8 Pelvimetry with Transvaginal Ultrasound

Cephalopelvic Disproportion

Increase. Skeletal deformities due to malnutrition have become extremely rare in the developed world. But during the past 20 years, the diagnosis of cephalopelvic disproportion has grown in frequency from 1.5% to 3.8% of all deliveries. It has been suggested that this is due to an average increase in birth weight by 100 g along with improved methods of perinatal surveillance (28).

Quantitative parameters. Several factors must be considered in predicting whether a spontaneous delivery can occur: the size and shape of the bony pelvis, the size and shape of the fetal head, fetal presentation and position, and uterine activity. It is not enough to consider only one piece of clinical information in predicting whether spontaneous delivery is feasible (30). Both fetal and maternal parameters should always be considered in order to exclude cephalopelvic disproportion.

X-Ray Pelvimetry

X-ray pelvimetry has been used for many years to supplement the clinical examination in the early detection of cephalopelvic disproportion (11). This method makes it possible to obtain and evaluate important obstetric measurements but should be used sparingly because of the radiation exposure to the fetus (26). Until 1970, up to 40% of all pregnant women underwent radiographic examination (10). Both the true conjugate and the inclination of the pelvic inlet plane can be measured radiographically. The transverse diameter of the pelvic inlet and the distance between the two ischial spines can also be determined.

Limited indications. Before a pregnant woman is selected for x-ray pelvimetry, it must be asked whether the information gained will significantly influence the subsequent management of the delivery (26).

Recent studies cast doubt on the importance of x-ray pelvimetry in terms of selecting patients for cesarean delivery (1, 21). Even if cephalopelvic disproportion is suspected, it does not imply a less favorable fetal outcome (24). X-ray pelvimetry in pregnancy does not make an important contribution to decision-making in patients who have had a previous cesarean section (20).

Increased risk of leukemia. The American College of Obstetricians and Gynecologists recommends that fetal radiation exposure be kept as low as possible, because so far there has been nothing to refute Stewart's studies showing an increased leukemia risk in children exposed to radiation in utero (2, 30). If radiographs are taken during pregnancy, the leukemia rate will increase depending on the timing of the examination and the radiation dose (3). The radiation exposure in x-ray pelvimetry is 0.15–0.9 rad, which is close to the maximum allowable dose in pregnancy (12).

Fetal-pelvic index. A breech presentation in primiparae is an indication for x-ray pelvimetry that is still being discussed today (9). When combined with prenatal ultrasound fetal weight estimation and x-ray pelvimetry, calculation of the "fetal-pelvic index" makes it possible to predict with some accuracy whether it will be necessary to perform a cesarean delivery for cephalopelvic disproportion. The accuracy of the prediction increases with the number of parameters that are evaluated. Studies in this area have shown a sensitivity of up to 86% and a specificity of up to 100% (22, 23).

Pelvimetry in the puerperium. X-ray pelvimetry can be used liberally in the puerperium following a protracted delivery or if there is suspicion of pelvic narrowing, as it can provide useful information on bony pelvic abnormalities that could affect a future pregnancy.

Ultrasound Pelvimetry

Abdominal ultrasound. Given the limited indications for x-ray use during pregnancy, it was only natural that early attempts would be made to obtain pelvic measurements using ultrasound (17, 18, 19). In earlier decades, compound scanners were the only instruments available for obstetric pelvimetry. With this method it was possible to measure the true conjugate, usually toward the end of the pregnancy, with an acceptable degree of accuracy (17). Measurements were taken from either B-mode or A-mode transabdominal scans, using frequencies in the range of 1–2 MHz. Large clinical series confirmed the accuracy of this method (27). Newer abdominal real-time scanners have proven unsatisfactory for obstetric pelvimetry. Only lately has an attempt been made to use real-time instruments with a transducer frequency of 3.5 MHz for pelvic measurements (15).

Vaginal ultrasound. The development of endovaginal scanners has opened up a new approach to pelvimetry. It was not long before vaginal scanners were used for the measurement of pelvic dimensions relevant to obstetrics. The results were compared with the results of compound scanners during pregnancy and of x-ray pelvimetry after the delivery (5, 7).

▬ *Method of Transvaginal Pelvimetry*

Transducer. Transvaginal pelvimetry is performed with a vaginal probe operating at a frequency of 5 MHz. Wide-angle sector scanners are superior to other types for this application (6). The ideal transducer is a panoramic end-fire probe with a 240° field of view.

Positioning and preparation. As in all vaginal ultrasound examinations, the lithotomy position is best as it gives the vaginal probe the greatest mobility. Transvaginal ultrasound measurements of the true conjugate can usually be performed without difficulty. In some cases, however, the examination must be repeated after evacuation of the bowel because a full rectum can cast an acoustic shadow that obscures the anterior border of the promontory.

Examination technique. The transvaginal probe is first positioned in the vagina to obtain a midsagittal scan. An accurate midsagittal position is confirmed by the simultaneous appearance of the pubic symphysis and sacral promontory in the same image (Figs. 8.**1**–8.**3**). For measurement of the true conjugate, the probe is lowered slightly to display the full height of the symphysis. The true conjugate is measured as the distance from the posterosuperior border of the symphysis to the promontory. Visualization of the end points of the true conjugate does not depend on fetal position. To measure the transverse pelvic diameter, the probe is rotated 90° and the probe handle is moved in the vertical plane until the linea terminalis on each side can be identified and measured (Fig. 8.**4**–8.**7**).

■ Results to Date

Patients. Transvaginal ultrasound pelvimetry was performed in 74 pregnant women using a panoramic scanner. Twenty-two of these cases were examined shortly before term. Preterm deliveries were excluded from analysis. In 58 cases the true conjugate was measured with a compound scanner, and in 36 cases a pelvic radiograph was obtained after delivery. The fetal presentation was cephalic in 65 of the cases examined. In 8 of 58 measurements taken with a compound scanner, no relevant results were obtained. Two of the eight cases were a transverse lie and three were breech. In one case the true conjugate could not be determined because of an oblique lie and in two cases because of maternal obesity.

True conjugate. Measurements of the true conjugate performed by vaginal ultrasound correlated well with compound scan measurements. The deviation from radiographic measurements was up to 5 mm (8).

Transverse diameter. Differences of 4 mm were found in measurements of the transverse diameter of the pelvic inlet. After 37 weeks, the greatest transverse pelvic diameter could not be measured in 7 primiparae because the fetal head was already too low in the pelvis. In the rest of the patients, the measurement could be performed without difficulty.

Ratio of true conjugate to BPD. One study documents the value of measuring the true conjugate alone in predicting cephalopelvic disproportion (Table 8.**1**). But because cephalopelvic disproportion is based on the relationship between the maternal pelvis and fetal head, the ratio between the true conjugate and fetal BPD should be calculated. This ratio averaged 1.29 in spontaneous deliveries. When cephalopelvic disproportion was present, the ratio averaged 1.17. Statistically, this difference was highly significant. It is interesting to note that there was no case of cephalopelvic disproportion in which the ratio was higher than 1.24. Cases with spontaneous delivery and cases delivered by cesarean section showed no significant differences with regard to BPD measured sonographically within 1 week before delivery or the weight of the newborn.

Advantages of transvaginal pelvimetry. The major advantages of vaginal ultrasound pelvimetry are its technical simplicity and lack of radiation exposure. It can also be used to determine the transverse diameter of the pelvic inlet, yielding information that is useful for evaluating the pelvic configuration in the inlet plane. The examination can be performed at any stage of pregnancy, and even severe obesity does not compromise the result. A full bladder is not required. Fetal position does not influence the result. Measurement of the transverse pelvic diameter can be difficult in primiparae after 37 weeks if the low fetal

head limits transducer mobility or if its acoustic shadow hampers identification of the lateral pelvic margin.

■ Comparison with CT and MRI

Computed tomography (CT). Digital radiography reduces radiation exposure by 15–30% compared with conventional radiography (4). The improved visualization of structures makes it considerably easier to interpret the results (16). The result can be more difficult to interpret in obese patients, however (4). The results of transvaginal ultrasound pelvimetry are not affected by obesity. Besides pelvic dimensions and fetal size, of course, the overall configuration and inclination of the pelvis and the angle of the pubic ramus are important in predicting the course of the delivery. The true conjugate and the transverse diameter of the pelvic inlet are the most important parameters, however, for making an overall assessment of the bony birth canal.

Capabilities of magnetic resonance imaging (MRI). While we have previously compared the results of vaginal ultrasound pelvimetry with measurements performed with a compound scanner and postpartum radiographs, it would also be desirable to compare the method with the results of computed tomography and magnetic resonance imaging. MRI can provide very high-quality images of the bony maternal pelvis, permitting accurate measurements to be taken (13, 14, 25). When MRI measurements of transverse pelvic diameter were compared with x-ray pelvimetry, discrepancies of up to 2 cm were found (25). For the present, MRI techniques are very costly and are not feasible for routine pelvimetry. Another drawback is that MRI is usually unavailable for acute examinations. Ultrasound equipment, on the other hand, is available in practically every obstetric department.

■ Conclusion

In primiparae with a suspected cephalopelvic disproportion, vaginal ultrasound pelvimetry could make an excellent routine study as it is well tolerated, involves no radiation exposure, and yields results comparable to those of other methods. Further improvements are likely to occur when 3-D technology can be applied to ultrasound pelvimetry.

Table 8.**1**   True conjugate, fetal weight, and fetal biparietal diameter in spontaneous deliveries and cesarean sections

Parameter	Spontaneous delivery (n = 49)	Cesarean section (n = 11)
True conjugate	11.8 cm (± 0,4)	10.9 cm (± 0.3)*
BPD	9.1 cm (± 0,3)	9.3 cm (± 0.2)
Weight	3340 g (± 440)	3470 g (± 450)

* P < 0.05. BPD: biparietal diameter

References

1. Alder, Ch., Aebi, S., Bernhard, M.: Der Stellenwert der radiologischen Beckenmessung. Geburtsh. Frauenheilk. 47 (1987) 483–486
2. American College of Obstetricians and Gynecologists: ACOG Bull 23 (1979) 10
3. Brent, R.L.: Irradiation in pregnancy, Gynecology and Obstetrics. 1981 edition. Edited by J. Sciarra. Philadelphia: Harper and Row, 1981
4. Claussen, C., Köhler, D., Christ, F., Golde, G., Lochner, B.: Pelvimetry by digital radiography and its dosimetry. J. Perinat. Med. 13 (1985) 287–292
5. Deutinger, J., Bernaschek, G.: Die vaginosonographische Pelvimetrie als neue Methode zur sonographischen Bestimmung der inneren Beckenmaße. Geburtsh. Frauenheilk. 46 (1986) 345–347
6. Deutinger, J., Bernaschek, G.: Die vaginosonographische Pelvimetrie – eine neue Methode zur sonographischen Bestimmung der inneren Beckenmaße. Ultraschalldiagnostik 85. Drei-Länder-Treffen Zürich. Otto, R.Ch., Schnaars, P. (Hrsg.): Thieme (1986) 2–3
7. Deutinger, J., Bernaschek, G.: Vaginosonographical Determination of the true conjugate and the transverse diameter of the pelvic inlet. Arch. Gynecol. Obstet. 240 (1987) 241–246
8. Deutinger, J.: Die vaginosonographische Beckenmessung. XII. Kongress der Deutschen Gesellschaft für Perinatale Medizin. Berlin 1.–4. Dezember 1987
9. Gimovsky, M.L., Willard, K., Neglio, M., Howard, Th., Zerne, S.: X-ray pelvimetry in a breech proctol: A comparison of digital radiography and conventional methods. Am. J. Obstet. Gynecol. 153 (1985) 887–888
10. Gordon, A., Pinchen, C., Walker, E., Tudor, J.: The changing place of radiology in obstetrics. Br. J. Radiol. 57 (1984) 891–893
11. Guthmann, H.: Die röntgenologische Messung der Conjugata vera. Fortschr. Röntgenstr. 36 (1929) 257
12. Hochuli, E.: Geburtshilfe, Gynäkologie und Grenzgebiete. Bern: Hans Huber 1985
13. Hricak, H., Albers, C., Crooks, L.E., Sheldon, P.E.: Magnetic resonance imaging of the female pelvis – initial experience. Am. J. Rad. 141 (1983) 1119–1128
14. Johnson, I.R., Symonds, E.M., Worthington, B.S., Broughton Pipkin, F., Hawkes, R.C., Gyngell, M.: Imaging the pregnant human uterus with nuclear magnetic resonance. Am. J. Obstet. Gynecol. 148 (1984) 1136–1139

15. Katanozaka, M., Yoshinaga, M., Fuchiwaki, K., Nagata, Y.: Measurement of obstetric conjugate by ultrasonic tomography and its significance. Am. J. Obstet. Gynecol. 180 (1999) 159–162
16. Kopelman, J.N., Duff, P., Karl, R.T., Schipul, A.H., Read, J.A.: Computed tomographic pelvimetry in the evaluation of breech presentation. Obstet. Gynecol. 68 (1986) 455–458
17. Kratochwil, A., Zeibekis, N.: Ultrasonic pelvimetry. Acta Obstet. Gynecol. Scand. 51 (1972) 357–362
18. Kratochwil, A., Jentsch, K., Brezina, K.F.: Ultraschallanatomie des weiblichen Beckens und ihre klinische Bedeutung. Arch. Gynecol. 214 (1973) 273–275
19. Kratochwil, A.: Ultraschalluntersuchung in der Geburtshilfe. In: Diethelm, L., Heuck, F., Olsson, O., Strnad, F., Vieten, H., Zuppinger, A. (Hrsg.): Handbuch der medizinischen Radiologie. Berlin: Springer 1980 S. 349–401
20. Mahmod, T.A., Grant, J.M.: The role of radiological pelvimetry in the management of patients who have had a previous caesarean section. J. Obstet. Gynaecol. 8 (1987) 24–28
21. Mandry, J., Grandjean, H., Reme, J.M., Pastor, J., Levade, C., Pontonnier, G.: Assessment of the predictive value of x-ray pelvimetry and biparietal diameter in cephalopelvic disproportion. Europ. J. Obstet. Gynec. Reprod. Biol. 15 (1983) 173–179
22. Morgan, M.A., Thurnau, G.R., Fishburne, J.I.jr.: The fetal-pelvic index as an indicator of fetal-pelvic disproportion: a preliminary report. Am. J. Obstet. Gynecol. 155 (1986) 608–613
23. Morgan, M.A., Thurnau, G.R.: Efficacy of the fetal-pelvic index in patients requiring labor induction. Am. J. Obstet. Gynecol. 159 (1988) 621–625
24. Parsons, M.T., Spellacy, W.N.: Prospective randomized study of x-ray pelvimetry in the primigravida. Obstet. Gynecol. 66 (1985) 76–79
25. Powell, M.C., Worthington, B.S., Buckley, J.M., Symonds, E.M.: Magnetic resonance imaging (MRI) in obstetrics. I. Maternal anatomy. Brit. J. Obstet. Gynaecol. 95 (1988) 31–37
26. Pritchard, J.A., MacDonald, P.C., Gant, N.F.: Williams Obstetrics. 17th edition. Norwalk, Connecticut: Appleton-Century-Crofts 1985; pp. 229–231
27. Schlensker, K.H.: Ultraschallmessungen der Conjugata vera obstetrica. Geburtsh. Frauenheilk. 39 (1979) 333–337
28. Silbar, E.L.: Factors related to the increasing section rates for cephalopelvic disproportion. Am. J. Obstet. Gynecol. 154 (1986) 1095–1098
29. Sporri, S., Gyr, T., Schollerer, A., Werlen, S., Schneider, H.: Methoden, Techniken und Anwendungsmöglichkeiten der geburtshilflichen Beckenmessung. Z. Geburtsh. Perinat. 198 (1994) 37–46
30. Stewart, A., Webb, J., Giles, D., Hewitt, D.: Malignant disease in childhood and diagnostic irradiation in utero. Lancet 2 (1956) 447–457

Fig. 8.**1** Transvaginal ultrasound pelvimetry (true conjugate), illustrated in a female skeleton. The vaginal probe is positioned in the pelvis so that the beam is in a vertical (sagittal) plane.

Fig. 8.**2** The true conjugate is measured from the posterosuperior edge of the pubic symphysis to the inner border of the sacral promontory.

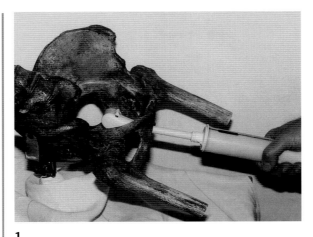

1

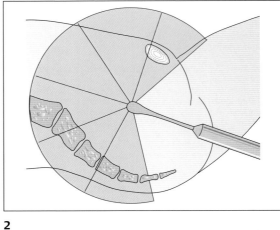

2

Fig. 8.**3** Measurement of the true conjugate by transvaginal ultrasound (S = symphysis, P = promontory, FLE = fetal lower extremity. The true conjugate in this case measures 117 mm.

Fig. 8.**4** Measurement of the transverse diameter of the pelvic inlet (transverse conjugate) by vaginal ultrasound, demonstrated on a female skeleton. The probe is rotated 90°, moving the beam to a coronal plane.

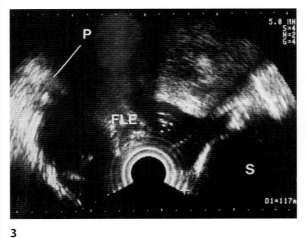

3

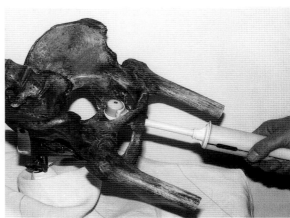

4

Fig. 8.**5** Diagram of the scan plane for measuring the transverse conjugate, viewed from the anterior aspect. The distance between the two ischial spines is measured.

Fig. 8.**6** Scan plane for measuring the transverse conjugate, viewed from the side.

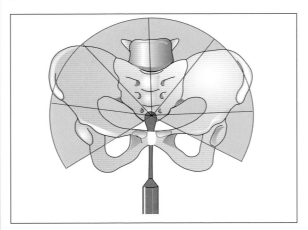

5

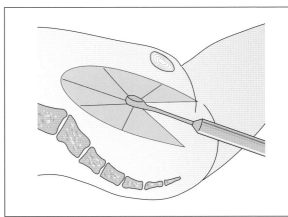

6

Fig. 8.**7** Measurement of the transverse conjugate by transvaginal ultrasound (S = symphysis, P = promontory). The transverse conjugate in this case measures 140 mm.

7

Abdominal Ultrasound

9 Normal Early Pregnancy, Biometry, and Gestational Age Assignment in the First Trimester

Basic Principles of Embryology (5, 15, 30)

From conception to implantation. About 12–24 hours after ovulation (about 14 days after menstruation), the ovum is fertilized in the ampullary portion of the fallopian tube. Over the next 3–4 days, the zygote migrates into the uterus. During this time the zygote undergoes mitotic division and segmentation, developing from a two-cell stage to a morula composed of 12–16 blastomeres. The zygote develops into a blastocyst, a fluid-filled cyst with an outer cell layer (trophoblast) and an inner cell mass (embryoblast), and implantation begins on the 20th postmenstrual day (= 6th day after conception).

Development of the embryonic disk. At implantation, the blastocyst burrows into the thick secretory endometrium. Implantation is completed by the 23rd day, at which time the blastocyst is deeply embedded in the endometrium. With the development of the trophoblast to the syncytiotrophoblast and cytotrophoblast and with further penetration of the syncytial cells into the stroma, the trophoblast gains attachment to the maternal sinusoids during the 4th postmenstrual week, establishing a primitive uteroplacental circulation. Meanwhile the embryoblast develops into a bilaminar embryonic disk composed of an ectoderm and endoderm, and the amniotic cavity and primary yolk sac are formed. By the end of the 4th week, the smaller secondary yolk sac forms, surrounded by the extraembryonic coelom, the chorionic cavity. The mesoderm forms during the 5th week, producing a trilaminar disk. The chorionic cavity enlarges, and by the end of 5 weeks the embryo is connected to the trophoblast only by a narrow connecting stalk (= future umbilical cord) (Fig. 9.**1**).

Organogenesis. Between 5 and 10 weeks' gestation, the organ rudiments develop from the 3 embryonic layers, and the embryonic body shape begins to appear. In the 7th week the extremities appear as paddle-shaped buds. In the 8th week the liver completely fills the abdominal cavity. The rapidly growing small intestine is extruded into the umbilical cord (physiologic umbilical hernia) and does not reenter the enlarged peritoneal cavity until the gut rotations are completed in the 12th week. By 10 weeks' gestation, the conceptus has acquired the distinctive appearance of a human embryo.

Development of the placenta. At 6 weeks' gestation the amniotic cavity enlarges at the expense of the chorionic cavity (Fig. 9.**2**), filling the entire chorionic sac by 12 weeks so that the chorion and amnion are apposed. The chorionic villi at the embryonic pole continue to grow and develop into the chorion frondosum, which combines with the decidua basalis to form the placenta. The chorionic villi at the anembryonic pole degenerate and form the chorion laeve. After degeneration of the decidua capsularis, the chorion laeve fuses with the decidua parietalis, obliterating the uterine cavity (Fig. 9.**3**).

Pregnancy Detection by Abdominal Ultrasound

Completed implantation. On average, 18–24 days pass between fertilization of the ovum and the time at which an intrauterine gestational sac can first be detected with abdominal ultrasound. Neither the transport of the fertilized ovum nor the early implantation of the blastocyst can be detected sonographically. It is not until the 5th week, when the conceptus is completely embedded in the endometrium and is beginning to grow, that the gestational sac can be identified within the uterine corpus as an echogenic ring with low-level internal echoes (3, 9, 11, 23).

Abdominal ultrasound cannot detect pregnancy as early as the serum β-hCG assay, which is positive just 7 days after conception. The advantage of ultrasound it that it can demonstrate the precise location of the gestational sac.

Implantation site. The implantation site is normally in the fundic portion of the uterine corpus (23), although implantation may also occur at a lower level. Kohorn and Kaufman (13) found no differences in the risk of spontaneous abortion associated with high, intermediate, and low implantations, whereas Hellman et al. (10) reported an increased abortion risk in low implantations. Cervical implantation is rare and is almost always associated with complications such as spontaneous abortion or, if the pregnancy continues, with risk of uterine rupture (31).

▬ *Gestational Sac*

By the 5th week of menstrual age, the gestational sac appears on both longitudinal and transverse scans as an echogenic ring-like structure with a hypoechoic cavity (Figs. 9.**4**–9.**6**).

Chorionic cavity. The hyperechoic ring of the gestational sac is formed by the chorion (11), and the hypoechoic cavity of the sac is formed initially by the extraembryonic coelom (= chorionic cavity) (23). In contrast to the pseudogestational sac of ectopic pregnancy (see Chapter 10), the gestational sac of an intrauterine pregnancy has an eccentric location (1) (Figs. 9.**4**–9.**8**). Initially round, the sac acquires an elliptical or reniform shape as growth proceeds (Figs. 9.**9**–9.**11**).

Amniotic cavity. The cavity of the gestational sac initially corresponds to the chorionic cavity. But as the amniotic cavity gradually expands (Fig. 9.**2**), it fills the entire chorionic sac (Fig. 9.**3**) and obliterates the chorionic cavity. By 11–12 weeks, then, the cavity of the gestational sac corresponds to the amniotic cavity.

The chorion laeve becomes less echogenic after 11 weeks. Hellman et al. (9) attribute this to the fusion of the decidua capsularis with the decidua parietalis, causing the reflective interfaces to disappear.

Implantation bleed. Between 6 and 8 weeks' gestation, it is common to see a hypoechoic streak next to the gestational sac or a triangular hypoechoic area below it. Lyons and Levi (16), who noted this feature in 60% of their patients, assume that it represents an implantation bleed that appears within the uterine cavity between the decidua capsularis and decidua parietalis (Fig. 9.**10**).

Embryo

Abdominal ultrasound can sometimes demonstrate the embryo as a small echogenic feature within the gestational sac as early as the 6th gestational week (Figs. 9.**7**, 9.**8**).

"Crouched in a corner." By the 7th gestational week, the embryo appears more clearly as an approximately 5-mm-long echogenic structure within the gestational sac, but occasionally it may be overlooked if it is "crouched in a corner" (Hackelöer [7]) of the chorionic cavity (Fig. 9.**9**). By the end of 7 weeks, the embryo has reached an average length of 10 mm and is consistently identifiable with abdominal ultrasound (Fig. 9.**10**).

Detection of Embryonic Heart Activity

Although rhythmic pulsations of the cardiac tube commence as early as the 6th gestational week (5), they can be detected with abdominal ultrasound no earlier than the 7th or 8th week. Robinson and Shaw-Dunn (25) could detect heart motion on the 45th postmenstrual day and Piiroinen (19) on the 42d day. Embryonic heart activity is most easily detected by M-mode scanning (Fig. 9.**11**).

Heart rate. The heart rate, according to Robinson and Shaw-Dunn (25), averages 123 bpm in the 7th week, rises to 177 bpm until the 9th week, and thereafter gradually declines until term (Fig. 9.**12**). The change in heart rate is related to the anatomic development of the heart.

Detection of Embryonic Movements

Active body movements by the embryo can sometimes be detected sonographically as early as 8 weeks' gestation and are consistently detected by 10 weeks (20, 22). If movements are not seen, they can sometimes be elicited by lightly tapping the maternal abdomen.

Brisk and sluggish movements. An intact pregnancy should be diagnosed only if embryonic body movements or heart activity can be positively detected. Reinold (20, 22) distinguishes two qualitative types of active movements: brisk and sluggish. If embryonic movements are sluggish or absent during a prolonged examination period, there is a greater likelihood of spontaneous abortion than when normal, brisk movements are present (22).

Schillinger (28) used M-mode scanning to quantify embryonic motor activity and found that the amplitude and speed of body movements increased between the 8th and 14th weeks of gestation.

Development in the First Trimester

Embryonic and Fetal Development

Head and trunk. While the embryo in the 7th and 8th weeks still appears sonographically as a uniform, echogenic structure within the gestational sac, a definite head and trunk can be identified starting in the 9th week (Fig. 9.**13**). The head at this stage comprises approximately 50% of the crown–rump length. The physiologic umbilical hernia may be discernible in a few cases (Fig. 9.**14**). Limbs can be seen next to the trunk by about 9 weeks' gestation (Figs. 9.**13**, 9.**15**).

Start of the fetal period. The start of the fetal period at the end of 10 weeks is marked by an increasing differentiation of the skull, trunk, extremities, and of the organs that began to form during the embryonic period (Figs. 9.**16**–9.**18**). As ossification progresses, the skull is recognized as consisting of a frontal bone, orbits, and a maxilla and mandible (Figs. 9.**16**–9.**18**). The first hyperechoic ossification centers in the limbs can also be discerned (Figs. 9.**17**, 9.**18**). By 12 weeks the spinal column can also be identified (Fig. 9.**19**).

Yolk Sac

The yolk sac appears by the 7th week as an echogenic, ring-like structure (2, 17) located close to the embryo within the gestational sac (Figs. 9.**14**, 9.**20**). Anatomically, the yolk sac is extra-amniotic, lying between the amnion and chorion (Fig. 9.**2**). Its diameter increases from 3 mm in the 7th week to 6 mm in the 11th week (2). By the 11th week, a yolk sac can rarely be identified (2). Apparently this relates to the union of the amnion and chorion (Fig. 9.**3**), causing obliteration of the chorionic cavity. The yolk sac and yolk duct then lie within the primitive umbilical cord bounded by the amnion and can no longer be detected with ultrasound.

Corpus Luteum of Pregnancy

It is common in early pregnancy to find a smooth-bordered, hypoechoic, cystic mass adjacent to the uterus. This represents the corpus luteum of pregnancy (Fig. 9.**6**, 9.**8**). It should not be mistaken for an abnormal cystic ovarian mass.

Biometry and Gestational Age Assignment in the First Trimester

The first parameters that are available for evaluating normal pregnancy development and determining gestational age in the first trimester are the gestational sac diameter and the crown–rump length. The biparietal diameter is also available at the end of the first trimester.

Gestational Sac Diameter

Linear growth. Several authors (9, 11, 12, 14, 21) performed ultrasound measurements of the gestational sac in early pregnancy and noted that the individual diameters showed a linear growth pattern.

Measurement technique. As an example, the values measured by Reinold (23) are shown graphically in Fig. 9.**21**. For practical biometry, the gestational sac should be measured from inner border to inner border—i.e., between the borders of the hypoechoic amniotic cavity. The outer borders are indistinct because of the decidual wall and would therefore yield an imprecise measurement. Also, the measurement should not be limited to a single diameter, because the shape of the gestational sac is markedly affected by bladder fullness and uterine contractions. When the longitudinal, transverse, and anteroposterior diameters have been measured, the mean sac diameter is determined by taking the arithmetic mean of the measurements.

Growth curves. Figure 9.22 shows the normal growth curves found by various investigators, in which mean gestational sac diameter is plotted as a function of gestational age.

Accuracy. When the gestational age is unknown, the mean gestational sac diameter provides the first measurable ultrasound parameter for gestational age assignment. This quantity is less precise than the crown–rump length, however. Holländer (11) determined gestational age to an accuracy of 1 week with 68% confidence as a function of the mean gestational sac diameter between the 6th and 14th weeks using the following formula:

Gestational age (weeks of menstrual age) =
1.384 · gestational sac diameter (cm) + 4.452.

Gestational sac volume. Robinson (26) determined gestational age with even greater accuracy by measuring the volume of the gestational sac. The sac volume increases exponentially from an average of 1 mL at 6 weeks to an average of 100 mL at 13 weeks. While the determination of gestational sac volume is too time-consuming to be applied in normal pregnancies, it can be of significant value in abnormal pregnancies and especially in the diagnosis of blighted ovum (26).

Crown–Rump Length

Accurate dating. Measurement of the crown–rump length (CRL) (24, 27), which can be performed as early as the 7th week (8), permits the most accurate determination of gestational age (Figs. 9.**10**, 9.**23**, 9.**24**). According to Robinson and Fleming (27), the CRL can estimate gestational age to an accuracy of ± 4.7 days with a single measurement and ± 2.7 days with three independent measurements at the 95% confidence level. Although other authors (4, 8, 18, 29) were unable to reproduce this degree of accuracy, there is no question that the CRL determined sonographically in the first trimester provides the most accurate estimate of gestational age during pregnancy.

Growth curves. Figures 9.**25** and 9.**26** show the grow curves for CRL versus gestational age determined by Hansmann et al. (8).

Guidelines. Table 9.**1** lists the guidelines that should be followed in abdominal ultrasound measurements of the CRL. Especially before 9 weeks' gestation, care should be taken that the CRL measurement does not include the adjacent yolk sac.

Toward the end of the first trimester, measurement of the CRL can be hampered by the tendency of the fetus to assume a curled posture. At this time is better to use other parameters such as biparietal diameter for gestational age assignment (see Chapter 13).

Summary of Key Parameters

Table 9.**2** shows the times at which the most important parameters can be detected with abdominal ultrasound in early pregnancy.

Table 9.1   Guidelines for the abdominal measurement of crown–rump length

> ➤ The embryo or fetus should be measured in its maximum craniocaudal extent.
> ➤ The embryo or fetus should be measured while in an extended position (Fig. 9.24).
> ➤ The points of measurement should be on the outer borders of the head and rump.

Table 9.2   Average times at which various parameters can first be detected by abdominal ultrasound in early pregnancy

1. Detection of the gestational sac	5 weeks
2. Detection of the yolk sac	6 weeks
3. Detection of the embryo	6 weeks
4. Measurement of crown–rump length	7 weeks
5. Detection of heart activity	7 weeks
6. Detection of embryonic movements	8 weeks
7. Differentiation of head, trunk, and limbs	9 weeks
8. Detection of the placenta	9 weeks

References

1. Abramovici, H., Auslender, R., Lewin, A., Faktor, J.H.: Gestational-pseudogestational sac: A new ultrasonic criterion for differential diagnosis. Amer. J. Obstet. Gynec. 145 (1983) 377–379
2. Crooij, M.J., Westhuis, M., Schoemaker, J., Exalto, N.: Ultrasonographic measurement of the yolk sac. Brit. J. Obstet. Gynaec. 89 (1982) 931–934
3. Donald, I.: Ultrasonic echo sounding in obstetrical and gynecological diagnosis. Amer. J. Obstet. Gynec. 93 (1965) 935–941
4. Drumm, J.E., Clinch, J., Mackenzie, G.: The ultrasonic measurement of fetal crown–rump length as a method of assessing gestational age. Brit. J. Obstet. Gynaec. 83 (1976) 417–421
5. England, M.A.: Farbatlas der Embryologie. Stuttgart: Schattauer 1985
6. Hackelöer, B.J., Hansmann, M.: Ultraschalldiagnostik in der Frühschwangerschaft. Gynäkologe 9 (1976) 108–122
7. Hackelöer, H.J.: Die Ultraschalluntersuchung im I. Trimester. In Holländer, H.J.: Die Ultraschalldiagnostik in der Schwangerschaft. München: Urban & Schwarzenberg 1984; S. 53
8. Hansmann, M., Schuhmacher, H., Foebus, J., Voigt, U.: Ultraschallbiometrie der fetalen Scheitelsteißlänge in der ersten Schwangerschaftshälfte. Geburtsh. u. Frauenheilk. 39 (1979) 656–666
9. Hellman, L.M., Kobayashi, M., Fillisti, L., Lavenhar, M., Cromb. E.: Growth and development of the human fetus prior to the twentieth week of gestation. Amer. J. Obstet. Gynec. 103 (1969) 789–800
10. Hellman, L.M., Kobayashi, M., Cromb, E.: Ultrasonic diagnosis of embryonic malformations. Amer. J. Obstet. Gynec. 115 (1973) 615–623
11. Holländer, H.J.: Die Ultraschalldiagnostik in der Schwangerschaft. München: Urban & Schwarzenberg 1972
12. Jouppila, P.: Ultrasound in the diagnosis of early pregnancy and its complications. Acta Obstet. Gynec. Scand. 50 Suppl. 15 (1971) 7–56
13. Kohorn, E.I., Kaufman, M.: Sonar in the first trimester of pregnancy. Obstet. Gynec. 44 (1974) 473–483
14. Kossoff, G., Garrett, W.J., Radavanovich, G.: Grey scale echography in obstetrics and gynecology. Aust. Radiol. 18 (1974) 62–111
15. Langman, J.: Medizinische Embryologie. Stuttgart: Thieme 1972
16. Lyons, E.A., Levi, C.S.: Ultrasound in the first trimester of pregnancy. Radiol. Clin. N. Amer. 20 (1982) 259–270
17. Mantoni, M., Pedersen, J.F.: Ultrasound visualization of the human yolk sac. J. clin. Ultrasound 7 (1979) 459–460
18. Moore, G.W., Hutchins, G.M., O'Rahilly, R.: The estimated age of staged human embryos and early fetuses. Amer. J. Obstet. Gynec. 139 (1981) 500–506
19. Piiroinen, O.: Detection of fetal heart activity during early pregnancy by combined B-Scan and Doppler examinations: A new application. Acta obstet. gynec. scand. 53 (1974) 231–233
20. Reinold, E.: Fetale Bewegungen in der Frühgravidität. Z. Geburtsh. Gynäk. 174 (1971) 220–225
21. Reinold, E.: Das Größenwachstum der Amnionhöhle in der ersten Hälfte der Gravidität. Wien. klin. Wschr. 84 (1972) 638–640
22. Reinold, E.: Clinical value of fetal spontaneous movements in early pregnancy. J. Perinat. Med. 1 (1973) 65–69
23. Reinold, E.: Ultrasonics in Early Pregnancy. Contributions to Gynecology and Obstetrics, Vol. 1. Series Editor: Keller, Basel: P.J. Karger 1976
24. Robinson, H.P.: Sonar measurement of fetal crown-rump length as means of assessing maturity in first trimester of pregnancy. Brit. med. J. 1973/IV, 28–31
25. Robinson, H.P., Shaw-Dunn, J.: Fetal heart rates as determined by sonar in early pregnancy. Brit. J. Obstet. Gynaec. 80 (1973) 805–809
26. Robinson, H.P.: "Gestation sac" volumes as determined by sonar in the first trimester of pregnancy. Brit. J. Obstet. Gynaec. 82 (1975) 100–107
27. Robinson, H.P., Fleming, J.E.: A critical evaluation of sonar "crown-rump length" measurements. Brit. J. Obstet. Gynaec. 82 (1975) 702–710
28. Schillinger, H.: Quantitative Untersuchungen zur embryonalen Motorik mit dem Ultraschall-time-motion-Verfahren. Arch. Gynäk. 222 (1977) 137–147
29. Schmidt, W., Hendrik, H.J., Kubli, F: Ultraschallfetometrie – die Scheitel-Steiß-Länge in der ersten Schwangerschaftshälfte. Z. Geburtsh. u. Perinat. 185 (1981) 327–335
30. Starck, D.: Embryologie. Stuttgart: Thieme 1975
31. Williams, R.S., Horger, E.O.: Ultrasonic diagnosis of cervical pregnancy. J. clin. Ultrasound 10 (1982) 454–456

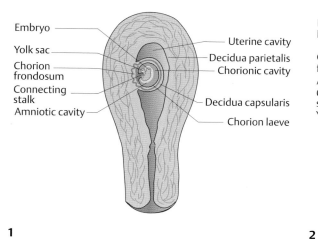

1

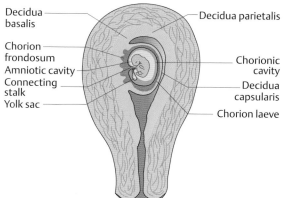

2

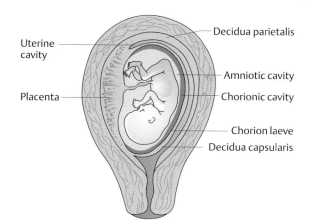

3

Normal early pregnancy

Fig. 9.**1**   Development of the embryo, membranes, and placenta at 5 weeks' gestation. Schematic representation of a longitudinal scan through the uterus.

Fig. 9.**2**   Development of the embryo, membranes, and placenta at 7 weeks' gestation. Schematic representation of a longitudinal scan through the uterus.

Fig. 9.**3**   Development of the fetus, membranes, and placenta at 12 weeks' gestation. Schematic representation of a longitudinal scan through the uterus.

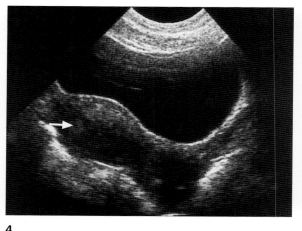

4

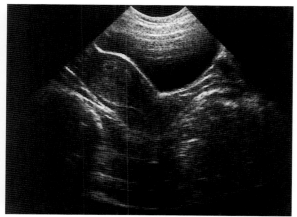

5

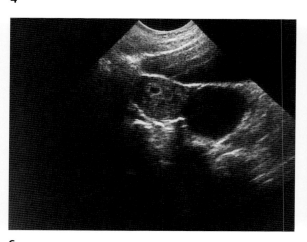

6

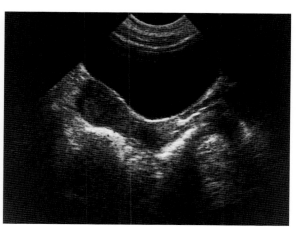

7

Detection of pregnancy

Fig. 9.**4**   Early pregnancy, day 32 of menstrual cycle. Longitudinal scan displays the intrauterine gestational sac as a small, eccentric, echogenic ring (arrow).

Fig. 9.**5**   Early pregnancy at 4 weeks, 6 days. Longitudinal scan shows a small, eccentric, echogenic intrauterine ring enclosing a hypoechoic cavity.

Fig. 9.**6**   Transverse scan of the same patient as in Fig. 9.**5** shows a large, sharply circumscribed corpus luteum cyst 4.6 cm in diameter to the left of the uterus.

Fig. 9.**7**   Early pregnancy at 5 weeks, 3 days. The embryo appears as a small, echogenic structure within the gestational sac. Longitudinal scan.

Fig. 9.**8**   Transverse scan of the patient in Fig. 9.**7** shows a sharply circumscribed corpus luteum cyst 3 cm in diameter to the right of the uterus.

Fig. 9.**9**   Early pregnancy at 6 weeks, 4 days, longitudinal scan. The embryo is lying against the wall of the gestational sac (arrow) and could easily be missed.

Fig. 9.**10**   Early pregnancy at 7 weeks, 3 days, longitudinal scan. The embryo is clearly visible within the gestational sac as an oblong echogenic structure. CRL 1.3 cm. The echo-free area below the sac (arrow) represents an implantation bleed.

Fig. 9.**11**   M-mode tracing at 8 weeks, 6 days, transverse scan. The scan indicates embryonic heart activity (arrow).

Fig. 9.**12**   Average embryonic/fetal heart rates between 6 and 15 weeks' gestation. After Robinson and Shaw-Dunn (25).

Fig. 9.**13**   Early pregnancy at 8 weeks, 4 days, longitudinal scan. The embryo consists of an identifiable head and trunk. Limb buds are also faintly visible.

Fig. 9.**14**   Physiologic umbilical hernia at 8 weeks, 6 days (long arrow), transverse scan. The small ring-like structure above the embryo is the yolk sac (arrowhead). Placenta (∗).

Fig. 9.**15**   Early pregnancy at 9 weeks, 3 days, longitudinal scan. The four limbs appear as bright echoes on the embryo. Placenta (∗).

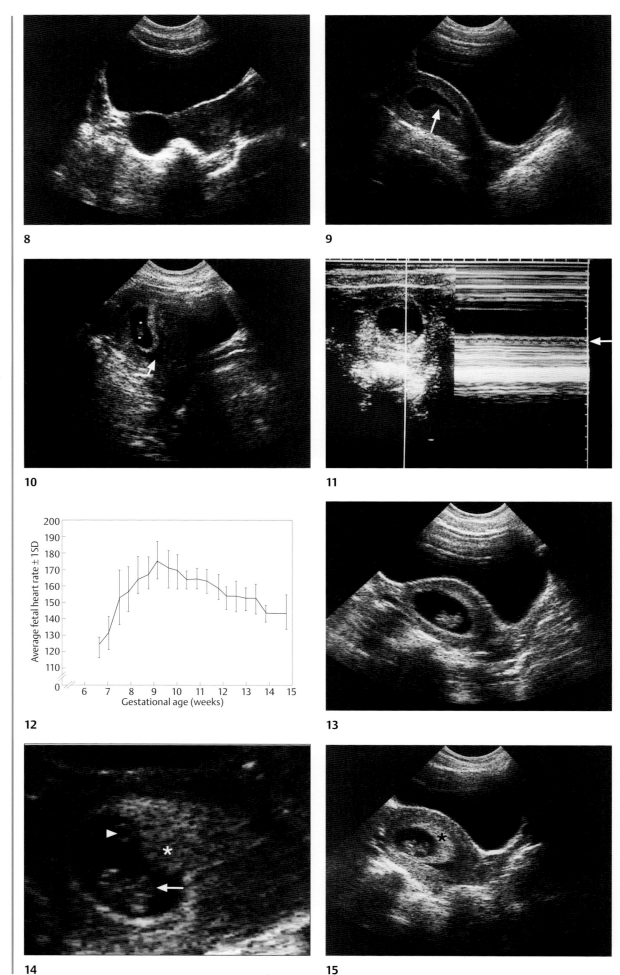

8

9

10

11

12

13

14

15

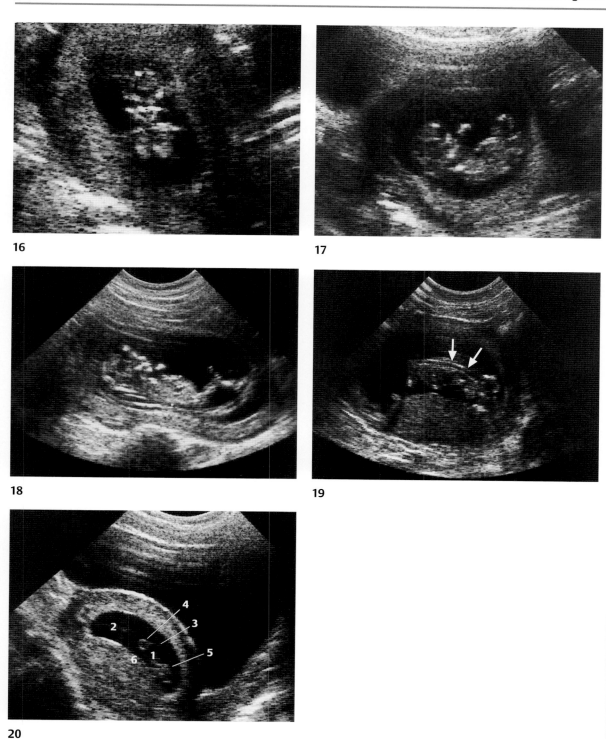

16

17

18

19

20

Fig. 9.**16** Early pregnancy at 10 weeks, 2 days, longitudinal scan. The fetus is displayed in coronal section. The main components of the skull—frontal bone, orbits, maxilla, and mandible—are plainly visible. The placenta is posterior.

Fig. 9.**17** Early pregnancy at 11 weeks, 5 days. Sagittal scan of the fetus demonstrates the face, trunk, and limbs. The early ossification centers in the limbs appear as bright echoes.

Fig. 9.**18** Fetal sagittal scan at 12 weeks, 6 days shows the head (profile), trunk, right leg, and a portion of one upper limb.

Fig. 9.**19** Early pregnancy at 12 weeks, 4 days, longitudinal scan. The fetal spine appears as a hyperechoic double line (arrows).

Fig. 9.**20** Early pregnancy at 8 weeks, 1 day, longitudinal scan. The amniotic cavity (1) and chorionic cavity (2) are separated from each other by a fine membrane, the amniotic epithelium (3). The yolk sac appears as an echogenic ring (4) close to the embryo (5). Placenta (6).

Biometry and gestational age

Fig. 9.21 Growth curves for mean gestational sac diameter as a function of gestational age (mean ± 95% confidence intervals). After Reinold (23).
a Longitudinal sac diameter.
b Transverse sac diameter.
c Anteroposterior sac diameter.

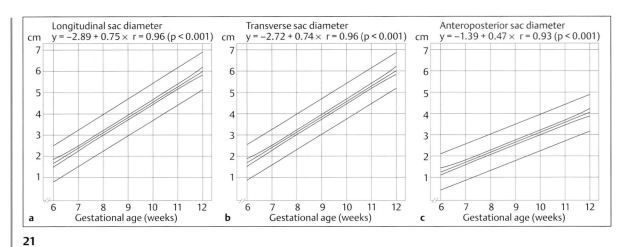

Longitudinal sac diameter
$y = -2.89 + 0.75 \times r = 0.96 (p < 0.001)$

Transverse sac diameter
$y = -2.72 + 0.74 \times r = 0.96 (p < 0.001)$

Anteroposterior sac diameter
$y = -1.39 + 0.47 \times r = 0.93 (p < 0.001)$

a Gestational age (weeks) **b** Gestational age (weeks) **c** Gestational age (weeks)

21

Fig. 9.22 Growth curves for mean gestational sac diameter as a function of gestational age (after Hackelöer and Hansmann [6]).
●–● Holländer: $y = 0.537 \cdot W - 1.401$ (11)
○–○ Hellman: $y = 0.702 \cdot W - 2.543$ (9)
▲–▲ Jouppila: $y = 0.58 \cdot W - 1.54$ (12)
△–△ Kohorn: $y = 0.74 \cdot W - 2.51$ (13)

Fig. 9.23 Early pregnancy, 9 weeks, longitudinal scan. The points for measuring the crown–rump length are shown (CRL = 25 mm).

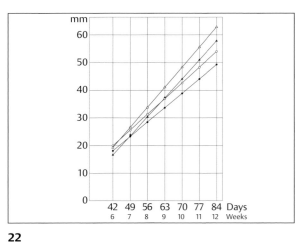

Days
Weeks

22

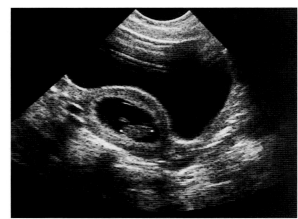

23

Fig. 9.24 Measurement of crown–rump length in a fetus with the body extended, 14th week, longitudinal scan. CRL = 76 mm.

Fig. 9.25 Crown–rump length plotted against gestational age (mean ± 2 SD; fifth-degree polynomial). Modified from Hansmann et al. (8).

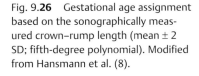

24

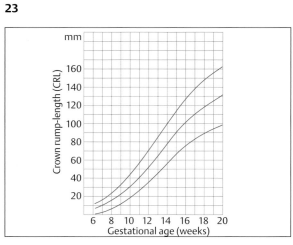

Crown rump-length (CRL)
Gestational age (weeks)

25

Fig. 9.26 Gestational age assignment based on the sonographically measured crown–rump length (mean ± 2 SD; fifth-degree polynomial). Modified from Hansmann et al. (8).

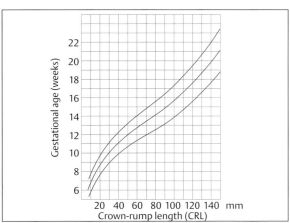

Gestational age (weeks)
Crown–rump length (CRL)

26

10 Abnormalities in the First Trimester

Although transvaginal ultrasound has now become the standard method for investigating abnormalities in the first trimester of pregnancy, abdominal ultrasound can also determine whether an early pregnancy is normal or abnormal in the majority of cases.

Full bladder. Before the uterus has enlarged to a significant degree, a full bladder is necessary to create an acoustic window for transabdominal scanning. If the bladder is not full and an acute examination is required (e.g., for a suspected ectopic pregnancy), scanning can be facilitated by inserting a catheter and distending the bladder with approximately 300 mL of physiologic saline.

Problems. Problems may be encountered in the abdominal ultrasound of obese patients and in patients with a retroflexed uterus. If the findings are equivocal, transvaginal ultrasound should be performed.

High-sited lesions. One advantage of abdominal ultrasound is that it can easily display lesions located relatively high in the pelvis, such as a pedunculated uterine fibroid or a high adnexal mass (cyst, dermoid). In women who have unexplained pain in early pregnancy, the abdominal transducer can also be used to inspect the kidneys for stones.

Spontaneous Abortion

First trimester bleeding is the most frequent complication of pregnancy, prompting a clinical diagnosis of "threatened abortion." According to Hackelöer and Hansmann (17), the majority of ultrasound findings can be assigned to one of the categories listed in Table 10.1.

Procedure. The following procedure is recommended for the ultrasound evaluation of an abnormal early pregnancy:
1. Obtain a full-length view of the uterus.
2. Identify or exclude an intrauterine gestational sac.
3. Locate the embryo, and perform necessary biometry on the embryo and gestational sac.
4. Check for embryonic heart activity or body movements.
5. Detect or exclude an adnexal mass or fluid in the cul-de-sac.

▰ Threatened Abortion

In approximately 50% of all patients with first trimester bleeding, ultrasound reveals a normally developed gestational sac for dates and a live embryo of normal size (17). It is not uncommon to find a partial separation of the membranes with an associated subchorionic hematoma (Figs. 10.**1**–10.**3**). This collection can mimic a second gesta-

Table 10.**1** Frequency of ultrasound diagnoses in threatened abortion (17)

1. Intact intrauterine pregnancy	50%
2. Blighted ovum	20–25%
3. Missed abortion	25–30%
4. Incomplete abortion	2–5%
5. Ectopic pregnancy	1–3%
6. Hydatidiform mole	1–3%

tional sac in the transverse scan (7, 19, 25, 53, 55), and so occasionally it is mistaken for a twin pregnancy (see Chapter 37). If embryonic heart activity can be detected in early pregnancy, there is less than a 10% likelihood that abortion will occur (24). Poor prognostic signs for continuation of the pregnancy are a gestational sac that is too small for dates, an embryo or fetus that is too small for gestational age, and a paucity of embryofetal movements.

▰ Inevitable Abortion

If ultrasound reveals marked deformation and descent of the gestational sac with dilatation of the cervical internal os, expulsion of the uterine contents is inevitable (Figs. 10.**4**–10.**6**).

▰ Complete Abortion

When the products of conception have been completely expelled, the uterine cavity will contain only narrow, band-like echogenic structures representing the decidual mucosa (Fig. 10.**7**).

▰ Incomplete Abortion

If the products of conception have already been partially expelled, ultrasound will not demonstrate the typical gestational sac and embryo. Instead, the uterus will be found to contain varying numbers of echogenic, irregularly shaped structures representing the retained abortion products (Fig. 10.**8**). Products retained in the cervical canal can occasionally mimic a cervical pregnancy (10, 17, 19).

▰ Blighted Ovum

Blighted ovum is the most common type of pregnancy failure, accounting for approximately 50% of all spontaneous abortions (19). It is a nonviable pregnancy in which the embryo and yolk sac are absent. Ultrasound reveals an empty gestational sac (2, 7, 13, 17, 24, 66), which usually enlarges normally during the initial weeks. But toward the end of the first trimester, the sac grows at a diminished rate or ceases to grow. Frequently the sac is misshapen and has ill-defined margins (Figs. 10.**9**–10.**11**).

Differential diagnosis. Differentiation is required from an intact early pregnancy in which the embryo cannot yet be identified. An embryo "crouched" in a corner of the sac is easily missed on cursory inspection (Hackelöer [18]).

Difficult imaging conditions. The examination is hampered by a retroflexed uterus. The increased distance between the abdominal wall and conceptus in these cases often prevents complete visualization of the gestational sac, and the embryo is easily missed. Similar problems can arise when the examination conditions are less than optimum due to extreme maternal obesity or an empty bladder. In cases of this kind, errors in diagnosis can be avoided by transvaginal scanning or, if a vaginal probe is not available, by performing serial scans at weekly intervals.

Confirming the diagnosis. If serial scans do not demonstrate either an embryo or a yolk sac in a gestational sac whose mean diameter is

Table 10.**2**   Unfavorable prognostic signs in abdominal ultrasound

> ➢ Gestational sac too small for dates
> ➢ Deformation of the gestational sac
> ➢ Nonvisualization of the embryo at 7 weeks' gestation
> ➢ No detectable heart activity at 8 weeks' gestation
> ➢ Mean gestational sac diameter ≥ 30 mm with no detectable embryo
>   or yolk sac
> ➢ Minimal increase in mean gestational sac diameter over a one-week period

30 mm or more, the diagnosis of blighted ovum is considered to be confirmed (10, 19).

Prognostic signs. The ultrasound findings listed in Table 10.**2** are considered poor prognostic signs with regard to the continuation and outcome of the pregnancy (10, 19, 49, 50, 52).

Missed Abortion

The ultrasound hallmark of a missed abortion (Figs. 10.**12**, 10.**13**) is an embryo that is too small for dates and shows no movements or cardiac pulsations. Abdominal percussion with the transducer elicits a typical, passive swaying motion of the dead embryo (17, 23, 24, 49, 55, 62). Since the embryo or fetus has probably been dead for some time, the structures that are still visible often appear ill-defined (Figs. 10.**12**, 10.**13**). Additionally, the embryo usually appears too small in relation to the gestational sac. An inexperienced examiner might mistake passive movements imparted to the fetus or embryo by transmitted maternal vascular pulsation, uterine contractions, or bowel motion for evidence of fetal life.

Early Pregnancy with an IUD in Place

Examination before 9 weeks. In women who become pregnant despite the use of an intrauterine device (IUD) for contraception, ultrasound can be used to define the exact location of the device in relation to the gestational sac. Whenever possible, this examination should be done before 9 completed weeks, while the IUD can still be defined separately from the gestational sac and has not yet been displaced cephalad by the enlarging sac. In most cases the IUD is located within the cervix (Fig. 10.**14**) or in the lower third of the uterine corpus. Although pregnancy can occur in association with a correctly positioned IUD, studies by Bernaschek et al. (6) showed that most pregnancies (78.4%) occur when the device is positioned too low.

Removing the IUD or leaving it in place. The relationship of the IUD to the gestational sac is of greatest interest when the patient desires to continue the pregnancy. If the IUD is in the cervix (Fig. 10.**14**) or lower uterine segment while the gestational sac is high in the uterus, it can be extracted without jeopardizing the pregnancy. Retrieval is recommended because pregnancies that continue with an IUD in place are at increased risk for spontaneous abortion (65). Conversely, in the rare cases where the IUD is located above or next to the gestational sac, the device should be left untouched because its removal would be associated with a high abortion risk (Fig. 10.**15**). These cases should still be monitored, however, by checking the position of the IUD sonographically at regular intervals (Figs. 10.**15**–10.**17**). There is no evidence that leaving and IUD in place increases the risk of fetal anomalies (6, 55).

Molar Pregnancy

The ultrasound appearance of a hydatidiform mole depends on the gestational age at which the patient is examined. A mole in the first trimester usually presents the ultrasound features of a missed abortion or incomplete abortion (31, 41, 48, 70). Scans show a gestational sac or residual sac that does not contain an embryo or fetus and is surrounded by a broad, echogenic rim of trophoblastic tissue. The sac does not grow with passage of time, and there is increasing trophoblastic proliferation (Figs. 10.**18**, 10.**19**).

Ultrasound appearance. The classic "snowstorm" pattern described by Donald (12) characterizes a fully developed mole as it might appear when scanned in the second trimester with older, lower-resolution equipment. With the high-resolution transducers in current use, this pattern is no longer seen. Instead, we observe a multitude of small vesicles up to 10 mm in size (41) within the uterus, which is too large for gestational age (Figs. 10.**20**, 10.**21**). A small residual sac can be found in most cases, but a fetus is not seen. Larger cystic areas within the molar tissue may represent gestational sac remnants or hemorrhagic areas (14).

Theca lutein cysts. Theca lutein cysts can be detected in approximately one-third of molar pregnancies (19, 41). Often they are bilateral. Their detection has prognostic significance because 50% of patients with theca lutein cysts larger than 5 cm will develop a choriocarcinoma (38).

β-hCG test. If there is doubt as to the presence of a molar pregnancy, a serum β-hCG assay will quickly confirm the diagnosis by showing elevated levels, although there have been reports of moles associated with low β-hCG titers (19).

Partial mole. A partial mole differs from the classic mole is that a gestational sac is present and the placenta contains numerous small cysts of varying size. Fetal parts often cannot be identified within the gestational sac (Figs. 10.**22**, 10.**23**) (41). If a fetus is seen, it is generally growth-retarded (41). Partial moles are commonly associated with chromosomal abnormalities such as triploidy or trisomy (41).

Invasive mole. Following treatment for a hydatidiform mole, 20% of patients develop a recurrence in the form of an invasive mole. Ultrasound in these cases shows a slightly enlarged uterus with focal areas of increased echogenicity within the myometrium. Vesicular changes are rarely found owing to the early diagnosis (new rise in serum β-hCG at follow-up) (Fig. 10.**24**) (41).

Incidence. The reported incidence of hydatidiform mole is one in 2000 pregnancies (41). The incidence of molar pregnancy with a live fetus is one in 100,000 to one in 1,000,000 (4, 22, 59). Most of these cases involve a partial mole (4, 22, 62).

Choriocarcinoma

Choriocarcinoma has a reported incidence of one in 40,000 pregnancies in the United States (41). Pathologically, it is characterized by a disordered growth of solid trophoblastic tissue with no sign of vesiculation. Typical lesions show aggressive invasion of the myometrium with associated hemorrhagic necrosis. Choriocarcinoma metastasizes predominantly to the lung, liver, gastrointestinal tract, and central nervous system (CNS).

Ultrasound appearance. Ultrasound reveals intensely echogenic intrauterine tissue containing cystic, hemorrhagic areas and showing no

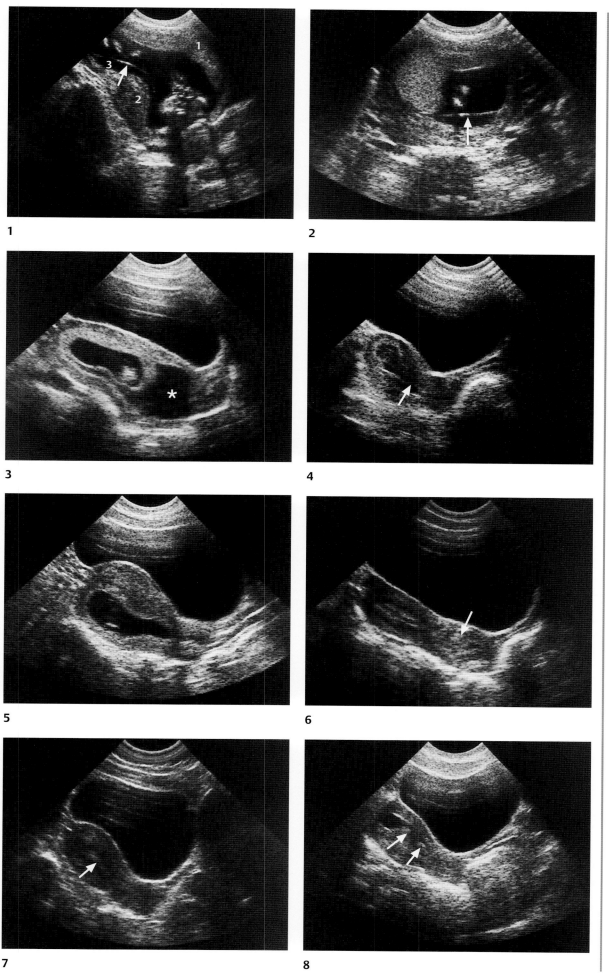

1

2

3

4

5

6

7

8

Spontaneous abortion

Fig. 10.**1**   Threatened abortion, 14 weeks. Longitudinal scan shows partial separation of the membranes (arrow) with a retrochorionic hematoma on the posterior uterine wall.
1 Placenta
2 Uterine contraction
3 Hematoma

Fig. 10.**2**   Threatened abortion, 14 weeks. Transverse scan shows separation of the membranes from the posterior uterine wall with a retrochorionic hematoma (arrow).

Fig. 10.**3**   Threatened abortion, 9 weeks. Longitudinal scan shows definite membrane separation from the posterior uterine wall with a large hematoma (∗) in the area of the lower fetal pole. The hematoma mimics a second gestational sac.

Fig. 10.**4**   Inevitable abortion, 10 weeks. Longitudinal scan shows marked distortion of the gestational sac with initial distal tracking of abortion products (arrow).

Fig. 10.**5**   Inevitable abortion, 11 weeks. Longitudinal scan shows conspicuous descent of the gestational sac with initial dilatation of the cervical internal os.

Fig. 10.**6**   Inevitable abortion, 10 weeks, longitudinal scan. The gestational products have already entered the cervical canal (arrow), leaving only the echogenic decidua within the uterine corpus.

Fig. 10.**7**   Complete abortion, 10 weeks, longitudinal scan. A gestational sac is no longer seen within the uterine cavity. The uterus contains only the decidua graviditatis, which appears as a hyperechoic band (arrow).

Fig. 10.**8**   Incomplete abortion, 7 weeks, longitudinal scan. The gestational sac is irregular and too small for gestational age. Inferior to it are irregular echogenic structures representing the retained products (arrows).

Fig. 10.**9**   Blighted ovum at 8 weeks, 6 days, longitudinal scan. The gestational sac is too small for dates, and an embryo is not visible.

Fig. 10.**10**   Blighted ovum, 11 weeks, longitudinal scan. The outline of the sac is indistinct, and fetal structures cannot be identified.

Fig. 10.**11**   Blighted ovum, 11 weeks. Transverse scan of the case in Fig. 10.10 shows the empty gestational sac.

Fig. 10.**12**   Missed abortion, 13 weeks, longitudinal scan. The gestational sac is too small for dates, and fetal structures are vaguely defined. There is no evidence of fetal heart activity.

Fig. 10.**13**   Missed abortion, 9 weeks, transverse scan. The embryo is too small in relation to the gestational sac. Its body structures are ill-defined, and there is no heart activity.

IUD in early pregnancy

Fig. 10.**14**   Intact early pregnancy (5 weeks) with an IUD in place, longitudinal scan. The displaced, echogenic IUD (Lippes loop) lies in the cervical canal (arrow).

Fig. 10.**15**   Early pregnancy (7 weeks) with an IUD in place, longitudinal scan of a retroflexed uterus. The echogenic IUD is adjacent to the gestational sac in the uterine corpus (arrow).

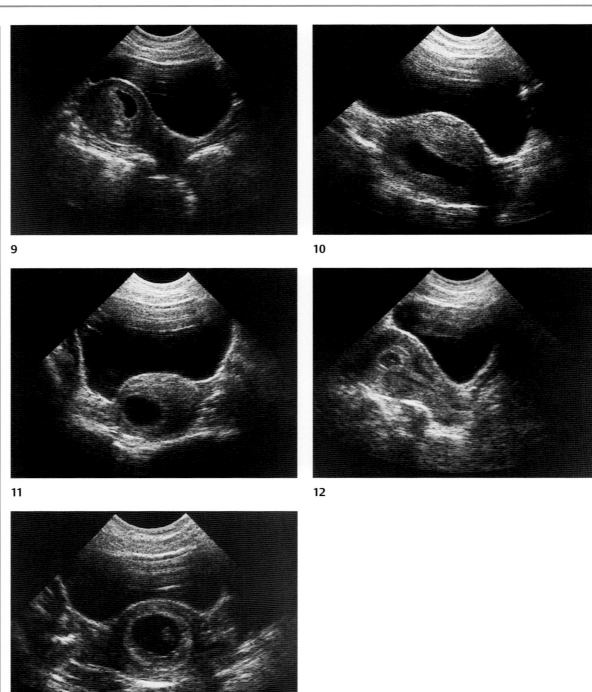

9

10

11

12

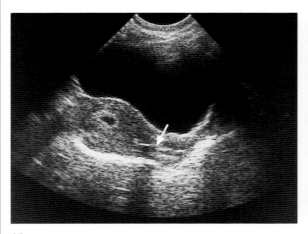

13

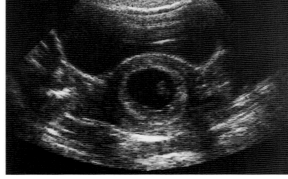

14

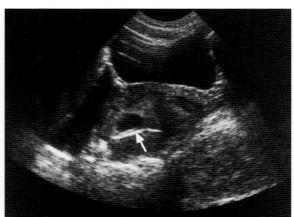

15

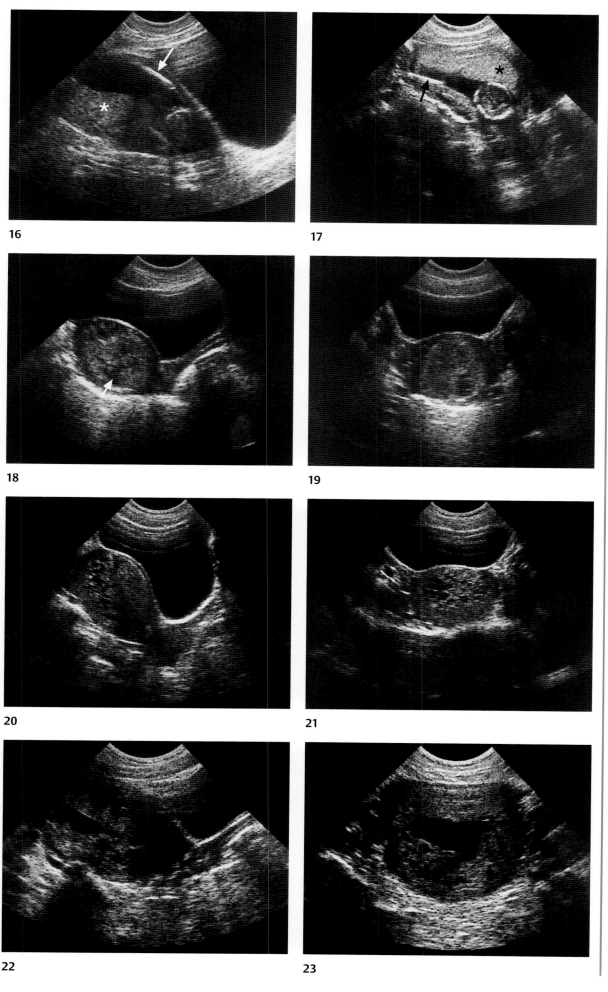

16

17

18

19

20

21

22

23

Fig. 10.**16** Intact pregnancy (14 weeks) with an IUD on the anterior uterine wall (arrow). Posterior wall placenta (∗). Longitudinal scan.

Fig. 10.**17** Intact pregnancy (14 weeks) with an IUD on the posterior wall of the uterine corpus (arrow). Abdominal wall placenta (∗). Longitudinal scan.

Molar pregnancy and choriocarcinoma

Fig. 10.**18** Hydatidiform mole (early finding) at 9 weeks. Longitudinal scan shows irregular, hyperechoic trophoblastic tissue within the enlarged uterus. Residual gestational sac (arrow).

Fig. 10.**19** Transverse scan of the case in Fig. 10.**18** shows the residual gestational sac in the left posterior half of the uterus, but an embryo cannot be positively identified.

Fig. 10.**20** Hydatidiform mole at 11 weeks, longitudinal scan. The uterine cavity is filled with hyperechoic trophoblastic tissue permeated by small cystic structures.

Fig. 10.**21** Transverse scan of the case in Fig. 10.**20**.

Fig. 10.**22** Partial mole at 16 weeks, longitudinal scan. The uterus contains a residual gestational sac with irregular borders and no evidence of fetal parts. Several vesicular, hyperechoic areas appear in the region of the placenta on the posterior uterine wall.

Fig. 10.**23** Transverse scan of the case in Fig. 10.**22**.

Fig. 10.**24**   Locally invasive mole, longitudinal scan. The patient underwent curettage on three previous occasions and had a markedly elevated β-hCG (86,900 ng/mL). Ultrasound shows focal hyperechoic areas extending into the myometrium.

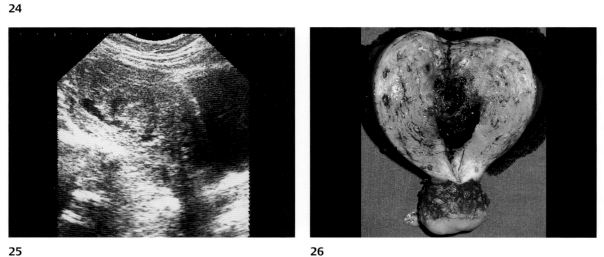

24

Fig. 10.**25**   Choriocarcinoma, longitudinal scan. The uterine cavity is filled with irregular, hyperechoic structures. Additionally there are hyperechoic cystic areas of varying size with no circumscribed vesicle formation.

Fig. 10.**26**   Surgical specimen corresponding to Fig. 10.**25**.

25   **26**

Ectopic pregnancy

Fig. 10.**27**   Left tubal pregnancy at 7 weeks, transverse scan. The ectopic pregnancy appears within the distended fallopian tube as an echogenic ring with a hypoechoic center (arrow). An intrauterine gestational sac cannot be detected.

Fig. 10.**28**   Intraoperative view of the tubal pregnancy in Fig. 10.**27**. The isthmic portion of the left tube is grossly distended (arrow).

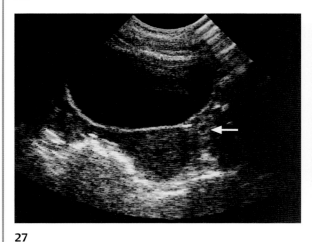
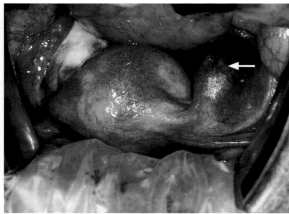

27   **28**

Fig. 10.**29**   Intact right tubal pregnancy at 5 weeks, transverse scan. The embryo appears as a bright, punctate echo within the ectopic gestational sac (arrow). An intrauterine sac is not seen.

Fig. 10.**30**   Intraoperative view of the tubal pregnancy in Fig. 10.**29**. The ampullary portion of the right tube is distended (arrow).

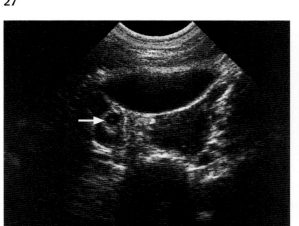
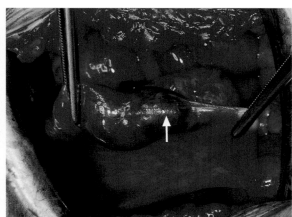

29   **30**

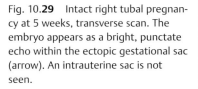

vesiculation (41) (Figs. 10.**25**, 10.**26**). Ultrasound is particularly valuable in the preoperative staging of disease and postoperative follow-up (exclusion of hepatic metastases).

Ectopic Pregnancy (Figs. 10.**27**–10.**46**)

The fact that ectopic pregnancy is responsible for up to 26% of maternal deaths (51, 57, 64) and is missed on initial examination in almost 70% of cases (20) accounts for the major importance of ultrasound in the early diagnosis of ectopic gestation. Ultrasound is definitely superior to bimanual examination in early ectopic pregnancy, when palpable abnormalities are not yet present in most cases.

Detection of ectopic pregnancy. There is much diversity of opinion in the literature regarding the clinical value of abdominal ultrasound in detecting ectopic pregnancy. While some authors claim that ultrasound is extremely precise (3, 32, 40), others are not convinced (12, 18, 30, 37). It is generally agreed that a direct, conclusive ultrasound diagnosis of ectopic pregnancy can be made only if a gestational sac with a live embryo can be identified outside the uterus (Figs. 10.**29**–10.**31**). This can be done only in a small percentage of cases, however. For the most part, the products of the ectopic pregnancy deteriorate at an early stage. As a result, the ectopic pregnancy often appears only as a mixed solid/cystic mass of variable size lying next to the uterus (36).

Location and frequency. Ninety-five percent of ectopic pregnancies occur within the fallopian tube, mostly in its ampullary segment (29). For many years the reported incidence of ectopic pregnancy was 1% of all pregnancies (11), but today it appears that the incidence is closer to 2%.

Signs of ectopic pregnancy. Since the pioneering work of Kobayashi et al. (27), the signs listed in Table 10.**3** are considered to be the most common ultrasound criteria of ectopic pregnancy (3, 9, 30, 37, 54, 56, 58). Published reports on the frequency of the individual signs vary considerably (Table 10.**4**). We investigated the diagnostic relevance of these parameters in a prospective study using abdominal ultrasound (16). The results of the study are summarized in Table 10.**5**.

β-hCG test. A pregnancy test should be performed whenever ectopic pregnancy is suspected. Only a positive test will allow a correct interpretation of the diverse ultrasound findings. If the urine test is negative or equivocally positive and the ultrasound findings are unclear, the more reliable serum β-hCG assay should be performed. Previous studies found a high false-negative rate of 12–50% for immunologic urine tests (16, 19, 29), but this is not a problem today owing to the much higher sensitivity of the test kits (Figs. 10.**39**, 10.**40**).

Diagnosis. Unless a live embryo is directly visualized outside the uterus, the following combination of factors must be present in order to establish a diagnosis of ectopic pregnancy:
- Positive β-hCG test
- Clinical findings (pain, spotting after 5–8 weeks of amenorrhea, palpable findings)
- Presence of suggestive ultrasound signs (see Table 10.**3**)

Detection or Exclusion of Intrauterine Pregnancy

The detection of an intrauterine pregnancy virtually rules out an ectopic pregnancy because coexisting intrauterine and extrauterine pregnancies (Fig. 10.**44**) occur in only one of 30,000 pregnancies (5, 47). However, if ultrasound shows no evidence of an intrauterine pregnancy and the patient has a positive pregnancy test, an empty uterus is the most common and important suggestive sign of ectopic pregnancy (16, 51). As for uterine size, we observed a normal-size uterus in almost half of the ectopic pregnancies in our series (16) (Table 10.**4**).

Differential diagnosis. If an isolated cyst is found in the adnexal region of a patient with a positive pregnancy test and the uterus is not enlarged, the differential diagnosis should include ectopic pregnancy as well as a corpus luteum cyst in an early intrauterine pregnancy that cannot yet be detected by abdominal ultrasound.

Pseudogestational Sac

Ultrasound demonstrates an intrauterine ring-like structure of high echogenicity in a number of ectopic pregnancies. This ring represents the decidual transformation of the endometrium lining the uterine cavity. The uterus may also contain secretions or blood that mimic the appearance of an intrauterine gestational sac, creating a "pseudogestational sac" (Figs. 10.**32**, 10.**33**) (33, 34, 39, 46, 67, 68). A similar ring-like structure is seen after ovulation (18). Abdominal ultrasound detects a pseudogestational sac in approximately 20% of ectopic pregnancies (16,

Table 10.**5** Ultrasound findings in 25 patients with ectopic pregnancy (after Goldhofer and Merz [16]).

Absence of an intrauterine gestational sac	24/25 (96%)
Adnexal mass	17/25 (68%)
Enlarged uterus without a gestational sac	13/25 (52%)
Retrouterine hematocele	13/25 (52%)
Decidual transformation of the endometrium	9/25 (36%)
Pseudogestational sac	5/25 (20%)
Intact extrauterine pregnancy	1/25 (4%)
Diagnosis confirmed	20/25 (80%)

Table 10.**3** Ultrasound signs that suggest ectopic pregnancy

- Enlarged uterus with no gestational sac
- Decidual transformation of the endometrium (intrauterine ring sign, central pseudogestational sac)
- Retrouterine hematocele
- Adnexal mass
- Detection of a (live) embryo outside the uterus

Table 10.**4** Ultrasound criteria for ectopic pregnancy (review of the literature)

Authors	Reference	n	Uterus enlarged	Adnexal mass	Retrouterine hematocele	Thick endometrium	Diagnosis confirmed
Schoenbaum et al. (58)	58	15	53%	93%	26%	20%	–
Lawson (30)	30	26	62%	81%	23%	23%	77%
Schmidt et al. (56)	56	60	42%	83%	72%	41%	85%
Müller und Leucht (40)	40	45	–	60%	95%	95%	93%
Baumgärtner et al. (3)	3	140	–	49%	50%	-	95%

Table 10.**6**   Features that distinguish a pseudogestational sac from a true intrauterine gestational sac

Pseudogestational sac	True gestational sac
➢ Central location	➢ Eccentric location
➢ Single ring structure (decidua)	➢ Double ring structure (decidua and trophoblast)

34). The size of the pseudosac is described as ranging from 1 to 5 cm (!) (1, 8, 19, 29, 43, 51). Table 10.**6** lists the ultrasound criteria that are useful in distinguishing a pseudogestational sac from a true gestational sac.

Retrouterine Hematocele

While tubal rupture can cause relatively large amounts of blood to collect in the abdomen and especially in the cul-de-sac, where they are easily visualized with ultrasound, smaller extravasations from a tubal abortion become distributed among the bowel loops and often cannot be detected sonographically. In an intact ectopic pregnancy, moreover, bleeding into the free peritoneal cavity often has not yet occurred at the time of ultrasound examination. It should also be considered that fluid in the cul-de-sac may occur physiologically (e.g., after ovulation) or as a result of intra-abdominal inflammatory disease.

Incidence. Reports vary greatly as to the incidence of retrouterine hematocele in ectopic pregnancies (Figs. 10.**34**, 10.**35**, 10.**39**), with figures ranging from 26% to 95% (3, 30, 40, 56, 58). In our own studies, we detected free fluid in the cul-de-sac in only 50% of ectopic pregnancies despite the use of a high-resolution abdominal transducer (16) (Table 10.**5**).

Tubal rupture. A tubal rupture, unlike a tubal abortion, is associated with copious fluid in the cul-de-sac. When the blood loss is relatively high, exceeding 1000 mL, the blood in the peritoneal cavity appears as a perihepatic, hypoechoic crescent on scans of the upper abdomen (Fig. 10.**36**).

Adnexal Mass

Variable appearance. Ectopic pregnancy can present with an extraordinary diversity of adnexal findings (Figs. 10.**37**–10.**43**). This is due to variations in the anatomic position of the ovary and fallopian tube, the variable size of the adnexal findings, and the heterogeneity of the pathoanatomic findings (intact ectopic pregnancy, tubal abortion, tubal rupture).

Intact tube. If the fallopian tube is still intact when the patient is scanned, the ectopic trophoblast can be identified in the adnexal region as a small, hyperechoic ring with a central, hypoechoic gestational sac (Figs. 10.**27**, 10.**29**, 10.**31**).

Tubal abortion. If a tubal abortion has occurred, ultrasound will reveal an irregular, partly cystic- and partly solid-appearing adnexal mass that may extend into the cul-de-sac, depending on the extent of the peritubal hematoma (Figs. 10.**41**–10.**43**). This finding can be particularly difficult to distinguish from an inflammatory adnexal mass (e.g., tubo-ovarian abscess) (see Fig. 10.**53**).

Differential diagnosis. Differentiation is also required from a hemorrhagic corpus luteum and from an ovarian cyst with a twisted pedicle. In our studies we observed adnexal changes in 68% of patients with ectopic pregnancy (16) (Table 10.**5**). Kadar et al. (26) found adnexal changes in only 40% of their cases.

Uncommon Sites of Ectopic Pregnancy

Interstitial Pregnancy

With an interstitial pregnancy (intramural portion of the fallopian tube), the gestational sac does not appear to be intrauterine or extrauterine at ultrasound. It displays a very eccentric location in the cornual region, with the myometrium only partially enclosing the sac (29).

Cervical Pregnancy

In the case of a cervical pregnancy, which occurs in 0.1% of all ectopic pregnancies (21), a gestational sac is found within the cervical canal. It can be difficult to recognize a complicated cervical pregnancy (Figs. 10.**45**, 10.**46**), as its features resemble those of an incomplete abortion with residual intracervical tissue.

Abdominal Pregnancy

An abdominal pregnancy can be confidently diagnosed with ultrasound only if a fetus and placenta are detected outside the small uterus. If the small uterus is displaced posteriorly, the pregnancy can be detected better by transvaginal scanning (Fig. 10.**47**) than abdominal scanning. Other notable features are the proximity of fetal parts to the maternal abdominal wall (29) and the absence of normal uterine wall thickness, especially in the area of the placental bed (Figs. 10.**47**, 10.**48**).

Role of Abdominal Ultrasound in the Diagnosis of Ectopic Pregnancy

High-risk patients. The risk of ectopic pregnancy is increased by recurrent adnexitis, antecedent ectopic pregnancy, and prior tubal surgery. In these patients, an effort should be made to detect ectopic pregnancy with ultrasound at the earliest possible stage—i.e., by 5–6 weeks' gestation.

Failure rates. According to reports in the literature, the diagnosis of ectopic pregnancy by abdominal ultrasound has a failure rate between 5% and 29% (3, 16, 19, 28, 30, 40). Because the various types of ectopic pregnancy may differ greatly in their ultrasound presentation, abdominal ultrasound alone cannot be considered an absolutely reliable method for the detection of ectopic pregnancy. Its accuracy is bound to improve as improvements are made in transducer resolution, as they have been in transvaginal ultrasound. Ultimately, both the transabdominal and transvaginal detection of ectopic pregnancy depend critically on the experience of the examiner.

Problem cases. The following cases can present problems in abdominal ultrasound examinations:
- A small tubal abortion less than 1.0 cm in diameter
- An old tubal abortion with a negative urinary β-hCG test
- An early intrauterine pregnancy in which the gestational sac is not yet detectable and there is a concomitant adnexal lesion (corpus luteum of pregnancy)

Conclusion. If ectopic pregnancy is suspected clinically in a patient who has a positive pregnancy test but no remarkable findings on abdominal ultrasound, the patient should be referred for transvaginal ultrasound and hospitalized for observation until the case can be resolved (intra- or extrauterine pregnancy or abortion). Serial ultrasound scans and (β-)hCG tests are recommended at two-day intervals during this time.

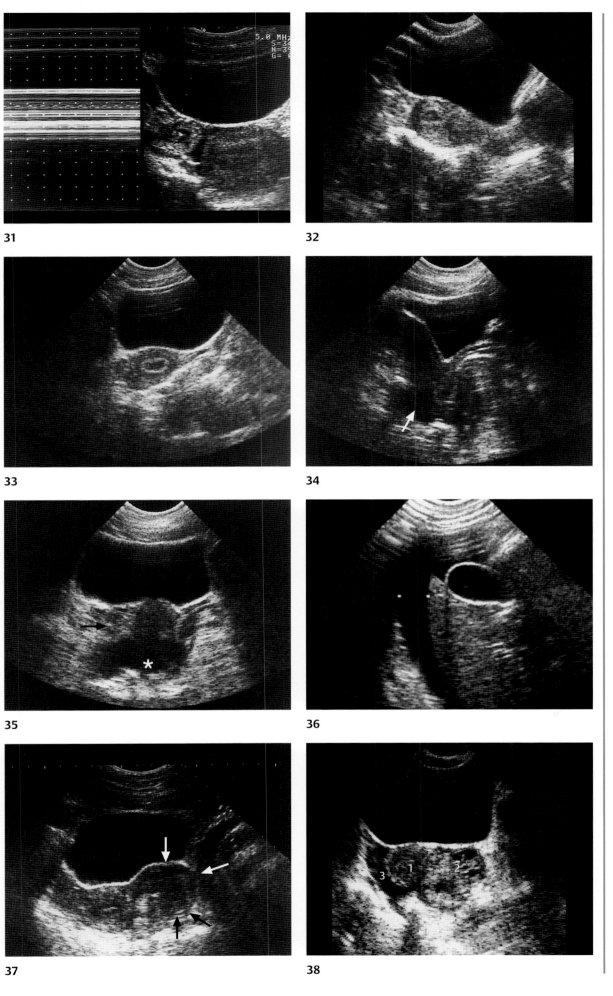

31

32

33

34

35

36

37

38

Fig. 10.**31** Intact right tubal pregnancy at 7 weeks. Transverse scan shows a gestational sac with a live embryo in the distended right tube, CRL 1.2 cm. The M-mode tracing demonstrates heart activity.

Fig. 10.**32** Uterus in a right tubal pregnancy, 6 weeks, longitudinal scan. At the center of the uterus is a pseudo-gestational sac. The hyperechoic decidua mimics an intrauterine pregnancy.

Fig. 10.**33** Central intrauterine pseudogestational sac and hyperechoic ring (decidua) in a left tubal pregnancy (not shown), 6 weeks, transverse scan.

Fig. 10.**34** Retrouterine hematocele (arrow) in a right tubal pregnancy, 7 weeks, longitudinal scan.

Fig. 10.**35** Transverse scan of the case in Fig. 10.**34** shows irregular distension of the right tube (arrow) and a retrouterine hematocele (∗).

Fig. 10.**36** Tubal rupture with copious free blood in the abdominal cavity. Perihepatic blood forms an echo-free crescent 2.1 cm long. Transverse scan.

Fig. 10.**37** Left tubal abortion at 7 weeks, transverse scan. The left tube is markedly distended by an intratubal hematoma (arrow).

Fig. 10.**38** Left tubal abortion at 11 weeks, transverse scan. The ectopic pregnancy appears here as a partly solid, partly cystic adnexal mass on the left side. 1 = Uterus, 2 = ectopic pregnancy, 3 = free fluid.

Fig. 10.**39**   Right tubal rupture at 7 weeks. Transverse scan shows the distended right tube and rupture site (arrow) and a small pseudogestational sac at the center of the uterus. Retrouterine hematocele (∗). Qualitative urine β-hCG test was negative!

Fig. 10.**40**   Intraoperative appearance of the rupture site in Fig. 10.**39**, viewed from the superior aspect.

Fig. 10.**41**   Old right tubal pregnancy at 7 weeks, 6 days, transverse scan. Status 3 weeks after elective termination. Note the marked distension of the right fallopian tube (arrow). In this case a typical echogenic ring-like structure cannot be identified within the tube.

Fig. 10.**42**   Small right tubal pregnancy at 4 weeks, 6 days, transverse scan. The ectopic pregnancy appears next to the unenlarged uterus as a hypoechoic structure 1.0 · 0.5 cm in size (arrow).

Fig. 10.**43**   Intraoperative view of the tubal pregnancy in Fig. 10.**42**. The isthmic portion of the right tube is slightly distended (arrow).

Fig. 10.**44**   Coexisting intrauterine and ectopic pregnancies at 6 weeks, 4 days. A hyperechoic chorionic ring is visible inside the uterus and also in the right fallopian tube. The first embryo is visible within the intrauterine gestational sac (arrowhead) (CRL 7 mm). The second embryo and yolk sac (arrow) are visible within the ectopic sac.

Fig. 10.**45**   Marked distension of the cervix in a complicated cervical pregnancy. The uterine corpus sits upon the cervix like a cap (arrow = endometrium).

Fig. 10.**46**   Surgical specimen of the complicated cervical pregnancy in Fig. 10.**45**. The uterine corpus has not been cut open.

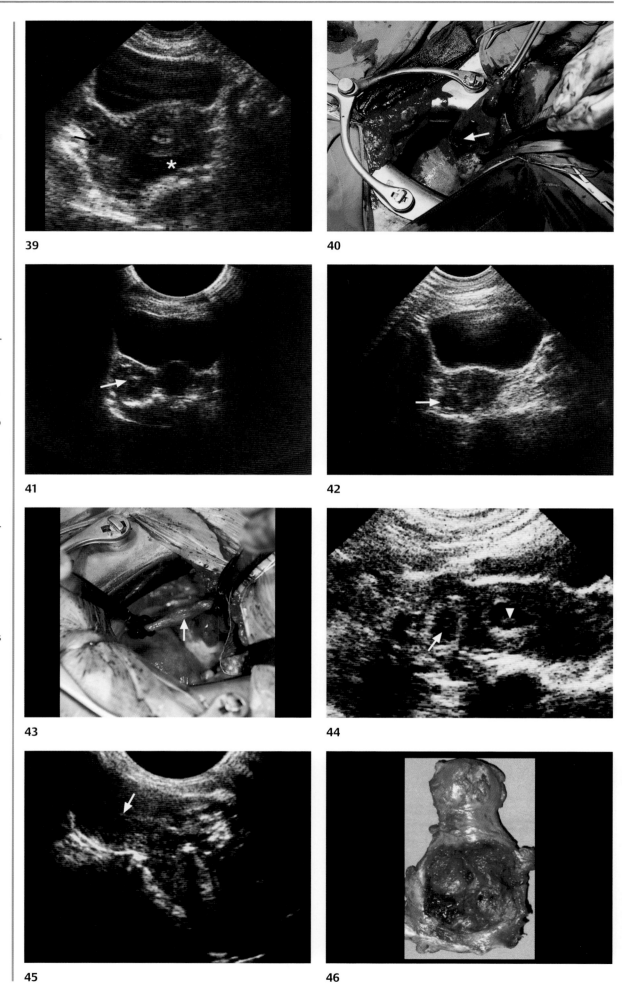

39

40

41

42

43

44

45

46

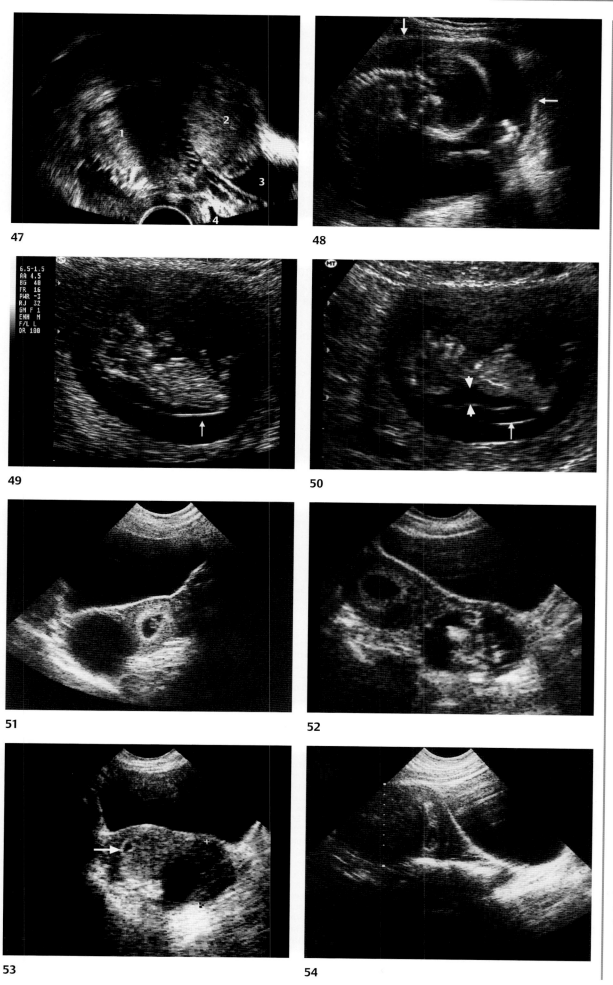

47

48

49

50

51

52

53

54

Fig. 10.**47** Abdominal pregnancy at 29 weeks. Transvaginal ultrasound shows a small, posteriorly displaced uterus in the lower pelvis (1). Anterior to the uterus is the placenta (2), bordered only by a thick membrane. Gestational sac (3), bladder (4).

Fig. 10.**48** Abdominal pregnancy at 20 weeks. The gestational sac extends anteriorly to the abdominal wall. A thick, echogenic membrane (arrows) is seen in place of a normally thick uterine wall.

Detection of fetal anomalies

Fig. 10.**49** Increased nuchal translucency thickness (7 mm) in a fetus at 11 weeks, 5 days. Because of its proximity to the amniotic membrane (arrow), the nuchal translucency is easily mistaken for the membrane itself.

Fig. 10.**50** Same fetus in Fig. 10.**49** after body movement. The nuchal translucency (7 mm, arrowheads) can now be clearly distinguished from the amniotic membrane (arrow).

Adnexal masses and fibroids

Fig. 10.**51** Intact early pregnancy, 7 weeks. Transverse scan shows a normal intrauterine gestational sac with a live embryo. To the right of the uterus is a 6 x 6.5-cm corpus luteum cyst with fine, diffuse internal echoes.

Fig. 10.**52** Early pregnancy, 8 weeks, transverse scan. To the left of the uterus is a 6.8 x 4.7-cm dermoid cyst with an irregular, bizarre, hyperechoic internal structure.

Fig. 10.**53** Early pregnancy, 5 weeks, transverse scan. To the left of the uterus is a 6 x 5-cm cystic structure, partially occupied by moderately coarse internal echoes of moderate intensity (= left tubo-ovarian abscess). Intrauterine gestational sac (arrow).

Fig. 10.**54** Early pregnancy, 8 weeks. Longitudinal scan shows an intramural fibroid on the posterior wall of the uterine fundus, just above the gestational sac. The tumor is 8 cm in diameter.

Early Detection of Fetal Anomalies in the First Trimester

▬ *Nuchal Translucency*

Transient sign. In early screening for fetal anomalies, the ultrasound detection of "nuchal translucency" (44) in the first trimester has emerged in recent years as an important suggestive sign. Usually seen between 11 and 14 weeks' gestation, this sign is considered pathologic if the translucent area is 3 mm or more in thickness.

Measurement. Nuchal translucency should be measured sonographically in a midsagittal plane through the fetus (Figs 10.**49**, 10.**50**). Its thickness is measured from the inner border of the skin to the inner border of the nuchal soft tissue (Fig. 10.**50**). The amniotic membrane can occasionally mimic increased nuchal translucency thickness when it is not in full contact with the chorionic membrane. The diagnosis is confirmed by defining the amniotic membrane as a separate and distinct structure from the nuchal translucency (Fig. 10.**50**).

Chromosomal abnormalities and structural defects. Increased thickness of the nuchal translucency is associated with a markedly increased risk of chromosomal abnormalities, especially trisomy 21 (45, 60) (see Chapter 2). If nuchal translucency is ≥ 3 mm in thickness, karyotyping should always be done by chorionic villus sampling or early amniocentesis. If a normal karyotype is found, the fetus should still be closely scrutinized for anomalies with ultrasound, since 4% of fetuses with a normal karyotype but increased nuchal translucency will be found to have structural defects such as cardiac anomalies, diaphragmatic defects, renal anomalies, or abdominal wall defects (45).

▬ *Major Anomalies*

Besides increased nuchal translucency, a careful search for fetal anomalies between 10 and 14 weeks' gestation may reveal various gross anomalies such an anencephaly, exencephaly, encephalocele, Meckel–Gruber syndrome, hydrocephalus, holoprosencephaly, renal anomalies, skeletal malformations, etc. (61). The early transvaginal detection of fetal anomalies is discussed in Chapter 6.

Adnexal Masses and Uterine Fibroids in Early Pregnancy

Corpus luteum cysts. It is relatively common to find masses of the adnexal region or uterus in ultrasound examinations of early pregnancy (15, 35, 63). The most common masses detected at this time are corpus luteum cysts (Fig. 10.**51**), which are seen in approximately 20% of all early pregnancies and generally resolve spontaneously by 14 weeks' gestation (17). Usually they can be clearly demarcated from the uterus with ultrasound. Most are unilocular, have smooth margins, and do not exceed 6–8 cm in size. Some contain fine internal echoes.

True ovarian tumors. True ovarian tumors such as dermoid cysts (Fig. 10.**52**) and cystomas usually contain additional internal structures (septa or solid components). Malignant ovarian tumors are extremely rare in association with pregnancy (19), as are inflammatory adnexal lesions such as tubo-ovarian abscess (Fig. 10.**53**).

Fibroids. Fibroids (leiomyomas) are the second most common tumor detected in pregnancy (42, 63). They can complicate the pregnancy in varying ways and degrees, depending on their size and location. In most cases the size and location of fibroids can be evaluated better with abdominal ultrasound than transvaginal ultrasound, since it is easier to scan cephalad with an abdominal probe (Figs. 10.**54**–10.**56**). Because of their rich blood supply, fibroids in pregnancy appear predominantly hypoechoic and are relatively easy to distinguish from the uterine musculature. There are cases, however, in which a well-perfused, pedunculated, subserosal fibroid can mimic an ovarian tumor (Fig. 10.**56**).

Serial examinations. Since the size and location of fibroids are accessible to early ultrasound evaluation, we can detect complications such as encroachment on the gestational sac at an early stage and, if necessary, plan appropriate treatment (e.g., fibroidectomy). It can also be determined whether a spontaneous delivery is feasible or whether a cesarean delivery is advised.

Local uterine contractions. Local uterine contractions can occasionally mimic a submucosal fibroid, as both may have a similar ultrasound appearance (Fig. 10.**57**) (69). Unlike a fibroid, however, the local uterine contraction is a transient feature that will disappear on follow-up scans (Fig. 10.**58**).

References

1. Abramovici, H., Auslender, R., Lewin, A., Faktor, J.H.: Gestational – pseudogestational sac: A new ultrasonic criterion for differential diagnosis. Amer. J. Obstet. Gynec. 145 (1983) 377–379
2. Anderson, S.G.: Management of threatened abortion with realtime sonography. Obstet. and Gynec. 55 (1980) 259–262
3. Baumgärtner, M., Lautenbacher, R., Ecke, A.: Neue Kriterien zur Erkennung der extrauterinen Gravidität durch Ultraschalldiagnostik. In Otto, R.C., Jann, F.X: Ultraschalldiagnostik 82. Stuttgart: Thieme 1983
4. Beischer, N.A.: Hydatiform mole with co-existent foetus. J. Obstet. Gynaec. Brit. Cwlth 68 (1961) 231–237
5. Berger, M.J., Taymor, M.L.: Simultaneous intrauterine and tubal pregnancies following ovulation induction. Amer. J. Obstet. Gynec. 113 (1972) 812–813
6. Bernaschek, G., Spernol, R., Beck, A.: IUD-Lage bei intrauterinen Schwangerschaften. Geburtsh. u. Frauenheilk. 41 (1981) 645–647
7. Boruto, F.: Alarmzeichen bei der sonographischen Beurteilung des Gestationssackes. Ultraschall 3 (1982) 140–141
8. Bradley, W.G., Fiske, C.E., Filly, R.A.: The double sac sign of early intrauterine pregnancy: Use in exclusion of ectopic pregnancy. Radiology 143 (1982) 223–226
9. Brown, T.W., Filly, R.A. Laing, F.C., Barton, J.: Analysis of ultrasonographic criteria in the evaluation of ectopic pregnancy. Amer. J. Roentgenol. 131 (1978) 967–971
10. DeCherney, A.H., Romero, R., Lake Polan, M.: Ultrasound in reproductive endocrinology. Fertil. and Steril. 37 (1982) 323–333
11. Dodson, M.G: Bleeding in pregnancy. In Aladjem, S. (ed.): Obstetrical Practice. St. Louis: Mosby, 1980; p. 451
12. Donald, I.: Ultrasonic echo sounding in obstetrical and gynecological diagnosis. Amer. J. Obstet. Gynec. 93 (1965) 935–941
13. Donald, I., Morley, P., Barnett, E.: The diagnosis of blighted ovum by sonar. J. Obstet. Gynaec. Brit. Cwlth 79 (1972) 304–310
14. Fleischer, A.C., James, A.E.jr., Krause, D.A., Illis, J. B.: Sonographic patterns in trophoblastic disease. Radiology 126 (1978) 215–220
15. Fleischer, A.C., Boehm, F.H., James, A.E.jr.: Sonographic evaluation of pelvic masses occurring during pregnancy. In Saunders, R., James, E. (eds.): The Principles and Practice of Ultrasonography in Obstetrics and Gynecology. New York: Appleton-Century-Crofts Medical 1980; p. 263
16. Goldhofer, W., Merz, E.: Extrauteringravidität: Sonographische Kriterien und ihre klinische Wertigkeit. Ultraschall 6 (1985) 194–199
17. Hackelöer, B.J., Hansmann, M.: Ultraschalldiagnostik in der Frühschwangerschaft. Gynäkologe 9 (1976) 108–122
18. Hackelöer, B.J.: Ultraschall-Untersuchungen im 1. Trimester. In Holländer, H. J.: Die Ultraschalldiagnostik in der Schwangerschaft. München: Urban & Schwarzenberg 1984
19. Hansmann, M., Hackelöer, B.J., Staudach, A.: Ultraschalldiagnostik in Geburtshilfe und Gynäkologie. Lehrbuch und Atlas. Berlin: Springer 1985
20. Hazekamp, J.T.: Ectopic pregnancy: Diagnostic dilemma and delay. Int. J. Gynaec. Obstet. 17 (1980) 598–600
21. Iffy, L.: Ectopic pregnancy, In Iffy, L., Kaminetzky, H.A. (eds.): Principles and Practice of Obstetrics and Perinatology. New York: Wiley 1981; p. 609
22. Jones, W.B., Lauersen, N.H.: Hydatidiform mole with co-existent fetus. Amer. J. Obstet Gynec. 122 (1975) 267–272
23. Jouppila, D.: Ultrasound in the diagnosis of early pregnancy and its complication. Acta obstet. gynec. scand. Suppl. 15 (1970) 50
24. Jouppila, P., Huntaniemi, I., Tapananen, J.: Early pregnancy failure: study by ultrasonic hormonal methods. Obstet. and Gynec. 55 (1980) 42–47
25. Jouppila, P.: Clinical consequences after ultrasonic diagnosis of intrauterine hematoma in threatened abortion. J. clin. Ultrasound 13 (1985) 107–111
26. Kadar, N., Taylor, K.J.W., Rosenfield, A.T., Romero, R.: Combined use of serum HCG and sonography in the diagnosis of ectopic pregnancy. Amer. J. Roentgenol. 141 (1983) 609–615

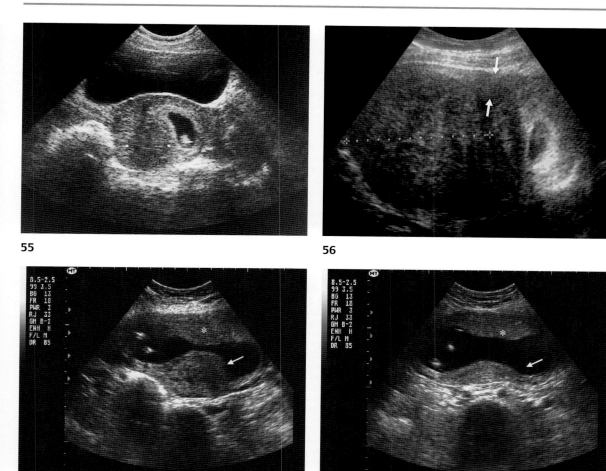

55

56

57

58

Fig. 10.**55** Early pregnancy, 9 weeks, transverse scan. The gestational sac is narrowed by an intramural fibroid 3.4 cm in diameter located just to the right of the sac.

Fig. 10.**56** Early pregnancy at 8 weeks, 6 days, longitudinal scan. Behind the uterus is a pedunculated, hypoechoic posterior wall fibroid measuring 8.1 cm in diameter. The tumor mimics an ovarian mass. Pedicle (arrows).

Fig. 10.**57** Intrauterine pregnancy at 15 weeks. Transverse scan demonstrates a contraction in the posterior uterine wall (arrow). Anterior wall placenta (*).

Fig. 10.**58** Same patient and scan plane as in Fig. 10.**57**. When the scan is repeated 20 minutes later, the wall contraction is no longer seen (arrow). Placenta (*).

27. Kobayashi, M., Hellman, L.M., Fillisti, L.P.: An aid in the diagnosis of ectopic pregnancy. Amer. J. Obstet. Gynec. 103 (1969) 1131–1140
28. Kobayashi, M., Hellman, L.M., Comb, E.: Atlas of ultrasonography in obstetrics and gynecology. London: Butterworths 1972
29. Laing, F.C., Jeffrey, R.B.: Ultrasound evaluation of ectopic pregnancy. Radiol. Clin. N. Amer. 20 (1982) 383–395
30. Lawson, T.L.: Ectopic pregnancy: criteria and accuracy of ultrasonic diagnosis. Amer. J. Roentgenol. 131 (1978) 153–156
31. MacVicar, J., Donald, I.: Sonar in the diagnosis of early pregnancy and its complication. J. Obstet. Gynaec. Brit. Cwlth 70 (1963) 387–395
32. Maklad, M.F., Wright, C.H.: Grey scale ultrasonography in the diagnosis of ectopic pregnancy. Radiology 126 (1978) 221–225
33. Mantoni, M., Pedersen, F.J.: Massive pseudogestational sac in ectopic pregnancy. J. clin. Ultrasound 11 (1983) 29–30
34. Marks, W.M., Filly, R.A., Callen, P.W., Laing, F.C.: The decidual cast of ectopic pregnancy: a confusing ultrasonographic appearance. Radiology 133 (1979) 451–454
35. Meinel, K.: Myome und Ovarialtumoren während der Schwangerschaft im Ultraschall-B-Bild. Zbl. Gynäk. 99 (1977) 180–186
36. Meinert, J.: Die fortgeschrittene Extrauterin-Gravidität (zugleich ein Beitrag zur kombinierten extra- und intrauterinen Schwangerschaft). Geburtsh. u. Frauenheilk. 41 (1981) 490–495
37. Meyenburg, M., Lange, J.: Ultraschall-Schnittbildtechnik – eine Methode zur Erfassung der ektopen Gravidität? Geburtsh. u. Frauenheilk. 38 (1978) 1032–1037
38. Morrow, C.P., Kletzky, O.A., Disaia, P.J. Townsend, D.E., Mishell D.R., Nakamura, R.M.: Clinical and laboratory correlates of molar pregnancy and trophoblastic disease. Amer. J. Obstet. Gynec. 128 (1977) 424–430
39. Mueller, C.E.: Intrauterine pseudogestational sac in ectopic pregnancy. J. clin. Ultrasound 7 (1979) 133–136
40. Müller, E., Leucht, W.: Ultraschalldiagnostik bei ektopen Schwangerschaften. Ultraschall 2 (1981) 158–168
41. Munyer, T.P., Callen, P.W., Filly, R.A.: Ultrasound of gestational trophoblastic disease. In Steel, W.B., Cochrane, W.J. (eds.): Gynecologic ultrasound. Clinics in Diagnostic Ultrasound 15, New York: Churchill Livingstone 1984; p. 105
42. Muram, D., Gillieson, M., Walters, J.H.: Myomas of the uterus in pregnancy: Ultrasonographic follow up. Amer. J. Obstet. Gynec. 138 (1980) 16–19
43. Nelson, P., Bowie, J.D., Rosenberg, E.: Early intrauterine pregnancy or decidual cast: An anatomic-sonographic approach. J. Ultrasound Med. 2 (1983) 543–547
44. Pandya, P.P., Snijders, R.J.M., Johnson S.P., Brizot, M., Nicolaides, K.H.: Screening for fetal trisomies by maternal age and fetal nuchal translucency thickness at 10 to 14 weeks of gestation. Br. J. Obstet. Gynaecol. 102 (1995) 957–962
45. Pandya, P.P., Kondylios, A., Hilbert, L., Snijders, R.J.M., Nicolaides, K.H.: Chromsomal defects and outcome in 1015 fetuses with increased nuchal translucency. Ultrasound Obstet. Gynecol. 5 (1995) 15–19
46. Pedersen, J.F.: Ultrasonic scanning in suspected ectopic pregnancy. Brit. J. Radiol. (1980) 1–4
47. Reece, E.A., Petrie, R.H., Sirmans, M.F., Finster, M., Todd, W.D.: Combined intrauterine and extrauterine gestations: A review. Amer. J. Obstet. Gynec. 146 (1983) 323–330
48. Reuter, K., Michlewitz, H., Kahn, P.C.: Early appearance of hydatiform mole by ultrasound. Amer. J. Roentgenol. 134 (1980) 588–589
49. Robinson, H.P.: Sonar in the management of abortion. J. Obstet. Gynaec. Brit. Cwlth 79 (1972) 90–94
50. Robinson, H.P.: The diagnosis of early pregnancy failure by sonar. Brit. J. Obstet. Gynaec. 82 (1975) 849–857
51. Romero, R., Taylor, K.J.W., Kadar, N., Hobbins, J.C.: The diagnosis of ectopic pregnancy. In Steel, W.B., Cochrane, W.J. (eds.): Gynecologic Ultrasound. New York: Churchill Livingstone 1984; p. 123
52. Sanders, R.C.: Ultrasound in the diagnosis of fetal death. In Sanders, R.C., Evette, J.jr.: The Principles and Practice of Ultrasonography in Obstetrics and Gynaecology. New York: Appleton-Century-Crofts 1980; p. 291
53. Schillinger, H.: Atlas der Ultraschalldiagnostik in der Schwangerschaft. Stuttgart: Schattauer 1984
54. Schlensker, K.H.: Ultraschalldiagnostik bei Verdacht auf Extrauteringravidität. Arch. Gynaekol. 219 (1975) 552–554
55. Schlensker, K.H.: Atlas der Ultraschalldiagnostik in Geburtshilfe und Gynäkologie. Stuttgart: Thieme 1984
56. Schmidt, W., Zaloumis, M., Heberling, D., Garoff, L., Runnebaum, B., Kubli, F.: Wertigkeit verschiedener Untersuchungsmethoden bei der präoperativen Abklärung der Extrauteringravidität. Geburtsh. Frauenheilk. 42 (1981) 829–834
57. Schneider, J., Berger, C.J., Cattell, C.: Maternal mortality due to ectopic pregnancy. A review of 1022 deaths. Obstet. Gynecol. 49 (1977) 557–561
58. Schoenbaum, S., Rosendorf, L., Kappelmann, N., Rowan, T.: Grayscale ultrasound in tubal pregnancy. Radiology 127 (1978) 757–761
59. Sicuranza, B.J., Tisdall, L.H.: Hydatidiform mole and eclampsia with co-existent living fetus in the second trimester of pregnancy. Amer. J. Obstet. Gynecol. 126 (1976) 513–514
60. Snijders, R.J.M., Pandya, P., Brizot, M.L., Nicolaides, K.H.: First trimester fetal nuchal translucency. In: Snijders, R.J.M., Nicolaides, K.H. (eds.): Ultrasound Markers For Fetal Chromosomal defects. The Parthenon Publishing Group 1996; p. 121–156
61. Souka, A.P., Nicolaides, K.H.: Diagnosis of fetal abnormalities at the 10-14-week scan. Ultrasound Obstet. Gynecol. 10 (1997) 429–442
62. Staudach, A.: Ultraschalldiagnostik in der Frühschwangerschaft: Methodik, Aussagewert und differentialdiagnostische Probleme. Zbl. Gynäk. 99 (1977) 979–984
63. Stein, W., Halberstadt, E., Leppien, G., Eckert, H.: Ultraschallkriterien zur Beurteilung der Gravidität bei Uterus myomatosus. Arch. Gynec. 219 (1975) 398–399
64. Tancer, M.L., Delke, I., Veridiano, N.P.: A fifteen year experience with ectopic pregnancy. Surg. Gynec. Obstet. 152 (1981) 179–182
65. Tatum, H.J., Schmidt, F.H., Jain, A.K.: Management and outcome of pregnancies associated with the Cooper T intrauterine contraceptive device. Amer. J. Obstet. Gynec. 126 (1976) 869–879
66. Terinde, R., Herberger, J., Wilke, J.: Ultraschalldiagnostik bei gestörter Frühschwangerschaft. Dtsch. med. Wschr. 104 (1979) 1629–1631
67. Weiner, C.P.: The pseudogestational sac in ectopic pregnancy. Amer. J. Obstet. Gynec. 139 (1981) 959–961
68. Weinraub, Z., Langer, R., Letko, Y., Bukovsky, I., Caspi, E.: Falscher intrauteriner Fruchtsack in der Ultraschalldiagnostik der Extrauteringravidität. Geburtsh. u. Frauenheilk. 41 (1981) 642–644
69. Wilson, R.L., Worthen, N.J.: Ultrasonic demonstration of myometrial contractions in intrauterine pregnancy. Amer. J. Roentgenol. 132 (1979) 243–247
70. Wittmann, B.K., Fulton, L., Cooperberg, P.L., Lyons, E.A., Miller, C., Shaw, D.: Molar pregnancy: Early diagnosis by ultrasound. J. clin. Ultrasound 9 (1981) 153–156

11 Normal Ultrasound Anatomy of the Fetus in the Second and Third Trimesters

Transvaginal ultrasound can define various anatomic details of the embryo or fetus during the first trimester (see Chapters 3 and 4). As the fetus continues to grow, abdominal ultrasound can be used during the second trimester to bring out further important details of fetal ultrasound anatomy. The period between 18 and 22 weeks' gestation is optimum for evaluating fetal anatomy, because by that time all the principal organs are well developed and can be visualized with ultrasound. It is also an opportune time to check for fetal abnormalities.

When ultrasound is used in the third trimester, examination of the normally developed fetus will essentially show only an increase in the size of the familiar organs. For our purposes, therefore, it is unnecessary to draw a distinction between scanning in the second and third trimesters.

Head

Embryology

Skull

The skull is composed of mesenchyma, which encases the developing brain. It consists of the neurocranium (calvaria, superior vault), which forms a protective covering for the brain, and the viscerocranium or facial skeleton, which consists mainly of the masticatory apparatus (11).

Neurocranium. The neurocranium (Fig. 11.**1**) is composed of two ontogenically distinct types of bone:
- Membrane bone (frontal bone, parietal bone), which develops by membranous ossification—i.e., the direct transformation of connective tissue to bone
- The primordial chondral bone of the superior floor. This bone develops by enchondral ossification, in which ossification centers form within the cartilaginous primordial cranium.

Individual superior bones like the occipital bone develop through the fusion of chondral bone and membrane bone. During fetal life and early childhood, the flat bones of the calvaria are united at their junctions by sutures composed of connective tissue (11) (Fig. 11.**1**).

Viscerocranium. The maxilla and mandible develop by membranous ossification, the hyoid bone by endochondral ossification.

Brain

Starting in the fifth week of embryonic life, the three primary brain vesicles (forebrain or prosencephalon, midbrain or mesencephalon, and hindbrain or rhombencephalon) develop into five secondary brain vesicles:
- Telencephalon (cerebral vesicle)
- Diencephalon (tween-brain vesicle)
- Mesencephalon (midbrain vesicle)
- Metencephalon (cerebellar vesicle)
- Myelencephalon (afterbrain vesicle)

Telencephalon and diencephalon. The telencephalon forms the cerebellar hemispheres, lateral ventricles, and lamina terminalis. The diencephalon forms the thalami, the posterior lobe of the pituitary, the infundibulum, and the epiphysis.

Mesencephalon. The mesencephalon lies between the diencephalon and metencephalon and is subject to much fewer morphologic changes than the other brain segments. Its lumen unites with the cerebral aqueduct, which interconnects the third and fourth ventricles (11).

Metencephalon. The metencephalon develops into a ventral portion, the pons, and a dorsal portion, the cerebellum. Its lumen develops into the fourth ventricle. The roof of the fourth ventricle remains thin and is closely related to the very vascular pia mater. The richly vascularized connective tissue of the pia mater, the tela choroidea, joins with the ependyma in the roof of the fourth ventricle to form the primordial choroid plexus. In similar fashion a choroid plexus develops in the roof of the third ventricle and on the medial walls of the lateral ventricles. Thus a total of four choroid plexuses are formed. They produce the cerebrospinal fluid, which then fills the ventricular system (11). In about the fourth month of embryonic development, the thin residual roof of the fourth ventricle bulges outward at three sites and ruptures. This creates three apertures: the unpaired foramen of Magendie in the median plane and the two foramina of Luschka on each side. These openings allow the cerebrospinal fluid to circulate from the fourth ventricle into the subarachnoid space that surrounds the brain.

Myelencephalon. The myelencephalon is the most inferior of the brain segments. It develops into the medulla oblongata.

Face and Ear

Facial development. It takes a relatively long times for the face to develop. At first the eyes are on the sides of the head and the nostrils are far apart. The nose is flat, and the ears are set level with the neck. Facial development is the result of changes in the positions and proportionalities of these structures. The eyes and nostrils move toward the midline while the ears move upward into the facial region (4).

Eyes. The eyes develop from protuberances in the prosencephalon. The lens and cornea are derived from the ectoderm of the lateral wall.

Nose and jaws. The nose develops from the medial nasal process and lateral nasal processes. The upper lip is formed from the two medial nasal eminences and both maxillary eminences. The mandibular processes fuse in the fourth week of embryonic development, while the maxillary processes and frontal process fuse in the sixth to seventh week (4).

Palate. The primitive palate is composed of three processes that are separated from the oral cavity by the nasal cavity:
- The medial primary palate
- The two lateral palatal processes of the "secondary palate"

The primary and secondary palates form between weeks 5 and 12 of embryonic development. Fusion of the palatal processes occurs mainly between weeks 7 and 12.

Tooth buds. Ten tooth buds arise from the dental lamina in each jaw. They give rise to the enamel organ from which the deciduous teeth are formed (4). In week 10 of embryonic development, buds for the permanent teeth form on the lingual aspect of the primordial milk teeth.

Ear. The auricle is formed from six auricular tubercles in the first and second branchial arches. After first appearing in the upper cervical region, the auricle migrates cephalad during the 10th week of embryonic development (4).

Ultrasound Anatomy

Three basic planes are available for scanning the fetal skull with ultrasound: transverse scans, sagittal scans, and coronal (frontal) scans. Transverse and sagittal scans are used principally in abdominal ultrasound, depending on fetal position and gestational age, while coronal and sagittal scans through the fetal head are most commonly used in transvaginal ultrasound.

The evaluation of head anatomy with transvaginal ultrasound is particularly important in early first trimester examinations (Fig. 11.**2**). It is also important in cases where the fetal head is very low in the lower pelvis and cannot be optimally visualized with abdominal ultrasound, but it is necessary to investigate a specific finding (Fig. 11.**3**).

Transverse Scans

During the second trimester, the fetal superior vault appears on transverse scan as a sharply marginated, hyperechoic, ellipsoidal structure (Figs. 11.**5**, 11.**11**). The skull generally presents a single contour line; there is little point in differentiating the skull from the galea at this time.

It is important to be familiar with the superior fontanels and sutures (Fig. 11.**1**), which form physiologic gaps and should not be misinterpreted as structural defects in the skull.

Midline echo. The midline echo is a hyperechoic line that runs along the fronto-occipital midline of the skull. It is formed anteriorly and posteriorly by the falx cerebri (5, 9, 14) and interhemispheric fissure (7) and centrally by the septum pellucidum (9) (Figs. 11.**2**, 11.**4**, 11.**5**, 11.**7**, 11.**9**, 11.**11**, 11.**13**, 11.**15**).

Lateral ventricles and cortex. At the end of the first trimester, the midline echo is still flanked by a pair of extremely wide lateral ventricles that occupy most of the superior interior. They are almost completely filled by the echogenic choroid plexus (5, 9) (Fig. 11.**2**). The brain mantle is sparsely developed at this stage and is difficult to appreciate because of its low echogenicity. As growth of the cortical brain tissue proceeds, the outer border of the lateral ventricles is displaced medially starting in about week 15, while the cortex becomes visible as a hypoechoic rim (Fig. 11.**4**). The posterior portion of the lateral ventricles is still occupied by choroid plexus, while the frontal horns contain only fluid (Fig. 11.**4**). By about week 19, the lateral ventricles display the characteristic pattern that is seen throughout the rest of the pregnancy (5). Because the hemispheres grow at a faster pace than the lateral ventricles (9), the latter occupy a relatively smaller intracranial volume while the individual brain structures become more prominent.

Head shape. Head shape varies considerably with fetal position, especially during the third trimester. While an elliptical head shape is seen in an oblique lie, the breech-presenting fetus has a more elongated "dolichocephalic" head shape (Fig. 11.**5**).

Depiction of brain anatomy. Brain anatomy, which has been described by several authors (3, 5, 6, 9, 10, 12, 14), is illustrated below for specific transverse and sagittal planes of section (Figs. 11.**6**, 11.**21**, 11.**37**). The ultrasound image shows marked structural differences between the portion of the hemisphere closer to the transducer and that farther from the transducer. The ventricular portion of the near hemisphere contains reverberation artifacts, which create the appearance of increased density in that region. The ventricular portion of the far hemisphere represents the true density and structural characteristics of that area (14).

Scan plane I (Figs. 11.**6**–11.**8**). This is the highest axial scan plane through the fetal head. It demonstrates the hypoechoic cerebral cortex located between the midline echo and the lateral calvaria. Parallel to the midline echo are the "periventricular lines," which should not be misinterpreted as the lateral ventricles. These echogenic lines (often only one line is seen in the far hemisphere) are either deep intracerebral veins (7) or periventricular white matter fibers (2). Anatomically, the periventricular lines are located just above the lateral ventricles.

Scan plane II (Figs. 11.**6**, 11.**9**, 11.**10**) demonstrates the hypoechoic lateral ventricles and part of the echogenic choroid plexus on each side. Through early measurement of the lateral ventricles (see Chapter 12), the development of hydrocephalus can be detected in its initial stage.

Scan plane III (Figs. 11.**6**, 11.**11**, 11.**12**) depicts the occipitofrontal plane. It is important for superior biometry (see Chapter 12), as both the biparietal diameter and the occipitofrontal diameter are measured on this plane.

The occipitofrontal midline echo is interrupted by a small echo-free area (Fig. 11.**11**). This represents the cavum septi pellucidi (9), not the third ventricle. The latter is situated between the two relatively hypoechoic thalamic nuclei and normally appears only as a streak or small slit. The frontal and occipital horns of the lateral ventricles can also be identified on this plane (Fig. 11.**11**).

Scan plane IV (Figs. 11.**6**, 11.**13**, 11.**14**) passes through the upper midbrain. The midline echo is only partially visible on this plane.

Scan plane V (Figs. 11.**6**, 11.**15**, 11.**16**) passes through the basal part of the midbrain and through the cerebellar hemispheres. The hypoechoic cerebral peduncles together form a butterfly-shaped figure at the center of the skull. The interpeduncular fossa can be seen between the peduncles.

Scan plane VI (Figs. 11.**6**, 11.**17**, 11.**18**) passes through the skull base and defines the anterior, middle, and posterior superior fossae. The sphenoid bone appears as a hyperechoic area at the junction of the anterior and middle fossae. A real-time scan will show the internal carotid artery pulsating at that location. The pons and lower cerebellum are visible in the posterior fossa.

Scan plane VII (Figs. 11.**6**, 11.**19**) is an oblique transverse scan that demonstrates the cavum septi pellucidi anteriorly and the cerebellum and cisterna magna posteriorly. The thickness of the nuchal fold can be measured on this plane between 16 and 24 weeks' gestation (see Chapter 12). Increased nuchal thickness is a ultrasound marker for trisomy 21.

A slightly lower scan plane will define the foramen magnum in the posteroinferior part of the skull (Fig. 11.**20**).

Sagittal Scans

Scan plane VIII is midsagittal (Fig. 11.**21**–11.**31**). A precise midsagittal scan will define the facial profile of a fetus lying in the occipitoposterior position. Facial structures can be identified by the start of the second trimester (Fig. 11.**22**). By about 18 weeks, ultrasound reveals a definite facial profile with a forehead, nose, upper jaw, mouth, and lower jaw. The profile becomes even more distinct as gestation progresses (Figs. 11.**23**–11.**26**).

The midsagittal scan is also useful for observing physiologic movements such as mouth opening and yawning (Figs. 11.**24**, 11.**25**). The tongue may even be definable, especially when the mouth is open (Figs. 11.**25**, 11.**27**). Fetal breathing movements can be observed on this plane, but the gray-scale image should be supplemented by color Doppler for this type of study (Figs. 11.**28**, 11.**29**).

If the fetus is in a favorable position, the midsagittal scan can also define various brain structures such as the cavum septi pellucidi, corpus callosum, lamina tecti, pons, and cerebellum (Figs. 11.**30**, 11.**31**). This scan plane is particularly useful for demonstrating the corpus callosum. It should be noted, however, that the corpus callosum probably cannot be defined sonographically until about 20 weeks' gestation. Given the timetable for its development, it is unlikely that this structure can be identified before 20 weeks (Fig. 11.**32**).

Scan plane IX is parasagittal (Figs. 11.**21**, 11.**33**). If the neurocranium can be defined in the parasagittal scan, it should be possible to identify the brain mantle, lateral ventricle, caudate nucleus, thalamus, and cerebellum. The relative positions of the cerebral ventricles are shown schematically in Fig. 11.**34**.

If the fetus is facing the transducer, the parasagittal scan will give a longitudinal section of the orbit and eye (Figs. 11.**33**, 11.**35**). With high-resolution equipment, the lens of the eye can be seen in the anterior part of the orbit by about 13 weeks' gestation (Fig. 11.**35**).

Scan plane X (Figs. 11.**21**, 11.**36**). A tangential sagittal scan defines the ear. This plane is useful for evaluating both the anatomy of the auricle and the level of its attachment.

Coronal Scans

Coronal images of the fetal face are most easily obtained when the fetus is lying on its side.

Scan plane XI (Figs. 11.**37**–11.**40**). An oblique coronal scan through the nasal tip and mandible defines the oronasal region. A cleft lip can be detected or excluded on this plane. The integrity of the upper lip can be confirmed, especially when the mouth is open (Fig. 11.**40**).

Scan plane XII (Figs. 11.**37**, 11.**41**). A tangential coronal scan through the fetal face, just anterior to the eye, defines the closed eyelids. This gives the impression of a "sleeping fetus."

Scan plane XIII (Figs. 11.**37**, 11.**42**, 11.**43**). This coronal scan through the facial skeleton can simultaneously delineate the orbits and jaw region. The ocular lens appears as an echogenic ring in the anterior part of the orbit. According to Staudach (14), the four echogenic points around the ring represent the four rectus muscles that encircle the eye. As gestation proceeds, both slow and rapid eye movements can be observed in this plane (1).

Scan plane XIV (Figs. 11.**37**, 11.**44**). This is an angled coronal plane, useful for making a general assessment of the orbits and nose.

Scan plane XV (Figs. 11.**37**, 11.**45**). This is a longitudinal coronal scan through the skull at the level of the cavum septi pellucidi. It can simultaneously define the brain mantle, corpus callosum, and lateral ventricles (Fig. 11.**46**) on both sides.

Scan plane XVI (Figs. 11.**37**, 11.**46**). On this plane the ear and the level of the auricular root can be evaluated outside the skull. Within the skull, this plane demonstrates the central part and inferior horn of the lateral ventricle (Fig. 11.**46**). The spinal column is seen below the skull.

Scan plane XVII (Figs. 11.**37**, 11.**47**, 11.**48**). This is a longitudinal coronal scan through the posterior fossa. It demonstrates the brain mantle, the lateral ventricle with the choroid plexus, and the cerebellum. The cerebellomedullary cistern can be seen below the cerebellum.

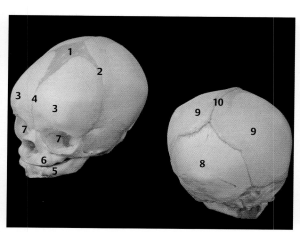

1

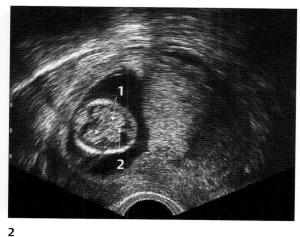

2

Skull

Fig. 11.**1**   Skull of a newborn. Anterior fontanel (1), coronal suture (2), frontal bone (3), frontal suture (4), mandible (5), maxilla (6), orbit (7), occipital bone (8), parietal bone (9), sagittal suture (10) (modified from 4).

Transverse scans

Fig. 11.**2**   Fetal skull at 12 weeks, 3 days. Hyperechoic choroid plexus (1) is already visible within both of the large lateral ventricles. Midline echo (2). Transvaginal ultrasound.

Fig. 11.**3**   Transvaginal scan of the normal brain surface at 35 weeks. The gyri are clearly defined. Coronal scan through the lower pelvis, with the fetus lying on its side.

Fig. 11.**4**   Left: axial scan of the fetal head, 18 weeks. The midline echo (1) is flanked by broad lateral ventricles (2) containing hyperechoic choroid plexus (3). Central part of the lateral ventricles (arrows). Cerebral cortex (4). Right: laterally angled oblique scan shows the C-shaped configuration of the choroid plexus.

Fig. 11.**5**   Elongated ("dolichocephalic") head shape of a breech-presenting fetus in the 1st position.

Fig. 11.**6**   Ultrasound scan planes through the fetal skull, shown in an anatomic model (planes I–VII, anatomic specimen from [4]).

Fig. 11.**7**   Scan plane I. The periventricular lines (arrows) run parallel to the midline echo. They do not represent the lateral ventricles.

Fig. 11.**8**   Anatomic section corresponding to Fig. 11.**7**.

Fig. 11.**9**   Scan plane II demonstrates the hypoechoic lateral ventricles (2) and the hyperechoic choroid plexus (3). Midline echo (1). Brain mantle (4).

Fig. 11.**10**   Anatomic section corresponding to Fig. 11.**9**.

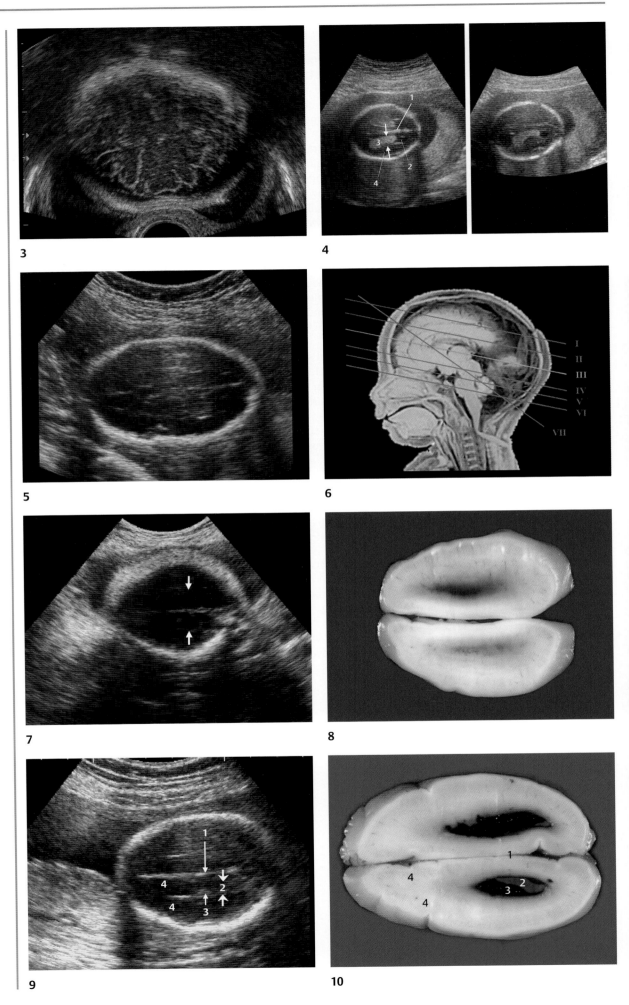

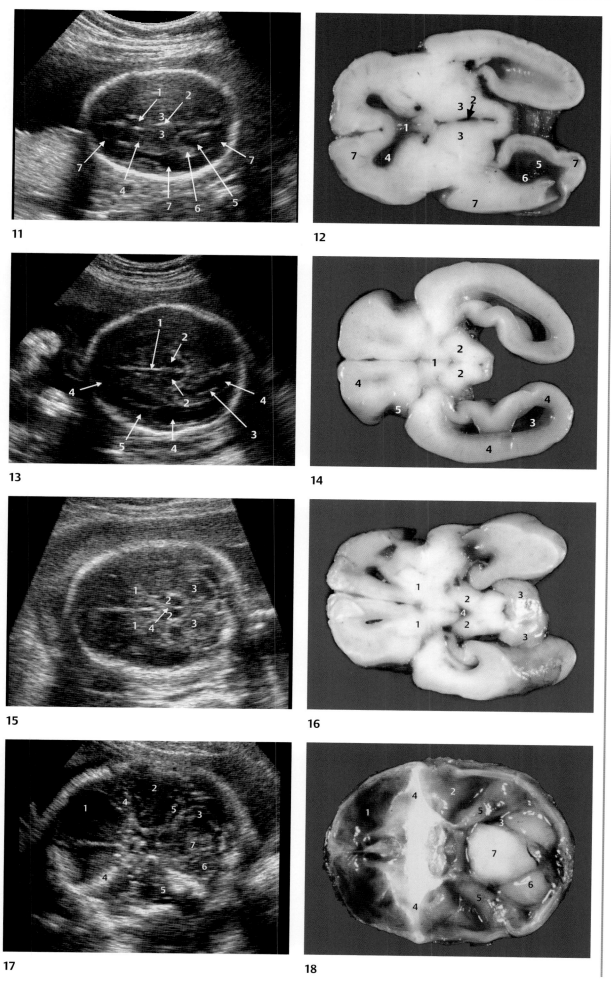

Fig. 11.11 Scan plane III (fronto-occipital plane): cavum septi pellucidi (1), midline echo (2), thalamus (3), frontal horn of lateral ventricle (4), occipital horn of lateral ventricle (5), choroid plexus (6), brain mantle (7).

Fig. 11.12 Anatomic section corresponding to Fig. 11.**11**.

Fig. 11.13 Scan plane IV: midline echo (1), upper midbrain (2), occipital horn (3), cerebral cortex (4), insula (5).

Fig. 11.14 Anatomic section corresponding to Fig. 11.**13**.

Fig. 11.15 Scan plane V: basal diencephalon (1), cerebral peduncles (2), cerebellum (3), interpeduncular fossa (4).

Fig. 11.16 Anatomic section corresponding to Fig. 11.**15**.

Fig. 11.17 Transverse scan through the base of the fetal skull (scan plane VI), 26 weeks: anterior fossa (1), middle fossa (2), posterior fossa (3), sphenoid bone (4), petrous temporal bone (5), cerebellum (6), pons (7).

Fig. 11.18 Anatomic section corresponding to Fig. 11.**17**.

11

12

13

14

15

16

17

18

Fig. 11.**19** Left: transverse scan angled posteriorly (scan plane VII) gives an optimum view of the cerebellum, 25 weeks. Left: cerebellar hemisphere (1), cerebellar vermis (2), cisterna magna (3), cavum septi pellucidi (4), brain mantle (5). Right: upper border of the cerebellum showing the cerebellar fissures (arrow).

Fig. 11.**20** Skull base viewed from below. Occipitoanterior breech presentation, 27 weeks. Occiput (1), foramen magnum (2).

Sagittal scans

Fig. 11.**21** Diagram of scan planes VIII–X. Left: viewed from the front. Right: viewed from above.

Fig. 11.**22** Sagittal scan through a fetus at 12 weeks, 6 days demonstrates the facial profile. Cephalic presentation.

Fig. 11.**23** Scan plane VIII at 22 weeks, 4 days. Midsagittal scan delineates the fetal facial profile.

Fig. 11.**24** Fetus with the mouth slightly open, 23 weeks.

Fig. 11.**25** Yawning fetus at 22 weeks. The tongue can be identified within the oral cavity.

Fig. 11.**26** Fetal facial profile at 29 weeks. Cephalic presentation.

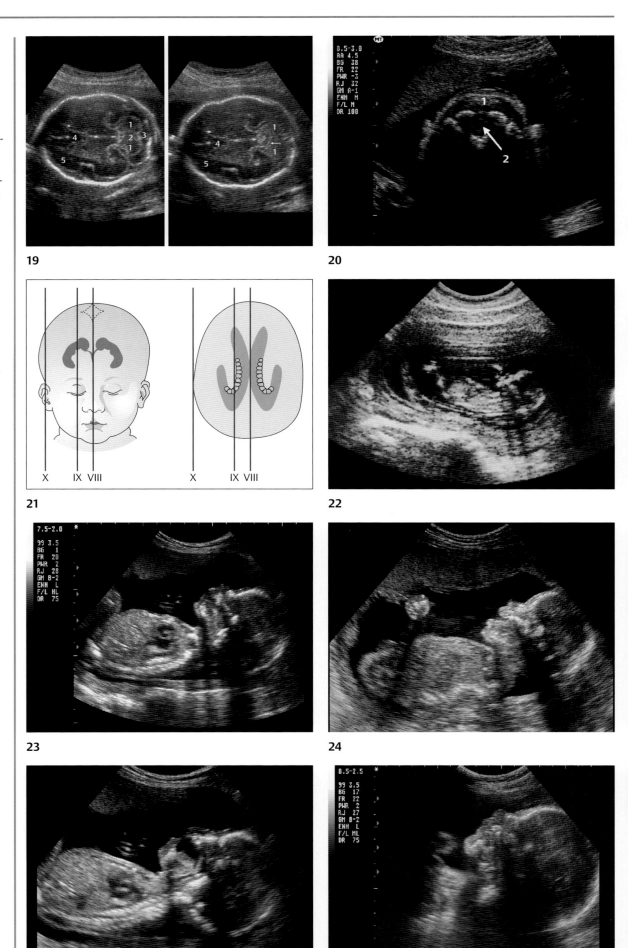

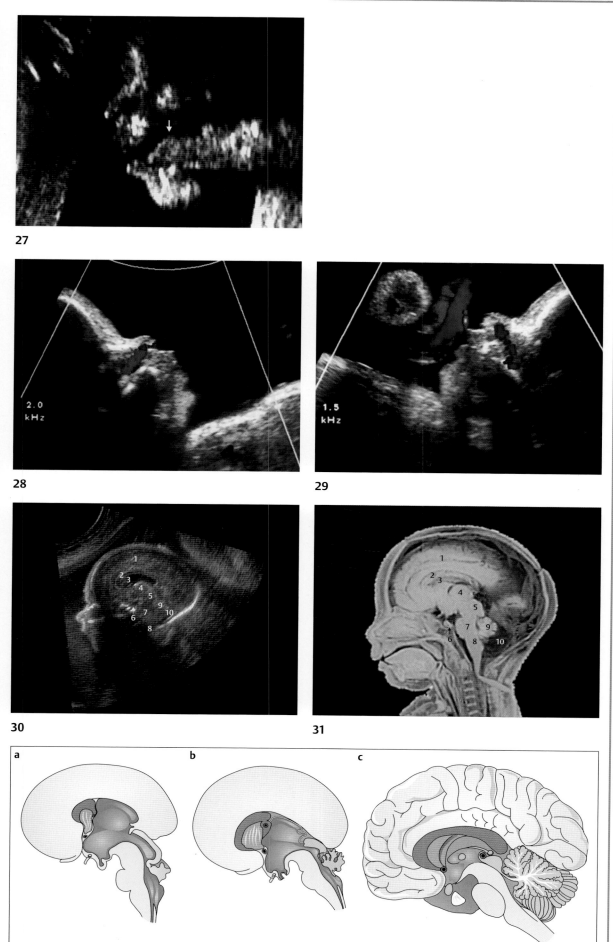

Fig. 11.**27** Fetal facial profile at 31 weeks, showing the nose, maxilla, mandible, and tongue (arrow).

Fig. 11.**28** Expiration: fetal breathing movement demonstrated by color Doppler (red).

Fig. 11.**29** Inspiration: breathing movement demonstrated by color Doppler (blue).

Fig. 11.**30** Midsagittal scan through the fetal brain (scan plane VIII, see Fig. 11.**21**): cerebrum (1), corpus callosum (2), cavum septi pellucidi (3), thalamus with third ventricle (4), lamina tecti (5), pituitary (6), pons (7), medulla oblongata (8), cerebellum (9), cisterna magna (10).

Fig. 11.**31** Anatomic section corresponding to Fig. 11.**30** (from [4]).

Fig. 11.**32** Development of the corpus callosum (after [8]).
a 16 weeks' gestation.
b 17 weeks' gestation.
c Adult.

Fig. 11.33 Parasagittal scan through the fetal skull (scan plane IX, see Fig. 11.21), 25 weeks. Brain mantle (1), lateral ventricle (2), caudate nucleus (3), thalamus (4), cerebellum (5).

Fig. 11.34 The cerebral ventricular system (after [15]).

Fig. 11.35 Sagittal scan through the left orbit at 19 weeks. The ocular lens (arrow) can be seen in the anterior part of the orbit.

Fig. 11.36 The right ear in a tangential scan (scan plane X, see Fig. 11.21).

Coronal scans

Fig. 11.37 Scan planes XI–XVI in an anatomic model (from [4]).

Fig. 11.38 Scan plane XI: an oblique coronal scan through the nasal tip and lower jaw.

Fig. 11.39 Scan plane XI: angled coronal scan through the fetal mouth, 32 weeks. The closed mouth is visible beneath the nose and nostrils.

Fig. 11.40 Scan plane XI. The mouth is open, and the tongue is visible between the parted lips.

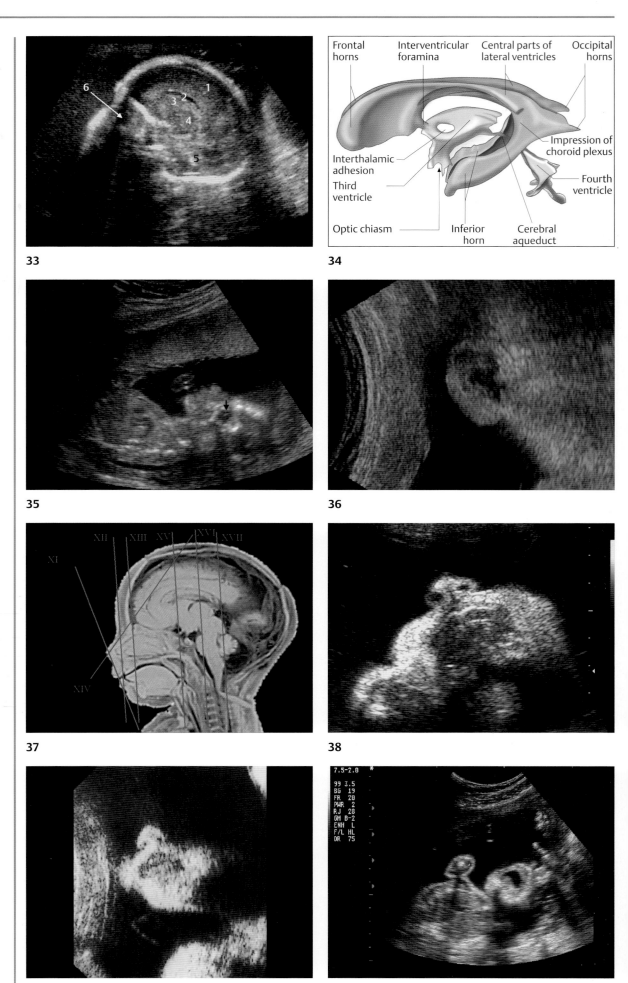

33

34
Frontal horns · Interventricular foramina · Central parts of lateral ventricles · Occipital horns · Impression of choroid plexus · Fourth ventricle · Cerebral aqueduct · Inferior horn · Optic chiasm · Third ventricle · Interthalamic adhesion

35

36

37

38

39

40

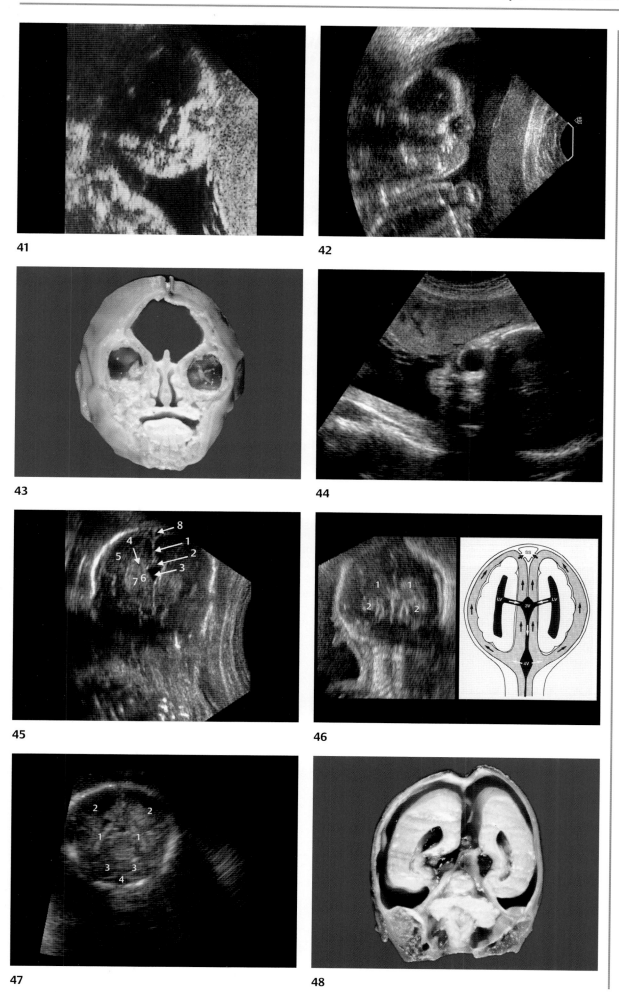

41

42

Fig. 11.41 Scan plane XII, 26 weeks. Frontal view of the fetal face showing the eyelid, nose, and mouth.

Fig. 11.42 Scan plane XIII (see Fig. 11.**37**). Frontal scan through the fetal skull permits the simultaneous evaluation of the orbits and jaws. The ocular lens can be seen within the left orbit.

43

44

Fig. 11.43 Anatomic section corresponding to Fig. 11.**42**.

Fig. 11.44 Oblique scan through the fetal face showing the orbits and nose.

45

46

Fig. 11.45 Scan plane XV: longitudinal coronal scan through the skull in the region of the cavum septi pellucidi. 1 = Falx cerebri, 2 = corpus callosum, 3 = cavum septi pellucidi, 4 = frontal horn of lateral ventricle, 5 = brain mantle, 6 = head of caudate nucleus, 7 = lentiform nucleus, 8 = sagittal sinus.

Fig. 11.46 Left: coronal scan plane XVI through the skull at the level of the auricular root. 1 = Lateral ventricle (central part), 2 = inferior horn of lateral ventricle. Right: diagram of the cerebral ventricular system in a coronal scan through the third and fourth ventricle. The arrows indicate the paths of CSF circulation (LV = lateral ventricle, 3V = third ventricle, 4V = fourth ventricle, SS = sagittal sinus) (modified from [13]).

Fig. 11.47 Scan plane XVII: longitudinal coronal scan through the posterior superior fossa shows the cerebellum and cerebellomedullary cistern, 19 weeks. Choroid plexus (1), brain mantle (2), cerebellum (3), cerebellomedullary cistern (4).

47

48

Fig. 11.48 Anatomic section corresponding to Fig. 11.**47**.

Spinal Column

Embryology

Ossification. The vertebrae form at the intersegmental levels from the primitive mesenchymatous vertebrae. These mesenchymatous models chondrify to produce a cartilaginous spinal column, which gradually ossifies (enchondral ossification). Toward the end of the embryonic period, three primary ossification centers appear: one in the vertebral body and two in the vertebral arch (3) (Fig. 11.**49a**). Ossification of the vertebral arches is apparent by the 8th week of embryonic development. In a fetus 10 cm long, the ossification extends from the 4th cervical vertebra to the 4th sacral vertebra (2). Approximately 95% of the population have seven cervical vertebrae, 12 thoracic vertebrae, five lumbar vertebrae, and five sacral vertebrae (2).

Unequal growth of the spinal cord and spinal column. Until the third month of embryonic life, the growth of the spinal cord parallels that of the spinal column, and the cord extends the full length of the spinal canal. But starting in the third month, the spine grows more rapidly than the inferior part of the spinal cord. As a result, the tapered part of the cord, the conus medullaris, terminates in the sacral part of the spinal canal, and the root fibers of the spinal nerves below the cervical level descend to their intervertebral foramina at an increasingly oblique angle. Because of the unequal growth of the spinal cord and spinal column, the tapered inferior end of the cord (conus medullaris) barely reaches the 3rd lumbar vertebra (Fig. 11.**50**) (2).

Ultrasound Anatomy

With transvaginal ultrasound, the fetal spine can be identified as a pair of fine, echogenic lines as early as 9 weeks' gestation (Fig. 11.**51**). With abdominal ultrasound, the entire spinal column can be seen by about 12 weeks' gestation, appearing as a continuous, echogenic double line that resembles a zipper.

Scan planes I and II. When the spine is imaged with the fetus lying exactly in an occipitoanterior position (scan plane I, Fig. 11.**49b**), only the anterior ossification center of the vertebral body will be seen (Fig. 11.**52**). If the scan is directed at a slightly oblique angle (scan plane II, Fig. 11.**49b**), however, it will define the ossification centers of the vertebral bodies and vertebral arches on one side (Figs. 11.**53**, 11.**54**). The two parallel lines taper to a pencil-like point in the sacral region while showing a slight amount of dorsiflexion (Figs. 11.**53**, 11.**55**). The hypoechoic band that runs between the two echogenic lines represents the vertebral canal with the spinal cord (Figs. 11.**52**–11.**55**). Because the spinal cord grows more slowly than the dura mater and spinal column, the inferior end of the cord eventually terminates at a higher level than the associated vertebrae. Thus, the cord terminates at S1 in the 25-week fetus but at L3 in the newborn (1). Observation of the occipitoanterior fetus simultaneously permits inspection of the fetal body surface (Fig. 11.**53**), which is particularly important in the detection of cleft anomalies.

Scan plane III. With the fetus lying on its side, a coronal scan through the vertebrae (Fig. 11.**49b**) will display the ossification centers of the vertebral arches as parallel rows of bright echoes (Figs 11.**56**–11.**59**). The normal spinal column appears slightly flared at the level of the craniocervical junction (Fig. 11.**56**), while its two echogenic lines converge in the sacral region (Fig. 11.**56**). In this position, the fetal iliac wing closer to the transducer will occasionally cast an acoustic shadow that mimics a defect in the lumbar spine (Figs. 11.**58**, 11.**59**).

Occipitoposterior position. The spine and dorsal body surface cannot be accurately evaluated when the fetus is occipitoposterior, because the fetal back is usually lying against the posterior uterine wall (Fig. 11.**60**) and portions of the spine may be shadowed by fetal extremities.

Transverse scan. A transverse scan of the spine clearly demonstrates the three ossification centers for the vertebral body and arch and the laterally placed centers for the ribs (Fig. 11.**61**). In late pregnancy when ossification is more advanced, the vertebra appears more like an echogenic ring in transverse section (Fig. 11.**62**). If the scan cuts the intervertebral space, it gives a clear view of the spinal canal and the ossification center anterior to it (Fig. 11.**63**). The intrinsic back muscles appear as oblique echoes behind the spinal column (Fig. 11.**64**).

Spine and spinal cord

Fig. 11.**49**   Diagram of the ossification centers in a fetal thoracic vertebra.
a 11 weeks.
b 19 weeks.
Scan plane I shows only the anterior ossification center of the vertebral body, while the slightly oblique plane II shows the ossification center of the vertebral body and vertebral arch. Plane III (coronal scan) displays both ossification centers of the vertebral arch (modified from [5]).

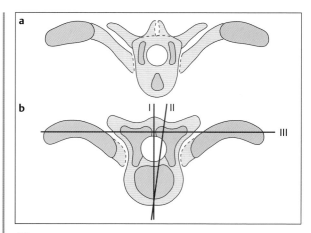

49

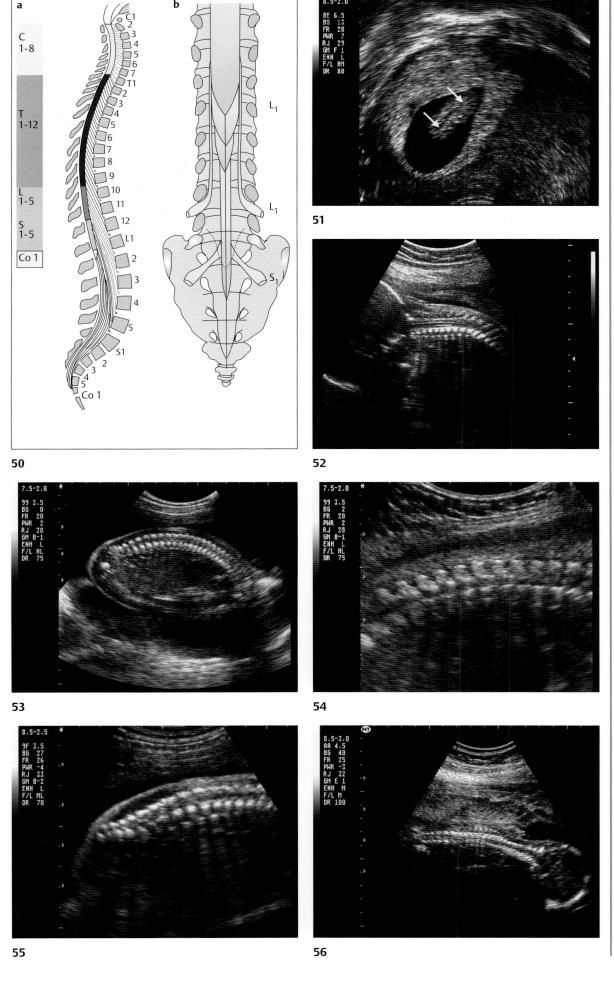

50

51

52

53

54

55

56

Fig. 11.**50** Vertebral bodies and spinal cord.
a Diagram of the human vertebral bodies, lateral aspect (modified from [4]). C = cervical, T = thoracic, L = lumbar, S = sacral, Co = coccygeal.
b Diagram of the spinal cord in relation to the spinal column, posterior aspect with the vertebral canal opened. The inferior end of the conus medullaris shows a relative ascent as gestation proceeds, ascending from the S4 level at 6 months' gestation to S3 at 7 months' gestation and to L3 in the newborn. The dashed line marks the end of the dural sac for the 6-month fetus and for adults (after [2]).

Fig. 11.**51** Spinal column at 9 weeks' gestation, coronal scan.

Fig. 11.**52** Superior portion of the spinal column, showing the spinal canal in sagittal section. Because the fetus is in an exact occipitoanterior position, only the anterior ossification centers of the cervical vertebrae are seen.

Fig. 11.**53** Full-length view of the fetal spine at 22 weeks, 4 days.

Fig. 11.**54** Dorsal ossification centers of the fetal spine at 32 weeks, 2 days.

Fig. 11.**55** Inferior end of the spinal column. The rows of ossification centers converge in the sacral region.

Fig. 11.**56** Coronal scan of the fetal spine (scan plane III, Fig. 11.**49b**) at 19 weeks. Note the physiologic expansion of the spinal column at the craniocervical junction and the convergence of the parallel rows of echogenic ossification centers in the sacral region.

Fig. 11.**57** The central canal in coronal section.

Fig. 11.**58** Coronal scan through the fetal spine (scan plane III, Fig. 11.**49b**) at 22 weeks. The echogenic iliac wing (arrow) appears on each side of the spine in the region of the lumbosacral junction. Shadowing from the upper iliac wing can mimic a defect in the spinal column.

Fig. 11.**59** Oblique coronal scan through the fetal spine at 22 weeks, 4 days. The acoustic shadow from the upper iliac wing mimics a defect in the spinal column.

Fig. 11.**60** Oblique sagittal scan through the spine of a fetus in an occipitoposterior breech presentation.

Fig. 11.**61** Transverse scan of the fetal spine at 22 weeks. The three ossification centers are clearly defined (1 = vertebral body, 2 = vertebral arch).

Fig. 11.**62** Transverse scan of the fetal spine in the third trimester.

Fig. 11.**63** View of the spinal canal and the ventral ossification center of the spinal column, 37 weeks.

Fig. 11.**64** Intrinsic back muscles (arrows) in a transverse scan.

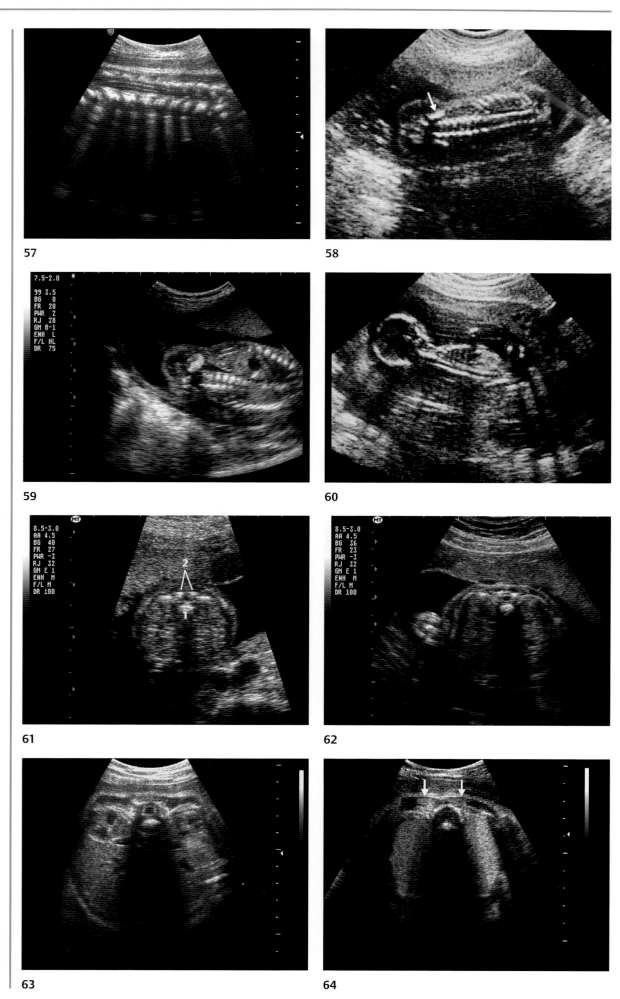

57

58

59

60

61

62

63

64

Neck Region

Although the neck is a relatively small body region, it is the setting for various complex and vital processes. Respiration, deglutition, and phonation all commence within this confined region immediately after birth. The neck also transmits the major neurovascular pathways that supply the brain with oxygen, nutrients, and neural information.

In the past, little was known about the antenatal development of this region. Our sparse knowledge of its prenatal anatomy came mainly from pathoanatomic studies or postnatal radiographic studies, even after the advent of ultrasonography (12). The first antenatal ultrasound studies on the anatomy and physiology of the fetal neck region became possible owing to the development of modern high-resolution ultrasound techniques (4, 6, 17, 19).

Embryology

Upper and lower respiratory tract. The respiratory tract is subdivided into an upper part consisting of the nasopharynx and a lower part consisting of the larynx, trachea, and lungs. This section deals with the development of the lower portions of the respiratory tract, which form as an outgrowths of the endoderm on the anterior side of the foregut and then separate from the digestive tract.

Fourth week. Initial signs of the developing respiratory system are already apparent in the fourth week of embryonic development (13). At this time a median groove called the laryngotracheal groove develops in the pharyngeal epithelium. The inferior portion of this groove already contains the lung rudiment. Shortly thereafter the unpaired lung rudiment descends by several somites and is no longer part of the pharyngeal region. Several days later, the inferior end of the embryonic trachea (called the laryngotracheal tube) forms two lateral outgrowths, the lung buds. The lung buds and embryonic trachea grow rapidly in the inferior direction into the mesenchymal tissue ventral to the foregut. The mesenchyma located between the foregut and laryngotracheal tube forms the tracheo-esophageal septum (14). As the trachea and esophagus lengthen caudally, the tracheo-esophageal septum also grows by adding tissue at its inferior end; it is bounded rostrally by the pharyngeal epithelium. The septum separates the laryngotracheal tube from the esophageal rudiment. In this way a progressive separation is established between the structures of the respiratory and digestive tracts. Errors in this process can lead to various malformations, the most common of which is tracheoesophageal fistula. Often the fistulas are combined with esophageal atresia.

Fifth to sixth week. By the fifth to sixth week, the trachea is completely surrounded by a mesenchymal border. At its superior end, the embryonic larynx begins to form during this period. During development of the internal structures of the larynx, there is a brief interval in which its lumen is occluded by epithelial adhesions. If this does not clear during subsequent development, it can lead to the rare anomaly of laryngeal atresia.

Seventh to eighth week. Starting in the seventh or eighth week, the embryonic pharynx and trachea communicate via a pharyngotracheal connection. Full communication is established between the pharyngeal and tracheal lumina by the end of the embryonic period. The first tracheal cartilages are differentiated in approximately the eighth week. The pharynx, trachea, and esophagus continue their rapid longitudinal growth during the rest of the embryonic period and also during the fetal period.

Ultrasound Anatomy

Coronal Scan

In our experience, coronal scans are best for evaluating the structures of the fetal neck.

Trachea, bifurcation, and main bronchi. The trachea, filled with lung fluid, is clearly visible in the coronal plane (Fig. 11.65). The echogenic tracheal cartilage rings are clearly delineated from the less echogenic surrounding tissue and from the echo-free lumen. In some cases the examiner may be able to define the tracheal bifurcation and the origin of the main bronchi (Fig. 11.66). Smaller bronchial divisions cannot be defined with equipment now available.

Larynx. The larynx is easily identified by locating the trachea and tracing it cephalad. Its junction with the hypopharynx is marked by a conical narrowing of the tracheal fluid band. The piriform recesses can be defined at this level by angling the transducer just 1–2° laterally (Fig. 11.67).

Epiglottis and aryepiglottis. Portions of the epiglottis can be visualized as small, echogenic structures projecting into the hypopharynx. When the transducer is directed 1–2 mm anteriorly, the epiglottis disappears and the aryepiglottis on each side comes into view (Fig. 11.68).

Esophagus. The esophagus is demonstrated by moving the transducer 1–2 mm posteriorly from a longitudinal view of the trachea. The proximal, collapsed portion of the esophagus cannot be seen in a normal fetus.

Cervical vessels. The large cervical vessels run parallel to the trachea. The common carotid artery springs from the brachiocephalic trunk on the right side and from the aortic arch on the left side. Lateral to the common carotid artery is the internal jugular vein.

Transverse Scan

Transverse scans at the level of the thyroid gland give an excellent view of the individual, echogenic tracheal cartilages, which are convex anteriorly and flattened posteriorly (Fig. 11.69). The thyroid gland appears as an echogenic structure on the anterior aspect of the trachea. Behind the trachea is the collapsed esophagus, which cannot be visualized. The internal jugular vein runs lateral to the common carotid artery at this level.

At the level of the larynx, the piriform recesses appear as deep indentations lateral to the epiglottis on each side (Fig. 11.70).

Sagittal Scan

This plane is considered the least favorable for the adequate evaluation of fetal neck structures. The upper respiratory tract can be defined only under optimum conditions. The fluid-filled pharynx can be seen behind the tongue only if the fetal neck is unflexed and the fetus is in an occipitoanterior position (Fig. 11.71). The epiglottis may be in contact with the uvula or several millimeters from it, depending on the contractile state of the pharyngeal muscles. The trachea is an echo-free structure that can be traced caudad to the level of the aortic arch.

Visualization of fetal neck structures. The immense diagnostic potential of high-resolution ultrasound has prompted a growing interest in the examination of fetal neck structures. Particular importance is placed on the upper airways and digestive tract. The few studies to date that have dealt with this subject have been limited exclusively to the visualization of these structures with B-mode ultrasound (4, 17, 19). The use of color Doppler imaging additionally permits an accurate description of functional processes in this region (respiration, deglutition) (6, 7, 19, 16). These studies have shown that the anatomy of the upper respiratory tract is strongly influenced by these physiologic processes.

Biometry

Normal values. To date, only two studies have reported normal values for the dimensions of the fetal upper airways, primarily the trachea (17, 19). But neither of these studies took into account the influence of functional processes on upper respiratory anatomy, and neither study defined reproducible planes for taking the measurements.

This prompted us to conduct a new study to determine normal dimensional values for the larynx, trachea, and pharynx. Specific inclusion and exclusion criteria were defined in addition to accurate and reproducible biometry planes. The biometry points were identified by anatomic characteristics that can be readily located with ultrasound (Fig. 11.**72**).

Normal Functional Processes

Deglutition

Fetal swallowing movements have been observed and described by many authors. These movements are believed to commence in the 11th week of gestation (5). Animal studies have proven that the fetus swallows a considerable amount of amniotic fluid daily and that this is an important mechanism of amniotic fluid circulation (18). Ultrasound has made it possible to observe fetal swallowing activity in vivo (3). The use of modern techniques, such as color Doppler combined with a cine loop system, has led to a better understanding of fetal swallowing (15, 16).

Stages of swallowing. The organs involved in the act of swallowing are the mouth, tongue, pharynx, larynx, trachea, and esophagus. Swallowing is almost always preceded by several sucking movements. Then the oral stage of swallowing begins. The amniotic fluid bolus that enters the open mouth is first pushed into the oropharynx by a posterior movement of the tongue. Next comes the pharyngeal stage in which the swallowed fluid bolus is directed toward the esophagus. This is accompanied by an upward movement of the larynx and a collapse of the oropharynx. Incomplete closure of the larynx by the glottis allows some of the amniotic fluid to enter the trachea. During the esophageal stage, the amniotic fluid bolus is conveyed into the stomach. This final stage of swallowing is not visible sonographically.

Breathing Movements

Recording intratracheal pressure changes. Fetal breathing movements can be observed as early as 11 weeks' gestation. The effect of this vital intrauterine activity on the growth and maturation of the lungs is still unclear. This is because most of our knowledge of fetal breathing movements comes from studies in experimental animals. At present the most widely used method for studying fetal breathing movements is to record intratracheal pressure variations in catheterized sheep fetuses. These data are applied to the human fetus, although they in no way correspond to in vivo conditions.

Ultrasound observation. With the development of modern ultrasound technology, it is now possible to observe fetal breathing movements in utero (11). Studies in human fetuses have so far dealt exclusively with the analysis of parameters relating to the frequency and duration of breathing episodes. The results of these studies have shown that fetal breathing movements are subject to considerable variability. As a result, possible clinical applications such as the prediction of fetal jeopardy are still controversial.

Analysis of inspiration and expiration. More recent studies have focused on analyzing the exact time parameters of the two phases of the individual respiratory cycle, consisting of inspiration and expiration. Badalian, Fox, and their colleagues laid the groundwork for fetal pulmonary Doppler ultrasound by using color and spectral Doppler imaging to record fetal perinasal fluid flow (1, 2). Animal studies are still necessary, however, for studying changes in fluid dynamics in deeper portions of the respiratory tract (e.g., in the trachea).

Pulmonary Doppler ultrasound. This stimulating question gave rise to the first standardized series of studies in which we recorded pulmonary fluid movements in the trachea generated by fetal breathing (7). We assume that the trachea is the best test object for detecting these fluid movements using pulmonary Doppler ultrasound. Tracheal flow patterns during the breathing movements are recorded by color Doppler. When alternating red and blue signals are recorded, indicating bidirectional flow (Fig. 11.**73**), the sample volume is positioned in the trachea (Fig. 11.**74**). Following appropriate angle correction, the Doppler spectra are recorded (Fig. 11.**75**). The spectra are characterized by alternating periods of positive and negative flow, corresponding to inspiration and expiration (Fig. 11.**75**). Another advantage of recording at the tracheal level is that it can detect all fluid motion toward and away from the lung. When the spectral traces were used to assess the time parameters of fetal breathing as well as tidal volumes, it was found that the calculated tidal volumes correlate with gestational age and, consequently, with pulmonary growth.

"Fetal pulmonary function test." Fetal pulmonary Doppler ultrasound (recording tracheal flow during breathing movements using color and spectral Doppler) (Fig. 11.**76**) is opening a new dimension in the analysis of human fetal breathing movements. It is providing new quantitative parameters, such as the fluid volume that is displaced during one respiratory cycle. In the future, a kind of "fetal pulmonary function test" could be developed to improve the diagnosis of pulmonary hypoplasia (8), since fetuses with fatal pulmonary hypoplasia have smaller tidal volumes than equal-age fetuses with normally developed lungs.

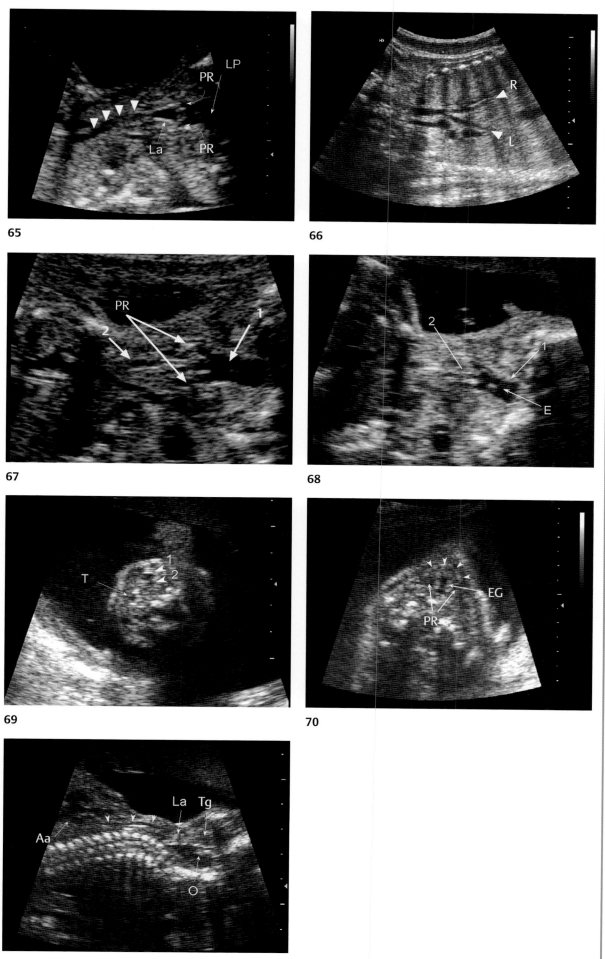

65

66

67

68

69

70

71

Ultrasound anatomy

Fig. 11.**65**   Coronal scan through the neck of a 21-week fetus. The trachea (arrowheads) appears as an echo-free structure in the midcervical region. The fluid-filled laryngopharynx (LP) is clearly visible. The piriform recesses (PR) appear as echo-free projections of the laryngopharynx around the larynx (La).

Fig. 11.**66**   Coronal scan through the thorax of a 31-week fetus. The trachea (arrowheads), filled with pulmonary fluid, can be traced to the origin of the right (R) and left (L) main bronchi.

Fig. 11.**67**   Coronal scan through the neck of a 31-week fetus. The piriform recesses (PR) can be defined by angling the transducer 1–2° laterally. Pharynx (1), larynx (2).

Fig. 11.**68**   Coronal scan through the neck of a 31-week fetus. The epiglottis (E) appears as an echogenic structure projecting into the hypopharynx. Pharynx (1), larynx (2).

Fig. 11.**69**   Transverse scan through the neck of a 25-week fetus at the level of the thyroid gland. Trachea (T), internal jugular vein (1) lateral to the common carotid artery (2).

Fig. 11.**70**   Transverse scan through the neck of a 24-week fetus at the level of the larynx (arrowheads). The piriform recesses (PR) are clearly demarcated lateral to the epiglottis (EG).

Fig. 11.**71**   Sagittal scan through the neck of a 24-week fetus. The trachea (arrowheads) is defined to the level of the aortic arch (Aa). The oropharynx (O) is behind the tongue (Tg) antenatally. Larynx (La).

Biometry and functional processes

Fig. 11.**72** Ultrasound biometry of the fetal upper airways. The pharyngeal diameter (PD) is measured at the level of the epiglottis. The laryngeal width (LW) is measured at the level of the piriform recesses. The site where the trachea is crossed by the brachiocephalic trunk (BT) is the landmark for measuring the tracheal diameter (TD). Ao (aorta) (after [9]).

Fig. 11.**73** Fetal breathing movements. Color Doppler images of one respiratory cycle. Fetal breathing movements generate a bidirectional pattern of fluid flow in the trachea, appearing blue in inspiration and red in expiration.

Fig. 11.**74** Fetal breathing movements. The sample volume is positioned on the fetal trachea, with appropriate angle correction. Imaged in coronal section, the trachea can be traced from the larynx (LA) to the tracheal bifurcation (TB) (from [8]).

Fig. 11.**75** Fetal breathing movements. Record of respiratory flow in the fetal trachea. The Doppler spectra vary with the phase of respiration (expiration, inspiration), alternating between positive and negative amplitudes.

Fig. 11.**76** Technique of pulmonary Doppler ultrasound in the fetus. As in vascular Doppler, the sample volume (SV) is positioned on the trachea (TR) with appropriate angle correction. P = pharynx, N = nasopharynx (after [7]).

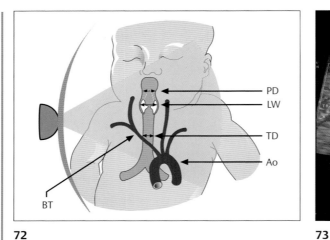

72

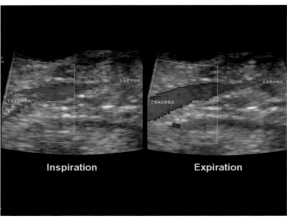

73

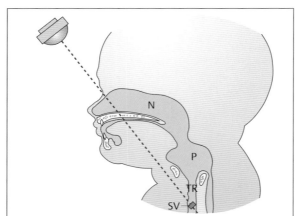

74

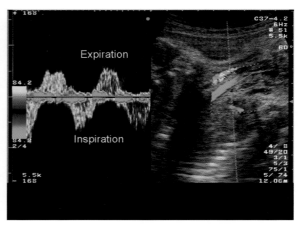

75

76

Thorax

■ *Bony Thorax, Clavicles, and Scapulae*

Embryology

The ribs develop from the costal processes of the thoracic vertebrae. They undergo chondrification and then ossification as the embryo develops (26). The primary ossification center in the body of the rib appears at about 14 weeks' gestation (12).

The clavicle, unlike the long tubular bones of the limbs, develops by membranous ossification. It is the first structure to be ossified, preceding the appearance of the first ossification centers in the femur (26).

The scapula undergoes enchondral ossification, which begins at the end of the second month of embryonic life. It is not completed until about 25 years of age.

Ultrasound Anatomy

Ribs. The thorax appears cone-shaped in longitudinal section (Fig. 11.**77**). It has a striated appearance due to shadowing from the ribs. A more tangential scan is useful for evaluating the ribs and especially their ossification (Fig. 11.**78**).

Clavicles. The clavicles are best demonstrated in a transverse plane below the neck (Fig. 11.**79**). An exact occipitoposterior or occipitoanterior position is most favorable, so that both clavicles can be defined in the same image and the sides can be directly compared.

Scapulae. The scapula is imaged by first defining the shoulder girdle in a lateral longitudinal scan. The probe is then angled slightly to obtain a posterior tangential view of the scapula in its full extent (Figs. 11.**80**, 11.**81**). In a transverse scan through the upper thorax, the scapula appears as a flat, echogenic feature posterolateral to the fetal spine (Fig. 11.**82**).

Heart. When the transverse scan is moved to a somewhat more inferior level, the pulsating fetal heart appears within the left hemithorax. Before obtaining more detailed views, the examiner should check the transverse scan to confirm that the heart is on the left side of the chest and that the cardiac axis is correct. Once this has been established, the examiner may proceed with a detailed inspection of the individual cardiac chambers (see Heart). It is important to note that the fetal heart has a more horizontal orientation than the neonatal heart due to the large size of the liver and the unexpanded lung (11).

■ *Lung and Diaphragm*

Embryology

Respiratory tract. The larynx, trachea, bronchial tree, and alveoli are derived from the endodermal alimentary tube. The main bronchi develop from the two lung buds. The right lung bud divides into three branches leading to the three pulmonary lobes on the right side. The left lung bud divides into two branches leading to the two left pulmonary lobes (Fig. 11.**83**). Throughout intrauterine development, the main bronchi undergo multiple dichotomous divisions. The mesoderm that surrounds the bronchial tree differentiates into cartilage, muscle tissue, and blood vessels.

Diaphragm. The diaphragm develops from several rudiments. The sternal and costal parts of the diaphragm arise from the septum transversum. A small part arises directly from the thoracic wall, and the posterolateral part of the diaphragm is formed from the pleuroperitoneal membrane (12).

Ultrasound Anatomy

Lungs. The lungs appear on transverse scans as uniformly echogenic structures located between the heart, spine, and ribs (Fig. 11.**84**). The echogenicity of the lungs changes with increasing gestational age. While the lung tissue is usually less echogenic than the liver in the second trimester, this pattern is reversed in the third trimester (2, 13). Some authors claim that the increased echogenicity of the lung provides an index of fetal lung maturity (13).

Diaphragm. When the diaphragm is intact, longitudinal scans show a curved, superiorly convex, hypoechoic line between the diaphragm and liver, representing the subphrenic space (Fig. 11.**85**). The diaphragm itself is moderately echogenic. It can be defined as a separate structure only in the presence of ascites or hydrothorax.

Fetal Breathing Movements

As early as 1888, Ahlfeld (1) described rhythmic movements of the fetal thorax that were detectable through the maternal abdominal wall in the final weeks of pregnancy. In 1970, Dawes et al. (9) and Merlet et al. (25) detected fetal breathing movements in experimental animals. In 1971, Body and Robinson (4) were the first to record respiratory movements of human fetuses by means of A-mode ultrasound. By using fast B-mode imaging and M-mode scanning, several authors (14, 24, 31, 33) were able to observe fetal breathing movements as early as 12–13 weeks' gestation (39).

Respiratory excursions. Fetal respiratory excursions start with a downward deflection of the diaphragm. The chest wall is drawn inward while the abdominal wall moves outward (Fig. 11.**86**). Then the diaphragm, chest wall, and abdominal wall return to their initial positions (31, 39). Neldam (28) published a nomogram relating the amplitudes of chest and abdominal wall excursions to gestational age. Fetal respiratory excursions are thought to be necessary for normal pulmonary development.

Frequency. Breathing movements occur episodically. They tend to be irregular in early pregnancy and become more regular by 34–36 weeks' gestation (37). Fetal breathing movements are greatly diminished or absent during delivery (5, 6, 8, 34).

Patrick et al. (30, 32) made continuous measurements of fetal breathing movements with real-time ultrasound for periods of 24 hours. They found a significant increase in fetal breathing movements during the second and third hours after meals and between 1:00 and 7:00 a.m. The longest period of fetal apnea lasted two hours (32). According to the authors, the breathing movement index, or the percentage of time in which breathing movements are observed in a healthy fetus, is approximately 30% during the last 10 weeks of pregnancy (32).

Factors that affect breathing activity. Various factors that can affect fetal breathing activity have been investigated. Hyperglycemia (3, 16, 19, 27) and hypercapnia (35, 38) were associated with an increase in the breathing movement index. Some authors also observed this in hyperoxia (38), whereas other authors (10, 36) found no significant change in fetal breathing activity (22). Nicotine use (17, 20, 21) and alcohol consumption (15, 18) caused a decrease in breathing movements. Fetal asphyxia in animal studies (7, 23, 29) was associated with decreased fetal breathing activity, including prolonged apnea. Intermittent or persistent abnormal breathing or gasping movements were noted as preterminal events.

No clinical implications. Despite numerous studies and discoveries in fetal physiology, researchers have not yet been able to draw clinical implications based on patterns of fetal respiratory movements because the physiologic range of breathing movements is extremely broad.

Bony thorax, clavicles, and scapulae

Fig. 11.**77**   Longitudinal scan of the fetal thorax, breech presentation, at 22 weeks. Acoustic shadows create a striate pattern behind the ribs.

Fig. 11.**78**   Fetal thorax, cephalic presentation, at 22 weeks, 4 days. The ossification of the ribs is easy to evaluate in this tangential scan of the thorax.

Fig. 11.**79**   Transverse scan through the fetal shoulder girdle at 26 weeks, 4 days demonstrates both of the curved clavicles.

Fig. 11.**80**   Dorsal tangential scan through the scapula, cephalic presentation, at 20 weeks.

Fig. 11.**81**   Tangential scan through the right scapula, breech presentation, 21 weeks.

Fig. 11.**82**   Transverse scan through the shoulder girdle, demonstrating both scapulae (arrows), 19 weeks. Lung and diaphragm

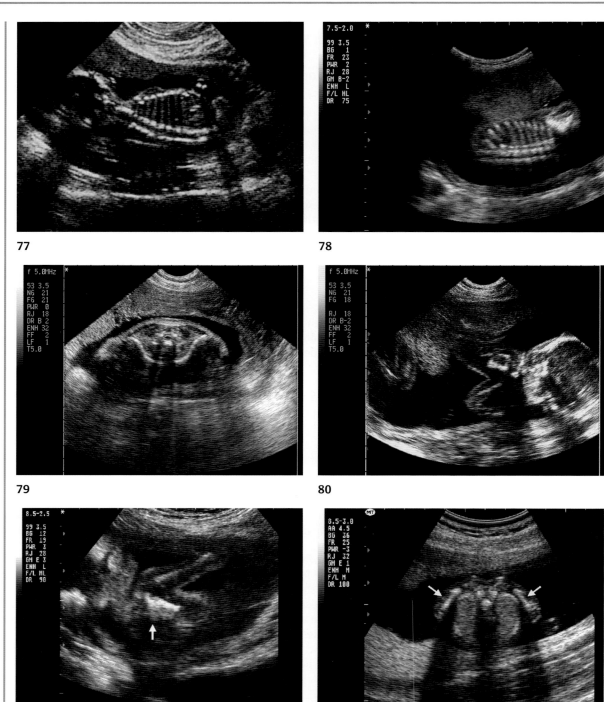

77

78

79

80

81

82

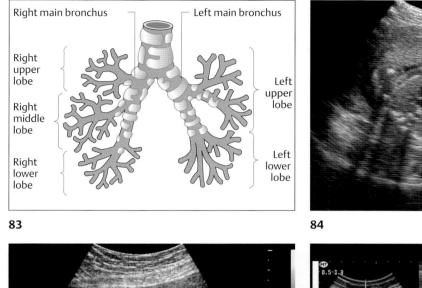

83

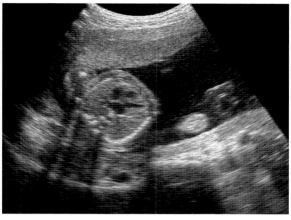

84

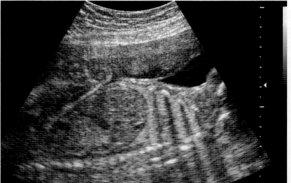

85

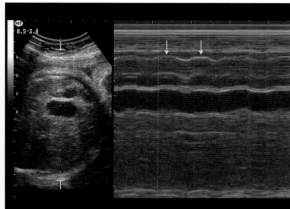

86

Fig. 11.**83**   Diagram of the fetal lower respiratory tract (after [26]).

Fig. 11.**84**   The lung at 20 weeks appears as a uniformly echogenic structure located obliquely behind the heart.

Fig. 11.**85**   Sagittal longitudinal scan through the thorax and abdomen at 20 weeks. The subphrenic space appears as a curved, hypoechoic line below the echogenic diaphragm.

Fig. 11.**86**   Transverse scan through the fetal abdomen at 37 weeks. M-mode trace demonstrates episodic fetal breathing movements (arrows).

Circulatory System (Fetal Circulation)

Embryology (2, 5)

Shortly before the end of 3 weeks' gestation, the primitive heart develops in the form of two endothelial tubes, which soon fuse to form a single heart tube. On about the 20th day of gestation, the heart tube gains attachment to the vascular network of the embryonic body, allantois, and yolk sac. A primitive cardiovascular system has developed by the end of the third week. Cardiac contractions arising from the sinus venosus begin on the 22nd day.

Circulation at 4 weeks

At the end of the fourth week, the initially arrhythmic contractions become regular enough to produce unidirectional flow.

Blood flow to the heart. The blood in the body of the embryo is conveyed to the embryonic heart by the anterior and posterior common cardinal veins. The umbilical veins carry blood from the placenta to the heart, and the omphalomesenteric veins carry blood from the yolk sac to the heart. All three vascular trunks communicate with one another in the area of the septum transversum before entering the sinus venosus (2) (Fig. 11.**87**).

Blood flow from the heart. The two aortic arches transport blood from the heart to the paired dorsal aortas, which unite inferiorly to form the unpaired abdominal aorta. Blood flows to the placenta via the umbilical arteries and to the yolk sac via the omphalomesenteric arteries (2) (Fig. 11.**87**).

Fully Developed Fetal Circulation

Blood flow to the heart. Following complete development of the fetal vascular system and the complex differentiation of the heart into two atria and two ventricles, oxygen-rich blood is carried from the placenta to the fetus by the umbilical vein. Of the two umbilical veins originally present, only the left vein is preserved (2). A small portion of the arterialized blood flows through the sinusoids of the liver, but most bypasses the liver and is carried by the ductus venosus to the inferior vena cava, where it mixes with venous blood from the lower extremity, pelvis, and abdominal cavity (Fig. 11.**88**).

Blood flow in and away from the heart. Blood then enters the right atrium, where it is routed toward the foramen ovale by the valve of the inferior vena cava. The inferior border of the septum secundum (crista dividens) separates the blood into two unequal parts. The greater part flows through the foramen ovale into the left atrium, mixes there with a small amount of blood from the lungs, flows into the left ventricle, and continues into the ascending aorta, whose branches principally supply the head, neck, and upper limbs (2).

The smaller part mixes with venous blood that passes through the superior vena cava into the right atrium and on into the right ventricle, flowing from there into the pulmonary trunk, ductus arteriosus, and aorta.

Only a relatively small portion of the arterialized blood is distributed to the internal organs and lower limbs. Very little blood flows into the lungs, because the pulmonary resistance is still very high.

Finally the blood flows back into the placenta via the umbilical arteries.

Changes during Birth

Closure of the foramen ovale. The foramen ovale, ductus arteriosus, umbilical arteries, and umbilical veins lose their functional significance at birth. When the vessels from the placenta are interrupted, the blood pressure in the inferior vena cava and right atrium falls precipitously. Meanwhile, the pressure in the left atrium rises swiftly as the lungs inflate with air and there is a sudden, strong increase in blood flow through the lungs. As a result, the blood pressure in the left atrium rapidly surpasses that in the right atrium, pressing the septum primum against the septum secundum and occluding the foramen ovale.

Ductus arteriosus, ductus venosus, and umbilical vessels. The ductus arteriosus and umbilical arteries become contracted at birth. The ductus arteriosus, ductus venosus, and umbilical vessels are rapidly obliterated due to proliferation of the vascular endothelium and perivascular connective tissue. The ligamentum teres of the liver persists as a remnant of the umbilical vein and often retains a small lumen initially. The distal segment of the umbilical artery in adults is located in the medial umbilical ligament. The proximal segment is preserved and gives rise to the superior vesical arteries.

The ligamentum venosum on the inferior surface of the liver is a remnant of the ductus venosus. The ligamentum arteriosum is derived from the ductus arteriosus. Transformation of the ductus arteriosus into a fibrous cord is completed in about the third postnatal month (2).

Ultrasound Anatomy

Color Doppler ultrasound. The large vessels of the fetal circulatory system are easily defined as hypoechoic bands by conventional B-mode imaging. Color Doppler ultrasound must be used to define smaller vessels, locate larger vessels more quickly, and determine their flow direction.

Transvaginal color Doppler ultrasound can detect umbilical and embryonic blood flow by the middle of the first trimester (Fig. 11.**89**). Abdominal ultrasound can provide a detailed study of the fetal circulation in the second and third trimesters.

Umbilical vein. From the cord insertion at the center of the abdomen (Fig. 11.**90**), the left umbilical vein (the right vein is obliterated in the 6th embryonic week [2]) runs obliquely upward to the liver at about a 45° angle, terminating at the portal sinus (3, 6) (Fig. 11.**88**).

Ductus venosus, portal vein, and inferior vena cava. Most of the oxygenated blood supplied by the umbilical vein flows into the ductus venosus after reaching the liver (Figs. 11.**88**, 11.**91**, 11.**92**). This routes the blood directly to the inferior vena cava, bypassing the hepatic capillary bed. The junction of the umbilical vein with the portal sinus is an important landmark for abdominal biometry (see Chapter 12) (3, 4, 6). A small portion of the umbilical venous blood mixes with the deoxygenated blood of the portal vein and flows through the hepatic sinusoids to the hepatic veins (Figs. 11.**91**, 11.**93**) and then to the inferior vena cava (7) (Fig. 11.**94**).

Heart. After entering the right atrium, most of the blood flows through the patent foramen ovale into the left atrium and then into the left ventricle (Fig. 11.**95**). A smaller amount passes through the right atrium into the right ventricle (Fig. 11.**95**).

Ascending aorta, pulmonary trunk, and ductus arteriosus. Blood flows from the left ventricle into the ascending aorta (Fig. 11.**96**) and from the right ventricle into the pulmonary trunk (Fig. 11.**97**) and the ductus arteriosus, which opens into the aorta. The crossing of the pulmonary trunk and ascending aorta can be clearly identified with color Doppler (Fig. 11.**98**).

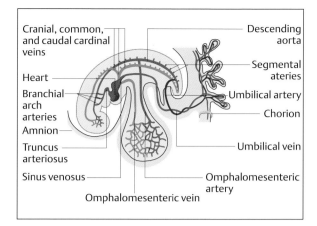

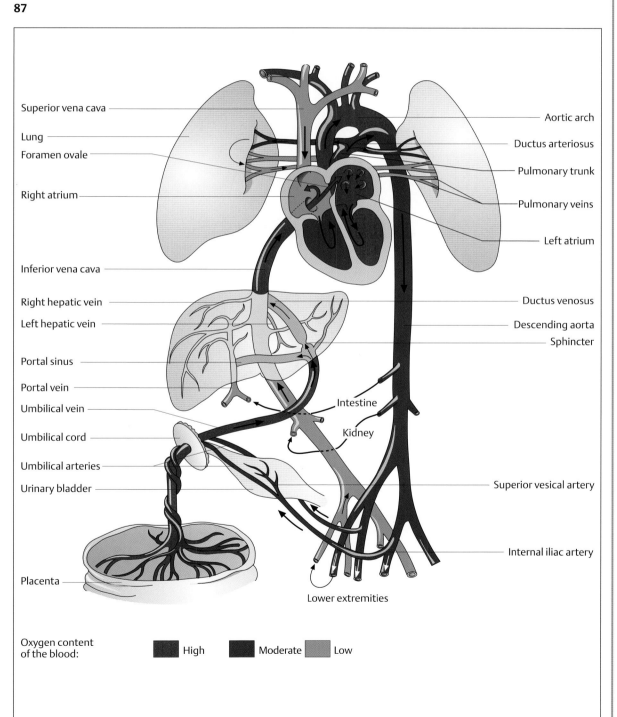

Placenta

Lower extremities

Oxygen content of the blood: High Moderate Low

Development of the fetal circulatory system

Fig. 11.**87** Diagram of the early embryonic circulation. Stage 12 (approximately 26th day of embryonic development) (after [5]).

Fig. 11.**88** Simplified diagram of the fetal circulation. The colors indicate the oxygen saturation of the blood. The arrows indicate the direction of blood flow. For simplicity, the organs are not drawn to scale (after [5]).

Aortic arch. A longitudinal oblique scan can define the aortic arch and the vessels arising from it (brachiocephalic trunk, left common carotid artery, left subclavian artery) (Fig. 11.**99**).

Cerebral blood flow. Cerebral blood flow is best evaluated by imaging the middle cerebral artery, which is usually oriented at a favorable angle relative to the transducer (Fig. 11.**100**).

Descending aorta. Tracing the aorta past the aortic arch (Figs. 11.**101**, 11.**102**), the examiner can identify the entire descending aorta as a pulsating band extending downward to its bifurcation into the iliac vessels (Fig. 11.**103**). In a transverse abdominal scan, the aorta and inferior vena cava appear as round, echo-free areas just anterior to the spine (1) (Fig. 11.**104**).

Intercostal arteries and renal vessels. With color Doppler, the intercostal arteries can be seen arising from the aorta at the level of the ribs (Fig. 11.**105**). The renal vessels can be seen arising from the aorta at a more inferior level (Figs. 11.**106**, 11.**107**).

Extremity vessels. The vessels supplying the upper and lower extremities can be defined with color Doppler (Figs. 11.**108**–11.**113**).

Umbilical arteries. Venous blood is returned to the placenta by the two umbilical arteries. If both umbilical arteries are present, one can be identified on each side of the urinary bladder (Fig. 11.**114**).

Fetal vessels

Fig. 11.**89**   The embryonic circulation at 9 weeks, 4 days demonstrated by color Doppler.

Fig. 11.**90**   Longitudinal scan of the fetus. The umbilical vein (arrow) runs upward to the liver at about a 45° angle. Cephalic presentation.

Fig. 11.**91**   Blood circulation within the fetal liver, anterior aspect. 1 = Umbilical vein, 2 = ductus venosus, 3 = portal sinus, 4 = portal vein, 5 = hepatic sinusoids, 6 = hepatic veins, 7 = inferior vena cava.

Fig. 11.**92**   Color Doppler view of the junction between the umbilical vein (1) and ductus venosus (2). Aorta (3), heart (4). Breech presentation.

Fig. 11.**93**   The liver and hepatic vessels, 22 weeks 6 days. Cephalic presentation, 1st position. Left: umbilical vein (1) and portal sinus (2). Right: right hepatic vein.

Fig. 11.**94**   Descending aorta (1) and inferior vena cava (2), 19 weeks, longitudinal scan.

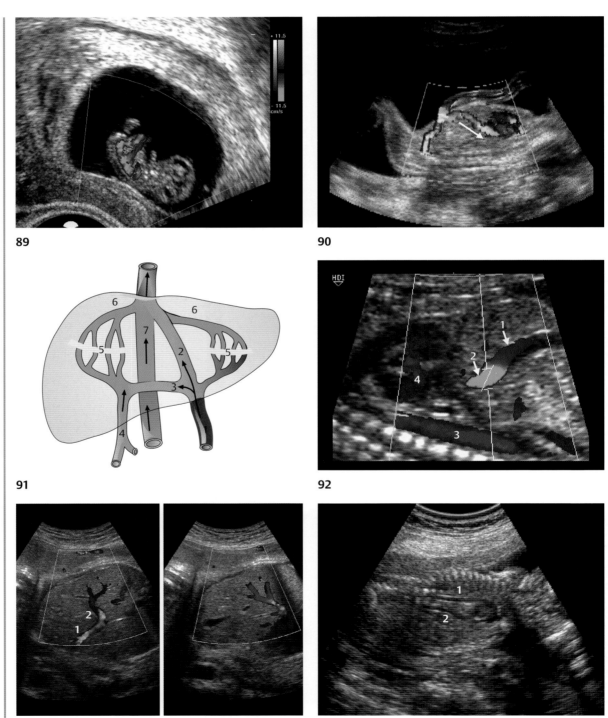

89

90

91

92

93

94

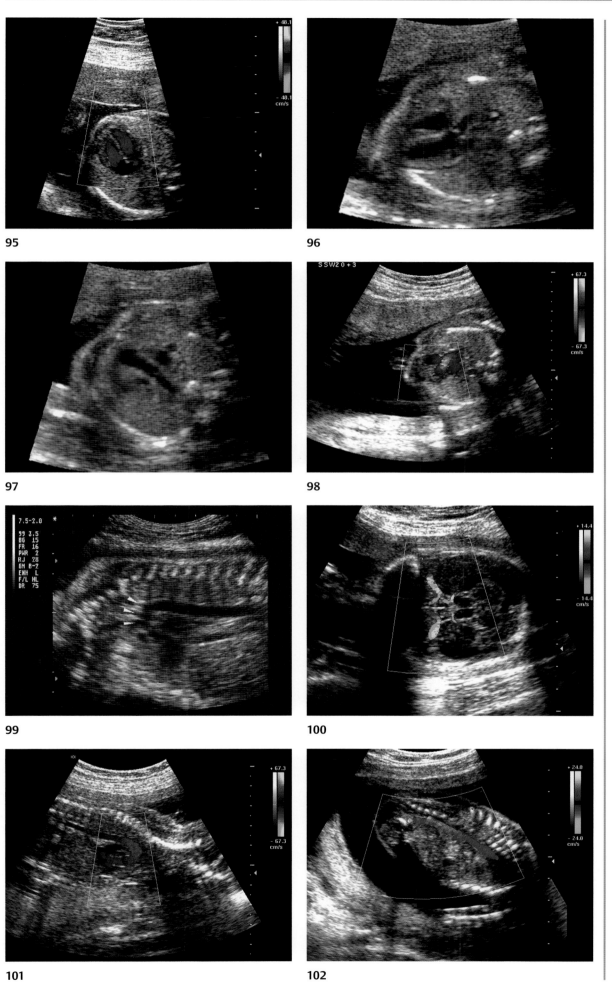

95

96

97

98

99

100

101

102

Fig. 11.**95** Color Doppler four-chamber view showing both ventricles. Breech presentation, 1st position.

Fig. 11.**96** Outflow tract of the aorta from the left ventricle at 23 weeks, 5 days. Cephalic presentation, 1st position.

Fig. 11.**97** Outflow tract of the pulmonary trunk from the right ventricle. Cephalic presentation, 1st position.

Fig. 11.**98** Color Doppler image of the site where the pulmonary trunk crosses the ascending aorta. 20 weeks, 3 days. Cephalic presentation, 1st position.

Fig. 11.**99** Aortic arch with the origins of the brachiocephalic trunk, left common carotid artery, and left subclavian artery (arrows). Breech presentation.

Fig. 11.**100** Color Doppler view of the middle cerebral artery.

Fig. 11.**101** Color Doppler view of the aortic arch and descending aorta. Cephalic presentation.

Fig. 11.**102** Distal portion of the aorta. Cephalic presentation.

Fig. 11.**103**   Bifurcation of the aorta into the iliac vessels (arrow).

Fig. 11.**104**   The descending aorta (1) and inferior vena cava (2) appear in a transverse scan as small, round, hypoechoic areas anterior to the spinal column. Umbilical vein (3), stomach (4). Cephalic presentation, 1st position. 22 weeks.

Fig. 11.**105**   Color Doppler image of the intercostal vessels.

Fig. 11.**106**   Origin of the renal arteries from the aorta. Cephalic presentation.

Fig. 11.**107**   Renal perfusion. Arrows indicate the borders of the kidney.

Fig. 11.**108**   Right axillary artery and vein.

Fig. 11.**109**   The brachial artery in the upper arm.

Fig. 11.**110**   The radial and ulnar arteries in the forearm.

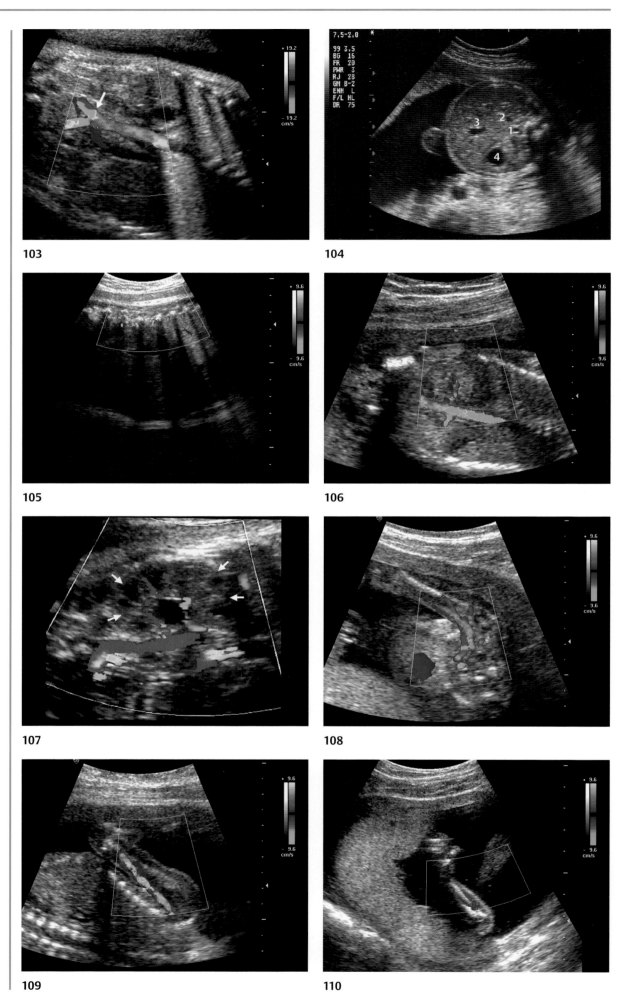

103

104

105

106

107

108

109

110

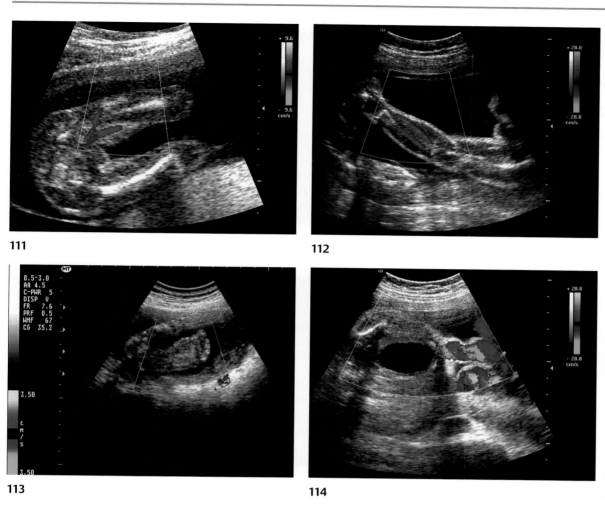

111

112

113

114

Fig. 11.111 Femoral artery and lateral femoral circumflex artery in the right lower extremity.

Fig. 11.112 Posterior tibial artery and peroneal artery in the lower leg.

Fig. 11.113 Left foot with medial plantar artery (plantar view), 27 weeks.

Fig. 11.114 When both umbilical arteries are present, one each can be identified on the right and left sides of the urinary bladder.

Heart

▬ *General Aspects of Fetal Heart Examination*

Indications and Technique

"Fetal heart examination" is a concept that is interpreted differently by different examiners. The spectrum ranges from one extreme, the detection of fetal heart activity ("positive heart activity"), to the other extreme involving the detailed scrutiny of all structures with B-mode and color Doppler, the measurement of all diameters, and a complete blood flow analysis based on Doppler spectra. For most examiners, a fetal cardiac scan consists of obtaining and evaluating a four-chamber B-mode image.

Content of the examination. The content of a fetal heart analysis depends mainly on the indication for the ultrasound examination. Far less is expected from a screening examination than from targeted imaging for fetal cardiac anomalies in high-risk cases (e.g., nonimmune hydrops).

Screening. The basic goal of screening at 20 weeks is to check for normal fetal development while systematically covering the most important fetal structures. In the heart, this means obtaining the four-chamber view and, ideally, evaluating the origin and course of the great vessels. Increasingly it is expected that screening at a level II center will include color Doppler imaging. Extensive biometric analysis and Doppler measurements are rarely necessary in screening and are more time-consuming than productive (4, 7, 8, 9).

Low-risk population. Studies on the systematic examination of the fetal heart have shown that after an initial learning period, the four-chamber view can be successfully defined in more than 90% of cases (25). It is estimated that obtaining the four-chamber view alone in a low-risk population results in a prenatal detection rate of 40% for congenital heart defects, and that this rate is increased to 70% when the great vessels are also scrutinized (21).

High-risk population. When a clear indication for fetal echocardiography exists in a high-risk population (see Chapter 25), an extended workup should be conducted that includes Doppler imaging. Veins, atria, ventricles, and great vessels should be selectively evaluated and cardiac defects excluded. Much greater attention is focused on the heart than in a screening examination. Quantitative and semiquantitative biometric and Doppler measurements are generally obtained and permit a detailed description for the exclusion or confirmation of a cardiac defect. A heart with a (complex) anomaly requires the most detailed scrutiny to provide the information necessary for prenatal follow-up and neonatal care.

Methods of examination. The various methods available for examining the fetal heart are covered in the sections below, and the techniques are described. The basic examination consists of B-mode images in various planes, supplemented by color Doppler imaging. The selective use of M-mode scanning will also be discussed along with Doppler spectral acquisition to evaluate blood flow in specific cardiac regions. Reference charts for various biometric and Doppler parameters are provided to help interpret the examination and distinguish between normal and pathologic findings (see Chapter 12). The basis for an optimum examination, however, is not a knowledge of cardiac anatomy and scan planes but the use of optimum equipment settings.

Imagers, Transducers, and Settings

Cine loop. Among the equipment features that are essential for fetal echocardiography are high B-mode resolution, zooming, an M-mode function, pulsed Doppler, and color-flow Doppler. Due to the high fetal heart rate (120–180 bpm), the system should also have a cine loop option for better evaluation of cardiac anatomy. With cine loop, the last 50–70 images can be stored in the system and retrieved for a detailed, frame-by-frame review.

Transducer. While linear and sector probes and convex arrays are all suitable for fetal echocardiography, most examiners prefer sector and convex probes because they are easier to handle. Transducers with high operating frequencies should be used. A 5.0-MHz probe can be used up to 25 weeks' gestation. In cases of maternal obesity (sound attenuation), polyhydramnios (heart deeper than 8 cm), or an occipitoanterior fetus in late pregnancy (rib shadows), a 3.5-MHz probe is more suitable for cardiac examinations.

The heart can be scanned transvaginally until about 15 weeks' gestation using probe frequencies of 5–7.5 MHz. Doppler flowmetry (spectral or color Doppler) requires lower Doppler frequencies in the range of 3.5–5.0 MHz. This permits the use of a higher pulse repetition frequency (q.v.), making it possible to record higher velocities.

Cardiac preset. If fetal echocardiography is performed frequently, it is advisable to store a "cardiac preset" (Table 11.**1**) that optimally matches the B-mode and Doppler functions and permits rapid switching from the general examination to a cardiac scan.

B-Mode Evaluation: Scan Planes in Fetal Echocardiography

Pediatric echocardiography. The scan planes used in pediatric echocardiography are based on the recommendations of the American Society of Echocardiography (22). These planes are imaged from the anterior side, allow for little flexibility, and are subject to the traditional limits imposed by the ribs and aerated lung. The nomenclature includes subcostal, apical, parasternal, and suprasternal transducer sites with long-axis, short-axis and four-chamber views.

Fetal echocardiography. In the fetus, the heart can be scanned from numerous sites because the lungs are not aerated and the ribs are not ossified. Indeed, these "flexible" planes are necessary because of continual fetal movements. As a result, examiners should not be limited to the classic echocardiographic planes but should develop their own planes that are both flexible and useful for fetal diagnosis (2, 12). Scan planes that are appropriate for the special requirements of fetal echocardiography (2) are illustrated in Figs. 11.**115**–11.**119**.

Four-chamber plane. The four-chamber plane is the basic cardiac screening plane, and adjacent transverse planes are visualized by shifting the transducer from the basic plane. If the fetus changes position during the examination, the four-chamber view can be reacquired as a basis for systematically continuing the examination (see Fig. 11.**121**).

Table 11.**1**   Requirements for optimum B-mode fetal cardiac examination

> Relatively high transducer frequency (e.g., 5.0 MHz)
> Hard image setting:
>   • Small dynamic range
>   • Hard contrast
>   • No smoothing
> Zoom feature
> Only one focal zone
> If available: narrow sector and high frame rate

All the subsequent planes are easily located even by a noncardiologist and, in our experience, provide maximum accuracy in the detection of malformations.

Systematic Analysis of Cardiac Structures: the Segmental Approach

Complexity of cardiac defects. During embryonic development, the heart undergoes a number of rotations, septations, and connections over a period of several weeks, explaining the complexity and variability of many cardiac defects. For example, complex cardiac defects can result from connection anomalies that may be associated with disturbances of lateralization. As a result, a number of cardiac anomalies feature not only septal defects or obstructed valves but also an anomalous connection of the cardiac chambers or vessels.

Three basic segments. To bring order into the classification of congenital heart disease, the pathologist van Praagh (26) proposed the "segmental approach," which was later expanded by other authors. In this system the three basic segments of the heart—the atria, the ventricles, and the great arteries near the heart—are identified according to anatomic criteria, and their connections and relationships to one another are analyzed. The individual cardiac structures have characteristic morphologic features and specific connections that are defined primarily on the basis of pathoanatomic and angiographic criteria.

Atria. The atria are recognized by the characteristic shape of their appendages, by the fossa ovalis of the right atrium, and by the entry of the systemic veins into the right atrium and the pulmonary veins into the left atrium. The valve of the septum primum (the "valve" of the foramen ovale) can be seen pulsating in the left atrium.

Ventricles. The right and left ventricles are distinguished by several features including their trabeculation, their atrioventricular valves, and their relationship to the semilunar valve of the artery arising from the ventricle.

Aorta and pulmonary trunk. The aorta and pulmonary trunk are easily distinguished by noting that while the aorta supplies the coronary arteries and systemic circulation (arterial trunks and descending aorta), the pulmonary trunk gives origin to the pulmonary arteries.

Visceroatrial situs. A segmental analysis of the heart involves checking the connections between the different segments. The atrial situs is determined first, since the atria and viscera are almost always on the same side of the body—i.e., atrial situs generally coincides with visceral situs. The visceroatrial situs—which may be normal (situs solitus), laterally transposed (situs inversus), or without sidedness (situs ambiguus)—is essential for making a diagnosis when abnormalities of rotation are present.

Atrioventricular and ventriculoarterial concordance. Next, atrioventricular concordance is assessed by determining whether the morphologic right (left) atrium is connected to the morphologic right (left) ventricle. Ventriculoarterial concordance is then checked by noting whether the right ventricle is connected to the pulmonary trunk and the left ventricle to the aorta. A D-transposition of the great vessels, for example, is defined as atrioventricular concordance with ventriculoarterial discordance.

Anatomic forms of cardiac structures. This approach, initially favored by pathologists, was later adopted for diagnostic imaging. Huhta et al. (23) introduced a segmental approach to echocardiography, but their system lacks many of the typical criteria. Also, many criteria cannot be evaluated in the fetus due to the minuscule size of the structures. We shall therefore examine the typical anatomic forms of the various cardiac structures as a supplement to analyzing the heart in the different planes of section.

Plane of the Upper Abdomen (Plane 0)

Visualization

Pathologists usually distinguish the right and left atria by evaluating the atrial appendages, but this method cannot be used with ultrasound. Knowing that the location of the abdominal organs, especially the inferior vena cava, correlates with the location of the atria, we can evaluate the atria by conducting a systematic analysis of the fetal upper abdomen (Table 11.**2**). Once the fetal position has been determined and the fetal spine located, the upper abdomen is scanned transversely at the level of the stomach and liver (Fig. 11.**120**).

Evaluation

The abdomen is divided into two halves by an imaginary anteroposterior line.

Left half (Fig. 11.**120**). This half contains the stomach, spleen, left hepatic border, and the descending aorta just anterior to the spine. The spleen can be identified between the border of the stomach and the ribs, but this is not important in fetal diagnosis because the definition of asplenia syndrome or polysplenia syndrome is no longer based on imaging the spleen (which cannot be done reliably) but on the visceroatrial situs.

Right half (Fig. 11.**120**). This half of the abdomen contains the liver and gallbladder (right), the umbilical vein (central, to the left of the gallbladder), and the star-shaped confluence of the hepatic veins toward the inferior vena cava. The latter structure is located anterior and to the right of the descending aorta. The hepatic veins and inferior vena cava open jointly into the right atrium.

After the abdominal situs has been evaluated, the transducer is angled cephalad to show the four-chamber view. The differential diagnosis of abnormalities in the upper abdomen is reviewed in Table 25.**6**.

Four-Chamber View (Plane 1)

Visualization (Figs. 11.115, 11.119, 11.121–123)

The four-chamber view lies in an anteroposterior plane that is directed obliquely upward. In the fetus, a four-chamber view can be obtained not just from the apical aspect but also from the right or left side of the chest and even from the dorsal aspect. In all cases an oblique plane is required to provide an optimum view. The advantage of the four-chamber plane is that it simultaneously depicts both atria, both ventricles, both atrioventricular valves, the interventricular and interatrial septum, and the foramen ovale between the septa (Fig. 11.**122**). The entrance of the pulmonary veins into the left atrium can also be seen in many cases. Cardiac defects that may be detected in this plane are listed in Table 11.**3**.

Table 11.**2** Checklist for evaluating the upper abdomen

> ➤ Full stomach on the left side
> ➤ Liver on the right side
> ➤ Aorta to the left of the spine
> ➤ Inferior vena cava to the right of the spine, anterior and to the right of the aorta

Scan planes in fetal echocardiography

Fig. 11.**115** The heart is examined in multiple planes. The basis is the four-chamber view, from which the other planes are derived.

Plane 1: Axial four-chamber view. This is the principal plane for evaluating the fetal heart (cf. Fig. 11.**122**).

Plane 2: From the four-chamber plane, the probe is angled slightly upward to define the origin of the aorta from the left ventricle (the long-axis or "five-chamber view") (cf. Fig. 11.**126**).

Plane 3: Angling the probe farther cephalad from plane 2 depicts the pulmonary trunk arising from the right ventricle, crossing the aorta at right angles. This plane gives a cross-sectional view of the ascending aorta and superior vena cava to the right of the pulmonary trunk (cf. Fig. 11.**127**) (from [2]).

Fig. 11.**116** Starting from the four-chamber view, the probe is moved cephalad to a parallel plane that will define the great vessels in the upper thorax.

Plane 4: From left to right, this axial plane crosses the pulmonary trunk, ascending aorta, and superior vena cava in the anterior thoracic cavity. It cuts across the descending aorta anterior to the spine.

Plane 5 is imaged by angling the probe upward from plane 4. In this view the ascending aorta and pulmonary trunk (from plane 4) pass simultaneously to the descending aorta on the left side of the spine, giving a tangential view of the pulmonary trunk and ductus arteriosus on one side and the aortic arch and aortic isthmus on the other side (cf. Fig. 11.**128**) (from [2]).

Fig. 11.**117** Plane 6 is a longitudinal scan, positioned here to define the aortic arch. The origins of the brachiocephalic vessels can be seen (cf. Figs. 11.**130** and 11.**142**).

Fig. 11.**118** The standard planes in pediatric and adult echocardiography besides the four- and two-chamber views are the parasagittal view (plane 7) and the short-axis view (plane 8). Plane 7 depicts the left ventricular inflow tract with the left atrium, mitral valve, and ventricle and the left ventricular outflow tract with the left ventricle, aortic valve, and aorta. The short-axis view (plane 8) is at the level of the aortic valve, perpendicular to the parasagittal plane. It shows the structures surrounding the aorta: the right ventricular inflow tract with the right atrium, tricuspid valve, and right

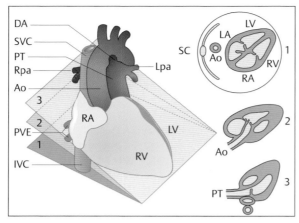

115

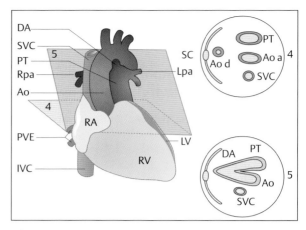

116

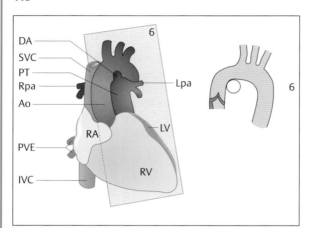

117

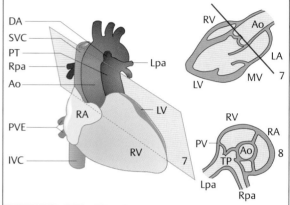

118

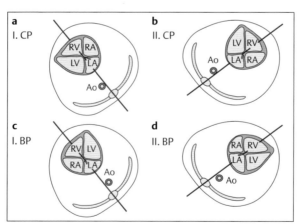

119

Abbreviations:

Ao	Aorta
BP	Breech presentation
CP	Cephalic presentation
DA	Ductus arteriosus
IVC	Inferior vena cava
LA	Left atrium
Lpa	Left pulmonary artery
LV	Left ventricle
MV	Mitral valve
PT	Pulmonary trunk
PV	Pulmonary valve
PVE	Pulmonary veins
RA	Right atrium
Rpa	Right pulmonary artery
RV	Right ventricle
SC	Spinal column
SVC	Superior vena cava

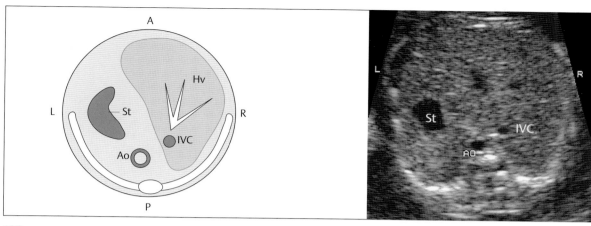

120

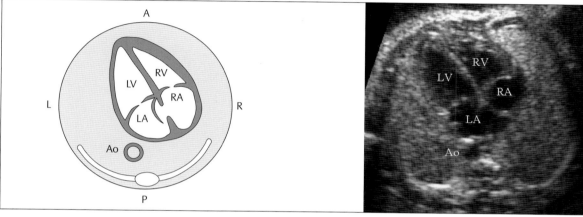

121

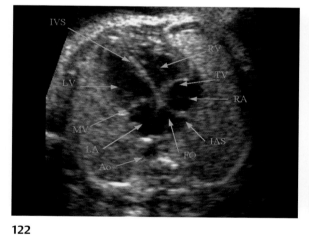

122

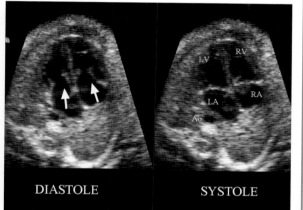

DIASTOLE SYSTOLE

123

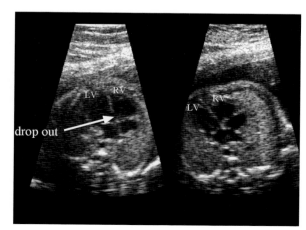

drop out

124

ventricle and the right ventricular out-flow tract with the right ventricle, pulmonary valve, pulmonary trunk, and the division of the pulmonary trunk into the right and left pulmonary arteries (cf. Fig. 11.**129**) (from [2]).

Fig. 11.**119** The four-chamber view can be obtained in various fetal positions: the first and second cephalic positions (a, b) and the first and second breech positions (c, d). Thus, fetal orientation should be determined at the start of the fetal heart examination.

Scan planes 0 to 8

Fig. 11.**120** A fetal cardiac scan starts with evaluation of the upper abdomen. After the fetal position has been determined and the spine located, the left and right sides of the abdomen are identified and provide further orientation. An imaginary line from the spine to the abdominal wall divides the transverse scan of the upper abdomen into two halves. On the left are the stomach (St) and, just anterior to the spine, the abdominal aorta. On the right are the liver with the hepatic veins (Hv) and the inferior vena cava (IVC), which is anterior and to the right of the aorta.

Fig. 11.**121** Apical four-chamber view. The view depicts both atria and ventricles, the interventricular and interatrial septum, and the descending aorta. Much information can be gained from the four-chamber view, and therefore this view should be systematically interpreted with the aid of a checklist. An important advantage of this plane is that it can be visualized in various fetal positions.

Fig. 11.**122** The apical four-chamber view (corresponding to plane 1) demonstrates the right and left ventricles, the right and left atria, the tricuspid and mitral valves, the interventricular septum (IVS), and the foramen ovale (FO) in the interatrial septum (IAS).

Fig. 11.**123** Apical four-chamber view in diastole (atrioventricular valves open) and in systole (valves closed). The cine loop technique permits a detailed analysis of the cardiac phases. Note the valve of the foramen ovale, which is clearly depicted in the scans.

Fig. 11.**124** In apical views of the ventricular septum, the "dropout effect" occurs when the thin membranous part of the septum does not produce an echo. This artifact creates the appearance of a septal defect. When the septum is scanned at a slightly more lateral angle, the continuity of the septum can be seen.

Fig. 11.**125**   "White spot" in the left ventricle. The echogenic papillary muscle is detectable in approximately 2–4% of all pregnancies. Although this phenomenon rarely has hemodynamic significance, the examiner should look for suggestive signs of cardiac and extracardiac anomalies (including chromosomal abnormalities) in targeted imaging.

Fig. 11.**126**   In the "five-chamber view," the origin of the aorta from the left ventricle can be seen in addition to both atria and ventricles. It corresponds to plane 2 in Fig. 11.**115**.

Fig. 11.**127**   Plane 3 shows the origin of the pulmonary trunk (PT) from the right ventricle. The ascending aorta and superior vena cava appear in cross section to the right of the PT.

Fig. 11.**128**   Plane 5 from an apical point of entry. This plane shows the V-shaped confluence of the pulmonary trunk and ductus arteriosus and of the aortic arch and aortic isthmus to the left of the spine. The superior vena cava appears in cross section on the right side. This view is very important in color Doppler studies (see Fig. 11.**116**).

Fig. 11.**129**   In the short-axis view, the aorta is encircled by the right ventricular inflow tract with the right atrium, tricuspid valve, and right ventricle and by the right outflow tract with the right ventricle, pulmonary valve, pulmonary trunk, and the division of the pulmonary trunk into the right pulmonary artery (Rpa) and left pulmonary artery (Lpa) ("circle and sausage" pattern, see drawing in Fig. 11.118).

Fig. 11.**130**   One of the most important longitudinal planes is the aortic arch view showing the origin of the brachiocephalic trunk (1), left common carotid artery (2) and left subclavian artery (3).

Fig. 11.**131**   The termination of the inferior and superior vena cava at the right atrium is evaluated in a longitudinal scan through the right side of the heart. The diaphragm (arrows, D) is seen separating the lung (Lu) from the liver (L).

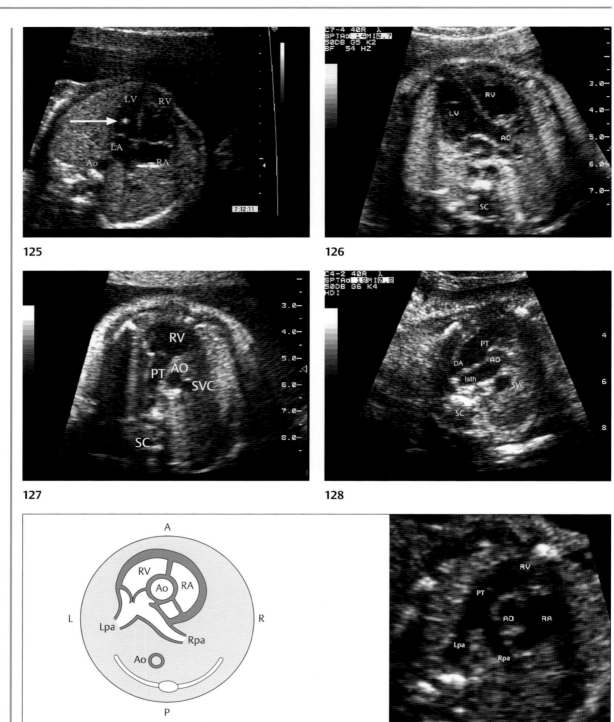

125

126

127

128

129

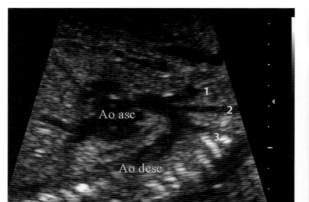

130

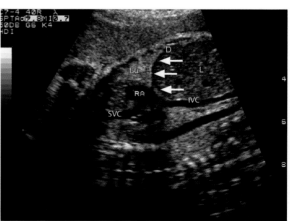

131

General Evaluation

According to recent studies, the four-chamber view does not have a 92% accuracy rate in the detection of congenital heart defects as was first believed (15). Its accuracy is more in the range of 40% (21). A checklist should be followed in interpreting the four-chamber view (Table 11.**4**). At each point in the list, possible or frequent pathologies should be excluded (Tables 25.**7**–25.**10**).

Location of the heart in the chest. The cardiac apex and the stomach should be located on the same (left) side. When an imaginary line is drawn from the spine to the sternum, one-third of the heart should be located in the right half of the chest and two-thirds in the left half.

Cardiac axis. The axis of the heart (direction of the septum) should be tilted toward the left side, forming a 45° angle (± 15°) with the midline.

Size of the heart. The heart occupies approximately one-third of the thoracic cavity. This can be checked by biometry: the CT ratio (ratio of cardiac and thoracic diameters) or CTA ratio (ratio of cardiac and thoracic areas).

Cardiac rhythm. Heart motions are evaluated in the real-time B-mode image.

Contractility. The contractility of the ventricles and atria is evaluated in the real-time B-mode image.

Table 11.**3**   Cardiac abnormalities that can be detected in the four-chamber view

> - Dextrocardia, mesocardia
> - Single ventricle
> - Ebstein anomaly (tricuspid valve dysplasia)
> - Left ventricular hypoplasia or hypertrophy
> - Right ventricular hypoplasia or hypertrophy
> - AV canal
> - Ventricular septal defect (large)
> - Atrial septal defect (large)
> - Coarctation of the aorta
> - Persistent left superior vena cava
> - Tetralogy of Fallot, double outlet ventricle or truncus arteriosus (only with large VSD in four-chamber view)
> - Anomalous pulmonary venous drainage*
> - Myocardial hypertrophy (due to various causes)
> - Pericardial effusion
> - Arrhythmias
> - Cardiac tumors
> - Ectopia cordis
> - Cardiomegaly (various causes)
> - Cardiomyopathy

* Detectable in some cases in the four-chamber view

Table 11.**4**   Checklist for interpreting the four-chamber view

> - Cardiac position in the chest and cardiac axis 45°
> - Size of the heart
> - Rhythm
> - Contractility
> - Size of left and right atrium
> - Size of let and right ventricle
> - Position and function of tricuspid and mitral valves
> - Continuity of interventricular septum
> - Position and form of interatrial septum or valve of foramen ovale
> - Normal termination of pulmonary veins

Evaluation of Specific Structures

Descending aorta. The descending aorta appears in cross section just to the left of the spine (Fig. 11.**121**). In front of the aorta is the left atrium. The (dilated) esophagus can sometimes be seen between them.

Left atrium. The valve of the foramen ovale (septum primum) can usually be seen beating in the left atrium. The valve appears as a line in an apical scan and often appears semicircular in a lateral scan. The pulmonary veins open into the left atrium. The left atrium opens into the left ventricle in the direction of the cardiac apex.

Left ventricle. This chamber has an elongated oval shape. Three morphologic characteristics distinguish it from the right ventricle:
- The lumen extends to the cardiac apex.
- There is no typical trabeculation of the myocardium (see Fig. 11.**125**).
- The mitral valve is at a more basal level than the tricuspid valve.

Right atrium. The left atrium communicates with the right atrium through the foramen ovale. The right atrium appears larger than the left atrium, and it does not contain a foramen ovale valve. Just inferior to the right atrium and close to the interatrial septum is the termination of the inferior vena cava (eustachian valve), which appears as a rounded vessel. The right atrium opens into the right ventricle in the direction of the cardiac apex.

Right ventricle. This ventricle has a somewhat rounded shape and is distinguished from the left ventricle by five characteristics:
- It is situated closer to the sternum.
- It contains prominent trabeculae.
- Its lumen does not extend to the cardiac apex like that of the left ventricle.
- The tricuspid valve is at a more apical level than the mitral valve.
- Between the cardiac apex and tricuspid valve is a thick papillary muscle (the moderator band), which is best seen in a lateral projection when the atrioventricular (AV) valve is closed.

Mitral valve and tricuspid valve. The anterior and posterior cusps of the mitral valve and the anterior and (postero)septal cusps of the tricuspid valve can be seen simultaneously, situated between the atria and ventricles. The tricuspid valve (right) and mitral valve (left) insert on the interventricular septum. The tricuspid valve insertion is located slightly closer to the apex than the mitral valve insertion.

Ventricular septum. The ventricular septum displays a narrow V shape in cross-section, with its broad apical attachment tapering to the attachment of the atrioventricular valves. The septum is best evaluated in a lateral scan, which can demonstrate its true thickness (2–4 mm) and its continuity (compare Fig. 11.**124** with Fig. 11.**122**).

Atrial septum. The atrial septum is interrupted centrally by the foramen ovale. The valve of the foramen ovale (septum primum) beats within the left atrium (Fig. 11.**123**).

Pulmonary veins. When the left atrium is closely scrutinized, the sites of entry of the pulmonary veins can often be seen. In most cases, the right pulmonary veins are clearly visualized in a basal view.

Pericardium. The pericardium is often visible as a thin border. A faint fluid crescent at the level of the AV plane is a normal finding and should not be misinterpreted as effusion.

Origin of the Aorta (Plane 2) and Pulmonary Trunk (Plane 3)

Visualization (Figs. 11.115, 11.116, 11.127)

Planes 2 and 3 are useful for evaluating ventriculoarterial concordance. **Five-chamber view.** The transducer is angled slightly more cephalad from the four-chamber view, pivoting at the apex, until the aorta is seen arising from the left ventricle (Fig. 11.**115**). This plane is also called the "five-chamber view" (Fig. 11.**126**).

Pulmonary trunk. The transducer is tilted slightly more cephalad from the previous plane to define the pulmonary trunk (Fig. 11.**115**). Attention is given to its connections with the right ventricle and descending aorta. The pulmonary trunk in this plane runs from the right ventricle toward the fetal spine (Fig. 11.**127**). It communicates with the ascending aorta via the ductus arteriosus. The pulmonary trunk appears on the left side of the image in this plane. Just to the right of the trunk is the central portion of the aortic arch. Farther to the right, the superior vena cava is displayed in cross section (Fig. 11.**127**).

Evaluation (Table 11.5)

Ventriculoarterial concordance. In planes 2 and 3, the examiner can check to see whether the aorta arises from the left ventricle and the pulmonary artery from the right ventricle and whether the aorta and pulmonary artery are perpendicular to each other.

Vascular caliber. The fetal pulmonary trunk has a larger caliber than the aorta. A discrepancy may signify hypoplasia of one vessel (e.g., in valvular atresia) or dilatation of the other.

Septoaortic continuity. The five-chamber view is excellent for assessing the continuity of the ventricular septum with the aorta to exclude most perimembranous ventricular septal defects and possible dextroposition of the aorta ("riding aorta").

Transverse and Tangential Scans of the Great Vessels and Superior Vena Cava (Planes 4 and 5)

Visualization (Fig. 11.116)

The transducer is shifted cephalad from its position in the four-chamber view to obtain a transverse view of the upper thorax (plane IV, Fig. 11.**116**). From this plane, the transducer is angled toward the fetal head (plane V) to obtain a tangential view of the aortic arch and aortic isthmus (right posterior) and the pulmonary trunk communicating with the aorta via the ductus arteriosus. In this plane, the pulmonary trunk and aorta form a V whose apex points toward the left lateral chest wall (Fig. 11.**128**). The superior vena cava is visualized in cross section to the right, and the trachea, with its echogenic border, is seen anteriorly in cross section.

Evaluation (Table 11.6)

Evaluation of the great vessels. These planes supplement planes 2 and 3 by demonstrating the great vessels. The examiner evaluates the posi-

Table 11.5 Checklist for evaluating the origins of the great vessels (planes 2 and 3)

> Normal site of origin
> Crossing of the vessels
> Compare calibers of both vessels
> Evaluate aortic and pulmonary valves
> Check continuity of ventricular septum

Table 11.6 Checklist for evaluating the great vessels (planes 4 and 5)

> Normal course and caliber of the great vessels and superior vena cava
> Evaluate aortic isthmus and ductus arteriosus
> Check for atypical vessels (e.g., persistent left superior vena cava)

tion of the vessels to check for transposition or malposition and also evaluates the vascular calibers, giving special attention to the aortic isthmus and ductus arteriosus. The great vessel plane is of major importance in color Doppler imaging (q.v.). If a (fourth) vessel is found just to the left of the pulmonary trunk, it may represent a persistent left superior vena cava (see Fig. 25.**48**), which is often present in complex cardiac defects or rotational anomalies.

Color Doppler. The great vessel plane is of key importance in color Doppler because blood flow through the aorta and pulmonary trunk should be of the same color (see Fig. 11.**143**). If there is a severe obstruction of the left or right ventricular outflow tract, retrograde flow will be found in the aorta or pulmonary trunk. This is helpful in detecting malformations of the aortic arch such as tubular hypoplasia, severe coarctation, or a discontinuity of the aortic arch. Also, plane V is excellent for evaluating the ductus arteriosus (e.g., for premature constriction of the duct) and detecting a right-sided aortic arch (trachea located to the left of the vessels or between the aorta and pulmonary trunk).

Longitudinal Scan Planes

The longitudinal scan planes are part of a complete examination of the fetal heart.

Right atrium. A sagittal scan through the right atrium can confirm normal termination of the superior and inferior vena cava at the right atrium (see Fig. 11.**131**). Angling the transducer slightly toward the fetal right side will demonstrate the umbilical vein, ductus venosus, and hepatic vein and their entry into the right atrium.

Aortic arch. An anteroposterior, paravertebral scan plane is tilted slightly to the left to obtain a parasagittal view of the aortic arch (Fig. 11.**117**). All three of the main vascular trunks—the brachiocephalic trunk, common carotid artery, and left subclavian artery—should be visualized (Fig. 11.**130**). This is most easily accomplished when the fetus is in an occipitoanterior lie.

Pulmonary trunk. The pulmonary trunk can be visualized in parasagittal section to the left of the aortic arch plane (16) (Fig. 11.**129**). It is identified by its junction with the ductus arteriosus, which enters the descending aorta. This is the optimum scan plane for Doppler flowmetry of the ductus arteriosus.

Conclusion

The complicated anatomy of the heart and the diversity of possible congenital heart defects make it difficult for examiners not trained in echocardiography to conduct an adequate evaluation of the fetal heart. While examination of the four-chamber view alone is relatively simple and can provide a large amount of information quickly, a complete and accurate evaluation requires a more systemic approach. Of course, all planes cannot be visualized in one sitting in every fetus. But it is important for examiners to know the various planes and the information they provide so that, when the fetus changes its position during the examination, they can reacquire orientation and locate the optimum planes. With this degree of flexibility, even less experienced examiners can achieve good results.

Biometry of the Fetal Heart

Cardiac dimensions. Biometric studies of the fetal heart can be very time-consuming and therefore are not performed in screening examinations. But fetal echocardiography involves more than just examining the four-chamber view or the origin of the great vessels. It includes the assessment of cardiac dimensions. Although an experienced examiner can visually evaluate the size of the heart, the cardiac chambers, the great vessels, and the interrelationships of the various structures, it is essential that reference charts be used whenever an apparent abnormality is found (see Chapter 12). Thus, measurements of the cardiac dimensions (e.g., length and width) are a part the "extended" biometry that should be performed in the investigation of fetal anomalies, intrauterine growth retardation, etc.

Screening for anomalies. While cardiac biometry is used mainly in screening for congenital heart disease, it can also be helpful in the diagnosis of pulmonary hypoplasia in cases of oligo- or anhydramnios or in fetuses with skeletal dysplasias, for example. It should be emphasized that dimensions that fall within normal limits do not necessarily exclude a cardiac defect, and that abnormal dimensions do not always correlate with a structural anomaly but may have a functional etiology.

Measurements in the B-mode image. The literature contains a large amount of biometric data on the heart, and some of these parameters are easily measured even by examiners not experienced in fetal echocardiography. In earlier studies, M-mode tracings were used to obtain biometric data on the fetal heart. But increasingly, M-mode scanning is becoming less important for biometric measurements in fetal echocardiography and is being superseded by B-mode imaging. Our current technique for fetal cardiac biometry consists of B-mode measurements in the four-chamber view, supplemented by the five-chamber view or pulmonary trunk view for measuring vascular diameters.

CT ratio. The cardiothoracic (CT) ratio is used to evaluate the size of the heart in relation to the thoracic cavity, as in cases of cardiomegaly or suspected pulmonary hypoplasia. Vascular diameters are measured at end systole, when the semilunar valve is closed. The caliber of the pulmonary valve is 1.2 times that of the aortic valve.

Table 11.**7** lists the abnormalities that should be considered when biometric parameters are found to be outside the normal range.

Spectral Doppler Echocardiography

Hemodynamics. The spectral Doppler examination permits a direct analysis of blood flow across the various cardiac valves and into the surrounding vessels. So besides evaluating morphologic features in the B-mode image, the examiner can also explore fetal intracardiac hemodynamics. Some of the data consist of absolute values such as flow velocities, stroke volumes, and cardiac output. But spectral Doppler can also provide blood flow ratios to assess the diastolic function of the atrioventricular valves (Tables 11.**8**, 11.**9**). The advent of color Doppler has made it easier to use spectral Doppler: first the region of interest is located in the color Doppler flow image, and then the sample volume is positioned at the desired site for recording Doppler spectra (Fig. 11.**132**).

Quantification of blood flow. The main advantage of spectral Doppler is its ability to quantify blood flow, providing a more valid basis for comparing data and monitoring changes in longitudinal follow-ups.

Aliasing. The main disadvantage of pulsed Doppler is the occurrence of aliasing at high velocities (e.g., due to valvular insufficiency or stenosis). Continuous-wave (CW) Doppler must be used for accurate quantification.

Applications. Pulsed Doppler echocardiography has been used for some years to investigate the cardiac valves (3). Additional applications have been devised in recent years, especially since the advent of color Doppler ultrasound. They include examination of the inferior (and su-

Table 11.**7** Signs of possible abnormalities in fetal cardiac biometry

Cardiac structure	Sign	Possible abnormalities
Aorta	Dilated	Tetralogy of Fallot, common trunk, pulmonary atresia with ventricular septal defect, Marfan syndrome, double outlet right ventricle, AV block
	Narrow	Aortic stenosis, aortic atresia, coarctation of aorta
Pulmonary trunk	Dilated	Hypoplastic left heart syndrome (compensatory), absent pulmonary valve, Marfan syndrome, AV block
	Narrow	Pulmonary atresia, pulmonary stenosis
Left ventricle	Dilated	Endocardial fibroelastosis, critical aortic stenosis, left ventricular aneurysm, aortic atresia with open mitral valve, dilated cardiomyopathy
	Narrow	Hypoplastic left heart syndrome, coarctation of aorta, mitral atresia with ventricular septal defect
Right ventricle	Dilated	Ebstein anomaly, dysplasia of tricuspid valve, pulmonary atresia, pulmonary stenosis, Uhl anomaly, dilated cardiomyopathy
	Narrow	Pulmonary atresia, pulmonary stenosis, tricuspid atresia with ventricular septal defect
Cardiac width	Dilated	All defects with tricuspid insufficiency, Ebstein anomaly, dysplasia of tricuspid valve, endocardial fibroelastosis, AV canal, cardiomyopathy, coarctation of aorta, AV block, tachycardia, heart failure
	Narrow	Intrathoracic compression (e.g., due to diaphragmatic defect), laryngeal atresia, cystic malformation of lung

Table 11.**8** Requirements for optimum pulsed spectral Doppler

> The beam–vessel angle should be as small as possible (0–15 °).
> The sample volume should be as narrow as possible (1–2 mm wide).
> A high-pass filter (between 150 and 200 Hz) should be used for examining valves.

Table 11.**9** Parameters that are evaluated in intracardiac Doppler echocardiography

Absolute velocities
> V_{max}
> $V_{diast.v}$ (end-diastolic)
> V_{max} in diastole

Absolute times
> Time to peak velocity
> Ejection time (e.g., duration of systole)

Calculation of areas, integrals, and volumes
> Mean velocity (cm/s)
> Time–velocity integral (cm)
> Stroke volume (SV) = TVI x vascular area x d2/4 (mL)
> Cardiac output (CO) = SV x heart rate (mL/min)

Ratios
> E/A for AV valves
> Pulsatility index
> Preload index and other venous indices

perior) vena cava, ductus arteriosus, pulmonary arteries and veins, and the foramen ovale region.

Doppler Measurements of Atrioventricular Valve Flow

Visualization. The atrioventricular valves are best visualized in the apical or basal four-chamber view. A narrow sample volume is selected (1–2 mm width of Doppler gate) and positioned in the ventricle just distal to the tricuspid or mitral valve (Fig. 11.**132**). If valve regurgitation is detected, the sample volume is placed more proximally in the adjacent atrium.

Two-peak configuration. The Doppler spectrum of flow across the AV valves in sinus rhythm typically shows two diastolic peaks (Fig. 11.**132**). The first peak, called the E peak, reflects passive blood flow from the atrium into the ventricle during early diastole. The second peak, called the A peak, is produced by atrial contraction at the end of diastole (9). The waveform of the mitral valve is often distinguishable from the tricuspid valve waveform by the reverse flow current to the aorta (3, 9). In contrast to the postnatal period, the A peak in the fetus is higher than the E peak, probably due to the stiffness of the myocardial wall.

Measurements of Semilunar Valve Flow

Visualization. Flow across the aortic valve is best measured in the apical five-chamber view, with the sample volume placed just distal to the valve (Fig. 11.**133**) (8). This plane allows for a beam–vessel angle < 15°.

Flow in the pulmonary trunk can be measured in the short-axis view or pulmonary trunk view, as we have described elsewhere (8). The use of color Doppler makes it considerably easier to position the sample volume (Fig. 11.**133**).

Parameters. The envelope curve of the Doppler spectrum is similar for both vessels, usually showing higher peaks and a sharper down slope in the aorta than in the pulmonary trunk. The peak and mean velocities, time-to-peak velocity, etc. can be measured over both vessels, and the stroke volumes and cardiac output can be determined when the vessel diameters and heart rate are known. The ratio of the stroke volumes of the right and left ventricles is 1.3 : 1, consistent with the fetal right ventricular dominance that has been documented in laboratory animal and Doppler studies.

Measurements in the Ductus Arteriosus

High blood flow velocity. The ductus arteriosus connects the pulmonary trunk to the descending aorta. It is a curved vessel whose diameter is slightly greater than that of the pulmonary trunk from which it arises but slightly less than that of the aorta to which it connects. This arrangement increases the blood flow velocity across the ductus arteriosus, and the highest flow velocities in the fetus are recorded in that vessel. The spectral waveform of the ductus arteriosus is distinguished by a typical high peak velocity (80–140 cm/s) in the second half of pregnancy, by a relatively long time to peak velocity (reaching Vmax almost at mid-systole), and by the typical diastolic peaks that follow a postsystolic notch (Fig. 11.**134**). The pulsatility index is normally greater than 2.

Visualization. The ductus arteriosus is visualized either in a longitudinal scan of the right ventricular outflow tract RV–PT–DA (right ventricle, pulmonary trunk, ductus arteriosus) or in scan plane V (Fig. 11.**116**). Color Doppler should be used in positioning the Doppler gate, since the best spectrum is obtained at the site where high velocities occur.

Measurements in the Inferior Vena Cava

Visualization. The inferior vena cava is best visualized in a longitudinal scan near the heart, or it may be scanned proximal to the termination of the ductus venosus (Fig. 11.**135**).

Three-peak configuration. While it is known that Doppler-recorded flow in the venous system normally shows a continuous spectrum, the veins about the heart are an exception. They are influenced by pressures that are transmitted to them from the atria during systole and diastole. As a result, the Doppler waveform of the inferior vena cava in sinus rhythm is characterized by three peaks labeled S, D, and A (Fig. 11.**136**). The first peak is caused by antegrade flow filling the atria during ventricular systole ("S"). It is followed by additional antegrade flow in early diastole ("D") that passively fills the ventricles after the AV valves have opened. This phase correlates with the E peak of the AV valves (see above). It is followed by atrial contraction ("A"), which correlates with the A peak of the AV valves. This third phase may not be evident in the Doppler spectrum of the inferior vena cava, or often it may appear as a small, retrograde peak.

Measurements in the Pulmonary Arteries

Visualization. For optimum Doppler examination, the right or left pulmonary artery should be scanned in a plane in which the vessels are parallel to the beam. As we have suggested elsewhere (10), the examination can be made more systematic by distinguishing three types of fetal position: fetal anterior side toward the maternal abdominal wall (i.e., facing the transducer) (type 1), fetal right side toward the maternal abdominal wall (type 2), and fetal left side toward the maternal abdominal wall (type 3). In these positions we found that the right and left pulmonary arteries could be optimally scanned (at a low angle) for Doppler interrogation, and we were able to record a spectrum from at least one artery in 88% of cases.

Typical Doppler waveform. Like the other cardiac structures, the pulmonary arteries display a typical Doppler waveform (13). The spectrum varies with the sampling site: the waveform recorded in the main stem of a pulmonary artery differs from that recorded in a peripheral branch (11). The Doppler waveform (13) is characterized by a sharp rise to peak velocity (Vmax) in early systole. After the Vmax peak, the velocity falls slightly to a second midsystolic peak. The end of systole is marked by a notch, which may fall below the baseline in the main stem. Next comes a period of low flow throughout diastole (Fig. 11.**137**), probably due to the windkessel function of the pulmonary trunk. The Doppler spectrum of the peripheral pulmonary arteries basically resembles that of the main stems but has lower peak velocities with a typical narrow systolic peak and a flat, uniform diastole.

Flow velocities. Flow in the main stem of the right pulmonary artery attains a peak velocity of 60 cm/s in the 20th week of gestation and reaches values up to 95 cm/s at term. The acceleration time (AT) in the right pulmonary artery is approximately 20–40 ms in the second half of pregnancy (11). During this period the AT is 30–50 ms over the pulmonary valve and 55–75 ms in the ductus arteriosus. The pulsatility index (PI) is diminished in the central and peripheral pulmonary arteries, presumably due to the vascular changes in the fetal pulmonary circulation. The potential clinical role of pulmonary Doppler is currently being investigated.

Measurements in the Pulmonary Veins

Visualization. The two right pulmonary veins terminate close to the septum primum and are best demonstrated by color Doppler in a plane between the four-chamber and five-chamber views from the apical or

Spectral Doppler echocardiography

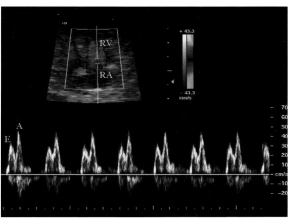

132

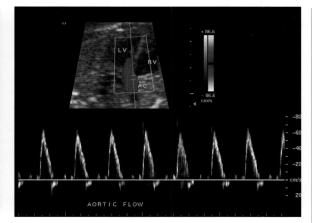

133

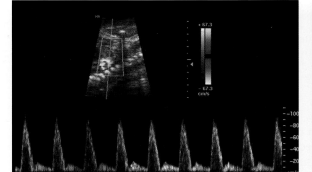

134

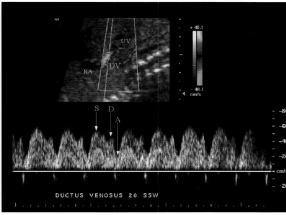

135

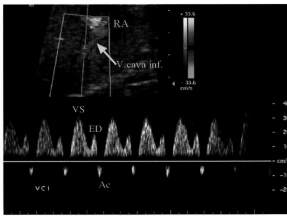

136

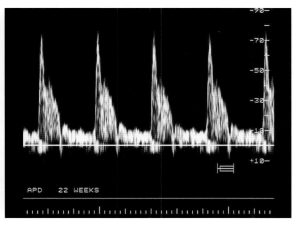

137

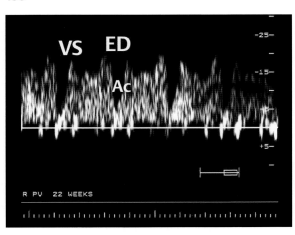

138

Fig. 11.**132** Doppler spectrum of the tricuspid valve (angle between AV perfusion and Doppler line < 10°). The Doppler waveform over the AV valves shows a characteristic two-peak configuration: early diastolic flow (E peak) and late diastolic flow produced by atrial contraction (A peak).

Fig. 11.**133** Doppler spectrum of the aortic valve at 26 weeks. The sample volume has been placed just distal to the aortic valve. Typical systolic Doppler spectrum with a sharp upstroke and downstroke (spectrum inverted). Vmax is 65 cm/s.

Fig. 11.**134** Doppler spectrum of the ductus arteriosus under normal conditions shows typical systolic peaks with intervals of diastolic flow. Vmax is 140 cm/s.

Fig. 11.**135** Doppler spectrum of the ductus venosus at 20 weeks shows the antegrade S, D and A waves that are typical of the veins around the heart.

Fig. 11.**136** Doppler spectrum of the inferior vena cava at 29 weeks shows typical antegrade S and D waves (VS = ventricular systole, ED = early diastole) and a small retrograde A wave (AC = atrial contraction) (explanation in text).

Fig. 11.**137** Doppler spectrum sampled from the main stem of a pulmonary artery (here: the right pulmonary artery) at 22 weeks.

Fig. 11.**138** The normal spectrum of a pulmonary vein at 26 weeks. Typical pulsatile waveform with three peaks: VS = ventricular systole, ED = early diastole, AC = atrial contraction.

basal aspect. They are most easily visualized when the fetal spine is down. Often only one of the two veins can be identified, usually the one that runs in line with the septum (Fig. 11.**141**). The left pulmonary veins open into the left atrium directly opposite the foramen ovale, so they are best visualized in a lateral plane. Again, the vein that enters the left atrium at a right angle is the easiest to define. In B-mode, however, it is easy to mistake a tapering pulmonary artery for a pulmonary vein. If doubt exists in a targeted examination, color Doppler can identify the veins by confirming their direct connection to the left atrium.

Three-peak configuration. The Doppler spectrum of the fetal pulmonary veins, like that of the other veins about the heart (superior and inferior vena cava, hepatic veins, ductus venosus), has a pulsatile waveform with three peaks designated S, D, and A (1). The spectrum of the pulmonary veins is most similar to that of the ductus venosus, showing antegrade flow throughout the cardiac cycle (Fig. 11.**138**). Animal studies and direct pressure measurements in humans have shown that postnatal pulmonary venous flow reflects the pressure changes in the left atrium during heart activity. The first peak occurs during ventricular systole (S). The Doppler waveform then shows a second peak during passive ventricular filling in early diastole (D). This diastolic peak reflects the relaxation of the left ventricle. During subsequent atrial contraction (A), the pressure in the left atrium rises against the closed valve of the foramen ovale. Meanwhile, flow in the pulmonary veins decreases slightly (A wave) but remains in the positive range.

Color Doppler Echocardiography

Basic Technical Principles

Principle. Color Doppler is used to map the temporal and spatial distribution of intracardiac blood flow. Its principle is based on the color-encoding of Doppler signals. Its technology can be described as "multigated pulsed Doppler," so it is actually an extension of the conventional pulsed system (18). The Doppler-shifted frequencies are measured in numerous (invisible) sample volumes distributed along the Doppler beam, and the instantaneous mean velocities are electronically calculated from those measurements. The velocities are then displayed as color-encoded pixels superimposed on the two-dimensional real-time image (5, 6, 17).

Role. Although fetal echocardiography was not introduced until the late 1980s, it has quickly gained an established place in prenatal diagnosis and has become a component of every fetal echocardiographic

Table 11.**10** Guidelines for optimum color Doppler examination of the fetal heart

Equipment settings
➤ Match the pulse repetition frequency (PRF, velocity scale) to the region: high for AV and semilunar valves (40 and 120 cm/s), low for veins (10–30 cm/s)
➤ Use a high refresh rate: persistence and smoothing should be reduced to a minimum
➤ Match the color filter and color sensitivity to the region: high filter and low sensitivity for most valves, low filter and high sensitivity for slow-flow regions like the pulmonary veins
➤ Set a higher line count and frame rate
➤ Increase color resolution at the expense of the B-mode image

Technique
➤ Use the highest possible frame rate: real-time image or narrow "box" setting in color Doppler mode
➤ Survey anatomy: start by analyzing cardiac anatomy in the B-mode image
➤ For an optimum color Doppler signal, use a beam–vessel angle close to 0° or 180° (e.g., scan the AV valves from the apex or base)
➤ Use zoom and cine loop functions as needed

Table 11.**11** Interpretation of the color Doppler image

➤ Blood flow **toward** the transducer (positive Doppler shift) is encoded in **red**
➤ Blood flow **away from** the transducer (negative Doppler shift) is encoded in **blue**
➤ **Turbulence** is indicated by green mixed with the red or blue. This creates a "mosaic pattern" that includes turquoise (blue + green) for negative Doppler shifts and yellow (red + green) for positive Doppler shifts. If the variance is not adjusted on the color scale, turbulence appears as aliasing
➤ The registered **velocities** are proportional to the **brightness levels**: as the velocity increases, the color becomes brighter (bright red or bright blue)
➤ Higher velocities that exceed the set velocity scale appear as **aliasing** (see below)

Table 11.**12** Types of information furnished by color Doppler in fetal echocardiography

➤ Detection of blood flow through structures (e.g., the perfusion of a hypoplastic ventricle, visualization of the pulmonary veins)
➤ Detection of blood flow direction (antegrade or retrograde) (e.g., in the great vessels)
➤ Detection of shunts and jets (e.g., in ventricular septal defects)
➤ Detection or confirmation of valvular stenosis or regurgitation based on the presence of turbulence
➤ Optimum valve localization for spectral Doppler interrogation

examination. In many ways, color Doppler imaging has become easier to use than spectral Doppler (18). It provides an immediate, general hemodynamic survey that conveys information quickly, making it possible to answer key diagnostic questions within a short time (17).

Procedure. The examiner must have a specific question to address if color Doppler is to furnish an optimum answer. If the imaged flows are to be quantified as well, spectral Doppler must be added. In these cases the color-flow image is helpful in positioning the sample volume to interrogate a specific area of interest. Important prerequisites in working with color Doppler, besides a knowledge of its basic physical principles, include optimum programming of the equipment (preset) (Table 11.**10**) and optimum visualization of the cardiac structure(s) of interest. The interpretation of color Doppler images and the principal types of information supplied in fetal echocardiography are reviewed in Tables 11.**11** and 11.**12**.

Aliasing

In color Doppler and in pulsed spectral Doppler, aliasing can occur at high velocities when the registered blood flow exceeds the set velocity range (5).

Prevention of aliasing. There are several ways to prevent aliasing:
- Know the range of the velocities that are to be sampled and set the pulse repetition frequency (PRF) accordingly: a high PRF for rapid flows (e.g., across the aortic valve, pulmonary valve, or ductus arteriosus), a low PRF for slow flows (pulmonary veins or inferior vena cava).
- Since PRF is influenced by tissue depth, use a lower-frequency transducer (1.5 or 3.5 MHz instead of 5 MHz).
- Lower the baseline and increase the velocity range to display flow in a single direction.

Color Doppler Evaluation of the Normal Fetal Heart

Color Doppler examination of the fetal heart is similar to B-mode and employs the same scan planes. Since Doppler is being used, the examiner should keep the beam at a low angle relative to the target vessel.

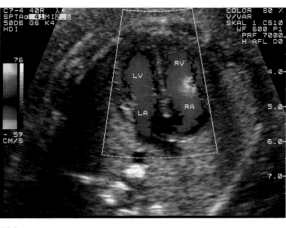

139

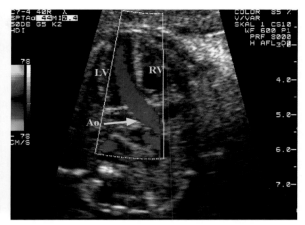

140

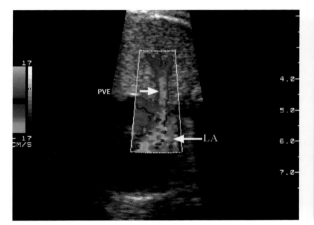

141

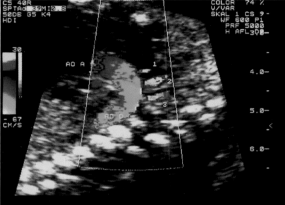

142

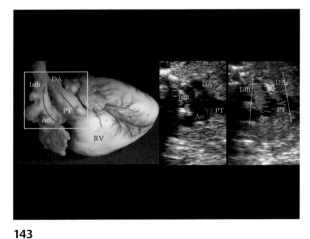

143

Color Doppler echocardiography

Fig. 11.**139** In the apical four-chamber view, diastolic blood flow is encoded in red (= flow toward the transducer), with clear separation of the right and left ventricular inflow tracts by the intact interventricular septum.

Fig. 11.**140** Apical five-chamber color Doppler view in systole demonstrates blood flow from the left ventricle across the aortic valve into the ascending aorta (blue = flow away from the transducer) (28 weeks).

Fig. 11.**141** Basal color Doppler view of the heart. The normal termination of a pulmonary vein is clearly visualized at this angle.

Fig. 11.**142** Ascending and descending aorta in an anterior longitudinal scan of the aortic arch at 30 weeks. As the blood is flowing away from the transducer, it is encoded in blue. Three arterial trunks arise in typical fashion from the aortic arch: the brachiocephalic trunk (1), left common carotid artery (2), and left subclavian artery (3). Blood entering these vessels flows toward the transducer, so it is encoded in red.

Fig. 11.**143** Three-vessel color Doppler view (plane 5 in Fig. 11.116) in a 23-week fetus. The left panel shows an anatomic view of the aorta and aortic isthmus, pulmonary trunk, and ductus arteriosus. In a fetus lying with the left side of the chest toward the transducer (center image), the great vessels are scanned tangentially and show a typical V-shaped pattern similar to that in the photo at left. The blood in both vessels is flowing toward the descending aorta, so both vessels are encoded in red (image at right).

Upper abdomen. In the segmental analysis of the upper abdomen, the aorta (left) can be distinguished from the inferior vena cava (right) by the contrasting colors of the different flow directions, provided an acceptable beam–vessel angle is maintained. Scanning the liver from the anterior side and angling the transducer cephalad will give an excellent color view of the hepatic veins draining into the inferior vena cava. A longitudinal scan can define the course of the umbilical veins through the liver, their junction with the ductus venosus, and the termination of the ductus at the inferior vena cava. The ductus venosus is distinguished from the other vessels by its higher blood flow velocities (brighter colors). The entry of the superior and inferior vena cava into the right atrium is easily evaluated in the longitudinal scan.

Four-chamber view. The apical or basal four-chamber view of the heart with color Doppler is the best view for assessing diastolic flow across the atrioventricular valves (Figs. 11.**139**, 11.**148**). It demonstrates the separate flows from the atria into the right and left ventricles, with both inflow tracts clearly separated by the interventricular septum. In the atria, color Doppler can demonstrate the physiologic right-to-left shunt through the patent foramen ovale, and in some circumstances (low PRF) it will show the normal drainage of the pulmonary veins into the left atrium (Fig. 11.**141**).

Five-chamber view. The transducer can be tilted cephalad from the apical four-chamber view to visualize the aortic root in the "five-chamber view." With color Doppler, the left ventricular inflow and outflow tracts can be simultaneously evaluated in this plane. Flow from the left ventricle into the aorta is observed during systole (Fig. 11.**140**), while blood encoded in the opposite color flows from the left atrium into the ventricle during diastole. This view not only permits the assessment of normal flow across the aortic valve but also demonstrates the continuity of the ventricular septum in the subaortic pars membranacea (ventricular septal defect?) with the aortic root (riding aorta?).

Origin of pulmonary trunk and short-axis view. From the five-chamber view, the transducer is angled further cephalad to define the origin of the pulmonary trunk, or the plane can be rotated to obtain the short-axis view (Fig. 11.**129**). The short-axis plane is best for evaluating flow in the right ventricular outflow tract across the pulmonary valve during systole (11).

Three-vessel view. Parallel and cephalad to the four-chamber view, this plane depicts the pulmonary trunk (left), aorta (center), and superior vena cava (right).

Course of the aortic arch and pulmonary trunk. The transducer is angled slightly more cephalad from the three-vessel view to define the course of the aortic arch, pulmonary trunk, and ductus arteriosus (Fig. 11.**143**). If there is an anomaly involving the great vessels, this plane will often show a distinct abnormality consisting of a marked caliber discrepancy between the aorta and pulmonary trunk, the nonvisualization of one vessel, or a color pattern indicating turbulence or retrograde flow due to valvular stenosis or atresia (6). In late pregnancy (approximately 33 weeks or later), it is common to find a mosaic pattern of turbulent flow at the ductus arteriosus due to initial narrowing in preparation for postnatal closure.

The aortic arch can be imaged in a longitudinal parasagittal scan to the left of the fetal spine. The origins of the three supraaortic vessels are easily identified in the color flow image (Fig. 11.**142**).

The color Doppler findings in various cardiac defects are explained in Chapter 25.

▬ *M-Mode Scanning (Time Motion)*

M-Mode Echocardiography

Principle. Because a fetal echocardiogram is difficult to record, the M-mode technique is used to record mechanical cardiac events and draw inferences about the electrical signals that have caused them. M-mode scanning was introduced into echocardiography many years ago, long before the advent of B-mode cardiac imaging. It could not be used in the fetus until high-resolution B-mode was available for accurately positioning the M-mode cursor so that the tracings could be assigned to specific structures.

Applications. M-mode has myriad uses, but its main applications are in cardiology. It is the optimum modality for taking fetal cardiac measurements such as septal and myocardial thickness, measuring the various luminal diameters in systole and diastole, evaluating the function of the atrioventricular valves, measuring the diameters of the aortic and pulmonary valves, and even assessing the patency of the foramen ovale. To obtain accurate measurements and findings, certain scan planes must be adhered to (perpendicular angle between the M-mode cursor and cardiac long axis). M-mode tracings cannot be precisely correlated with the cardiac cycle, however, due to the lack of a concomitant fetal electrocardiography (ECG) trace. M-mode is an effective tool for detecting and documenting reduced myocardial contractility, as in endocardial fibroelastosis or cardiomyopathy. It is also the best technique for analyzing fetal arrhythmias. When the cursor is directed simultaneously through an atrium and ventricle (Figs. 11.**144**, 11.**145**), fetal dysrhythmias can be accurately classified.

In fetal echocardiography, the M-mode evaluation of cardiac functions and dimensions has become less important in recent years owing to the availability of Doppler imaging and cine loop analysis. It is still an essential modality, however, in the diagnosis and differential diagnosis of arrhythmias.

M-Mode Color Doppler Echocardiography

Principle. In conventional M-mode echocardiography, the movements of structures along an examiner-placed M-mode cursor are traced as a function of time. This permits cardiac contractions to be imaged with a high degree of temporal resolution. If color flow is also switched on when the cursor has been optimally positioned, the hemodynamic changes that accompany the mechanical contractions will be displayed in color along the designated line (Fig. 11.**146**) (19).

Applications. This technique, known also as color-coded M-mode echocardiography, is useful for analyzing atrioventricular conduction in the diagnosis of arrhythmias and for the temporal analysis of hemodynamic events at incompetent AV valves, for example, to evaluate both the timing and duration of valvular insufficiency. Another application is in analyzing the temporal relationship of the systolic and diastolic phases in physiologic shunts (foramen ovale) and pathologic shunts (VSD, ASD II) in the fetus. Although little has been reported in the literature on the use of this method in fetal echocardiography, experienced examiners have found it to be an essential tool for selected investigations in fetal cardiology.

▬ *New Diagnostic Methods and Trends in Fetal Echocardiography*

Transvaginal Ultrasound

In the late 1980s, improvements in B-mode resolution and the introduction of color Doppler in transvaginal ultrasound led to the development of transvaginal fetal echocardiography (20).

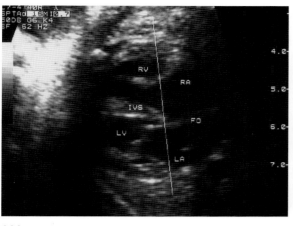

144

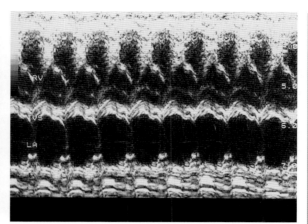

145

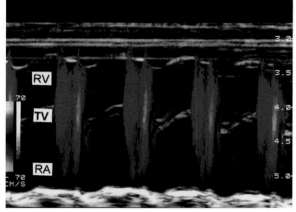

146

M-mode evaluation

Fig. 11.**144** For M-mode echocardiography, the M-mode cursor is positioned under B-mode guidance. Here it is directed through the right ventricle, septum, and left atrium.

Fig. 11.**145** The M-mode tracing records the movements of the corresponding structures as a function of time.

Fig. 11.**146** Color Doppler M-mode at 28 weeks. The M-mode cursor has been placed through the right atrium and right ventricle across the tricuspid valve. Perfusion and length of diastole are normal, and the valve is competent during systole.

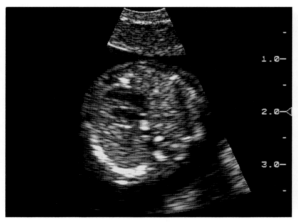

147

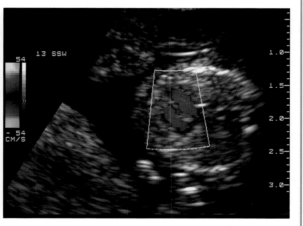

148

Transvaginal fetal echocardiography

Fig. 11.**147** Four-chamber view in B-mode at 13 weeks. The atria, ventricles, and interventricular septum are clearly visualized.

Fig. 11.**148** Four-chamber view at 13 weeks. Color Doppler demonstrates the separate diastolic perfusion of both ventricles.

Fig. 11.**149** Short-axis color Doppler view at 12 weeks, 4 days demonstrates the aorta in cross section, the pulmonary trunk (PT), the right pulmonary artery (Rpa), and the ductus arteriosus (DA).

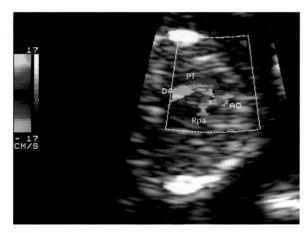

149

Diagnostic capabilities. With the ability to use a higher transducer frequency (better resolution) and shorter coupling path (proximity of the transducer to the object of interest), transvaginal ultrasound can be used even in early pregnancy to define fetal cardiac structures and check for normal hemodynamics (color Doppler). The examination is performed between 12 and 16 weeks' gestation. By 13–14 weeks, it is always possible to conduct a complete analysis of cardiac anatomy with B-mode and color Doppler imaging. Four-chamber anatomy can be optimally evaluated (Figs. 11.**147**, 11.**148**), and color Doppler can be used to define the origins and crossings of the great vessels (Fig. 11.**149**). Even at this early stage, it is possible to detect complex cardiac defects. But because this early examination is costly and time-consuming, it is reserved for high-risk cases (especially those with a positive history), cases where a fetal abnormality has been noted (e.g., nuchal edema, bradycardia, omphalocele), or cases with a high maternal risk (diabetes mellitus, drug use, maternal age).

Limitations. Despite the reliability of an early diagnosis, transvaginal ultrasound also has its limitations. First, the capabilities of the examination are limited by an unfavorable fetal position or an unfavorable beam angle, due in part to the limited maneuverability of the rigid probe. Second, the heart is still very small at this stage, and small defects are easily overlooked (cardiac width is approximately 5 mm at 12 weeks, 6 mm at 13 weeks, and 7.5 mm at 14 weeks!). Another major drawback of the method is the fact that a number of "congenital" heart defects are not yet fully developed at this stage, particularly defects that involve outflow tract obstructions (ventricular hypoplasia or hypertrophy, hypoplasia of a major vessel). It is recommended, therefore, that a second follow-up examination (transabdominal) be scheduled at 20 weeks to reevaluate cardiac anatomy. We caution the less experienced examiner against making a hasty diagnosis and drawing hasty conclusions.

Outlook. Besides permitting the early diagnosis of cardiac abnormalities, fetal transvaginal echocardiography will yield new insights on the intrauterine "in vivo" development of the various cardiac defects and shed light on new pathogenic aspects of fetal hemodynamics.

Power Color Doppler

Principle. Power color Doppler (PCD, power Doppler) is a new method in vascular diagnosis that employs a different means of processing the displaying the Doppler signals than in color Doppler. Instead of analyzing flow signals for positive or negative Doppler shifts, PCD evaluates their amplitudes independently of their direction.

Advantages and disadvantages. The main advantages of PCD are its ability to detect slow flow (in small vessels) and especially its lack of

angle dependence, enabling it to visualize flows independently of the beam–vessel angle. The disadvantages are its inability to detect flow direction (arteries and veins are indistinguishable) and the fact that all flows, whether fast or slow, are displayed simultaneously and superimposed over the B-mode image as in color Doppler, except that all flows are encoded in the same color (usually yellow-orange) (14, 24). Thus the image resembles an angiogram, accounting for the alternate term "color power angiography" for this technique. A major drawback of PCD for cardiac scanning is the need to use optimum equipment settings, which requires some experience.

Applications. Although PCD is not designed primarily for fetal cardiac studies, we have found that its selective use can yield important information in many cases (Figs. 11.**150**–11.**152**). Particularly when acoustic conditions are unfavorable because the fetus is lying on its side, PCD can demonstrate the perfusion of two separate ventricles to exclude ventricular hypoplasia or a complete AV canal (Fig. 11.**150**). Since the aorta is usually oriented parallel to the surface in a typical fetal lie (not optimum for color Doppler scanning), PCD can help confirm the continuity of the aortic arch from the heart to the abdomen (Fig. 11.**151**). We have also found that small muscular ventricular septal defects are sometimes easier to detect with PCD. Because flows are displayed independently of the flow velocity, a hypoplastic vessel (e.g., in pulmonary atresia) is clearly imaged adjacent to a different, dilated vessel so that a specific diagnosis can be made.

PCD cannot detect turbulence, valve regurgitation, or retrograde flow. Consequently, its future role may be limited to that of a useful adjunct to color Doppler ultrasound in selected cases.

Three-Dimensional Imaging of the Fetal Heart

The main problem in three-dimensional cardiac imaging is the fourth dimension (time). All of the cardiac structures assume various shapes and positions during one cardiac cycle, and so the unit can generate a 3-D image only as a function of the cardiac phase—i.e., in relation to systole or diastole. In cardiology, these phases can be defined rather precisely by ECG triggering, but at present this method cannot be used in the fetus. Postmortem 3-D examinations have been done in fetuses as well as studies in which M-mode was used to identify the individual cardiac phases. It is reasonable to expect that further developments in this area will be forthcoming.

On some units, PCD can be used to generate a three-dimensional view of the vascular tree without displaying a simultaneous B-mode image (14) (Fig. 11.**153**). This can provide a better appreciation of the position of the vascular tree in space and, in the future, may become a helpful tool in cardiac diagnosis (14) (Fig. 11.**154**).

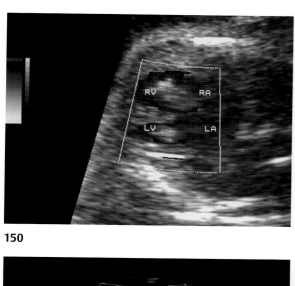

150

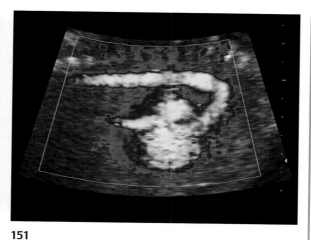

151

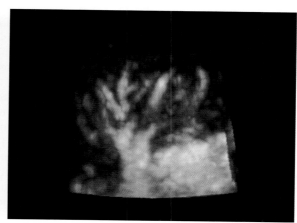

152

153

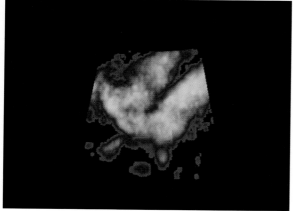

154

Power color Doppler

Fig. 11.**150** The main advantages of PCD are its sensitivity in detecting flows and its insensitivity to beam-vessel angle. It was very difficult to evaluate the fetal heart in this obese patient (9 cm deep!). This lateral scan shows the perfusion of both atrioventricular tracts, sparing the septum. This finding excludes ventricular hypoplasia and large septal defects.

Fig. 11.**151** In this case the aorta runs parallel to the surface and is poorly visualized by color Doppler. With PCD, the descending aorta is defined over its entire length.

Fig. 11.**152** PCD optimally demonstrates the perfusion of both ventricles in this four-chamber view. The termination of the pulmonary veins is also seen.

Fig. 11.**153** Three-dimensional PCD image of the left pulmonary vascular tree in a 27-week fetus. In the future, this method could yield new information on the development of the pulmonary vascular bed.

Fig. 11.**154** Three-dimensional PCD mode in a 29-week fetus demonstrates the heart with both ventricles and the pulmonary veins. The technique of 3-D cardiac power Doppler is still in the developmental stage.

Abdomen

Embryology (1, 3, 5)

Liver. The liver develops as an outgrowth of the embryonic foregut during the fourth month of intrauterine development. The right and left lobes of the liver are originally the same size. But from the sixth week on, the right lobe grows considerably more than the left lobe. The caudate and quadrate lobes are differentiated later in the area of the right hepatic lobe. In the sixth week of embryonic development, hematopoiesis commences in the liver. It is maximal between the 12th and 24th weeks and then gradually declines until term (1).

Gallbladder. The gallbladder develops during the fourth embryonic week as a compact endodermal outgrowth of the hepatic rudiment. The gallbladder is initially on the midline and later migrates laterally (1). Bile production commences between the 13th and 16th weeks (5).

Spleen. The spleen is derived from the mesoderm, developing from the area of the dorsal mesogastrium (1). Erythropoiesis in the spleen ceases in about the 28th week of embryonic development and thereafter occurs in the bone marrow (5).

Pancreas. The pancreas develops during the 5th to 8th week from two epithelial buds of the foregut, one dorsal bud and one ventral endodermal bud. A bipartite pancreatic rudiment may grow around the duodenum (annular pancreas), leading to duodenal obstruction (5). Development of the exocrine pancreas occurs during the 12th week, and insulin synthesis begins in the 20th week (1).

Bowel. The primitive bowel is subdivided into three segments:
- Foregut
- Midgut
- Hindgut

The foregut gives rise to the pharynx, lower respiratory tract, esophagus, stomach, and the duodenum as far as the bile duct orifice.

Structures derived from the midgut are the small intestine except for the upper duodenal segment, the cecum, appendix, ascending colon, and the right half of the transverse colon.

Structures derived from the hindgut are the left half of the transverse colon, the descending colon, the sigmoid colon, the rectum, the upper part of the anal canal, and the inferior portions of the urogenital tract (5).

The anal canal is composed of two rudiments: the upper two-thirds develop from the colon, the lower third from the proctodeum.

Physiologic umbilical hernia. During the rotation of the midgut, the fast-growing small bowel is extruded outside the embryo into the umbilical cord. This "physiologic umbilical hernia" occurs in the sixth week of embryonic development. Following a 270° clockwise rotation of the umbilical cord, the loops of small bowel reenter the body cavity at 10 weeks' gestation (1, 5) (Fig. 11.**155**).

Ultrasound Anatomy

The physiologic umbilical hernia can be observed between 8 and 12 weeks' gestation by transvaginal ultrasound (Fig. 11.**156**). Normally it is no longer detectable by the start of the second trimester. If a protrusion is still seen at that location, an omphalocele should be suspected.

Of the intra-abdominal organs that can be visualized with ultrasound, the most important are the liver with the umbilical vein, the stomach, and the bowel.

Longitudinal Scans

Midsagittal longitudinal scan. The abdominal wall appears in the midsagittal longitudinal scan as a continuous, anteriorly convex line (Fig. 11.**157**) that is interrupted only by the umbilical cord insertion (Fig. 11.**158**).

Parasagittal longitudinal scan. The transducer is shifted to the left to obtain a parasagittal longitudinal scan showing the stomach as a hypoechoic, oblong anteroposterior structure within the abdomen (Fig. 11.**159**).

Transverse Scans

Liver. A transverse scan through the upper abdomen demonstrates the liver, whose large size is commensurate with its function as a blood-forming organ in the fetus. The liver has a relatively homogeneous, moderately echogenic structure (Fig. 11.**160**). The site where the umbilical vein enters the portal sinus can be identified within the liver (Fig. 11.**160**). This site is an important reference point for abdominal biometry (4) (see Chapter 12).

Stomach. The stomach appears in transverse section as a round or oval area, usually devoid of echoes, in the left upper abdomen (Fig. 11.**160**). Stomach contents are occasionally observed, particularly in the third trimester (Fig. 11.**161**). This material consists of vernix flakes that have entered the stomach by swallowing. Wladimiroff et al. (9) studied the filling and emptying times of the fetal stomach. While it generally took less than 45 minutes for the stomach to fill, the gastric emptying times ranged from a few minutes to 45 minutes.

It is important to check the topographic location of the stomach when evaluating fetal anatomy with ultrasound. In transverse scans it appears at various sites on the monitor depending on the fetal position (Fig. 11.**162**).

Gallbladder. Since bile production commences at an early stage, the gallbladder can be recognized as an oblong, fluid-filled organ in the area of the right hepatic lobe as early as the second trimester on a transverse scan angled slightly anteriorly (Fig. 11.**163**). With its oblong shape, it may be confused with the umbilical vein. But in contrast to the umbilical vein, the hypoechoic gallbladder cannot be traced past the boundaries of the liver.

Spleen. The spleen is located obliquely behind the stomach in the transverse scan (7, 8) (Fig. 11.**164**). It is often indistinguishable from the liver, however, because of their similar echogenicities.

Pseudoascites. A hypoechoic space is occasionally seen between the liver and anterior abdominal wall of the fetus (Fig. 11.**165**). Rosenthal et al. (6) called this finding pseudoascites because it mimics early ascites. It may be caused by the abdominal wall muscle (2) or a conspicuous fat layer.

Umbilical cord insertion. The transverse scan plane is shifted slightly caudad to show a cross-sectional view of the umbilical cord insertion (Fig. 11.**166**).

Bowel. The bowel appears in the lower abdomen as a relatively homogeneous, convoluted structure of moderate echogenicity. Especially in late pregnancy, both the small and large bowel may contain scattered fluid-filled areas appearing as elongated hypoechoic zones (Fig. 11.**167**). Fine internal echoes may be seen within some of these fluid-filled areas.

Individual fluid-filled bowel loops are considered a normal finding, especially in the third trimester, and should not be interpreted as intestinal or anal atresia without additional follow-up (Fig. 11.**168**).

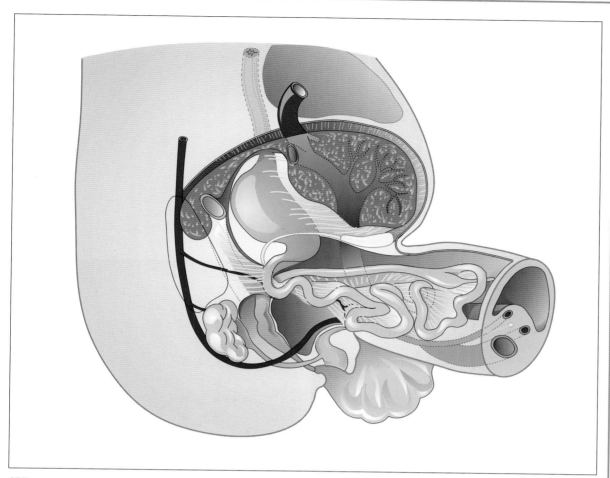

155

Fig. 11.**155**   Diagram of the physiologic umbilical hernia (after [2]).

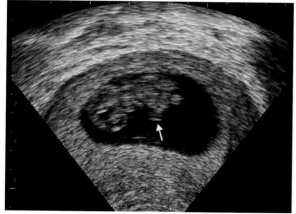

156

Fig. 11.**156**   Sagittal scan of the physiologic umbilical hernia in a 9-week embryo.

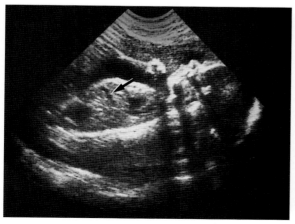

157

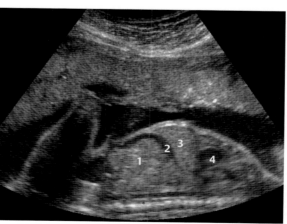

158

Fig. 11.**157**   Longitudinal sagittal scan of a 23-week fetus in a cephalic presentation. The bowel appears as a moderately echogenic structure below the liver and umbilical vein (arrow).

Fig. 11.**158**   Fetal longitudinal scan demonstrates the umbilical cord insertion and the umbilical vein, which runs obliquely upward to the liver at about a 45° angle. Cephalic presentation. Bowel (1), umbilical vein (2), liver (3), heart (4).

Fig. 11.**159**   Longitudinal scan of the stomach at 29 weeks. Cephalic presentation.

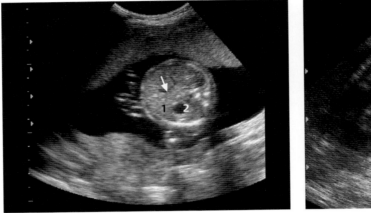

159

Transverse scans

Fig. 11.**160**   Transverse scan through the fetal abdomen. Cephalic presentation, 1st position. 1 = Liver, 2 = stomach, arrow = termination of umbilical vein at portal sinus.

Fig. 11.**161**   Full fetal stomach at 27 weeks.

160

161

Fig. 11.**162**   Position of the stomach in various fetal presentations (photo montage). Transverse scans through the fetal abdomen, 22 weeks.
a Cephalic presentation, 1st position.
b Cephalic presentation, 2nd position.
c Breech presentation, 1st position.
d Breech presentation, 2nd position.

Fig. 11.**163**   Fetal gallbladder (arrow) in a transverse abdominal scan at 22 weeks. Cephalic presentation, 1st position.

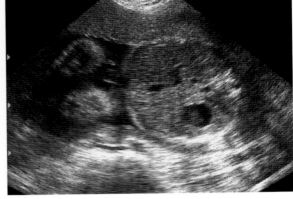

I. CP	II. CP
a	b
I. BP	II. BP
c	d

162

163

Fig. 11.**164**   Spleen (arrow), 3.1 · 1.6 cm, 34 weeks. Cephalic presentation, 2nd position.

Fig. 11.**165**   Pseudoascites (arrow), 25 weeks. Transverse abdominal scan.

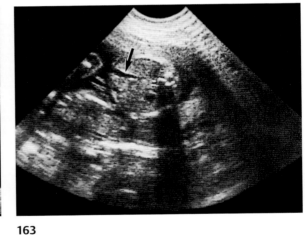

164

165

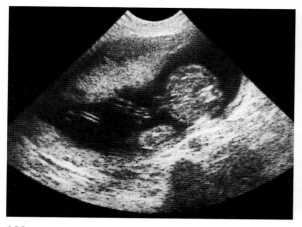

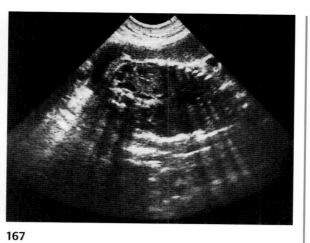

166

167

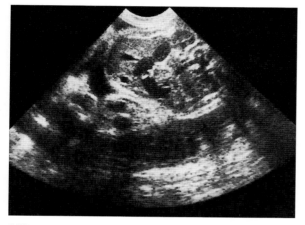

168

Fig. 11.**166** Transverse scan through the fetal abdomen at the level of the umbilical cord insertion, 22 weeks.

Fig. 11.**167** Physiologic fluid collection in the small bowel and colon, 33 weeks. Longitudinal scan.

Fig. 11.**168** Transverse abdominal scan demonstrates the fluid-filled colon at 39 weeks. This does not signify anal atresia!

Urinary Tract, Adrenal Glands, and Pelvis

Embryology

Kidneys. In about the fifth week of embryonic development, the ureteral bud separates from the mesonephric duct and grows dorsally. Its blind extremity penetrates the metanephrogenic blastema, which then condenses around the ureteral bud, forming a kind of capsule. The ureter, renal pelvis, calices, and collecting tubules develop from the stalk of the ureteral bud, while the nephrons differentiate from the metanephrogenic tissue. The glomerular capillaries develop in situ within the Bowman capsule. As early as the 8th week of gestation, urine is formed and excreted into the amniotic cavity (3).

Migration of the kidney. The kidney undergoes a marked change of position during intrauterine development. After developing in the lower pelvis in the fifth embryonic week, it migrates cephalad along the dorsal abdominal wall. By weeks 34 to 36, it has reached the approximate level of the second lumbar vertebra. The renal pelvis, which initially is directed ventrally, later rotates to face medially. The upward migration is complete when the kidney has reached the level of the adrenal gland (3). The vascular supply to the kidneys changes during their migration. The definitive renal arteries do not develop before the ninth embryonic week (7). The constantly changing blood supply of the kidneys during their migration explains why anatomic variations in the renal arteries are relatively common.

Adrenal gland. The adrenal gland develops from two primordia: the medulla from the neuroectoderm and the cortex from the mesoderm (3). The fetal adrenal gland is quite large compared with the kidney as a result of brisk cortical growth. After birth, the adrenal glands rapidly diminish in size, due mainly to regression of the fetal cortex. The adrenal gland loses approximately one-third of its weight during the first 2–3 weeks after birth (7).

Urinary bladder. After the endodermal cloaca has been divided by the urorectal septum into the urogenital sinus and the rectum, the bladder develops from the superior portion of the urogenital sinus.

Pelvic bones. Three ossification centers appear on each side of the cartilaginous pelvis in the third, fourth, and fifth months of embryonic life. The center for the ilium appears first, followed by the center for the ischium and finally the pubis. The centers enlarge at the expense of the cartilage and converge. The three bones do not fuse together until about 20 years of age. At birth, the three ossification centers are still widely separated by cartilaginous plates.

Ultrasound Anatomy

Kidneys

Transverse scan. Under favorable conditions, the retroperitoneal kidneys can be identified in transverse scans as early as 13 weeks' gestation but are not consistently found until 17 weeks. Lawson et al. (5) were able to detect the kidneys in fewer than 50% of cases before 17 weeks (Fig. 11.**169**) but could demonstrate one or both kidneys in 90% of cases between 17 and 22 weeks (Fig. 11.**170**).

Physiologic renal pelvic expansion. Occasionally a slight expansion of the renal pelvis by up to 5 mm in its anteroposterior dimension is noted during the second trimester (Fig. 11.**171**). Usually this represents a physiologic widening of the renal pelvis, but slight bilateral expansion may signify trisomy 21 in rare cases.

Fetal position. On transverse scans, the kidneys are easily identified on both sides of the spine in the occipitoanterior or occipitoposterior fetus (Fig. 11.**172**). A hypoechoic, slit-like lumen in the renal pelvis is a normal finding and does not indicate an outflow obstruction. If the fetus is in a lateral position, the kidney farther from the transducer is obscured by the acoustic shadow of the spine and cannot be evaluated (Fig. 11.**173**).

Paravertebral longitudinal scan. The kidney appears on the paravertebral longitudinal scan as a well-defined oval structure with a hypoechoic parenchymal rim and a more echogenic renal pelvis (Fig. 11.**174**).

Renal size. The kidneys show a linear rate of growth throughout pregnancy (see Chapter 12) (1, 4). The evaluation of renal size should not rely on absolute renal dimensions alone but also on the relationship of kidney size to abdominal growth (4). The ratio of renal circumference to abdominal circumference remains a fairly constant 0.27–0.30 throughout pregnancy (4).

Adrenal Glands

Delineation. The adrenal gland is difficult to distinguish from the kidney, because both have a similar echo pattern and the adrenal gland lies directly on the superior pole of the kidney.

Size. While the adrenal gland is still significantly larger than the kidney in the second month of pregnancy, this relationship gradually changes in favor of the kidney until, at term, the ratio of adrenal weight to renal weight is approximately 1 : 3 (8). On a transverse abdominal scan above the kidneys, the adrenal glands appear adjacent to the spine as elliptical, disk-shaped organs with a hypoechoic cortex and hyperechoic medulla (2) (Fig. 11.**175**).

Bladder and Pelvic Bones

Longitudinal and coronal scans. The fetal bladder can be identified as early as 12 weeks' gestation by transvaginal scanning (Fig. 11.**176**). In the second and third trimesters, it appears on transabdominal sagittal scans as a cystic, echogenic, round-to-oval structure in the lower pelvis, depending on its degree of fullness (Fig. 11.**177**). A coronal scan simultaneously demonstrates the echogenic pelvic bones situated lateral to the bladder (Fig. 11.**178**). The ossified iliac wing is best visualized in an oblique coronal scan (Fig. 11.**179**).

Transverse scan. The bladder appears in the anterior half of the lower pelvis in the transverse scan (Fig. 11.**180**).

Exclusion of anomalies. Because the fetal bladder empties at regular intervals (2), it cannot be seen in every ultrasound examination. If the bladder is still not visualized in one or two follow-up examinations, targeted imaging should be performed to exclude a urinary tract anomaly (e.g., exstrophy of the bladder).

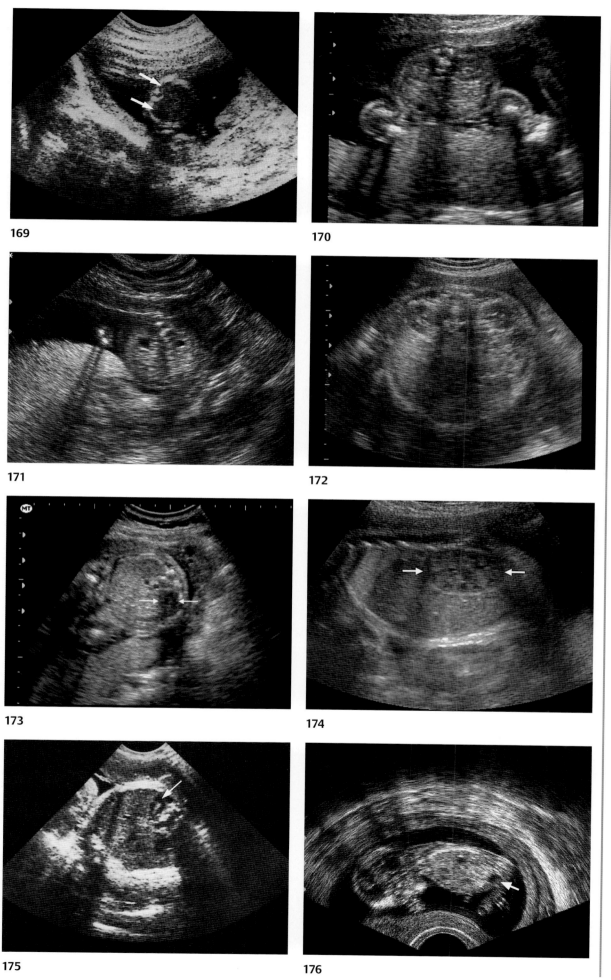

169

170

171

172

173

174

175

176

Kidneys

Fig. 11.**169** Transverse scan of the fetal kidneys (arrow) at 15 weeks.

Fig. 11.**170** Transverse scan of the kidneys in an occipitoanterior fetus at 20 weeks.

Fig. 11.**171** Slight expansion of the fetal pyelocaliceal system in the second trimester.

Fig. 11.**172** Slight, bilateral widening of the pyelocaliceal system at 36 weeks.

Fig. 11.**173** With the fetus in a lateral position, the kidney farther from the transducer (here, the left kidney in a cephalic presentation with the spine to the left) is obscured by shadowing from the spine (arrows), 23 weeks.

Fig. 11.**174** Longitudinal view of the kidney (arrows) at 30 weeks. Note the relatively hypoechoic cortex. The calices appear as echo-free areas.

Adrenal glands and bladder

Fig. 11.**175** Transverse scan of the adrenal gland at 36 weeks demonstrates the hypoechoic cortex and hyperechoic medulla (arrow).

Fig. 11.**176** Fetal bladder in a transvaginal scan (arrow) at 12 weeks.

Fig. 11.**177** Longitudinal sagittal scan of the fetal bladder at 29 weeks.

Fig. 11.**178** Longitudinal coronal scan of the fetal bladder, cephalic presentation, 22 weeks.

Fig. 11.**179** Slightly oblique coronal scan demonstrates the ossified iliac wing (arrow) at 22 weeks, 4 days.

Fig. 11.**180** Transverse scan of the bladder at 24 weeks.

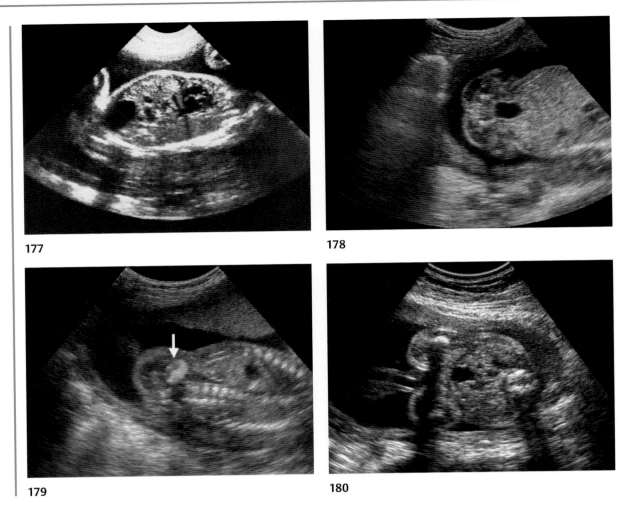

177

178

179

180

Genitalia

Embryology (4, 6, 12)

External genitalia. The early development of the external genitalia is initially the same in both sexes. Differentiation begins in the 9th week of embryonic development and continues until the 12th week (6). Masculinization of the indifferent stage is triggered by androgens produced in the testis. The phallus lengthens to form a penis. If sufficient androgens are not produced, feminization of the genital organs occurs. The initially rapid growth of the phallus gradually slows, and the relatively small clitoris is formed. The scrotal sac is formed by fusion of the genital swellings. The labia minora develop from the genital folds, the labia majora from the genital swellings (6).

Gonads. The ovaries and testes develop from the primordial gonads, which are comprised of a cortex and medulla. The Y chromosome exerts a potent testicularizing effect on the medulla of the indifferent gonad. The absence of a Y chromosome leads to the formation of an ovary. In embryos with an XX chromosome makeup, the cortex normally differentiates into an ovary while the medulla degenerates. Conversely, in embryos with an XY chromosome makeup, the medulla continues to differentiate into a male gonad while the cortical zone degenerates (6).

Genital tract. The development of the genital tract in both sexes begins with the formation of two tubes on each side: the wolffian (mesonephric) duct and the müllerian (paramesonephric) duct. In male embryos, the wolffian ducts differentiate into the male genital tract while development of the müllerian ducts is suppressed. In female embryos, the wolffian ducts degenerate while the müllerian ducts develop into the internal genital organs (7) (Fig. 11.**181**).

By 18 weeks' gestation in the female fetus, a complete uterus has formed and the vagina has a discernible lumen. In the male fetus, descent of the testis commences in the 20th week of gestation. The testis still lies on the posterior abdominal wall at this time (6).

Ultrasound Anatomy

Sex Identification

In most cases, antenatal sex identification is of interest only to the parents. But the ultrasound determination of fetal gender can assume clinical importance in sex-linked hereditary disorders (e.g., Hunter syndrome) and in fetuses with cystic masses of the lower abdomen (e.g., ovarian cyst, peritoneal cyst, prune belly syndrome).

Timing. Reports on the gestational age at which fetal sex can be sonographically determined range from 11 weeks (5) to 12 weeks (7). It is unlikely that sex identification is possible at an earlier stage because the external genitalia of both sexes show the same morphologic development until 11 weeks. After that time, sexual differentiation proceeds at a rapid pace (1). Mielke et al. (5) report an overall fetal sex determination rate of 80.3% between 11 and 16 weeks' gestation. It was found, however, that the sex determination rate depended markedly on gestational age, ranging from just 53% at 11–12 weeks (10 of 19) to 97% at 15–16 weeks (32 of 33).

Natsuyama (7) reported an overall fetal sex determination rate of 97.1% between 12 and 40 weeks. Accuracy rates of 97% (8) to 100% (7) have been reported for sex prediction in male fetuses and 78% (9) to 99.9% (8) in female fetuses.

Several groups of authors have published studies on ultrasound sex determination (3, 8, 9, 10, 13). Most of these studies were done in the middle or late second trimester, however. Bronshtein et al. (2) reported on early sex assignment by transvaginal ultrasound in 1990.

Determining factors. The success of antenatal sex identification depends on several factors:
- The experience of the examiner
- The quality of the ultrasound equipment
- Gestational age
- Fetal position

If the fetus is in a breech presentation with a low-lying rump, is in an occipitoanterior position, has its legs crossed, or if there is a paucity of amniotic fluid, sex identification may not be possible or may require multiple examinations.

Various criteria can be used in the ultrasound differentiation of males and females.

Male Genitalia

In males, the penis and scrotum can be defined separately or simultaneously, depending on the fetal position (Figs. 11.**182**–11.**186**). The testes are definable within the scrotal sac only after descent has occurred, and so usually they cannot be seen until the third trimester (Fig. 11.**185**). If the genitalia are observed with color Doppler for an extended period when the fetal bladder is full, a fluid jet may be seen indicating micturition (Fig. 11.**186**).

Occasionally, the umbilical cord between the legs can mimic the male organ. Color Doppler can quickly resolve any doubts by identifying the two umbilical arteries and the umbilical vein.

Female Genitalia

Labia. In females, the labia majora and minora appear initially as three parallel, echogenic streaks (Fig. 11.**187**). The labia majora become more distinct later in the pregnancy (Fig. 11.**188**). The female gender is most easily identified when the fetus is in an occipitoposterior position with its legs abducted.

Normally the ovaries cannot be detected with prenatal ultrasound because of their small size. Similarly, the uterus is virtually indistinguishable from its surroundings due to its small size and moderate echogenicity.

Differential Diagnostic Criteria

In girls, it should be considered that the phallus-like clitoris can mimic a penis on transverse scans obtained during the second trimester. To aid differentiation, several authors (2, 5) recommend evaluating the direction of the phallus in a longitudinal sagittal scan: the clitoris is directed inferiorly (Fig. 11.**189**) while the penis is directed superiorly (Fig. 11.**183**).

If the labia majora are well developed, they can sometimes be mistaken for a scrotum. This is especially true when the fetus is examined before the testes have descended (11). Differentiation is aided in these cases by tapping the maternal abdomen sharply with the transducer. In males, this will impart a swaying motion to the scrotum.

Development of the genital organs

Fig. 11.**181** Genital development.
a Genital organs in the indifferent bisexual stage.
b Male differentiation of the genital organs.
c Female differentiation of the genital organs.
1 = Kidney, 2 = ureter, 3 = Gonadal/ovarian suspensory ligament, 4 = rete testis/rete ovarii, 5 = efferent ductules/epoophoron, 6 = appendix epididymis/appendix vesicularis, 7 = ductus aberrans inferior, 8 = paradidymis/paroophoron, 9 = wolffian duct (ductus deferens), 10 = muellerian duct/appendix testis (uterine tube), 11 = mesonephros, 12 = urogenital sinus, 13 = inferior gonadal ligament/gubernaculum/uterine round ligament, 14 = uterus, 15 = Gartner's duct, 16 = vagina, 17 = urinary bladder, 18 = Mueller's tubercle/prostatic utricle on seminal colliculus, 19 = orifice of wolffian duct (ejaculatory duct), 20 = prostate, 21 = genital tubercle/penis/clitoris, 22 = opening of urogenital sinus/urethra/urethral orifice, 23 = vaginal orifice, 24 = anus (modified from [12])

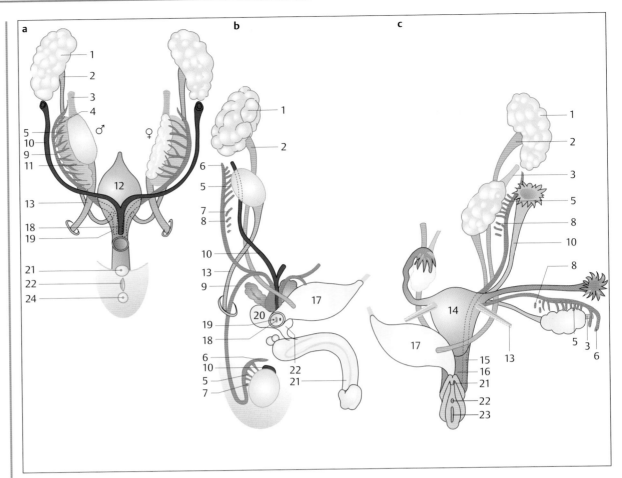

181

Male genitalia

Fig. 11.**182** Penis demonstrated by transvaginal ultrasound at 12 weeks, 3 days. Transverse scan through the fetal pelvis.

Fig. 11.**183** Early demonstration of the penis by abdominal ultrasound at 13 weeks, 4 days. Midsagittal scan. The penis is directed superiorly.

Fig. 11.**184** Longitudinal sagittal scan of male genitalia at 39 weeks.

Fig. 11.**185** Descended testes within the scrotum at 34 weeks.

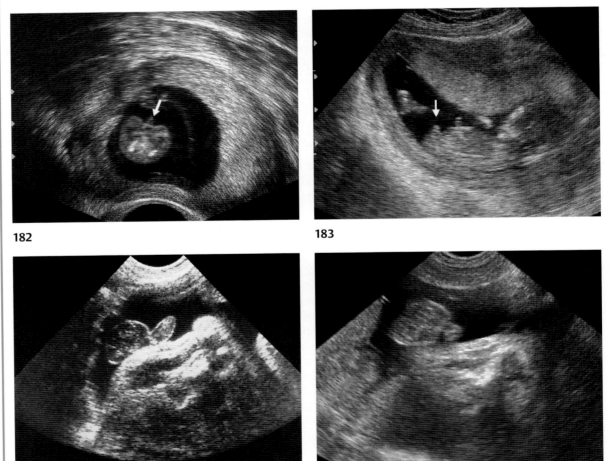

182

183

184

185

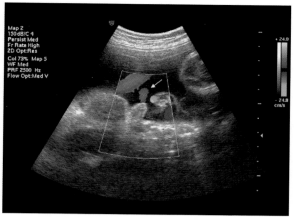

186

Fig. 11.**186** Color Doppler image of the fluid jet caused by fetal micturition (arrow).

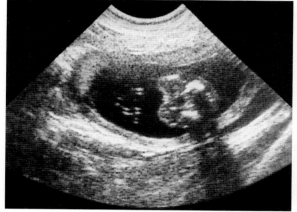

187

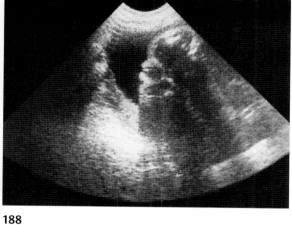

188

Female genitalia

Fig. 11.**187** Female genitalia at 18 weeks. Transverse scan through the fetal pelvis.

Fig. 11.**188** Female genitalia (labia majora and minora) at 32 weeks. Longitudinal coronal scan.

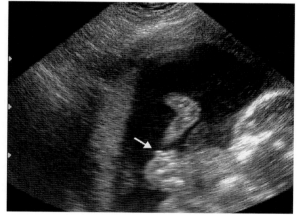

189

Fig. 11.**189** Female genitalia at 17 weeks, 5 days. Longitudinal sagittal scan of a fetus in cephalic presentation. The clitoris is directed inferiorly (arrow), distinguishing it from a penis.

Limbs

Embryology (3, 5, 7, 12)

Limb buds. The upper limb of the human embryo starts to develop at the end of Carnegie stage 12 (about the 26th day of gestation, 3–5 mm) as a bud-like outgrowth from the lateral body wall. The lower limb bud does not appear until stage 13 (28th day, 5.5 mm). During the 6th week (stages 16 and 17), the limb buds show a greater degree of differentiation. The upper portion of the upper limb buds develops into the shoulder, the central portion into the upper arm and forearm, and the lower portion into the hand. Similarly, the hip develops from the upper portion of the lower limb buds, the thigh and lower leg from the central portion, and the foot from the distal portion. On the whole, the lower limb differentiates somewhat later than the upper limb.

Bone tissue. Bone tissue always develops from connective tissue, either directly from the mesenchyma or by the transformation or replacement of cartilaginous tissue.

Membranous ossification. In membranous ossification, mesenchymal connective tissue is transformed directly into bone. An example of membranous ossification is the clavicle, which ossifies during the sixth week of embryonic development.

Enchondral and perichondral ossification. In enchondral ossification, which is the predominant mechanism in the skeleton of the limbs, the bone is first modeled in cartilage and later ossifies.

Two ossification mechanisms occur in the limbs. The small, short bones of the hands and feet ossify entirely through internal ossification (enchondral ossification). This process also occurs in the long tubular bones but is supplemented by perichondral ossification, in which new bone is laid down on the outer surface.

Longitudinal growth. Longitudinal growth of the long tubular bones is sustained by the epiphyseal plate, a narrow zone of cartilage placed between the diaphysis and epiphysis of the bone. The zone of bone formation located within the diaphysis is called the primary diaphyseal ossification center. The diaphyses are mostly ossified at birth, while the epiphyses are still mostly cartilaginous (Fig. 11.**190**). Small, secondary ossification centers develop in the epiphyses after birth, separate from the distal epiphyseal center of the femur (= first epiphyseal center) and the proximal epiphyseal center of the tibia (Fig. 11.**190**). The epiphyseal plate fuses at about 20 years of age, marking the completion of longitudinal growth.

Ultrasound Anatomy

Long tubular bones. After the long fetal limb bones have acquired a primary ossification center in the diaphysis, they can be visualized with ultrasound. Transvaginal scanning can detect the first ossification centers as early as 9 weeks' gestation. The ossified shafts can be measured transvaginally by 9–10 weeks (Fig. 11.**191**).

With transabdominal ultrasound, the ossified shafts of the long limb bones can consistently be detected by 12 weeks' gestation (10, 13) (see Chapter 12).

Cartilaginous epiphyses. The only parts of the long bones in the fetus that are detectable sonographically are the ossified shafts. The cartilaginous ends of the long bones normally are not visible, although high-resolution scanners can often detect the cartilaginous epiphyses, especially in the late second trimester and third trimester. They appear hypoechoic in relation to the echogenic shaft (Fig. 11.**192**).

Determining factors. Ultrasound visualization of the four limbs depends mainly on gestational age and fetal movements. While it is often simple to demonstrate whole fetal limbs in early pregnancy (Figs. 11.**193**, 11.**194**), this is rarely possible in late pregnancy due to the greater lengths and flexed positions of the extremities. If the fetus happens to be stationary, it is not difficult to define the individual segments of the upper and lower limbs. But to visualize the limb segments in an actively moving fetus, the examiner must be able to adjust the scan plane quickly while the limb is moving or when it briefly comes to rest. A large cine loop memory is useful in these cases, as it permits the unhurried analysis of selected limb segments even when they are in motion.

Lower Limb

Femoral shaft. The femur is the easiest limb bone to visualize because the thigh has only a limited range of motion (Figs. 11.**191**–11.**197**). The femur may be found in front of the trunk or in line with it, depending on its degree of flexion or extension. Some degree of bowing may be seen, depending on the relation of the femur to the transducer (11) (Fig. 11.**196**). Bowing is disregarded during the measurement of femur length (see Chapter 12).

Tibia and fibula. If the leg is extended, the tibia and fibula will appear in line with the distal femur. But if the leg is flexed, the scan plane must be adjusted according to the flexion angle at the knee (Figs. 11.**194**, 11.**198**). When imaged concurrently, the tibia and fibula can be distinguished by their position and by the thickness of the ossified portion of the bone. The laterally situated fibula is somewhat shorter and thinner than the tibia and occupies a slightly more distal position (7, 9).

Ossification centers of the distal femur and proximal tibia. The femur and tibia are the only two bones with a secondary ossification center that can be detected sonographically during the third trimester. The distal femoral ossification center (Figs. 11.**190**, 11.**197**) can be identified by 32–33 weeks on average (1, 2, 8) and the proximal tibial ossification center (Fig. 11.**199**) by 36–37 weeks (1, 2).

Foot. The foot may be seen in direct continuity with the lower leg in a sagittal section (Fig. 11.**200**), or it may be viewed from the plantar aspect (Fig. 11.**201**). The plantar view is more rewarding since it defines all five toes, but it can be time-consuming. It is acquired by obtaining a sagittal view of the lower leg and foot and then rotating the transducer 90°. This will give a plantar view of the foot unless angular deformity is present.

Starting at about 22 weeks, the ossification centers in the calcaneus, talus, metatarsals, and phalanges can be identified with ultrasound.

Upper Limb

As with the lower limb, it is usually easiest to visualize the upper limb in early pregnancy (Figs. 11.**202**, 11.**203**).

Humerus. The humerus is the easiest of the upper limb bones to define with ultrasound, as it has less freedom of movement than the forearm. To locate the humerus, start with a transverse scan of the shoulder girdle. This will define the proximal end of the humerus in cross section. Then rotate the transducer 90°. If the arm is adducted, this will give a long-axis view of the humeral shaft parallel to the thorax (Fig. 11.**204**). If the arm is abducted, pivot the scan plane at the shoulder until the full length of the humeral shaft is defined.

Radius and ulna. If the arm is extended, the radius and ulna appear in direct continuity with the humerus. If the forearm is flexed, the scan plane must be redirected according to the flexion angle at the elbow. If the forearm is supinated, the two bones will be adjacent and parallel (Fig. 11.**205**). The proximal end of the ulna will always be longer than that of the radius. If the forearm is pronated, the radius and ulna will be crossed (Fig. 11.**206**). The transducer must be rotated approximately 20° to image the second bone (9) (Figs. 11.**206**, 11.**207**).

Metacarpals and fingers. In contrast to the long arm bones, it usually takes considerable time to define the metacarpal bones and all five fin-

gers unless they are seen fortuitously. In the second trimester, the hand can often be visualized in an open position with the fingers extended (Fig. 11.**208**). By the third trimester, the hand is typically curled into a fist (Fig. 11.**209**). The thumb is often adducted at this time and cannot be clearly visualized.

The ossified metacarpals and phalanges can be detected sonographically starting in the second trimester. The carpal bones do not ossify until after birth, and prenatally they appear only as hypoechoic structures.

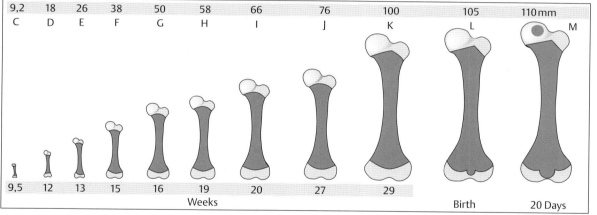

190

Ossification

Fig. 11.**190** Development of the human femur from the first trimester until term (after [6], modified from [4]). The ossification centers are dark, the epiphyses white.

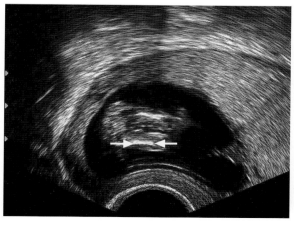

191

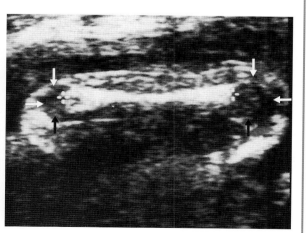

192

Lower limb

Fig. 11.**191** Transvaginal scan of the ossified femoral shaft (arrows) at 10 weeks + 6 days.

Fig. 11.**192** Femur at 25 weeks. The length of the ossified shaft is 4.3 cm. The cartilaginous epiphyses appear as hypoechoic areas extending past the cursors (arrows).

Fig. 11.**193** Both lower limbs are in the extended position, 13 weeks.

Fig. 11.**194** Extended left leg at 19 weeks. 1 = Ilium, 2 = femur, 3 = tibia, 4 = foot.

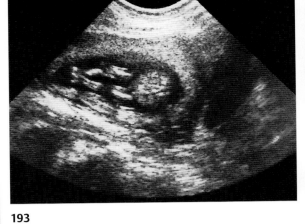

193

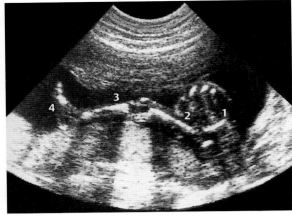

194

Fig. 11.**195** Ossified femoral shaft at 27 weeks, 4 days.

Fig. 11.**196** Anatomic and ultrasound (water-path) comparison of the femur (from [11]). A variable degree of physiologic bowing is seen, depending on the relation of the bone to the transducer. Bowing is greatest when the bone is scanned from the dorsal or medial aspect.

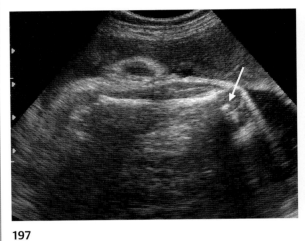

195

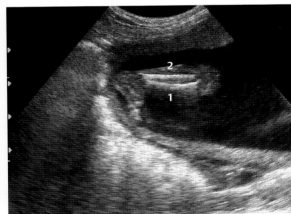

196

Fig. 11.**197** View of the femur showing the distal femoral ossification center (arrow) at 36 weeks.

Fig. 11.**198** Lower leg with tibia (1) and fibula (2) at 22 weeks.

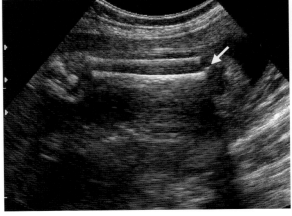

197

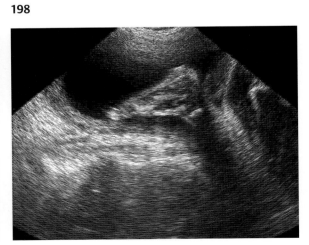

198

Fig. 11.**199** Proximal tibial ossification center at 36 weeks.

Fig. 11.**200** Sagittal view of the foot at 25 weeks.

199

200

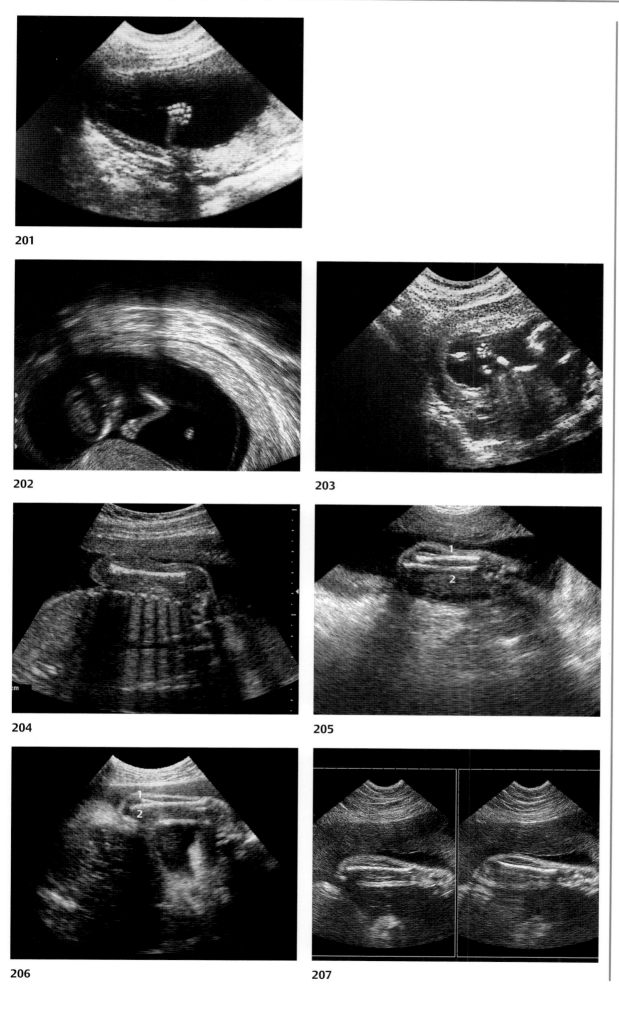

201

202

203

204

205

206

207

Fig. 11.**201**   Right foot at 19 weeks, imaged from the plantar aspect.

Upper limb

Fig. 11.**202**   Transvaginal scan of the flexed left arm at 12 weeks.

Fig. 11.**203**   Full-length view of the left upper limb at 13 weeks.

Fig. 11.**204**   Humerus at 20 weeks, 3 days.

Fig. 11.**205**   Supinated forearm at 26 weeks, 4 days. The radius and ulna are parallel to each other. 1 = Radius, 2 = ulna.

Fig. 11.**206**   Pronated forearm at 31 weeks, 3 days. The radius and ulna and crossed. 1 = Radius, 2 = ulna. The wrist is flexed.

Fig. 11.**207**   Separate views of the ulna (left) and radius (right). The transducer is rotated approximately 20° to move from the long axis of the ulna to that of the radius.

Fig. 11.**208** Extended left hand at 17 weeks, 6 days. The carpal bones and the ossification centers of the phalanges are clearly defined.

Fig. 11.**209** Right hand (fist) at 26 weeks. The thumb (arrow) is adducted.

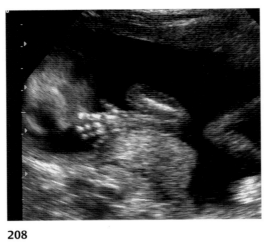

208

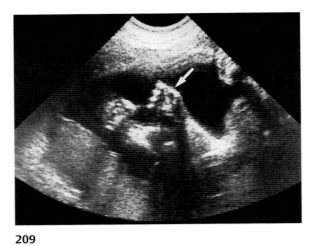

209

References Chapter 11

Head

1. Birnholz, J.C.: The development of human fetal eye movement patterns. Science 213 (1981) 679–681
2. Bowerman, R., DiPietro, M. Errorneous sonographic identification of fetal lateral ventricles: Relationship to the echogenic perventricular „blush". AJNR 8 (1987) 661–664
3. Denkhaus, H., Winsberg, F.: Ultrasonic measurement of the fetal ventricular system. Radiology 131 (1979) 781–787
4. England, M.A.: Farbatlas der Embryologie. Stuttgart: Schattauer 1985
5. Fiske, C.E., Filly, R.A.: Ultrasound evaluation of the normal and abnormal fetal neural axis. Radiol. Clin. N. Amer. 20 (1982) 285–296
6. Hadlock, F.P., Deter, R.L., Park, S.K.: Real-time sonography: Ventricular und vascular anatomy of the fetal brain in utero. Amer. J. Roentgenol. 136 (1981) 133–137
7. Hertzberg, B.S., Bowie, J.D., Burger, P.C., Marshburn, P.B., Djang, W.T.: The three lines: Origin of sonographic landmarks in the fetal head. AJR 149 (1987) 1009–1012
8. Hinrichsen, K.V.: Human-Embryologie. Berlin: Springer 1990
9. Johnson, M.L., Dunne, M.G., Mack, L.A., Rashbaum, C.L.: Evaluation of fetal intracranial anatomy by static and real-time ultrasound. J. clin. Ultrasound 8 (1980) 311–318
10. Kossoff, G., Garrett, W.J.: Intracranial detail in fetal echograms. Invest. Radiol. 7 (1972) 159–163
11. Moore, K.L.: Embryologie. Stuttgart: Schattauer 1985
12. Pigadas, A., Thompson, J.R., Grube, G.L.: Normal infant brain anatomy: Correlated real-time sonograms and brain speciments. Amer. J. Roentgenol. 137 (1981) 815–820
13. Romero, R., Pilu, G., Jeanty, P., Ghidini, A., Hobbins, J.C.: Prenatal diagnosis of congenital anomalies. Norwalk: Appleton & Lange, 1988
14. Staudach, A.: Fetale Anatomie im Ultraschall. Berlin: Springer 1986
15. Waldeyer, A.: Anatomie des Menschen II. Berlin: De Gruyter & Co 1970; S. 347

Spinal Column

1. England, M.A.: Farbatlas der Embryologie. Stuttgart: Schattauer 1985
2. Hinrichsen, K.V.: Human-Embryologie. Berlin: Springer 1990
3. Moore, K.L.: Embryologie. Stuttgart: Schattauer 1985
4. Sobotta, J., Becher, H.: Atlas der Anatomie des Menschen. 3. Teil. München: Urban & Schwarzenberg 1971
5. Staudach, A.: Fetale Anatomie im Ultraschall. Berlin: Springer 1986

Neck

1. Badalian, S.S., Chao, C., Fox, H., Timor-Tritsch, I.E.: Fetal breathing-related nasal fluid flow velocity in uncomplicated pregnancies. Am. J. Obstet. Gynecol. 169 (1993) 563–567
2. Badalian, S.S., Fox, H.E., Zimmer, E.Z., Fifer, W.P., Stark, R.I.: Patterns of perinasal fluid flow and contraction of the diaphragm in the human fetus. Ultrasound Obstet. Gynecol. 8 (1996) 109–113
3. Bowie, J.D., Clair, M.R.: Fetal swallowing and regurgitation: Observation of normal and abnormal activity: Radiology 44 (1982) 877–878
4. Cooper, C., Barry, S.M., Bowie, J.D., Albright, T.O., Callen, P.W.: Ultrasound evaluation of the normal fetal upper airway and esophagus. J. Ultrasound Med. 4 (1985) 343–345
5. Diamant, N.E.: Development of the esophageal function: Am. Rev. Respir. Dis. 131(suppl) (1985) 29–32
6. Isaacson, G., Birnholz, J.C.: Human fetal upper respiratory tract function as revealed by ultrasonography. Ann. Otol. Rhinol. Laryngol. 100 (1991)743–747
7. Kalache, K.D., Chaoui, R., Bollmann, R.: Doppler assessment of tracheal and nasal fluid flow during fetal breathing movements: preliminary observations. Ultrasound Obst. Gynecol. 9 (1997) 257–261
8. Kalache, K.D., Chaoui, R., Hartung, J., Bollmann, R.: Doppler assessment of tracheal fluid flow during fetal breathing movements in cases of congenital diaphragmatic hernia. Ultrasound Obstet. Gynecol. (1998) 27–32
9. Kalache, K.D., Franz, M., Chaoui, R., Bollmann, R.: Ultrasound measurements of the diameter of the fetal trachea, larynx and pharynx throughout gestation: applicability to prenatal diagnosis of obstructive anomalies of the upper respiratory-digestive tract. Prenatal Diagnosis 19 (1999) 211–218
10. López Ramón y Cajal, C.: Description of human laryngeal functions: phonation. Early Hum. Dev. 45 (1996) 63–72
11. Marsal, K., Gennser, G., Lindstrom, K.: Real-time ultrasonography for quantified analysis of fetal breathing movements. Lancet 2 (1976) 718–719
12. Moore, S.M., Laitman, J.T.: Development of the fetal upper respiratory tract during the second trimester. Am. J. Phys. Anthrop. 78 (1989) 274–275
13. O'Rahilly, R., Tucker, J.A.: The early development of the larynx in staged human embryos. Ann. Otol. Rhinol. Laryngol. 82 (Suppl 7) (1973) 1–27
14. O'Rahilly, R., Müller, F.: Respiratory and alimentary relations in staged human embryos. New embryological data and congenital anomalies. Ann. Otol. Rhinol. Laryngol. 93 (1984) 421–429
15. Petrikovsky, B.M., Kaplan, G.P., Pestrak, H.: The application of color doppler technology to the study of fetal swallowing. Obstet. Gynecol. 86 (1995) 605–608
16. Petrikovsky, B., Gross, B., Kaplan, G.: Fetal pharyngeal distention – Is it a normal component of fetal swallowing? Early Hum. Dev. 46 (1996) 77–81
17. Richards, D.S., Farah, L.A.: Sonographic visualization of the fetal upper airway. Ultrasound Obstet. Gynecol. 4 (1994) 21–23
18. Sherman, D.J., Ross, M.G., Day, L., Ervin, M.G.: Fetal swallowing: Correlation of electromyography and esophageal fluid flow. (1990). Am. J. Physiol. 258 (1990) R1386–1394
19. Wolfson, V.P., Laitman, J.T.: Ultrasound investigation of fetal human upper respiratory anatomy. The antomical record 227 (1990) 363–372

Thorax

1. Ahlfeld, F.: Über bisher noch nicht beschriebene intrauterine Bewegungen des Kindes. Verh. Dtsch. Ges. Gynäk. 2 (1888) 203–210
2. Benson, D.M., Waldroup, L.D., Kurtz, A.B., Rose, J.L., Rifkin, M.D., Goldberg, B.B.: Ultrasonic tissue characterization of fetal lung, liver and placenta for the purpose of assessing fetal maturity. J. Ultrasound Med. 2 (1983) 489–494
3. Bocking, A., Adamson, L., Cousin, A. et al.: Effects of intravenous glucose injections of human fetal breathing movements and gross fetal body movements at 38 to 40 weeks gestational age. Amer. J. Obstet. Gynecol. 142 (1982) 606–611
4. Boddy, K., Robinson, J.S.: External method for detection of fetal breathing in utero. Lancet 1971/II, 1231–1233
5. Boylan, P., Lewis, P.J.: Fetal breathing in labor. Obstet. Gynecol. 56 (1980) 35–38
6. Boylan, P., O'Donovan, P., Owens, O.J.: Fetal breathing movements and the diagnosis of labor: A prospective analysis of 100 cases. Obstet. Gynecol. 66 (1985) 517–520
7. Capman, R.L., Dawes, G.S., Rurak, D.W., Richards, R.T.: Intermittent breathing before death in fetal lambs. Amer. J. Obstet. Gynecol. 131 (1978) 894–898
8. Carmichael, L., Campbell, K., Patrick, J.: Fetal breathing, gross fetal body movements, and maternal and fetal heart rates before spontaneous labor at term. Amer. J. Obstet. Gynecol. 148 (1984) 675–679
9. Dawes, G.S., Fox, H.E., Leduc, B. M., Liggins, G.C., Richards, R.T.: Respiratory movements and paradoxal sleep in the fetal lamb. J. Physiol. 210 (1970) 47P–48P
10. Devoe, L.D., Abduljabbar, H., Carmichael, L., Probert, C., Patrick, J.: The effects of maternal hyperoxia on fetal breathing movements in third-trimester pregnancies. Amer. J. Obstet. Gynecol. 148 (1984) 790–794
11. DeVore, G.R., Donnerstein, R.L., Kleinmann, C.D., Hobbins, J.C.: Fetal echocardiography. I. Normal anatomy as determined by real-time-directed M-mode ultrasound. Amer. J. Obstet. Gynec. 144 (1982) 249–260
12. England, M.A.: Farbatlas der Embryologie. Stuttgart: Schattauer 1985
13. Fendel, H., Fendel, M.: Ultraschallechographische Intensitätsänderung der fetalen Lunge im letzten Trimenon als möglicher Hinweis für die Lungenreife. Z. Geburtsh. Perinat. 188 (1984) 269–271
14. Fox, H.E., Hohler, C.W.: Fetal evaluation by real-time imaging. Clin. Obstet. Gynecol. 20 (1977) 339–349
15. Fox, H.E., Steinbrecher, M., Pessel, D., Inglis, J., Medvid, L., Angel, E.: Maternal ethanol ingestion and the occurence of human fetal breathing movements. Amer. J. Obstet. Gynecol. 132 (1978) 354–358
16. Fox, H.E., Hohler, C.W., Steinbrecher, M.: Human fetal breathing movements after carbohydrate ingestion in fasting and nonfasting subjects. Amer. J. Obstet. Gynecol. 144 (1982) 213–217
17. Gennser, G., Marsál, K., Brantmark, K.: Maternal smoking in fetal breathing movements. Amer. J. Obstet. Gynecol. 123 (1975) 861–867
18. Lewis, P.J., Boylan, P.: Alcohol and fetal breathing. Lancet 1979/I, 388
19. Luther, E.R., Gray, J., Stinson, D., Allen, A.: Characteristics of glucose-stimulated breathing movements in human fetuses with intrauterine growth retardation. Amer. J. Obstet. Gynecol. 148 (1984) 640–643
20. Manning, F.A., Pugh, E.W., Boddy, K.: Effect of cigarette smoking on fetal breathing movements in normal pregnancies. Brit. med. J. 1975/II, 552–553
21. Manning, F.A., Feyerabend, C.: Cigarette smoking and fetal breathing movements. Brit. J. Obstet. Gynaec. 83 (1976) 262–270
22. Manning, F.A., Platt, L.D.: Maternal hypoxaemia and fetal breathing movements. Obstet. Gynecol. 53 (1979) 758–760
23. Manning, F.A., Martin, C.M.jr., Murata, Y., Miyaki, K., Danzler, G.: Breathing movements before death in the primate fetus (Macaca mulatta). Amer. J. Obstet. Gynecol. 135 (1979) 71–76
24. Marsál, K., Gennser, G., Lindstrom, K.: Real-time ultrasonography for quantified analysis of fetal breathing movement. Lancet 1976/II, 718–719
25. Merlet, C., Hoerter, J., Devilleneuve, C., Tchobroutsky, C.: Mise en évidence de mouvements respiratoires chez le foetus d'agneau in utero au cours du dernier mois de la gestation. Comptes Rendus Hebd. Séances Acad. Sci. (Paris) (ser. D.) 270 (1970) 2462–2464
26. Moore, K.L.: Embryologie. Stuttgart: Schattauer 1985
27. Natale, R., Richardson, B., Patrick, J.: Effects of intravenous glucose infusion of human fetal breathing activity. Obstet. Gynecol. 59 (1981) 320–324
28. Neldam, S.: Fetal respiratory movements: A nomogram for fetal thoracic and abdominal respiratory movements. Amer. J. Obstet. Gynecol. 142 (1982) 867–869
29. Patrick, J.E., Dalton, K.J., Dawes, G.S.: Breathing patterns before death in fetal lambs. Amer. J. Obstet. Gynecol. 125 (1976) 73–78
30. Patrick, J., Natale, R., Richardson, B.: Patterns of human fetal breathing activity at 34 to 35 weeks gestational age. Amer. J. Obstet. Gynecol. 132 (1978) 507–513
31. Patrick, J., Fetherston, W., Vick, H., Voegelin, R.: Human fetal breathing movements and gross fetal body movements at weeks 34 to 35 of gestation. Amer. J. Obstet. Gynecol. 130 (1978) 693–699
32. Patrick, J., Campbell, K., Carmichael, L., Natale, R., Richardson, B.: Patterns of human breathing during the last 10 weeks of pregnancy. Obstet. and Gynecol. 56 (1980) 24–30
33. Platt, L.D., Manning, F.A., Lemay, M., Sipos, L.: Human fetal breathing: Relationship to fetal condition. Amer. J. Obstet. Gynecol. 132 (1978) 514–518
34. Richardson, B., Natale, R., Patrick, J.: Human fetal breathing activity during electivly induced labor at term. Amer. J. Obstet. Gynecol. 133 (1979) 247–255
35. Ritchie, J.W.K., Lakhani, K.: Fetal breathing movements on response to maternal inhalation of 5% carbon dioxide. Amer. J. Obstet. Gynecol. 136 (1980) 386–388
36. Ritchie, J.W., Lakhani, K.: Fetal breathing movements and maternal hyperoxia. Brit. J. Obstet. Gynaec. 97 (1980) 1084–1086
37. Trudinger, B.J., Knight, P.C.: Fetal age and patterns of human fetal breathing movements. Amer. J. Obstet. Gynecol. 137 (1980) 724–728
38. Van Weering, H.K., Wladimiroff, J.W., Roodenburg, P.J.: Effect of changes in maternal blood gases on fetal breathing movements. Contr. Gynecol. Obstet. 6 (1979) 88–91
39. Wladimiroff, J.W., Haller, U.: Fetale Atembewegungen. Swiss Med. 4 (1982) 131

Circulatory System

1. Bernaschek, G., Dadak, C., Kratochwil, A.: Echographische Darstellung der großen fetalen Gefäße. Ultraschall 1 (1980) 101–105
2. England, M.A.: Farbatlas der Embryologie. Stuttgart: Schattauer 1985
3. Hansmann, M.: Ultraschallbiometrie im II. und III. Trimester der Schwangerschaft. Gynäkologe 9 (1976) 133
4. Kugener, H., Hansmann, M.: Zur Topographie einer Referenzebene für die Ultraschallthorakometrie. Z. Geburtsh. Perinat. 180 (1976) 313–319
5. Moore, K.L.: Embryologie. Stuttgart: Schattauer 1985
6. Morin, F.R., Winsberg, F.: Ultrasonic and radiographic study of the vessels of the fetal liver. J. clin. Ultrasound 6 (1978) 409–411
7. Starck, D.: Embryologie. Stuttgart: Thieme 1975

Heart

1. Better, D.J., Kaufman, S., Allan, L.D.: The normal pattern of pulmonary venous flow on pulsed Doppler examination of the human fetus. J Am Soc Echocardiol 9 (1996) 281–285
2. Chaoui, R., Bollmann, R., Hoffmann, H., Heling, K.S.: Sonoanatomie des fetalen Herzens – Vorschlag einfacher Schnittebenen für den Nichtkardiologen Ultraschall Klin Prax 6 (1991) 59–67
3. Chaoui, R., Heling, K.S., Bollmann, R., Kalache, K.: Die fetale Doppler-Echokardiographie. Ultraschall Klin Prax 8 (1993) 1–11
4. Chaoui, R., Heling, K.S., Bollmann, R.: Sonographische Messungen am fetalen Herzen in der Vierkammerblick-Ebene. Geburtsh Frauenheilk 54 (1994) 92–97
5. Chaoui, R., Bollmann, R.: Die fetale Farb-Doppler-Echokardiographie: Teil 1: Grundlagen und normale Befunde. Ultraschall Med. 15 (1994) 100–104
6. Chaoui, R., Bollmann, R.: Die fetale Farb-Doppler-Echokardiographie: Teil 2: Fehlbildungen des Herzens und der großen Gefäße. Ultraschall Med. 15 (1994) 105–112
7. Chaoui, R., Heling, K.S., Bollmann, R.: Sonographische Messungen der Durchmesser der Aorta und des Truncus pulmonalis beim Feten. Gynäkol. Geburtshilfliche Rundsch. 34 (1994) 145–151
8. Chaoui, R., Heling, K.S., Taddei, F., Bollmann, R.: Doppler-echokardiographische Analyse des Blutflusses über den fetalen Aorten- und Pulmonalklappen in der zweiten Hälfte der Schwangerschaft. Geburtsh. u. Frauenheilk. 55 (1995) 207–217
9. Chaoui, R., Heling, K.S., Taddei, F., Bollmann, R.: Fetale atrioventrikuläre Geschwindigkeiten in der zweiten Hälfte der Schwangerschaft: eine Dopplerechokardiographische Studie. Z Geburtsh u Neonat. 200 (1996) 13–20
10. Chaoui, R., Taddei, F., Bast, C. et al.: Standardisierte Ebenen zur Dopplersonographie der fetalen Lungenarterien. Ultraschall Klin Prax. 10 (1996) 118–123
11. Chaoui, R., Taddei, F., Bast, C. et al.: Sonographische Untersuchung des fetalen Lungenkreislaufs. Gynäkologe 30 (1997) 230–239
12. Chaoui, R., Heling, K.S., Bollmann, R.: B-Bild Sonographie des fetalen Herzens. In: Schmidt, W. (Hrsg.): Jahrbuch der Gynäkologie und Geburtshilfe 1997/1998. Biermann; S.103–113
13. Chaoui, R., Taddei, F., Rizzo, G., Bast, C., Lenz, F., Bollmann, R.: Doppler echocardiography of the main stems of the pulmonary arteries in the normal human fetus. Ultrasound Obstet Gynecol 11 (1998) 173–179
14. Chaoui, R., Kalache, K.: Three-Dimensional Color Power Imaging: Principles and First Experience in Prenatal Diagnosis. In: Merz, E. (Hrsg.): 3D Ultrasonography in Obstetrics and Gynecology. Philadelphia: Lippincott Williams & Wilkins 1998; pp.135–142
15. Copel, J.A., Pilu, G., Green, J., Hobbins, J.C., Kleinman, C.S.: Fetal echocardiographic screening for congenital heart disease: the importance of the four-chamber view. Am J Obstet Gynecol. 157 (1987) 648–655
16. DeVore, G.R.: The prenatal diagnosis of congenital heart disease – a practical approach for the fetal sonographer. J Clin Ultrasound 13 (1985) 229–245
17. DeVore, G.R.: The use of color Doppler imaging to examine the fetal heart. Normal and pathologic anatomy; In: Jaffe, R., Warsof, S.L. (eds.): Color Doppler imaging in obstetrics and gynecology. New York: McGraw-Hill Inc. 1992; pp. 121–154
18. Gembruch, U., Hansmann, M., Redel, D.A., Bald, R.: Zweidimensionale farbkodierte fetale Doppler-Echokardiographie – ihr Stellenwert in der pränatalen Diagnostik. Geburtsh Frauenheilk 48 (1988) 381–388
19. Gembruch, U., Bald, R., Hansmann, M.: Die farbkodierte M-Mode-Doppler-Echokardiographie bei der Diagnostik fetaler Arrhythmien. Geburtsh. Frauenheilk. 50 (1990) 286–290
20. Gembruch, U., Knöpfle, G., Bald, R., Hansmann, M.: Early diagnosis of fetal congenital heart disease by transvaginal echocardiography. Ultrasound Obstet. Gynecol. 3 (1993) 310–317
21. Gembruch, U., Chaoui, R.: Pränatale Diagnostik fetaler Herzfehler durch Untersuchung von „high-risk"- und „low-risk"-Kollektiven – Möglichkeiten und Grenzen eines Screening-Programms. Gynäkologe 30 (1997) 191–199
22. Henry, W.L., DeMaria, A., Gramiak, R. et al.: Report of the American Society of Echocardiography Committee on nomenclature and standards in two-dimensional echocardiography. Circulation 62 (1980) 212–217
23. Huhta, J.C., Smallhorn, J.F., McCartney, F.J.: Two-dimensional echocardiographic diagnosis of situs. Br. Heart J. 48 (1982) 97–103
24. Kalache, K.D, Nguyen-Dobinsky, T.N., Chaoui, R., Bollmarn, R.: CD-ROM Ultraschall Angiographie in der Geburtshilfe. Berlin: W. de Gruyter (1998)
25. Tegnander, E., Eik-Nes, S.H., Linker, D.T.: Incorporating the four-chamber view of the fetal heart into the second-trimester routine fetal examination. Ultrasound Obstet Gynecol 4 (1994) 24–28
26. Van Praagh, R.: The segmental approach to diagnosis in congenital heart disease. Birth Defects 8 (1972) 4–23

Abdomen

1. England, M.A.: Farbatlas der Embryologie. Stuttgart: Schattauer 1985
2. Hashimoto, B.E., Filly, R.A., Callen, P.W.: Fetal pseudoascites: further anatomic observations. J. Ultrasound Med. 5 (1986) 151–152
3. Hinrichsen, K.V.: Human-Embryologie. Berlin: Springer 1990

4. Kugener, H., Hansmann, M.: Zur Topographie einer Referenzebene für die Ultraschallthorakometrie. Z. Geburtsh. Perinat. 180 (1976) 313–319
5. Moore, K.L.: Embryologie. Stuttgart: Schattauer 1985
6. Rosenthal, S.J., Filly, R.A., Callen, P.W., Sommer, F.G.: Fetal pseudo-ascites. Radiology 131 (1979) 195–197
7. Schmidt, W., Yarkoni, S., Jeanty, P., Grannum, P., Hobbins, J.C.: Sonographic measurements of the fetal spleen: Clinical implications. J. Ultrasound Med. 4 (1985) 667
8. Staudach, A.: Fetale Anatomie im Ultraschall. Berlin: Springer 1986
9. Wladimiroff, J.W., Leijs, R., Smit, B.: Human fetal stomach profiles. In: Kurjak, A. (ed.): Recent advances in ultrasound diagnosis. 2. Excerpta Medica International Congress Series 498 (1980)

Urinary Tract, Adrenal Glands, and Pelvis

1. Bernaschek, G., Kratochwil, A.: Echographische Studie über das Wachstum der fetalen Niere in der zweiten Schwangerschaftshälfte. Geburtsh. u. Frauenheilk. 40 (1980) 1059–1064
2. Campbell, S., Wladimiroff, J.W., Dewhurst, C.J.: The antenatal measurement of fetal urine production. Brit. J. Obstet. Gynaec. 80 (1973) 680–686
3. England, M.A.: Farbatlas der Embryologie. Stuttgart: Schattauer 1985
4. Grannum, P., Bracken, M., Silverman, R., Hobbins, J.C.: Assessment of fetal kidney size in normal gestation by comparison of ratio or kidney circumference to abdominal circumference. Amer. J. Obstet. Gynec. 136 (1980) 249–254
5. Lawson, T.L., Foley, W.D., Berland, L.L., Clark, K.E.: Ultrasonic evaluation of fetal kidneys. Radiology 138 (1981) 153–156
6. Lewis, E., Kurtz, A.B., Dubbins, P.A., Wapner, R.J., Goldberg, B.B.: Real-time ultrasonographic evaluation of normal fetal adrenal glands. J. Ultrasound Med. 1 (1982) 265–270
7. Moore, K.L.: Embryologie. Stuttgart: Schattauer 1985
8. Starck, D.: Embryologie. Stuttgart: Thieme 1975

Genitalia

1. Ammini, A.C., Pandey, J., Vijyaraghavan, M., Sabherwal, U.: Human female phenotypic development: role of fetal ovaries. J. Clin. Endocrinol. Metab. 79 (1994) 604–608
2. Bronsthein, M., Rottem, S., Yoffe, N., Blumenfeld, Z., Brandes, J.M.: Early determination of fetal sex using transvaginal sonography: technique and pitfalls. J. Clin. Ultrasound 18 (1990) 302–306
3. Elejalde, B.R., de Elejalde, M.M., Heitman, T.: Visualization of the fetal genitalia by ultrasonography: A review of the literature and analysis of its accuracy and ethical implication. J. Ultrasound Med. 4 (1985) 633–639
4. England, M. A.: Farbatlas der Embryologie. Stuttgart: Schattauer 1985
5. Mielke, G., Kiesel, L., Backsch, C., Erz, W., Gonser, M.: Fetal sex determination by high resolution ultrasound in early pregnancy. Europ. J. Obstet. Gynecol. & Reprod. Biol. 7 (1998) 109–114
6. Moore, K.L.: Embryologie. Stuttgart: Schattauer 1985
7. Natsuyama, E.: Sonographic determination of fetal sex from twelve weeks of gestation. Amer. J. Obstet. Gynec. 149 (1984) 748–757
8. Schotten, A., Giese, C.: Fetale Geschlechtsdiagnostik mit Ultraschall. Ultraschall 2 (1981) 262–263
9. Shalev, E., Weiner, E., Zuckerman, H.: Ultrasound determination of fetal sex. Amer. J. Obstet. Gynec. 141 (1981) 582–583
10. Smulian, J.C., Feeney, L.D., Fabbri, E.L., Rodis, J.F., Campbell, W.A.: Second trimester sonographic prediction of fetal gender. J. Mat. Fetal Invest. 6 (1996) 67–69
11. Starck, D.: Embryologie. Stuttgart: Thieme 1975
12. Wartenberg, H.: Entwicklung der Genitalorgane und Bildung der Gameten. In: Hinrichsen, K.V. (Hrsg.): Human-Embryologie. Berlin: Springer 1990; S. 745–822
13. Watson, W.J.: Early-second-trimester fetal sex determination with ultrasound. J. Reprod. Med. 35 (1990) 247–249

Limbs

1. Bernaschek, G.: Die Besonderheiten einer neuartigen echographischen Bestimmung der Kniegelenkskerne des Feten. Geburtsh. u. Frauenheilk. 42 (1982) 94–97
2. Bernaschek, G., Bartl, W., Wolf, G.: Epiphysenzentren im Kniebereich – ein sonographisch-radiologischer Vergleich. Z. Geburtsh. Perinat. 187 (1983) 250–253
3. England, M.A.: Farbatlas der Embryologie. Stuttgart: Schattauer 1985
4. Felts, W.J.L.: The prenatal development of the human femur. Am. J. Anat. 94 (1954) 1–44
5. Hinrichsen, K.V.: Human-Embryologie. Berlin: Springer 1990
6. Knese, K.H.: Handbuch der mikroskopischen Anatomie des Menschen. Stützgewebe und Skelettsystem II/5. Berlin: Springer 1979
7. Langmann, J.: Medizinische Embryologie. 2. Aufl. Stuttgart: Thieme 1972; S. 216
8. Mahony, B.S., Callen, P.W., Filly, R.A.: The distal femoral epiphyseal ossification center in the assessment of third-trimester menstrual age: Sonographic identification and measurement. Radiology 155 (1985) 201–204
9. Merz, E., Pehl, S., Goldhofer, W., Hoffmann, G.: Biometrie der großen fetalen Extremitätenknochen im III. Trimenon. Ultraschall 5 (1984) 136–143
10. Merz, E., Kim-Kern, M.S., Pehl, S.: Ultrasonic mensuration of fetal limb bones in the second and third trimesters. J. Clin. Ultrasound 15 (1987) 175–183
11. Merz, E.: Sonographische Überwachung der fetalen Knochenentwicklung im II. und III. Trimenon. Eine Studie über das Wachstum der langen Röhrenknochen im Vergleich zum Kopf- und Rumpfwachstum sowie über die Verwendungsmöglichkeiten der fetalen Knochenlänge im Rahmen der geburtshilflichen Ultraschalluntersuchung. Habilitationsschrift, Universitäts-Frauenklinik Mainz (1988)
12. Moore, K.L.: Embryologie. Stuttgart: Schattauer 1985
13. Schlensker, K.H.: Die sonographische Darstellung der fetalen Extremitäten im mittleren Trimenon. Geburtsh. u. Frauenheilk. 41 (1981) 366–373
14. Starck, D.: Embryologie. Stuttgart: Thieme 1975

12 Fetal Biometry in the Second and Third Trimesters

Since the introduction of ultrasound into obstetrics, fetal biometry has become an established part of prenatal diagnosis. The accurate measurement and documentation of biometric parameters in the second and third trimesters have become an essential basis for the evaluation of fetal growth. Besides confirming normal fetal development, the ultrasound measurements can be compared with standard reference charts to detect early abnormalities of fetal growth. Growth disturbances (e.g., intrauterine growth retardation [IUGR], macrosomia) as well as various malformations (e.g., hydrocephalus or dwarfism) can be specifically detected and their degree of severity assessed.

Indications. Besides monitoring fetal growth and detecting malformations, biometric parameters are also used to provide a baseline for "late" pregnancy dating and fetal weight estimation (Table 12.**1**).

Table 12.**1**   Applications of fetal biometry in the second and third trimesters

> Monitoring fetal growth to confirm normal growth or detect discrepancies at an early stage (IUG, macrosomia)
> Detection of fetal anomalies
> Late gestational age assignment
> Fetal weight estimation

Prerequisites

Table 12.**2** lists several factors that are important in the accurate measurement of fetal biometric parameters.

Table 12.**2**   Important factors in fetal biometry

> Definition of gestational age (completed weeks)
> Equipment settings (sound velocity, gain)
> Definition of the reference plane
> Definition of biometry points
> Definition of growth curves

▧ Gestational Age

Completed or current week of gestation. To compare ultrasound measurements with growth charts, a uniform method of defining gestational age is required. This means stating whether the normal values for a given week of gestation are based on the completed week or the current week. If the notation method is ignored, the difference resulting from a partial week can sometimes lead to the erroneous evaluation of fetal growth. To eliminate this problem, gestational age should be stated in completed weeks whenever possible (22, 125).

Redating. Assigning a new date should be done early in the pregnancy if at all, and it should be done only once. Redating the pregnancy several times can lead to great confusion and can cause growth disturbances to be missed or detected too late.

▧ Equipment Settings

Velocity calibration. Contrary to the 1975 recommendation of the European Study Group in Dubrovnik that machines be calibrated to a sound velocity of 1600 m/s for A-mode measurements of BPD, the real-time scanners in current use are calibrated to a velocity of 1540 m/s. This corresponds to the mean propagation velocity of ultrasound in human tissue at 37° C.

Since measurements are affected by velocity calibration (a dimension measuring 8.0 cm at 1540 m/s would measure 8.3 cm at 1600 m/s), there was a time when measurements taken at different velocities could not be directly compared with each other and had to be converted using the following formula:

$$\frac{\text{Sound velocity of machine A}}{\text{Sound velocity of machine B}} \cdot \text{Measurement with machine B} = \text{Measurement}$$

Since all ultrasound equipment in current use is calibrated to the same velocity, this problem no longer exists.

Gain setting. Unlike sound velocity, the gain setting is still an important factor in modern scanners. As the gain is increased, contours on the ultrasound image become broader, and therefore longer measurements are obtained. Thus, Hughey and Sabbagha (57) found an average difference of 3 mm in outer-to-outer BPDs that were measured at moderate and high gain settings. It is recommended that a medium gain setting be used for all measurements.

Scale calibration. Systemic errors can occur in ultrasound machines that have poorly calibrated scales. These problems can be detected only by running a test program created for the particular machine.

▧ Defining the Reference Plane

Accurate biometry requires the consistent use of standard reference planes. Taking measurements above or below the proper plane will lead to errors. The same applies to oblique measurements. If it is discovered that an oblique plane has been used, an attempt should be made to establish a correct plane before any additional follow-up measurements are taken.

▧ Defining the Biometry Points

With present-day scanners, the points for taking measurements in fetal biometry are usually defined with electronic cursors in the stored image. It is critical whether the calipers are placed for an outer-to-outer, outer-to-inner, or inner-to-inner measurement.

Outer-to-inner and outer-to-outer measurements. The outer-to-inner BPD is most commonly used in English-speaking countries. This means that the BPD is measured from the proximal outer wall of the skull to the distal inner wall. In European countries (41, 55, 56), it is customary to use the outer-to-outer BPD measured between the outer aspects of the fetal skull. Hughey and Sabbagha (57) showed in babies delivered by cesarean section that the outer-to-outer BPD measured at a sound velocity of 1540 m/s corresponds most closely to the true anatomic biparietal diameter.

Measurements in late pregnancy. Transducers used in late pregnancy should be able to handle measurements up to 12 cm in length. This is necessary to ensure that measurements of the occipitofrontal diameter, for example, can still be performed.

Use of Growth Charts

Criticism of growth charts. Growth charts published by various authors are available for evaluating a variety of fetal growth parameters (10, 12, 17, 18, 20, 24, 28, 35, 37, 38, 39, 40, 49, 55, 80, 84, 115). In a 1993 review of biometric studies, Altman and Chitty (4) state that a number of published fetal growth charts do not conform to the desired standards. Their criticisms relate both to study design and to data analysis:

1. Some studies were flawed (or unclear) in their method of patient selection.
2. Some fetuses were measured more than once (or it is unclear how often they were measured).
3. The inclusion or exclusion criteria were faulty (or unclear).
4. The case numbers were too small.
5. The method of pregnancy dating was unclear.
6. It cannot be determined whether single measurements were used or whether several measurements were averaged together.

A valid result can be achieved only if the study is designed in such a way that the construction of growth charts is its primary goal.

Cross-sectional and longitudinal studies. In principle, a study of this kind may have a cross-sectional (80, 82, 83, 84) or longitudinal design (19, 27, 104). The advantage of a longitudinal study is that it can detect typical growth patterns that occur during pregnancy. The disadvantage is that, in most cases, not enough patients are available for the study. As a result, longitudinal studies are not ideal for the creation of fetal growth charts. A large-scale cross-sectional study can provide a much greater volume of data, making it a more suitable design for creating normal growth charts. Care must be taken, however, that the case numbers in these studies are reasonably well distributed between different age groups.

Polynomials and growth models. At present, higher-order polynomials are the method most commonly used in statistics for fitting curves to a set of data points. The drawback of this method is that it places too much weight on irrelevant data fluctuations. Also, polynomials generally do not follow a monotonic path over the entire observation period. For this reason, a number of authors prefer to use a growth model (3, 82, 83, 84, 103). This offers several advantages over the use of higher-order polynomials:

- A single model function can accurately describe the growth curve of multiple fetal parameters.
- Smooth curves are generated for all biometric parameters.
- The upper and lower limits for all parameter are calculated according to a uniform procedure (123).
- The resulting growth curves can easily be integrated into commercially available ultrasound equipment.

Upper and lower limits. The upper and lower limits of growth curves may be represented by two standard deviations (± 2 SD) or by percentile curves. When percentile curves are used, the 95th and 5th percentiles usually define the limits of the normal range. This means that 5% of normal children fall above the upper limit of the central 90% range and another 5% of normals fall below the lower limit.

Documentation

All measured biometric data should be properly documented. The more detailed the documentation, the easier it will be to recognize growth disturbances in subsequent follow-ups. Computer programs are of great value in this regard, as they permit a direct comparison of measurements with normal growth curves as well as the direct monitoring of progression by displaying previous data alongside current measurements.

Basic Biometry

Basic biometry is a part of the screening examinations that are performed during the second and third trimesters. It includes the parameters listed in Table 12.3. All additional parameters fall under the heading of extended biometry.

Table 12.**3** Parameters measured in basic biometry

Head	Biparietal diameter (BPD) Occipitofrontal diameter (OFD) Head circumference (HC)
Abdomen	Abdominal transverse diameter (ATD) Abdominal sagittal diameter (ASD Abdominal circumference (AC)
Limbs	Femur or humerus length (FL, HL)

Cephalometry

Parameters. The parameters available for biometry of the fetal head are the biparietal diameter (BPD), the occipitofrontal diameter (OFD), and head circumference (HC). When the correct anatomic reference plane is selected, all three of these parameters can be measured simultaneously.

Reference plane. The correct reference plane for fetal cephalometry is the transverse occipitofrontal plane. It is recognized by its symmetrical ovoid shape, the presence of a distinct midline echo, and the cavum septi pellucidi in the anterior third of the skull (12, 38) (Figs. 12.**1**–12.**3**). This plane also cuts both thalamic nuclei, which appear as central hypoechoic structures flanking the midline echo.

Technique. Both the BPD and the OFD are outer-to-outer measurements taken from skin to skin. With modern equipment, the HC can be measured directly by tracing around it with a light pen on the screen, or it can be calculated from the BPD and OFD by using the modified formula for an ellipse, as recommended by Hansmann (42):

$$HC = 2{,}325 \times \sqrt{BPD^2 + OFD^2}$$

For convenience, charts are provided in the Appendix that permit the HC to be read directly from the BPD and OFD.

Dolichocephalic head shape. Measurement of the HC is particularly recommended when the fetal head shape is dolichocephalic (Fig. 12.**3**). Because the dolichocephalic BPD is frequently below the 5th percentile (while the OFD comes out too large), measuring the BPD alone could falsely imply that head growth is deficient. But when the head circumference is used, both the BPD and OFD enter into the calculation, canceling out the effects of the dolichocephaly.

Growth curves. Numerous growth charts have been published in recent years for BPD (10, 38, 41, 53, 55, 72, 80, 105, 115, 124, 127), OFD (41, 53, 72, 80, 115), and HC (18, 37, 41, 53, 80, 96, 115). The charts differ with regard to case numbers, calibrated sound velocity, and the points that were used in taking the measurements.

The growth curves for BPD, OFD, and HC shown in Fig. 12.**4** were derived from a prospective cross-sectional study of 2032 healthy women with uncomplicated pregnancies and sonographically confirmed dates (84). The observation period was from 12 to 41 completed weeks of gestation. All the measurements were outer-to-outer.

Taking the normal population as our data base, we developed a growth model in which we could characterize the growth of all measured parameters by constructing a 90% reference band with a single basic formula. This enabled us to plot growth curves defining a smooth, consistent normal range of values. All the parameters investigated display a nonlinear growth pattern that levels off in the third trimester.

The normal data related to gestational age (5th, 50th, and 95th percentiles) are presented in tables in the Appendix.

Abdominometry

Reference plane. Hansmann (8) defines the reference plane for fetal trunk measurements as the plane in which the umbilical vein enters the portal sinus. He devised a simplified model of the fetal trunk (41, 68) consisting of two truncated cones turned base-to-base and separated by an approximately cylindrical segment of variable thickness (Fig. 12.**5**). The upper truncated cone in this model represents the thorax containing the heart, thymus, lungs, and the upper portion of the liver. The cylindrical segment represents the upper abdomen with the liver, spleen, and pancreas. The lower truncated cone represents the mid and lower abdomen with the bowel loops, kidneys, and bladder. Because the trunk diameter is greatest in the middle segment and also shows the least variation craniocaudally (Fig. 12.**5**), that is the best region for obtaining stable, reproducible trunk measurements. Thus, the anatomic target area is the liver, which is partially intrathoracic due to the unexpanded state of the fetal lungs (41). Kugener and Hansmann (68) and later Morin and Winsberg (89) found that the junction of the umbilical vein with the portal sinus was the most stable reference point within the liver. In the fetus this point is located at the level of the thoracic outlet (Fig. 12.**6**). This led Hansmann (41) to recommend the thoracic outlet as the reference plane for fetal "thoracometry." Today, however, the term "thoracometry" has been replaced by "abdominometry," since the measurement is actually performed in the upper abdomen. The term "thoracometry" is used only for thoracic measurements taken in the plane of the cardiac valves.

Locating the reference plane. The reference plane for abdominometry is located by first defining the fetal trunk in a transverse scan perpendicular to the long axis. The liver, stomach, and umbilical vein are identified. The scan plane is then moved a short distance cephalad until the trunk appears approximately circular and the umbilical vein appears only as a short vascular segment within the liver, well back from the anterior abdominal wall (Fig. 12.**7**). This is the level at which the umbilical vein enters the portal sinus (41, 68, 89), so it represents the desired reference plane for trunk measurements.

Pitfalls. If the scan defines the full length of the umbilical vein (Fig. 12.**7**), the plane must be oblique due to the anatomic course of the umbilical vein (Fig. 12.**6**). This scan (which Hansmann called the "salami scan" [41]) causes the abdomen to appear too large in its anteroposterior dimension.

Trunk measurements can also be altered by pressing too hard on the maternal abdomen with the transducer, distorting the shape of the fetal abdomen.

Parameters. When the correct reference plane has been located, both trunk parameters—the abdominal transverse diameter (ATD) and abdominal sagittal diameter (ASD)—are measured as outer-to-outer dimensions (Figs. 12.**7**, 12.**8**). The abdominal circumference (AC) can be measured electronically by tracing around it with a light pen, or it can be calculated from the ATD and ASD using the formula for an ellipse (84) (Fig. 12.**8**):

$$AC = \frac{ATD + ASD}{2} \times 3{,}142$$

Growth curves. The abdominal growth charts that have been published in the literature (18, 40, 41, 53, 55, 56, 80, 84, 115, 118) are based on varying case numbers and show considerable variation among different studies.

The growth curves for the abdominal parameters shown in Fig. 12.**4** were derived from a prospective cross-sectional study of 2032 healthy women with uncomplicated pregnancies and sonographically confirmed dates. The observation period was from 12 to 41 completed gestational weeks. The curves were plotted using the growth model described above (84). All the measurements were outer-to-outer.

In contrast to an earlier study in which we obtained a linear growth curve for the abdominal parameters (80), the larger and more recent study showed that abdominal growth, like superior growth, leveled off in the third trimester.

Tables relating the normal values for ATD, ASD, and AC to gestational age (5th, 50th, and 95th percentiles) are presented in the Appendix.

Head/trunk ratio. The head/trunk ratio can be used to detect proportional or disproportional growth retardation as well as micro- or macrocephalic development of the head. The ratio may be expressed as the ratio of BPD to ATD (41) or as the ratio of HC to AC (81) (Fig. 12.**9**).

Measuring the Long Tubular Bones

Indications. Besides confirming normal fetal development, ultrasound measurements of the long limb bones (23, 25, 26, 51, 61, 62, 84, 108, 115, 119) are done mainly for the early detection or exclusion of skeletal dysplasias. Skeletal biometry also serves as an adjunct to superior and abdominal measurements for the assessment of gestational age (39, 63, 81, 94, 109). When related to biparietal diameter, it can also be helpful in the diagnosis of microcephaly (54). In cases of intrauterine fetal death where there is already deformation of the fetal skull, the length of the limb bones can be used to estimate the age of the fetus, provided there is no significant growth retardation or skeletal dysplasia.

Parameters. The ossified shaft of the selected long bone, consisting of the diaphysis and metaphysis, is measured. The proximal and distal epiphyses are ignored (Fig. 12.**10**). The curvature of the bone is also ignored when taking the measurement.

Technique. The sound beam should be perpendicular to the long axis of the bone if possible (Figs. 12.**11**–12.**15**), because with a parallel beam, the high sound conduction velocity in bone (approximately 3360 m/s) can cause a foreshortening effect (51). Oblique scans also lead to underestimation of length, so care should be taken that the bone is imaged and measured in its true axial length. Also, the examiner should make certain that the ends of the bones are sharply defined and that part of another bone is not superimposed over the bone end being measured. For example, part of the ischium overlying the femur or part of the ulna overlying the humerus will make the measurement too large. The length of the femur or tibia will also be overstated if the proximal or distal epiphysis is included in the measurement.

Growth curves. The femur has the longest shaft of any of the long tubular bones. Accordingly, the majority of growth curves have been plotted for the femur (24, 53, 95, 100, 109, 115, 119, 122), while only a few have been published for other limb bones (24, 100, 108, 119, 131).

While measurement of the femur or humerus has become an established part of screening examinations, measurements of the other long tubular bones is still reserved for extended biometry. To date, Jeanty et al. (59, 61, 62), Merz et al. (78, 79, 81, 84), and Exacoustos et al. (23) have reported on systematic measurements of all six of the fetal long bones.

Analogous to the growth models developed for head and trunk dimensions, we have also used our study data to create a growth model for the long limb bones (84). The growth curves derived from this model are shown in Fig. 12.**16**. Tables in the Appendix list the corresponding data for the 5th, 50th, and 95th percentiles. Like the superior parameters, all six of the measured limb bones show an almost linear growth rate in the second trimester, followed by a declining rate in the third trimester.

Bone disorders. The selective ultrasound imaging of all the long tubular bones yields a skeletal growth pattern that can be used for the intrauterine diagnosis of various bone disorders. Conversely, if ultrasound confirms normal bone length and structure in cases that are at risk for the recurrence of a particular fetal bone disease, that disease can be excluded with a high degree of confidence.

Extended Biometry (Organ Biometry)

Unlike basic biometry, extended biometry involves the measurement of detailed parameters for the purpose of addressing a specific issue. Measurements of the distal long tubular bones (tibia, fibula, radius, ulna), discussed above, are included in the concept of extended biometry.

Head and Neck

Cerebral Ventricles

Biometry points. Hydrocephalus can be diagnosed with ultrasound at an early stage by detecting incipient dilatation of the cerebral ventricles. Measurements of the lateral ventricles can be taken at the level of the frontal horns (Figs. 12.**17**, 12.**19**), pars centralis, or occipital horns (Figs. 12.**18**, 12.**19**) (17, 99, 65, 115, 126). The frontal measurements are the easiest to perform.

Technique. At one time it was customary to measure the frontal horn, pars centralis, and occipital horn from the midline echo to the lateral ventricular margin (Fig. 12.**17**). Today, with the improved resolution of modern scanners, the lateral ventricles can be measured directly (Fig. 12.**18**).

Normal values. According to the normal values measured by Johnson et al. (65), the lateral ventricles (pars centralis) of a normally developed fetus should not exceed a width of 1.3 cm at any time during pregnancy (see table in Appendix). Denkhaus and Winsberg (17) measured both frontal horns together to obtain the bifrontal ventricular width, which averaged 1.1 cm at 13 weeks' gestation and increased to 2.4 cm at term. The ratio of bifrontal ventricular width to BPD was 0.48 at 13 weeks and decreased to 0.25 by term. Prenzlau and Bildge (99) reported in 1985 on measurements of the occipital and inferior horns of the fetal ventricular system. Snijders and Nicolaides (115) published more recent data on normal frontal and occipital horn widths.

Cerebral Hemispheres

Hemispheric width. Measurements of hemispheric width were published by Johnson et al. (65) and Snijders and Nicolaides (115)

(Fig. 12.**19**). These authors measured the distance from the midline echo to the inner table of the calvaria (Fig. 12.**17**).

Ventricular–hemispheric ratio. Various authors (13, 28, 65, 115) have related the ventricular width at the pars centralis to the hemispheric width measured from the midline echo to the inner table of the skull (Fig. 12.**17**) and have calculated the ventricular–hemispheric ratio (V/H ratio) as a function of gestational age (Fig. 12.**20**). According to Johnson et al. (65), the normal V/H ratio decreases from an average of 0.56 at 15 weeks to 0.28 at term. Garrett (28) states that a V/H ratio greater than 0.5 after 18 weeks is proof of hydrocephalus. However, the data of Johnson et al. (65) indicate that this evidence for hydrocephalus is not conclusive until 21 weeks.

Cavum Septi Pellucidi

The cavum septi pellucidi is a slit-like hypoechoic cavity located on the anterior midline of the brain, inferior to the corpus callosum, and bordered by the two layers of the septum pellucidum. The septum pellucidum separates the frontal horns of the lateral ventricles (Fig. 12.**21**).

Normal values. Jou et al. (67) measured the cavum septi pellucidi in 608 fetuses between 19 and 42 weeks' gestation. The cavum septi pellucidi showed a uniform increase in size between 19 and 27 weeks, followed by a plateau that continued until term (Figs. 12.**19**, 12.**21**).

Cerebral dysfunction. A broad cavum septi pellucidi in childhood (>10 mm) is suggestive of cerebral dysfunction and may be associated with an increased risk of mental retardation, developmental delay, and neuropsychiatric disorders (9, 74, 106). It is still unclear whether the intrauterine detection of a large cavum septi pellucidi has similar implications.

Cerebellum

Transverse cerebellar diameter. Measurements of the transverse cerebellar diameter (TCD) (Figs. 12.**19**, 12.**22**, 12.**23**) have been published by various authors (29, 47, 50, 88, 114, 115).

Reference plane. The TCD is measured by tilting the occipitofrontal plane downward until the cerebellum appears as a bilobed structure in the posterior fossa. The cavum septi pellucidi can still be seen anteriorly in this plane. Goldstein et al. (29) found a nonlinear relationship between TCD and gestational age, while the other authors found a more linear relationship. Since the value of the TCD is approximately equal to the week of gestation between 12 and 22 weeks, this parameter is also useful for gestational age assignment.

Cisterna Magna

The cisterna magna is measured in the same plane as the cerebellum (Fig. 12.**24**). The growth curve is initially linear and declines toward the end of the pregnancy. Figure 12.**19** shows the data of Snijders and Nicolaides (115). Widening of the cisterna magna may be considered a suggestive sign of trisomy 18 (116) or trisomy 13 (70). The differential diagnosis includes Dandy–Walker malformation.

Nuchal Fold in the Second Trimester

The skin and subcutaneous tissue in the nuchal area, called the "nuchal fold," should not exceed 5 mm in diameter between 15 and 20 weeks' gestation. If it does, it implies an increased risk of trisomy 21 (6). The nuchal fold should not be confused with "nuchal translucency" at the end of the first trimester, which is caused by a fluid collection. The nuchal fold is measured in the posteriorly angled transverse scan through the fetal head that is also used to define and measure the cerebellum (Figs. 12.**25**, 12.**26**).

Orbital Diameters, Inner and Outer Interorbital Distance

Reference planes. The orbital diameters and the inner and outer interorbital distances can be measured as early as 13 weeks in a coronal scan, angled coronal scan, or transverse scan (Fig. 12.**27**). To detect or exclude certain syndromes that are associated with facial dysmorphia in the form of orbital asymmetry or hypo- or hypertelorism, it is essential to know the normal growth of the various orbital parameters as a function of gestational age.

Growth curves. Mayden et al. (75), Jeanty et al. (60), and Merz et al. (82) have published growth curves for orbital diameters or interorbital distances. Figure 12.**28** shows the growth curves for orbital diameters and interorbital distances that Merz et al. (82) established for 1090 normal fetuses between 12 and 41 weeks. On the whole, all of the orbital dimensions showed a nonlinear pattern of growth.

Ear

Ear length. Lettieri et al. (71) published a growth curve for fetal ear length in 1993 (Figs. 12.**29**, 12.**30**). Ear lengths at or below the tenth percentile are considered useful in identifying aneuploid fetuses with ultrasound (71).

Thyroid Gland

The thyroid gland is a relatively small structure that can be defined only by a high-resolution scanner with a zoom feature (Fig. 12.**31**).

Technique. Meinel and Döring (76) recommend the following technique for imaging the plane of the thyroid gland: Start with a longitudinal scan through the fetal neck showing the pharynx, larynx, and upper trachea. Then rotate the transducer 90° over the trachea to obtain a circular cross section of the neck with the vertebral ossification centers posterior. Next, shift the transducer cranially or caudally to locate a transverse plane that meets the following criteria:
- The circular, echo-free trachea is in the anterior midline of the neck.
- Lateral to the trachea, both thyroid lobes appear in their greatest transverse dimension.
- The echo-free cross sections of both carotid arteries and jugular veins appear lateral and posterior to the thyroid gland. These vessels are easily located with color Doppler.

Normal values. The transverse diameter of both thyroid lobes (including the trachea), the transverse diameters of the right and left lobes, and the AP diameters of the right and left lobes are shown in the Appendix as a function of gestational age based on data from Meinel and Döring (76).

A simple rule of thumb for routine studies is that the transverse diameter of both thyroid lobes, including the trachea, increases from 10 mm at 20 weeks to 20 mm at term (76).

Early detection. Measurement of the fetal thyroid gland can be useful in the early detection of fetal thyroid abnormalities. Initial prenatal treatment approaches are available in cases where a hypothyroid goiter is detected.

Thorax

Thoracometry

Schlensker (107), Stöger and Kratochwil (117), Levi and Erbsman (72), and Merz et al. (83) are among the few authors who have performed fetal thoracic measurements on the cardiac plane (Fig. 12.**32**). This type of thoracometry should not be confused with the older term "thoracometry" that was applied to abdominal measurements (41).

Growth curves. Figure 12.**23** shows the growth curves published by Merz et al. (83) for the bony thorax and oblique lung diameter. The bony thoracic parameters initially show a linear growth pattern, which levels off in the third trimester. By contrast, the growth rate of the oblique lung diameter shows a slight decline by just 12 weeks' gestation.

Pulmonary hypoplasia. Pulmonary hypoplasia can be detected as early as 24 weeks by means of thoracometry and lung measurements (85). Both thoracic and pulmonary biometry can detect this condition in fetuses with skeletal dysplasias (e.g., thanatophoric dysplasia) or bilateral renal agenesis, but only pulmonary biometry can detect it in fetuses with a diaphragmatic hernia or hydrothorax (85).

Heart

Parameters. The real-time four-chamber view provides a good general impression of fetal heart size and the width of the cardiac ventricles. The transverse cardiac diameter can be measured at the level of the valve plane and related to the transverse thoracic diameter. According to Garrett (28), the ratio of transverse cardiac diameter to transverse thoracic diameter is 0.52 in a normal fetus.

M-mode or cine loop. Either M-mode imaging or a cine loop is necessary for a precise evaluation of ventricular width during diastole and systole. The first step in both techniques is to obtain a four-chamber cardiac view in the two-dimensional real-time scan. If M-mode is used, a tracing is obtained at the level of the atrioventricular valves, perpendicular to the interventricular septum (20, 129, 130). If a cine loop is used, the four-chamber view is acquired, and then the image is zoomed and frozen. The cine loop is then reviewed to locate the cardiac phase in which the AV valves are closed at the end of diastole (Fig. 12.**34**).

Normal values for diameters. Wladimiroff et al. (129, 130) state that the end-diastolic transverse diameter of the right ventricle increases from 11 mm at 28 weeks to 18 mm at 40 weeks, while the end-systolic transverse diameter increases from 8 mm to 14 mm during the same period. The same progression is seen in the end-diastolic and end-systolic diameters of the left ventricle (see ventricular dimensions in Appendix), resulting in a right-to-left ratio of 1 : 1. DeVore et al. (20) found the same, constant right-to-left ratio (0.98 ± 0.08 [s]) in normal fetuses as early as 18 weeks' gestation.

Cardiac output. According to Wladimiroff et al. (130), the ventricular volumes in the end-diastolic and end-systolic phases can be determined by simultaneously measuring the transverse and longitudinal diameters of the left ventricle in the two-dimensional real-time image. Then the fetal heart rate and cardiac output can be calculated from the difference between these volumes (= stroke volume).

Other cardiac parameters. DeVore et al. (20, 21) reported on other cardiac parameters such as ventricular wall thickness and on M-mode measurements at the level of the aortic arch.

Figure 12.**35** shows the growth charts published by Chaoui et al. (15, 16) for cardiac length, cardiac width, cardiothoracic ratio, the diameters of the aorta (Fig. 12.**36**) and pulmonary trunk (Fig. 12.**37**), and the ratio of the pulmonary trunk and aortic diameters. Sharland and Allan (112) published additional growth charts for the fetal heart in 1992.

Abdomen and Pelvis

Liver

Growth curves. Growth curves for the fetal liver have been published by Vinzileos et al. (120), Murao et al. (90), and Roberts et al. (102). The length of the right lobe of the liver is measured from the diaphragm at the right cardiopulmonary boundary to the inferior hepatic border (Fig. 12.**38**). Roberts et al. (102) found that the growth in liver length flattens during the third trimester, whereas Murao et al. (90) observed a linear growth rate. The growth curve for fetal liver length shown in Fig. 12.**39** is based on the normal values published by Vinzileos et al. (120). Murao et al. (90) published normal data for the left lobe of the liver.

Gallbladder

The gallbladder is located at the inferior border of the right lobe of the liver, lateral to the entry of the umbilical vein (Fig. 12.**40**). Measurements of gallbladder length and width have been published by Goldstein et al. (33) and Hata et al. (44). The normal values for longitudinal and transverse gallbladder dimensions published in 1994 by Goldstein et al. (33) are listed in a table in the Appendix.

Spleen

Growth curves. Fetal spleen measurements have been published by Hobbins (52), Schmidt et al. (110), and Hata et al. (48). Figure 12.**39** shows the normal growth curves for longitudinal, sagittal, and transverse diameters and for the circumference and volume of the spleen based on data from Schmidt et al. (110).

Technique. The spleen is imaged posterolateral to the fluid-filled stomach in a transverse abdominal scan. The longitudinal diameter of the spleen is measured from its highest point lateral to the spine to its highest point bordering the abdominal wall (Fig. 12.**41**). The transverse splenic diameter is the maximum dimension measured perpendicular to the long diameter. The sagittal diameter of the spleen is defined by rotating the transducer 90° (longitudinal abdominal scan) and is measured perpendicular to the transverse diameter (110).

Splenomegaly. Splenomegaly is found in hemolytic anemias, chronic intrauterine infections, and in various metabolic disorders such as Gaucher disease and Niemann-Pick disease.

Pancreas

Hata et al. (45) investigated the head-to-tail length of the fetal pancreas between 20 and 40 weeks' gestation. Pancreas length was measured in a slightly oblique transverse scan through the fetal abdomen (Fig. 12.**42**). Pancreas length showed an almost linear growth pattern during pregnancy.

Stomach

The stomach is identified as a hypoechoic structure in the left upper abdomen. It appears elliptical in longitudinal section and round to oval in transverse section (Fig. 12.**43**).

Growth curves. Fetal stomach measurements have been published by Goldstein et al. (30), Nagata et al. (91), and Wilhelm et al. (126). Goldstein et al. (30) investigated the longitudinal, AP and transverse diameters of the fetal stomach between 9 and 40 weeks and found a linear growth pattern for all of the parameters. But when Nagata et al. (91) measured the longitudinal and AP gastric diameters, they found that these dimensions grew between 16–17 and 26–27 weeks, ceased to grow between 26–27 and 32–33 weeks, resumed growth between 32–33 and 36–37 weeks, and began to decline at 36–37 weeks.

On the whole, measurements of the fetal stomach are of little importance in biometry due to the normal daily fluctuations in the fullness and dimensions of the stomach. Goldstein et al. (30) reported, however, that they could detect very little change in gastric size over a three-hour observation period.

Bowel

Small-bowel loops. Nyberg et al. (93) reported on the measurement of small-bowel loops. They found that the small bowel never exceeded 7 mm in diameter after 34 weeks' gestation.

Colon loops. Especially in the third trimester, it is not uncommon to find fluid-distended colon loops in the fetal abdomen (Fig. 12.**44**). They are considered a normal finding. Various authors have measured the colon diameter (5, 31, 93). Goldstein et al. (31) measured the outer-to-outer colon diameter while Nyberg et al. (93) and Aoki et al. (5) measured the inner-to-inner diameter. The Appendix includes a chart showing the transverse colon diameters determined by Goldstein et al. (31) as a function of gestational age.

Kidneys

Renal diameters. Measurements of the various renal diameters were performed by Grannum et al. (13) and by Bernaschek and Kratochwil (7). Both groups found a steady increase in all three renal diameters until term. Measurements by Bernaschek and Kratochwil (7) between 20 and 40 weeks of gestation showed that the average longitudinal diameter of the fetal kidney increased from 22 to 44 mm, the transverse diameter from 15 to 31 mm, and the AP diameter from 10 to 20 mm.

Technique. The longitudinal renal diameter is measured in a paravertebral longitudinal scan (Fig. 12.**45**) and the transverse and AP diameters in a transverse scan (Fig. 12.**46**).

Growth curves. The growth curves for longitudinal and AP renal diameters shown in Fig. 12.**39** are based on reference data published by Bertagnoli et al. (8).

Renal circumference. Granuum et al. (35) also related renal circumference to abdominal circumference and found a constant ratio of 0.27 to 0.30 throughout pregnancy.

Adrenal Glands

The adrenal glands appear in transverse section (Fig. 12.**47**) as hypoechoic disk-shaped structures with an echogenic center located medial to the kidneys. In longitudinal section (Fig. 12.**47**), the adrenal gland appears as a heart-shaped structure located lateral to the spine and superomedial to the kidneys. Measurements of the adrenal glands have been published by Lewis et al. (73), Jeanty (64), and Hata (43, 46).

Bladder

Bladder volume. The capacity of the fetal bladder increases with gestational age. At 32 weeks the maximum bladder volume is still about

Table 12.4 Hourly fetal urine production rate versus gestational age. Synopsis of several studies (after [49])

Weeks	Campbell et al. (11) mL/h	Wladimiroff et al. (128) mL/h	Kurjak et al. (69) mL/h	Nakai (92) mL/h	Shin et al. (113) mL/h	Rabinowitz et al. (101) mL/h
20	–	–	–	2	2	5
21	–	–	–	2	–	–
22	–	–	2	3	–	–
23	–	–	3	3	–	–
24	–	–	4	4	–	9
25	–	–	5	4	–	–
26	–	–	6	5	–	–
27	–	–	7	6	–	–
28	–	–	8	7	11	14
29	–	–	8	8	–	–
30	–	10	10	9	–	18
31	–	11	11	10	–	–
32	12	12	12	12	–	22
33	14	14	13	14	–	–
34	15	15	14	16	–	27
35	17	18	18	18	32	–
36	18	18	19	21	–	33
37	21	21	21	24	42	–
38	23	24	24	28	43	41
39	25	26	25	33	–	–
40	28	27	26	38	35	51
41	26	26	27	44	34	–

10 mL, while at 40 weeks it is approximately 35 mL (11). The bladder volume (BV) (Fig. 12.**48**) is determined from the maximum bladder length, AP diameter, and transverse diameter using the following formula for an ellipsoidal body:

$$BV = {}^4\!/_3 \, \pi \times \text{longitudinal diameter}/2 \times \text{AP diameter}/2 \times \text{transverse diameter}/2$$

Hourly urine production rate. Measurements of fetal bladder volume have been used to calculate the hourly fetal urine production rate (11, 69, 92, 101, 113, 128). When several volume measurements are taken at intervals of 15–30 minutes, the hourly urine production rate can be calculated from the difference between the empty and full bladder. Bladder filling is a continuous process that has an average duration of 110 minutes (50–155 minutes) (11).

Hourly urine production increases with gestational age from an average of 9.6 mL/h at 30 weeks to 27.3 mL/h at 40 weeks (128). Table 12.**4** shows a synopsis of the hourly urine production rates determined by various groups of authors as a function of gestational age. It is apparent that the rates determined by Shin et al. (113) and Rabinowitz et al. (101) are markedly higher than those found by other authors (11, 69, 92, 128).

Growth retardation. Wladimiroff and Campbell (128) compared the hourly urine production rates of normally developed fetuses with those of growth-retarded fetuses and found that hourly fetal urine production was markedly lower in the growth-retarded fetuses.

Bladder emptying. The process of fetal bladder emptying is variable and may occur in a few seconds or may occur gradually over a period of 30 minutes (11). Bladder emptying is usually incomplete, leaving a small residual volume. According to Visser et al. (121), bladder emptying in 95% of cases occurs at the start of a strong oscillatory phase of fetal heart activity.

Specific Bone Measurements

Clavicle

Growth curves. Yarkoni et al. (132) published growth measurements of the normal fetal clavicle (Fig. 12.**49**). They found a linear growth rate between 15 and 40 weeks' gestation. Figure 12.**50** shows the growth curve for the clavicle based on the authors" data.

Diseases. The measurement of clavicular length is important in the prenatal detection of various diseases such cleidocranial dysplasia, Holt–Oram syndrome, Goltz syndrome, and Melnick–Needles syndrome.

Rib Length

Normal values. Abuhamad et al. (1) in 1996 published data on normal fetal rib length at the level of the four-chamber view. The authors observed linear growth from 14 to 40 weeks' gestation. The data from this study are the basis for the growth curve plotted in Fig. 12.**50**. The corresponding numerical data are listed in a table in the Appendix.

Technique. Rib length is measured in a transverse scan through the thorax at the level of the four-chamber view (Fig. 12.**51**). The rib closest to the transducer is measured. This is done by starting at the distal end of the ossified rib and moving the cursor along the curve of the rib and past the visible proximal end of the rib to the lateral border of the thoracic vertebral body.

Skeletal dysplasias. Fetal rib length can be used in the diagnosis of skeletal dysplasias such as the short rib–polydactyly syndrome.

Vertebral Bodies

Growth curves. Issel (58) published measurements of multiple fetal vertebrae in 1989. He measured the height of the five lumbar vertebrae plus the height of the T12 vertebral body in 2088 fetuses between 13 and 41 weeks' gestation (Fig. 12.**52**). It was found that the total height of the six vertebral bodies increased rather uniformly from 1.3 cm at 13 weeks to 6.3 cm at 41 weeks. Issel's data are shown graphically in Fig. 12.**50**.

Skeletal dysplasia. The ultrasound measurement of these six vertebral bodies could be important in cases where ossification of the fetal spinal column is impaired due to skeletal dysplasia.

Foot

The fetal foot can be measured in a lateral view or from the plantar aspect (Fig. 12.**53**).

Growth curves. Various ultrasound growth studies on the fetal foot were published during the 1980s (32, 66, 77, 87, 97). Most of these studies were based on relatively small case numbers and are difficult to compare with one another due to differences in methodology. The growth chart for fetal foot length shown in Fig. 12.**50** is based on data published by Merz et al. (86) in the year 2000. This was a prospective cross-sectional study done in 610 pregnant women with sonographically confirmed gestational ages between 12 and 41 completed weeks. It was found that the growth rate of the foot leveled off slightly up to 24 weeks and thereafter increased at an almost linear rate.

Comparative parameter. Fetal foot length is a good parameter for comparing with femur length, as the latter exhibits a similar growth pattern (Fig. 12.**54**). If the foot length is normal for dates while the femur is too short, this may indicate a disturbance of skeletal growth. Fetal foot length is also a very reliable parameter for determining gestational age (111).

Femur–foot ratio. The ratio of femur length to foot length averages approximately 1 up to 28 weeks' gestation. Thereafter it declines, slightly at first and then at a faster rate (Fig. 12.**50**) (86). On the whole, few studies have been published on the relationship between femur length and foot length (14, 32, 86, 97). Campbell et al. (14), who studied cases of skeletal dysplasia, state that a femur–foot ratio less than 1 is pathological. Goldstein et al. (32) and Platt et al. (97) reported on the foot-to-femur ratio.

Other Measurements

In addition to the parameters already described, other fetal growth parameters have been investigated and published in recent years. They include nasal width (34), bony nasal length (36), tongue circumference (2), shoulder-rump length (53, 98), the length and circumference of the thigh and lower leg (53), etc. Such parameters can be useful in selected investigations, but they are of minor importance compared with the parameters described above.

References

1. Abuhamad, A.Z., Sedule-Murphy, S.J., Dolm, P., Youssef, H., Warsof, S.L., Evans, A.T.: Prenatal ultrasonographic fetal rib length measurement: correlation with gestational age. Ultrasound Obstet. Gynecol. 7 (1996) 193–196
2. Achiron, R., Ben Arie, A., Gabbay, U., Mashiach, S., Roststein, Z., Lipitz, S.: Development of fetal tongue between 14 and 26 weeks of gestation: in utero ultrasonographic measurements. Ultrasound Obstet. Gynecol. 9 (1997) 39–41
3. Altman, D.G.: Constructing age-related reference centiles using absolute residuals. Stat. Med. 12 (1993) 917–924
4. Altman, D.G., Chitty, L.S.: Design and analysis of studies to derive charts of fetal size. Ultrasound Obstet. Gynecol. 3 (1993) 378–383
5. Aoki, S., Hata, T., Senoh, D. et al.: Ultrasonographic measurement of fetal colon. Acta Neanatol. Jpn. 25 (1989) 559–562
6. Benacerraf, B.R., Gelman, R., Frigoletto, F.D.: Sonographic identification of second trimester fetuses with Down's syndrome. N. Engl. J. Med. 317 (1987) 1371–1376
7. Bernaschek, G., Kratochwil, A.: Echographische Studie über das Wachstum der fetalen Niere in der zweiten Schwangerschaftshälfte. Geburtsh. u. Frauenheilk. 40 (1980) 1059–1064
8. Bertagnoli, L., Lalatta, F., Galliechio, R. et al.: Quantitative characterization of the growth of the fetal kidney. J. clin. Ultrasound 11 (1983) 349–356
9. Bodensteiner, J.B., Schaefer, G.B., Craft, J.M.: Cavum septi pellucidi and cavum vergae in normal and developmentally delayed populations. J. Child. Neurol. 13 (1998) 120–121
10. Campbell, S., Newman, G.B.: Growth of the fetal biparietal diameter during normal pregnancy. J. Obstet. Gynaec. Brit. Cwlth 78 (1971) 513–519
11. Campbell, S., Wladimiroff, J.W., Dewhurst, C.J.: The antenatal measurement of fetal urine production. J. Obstet. Gynaec. Brit. Cwlth 80 (1973) 680–686
12. Campbell, S., Thoms, A.: Ultrasound measurement of the fetal head to abdomen circumference ratio in the assessment of growth retardation. Brit. J. Obstet. Gynaec. 84 (1977) 165–174
13. Campbell, S.: Early prenatal diagnosis of fetal abnormality by ultrasound scanning. In Murken, J.D., Rutkowski, S., Schwinger, E.: Prenatal Diagnosis. Stuttgart: Enke 1979; p. 183
14. Campbell, J., Henderson, A., Campbell, S.: The fetal femur/foot length ratio: a new parameter to assess dysplastic limb reduction. Obstet. Gynecol. 72 (1988) 181–184
15. Chaoui, R., Heling, K.S., Bollmann, R.: Sonographische Messungen am fetalen Herzen in der Vierkammerblick-Ebene. Geburtsh. Frauenheilk. 54 (1994) 92–97
16. Chaoui, R., Heling, K.S., Bollmann, R.: Sonographische Messungen der Durchmesser der Aorta und des Truncus pulmonalis beim Feten. Gynäkol. Geburtshilfl. Rundschau 34 (1994) 145–151
17. Denkhaus, H., Winsberg, F.: Ultrasonic measurement of the fetal ventricular system. Radiology 131 (1979) 781–787
18. Deter, R.L., Harrist, R.B., Hadlock, F.P., Carpenter, R.J.: Fetal head and abdominal circumferences: II. A critical re-evaluation of the relationship to menstrual age. J. clin. Ultrasound 10 (1982) 365–372
19. Deter, R.L., Harrist, R.B.: Growth standards for anatomic measurements and growth rates derived from longitudinal studies of normal fetal growth. J. clin. Ultrasound 20 (1992) 381–388
20. DeVore, G.R., Siassi, B., Platt, L.D.: Fetal echocardiography IV. M-mode assessment of ventricular size and contractility during the second and third trimesters of prengnancy in the normal fetus. Amer. J. Obstet. Gynec. 150 (1984) 981–988
21. DeVore, G.R., Siassi, B., Platt, L.D.: Fetal echocardiography I. M-mode measurements of the aortic root and aortic valve in second- and third-trimester normal human fetus. Amer. J. Obstet. Gynec. 152 (1985) 543–550
22. European Congress on Perinatal Medicine: Suggestions concerning the nomenclature of birthweight and gestational age. Acta Paediatr. Scand. 59 (1970) 480
23. Exacoustos, C., Rosati, P., Rizzo, G., Arduini, D.: Ultrasound measurements of fetal limb bones. Ultrasound Obstet. Gynecol. 1 (1991) 325–330
24. Farrant, P., Meire, H.B.: Ultrasound measurement of fetal limb length. Brit. J. Radiol. 54 (1981) 660–664
25. Filly, R.A., Golbus, M.S., Carey, J.C. Hall, J.G.: Short-limbed dwarfism: Ultrasonographic diagnosis by mensuration of fetal femoral length. Radiology 138 (1981) 653–656
26. Filly, R.A., Golbus, M.S.: Ultrasonography of the normal and the pathologic fetal skeleton. Radiol. clin. N. Amer. 20 (1982) 311–323
27. Gallivan, S., Robson, S.C., Chang, T.C., Vaughan, J., Spencer, J.A.D.: An investigation of fetal growth using serial ultrasound data. Ultrasound Obstet. Gynecol. 3 (1993) 109–114
28. Garrett, W.J.: Ultrasound in discerning normal fetal anatomy. In: Hobbins, J.C. (ed.): Diagnostik Ultrasound in Obstetrics. New York: Churchill Livingstone 1979; p. 57
29. Goldstein, I., Reece, E.A., Pilu, G., Bovicelli, L., Hobbins, J.C.: Cerebellar measurements with ultrasonography in the evaluation of fetal growth and development. Am. J. Obstet. Gynecol. 156 (1987)1065–1069
30. Goldstein, I., Reece, E.A., Yarkoni, S., Wan, M., Green, J.L.J., Hobbins, J.C.: Growth of the fetal stomach in normal pregnancies. Obstet. Gynecol. 70 (1987) 641–644
31. Goldstein, I., Lockwood, C., Hobins, J.C.: Ultrasound assessment of fetal intestinal development in the evaluation of gestational age. Obstet. Gynecol. 70 (1987) 682–686
32. Goldstein, I., Reece, E.A., Hobbins, J.C.: Sonographic appearance of the fetal heel ossification centers and foot length measurements provide independent markers for gestational age estimation. Amer. J. Obstet. Gynecol. 159(4) (1988) 923–926
33. Goldstein, I., Tamir, A., Weisman, A., Jakobi, P. Copel, J.A.: Growth of the fetal gall bladder in normal pregnancies. Ultrasound Obstet. Gynecol. 4 (1994) 289–293
34. Goldstein, I., Tamir, A., Itskovitz-Eldor, J., Zimmer, E.Z.: Growth of the fetal nose width and nostril distance in normal pregnancies. Ultrasound Obstet. Gynecol. 9 (1997) 35–38
35. Grannum, P., Bracken, M., Silverman, R., Hobbins, J.C.: Assessment of fetal kidney size in normal gestation by comparison of ratio of kidney circumference to abdominal circumference. Amer. J. Obstet. Gynec. 136 (1980) 249–254
36. Guis, F., Ville, Y., Vincent, Y., Doumerc, S., Pons, J.C., Frydman, R.: Ultrasound evaluation of the length of the fetal nasal bones throughout gestation. Ultrasound Obstet. Gynecol. 5 (1995) 304–307
37. Hadlock, F.P., Deter, R.L., Harrist, R.B., Park, S.K.: Fetal head circumference: Relation to menstrual age. Amer. J. Roentgenol. 138 (1982) 649–653
38. Hadlock, F.P., Deter, R.L., Harrist, R.B., Park, S.K.: Fetal biparietal diameter: Rational choice of plane of section for sonographic measurement. Amer. J. Roentgenol. 138 (1982) 871–874
39. Hadlock, F.P., Harrist, R.B., Deter, R.L., Park, S.K.: Fetal femur length as a predictor of menstrual age: Sonographically measured. Amer. J. Roentgenol. 138 (1982) 875–878
40. Hadlock, F.P., Deter, R.L., Harrist, R.B., Park, S.K.: Fetal abdominal circumference as a predictor of menstrual age. Amer. J. Roentgenol. 139 (1982) 367–370
41. Hansmann, M.: Ultraschallbiometrie im II. und III. Trimester der Schwangerschaft. Gynäkologe 9 (1976) 133–155
42. Hansmann, M.: Bestimmung des Gestationsalters und -gewichts und die Bedeutung für das klinische Management. In: Huch, A., Huch, R., Duc, G., Rooth, G.: Klinisches Management des kleinen Frühgeborenen. Stuttgart: Thieme 1982; S. 31
43. Hata, K., Hata, T., Kitao, M.: Ultrasonographic identification and measurement of the human fetal adrenal gland in utero. Int. J. Gynecol. Obstet. 23 (1985) 355–359
44. Hata, K., Aoki, S., Hata, T., Murao, F., Kitao, M.: Ultrasonographic identification of the human fetal gallbladder in utero. Gynecol. Obstet. Invest. 23 (1987) 79–83
45. Hata, K., Hata, T., Kitao, M.: Ultrasonographic identification and measurement of the human fetal pancreas in utero. Int. J. Gynecol. Obstet. 26 (1988) 61–64
46. Hata, K., Hata, T., Kitao, M.: Ultrasonographic identification and measurement of the human fetal adrenal gland in utero: Clinical application. Gynecol. Obstet. Invest. 25 (1988) 16–22
47. Hata, K., Hata, T., Senoh, D. et al.: Ultrasonographic measurement of the fetal transverse cerebellum in utero. Gynecol. Obstet. Invest. 28 (1989) 111–112
48. Hata, T., Aoki, S., Takamori, H., Hata, K., Murao, F., Kitao, M.: Ultrasonographic in utero identification and measurement of the normal fetal spleen. Gynecol. Obstet. Invest. 23 (1987) 124–128
49. Hata, T., Deter, R.L.: A review of fetal organ measurements obtained with ultrasound: normal growth. J. clin. Ultrasound 20 (1992) 155–174
50. Hill, L.M., Guzick, D., Fries, J., Hixson, J., Rivello, D.: The transverse cerebellar diameter in estimating gestational age in the large for gestational age fetus. Obstet. Gynecol. 75 (1990) 981–985
51. Hobbins, J.C., Bracken, M.B., Mahoney, M.J.: Diagnosis of fetal skeletal dysplasias with ultrasound. Amer. J. Obstet. Gynec.142 (1982) 306–312
52. Hobbins, J.C.: Sonographic measurements of the fetal spleen: Clinical implications. J. Ultrasound Med. 4 (1985) 667–672
53. Hoffbauer, H., Arabin, B., Pachaly, J.: Über die sonographische Messung multipler fetaler Körperparameter. Ultraschall 1 (1980) 84–100
54. Hohler, C.W., Quetel, T.A.: Comparison of ultrasound femur length and biparietal diameter in late pregnancy. Amer. J. Obstet. Gynec. 141 (1981) 759–760
55. Holländer, H.J.: Die Ultraschalldiagnostik in der Schwangerschaft. München: Urban & Schwarzenberg 1972
56. Holländer, H.J.: Die Ultraschalldiagnostik in der Schwangerschaft. München: Urban & Schwarzenberg 1984
57. Hughey, M., Sabbagha, R.E.: Cephalometry by real-time imaging: A critical evaluation. Amer. J. Obstet. Gynec. 131 (1978) 825–830
58. Issel, E.P.: Die Messung der Höhe von 6 Wirbelkörpern als neuer Parameter in der Fetometrie. Ultraschall Klin. Prax. 4 (1989) 21–25

Continued on page 159

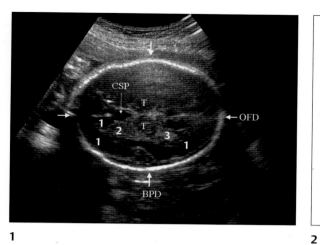

1

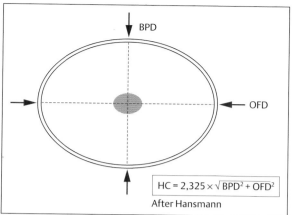

$$HC = 2,325 \times \sqrt{BPD^2 + OFD^2}$$

After Hansmann

2

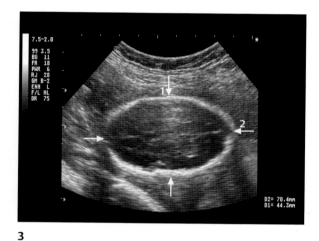

3

Cephalometry

Fig. 12.**1**   Correct ultrasound plane for measuring the biparietal and occipitofrontal diameters. Outer-to-outer (skin-to-skin) measurements (BPD 66 mm, OFD 78 mm) at 25 weeks. Cephalic presentation, 1st position. CSP = cavum septi pellucidi, T = thalamus, 1 = brain mantle, 2 = frontal horn of lateral ventricle, 3 = occipital horn of lateral ventricle.

Fig. 12.**2**   Calculating head circumference (HC) from BPD and OFD (after [42]).

Fig. 12.**3**   Dolichocephalic head shape in a breech-presenting fetus at 22 weeks, 1 day. BPD (1) 44 mm, OFD (2) 70 mm.

Fig. 12.**4** Growth curves for the fetal head and abdomen as a function of gestational age (in completed weeks). The 5th, 50th, and 95th percentiles are shown (after [84]).

a Biparietal diameter (BPD).
b Occipitofrontal diameter (OFD).
c Head circumference (HC).
d Abdominal transverse diameter (ATD).
e Abdominal sagittal diameter (ASD).
f Abdominal circumference (AC).

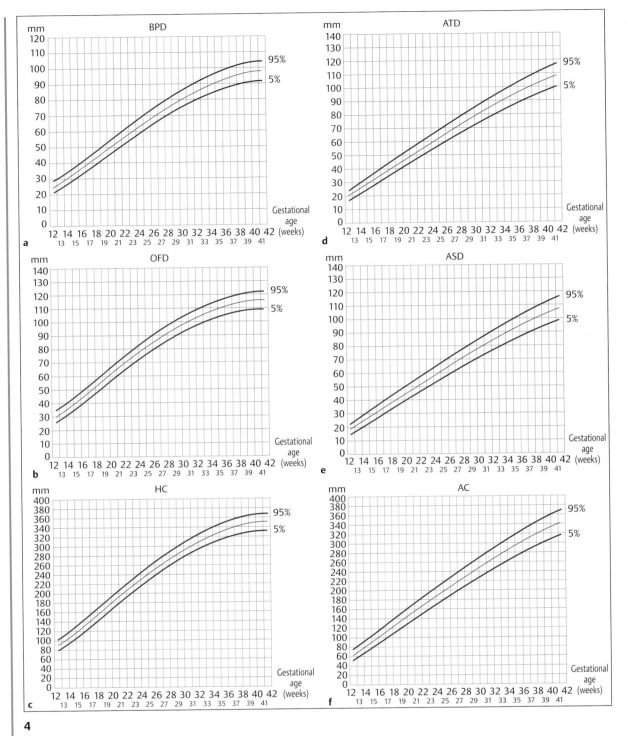

4

Abdominal Biometry

Fig. 12.**5** Radiograph of a fetal trunk indicating the superior and inferior "cones" and the interposed upper abdominal cylinder (after [68]).

Fig. 12.**6** Scan plane 1 = standard reference plane for abdominometry. → = Entry of the umbilical vein into the portal sinus. Plane 2 shows an extended intra-abdominal segment of the umbilical vein (approximately 45–60° oblique, the "salami scan"). Fetus is in a cephalic presentation.

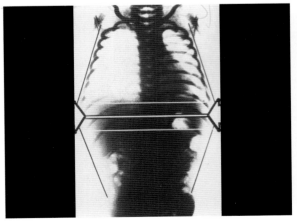

5

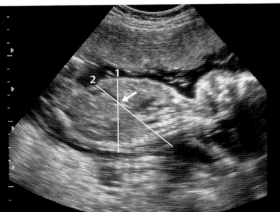

6

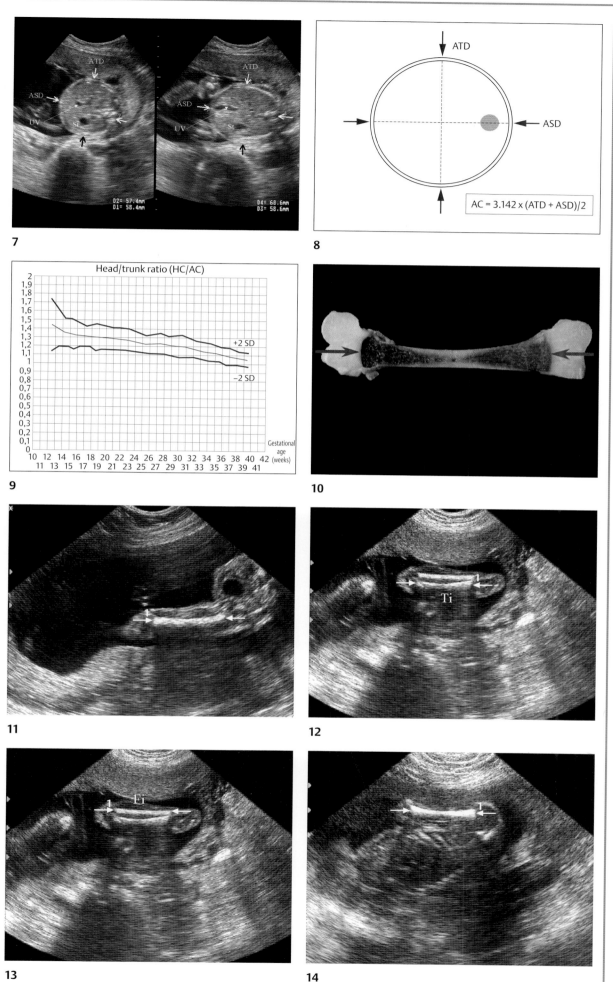

7

8

9

10

11

12

13

14

Head/trunk ratio (HC/AC)

AC = 3.142 x (ATD + ASD)/2

Fig. 12.**7** Left: correct reference plane for abdominometry. The abdomen has a circular cross section, and only a short segment of the umbilical vein is visible within the abdomen. St = stomach. ATD 58 mm, ASD 57 mm, 24 weeks.
Right: oblique scan through the fetal abdomen, incorrect for abdominometry. A long segment of the umbilical vein (UV) can be traced inward from the abdominal wall ("salami scan"). The sagittal abdominal diameter in this plane appears too large (ATD 59 mm, ASD 69 mm).

Fig. 12.**8** The abdominal circumference is calculated from the two abdominal diameters, ATD and ASD, using the formula for an ellipse.
Key: AC = 3.142 · (ATD + ASD)/2

Fig. 12.**9** Head/trunk ratio versus gestational age in completed weeks (after [81]).

Long Tubular Bones

Fig. 12.**10** Specimen of a fetal femur. The length of long tubular bones is determined by measuring the ossified shaft, consisting of the diaphysis and metaphysis. The cartilaginous epiphyses are disregarded.

Fig. 12.**11** Measurement of the ossified femoral shaft. The femur length measures 37 mm at 22 weeks. The longest ossified segment is measured, ignoring the curvature of the bone. The measurement does not include the femoral ossification center that appears in the third trimester.

Fig. 12.**12** Tibia length measures 34 mm at 21 weeks.

Fig. 12.**13** Fibula length measures 33 mm at 21 weeks, 6 days. The fibular shaft is slightly thinner than the tibial shaft.

Fig. 12.**14** Humeral length measures 34 mm at 21 weeks.

Fig. 12.**15** Measurement of radial and ulnar length at 31 weeks. The radius, which measures 44 mm, is considerably shorter than the ulna, which measures 50 mm.

Fig. 12.**16** Growth curves for the fetal long limb bones as a function of gestational age (in completed weeks). The 5th, 50th, and 95th percentiles are shown (after [84]).
a Femur.
b Tibia.
c Fibula.
d Humerus.
e Radius.
f Ulna.

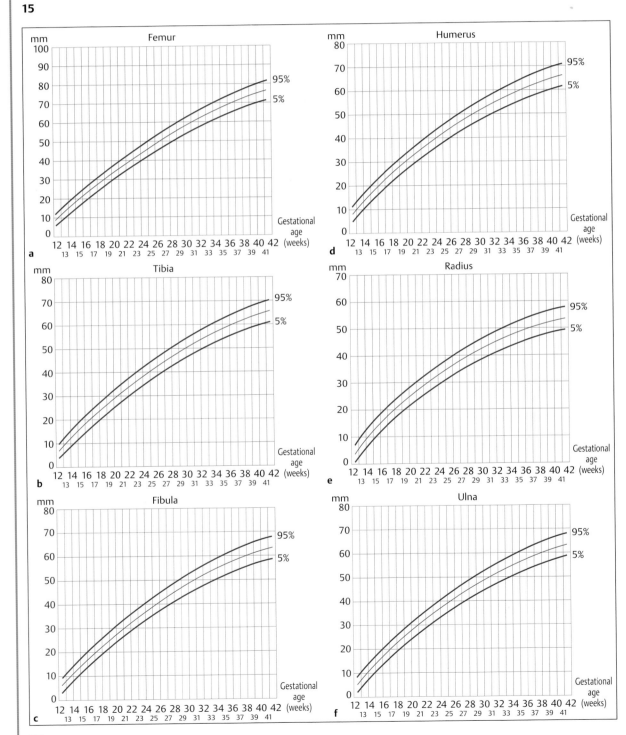

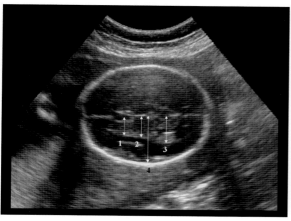

17

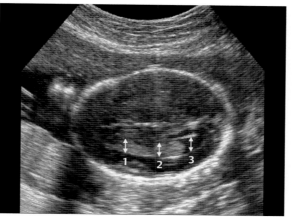

18

Fig. 12.**17** The width of the lateral ventricle is measured at various points from the midline echo: (1) frontal horn, (2) pars centralis, (3) occipital horn. The hemispheric width (HW) is measured from the midline echo to the inner border of the calvaria (4).

Fig. 12.**18** Measurement of the exact anatomic width of the lateral ventricle: (1) frontal horn, (2) pars centralis, (3) occipital horn (7 mm). 20 weeks, 5 days.

Fig. 12.**19** Organ biometry. Growth of intracranial structures versus gestational age (in completed weeks). The 5th, 50th, and 95th percentiles are shown (a, b, c, e, and f based on data from [115], d based on data from [67]).
- **a** Lateral ventricle, frontal horn.
- **b** Lateral ventricle, occipital horn.
- **c** Cerebral hemisphere.
- **d** Cavum septi pellucidi (transverse diameter).
- **e** Transverse cerebellar diameter.
- **f** Width of cisterna magna (AP diameter).

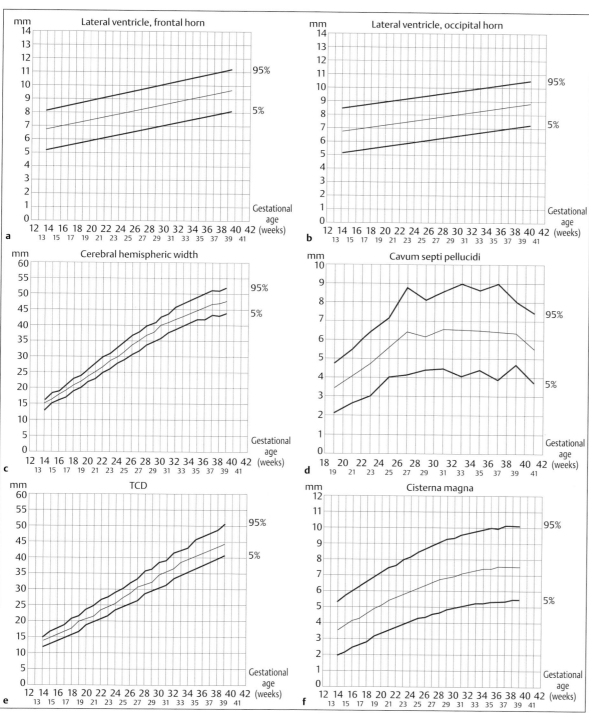

19

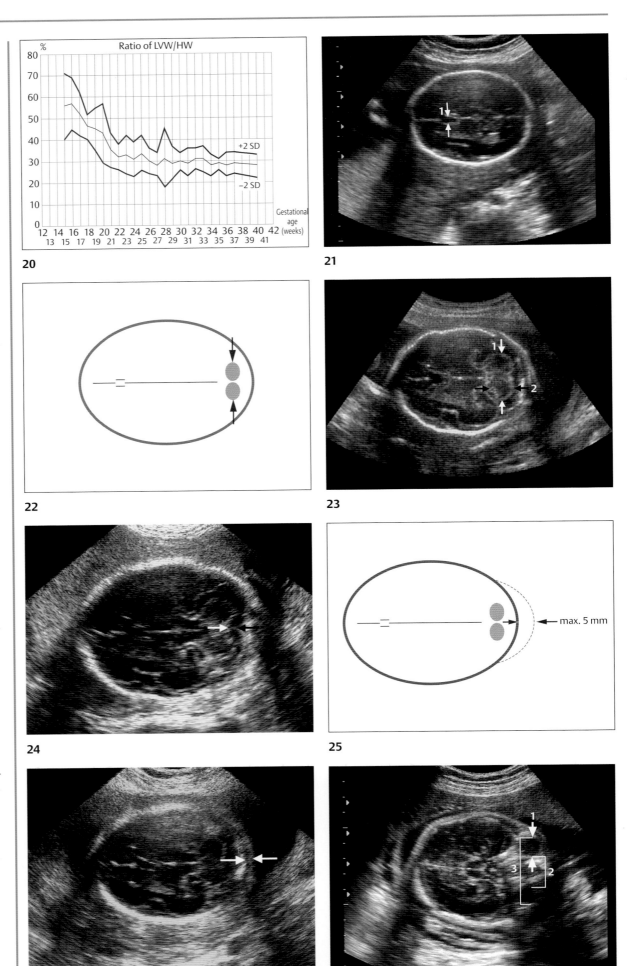

Fig. 12.**20**   Ventricular-hemispheric ratio versus gestational age (in completed weeks). LVW = lateral ventricular width, HW = hemispheric width. Mean values ± 2 SD (based on data from [65]).

Fig. 12.**21**   Inner-to-inner measurement of the cavum septi pellucidi (5 mm) at 28 weeks.

Fig. 12.**22**   Schematic representation of the points used in measuring the transverse cerebellar diameter (TCD).

Fig. 12.**23**   Measurement of the transverse (1) and sagittal cerebellar diameters (2), 25 weeks.

Fig. 12.**24**   Scan plane VI (see Fig. 11.**6**) is tilted for measurement of the cisterna magna (6 mm at 26 weeks).

Fig. 12.**25**   Measurement of the "nuchal fold" in the second trimester. The measurement is taken in scan plane VII (see Fig. 11.**6**), which demonstrates the cerebellum posteriorly and the cavum septi pellucidi anteriorly.

Fig. 12.**26**   The "nuchal fold" is measured between the skull and outer skin. A fold up to 5 mm thick is a normal finding.

Fig. 12.**27**   Measurement of the orbital diameter (D1 = 15 mm), inner interorbital distance (D2 = 15 mm), and outer interorbital distance (D3 = 45 mm) at 28 weeks.

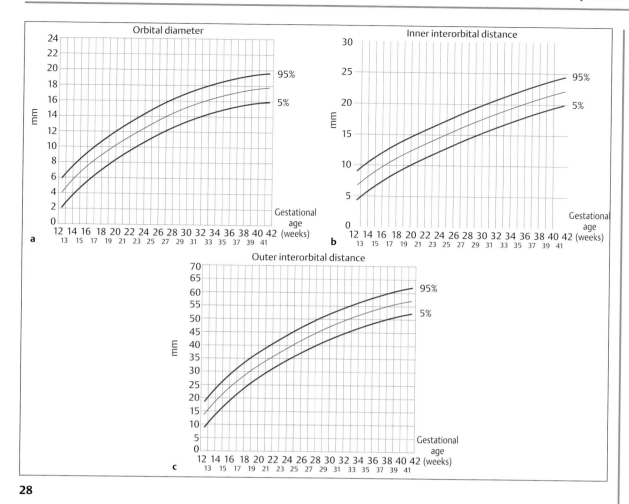

28

Fig. 12.**28** Growth curves for the fetal orbital diameter (**a**), inner interorbital distance (**b**), and outer interorbital distance (**c**) as a function of gestational age (in completed weeks). The 5th, 50th, and 95th percentiles are shown (after [82]).

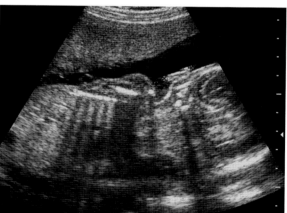

29

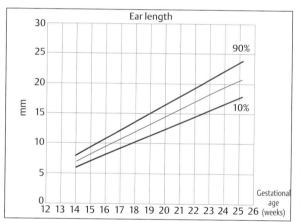

30

Fig. 12.**29** Measurement of ear length in a fetus lying on its side (15 mm) at 20 weeks.

Fig. 12.**30** Growth curve for the fetal ear length as a function of gestational age (in completed weeks). The 10th, 50th, and 95th percentiles are shown (after [71]).

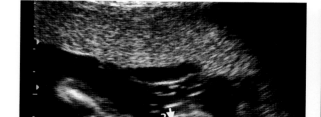

31

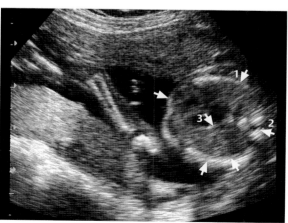

32

Fig. 12.**31** Measurement of the transverse diameter of both thyroid lobes (1) (D = 21 mm) and the AP diameter of the left lobe (2) (D = 10 mm) at 20 weeks. The fetus is in a cephalic presentation with the spine down.

Thoracometry

Fig. 12.**32** Measurement of the transverse and sagittal bony thoracic diameters (BTTD [1] = 41 mm, BTSD [2] = 42 mm) and of the oblique lung diameter in continuity with the long axis of the heart (LD [3] = 16 mm). 20 weeks, 5 days. Breech presentation, 1st position.

Fig. 12.**33** Thoracometry.
a Diagram showing the correct measurement of the bony thoracic transverse diameter (BTTD), the bony thoracic sagittal diameter (BTSD), and the oblique lung diameter (LD).
b–f Growth charts for the BTTD (**b**), BTSD (**c**), bony thoracic circumference (BTC, **d**), LD (**e**), and the ratio of LD to BTC (**f**) versus gestational age (in completed weeks). The 5th, 50th, and 95th percentiles are shown (after [83]).

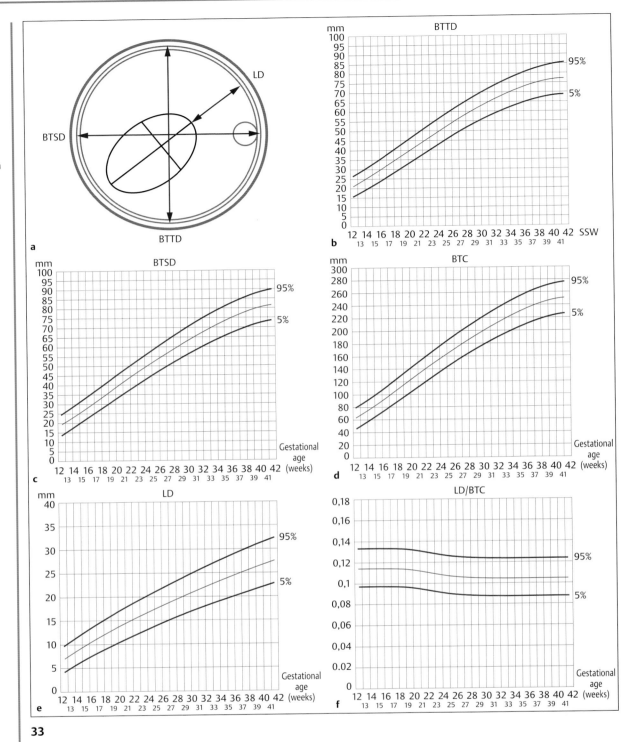

33

Fig. 12.**34** Measurement of cardiac length (D1) and cardiac width (D2) in the four-chamber view with the AV valves closed.

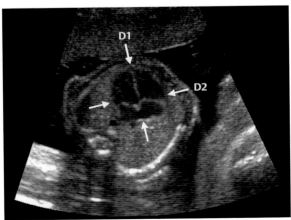

34

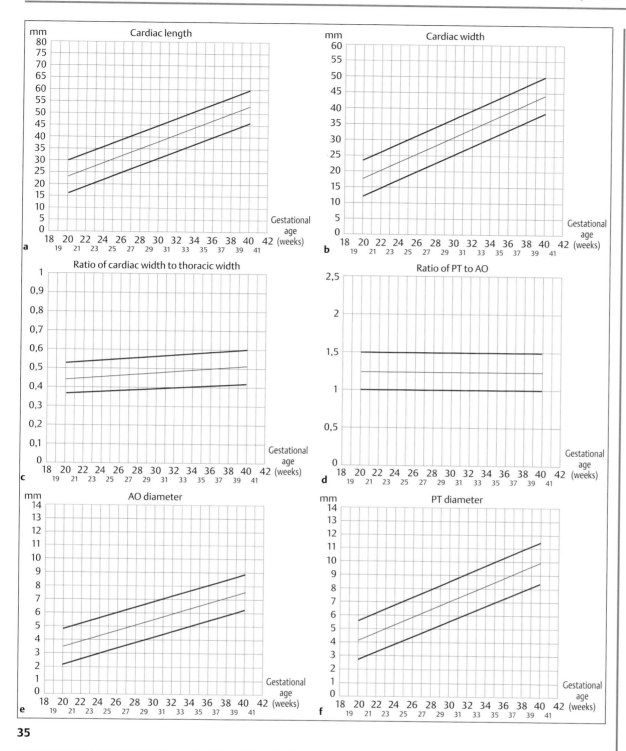

Fig. 12.**35** Growth curves for various cardiac parameters as a function of gestational age (in completed weeks). The 95% confidence interval is shown (a–c based on data from [15], **d–f** based on data from [16]).

a Cardiac length.

b Cardiac width.

c Ratio of cardiac width to thoracic width.

d Ratio of pulmonary trunk diameter (PT) to aortic diameter (AO).

e Aortic (AO) diameter.

f Pulmonary trunk (PT) diameter.

35

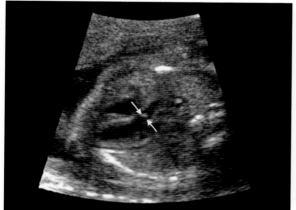

36

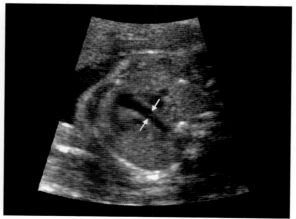

37

Fig. 12.**36** Inner-to-inner measurement of the aortic diameter (4.5 mm), 23 weeks. The best measurement is obtained at the start of diastole when the aortic valve is closed.

Fig. 12.**37** Measurement of the pulmonary trunk diameter (5.6 mm), 23 weeks. Like the aortic diameter, this is an inner-to-inner measurement taken at the start of diastole when the valve is closed.

Organ Biometry: Abdominal and Pelvis

Fig. 12.**38** The length of the fetal liver (right lobe) is measured from the diaphragm to the inferior hepatic border. A length of 45 mm at 34 weeks is in the mid-normal range.

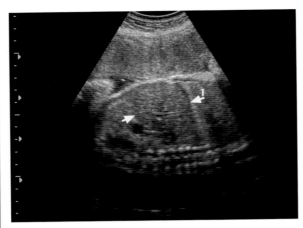

38

Fig. 12.**39** Growth curves for liver length (**a**), spleen length (**b**), transverse spleen diameter (**c**), sagittal spleen diameter (**d**), kidney length (**e**), and kidney AP diameter (**f**) as a function of gestational age (in completed weeks). The curves are shown as percentiles (5th, 50th, and 95th) or as the mean ± 2 SD (a based on data from [120], b–d based on data from [110], e–f based on data from [8]).

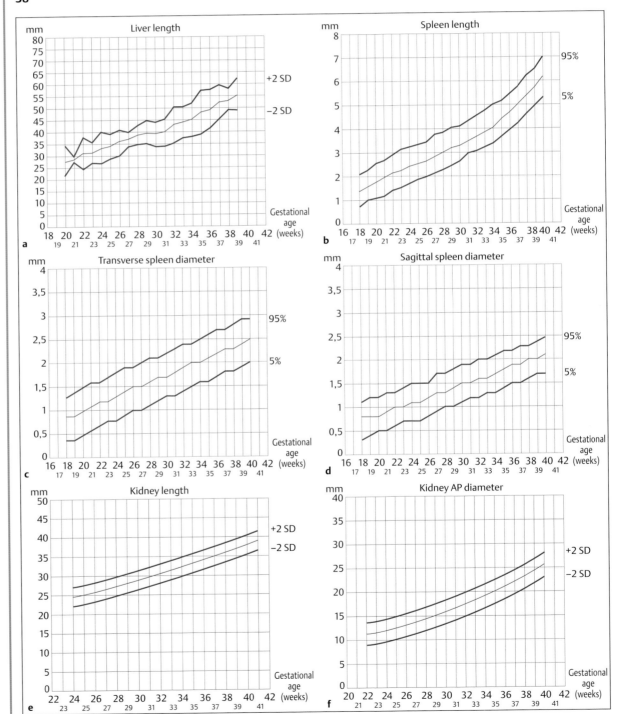

39

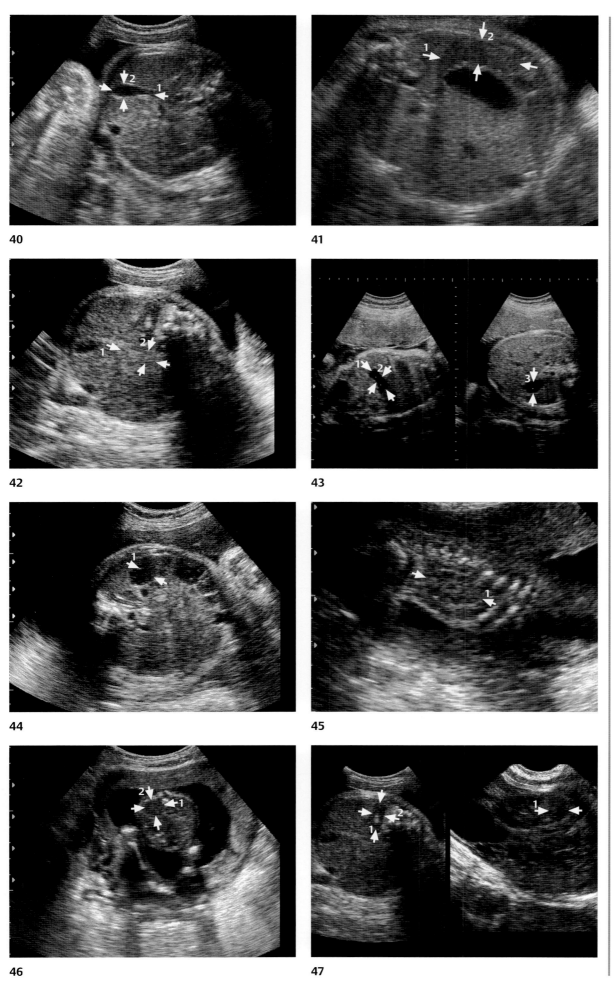

40

41

42

43

44

45

46

47

Fig. 12.**40**   Inner-to-inner measurement of gallbladder length and width (length: 28 mm, width: 10 mm) at 35 weeks, 4 days. Cephalic presentation, 2nd position.

Fig. 12.**41**   Measurement of the length and width of the fetal spleen in a transverse abdominal scan (length: 35 mm, width: 13 mm) at 35 weeks. The sagittal spleen diameter is measured in a longitudinal abdominal scan.

Fig. 12.**42**   Measurement of the length and width of the pancreas in a slightly oblique transverse scan (length: 26 mm, width: 9 mm) at 35 weeks.

Fig. 12.**43**   Measurement of the fetal stomach in a longitudinal abdominal scan (left image) and transverse abdominal scan (right image) at 32 weeks. The gastric volume is 2.3 mL.

Fig. 12.**44**   The diameter of fluid-filled colon loops is measured from inner-to-inner margin (luminal width 17 mm).

Fig. 12.**45**   Measurement of longitudinal renal diameter in a paravertebral longitudinal scan (25 mm) at 22 weeks.

Fig. 12.**46**   Measurement of the transverse and AP renal diameters in a transverse scan at 17 weeks, 6 days. Transverse diameter of the left kidney (1): 11 mm. AP diameter of the left kidney (2): 10 mm. The fetus is in a breech presentation with the spine up.

Fig. 12.**47**   Left: measurement of the right adrenal gland in transverse section (21 x 11 mm) at 35 weeks, 4 days. Right: measurement of the length of the adrenal gland at the superior border of the kidney (arrows).

Fig. 12.**48** Measurement of the three mutually perpendicular diameters of the fetal bladder. Left: coronal scan showing the longitudinal diameter (25 mm) and transverse diameter (19 mm). Right: transverse scan showing the AP diameter (17 mm). The three diameters indicate a bladder volume of 4.2 mL. 30 weeks.

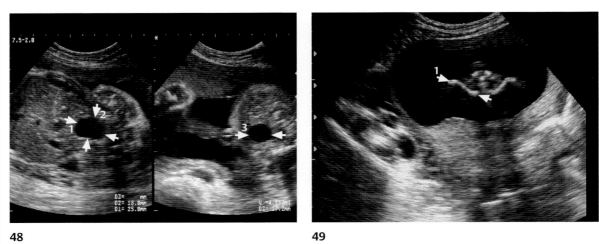

48　　　　　　　　　　　**49**

Specific Bone Measurements

Fig. 12.**49** Measurement of clavicle length (20 mm) at 17 weeks. The curvature of the bone is ignored.

Fig. 12.**50** Growth curves for clavicle length (**a**), rib length (**b**), the length of six vertebral bodies (**c**), foot length (**d**), and the ratio of femur to foot length (**e**) as a function of gestational age (in completed weeks). The curves are shown as percentiles (5th, 50th, and 95th) or as the mean ± 2 SD (a based on data from [132], **b** based on data from [1], **c** based on data from [58], **d** and **e** based on data from [86]).

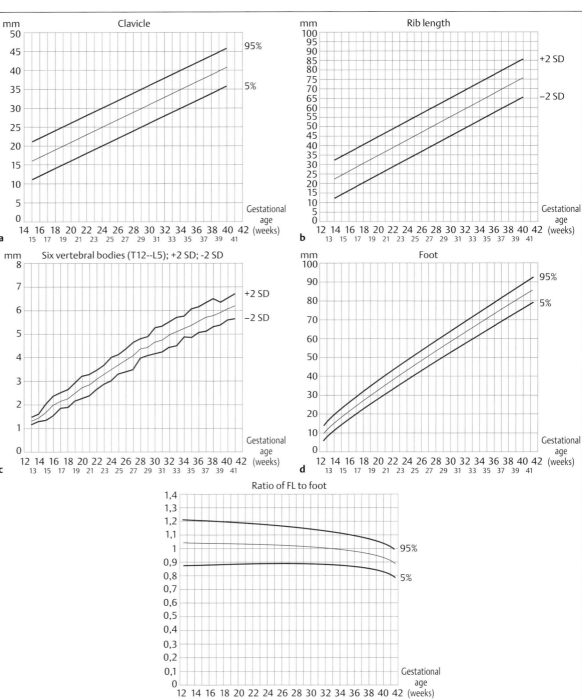

50

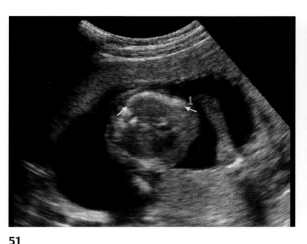

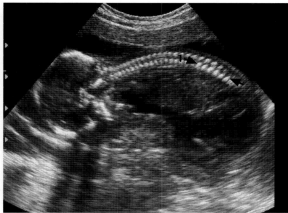

Fig. 12.**51** Rib length measured in a transverse thoracic scan at the level of the four-chamber view. The measurement extends from the distal end of the ossified rib along the curve of the rib to the lateral margin of the associated thoracic vertebral body. Vertebral length = 28 mm at 18 weeks.

Fig. 12.**52** Vertebral measurement described by Iseel (58). The segment comprising the 5 lumbar vertebrae and 12th thoracic vertebra is measured. Length = 22 mm at 17 weeks.

Fig. 12.**53** Measurement of the foot from the plantar aspect. Foot length = 47 mm at 28 weeks.

Fig. 12.**54** Comparative measurements of the foot and femur at 28 weeks. If growth is normal, the two measurements will be similar up to 28 weeks. Femur length = 44 mm, foot length = 49 mm.

51

52

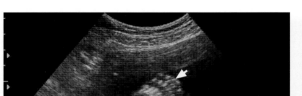

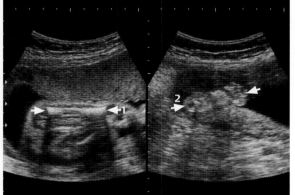

53

54

Continued from page 146

59. Jeanty, P., Kirkpatrick, C., Dramaix-Wilmet, M., Struyven, J.: Ultrasonic evaluation of fetal limb growth. Radiology 140 (1981) 165–168
60. Jeanty, P., Dramaix-Wilmet, M., van Gansbeke, D., van Regemorter, M., Roedesch, F.: Fetal ocular biometry by ultrasound. Radiology 142 (1982) 513–516
61. Jeanty, P., Dramaix-Wilmet, M., van Kerkem, J., Petroons, P., Schwers, J.: Ultrasonic evaluation of fetal limb growth. Radiology 143 (1982) 751–754
62. Jeanty, P.: Fetal limb biometry. Radiology 147 (1983) 601–602
63. Jeanty, P., Rodesch, F., Delbeke, D., Dumont, J.E.: Estimation of gestational age from measurement of fetal long bones. J. Ultrasound Med. 3 (1984) 75–79
64. Jeanty, P., Chervenak, F., Grannum, P., Hobbins; J.C.: Normal ultrasonic size and characteristics of the fetal adrenal glands. Prenat. Diagn. 4 (1984) 21–28
65. Johnson, M.L., Dunne, M.G., Mack, L.A., Rashbaum, C.L.: Evaluation of fetal intracranial anatomy by static and real-time ultrasound. J. clin. Ultrasound 8 (1980) 311–318
66. Jordaan, H.V.: Fetal foot length. S. Afr. Med. J. 62(14) (1982) 473–475
67. Jou, H.-J., Shyu, M.-K., Wu, S.-C., Chen, S.-M., Su, C.-H., Hsieh, F.-J.: Ultrasound measurement of the fetal cavum septi pellucidi. Ultrasound Obstet. Gynecol. 12 (1998) 419–421
68. Kugener, H., Hansmann, M.: Zur Topographie einer Referenzebene für die Ultraschallthorakometrie. Z. Geburtsh. Perinat. 180 (1976) 313–319
69. Kurjak, A., Kirkinen, P., Latin, V., Ivankovic, D.: Ultrasonic assessment of fetal kidney function in normal and complicated pregnancies. Amer. J. Obstet. Gynecol. 141 (1981) 266–270
70. Lehman, C.D., Nyberg, D.A., Winter, T.C.3rd, Kapur, R.P., Resta, R.G., Luthy, D.A.: Trisomy 13 syndrome: prenatal US findings in a review of 33 cases. Radiology 194 (1995) 217–222
71. Lettieri, L., Rodis, J.F., Vintzileos, A.M., Feeney, L., Ciarleglio, L., Craffey, A.: Ear length in second-trimester aneuploid fetuses. Obstet. Gynecol. 81 (1993) 57–60
72. Levi, S., Erbsman, F.: Antenatal fetal growth from the nineteenth week. Amer. J. Obstet. Gynec. 121 (1975) 262–268
73. Lewis, E., Jurtz, A.B., Dubbins, P.A., Wapner, R.J., Goldberg, B.B.: Real-time ultrasonographic evaluation of normal fetal adrenal glands. J. Ultrasound Med. 1 (1982) 265–270
74. Lewis, S.W., Mezey, G.C.: Clinical correlates of septum pellucidum cavities: an unusual association with psychosis. Psychol. Med. 15 (1985) 43–54
75. Mayden, K.L., Tortora, M., Berkowitz, R.L., Bracken, M., Hobbins, J.C.: Orbital diameters: A new parameter for prenatal diagnosis and dating. Amer. J. Obstet. Gynec. 144 (1982) 289–297
76. Meinel, K., Döring, K.: Wachstum der fetalen Schilddrüse in der II. Schwangerschaftshälfte – Sonographisch-biometrische Untersuchungen. Ultraschall in Med. 18 (1997) 258–261

77. Mercer, B.M., Sklar, S., Shariatmadar, A., Gillieson, M.S., D'Alton, M.E.: Fetal foot length as a predicator of gestational age. Amer. J. Obstet. Gynecol. 156(2) (1987) 350–355
78. Merz, E., Pehl, S., Goldhofer, W., Hoffmann, G.: Biometrie der großen Extremitätenknochen im III. Trimenon. Ultraschall 5 (1984) 136–143
79. Merz, E., Kim-Kern, M.S., Pehl, S.: Ultrasonic mensuration of fetal limb bones in the second and third trimesters. J. Clin. Ultrasound 15 (1987) 175–183
80. Merz, E., Grüssner, A., Kern, F.: Entwicklung eines Wachstumsmodells für fetale Kopf- und Rumpfmaße. Geburtsh. u. Frauenheilk. 47 (1987) 738–741
81. Merz, E.: Habilitationsschrift: Sonographische Überwachung der fetalen Knochenentwicklung im II. und III. Trimenon. Eine Studie über das Wachstum der langen Röhrenknochen im Vergleich zum Kopf- und Rumpfwachstum sowie über die Verwendungsmöglichkeiten der fetalen Knochenlänge im Rahmen der geburtshilflichen Ultraschalluntersuchung. Mainz (1988)
82. Merz, E., Wellek, S., Püttmann, S., Bahlmann, F., Weber, G.: Orbitadurchmesser, innerer und äußerer Orbitaabstand. Ein Wachstumsmodell für die fetalen Orbitamaße. Ultraschall in Med. 16 (1995) 12–17
83. Merz, E., Wellek, S., Bahlmann, F., Weber, G.: Sonographische Normkurven des fetalen knöchernen Thorax und der fetalen Lunge. Geburtsh. u. Frauenheilk. 55 (1995) 77–82
84. Merz, E., Wellek, S.: Das normale fetale Wachstumsprofil – ein einheitliches Modell zur Berechnung von Normkurven für die gängigen Kopf- und Abdomenparameter sowie die großen Extremitätenknochen. Ultraschall in Med. 17 (1996) 153–162
85. Merz, E., Miric-Tesanic, D., Bahlmann, F., Weber, G., Hallermann, C.: Prenatal sonographic chest and lung measurements for predicting severe pulmonary hypoplasia. Prenatal Diagnosis 19 (1999) 614–619
86. Merz, E., Oberstein, A., Wellek, S.: Age-related reference ranges for the fetal footlength. Ultraschall in Med. 21 (2000) 79–85
87. Mhaskar, R., Agarwal, N., Takkar, D. et al.: Fetal foot length – a new parameter for assesment of gestational age. Int. J. Gynaecol. Obstet. 29(1) (1989) 35–38
88. Montenegro, N.A., Leite, L.P.: Fetal cerebellar measurements in second trimester ultrasonography: Clinical value. J. Perinat. Med. 17 (1989) 365–369
89. Morin, F., Winsberg, F.: Ultrasonic and radiographic study of the vessels of the fetal liver. J. clin. Ultrasound 6 (1978) 409–411
90. Murao, F., Takamori, H., Hata, X., Hata, T., Kitao, M.: Fetal liver measurements by ultrasonography. Int. J. Gynecol. Obstet. 25 (1987) 381–385
91. Nagata, S., Koyanagi, T., Horimoto, N., Satoh. S., Nakano, H.: Chronological development of the fetal stomach assessed using real-time ultrasound. Early Hum. Dev. 22 (1990) 15–20
92. Nakai, A.: Ultrasonographic evaluation of fetal renal function. Acta Neonatol. Jpn. 22 (1986) 887–895
93. Nyberg, D.A., Mack, L.A., Patten, R.M., Cyr, D.R.: Fetal bowel – Normal sonographic findings. J. Ultrasound Med. 6 (1987) 3–6

94. O'Brien, G.D., Queenan, J.T., Campbell, S.: Assessment of gestational age in the second trimester by real-time ultrasound measurement of the femur length. Amer. J. Obstet. Gynec. 139 (1981) 540–545

95. O'Brien, G.D., Queenan, J.T.: Ultrasound fetal femur length in relation to intrauterine growth retardation. Amer. J. Obstet. Gynec. 144 (1982) 35–39

96. Ott, W.J.: The use of ultrasonic fetal head circumference for predicting expected date of confinement. J. Clin. Ultrasound 12 (1984) 411–415

97. Platt, L.D., Medearis, A.L., DeVore, G.R., Horenstein, J.M., Carlson, D.E., Brar, H.S.: Fetal foot length: relationship to menstrual age and fetal measurements in the second trimester. Obstet. Gynecol. 71 (1988) 526–531

98. Prenzlau, P., Issel, E.P.: Die praktische Bedeutung der Messung der Schulter-Steiß-Länge (Trunkometrie) beim Feten mittels Ultraschall. Zbl. Gynäk. 95 (1973) 1421–1426

99. Prenzlau, P., Bildge, M.: Die Entwicklung der fetalen Lateralventrikel und ihre Identifizierung im Laufe der Schwangerschaft durch Sonographie – I. Mitteilung. Ultraschall 6 (1985) 215–220

100. Queenan, J.T., O'Brien, G.D., Campbell, S.: Ultrasound measurement of fetal limb bones. Amer. J. Obstet. Gynec. 138 (1980) 297–302

101. Rabinowitz, R., Peters, M.T., Vyas, S., Campbell, S., Nicolaides, K.H.: Measurement of fetal urine production in normal pregnancy by real-time ultrasonography. Amer. J. Obstet. Gynecol. 161 (1989) 1264–1266

102. Roberts, A.B., Mitchell, J.M., Pattison, N.S.: Fetal liver length in normal and isoimmunized pregnancies. Amer. J. Obstet. Gynecol. 161 (1989) 42–46

103. Rossavik, I.K., Deter, R.L.: Mathematical modeling of fetal growth: I. Basic principles. J. clin. Ultrasound 12 (1984) 529–533

104. Royston, P., Altmann, D.G.: Design and analysis of longitudinal studies of fetal size. Ultrasound Obstet. Gynecol. 6 (1995) 307–312

105. Sabbagha, R.E., Barton, F.B., Barton, B.A.: Sonar biparietal diameter. I. Analysis of percentile growth differences in two normal populations using same methodology. Amer. J. Obstet. Gynec. 126 (1976) 479–484

106. Schaefer, G.B., Bodensteiner, J.B., Thompson, J.N.: Subtle anomalies of the septum pellucidum and neurodevelopmental deficits. Dev. Med. Child. Neurol. 36 (1994) 554–559

107. Schlensker, K.H.: Eine Ultraschallmethodik zur Thorakometrie beim Feten. Geburtsh. u. Frauenheilk. 33 (1973) 440–446

108. Schlensker, K.H.: Die sonographische Darstellung der fetalen Extremitäten im mittleren Trimenon. Geburtsh. u. Frauenheilk. 41 (1981) 366–373

109. Schmidt, W., Hendrik, H.: Fetale Femurlänge im zweiten und dritten Schwangerschaftstrimenon. Geburtsh. u. Frauenheilk. 45 (1985) 91–97

110. Schmidt, W., Yarkoni, S., Jeanty, P., Grannum, P., Hobbins, J.C.: Sonographic measurements of the fetal spleen: Clinical implications. J. Ultrasound Med. 4 (1985) 667–672

111. Shalev, E., Weiner, E., Zuckermann, H., Megory, E.: Reliability of sonographic measurement of the fetal foot. J. Ultrasound Med. 8 (1989) 259–262

112. Sharland, G.K., Allan, L.D.: Normal fetal cardiac measurements derived by cross-sectional echocardiography. Ultrasound Obstet. Gynecol. 2 (1992) 175–181

113. Shin, T., Koyanagi, T., Hara, K., Kubota, S., Nakano, H.: Development of urine production and urination in the human fetus assessed by real-time ultrasound. Asia-Oceania J. Obstet. Gynaecol. 13 (1987) 473–479

114. Smith, P.A., Johansson, D., Tzannatos, C., Campbell, S.: Prenatal measurement of the fetal cerebellum and cisterna cerebellomedullaris by ultrasound. Prenat. Diagn. 6 (1986) 133–141

115. Snijders, R.J.M., Nicolaides, K.H.: Fetal biometry at 14-40 weeks' gestation. Ultrasound Obstet. Gynecol. 4 (1994) 34–48

116. Steiger, R.M., Porto, M., Lagrew, D.C., Randall, R.: Biometry of the fetal cisterna magna: estimates of the ability to detect trisomy 18. Ultrasound Obstet. Gynecol. 5 (1995) 384–390

117. Stöger, H., Kratochwil, A.: Ultraschallbiometrie des fetalen Wachstums. Geburtsh. u. Frauenheilk. 34 (1974) 611–616

118. Tamura, R.K., Sabbagha, R.E.: Percentile ranks of sonor fetal abdominal circumference measurements. Amer. J. Obstet. Gynec. 138 (1980) 475–479

119. Terinde, R., Driedger, E., Müller, J.E.A., Kozlowski, P., Schadewaldt, L.: Extremitätenwachstum, Gestationsalterschätzung und Mißbildungsdiagnostik durch Ultraschall-Vermessung fetaler Knochen im II. Trimenon. Z. Geburtsh. Perinat. 186 (1982) 125–132

120. Vintzileos, A.M., Neckles, S., Campbell, W.A., Andreoli, J.W.jr., Kaplan, B.M., Nochimson, D.J.: Fetal liver ultrasound measurements during normal pregnancy. Obstet. and Gynec. 66 (1985) 477–480

121. Visser, G.H., Goodman, J.D., Levine, D.H., Dawes, G.S.: Micturition and the heart period cycle in the human fetus. Brit. J. Obstet. Gynaecol. 88 (1981) 803–805

122. Warda, A.H., Deter, R.L., Rossavik, I.K., Carpenter, R.J., Hadlock, F.P.: Fetal femur length: A critical reevaluation of the relationship to menstrual age. Obstet. and Gynecol. 66 (1985) 69–75

123. Wellek, S., Merz, E.: Age-related reference ranges for growth parameters. Meth. Inform. Med. 34 (1995) 523–528

124. Wexler, S, Fuchs, C., Golan, A., David, M.P.: Tolerance interval for standards in ultrasound measurements: Determination of BPD standards. J. Clin. Ultrasound 14 (1986) 243–250

125. WHO Manual of the International Statistical Classification of Diseases, Injuries and Causes of Death, Geneva (1967)

126. Wilhelm, C., Prömpeler, H., Räfle, P., Schillinger, H.: Sonographische Biometrie fetaler Organe. Z. Geburtsh. u. Perinat. 195 (1991) 123–130

127. Willocks, J., Donald, I., Duggan, T.C., Day, N.: Foetal cephalometry by ultrasound. Brit. J. Obstet. Gynaec. 71 (1964) 11–20

128. Wladimiroff, J.W., Campbell, S.: Fetal urine production rates in normal and complicated pregnancy. Lancet I (1974) 151–154

129. Wladimiroff, J.W.: Ultraschalluntersuchung des fetalen und neonatalen Herzens und des kardiovaskulären Systems. Ultraschall 2 (1981) 221–225

130. Wladimiroff, J.W., Vosters, R., McGhie, J.S.: Normal cardiac ventricular geometry and function during the last trimesters of pregnancy and early neonatal period. Brit. J. Obstet. Gynaec. 89 (1982) 839–844

131. Wladimiroff, J.W., Niermeijer, M.F., Laar, J., Jahoda, M., Stewart, P.A.: Prenatal diagnosis of skeletal dysplasia by real-time ultrasound. Obstet. and Gynec. 63 (1984) 360–364

132. Yarkoni, S., Schmidt, W., Jeanty, P., Reece, E., Hobbins, J.C.: Clavicular measurement: a new biometric parameter for fetal evaluation. J. Ultrasound Med. 4 (1985) 467–470

13 Gestational Age Assignment in the Second and Third Trimesters

Importance of Estimating Gestational Age

Prenatal care. The early, accurate dating of a pregnancy is an important prerequisite for the continued surveillance of the pregnancy. Fetal growth as well as certain laboratory findings (e.g., serum or amniotic fluid AFP, triple test [28]) can be correctly interpreted only when the gestational age is known.

When the gestational age is established in early pregnancy, it provides a baseline for detecting early fetal growth retardation in the second trimester so that there is still sufficient time for karyotyping. Also, if the gravida goes past her calculated due date, postmaturity can be diagnosed with a high degree of confidence. By the same token, unnecessary induction of labor can be avoided if it is uncertain that the pregnancy is actually postmature.

Ultrasound pregnancy dating. In approximately 20% of all pregnancies (17–22% [2, 13, 16]), the gestational age cannot be determined from the patient's history. It is in just such cases that ultrasound dating of the pregnancy becomes tremendously important. Various ultrasound parameters can be used to estimate gestational age, depending on how far the pregnancy has progressed (Table 13.1, Fig. 13.**1**).

Curves for Estimating Gestational Age

When gestational age is estimated, it should be understood that the gestational age is not simply read from the standard growth chart for a given biometric parameter. Instead, special curves should be used in which the selected growth parameter is plotted as an independent variable on the x axis and time is plotted as a dependent variable on the y axis. This is a coordinate system in which the axes are switched compared with growth charts (1, 10, 15, 19). Only this type of representation can provide a statistically accurate mean value and standard deviation for determining the age of a pregnancy (see also tables in the Appendix).

Second Trimester

Superior and femoral dimensions. Starting in the second trimester, the crown–rump length is a less reliable predictor of gestational age be-

Table 13.1   Ultrasound parameters used in estimating gestational age

First trimester
> Mean diameter of gestational sac (10, 16, 19)
> Crown–rump length (9, 16, 19, 20, 21, 25, 29)

Second and third trimesters
> Crown–rump length (only until the mid-second trimester [9, 16, 25])
> Superior dimensions (BPD, OFD, HC) (1, 4, 7, 8, 11, 12, 14, 15, 16, 18, 22, 23, 24)
> Abdominal dimensions (ATD, ASD, AC) (6, 7, 15, 16)
> Limb bones (usually the femur) (1, 5, 7, 14, 15, 17, 26, 27, 30)
> Cerebellum (1)

cause the fetus often assumes a curved posture. Thus the CRL becomes more difficult to measure, and it cannot be measured as accurately as in early pregnancy. Table 13.**1** lists the parameters that provide more accurate estimates of gestational age in the second and third trimesters. The most important of these are biparietal diameter, head circumference, and femur length. During the first half of the second trimester, gestational age can be estimated to an accuracy of ± 7 to ± 10 days (2 SD) using the biparietal diameter (8, 24) or femur length (5, 17, 26). An accuracy of ± 10 days (2 SD) has been reported for head circumference (4) and ± 13 days (2 SD) for abdominal circumference (6) during this period.

Regardless of the parameter used, it is essential that it be measured on the correct ultrasound reference plane.

Abdominal dimensions. Because the fetal trunk is deformable, abdominal measurements are more subject to errors than other parameters. Consequently, they are less suitable for the assessment of gestational age.

Transverse cerebellar diameter. If the gestational age is uncertain, it can be helpful to measure the transverse cerebellar diameter. Between 17 and 22 mm, the transverse diameter of the cerebellum is approximately equal to the mean value of the gestational age in weeks (see table in Appendix [1]).

Third Trimester

Less precise. The estimation of gestational age is much less precise in the third trimester than earlier in the pregnancy. Estimates based on the biparietal diameter (8, 24), head circumference (4), abdominal circumference (6), and femur length (5, 26) in the third trimester are accurate to only about ± 3 weeks (2 SD). We were able to achieve a somewhat better accuracy of ± 17 days (2 SD) in our third-trimester patients (14) based on the individual parameters of head circumference and femur length, but the scatter for biparietal diameter was still ± 20 days. The use of head circumference for estimating gestational age is most advantageous over the biparietal diameter when the fetus has a dolichocephalic or brachycephalic head shape (3, 18).

Femur length. If measurement of both the biparietal diameter and head circumference is seriously hampered by a deeply engaged head following membrane rupture or by an oblique head position in a breech-presenting fetus, an equally good gestational age assignment can be made on the basis of femur length.

Use of multiple parameters. Gestational age can be estimated somewhat more accurately in the third trimester by using multiple fetal growth parameters (7) instead of single parameters. However, an accuracy comparable to that based on the crown–rump length, biparietal diameter, or femur length during the first trimester cannot be achieved in late pregnancy due to the increasing biological variability of the growth parameters. Thus, if the dates of a pregnancy are uncertain, the first ultrasound examination should be performed early—preferably during the first 10 weeks—so that the estimate will be as accurate as possible.

Fig. 13.**1** Gestational age estimation. The curves for the 5th, 50th, and 95th percentiles are shown (based on data from [15]).

a Based on biparietal diameter.
b Based on head circumference.
c Based on abdominal circumference.
d Based on femur length.

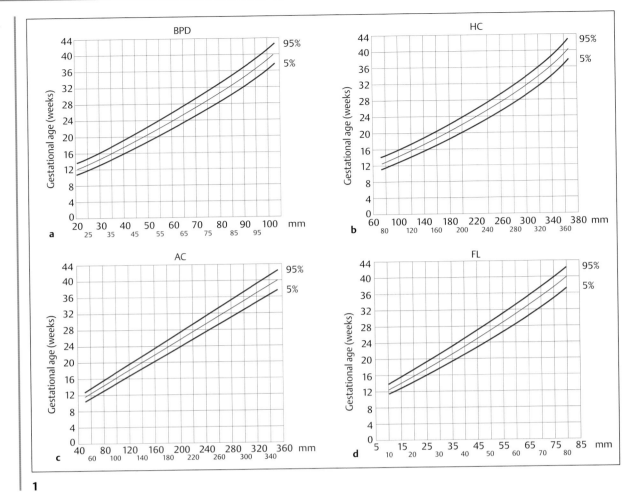

1

References

1. Altman, D.G., Chitty, L.S.: New charts for ultrasound dating of pregnancy. Ultrasound Obstet. Gynecol. 10 (1997) 174–191
2. Dewhurst, C.J., Beazley, J.M., Campbell, S.: Assessment of fetal maturity and dysmaturity. Amer. J. Obstet. Gynec. 113 (1972) 141–149
3. Hadlock, F.P., Deter, R.L., Carpenter, R.J., Park, S.K.: Estimating fetal age: Effect of head shape on BPD. Amer. J. Roentgenol.137 (1981) 83–85
4. Hadlock, F.P., Deter, R., Harrist, R.B., Park, S.K.: Fetal head circumference: Relation to menstrual age. Amer. J. Roentgenol. 138 (1982) 649–653
5. Hadlock, F.P., Deter, R.L., Park, S.K.: Fetal femur length as a predictor of menstrual age: Sonographically measured. Amer. J. Roentgenol. 138 (1982) 875–878
6. Hadlock, F.P., Deter, R.L. , Harrist, R.B., Park, S.K.: Fetal abdominal circumference as a predictor of menstrual age. Amer. J. Roentgenol. 139 (1982) 367–370
7. Hadlock, F.P., Deter, R.L. , Harrist, R.B., Park, S.K.: Computer assisted analysis of fetal age in the third trimester using multiple fetal growth parameters. J. Clin. Ultrasound 11 (1983) 313–316
8. Hansmann, M.: Ultraschallbiometrie im II. und III. Trimester der Schwangerschaft. Gynäkologe 9 (1976) 133–155
9. Hansmann, M., Schuhmacher, H., Foebus, J.: Ultraschallbiometrie der fetalen Scheitel-steißlänge in der ersten Schwangerschaftshälfte. Geburtsh. u. Frauenheilk. 39 (1979) 656–666
10. Holländer, H.J.: Die Ultraschalldiagnostik in der Schwangerschaft. München: Urban & Schwarzenberg 1972
11. Kopta, M.M., May, R.R., Crane, J.P.: A comparison of the reliability of the estimated date of confinement predicted by crown rump length and biparietal diameter. Amer. J. Obstet. Gynec. 145 (1983) 562–565
12. Kurtz, A.B., Wapner, R.J., Kurtz, R.J. et al.: Analysis of biparietal diameter as an accurate indicator of gestational age. J. clin. Ultrasound 8 (1980) 319–326
13. Lind, T., Billewicz, W.Z.: A point-scoring system for estimating gestational age from examination of amniotic fluid. Brit. J. Hosp. Med. 4 (1971) 681–685
14. Merz, E., Pehl, S., Goldhofer, W., Hoffmann, G.: Sonographische Vermessung fetaler Extremitätenknochen zur Gestationsalterschätzung im III. Trimenon. Arch. Gynec. 238 (1985) 190
15. Merz, E.: Standardisierung der fetalen Biometrie. Gynäkologie u. Geburtshilfe 1 (1991) 29–35
16. Müller, J.E.A.: Erstellung und Nutzung von Ultraschallkurven und Ultraschalltabellen an der Universitäts-Frauenklinik Düsseldorf. Inauguraldissertation, Düsseldorf 1980

17. O'Brien, G.D., Queenan, J.T., Campbell, S.: Assessment of gestational age in the second trimester by real-time ultrasound measurement of the femur length. Amer. J. Obstet. Gynec. 139 (1981) 540–545
18. Ott, W.J.: The use of ultrasonic fetal head circumference for predicting expected date of confinement. J. clin. Ultrasound 12 (1984) 411–415
19. Rempen, A.: Biometrie in der Frühgravidität (I. Trimenon). Gynäkologie u. Geburtshilfe 1 (1991) 23–28
20. Rempen, A.: Vaginale Sonographie im I. Trimenon. II. Quantitative Parameter. Z. Geburtsh. u. Perinat. 195 (1991) 163–171
21. Robinson, H.P., Fleming, J.E.E.: A critical evaluation of sonar crown-rump-length-measurements. Brit. J. Obstet. Gynaec. 82 (1975) 702–710
22. Sabbagha, R.E., Barton, F.B., Barton, B.A.: Sonar biparietal diameter. I. Analysis of percentile growth differences in two normal populations using same methology. Amer. J. Obstet. Gynec. 126 (1976) 479–484
23. Sabbagha, R.E., Barton, B.A., Barton, F.B., Kingas, E., Orgill, J., Turner, J.H.: Sonar biparietal diameter. II. Predictive of three fetal growth pattern leading to a closer assessment of gestational age and neonatal weight. Amer. J. Obstet. Gynec. 126 (1976) 485–490
24. Sabbagha, R.E., Hughey, M.: Standardization of sonar cephalometry and gestational age. Obstet. and Gynec. 52 (1978) 402–406
25. Schmidt, W., Hendrik, H.J., Kubli, F.: Ultraschallfetometrie – die Scheitel-Steißlänge in der ersten Schwangerschaftshälfte. Z. Geburtsh. Perinat. 185 (1981) 327–335
26. Schmidt, W., Hendrik, H.J.: Fetale Femurlänge im zweiten und dritten Schwangerschaftstrimenon. Geburtsh. u. Frauenheilk. 45 (1985) 91–97
27. Terinde, R., Driedger, E., Müller, J.E.A., Kozlowski, P., Schadewaldt, I.: Extremitätenwachstum, Gestationsalter-Schätzung und Mißbildungsdiagnostik durch Ultraschall-Vermessung fetaler Knochen im II. Trimenon. Z. Geburtsh. Perinat. 186 (1982) 125–132
28. Wald, N.J., Cuckle, H.S., Densem, J.W, Kennard, A., Smith, D.: Maternal serum screening for Down's syndrome: the effect of routine ultrasound scan determination of gestational age and adjustment for maternal weight. Br. J. Obstet. Gynaecol. 99 (1992) 144–149
29. Wisser, J., Dirschedl, P., Krone, S.: Estimation of gestational age by tranvaginal sonogrphic measurement of greatest embryonic length in dated human embryos. Ultrasound Obstet. Gynecol. 4 (1994) 457–462
30. Yeh, M.N., Bracero, L., Reilly, K.B., Murtha, L., Aboulafia, M., Barron, B.A.: Ultrasonic measurement of the femur length as an index of fetal gestational age. Amer. J. Obstet. Gynec. 144 (1982) 519–522

14 Fetal Weight Estimation

Importance of Fetal Weight Estimation

Obstetric management. The estimation of fetal body weight is becoming increasingly important in modern obstetrics. This particularly applies to the clinical management of impending prematurity, fetal growth retardation, and fetal macrosomia.

Because neonatal mortality rates rise with declining birth weight (4, 64), it is prudent to delay a preterm delivery whenever possible until it appears reasonably certain that a viable infant can be delivered.

Macrosomia is likewise associated with increased neonatal mortality and morbidity (47). When this condition is recognized, an elective cesarean section can be scheduled to reduce the risk of shoulder dystocia and brachial palsy. Another option would be preterm induction in cases where the fetus has reached sufficient maturity but still has a low estimated weight.

Normal Curves and Definitions

Factors affecting fetal weight. The intrauterine pattern of fetal growth and the progression of fetal weight are influenced by various factors. The most important of these are genetic, ethnic, climatic, and socioeconomic.

Based on anthropometric data gathered in newborns, various charts for normal fetal weight gain have been published in the U.S. (20, 21, 24), England and Scotland (12, 60), France (19), Italy (17), Sweden (16, 59), Austria (26), Switzerland (66), Hungary (5), and Germany (27, 34, 37, 65). Differences in the makeup of the various statistical groups (different populations, nonhomogeneous distributions, inclusion of dead or malformed newborns, uncertain dates) resulted in a large range of variation in the birth weights that were defined as normal. It has also been found that curves established in one continent could not always be applied to another. For example, normal birth weights recorded in Colorado (41) are generally lower than those recorded in Europe (see above) because of Colorado's higher altitude (1584 m) above sea level.

Fetal weight. Figure 14.**1** shows a percentile curve for fetal weight based on data published by Gallivan et al. (1993). These authors performed serial ultrasound examinations in 67 Caucasian women and used the Hadlock formula (23) and a mathematical model to calculate normal data for fetal weight. It should be noted that the biparietal diameter used in this ultrasound weight calculation was an outer-to-inner measurement.

Birth weight and length. Figures 14.**2**–14.**4** show the normal values for birth weight and body length that were recorded between 23 and 43 weeks in 563,480 singleton pregnancies in Germany in 1992 (Voigt et al. [65]). The data were analyzed separately for males and females. A direct comparison shows that the birth weight of girls was consistently slightly lower than that of boys (Fig. 14.**2**).

Phases of weight gain. Four different phases of fetal weight gain have been identified (11):

1. Slow phase
2. Accelerated phase
3. Maximum growth phase
4. Declining growth phase

Definitions. A fetus whose body weight is between the 10th and 90th percentile curves is defined as eutrophic. A percentile curve is the boundary line indicating the percentage of the population which falls above or below that line.

Fetuses below the 10th percentile for body weight are generally classified as small for gestational age (SGA) while fetuses above the 90th percentile are classified as hypertrophic.

Infants born earlier than 37 weeks are classified as premature. Those born after 42 weeks are postmature.

Ultrasound Estimation of Fetal Weight

With the introduction of ultrasound into obstetrics, a method has become available for estimating fetal weight on the basis of designated fetal growth parameters.

Biparietal diameter. The earliest ultrasound weight estimates, which were based entirely on biparietal diameter (28, 30, 35, 36, 39, 52, 62, 68), were not significantly more accurate than clinical weight estimation based on inspection and palpation. While the clinical estimate was accurate to within ± 500 g of the actual weight in 79.9% (40) and 82.5% (49) of cases, the accuracy of ultrasound estimates ranged from ± 350 g to ± 500 g, depending on the formula used. Initially, therefore, efforts were limited to determining the birth weight that could reasonably be expected when the biparietal diameter was greater than or equal to a given value. For example, Holländer (28) found that a birth weight of 2500 g could be predicted with 98.5% confidence when the BPD measured 9.2 cm or more. Schlensker and Decker (53) found that this birth weight was consistently achieved only when the BPD was at least 9.4 cm.

Head and trunk parameters. The only way to estimate fetal weight to an accuracy better than ± 300 g is by taking into account abdominal parameters or by combining head and trunk parameters. Using abdominal circumference alone, Campbell and Wilkin (10) and Higginbottom et al. (25) were able to obtain better estimates than with the BPD. When Hansmann (24) used both the BPD and ATD, he was able to estimate fetal weight to an accuracy of ± 240 g. Schillinger et al. (52) estimated fetal weight from the BPD and mean abdominal diameter (AM = [ATD + ASD] / 2) as well as from HC, AC, and the corresponding cross-sectional areas. They achieved their best results (standard deviation 233 g) by the planimetric measurement of areas.

Other approaches. Various other methods and parameters have also been used. Issel and Prenzlau (30) and Miller (46) factored trunk length into their calculation of fetal weight. Morrison and McLennan (48) used planimetric volume measurements to predict fetal weight, and Brinkley et al. (9) used a three-dimensional reconstruction of the head and trunk.

Bernaschek and Kratochwil (2) did not employ superior or abdominal measurements at all, but used fetal renal volume as a means of estimating fetal weight.

Newer formulas for fetal weight estimation employ other parameters such as thigh circumference (3), chest circumference (69), and cheek-to-cheek distance (1).

Weight estimation formulas. Most formulas in current use are based on measurements of the fetal head and abdomen (14, 24, 29, 33, 43, 50, 57, 63, 67). Some formulas also include femur length (23, 50). Schuhmacher (54) added gestational age as a factor. Seeds et al. (56) used femur length instead of BPD for fetal weight estimation.

The various formulas that are used in fetal weight estimation are listed in Table 14.1. The spectrum ranges from simple to complicated formulas. The estimated weight is relatively easy to calculate from formulas that have just one or two parameters, and the result can easily be read from a table. Formulas that contain more than two parameters require computer calculation.

Confidence and accuracy of estimates. The quality of a fetal weight estimate can be evaluated by considering both the confidence of the estimate (the percentage of cases in which the true weight is within ± 10% of the estimated weight) and the accuracy of the estimate (the percentage of cases in which the estimated weight is within ± 10% of the true weight). The error of an estimate can be measured by stating the mean absolute difference between the estimated and true weights or by stating the percentage of extreme estimates that are in error by more than 500 g or 1000 g (43).

No ideal formula. Both the diversity of the formulas and the revisions that are continually proposed for weight estimations (13, 31, 44, 51) show that there is no formula that can provide an absolutely reliable weight estimation in all cases. Also, comparative studies by Bernaschek

and Kratochwil (7) and by Merz et al. (43) have shown that there is no single formula that is ideally suited for estimating weight in all fetal weight classes. Another difficulty is that changes in the amniotic fluid volume (e.g., oligohydramnios) can prevent an accurate measurement of abdominal circumference, with a corresponding error in weight estimation. On the other hand, Meyer et al. (44) found that the accuracy of ultrasound fetal weight estimation was independent of the amniotic fluid volume.

Weight Estimation in Normal-Weight Infants

When Bernaschek and Kratochwil (3) tested the formulas of Hansmann (24), Campbell and Wilkin (10), and Schillinger et al. (52), they found that the method of Hansmann (24) provided the best estimate for normal-weight infants at term. The estimated weight differed from the true birth weight by an average of only 139.97 g.

In our own study of normal-weight infants (2500–3499 g) (43), we found that the formula of Shepard et al. (57) was 72.6% accurate in predicting birth weight. The formula of Hansmann (24) was 67.9% accurate, and the formula of Merz (43) was 61.9% accurate.

Rough estimate. The following simple formula is used by Merz (43):

$$W \text{ (g)} = 0.1 \times AC^3 \text{ (cm)}$$

This equation can provide a fast, reasonably good estimate of fetal weight in the range from 1200 to 3800 g (AC = 22.9–33.6 cm). Within this range, the estimated weight curve is very close to the actual weight curve. This formula underestimates weight in fetuses less than 1200 g and overestimates weight above 3800 g.

Weight Estimation in Low-Weight Fetuses

Campbell–Wilkin formula. According to Bernaschek and Kratochwil (7), the formula of Campbell and Wilkin (10) yields the best results in premature and small-for-date infants. Using this formula, which is based entirely on abdominal circumference, they estimated fetal weight to an accuracy of ± 152.5 g.

Shepard formula. In a prospective study, Merz et al. (43) tested the weight estimation formulas of other authors (Hansmann [24], Schillinger et al. [52], Campbell and Wilkin [10], Warsof et al. [67], Shepard et al. [57], Higginbottom et al. [25], Thurnau et al. [63]) and their own formula (Merz 1982 [43]) (see formulas in Table 14.1) in a total of 196 fetuses weighing between 610 and 4520 g. It was found that in small fetuses weighing less than 2500 g, the formula of Shepard et al. (57) estimated weight with the highest accuracy (72%)—i.e., the birth weight was within ± 10% of the estimated weight in 72% of cases.

Contradictory results. Recent comparative studies have yielded contradictory results on the weight estimation formula that is best for low-weight fetuses (< 2500 g). When Larsen et al. (38) tested the formulas of Warsof (67), Shepard (57), and Hadlock (23), they found that only the Warsof equation yielded reliable results, whereas the Shepard and Hadlock equations led to significant overestimation in the low-weight group. On the other hand, Scott et al. (55) found that the Warsof formula was not suitable for fetal weights < 1000 g, as 80% of the infants in their study were underestimated and only 61% of cases were within 15% of the estimated weight.

Growth-retarded and extremely immature fetuses. According to Guidetti et al. (22), the best results in growth-retarded fetuses are obtained by including femur length in the formula. Mielke et al. (45) described a new weight estimation formula that is specifically designed for extremely immature fetuses.

Table 14.1 Formulas used by various authors for fetal weight estimation

Author	Formula
Campbell und Wilkin (10)	$\log_e W = -4.564 + 0.282 \times AC - 0.00331 \times AC^2$ (cm, kg)
Eik-Nes (14)	$W = BPD^{1.85628} \times ATD^{1.34008} \times 1.43149 \times 10^{-3}$ (mm, g)
Hadlock et al. (23)	$W = 1.5622 - 0.01080 \times HC + 0.04680 \times AC + 0.171 \times FL + 0.00034 \times HC^2 - 0.003685 \times AC \times FL$ (cm, kg)
Hansmann (24)	$W = -1.05775 \times BPD + 0.649145 \times ATD + 0.0930707 \times BPD^2 - 0.020562 \times ATD^2 + 0.515263$ (cm, kg)
Higginbottom et al. (25)	$W = 0.0816 \times AC^3$ (cm, g)
Holländer (29)	$W = 7.344 \times BPD + 55.056 \times AM - 3270$ (mm, g)
Merz (43)	$W = 0.1 \times AC^3$ (cm, g)
Merz et al. (43)	$W = -3200.40479 + 157.07186 \times AC + 15.90391 \times BPD^2$ (cm, g)
Ott et al. (50)	$W = 2.0660 + 0.04355 \times HC + 0.05394 \times AC - 0.000858 \times HC \times AC + 1.2594 \times FL/AC$ (cm, kg)
Schillinger et al. (52)	$W = 397.7 \times (BPD + AM/2) - 4387$ (cm, g)
Schuhmacher (54)	$W = -0.001665958 \times ATD^3 + 0.4133629 \times ATD^2 - 0.5580294 \times ATD - 0.01231535 \times BPD^3 + 3.702 \times BPD^2 - 330.18110 \times BPD - 0.49371990 \times weeks^3 + 55.958061 \times weeks^2 - 2034.3901 \times weeks + 32768.19$ (mm, g)
Shepard et al. (57)	$\log_{10} W = -1.7492 + 0.166 \times BPD + 0.046 \times AC - 2.646 \times (AC \times BPD)/1000$ (cm, kg)
Thurnau et al. (63)	$W = (BPD \times AC \times 9.337) - 299.076$ (cm, g)
Warsof et al. (67)	$\log_{10} W = -1.599 + 0.144 \times BPD + 0.032 \times AC - 0.111 \times (BPD^2 \times AC)/1000$ (cm, kg)

BPD = biparietal diameter, HC = head circumference, ATD = abdominal transverse diameter, ASD = abdominal sagittal diameter, AM = mean abdominal diameter (AM = [ATD + ASD]/2), AC = abdominal circumference, FL = femur length, weeks = weeks' gestation

Weight Estimation in Macrosomic Fetuses

Schillinger formula. In comparative studies by Bernaschek and Kratochwil (7) in macrosomic fetuses, the best results were achieved with head and abdominal measurements using the formula of Schillinger et al. (52). This method gave an average underestimate of 286.2 g. In comparative studies by Merz et al. (43) in fetuses weighing more than 3500 g, the Schillinger formula based on BPD and abdominal diameter (52) provided the highest accuracy rate of 91.9%, followed by the Hansmann formula (24) at 83.9%, the formula of Shepard et al. (57) at 72.6%, and the formula of Merz (43) at 69.4%. Smith et al. (58) described good results in macrosomic fetuses using the Hadlock formula (23) based on abdominal circumference and femur length.

Fetal body fat. Alsulyman et al. (2) found that the percentage error of fetal weight estimates in macrosomic fetuses (birth weight $\geq$ 4500 g) was significantly greater than that observed in fetuses with a lower birth weight. Bernstein and Catalano (8) report that body fat in the fetuses of diabetic mothers leads to an overestimation of fetal weight.

Weight Estimation in all Weight Classes

When we tested several weight estimation formulas (43), we found that only the formula of Shepard et al. (57) yielded acceptable results for all three of the weight classes that were investigated.

Merz formula for all weight classes. In the search for a formula that can give a reliable weight estimation (accurate to within ± 10% of the true weight) in all weight classes regardless of gestational age, we performed a computer analysis of the ultrasound measurements and birth weights of 167 fetuses weighing between 2000 and 4520 g (43). Using correlation analysis and comparing linear, logarithmic, and polynomial statements, we were able to derive an optimum formula for estimating fetal weight in all categories:

$$W\ (g) = -3200.40479 + 157.07186 \times AC\ (cm) + 15.90391 \times BPD^2\ (cm)$$

Using this formula, we were able to estimate weights in our total population with a mean absolute error of 221 g with 71.4% confidence. Although this formula was derived only for fetal weights ranging from 2000 to 4520 g (BPD 8–10.5 cm, AC 26.4–36.5 cm), it can also be applied to fetuses weighing as little as 1000 g (BPD 7.0 cm, AC 21.8 cm). Below 1000 g, fetal weight is underestimated.

Tables in the Appendix. Data calculated from this formula have been tabulated in the Appendix to simplify fetal weight estimation for given values of BPD and AC. The Appendix also contains a weight table for low-weight fetuses based on the formula of Shepard et al. (57) and a table for macrosomic fetuses based on the formula of Schillinger et al. (52).

3D ultrasound. 3D ultrasound has led to new approaches for fetal weight estimation, promising further improvements in weight prediction based on the determination of volumes. Chang et al. (12) described weight estimation by 3D ultrasound volumetry of the fetal thigh. Favre et al. (15) described fetal weight estimation using arm and leg circumferences obtained by 3D ultrasound.

Weight Estimation in Multiple Pregnancies

Jensen et al. (32) and Lynch et al. (42) reported on fetal weight estimation in twins, and Lynch et al. (42) described weight estimation in triplets.

References

1. Abramowicz, J.S., Robischon, K., Cox, C.: Incorporating sonographic cheek-to-cheek diameter, biparietal diameter and abdominal circumference improves weight estimation in the macrosomic fetus. Ultrasound Obstet. Gynecol. 9 (1997) 409–413
2. Alsulyman, O.M., Ouzounian, J.G., Kjos, S.L.: The accuracy of intrapartum ultrasonographic fetal weight estimation in diabetic pregnancies. Amer. J. Obstet. Gynecol. 177 (1997) 503–506
3. Balouet, P., Hamel, P., Domessent, D. et al.: Estimation du poids foetal par la mesure de la graisse des membres. Application au diagnostic de l'hypotrophie. J. Gynecol. Obstet. Biol. Reprod. Paris 23 (1994) 64–68
4. Battaglia, F.C., Lubchenco, L.O.: A practical classification of newborn infants by weight and gestational age. J. Pediat. 71 (1967) 159–163
5. Bazso, J., Vachter, J., Lnyi, I.: Die Schätzung der fetalen Gewichtszunahme und ihre Variationen aus dem Geburtsgewicht bei ungarischen Neugeborenen. Geburtsh. u. Frauenheilk. 29 (1969) 845–852
6. Bernaschek, G., Kratochwil, A.: Die Möglichkeit der intrauterinen Gewichtsschätzung aus dem fetalen Nierenvolumen. Ultraschall 1 (1980) 223–227
7. Bernaschek, G., Kratochwil, A.: Vergleich von Gewichtsschätzungsmethoden aus Kephalo- und Abdominometrie. Geburtsh. u. Frauenheilk. 41 (1981) 114–117
8. Bernstein, I.M., Catalano, P.M.: Influence of fetal fat on the ultrasound estimation of fetal weight in diabetic mothers. Obstet. Gynecol. 79 (1992) 561–563
9. Brinkley, J.F., McCallum, W.D., Liu, D.Y.: Fetal weight estimation from ultrasonic three-dimensional head and trunk reconstructions: Evaluation in vitro. Amer. J. Obstet. Gynec. 144 (1982) 715–721
10. Campbell, S., Wilkin, D.: Ultrasonic measurement of fetal abdomen circumference in the estimation of fetal weight. Brit. J. Obstet. Gynaec. 82 (1975) 689–697
11. Carrera, J.M., Devesa, R., Carrera, M.: Dynamics of fetal growth. In: Kurjak, A. (ed.): Textbook of Perinatal Medicine. Vol. 2 (1998) 1140–1147
12. Chang, F.M., Liang, R.I., Ko, H.C., Yao, B.L., Chang, C.H., Yu, C.H.: Three-dimensional ultrasound-assessed fetal thigh volumetry in predicting birth weight. Obstet. Gynecol. (90) 1997 331–339
13. Dudley, N.J.: Selection of appropriate ultrasound methods for the estimation of fetal weight. Br. J. Radiol. 68 (1995) 385–388
14. Eik-Nes, S.H.: Ultrasonic assessment of human fetal weight, growth and blood flow. Habilitationsschrift, Malmö 1980
15. Favre, R., Bader, A.M., Nisand, G.: Prospective study on fetal weight estimation using limb circumferences obtained by three-dimensional ultrasound. Ultrasound Obstet. Gynecol. 6 (1995) 140–144
16. Finnström, O.: Studies on maturity in newborn infants. Acta pediat. Scand. 60 (1971) 685–694
17. Fraccaro, M.: A contribution to the study of birth weight based on an Italian sample. Ann. Hum. Genet. 20 (1956) 282–298
18. Gallivan, S., Robson, S.C., Chang, T.C., Vaugham, J., Spencer, J.A.D.: An investigation of fetal growth using serial ultrasound data. Ultrasound Obstet. Gynecol. 3 (1993) 109–114
19. Goujard, J., Kaminski, M., Rumeau-Rougette, C.: Moyenne pondérale et age gestationnel en relation avec quelques caractéristiques maternelles. Arch. Franc. Ped. 30 (1973) 341
20. Gruenwald, P.: The fetus in prolonged pregnancy. Amer. J. Obstet. Gynecol. 1964 (1964) 503–509
21. Gruenwald, P.: Infants of low birth weight among 5000 deliveries. Pediatrics 34 (1964) 157–162
22. Guidetti, D.A., Divon, M.Y., Braverman, J.J., Langer, O., Merkatz, I.R.: Sonographic estimates of fetal weight in the intrauterine growth retardation population. Amer. J. Perinatol. 7 (1990) 5–7
23. Hadlock, F.P., Harrist, R.B., Martinez-Poyer, J.: In utero analysis of fetal growth: a sonographic weight standard. Radiology 181 (1991) 129–133
24. Hansmann, M.: Ultraschallbiometrie im II. und III. Trimester der Schwangerschaft. Gynäkologe 9 (1976) 133–155
25. Higginbottom, J., Slater, J., Porter, G., Whitfield, C.R.: Estimation of fetal weight from ultrasonic measurement of trunk circumference. Brit. J. Obstet. Gynaec. 82 (1975) 698–701
26. Hohenauer, L.: Intrauterines Längen- und Gewichtswachstum. Pädiatr. Pädol. 8 (1973) 195–205
27. Hohenauer, L.: Intrauterine Wachtumskurven für den Deutschen Sprachraum. Z. Geburtsh. u. Perinat. 184 (1980) 167–179
28. Holländer, H.J.: Die Ultraschalldiagnostik in der Schwangerschaft. München: Urban & Schwarzenberg 1972
29. Holländer, H.J.: Die Ultraschalldiagnostik in der Schwangerschaft. München: Urban & Schwarzenberg 1984
30. Issel, E.P., Prenzlau, P.: Eine neue Methode zur Berechnung des fetalen Gewichtes mittels Ultraschall-B-Bild Technik. Zbl. Gynäk. 96 (1974) 419–429
31. Jackson, D.W., Pitts, D.K., Kushner, R.: Estimation of fetal weight by means of ultrasound: a comparison of methods. J. Am. Osteopath. Assoc. 90 (1990) 1071–1080
32. Jensen, O.H., Jenssen, H.: Prediction of fetal weights in twins. Acta Obstet. Gynecol. Scand. 74 (1995) 177–180
33. Jordan, H.B.F.: Estimation of fetal weight by ultrasound. J. Clin. Ultrasound 11 (1983) 59–66
34. Kattner, E., Metze, B., Keen, D.V., Pearse, R.G., Dudenhausen, J.W.: Perzentilenkurven für Geburtsgewicht, Länge und Kopfumfang unter besonderer Berücksichtigung sehr unreifer Frühgeborener. Perinatalmedizin 4 (1992) 118–121
35. Kohorn, E.I.: An evaluation of ultrasonic fetal cephalometry. Amer. J. Obstet. Gynec. 97 (1967) 553–559
36. Kratochwil, A.: Ultraschalldiagnostik in Geburtshilfe und Gynäkologie. Stuttgart: Thieme 1968

Fig. 14.**1** Percentile curves for fetal weight (5th, 10th, 50th, 90th, and 95th percentiles), calculated from a mathematical model based on measured ultrasound parameters (data from [18]).

Fig. 14.**2** Weight comparisons of male and female newborns in Germany (10th, 50th, 90th percentiles) (after Voigt et al. [65]).

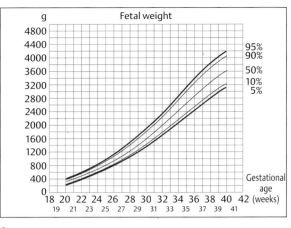

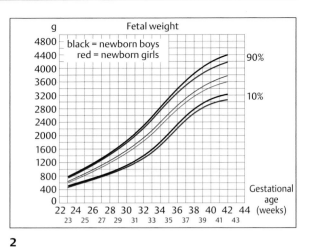

Fig. 14.**3** Percentile curves for birth-weight (5th, 10th, 50th, 90th, and 95th percentiles), by gender, in Germany in 1992 (after [65]).
a Male newborns.
b Female newborns.

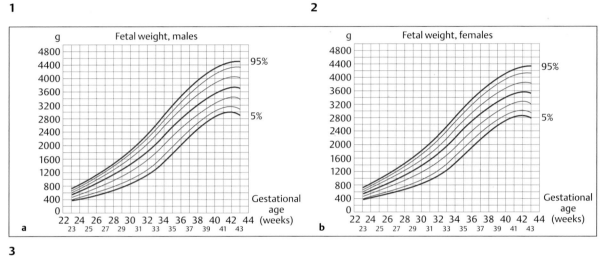

Fig. 14.**4** Percentiles of newborn length (singletons) in Germany in 1992 (after [65]).
a Male newborns.
b Female newborns.

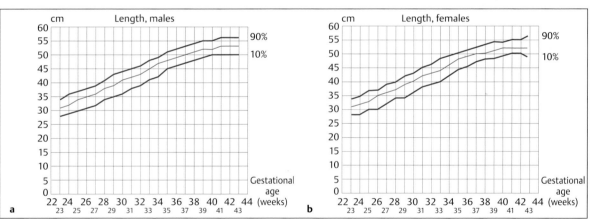

37. Kyank, H., Kruse, H.J., Adomszent, S., Plesse, R.: Standardwerte für Geburtsgewichte und Geburtslängen von Neugeborenen in der DDR. Zentralbl. Gynäkol. 99 (1977) 461–465
38. Larsen, T., Petersen, S., Greisen, G., Larsen, J.F.: Normal fetal growth evaluated by longitudinal ultrasound examinations. Early Hum. Dev. 24 (1990) 37–45
39. Levi, S.: Ultrasonodiagnostic en obstétrique: Intérêt clinique de la mesure du diamètre biparétal du foetus. Gynéc. et Obstét. 69 (1970) 227–238
40. Loeffler, F.E.: Clinical foetal weight prediction. Brit. J. Obstet. Gynaec. 74 (1967) 657–677
41. Lubchenco, L.O., Hansman, C., Dressler, M., Boyd, E.: Intrauterine growth as estimated from live-born weight data at 24–42 weeks of gestation. Pediatrics 32 (1963) 793–801
42. Lynch, L., Lapinski, R., Alvarez, M., Lockwood, C.J.: Accuracy of ultrasound estimation of fetal weight in multiple pregnancies. Ultrasound Obstet. Gynecol. 6 (1995) 349–352
43. Merz, E., Lieser, H., Schicketanz, K.H., Härle, J.: Intrauterine Gewichtsschätzung mittels Ultraschall. Ein Vergleich mehrerer Gewichtsschätzungsmethoden sowie die Entwicklung einer neuen Formel zur Bestimmung des Fetalgewichtes. Ultraschall 9 (1988) 15–24
44. Meyer, W.J., Font, G.E., Gauthier, D.W., Myles, T.D., Bieniarz, A., Rodriguez, A.: Effect of amniotic fluid volume on ultrasonic fetal weight estimation. J. Ultrasound Med. 14 (1995) 193–197
45. Mielke, G., Pietsch-Breitfeld, B., Salinass, R., Risse, T., Marzusch, K.: A new formula for prenatal ultrasonographic weight estimation in extremely preterm fetuses. Gynecol. Obstet. Invest. 40 (1995) 84–88
46. Miller, E.C.: Zum Problem der Gewichtsbestimmung des Feten durch Ultraschallbiometrie. Zbl. Gynäk. 5 (1980) 272–282
47. Modanlou, H.D., Dorchester, W.L., Thorosian, A., Freeman, R.K.: Macrosomia – Maternal, fetal, and neonatal implications. Obstet. Gynec. 55 (1980) 420–424
48. Morrison, J., McLennan, M.J.: The theory, feasibility and accuracy of an ultrasonic method of estimating fetal weight. Brit. J. Obstet. Gynaec. 83 (1976) 833–837
49. Ong, H.C., Sen, D.K.: Clinical estimation of fetal weight. Amer. J. Obstet. Gynec. 112 (1972) 877–880
50. Ott, W.J.: Clinical application of fetal weight determination by real-time ultrasound measurement. Obstet. and Gynec. 57 (1981) 758–762
51. Pedersen, J.F., Molsted-Pedersen, L.: Sonographic estimation of fetal weight in diabetic pregnancy. Brit J. Obstet. Gynaecol. 99 (1992) 475–478
52. Schillinger, H., Müller, R., Kretzschmar, M., Wode, J.: Gewichtsbestimmung des Feten durch Ultraschall. Geburtsh. u. Frauenheilk. 35 (1975) 858–865
53. Schlensker, K.H., Decker, I.: Voraussagen des kindlichen Geburtsgewichtes auf Grund der Ultraschallkephalometrie und -thorakometrie am Feten. Geburtsh. u. Frauenheilk. 33 (1973) 859–867
54. Schuhmacher, H.: Mehrparametrische nichtlineare fetale Gewichtsschätzung aus Ultraschallmeßwerten unter Berücksichtigung des Gestationsalters. Inaugural-Dissertation, Bonn 1979
55. Scott, F., Beeby, P., Abbott, J.: Accuracy of estimated fetal weight below 1000 g. Aust. N. Z. J. Obstet. Gynaecol. 36 (1996) 129–132
56. Seeds, J.W., Cefalo, R.C., Bowes, W.A.: Femur length in the estimation of fetal weight less than 1500 grams. Amer. J. Obstet. Gynec. 149 (1984) 233–235
57. Shepard, M.J., Richards, V.A., Berkowitz, R.L., Warsof, S.L., Hobbins, J.C.: An evaluation of two equations for predicting fetal weight by ultrasound. Amer. J. Obstet. Gynec. 142 (1982) 47–54
58. Smith, G.C., Smith, M.F., McNay, M.B., Fleming, J.E.: The relation between fetal abdominal circumference and birthweight: findings in 3512 pregnancies. Brit. J. Obstet. Gynaecol. 104 (1997) 186–190
59. Sterky, G.: Swedish standard curves for intrauterine growth. Pediatrics 46 (1970) 7–8
60. Tanner, J.M.: Standards for birth weight or intrauterine growth. Pediatrics 46 (1970) 1–6
61. Thomson, A.M., Billewicz, W.Z., Hytten, F.E.: The assessment of fetal growth. J. Obstet. Gynaec. Brit. Cwlth. 75 (1968) 903–916
62. Thompson, H.E., Holmes, J.H., Gottesfeld, K.R., Taylor, E.S.: Fetal development as determined by ultrasonic pulse echo techniques. Amer. J. Obstet. Gynec. 92 (1965) 44–52
63. Thurnau, G.E., Tamura, R.K., Sabbagha, R. et al.: A simple estimated fetal weight equation based on real-time ultrasound measurements of fetuses less than thirty-four weeks gestation. Amer. J. Obstet. Gynec. 145 (1983) 557–561
64. Usher, R.H., McLean, F.H.: Normal fetal growth and the significance of fetal growth retardation. In Davis, J.A., Dobbing, J.: Scientific Foundations of Paediatrics. London: Heinemann 1974; p. 69
65. Voigt, M., Schneider, K.T.M., Jährig, K.: Analyse des Geburtengutes des Jahrganges 1992 der Bundesrepublik Deutschland. Teil 1: Neue Perzentilwerte für die Körpermaße von Neugeborenen. Geburtsh. u. Frauenheilk. 56 (1996) 550–558
66. Wälli, R.: Gewicht, Länge und Kopfumfang neugeborener Kinder (Einlinge und Zwillinge) und ihre Abhängigkeit von mütterlichen Faktoren. Inauguraldissertation Med. Fakultät der Univ. Zürich 1978
67. Warsof, S.L., Gohari, P., Berkowitz, R.L., Hobbins, J.C.: The estimate of fetal weight by computer-assisted analysis. Amer. J. Obstet. Gynec. 128 (1977) 881–892
68. Willocks, J., Donald, I., Duggan, T.C., Day, N.: Foetal cephalometry by ultrasound. J. Obstet. Gynaec. Brit. Cwlth 71 (1964) 11–20
69. Winn, H.N., Rauk, P.N., Petrie, R.H.: Use of the fetal chest in estimating fetal weight. Amer. J. Obstet. Gynecol. 167 (1992) 448–450

15 Fetal Behavior

The use of ultrasonography in the field of obstetrics started with the introduction of compound B-scanning, and fetal biometry was the first goal. With improving ultrasound resolution and the introduction of real-time ultrasonography, interest in fetal motility also developed.

Influencing factors. The description of fetal movements underwent a further substantial change when the concept of fetal behavior and fetal behavioral states was developed—starting an avalanche of studies on fetal behavior (44). Rapidly, however, it became clear that fetal behavior could only be studied in a very general fashion, since a large number of variables—such as the time of the day, meals, smoking, etc.—can have a significant influence on fetal behavior. The most important factor appeared to be gestational age, and it became clear that the fetus's behavior at 20 weeks bears few resemblances to the behavior of the fetus near term.

Fetal behavior can be regarded as the output of the activity of the fetal central nervous system (CNS), and abnormal behavior can sometimes be observed in fetuses with severe brain damage. It has become apparent that the intrauterine environment is not always 100% safe. The fetus is only a human being and is just as prone as a child or an adult to have an accident, develop a disease or suffer an iatrogenic problem (45).

This chapter reviews the most important data on isolated fetal behavioral variables such as body, eye and mouth movements, followed by the description of fetal behavioral states and a discussion of applications of the concept of fetal behavior in clinical practice.

Fetal Behavioral Patterns and States in Detail

▰ Fetal Movements

Movements During the First Half of Pregnancy

One of the very first descriptions of fetal movements can be found in the Bible: "And the children struggled together within her" (Genesis 25:22). However, it was not until 1976 that Reinold showed that the fetus does in fact move spontaneously, even during the first trimester of pregnancy. He also showed that an absence of body movements may indicate impending fetal death, while the presence of body movements is reassuring.

Categorization. In 1982, de Vries et al. published their results on the observation of fetal somatic activity in the first half of pregnancy. They introduced a classification of movement patterns and described how the individual movements take place in terms of speed, force and amplitude.

Startles. This is how de Vries et al. describe a startle, for example: "abrupt flexion and/or extension of both arms and legs at the same time. The amplitude of the movement is mostly large but can also be small, and even just discernible" (74).

First occurrence. De Vries et al. also clearly showed that most of the repertoire of movements that can be distinguished in the third trimester and after birth are already present at 14 weeks of gestation. The time of first occurrence of several fetal movements is indicated In Table 15.**1**.

Quiescent phases. It is not only the different types of movement that are important, but also the periods of quiescence between movements. The longest period of quiescence at 8 weeks is 260 seconds (range 108–780 s) and at 19 weeks 127 s (range 77–306 s) (77). Periods of quiescence rapidly increase in duration in the second half of pregnancy (Fig. 15.**1**).

Movements During the Second Half of Pregnancy

Longer phases. Considerable attention has been given to the presence of gross body movements in the second and third trimesters (69), but it is only in the last weeks of pregnancy that the fetus shows quite clearly prolonged periods in which movements are either present or absent. As the gestational age progresses, the periods in which body movements can be absent become dramatically longer. In the near-term fetus, fetal movements can be absent for up to 45 min (Fig. 15.**1**). This observation again shows the importance of taking fetal age into account; what is normal in a fetus at 20 weeks may be abnormal in the same fetus at 38 weeks.

Quality assessment. During the past 10 years, it has also become clear that counting the number of movements is not particularly useful in the clinical setting. Even a fetus with mild hypoxic growth retardation still makes body movements. Examining the quality of the movements and their speed and amplitude appears to be much more important. De Vries et al. (74, 75) introduced the concept of quality of movements in the first trimester, and Bekedam et al. (8) assessed this aspect in 10 intrauterine growth-retarded fetuses between 29 and 35 weeks. However, it is still not feasible to use the quality of movements in a single case as a tool for clinical decision-making.

▰ Fetal Breathing Movements and Hiccups

The first observation of fetal breathing movements was reported by Ahlfeld in Germany in 1888 (1). At that time he was not believed, and his observations were almost universally ignored until Dawes et al. (15) described breathing movements in fetal lambs in 1970, followed by observations by Boddy and Robinson (10) in the human fetus in 1971.

Paradoxical movement. A detailed M-mode analysis of human fetal breathing movements was published in 1978 by Bots et al. (11). They described breathing movements as being "paradoxical," as the ribcage made an inward movement during "inspiration," while the diaphragm made a downward movement.

Influencing factors. With modern ultrasound equipment, breathing movements can be easily detected from around 11 weeks of gestation (Table 15.**1**). Immediately after the discovery of these movements, it was hoped that it would be possible to use them as a sensitive indicator for the detection of fetal distress. However, it soon became apparent that breathing movements are not continuously present and are influenced by many conditions:

- For example, a postprandial increase in breathing movements from 20–22 weeks onward is reported by de Vries et al. (76).
- Nijhuis et al. (39) showed that there is an increase after glucose intake by the mother at 24 weeks.
- Smoking reduces the incidence of fetal breathing (31).
- During fetal rest periods (71), breathing is much more likely to be absent, and is also likely to be much more regular (37, 63).
- The duration of periods in which breathing movements may be absent increases substantially during pregnancy, and near term it is not unusual for breathing movements to be absent for as long as 120 min (50).

In general, fetal breathing should not be investigated in behavioral studies as an independent variable, but should always be examined in combination with other variables and preferably in highly standardized conditions.

Reduction toward the end of pregnancy. In the final weeks of pregnancy, the incidence of fetal breathing decreases, and breathing movements are absent during labor (14). On the basis of these observations, it was suggested that it might be possible to use an absence of breathing as an indicator of imminent preterm labor. However, the method does not appear to be sufficiently specific.

Fetal hiccups can also be observed from 8–10 weeks of gestation (Table 15.**1**). These short and powerful contractions of the diaphragm are easily distinguished from breathing movements. Periods in which hiccups occur every 2–3 seconds can be observed quite regularly in the first trimester, while in the third trimester only two to four episodes of hiccups per 24 hours are seen.

Fetal Mouth Movements

Sucking and swallowing movements. The fetal mouth is easily visualized with modern ultrasound equipment, and sucking and swallowing can be observed from 12 weeks of gestation onward. Specific mouth and sucking behavior can be observed: recurrent clusters of regular mouth movements are seen during quiet states (state 1F), while in the 3F state more powerful sucking movements can be observed (for an overview, see Van Woerden and Van Geijn [80]). Both regular mouth movements and sucking movements may be associated with sinusoidal fetal heart rate patterns, which may confuse the clinician (38, 78).

Gastric filling. The fetus also swallows amniotic fluid. A normal amount of amniotic fluid is the result of fetal swallowing and fetal micturition. Ultrasonography may show gastric filling as a result of fetal swallowing

(65). An absence of gastric filling may be important when certain anomalies are suspected (e.g., esophageal atresia), but the formulas developed to calculate the volume of the stomach have not been accepted in clinical practice (see also Chapter 12).

Fetal Eye Movements

In 1981, Bots and co-workers (12) published the first observation of fetal eye movements using ultrasound and recorded them using M-mode ultrasonography. In the same year, Birnholz (9) also described eye movements and made a distinction between slow eye movements, which can be observed from 16 weeks of gestation onward, and rapid eye movements, which are present from 23 weeks onward. The ability to observe and record eye movements added a new variable in the study of fetal motility. At this stage, fetal and neonatal data appeared to be rather similar. However, it is not always possible to compare fetal data with those in the neonate, since in the neonate it is not eye movements that are used in behavioral studies but rather the criterion "eyes open" or "eyes closed" (52).

Behavioral studies. The presence or absence of fetal eye movements has not so far been used to assess the condition of the fetus, except in the context of behavioral studies. In growth-retarded fetuses and hydrocephalic fetuses, Arduini et al. observed less rapid eye movements than in normal fetuses (4,5).

Fetal Urine Production

Linear increase. The fetal bladder (and kidneys) can be visualized from 10–11 weeks of gestation onward. On the basis of ultrasonographic measurements of the filling of the bladder, fetal urine production appears to increase in a linear fashion from a few milliliters per hour up to 25–50 mL/h in the term fetus. A reduction in urine production may be observed in the post-term fetus. Visser et al. (67) showed that in the term fetus, fetal voiding often occurs quickly after a transition from behavioral state 1F to 2F. In clinical practice, it is mainly the presence or absence of bladder filling that is important, while measurements of bladder volume or of the filling rate are only used rarely.

Fetal Heart Rate Patterns

The fetal heartbeat is actually the first form of activity that can be observed using transvaginal ultrasonography. Heart activity can already be visualized at 5–6 weeks of gestation. The initial rate of 100 beats per minute (bpm) increases to a mean rate of 167 bpm at 9 weeks, followed by a gradual decrease to 156 bpm at 12 weeks (22).

Cardiotocography (CTG). Electronic monitoring of the fetal heart rate (FHR) in combination with contractions, known as cardiotocography, was developed for intrapartum use by Caldeyro-Barcia et al. in 1966 (13) and by Hamm-Macher and Werners (21) and Hon (24) in 1968. In 1969, Kubli et al. (28) also first described the antepartum use of the technique. The various scoring systems that have been developed all show wide intraobserver and interobserver variability. However, their specificity is such that clinicians rely on the method (30, 64). Their sensitivity for predicting fetal distress is fairly poor. Perhaps due to the lack of a better tool, fetal heart rate monitoring has become the gold standard for fetal monitoring.

Variability and accelerations. In general, good bandwidth or beat-to-beat variability and accelerations indicate a good fetal condition, while a silent pattern (small bandwidth, no accelerations) is indicative of fetal distress, certainly in the presence of severe variable or late decelerations. One of the problems is that many scores that were developed to improve the interpretation of CTG did not take the age of the fetus into

Table 15.1 First appearance of several movements during the first trimester

Type of movement	Weeks
Fetal heart activity*	5.5–6.5
Just-discernible movement	7.5–8.5
Startles	8.0–9.5
General movement	8.5–9.5
Stretching	10.5–15.5
Rotation	10.0–11.0
Isolated arm/leg movement	9.5–10.5
Jaw opening	10.5–12.5
Sucking and swallowing	12.5–14.5
Yawning	11.5–15.5
Breathing movements	10.5–11.5
Hiccups	8.5–10.5
Eye movements**	
- Slow	16.0
- Rapid	23.0

Adapted from de Vries 1992 (77), * after van Heesvvijk 1990 (22), ** after Birnholz 1981 (9)

account. Visser et al. (66) showed a clear developmental trend during gestation in the amplitude and duration of the accelerations. Computer analysis has been introduced to overcome interobserver and intraobserver variation by providing an objective numerical analysis of basal FHR, FHR variability, accelerations and decelerations (Sonicaid system; Dawes et al. [16]).

In normal fetuses, basal FHR has been found to decrease with increasing gestational age, while long-term and short-term FHR variability increase (46, 54, 58). The normal baseline FHR near term varies between 110 and 150 bpm (46, 57). The lower limit (P = 2.5) of the normal range of FHR variability increases till 30 weeks of gestation in recordings of 1 h duration and stabilizes thereafter at around 30 and 5.5 ms for long-term and short-term FHR variability, respectively, despite an overall increase in FHR variability and a widening of the normal range (46).

Considerable differences between reference ranges based on 1-h recordings and those based on shorter recordings have been described. A certain degree of intrafetal consistency was found to be present from 24 weeks of gestation, indicated by an intrafetal variance of only 19–55% of the total FHR variation. For monitoring trends—e.g., in growth-retarded fetuses, each fetus should therefore serve as its own control, using recordings of standardized duration and appropriate reference ranges (46).

Fetal heart rate patterns A–D. In 1979, Timor-Tritsch et al. (62) pointed out that the fetal heart rate pattern (FHRP) was dependent on the fetal behavioral state. In 1982, definitions of four different fetal heart rate patterns—FHRP A through D—were introduced and used to define behavioral states in combination with the presence or absence of body and eye movements (36) (Fig. 15.**2**). On this basis, the following changes during the course of pregnancy were described:

- It was found that not only does the form of the accelerations change during gestation, but also that the length of silent heart rate patterns (FHRP A) increases during gestation without any sign of fetal distress (36, 42).
- During gestation, normal basal FHR decreases both in FHRP A and B.
- Long-term and short-term FHR variability increases during FHRP B and slightly decreases during FHRP A near term (47).
- During FHRP A, FHR variability was below the normal range of overall FHR variation in 50% of cases, hampering adequate assessment of the fetal condition. It is therefore important to include B patterns in the analysis.

It did not appear to be possible to identify FHRP A and B adequately using Sonicaid System 8002. However, Nijhuis et al. (47) described techniques with which computerized identification of patterns A and B may be possible.

▬ *Fetal Behavioral States*

Definitions

Assessment of fetal behavior. A combination of ultrasonographic observation of fetal activity and simultaneous recording of the FHRP is called the assessment of fetal behavior.

During the first half of pregnancy, all of the movements appear to occur more or less independently of each another and do not elicit a specific FHRP.

Behavioral states. It is necessary to link variables (e.g., absence of movements, absence of eye movements and FHRP A) in order to recognize behavioral patterns (43). Linkage between variables of this type has been reported from 25–30 weeks (17), and also at 30–32 weeks (68).

Behavioral states near term. Near term, linkage is such that fetal behavioral states can be described—constellations of physiological and behavioral variables (e.g., no eye movements, no body movements, FHRP A) that are stable over time and recur repeatedly, not only in the same infant, but also in similar forms in all infants (52).

Prerequisites

Three major prerequisites need to be met before a behavioral state can be recognized:

Coincidence, linkage. Firstly, a specific combination of certain variables has to occur at the same time (coincidence, linkage).

Three-minute threshold. Secondly, for a combination of this type to be identified, it has to be stable over time (by definition, at least 3 min).

State transition. Thirdly, it has to be possible to observe a clear change from one state to another, a "state transition." By definition, this transition should be completed within 3 min.

Behavioral states 1F to 4F

Based on recordings of fetal behavior with two ultrasound scanners and a simultaneous registration of the FHRP, four behavioral states—1F through 4F—have been defined. The suffix "F" for "fetal" was added to indicate the close relationship with the neonatal states.

State 1F (similar to state 1 or non-REM sleep in the neonate): quiescence, which can be regularly interrupted by brief gross body movements, mostly startles. Eye movements are absent. FHRP A is a stable pattern with a small oscillation bandwidth and no accelerations, except in combination with a startle (Fig. 15.**2**).

State 2F (similar to state 2 or REM sleep in the neonate): frequent and periodic gross body movements, mainly stretches and retroflexions, and movements of the extremities. Eye movements are present. FHRP B has a wider oscillation bandwidth and frequent accelerations during movements (Fig. 15.**2**).

State 3F (similar to state 3 or quiet wakefulness in the neonate): gross body movements absent. Eye movements present. FHRP C is stable, but with a wider oscillation bandwidth than FHRP A and no accelerations (Fig. 15.**2**).

State 4F (similar to state 4 or active wakefulness in the neonate): vigorous, continual activity, including many trunk rotations. Eye movements are present. FHRP D is unstable, with large and long-lasting accelerations, often merging into sustained tachycardia (Fig. 15.**2**).

Research results. After the introduction of these definitions, many other research groups were able to confirm the same findings (e.g., van Vliet et al. 1985 [72], van Woerden et al. 1989 [79], Arduini et al. 1985 [3]). The introduction of the concept of states had a considerable influence on both animal and human research. For example, it appeared that breathing movements were largely absent in state 1F (71), but that if they were present they were much more regular (37). Many studies have been conducted to search for changes in behavior in growth-retarded fetuses (7, 8, 73), fetuses in diabetic mothers (33) and in mothers taking antiepileptic drugs (19), cocaine (25), methadone (2), or corticosteroids (34, 35). For reviews, see Nijhuis 1992 (44), Richardson 1992 (55), Groome and Watson 1992 (20), Koyanagi et al. 1995 (27), Romanini and Rizzo 1995 (56), and James 1997 (26).

In post-term fetuses, van de Pas et al. (49) showed an increase in the percentage of time spent by the fetus in states 3F and 4F, mainly at the expense of state 2F, implying that the fetus is more "awake" in utero.

In addition, Doppler measurements in several fetal vessels appeared to be state-related, although in compromised fetuses this state dependency plays a minor role (18).

Biophysical Profile

The biophysical profile was introduced in 1980 by Manning et al. (32) as a clinical tool for assessing fetal well-being. The profile consists of five items that need to be observed over a period of 30 min. Each item can be scored as 0 or 2, with a maximum score of 10 points (Table 15.**2**).

Good fetal condition. A good fetal condition is supposed to be present with a score of 8–10.

Fetal asphyxia. There is a high probability of fetal asphyxia with a score of 4 or 6, and with a score of 0 or 2 points, fetal asphyxia is almost certain.

Influence of gestational age. When the biophysical test is used, gestational age needs to be taken into account. For example, during a period of 1F, a healthy fetus at 40 weeks would get 2 points for a normal amount of amniotic fluid.

Acute and chronic criteria. It should also be noted realize that the first four items are acute variables, while amniotic fluid represents a more chronic variable.

Clinical Applications

Silent and sinusoidal heart tone pattern. Insight into fetal behavior and fetal biophysics has also influenced the interpretation of CTGs. The two most important examples are the "silent" heart rate pattern and the "sinusoidal" heart rate pattern. Clearly, a silent FHR pattern may indicate fetal distress, but it may also reflect a physiological 1F behavioral state. It is therefore crucially important for a differential diagnosis to be considered if a silent heart rate pattern is recorded (42) (Table 15.**3**).

Intrauterine brain death syndrome. The most extreme example of a silent heart rate pattern is the intrauterine brain death syndrome, which is thought to result from a severe hypoxic accident with subsequent fetal recovery. The FHRP is persistently silent, with a somewhat elevated baseline, and the fetus does not move (Fig. 15.**3**). The absence of decelerations excludes asphyxia, and a cordocentesis would reveal a normal pH value. At birth—usually by caesarean section because of "fetal distress"—a floppy infant is born and artificial ventilation is needed. The electroencephalogram is isoelectric, and a diagnosis of brain death is then finally made (40, 41).

Differential diagnosis. As mentioned above, regular mouthing and sucking movements may lead to a "sinusoidal" FHRP, a heart rate pattern that may also be recorded in combination with severe fetal anemia. Differential diagnoses for this FHRP are given in Table 15.**3**.

Effect of corticosteroids. The studies by Mulder et al. (34, 35) are important for clinical practice, as they show a clear effect of betamethasone on fetal behavior. This drug, which is used to stimulate fetal lung maturation, decreases heart rate variability and the numbers of movements. Dexamethasone, which is used for the same purpose, appears to increase short-term FHR variability in particular (35).

Sequential changes. Finally, Visser et al. (70) examined sequential

Table 15.**2** Biophysikalisches nach Manning et al. (32)

Criteria	2	0
Fetal movements	Three or more episodes of movement of the trunk and limbs, either in concert or separately (in 30 min)	≥ 2 episodes in 30 min
Fetal tone	One or more episodes of extension–flexion movements of the limbs, or the the presence of opening and closing of the fetal hand	Only slow extension with subsequent partial flexion; absence of movements
Fetal breathing movements	One or more episodes of of chest and abdominal wall movements lasting for at least 30 s	No such episodes or lasting less than 30 s (in 30 min)
Fetal heart rate (FHR)	At least two episodes of fetal acceleration of more than 15 bpm and lasting longer than 15 s	More than two episodes of acceleration, or accelerations less than 15 bpm (in 20 min)
Amniotic fluid	At least one pocket that measures at least 1 cm in two perpendicular planes	No evidence of an amniotic fluid pocket or a pocket less than 1 cm in size in two perpendicular planes

changes in variables observed in deteriorating fetal conditions. The authors suggest that changes in fetal behavior and in the quality of fetal movements are among the initial signs, while a terminal heart rate pattern is of course the final step.

Fetal Neurology

Fetal behavior reflects the activity of the fetal CNS, and a major research goal is to achieve more direct insight into the fetal CNS by developing a method of intrauterine neurological examination.

Observations and tests. There are as yet few examples of this type of examination. Fetuses with congenital anomalies may show bizarre behavior (51) or dissociation between heart rate and movements (60). Other groups have investigated state transitions rather than behavioral states (6, 48), but it is still difficult to draw conclusions from a single behavioral recording in a single fetus. Tas et al. (59) were able to evoke an intercostal-to-phrenic inhibitory reflex (IPIR): compression of the ribcage results in an apnea. This appears to be an interesting approach, but the authors did not observe any significantly different results in a group of growth-retarded fetuses (61).

Fetal habituation—i.e., the cessation of response to a repeated stimulus—is another test. Hepper and Shahidiullah (23) demonstrated that fetuses with Down syndrome take longer to habituate than normal fetuses, for example.

Fetal neurological examination. In 1995, Leader commented (29), "It seems likely that no single, isolated aspect of behavior alone will evolve but rather a combination of behaviors to form a prenatal neurological examination."

Conclusion

Value of behavioral observations. Insight into fetal behavior is crucial for understanding normal fetal well-being and evaluating the potentially compromised fetus. It has introduced a completely new way of looking at the developing human being. But it is also clear that no sin-

Table 15.**3** Differential diagnosis and suggested management when there is evidence of a silent or sinusoidal heart rate pattern

Silent heart rate pattern	
Differential diagnosis	**Management**
State 1F	Extension of the recording time
Effect of drugs	Exclusion of use of drugs
Tachycardia	Inspection of baseline
Anomalies	Ultrasonographic examination
	Behavioral study
Hypoxia	Contraction stress test (CST)
Brain death	Cordocentesis

Sinusoidal heart rate pattern	
Differential diagnosis	**Management**
Fetal mouth movements	Behavioral study
- Sucking ("major" or "marked")	
- Regular mouthing ("minor")	
Effect of drugs	Exclusion of drug abuse
Congenital anomalies	Ultrasonographic examination
Fetal asphyxia	Biophysical profile testing
Fetal anemia	Cordocentesis

gle test is able to predict with certainty whether the fetus is compromised and/or what the optimal timing is for delivery. In addition, and much more importantly, we have no methods of ascertaining which fetuses are likely to develop minor or major handicaps after birth.

Goal. Studying fetal behavior is still very time-consuming and is therefore mostly conducted in research conditions. The aim in the coming years should be to develop more appropriate methods of analyzing fetal behavior, in order to obtain better insights into the condition of the endangered fetus. To obtain better insights into the quality of the fetal CNS, the development of a sensitive and practical method of intrauterine neurological examination should have high priority in clinical perinatology.

References

1. Ahlfeld, F.: Über intrauterine Atembewegungen des Kindes. Ver. Dsch. Ges. Gynäk., 2 (1888) 203–210
2. Archie, C.L., Milton, I.L., Sokol, R.J., Norman, G.: The effects of Methadone treatment on the reactivity of the nonstress test. Obstet. Gynecol. 74 (1989) 254–255
3. Arduini, D., Rizzo, G., Giorlandino, C., Vizzone, A., Nava, S., Dell'Aqua, S.: The fetal behavioural states: an ultrasonic study. Prenatal Diagnosis 5 (1985) 269–276
4. Arduini, D., Rizzo, G., Caforio, L., Mancuso, S.: Development of behavioural states in hydrocephalic fetuses. Fetal Ther. 2 (1987) 135–143
5. Arduini, D., Rizzo, G., Caforio, L., Boccolini, M.R., Romanini, C., Mancuso, S.: Behavioural state transitions in healthy and growth retarded fetuses. Early Hum. Dev., 19 (1989) 155–165
6. Arduini, D., Rizzo G., Massacesi M., Boccolini M.R., Romanini, C., Mancuso, S.: Longitudinal assessment of behavioural transitions in healthy fetuses during the last trimester of pregnancy. J Perinat. Med. 1 (1991) 67–72
7. Arduini, D., Rizzo, G., Romanini, C.: Growth retardation. In: Nijhuis, J.G. (ed.): Fetal behaviour, developmental and perinatal aspects. Oxford: Oxford University Press 1992; pp 181–208
8. Bekedam, D.J., Visser, G.H.A., de Vries, J.J., Prechtl, H.F.R.: Motor behaviour in the growth-retarded fetus. Early Hum. Dev. 12 (1985) 155–165
9. Birnholz, J.C.: The development of human fetal eye movement patterns. Science 213 (1981) 679–681
10. Boddy, K., Robinson, J.S.: External method for detection of fetal breathing in utero. Lancet, 2 (1971) 1231–1233
11. Bots, R.S.G.M., Broeders, G.H.B., Farman, D.J., Haverkorn, M.J., Stolte, L.A.M.: Fetal breathing movements in the normal and growth-retarded fetus: a multiscan/M-mode echofetographic study. Eur. J. Obstet. Gynaecol. Reprod. Biol. 8 (1978) 21–29
12. Bots, R.S.G.M., Nijhuis, J.G., Martin Jr., C.B., Prechtl, H.F.R.: Human fetal eye movements: detection in utero by ultrasonography. Early Hum. Dev. 5 (1981) 87–94
13. Caldeyro-Barcia, R., Mendez-Bauer, C., Poseiro, J.J. et al.: Control of human fetal heart rate during labor. In: Cassels, D.E. (ed.): The heart rate and circulation in the new-born and infant. New York: Grune and Stratton 1966
14. Carmichael, L., Campbell, K., Patrick, J.: Fetal breathing, gross fetal body movements, and maternal and fetal heart rates before spontaneous labor at term. Amer. J. Obstet. Gynecol. 148 (1984) 675–679
15. Dawes, G.S., Leduc, H.E., Liggins, G.C., Richards, R.T.: Respiratory movements and paradoxal sleep in the foetal lamb. J. Physiol. 21 (1970) 47p–48p
16. Dawes, G.S., Moulden, M., Redman, C.W.G.: System 8000. Computerized antenatal FHR analysis. J. Perinat. Med. 19 (1991) 47–51

17. Drogtrop, A.P., Ubels, R., Nijhuis, J.G.: The association between fetal body movements, eye movements, and heart rate patterns between 25 and 30 weeks of gestation. Early Hum. Dev. 23 (1990) 67–73
18. Eyck, J. van, Wladimiroff, J.W.: Doppler flow measurements. In: Nijhuis, J.G. (ed.): Fetal behaviour, developmental and perinatal aspects. Oxford: Oxford University Press 1992; pp 227–241
19. Geijn, H.P. van, Swartjes, J.M., van Woerden, E.E., Caron, F.J.M., Brons, J.T.J., Arts, N.F.T.: Fetal behavioural states in epileptic pregnancies. Europ. J. Obstet. Gynecol. Reprod. Biol. 21 (1986) 309–314
20. Groome, L.J., Watson, J.E.: Assessment of in utero neurobehavioural development. I. Fetal behavioural states. J. Matern. Fetal Invest. 2 (1992) 183–194
21. Hamm-Macher, K., Werners, P.H.: Über die Auswertung und Dokumentation von CTG-Ergebnissen. Gynaecologia 166 (1968) 410–423
22. Heeswijk, M. van, Nijhuis, J.G., Hollanders, H.M.G.: Fetal heart rate in early pregnancy. Early Hum. Dev. 22 (1990) 151–156
23. Hepper, P., Shahidullah, S.: Abnormal fetal behaviour in Down's syndrome fetuses. Quarterly J. Clin. Psych. 44B (1992) 305–317
24. Hon, E.H.: An atlas of fetal heart rate patterns. New Haven, USA: Harty Press Inc. 1968
25. Hume, R.F.jr., O'Donnell, K.J., Stanger, C.L., Killam, A.P., Gingras, J.L.: In utero cocaine exposure: observations of fetal behavioural state may predict neonatal outcome. Amer. J. Obstet. Gynecol. 161 (1989) 685–690
26. James, D.: Fetal behaviour. Current Obstet. Gynaecol. 7 (1997) 30–35
27. Koyanagi, T., Nabekura, J., Nakano, H.: Brain function in utero unique to the developing fetus. Fetal and Maternal Med. Rev. 7 (1995) 129–141
28. Kubli, F.W., Käser, O., Hinselmann, M.: Diagnostic management of chronic placental insufficiency. In: Pecile, A., Finzi, C. (eds.): The foeto-placental unit. Excerpta Medica Foundation, Amsterdam (1969) 323–339
29. Leader, l.R.: Studies in fetal behaviour. Brit. J. Obstet. Gynaecol. 102 (1995) 595–597
30. Lotgering, F.K., Wallenburg, H.C.S., Schouten, H.J.A.: Interobserver and intraobserver variation in the assessment of antepartum cardiotocograms. Amer. J. Obstet. Gynecol. 144 (1982) 701–705
31. Manning, F.A., Pugh, E.W., Boddy, K.: Effect of cigarette smoking on fetal breathing movements in normal pregnancies. Brit. J. Obstet. Gynaecol. 82 (1975) 552–555
32. Manning, F.A., Platt, L.D., Sipos, L.: Antepartum evaluation: development of a fetal biophysical profile scoring. Amer. J. Obstet. Gynecol. 136 (1980) 787–795
33. Mulder, E.J.H., Visser, G.H.A., Bekedam, D.J., Prechtl, H.F.R.: Emergence of behavioural states in fetuses of type-I diabetic women. Early Hum. Dev. 15 (1987) 231–252
34. Mulder, E.J.H., Derks, J.B., Zonneveld, M.F., Bruinse, H.W., Visser, G.H.A.: Transient reduction in fetal activity and heart rate variation after maternal betamethasone administration. Early Hum. Dev. 36 (1994) 49–60
35. Mulder, E.J.H., Derks, J.B., Visser, G.H.A.: Antenatal corticosteroid therapy and fetal behaviour: a randomised study of the effects of betamethasone and dexamethasone. Brit. J. Obstet. Gynaecol. 104 (1997) 1239–1247
36. Nijhuis, J.G., Bots, R.S.G.M., Martin, C.B. jr., Prechtl, H.F.R.: Are there behavioural states in the human fetus? Early Hum. Dev. 6 (1982) 177–195
37. Nijhuis, J.G., Martin, Jr. C.B., Gommers, S., Bouws, P., Bots, R.S.G.M., Jongsma, H.W.: The rhythmicity of fetal breathing varies with behavioural state in the human fetus. Early Hum. Dev. 9 (1983) 1–7
38. Nijhuis, J.G., Staisch, K.J., Martin, C.B.jr., Prechtl, H.F.R: A sinusoidal-like fetal heart-rate pattern in association with fetal sucking – report of 2 cases. Europ. J. Obstet. Gynecol. Reprod. Biol. 16 (1984) 353–358
39. Nijhuis, J.G., Jongsma, H.W., Crijns, I.J.M.J., Valk, I.M.G.M. de, Velden, J.W.H.J. van der: Effects of maternal glucose ingestion on human fetal breathing movements at weeks 24, and 28 of gestation. Early Hum. Dev. 13 (1986) 183–188
40. Nijhuis, J.G., Kruyt, N., Wijck, J.A.M. van: Fetal brain death. Two case reports. Brit. J. Obstet. Gynaecol., 95 (1988) 197–200
41. Nijhuis, J.G., Crevels, A.J., Dongen, P.W.J. van: Fetal brain death: The definition of a fetal heart rate pattern and its clinical consequenses. Obstet. Gynecol. Survey 46 (1990) 229–232
42. Nijhuis, J.G., Tas, B.A.P.J.: Physiological and clinical aspects of the development of fetal behaviour. In: Hanson, M.A. (ed.): The fetal and neonatal brainstem, developmental and clinical issues. Cambridge: Cambridge University Press 1991; pp. 268–281
43. Nijhuis, J.G., Pas, M. van de: Behavioural states and their ontogeny. Human studies. Seminars in Perinatology 16 (1992) 206–210
44. Nijhuis, J.G. (ed.): Fetal behaviour, developmental and perinatal aspects. Oxford: Oxford University Press 1992
45. Nijhuis, J.G.: Physiological and clinical consequences in relation to the development of fetal behaviour and fetal behavioural states. In: Krasnegor, N.A., Lecanuet, P., Fifer, W.P., Smotherman W.P. (eds.): Fetal Development: A psychobiological perspective. Hillsdale, New Jersey, USA: Lawrence Erlbaum Ass. Publishers 1995; pp. 67–82
46. Nijhuis, I.J.M., Ten Hof, J., Mulder, E.J.H. et al.: Numerical fetal heart rate analysis: normograms, minimal duration of recording and intrafetal consistency. Prenat. Neonat. Med. 3 (1998) 314–322
47. Nijhuis, I.J.M., Ten Hof, J., Mulder, E.J.H. et al.: Fetal Heart Rate (FHR) parameters during FHR patterns A and B: a longitudinal study from 24 weeks' gestation. Prenat. Neonat. Med. 3 (1998) 383–399
48. Nijhuis, J.G., Pas, M. van de, Jongsma, H.W.: Fetal behavioural state transitions in uncomplicated pregnancies after 41 weeks of gestation. Early Hum. Dev. 52 (1998) 125–133
49. Pas, M. van de, Niihuis, J.G., Jongsma, H.W.: Fetal behaviour in uncomplicated pregnancies after 41 weeks of gestation. Early Hum. Dev. 40 (1994) 29–38
50. Patrick, J., Campbell, K., Carmichael, L., Natale, R., Richardson, B.: Patterns of human fetal breathing during the last 10 weeks of pregnancy. Obstet. Gynecol. 56 (1980) 24–30
51. Pillai, M., Garrett, C., James, D.: Bizarre fetal behaviour associated with lethal congenital anomalies: a case report. Europ. J. Obstet. Gynecol. Reprod. Biol. 39 (1991) 215–218
52. Prechtl, H.F.R., Weinmann, H.M., Akiyama, Y.: Organization of physiological parameters in normal and neurologically abnormal infants. Neuropädiatrie 1 (1969) 101–129

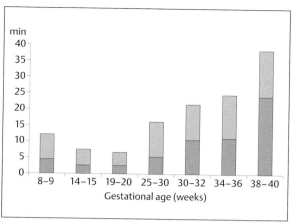

Fig. 15.**1** Maximum and mean duration (in minutes) of periods in which body movements can be absent at different gestational ages.

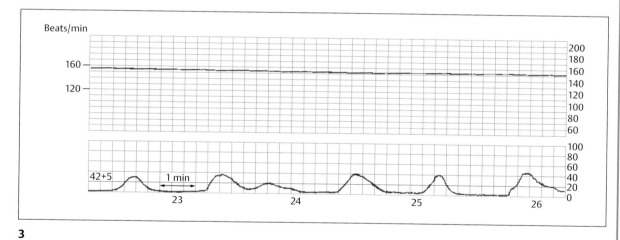

	Criteria			
	FHRP	Body movements	Eye movements	Breathing movements
Behavioral state 1F	A	--	--	Regular
Behavioral state 2F	B	++	++	Irregular
Behavioral state 3F	C	--	++	Regular
Behavioral state 4F	D	++	++	Irregular

Fig. 15.**2** Schematic diagram of the definition of the four behavioral states and their relation to breathing (if present). In the lower part, an example is given of each of the heart rate patterns (A through D), at a recording speed of 3 cm/min. FHRP = fetal heart rate pattern.

Fig. 15.**3** An example of a persistent, absolutely silent fetal heart rate pattern and absence of fetal activity. Note the relatively high baseline of 155 bpm. This recording indicates fetal brain death (reproduced with kind permission from Tas and Nijhuis, 1992 [60]).

53. Reinold, E.: Beobachtung fetaler Aktivität in der ersten Hälfte der Gravidität mit dem Ultraschall. Pädiatr. Pädol. 6 (1976) 274–279
54. Ribbert, L.S.M., Fidier, V., Visser, G.H.A.: Computer-assisted analysis of normal second trimester fetal heart rate patterns. J. Perinat. Med. 19 (1991) 53–59
55. Richardson, B.S.: (Guest editor) Fetal behavioural states. Seminars in Perinatology 16 (1992) 4
56. Romanini, C., Rizzo, G.: Fetal behaviour in normal and compromised fetuses. An overview. Early Hum. Dev. 43 (1995) 117–131
57. Rooth, G., Huch, A., Huch, R.: Guidelines for the use of fetal monitoring. Int. J. of Gynecol. Obstet. 25 (1987) 159–167
58. Snijders, R.J.M., Ribbert, L.S.M., Visser, G.H.A., Mulder, E.J.H.: Numeric analysis of heart rate variation in intrauterine growth-retarded fetuses: A longitudinal study. Amer. J. Obstet. Gynecol. 166 (1992) 22–27
59. Tas, B.A.P.J., Nijhuis, J.G., Lucas, A.J. et al.: The intercostal-to-phrenic inhibitory reflex in the human fetus near term. Early Hum. Dev. 22 (1991) 145–149
60. Tas, B.A.P.J., Nijhuis, J.G.: Consequences for fetal monitoring. In: Nijhuis, J.G. (ed.): Fetal behaviour, developmental and perinatal aspects. Oxford: Oxford University Press 1992; pp. 258–269
61. Tas, B.A.P.J., Nijhuis, J.G., Nelen, W., Willems, E.: The intercostal-to-phrenic inhibitory reflex in normal and intra-uterine growth-retarded (IUGR) human fetuses from 26 to 40 weeks of gestation. Early Hum. Dev. 32 (1993) 177–182
62. Timor-Tritsch, I.E., Dierker, L.J., Hertz, R.H., Deagan, C., Rosen, M.G.: Studies of antepartum behavioural states in the human fetus at term. Amer. J. Obstet. Gynecol. 132 (1979) 524–528
63. Timor-Tritsch, I.E., Dierker, L.J., Hertz, R.H., Chik, L., Rosen, M.G.: Regular and irregular human fetal respiratory movements. Early Hum. Dev. 4 (1980) 315–324
64. Trimbos, J.B., Keirse, M.J.C.N.: Observer variability in assessment of antepartum cardiotocograms. Brit. J. Obstet. Gynaecol. 85 (1978) 900–906
65. Vandenberghe, K, de Wolf, K.: Intrauterine assessment of fetal stomach function. Physiology and clinic. In: Kurjak, A. (ed.): Recent advances in Ultrasound Diagnosis. 2nd ed. Excerpta Medica, Amsterdam. Internat. Congress Series 498 (1980) 417–421
66. Visser, G.H.A., Dawes, G.S., Redman, C.W.G.: Numerical analysis of the normal human antenatal fetal heart rate. Brit. J. Obstet. Gynaecol. 88 (1981) 792–802
67. Visser, G.H.A., Goodman, J.D.S., Levine, D.H. et al.: Micturition and the heart rate period cycle in the human fetus. Brit. J. Obstet. Gynaecol. 153 (1981) 803–805
68. Visser, G.H.A., Poelman-Weesjes, G., Cohen, T.M.N. et al.: Fetal behaviour at 30 to 32 weeks of gestation. Ped. Res. 22 (1987) 655–658
69. Visser, G.H.A.: The second trimester. In: Nijhuis, J.G. (ed.): Fetal behaviour, developmental and perinatal aspects. Oxford: Oxford University Press 1992; pp. 17–26
70. Visser, G.H.A., Ribbert, L.S.M., Bekedam, D.J.: Sequential changes in Doppler waveform, fetal heart rate and movements patterns in IUGR fetuses. In: van Geijn, H.P., Copray, F.J.A. (eds.): A critical appraisal of fetal surveillance. Amsterdam: Elsevier Science b.v. 1994; pp. 193–200
71. Vliet M.A.T. van, Martin, C.B. jr., Nijhuis, J.G., Prechtl, H.F.: The relationship between fetal activity, and behavioural states and fetal breathing movements in normal and growth-retarded fetuses. Amer. J. Obstet. Gynecol. 153 (1985) 582–588
72. Vliet, M.A. van, Martin, C.B. jr., Nijhuis, J.G., Prechtl, H.F.: Behavioural states in fetuses of nulliparous women. Early Hum. Dev. 12 (1985) 121–135
73. Vliet, M.A. van, Martin, C.B. jr., Nijhuis, J.G., Prechtl, H.F.: Behavioural states in growth retarded human fetuses. Early Hum. Dev. 12 (1985) 183–197
74. Vries, J.I.P. de, Visser, G.H.A., Prechtl, H.F.R.: The emergence of fetal behaviour. I. Qualitative aspects. Early Hum. Dev. 7 (1982) 301–322
75. Vries, J.I.P. de, Visser, G.H.A., Prechtl, H.F.R.: The emergence of fetal behaviour. II. Quantitative aspects. Early Hum. Dev. 12 (1985) 99–120
76. Vries, J.I.P. de, Visser, G.H.A., Mulder, E.J.H., Prechtl, H.F.R.: Diurnal and other variations in fetal movement, and heart rate patterns at 20–22 weeks. Early Hum. Dev. 15 (1987) 333–348
77. Vries J.I.P., de: The first trimester. In: Nijhuis, J.G. (ed.): Fetal behaviour, developmental and perinatal aspects. Oxford: Oxford University Press 1992; pp. 3–16
78. Woerden, E.E. van, Geijn, H.P. van, Svvartjes, J.M., Caron, F.J.M., Brons, J.T.J., Arts, N.F.Th.: Fetal heart rhythms during behavioural state 1F. Europ. J. Obstet. Gynecol. Reprod. Biol. 28 (1988) 29–38
79. Woerden, E.E. van, Geijn, H.P. van, Caron, F.J.M., Mantel, R., Swartjes, J.M., Arts, N.F.Th.: Automated assignment of fetal behavioural states near term. Hum. Dev. 19 (1989) 137–146
80. Woerden, E.E. van, Geijn, H.P. van: Heart-rate patterns and fetal movements. In: Nijhuis, J.G. (ed.): Fetal behaviour, developmental and perinatal aspects. Oxford: Oxford University Press 1992; pp 41–56

16 Fetal Growth Disturbances in the Second and Third Trimesters

Biometry. As explained in Chapter 12, the accurate measurement and documentation of fetal biometric parameters in the second and third trimesters forms an essential basis for the evaluation of fetal growth. By comparing the ultrasound measurements with standard growth charts, one can recognize normal fetal development (Fig. 16.**1**) or detect growth discrepancies at an early stage. It is essential, however, that the gestational age be established or confirmed as accurate by ultrasound measurements during the first trimester.

Late initial examination. If the initial ultrasound examination is not performed until 20 weeks or later and the dates are uncertain, fetal growth cannot be accurately evaluated based on a single examination (Fig. 16.3). This type of case requires serial examinations as well as a specific comparison of how closely the individual growth parameters match the assumed gestational age.

Redating. It is not good practice to adjust the gestational age repeatedly due to discrepancies in ultrasound measurements, as this will prevent the early detection of a growth disturbance.

Error in Dates

If the dates are uncertain and an initial ultrasound examination in the second trimester shows that both head and abdominal growth are below the 5th percentile, either there is an error in dates of days or weeks (Fig. 16.**2**) or the fetus is manifesting early proportional growth retardation.

Clues. An error in dates can be recognized by noting that all growth parameters show the same, consistent time lag in serial examinations. This can also occur with a genetically small fetus, but this type of fetus would exhibit normal growth during the first trimester (Fig. 16.3), whereas a true error in dates would already produce a growth discrepancy in the first trimester.

Intrauterine Growth Retardation

Prognosis. Intrauterine growth retardation (IUGR), known also as small for gestational age (SGA) status, is associated with a marked increase in perinatal morbidity and mortality. As various investigators have shown, the mortality rate in growth-retarded infants is 3–8 times higher than in newborns of normal weight (46, 67, 83). Live-born growth-retarded infants are more prone to disturbances of adaptation and development than normal-weight babies (6, 20, 21), and follow-up studies, particularly in twins, have shown that some of these effects are permanent (1, 6, 36). As Usher and McLean (70) point out, 70% of deaths in growth-retarded fetuses are preventable if IUGR can be diagnosed by 34 weeks' gestation. This underscores the importance of the early detection of IUGR so that appropriate diagnostic and therapeutic measures can be implemented.

Diagnosis. Ultrasound has become the foremost method for the early detection of IUGR (17), superseding other less reliable methods such as palpation, abdominal girth measurement (78), and measurement of the symphyseal-fundal distance (7, 78). Especially in obese patients or in patients with an abnormal amniotic fluid volume (oligo- or polyhydramnios), the ultrasound evaluation of fetal growth is definitely superior to clinical assessment.

Definitions and growth parameters. By definition, an infant is classified as growth-retarded if its birth weight is below the 10th percentile of the weight that is appropriate for its gestational age (6, 24). But prenatal ultrasound permits only an indirect estimation of fetal weight based on the evaluation of individual parameters, and the calculations are affected by measurement errors. A better approach is to identify specific, sonographically measurable body parameters (biparietal diameter, head circumference, abdominal transverse diameter, abdominal circumference) and apply these parameters directly to the evaluation of fetal growth.

The fifth percentile is most commonly used as the cutoff point for making a diagnosis of IUGR (49). Thus, IUGR is considered to be present if the fetal parameter in question is below the fifth percentile of the growth curve. Other authors use two standard deviations (2 SD) as the cutoff for IUGR, and a few authors use the tenth percentile.

▬ *Types of IUGR*

Basic types. Two principal types of IUGR can be distinguished on the basis of their distinctive ultrasound growth patterns (8, 19, 31, 32):
1. Proportional (symmetrical) IUGR (Figs. 16.**4**, 16.**14**)
2. Disproportional (asymmetrical) IUGR (Figs. 16.**5**, 16.**6**, 16.**15**)

Dependence on growth phases. The type of IUGR that develops appears to depend on the timing and duration of the growth disturbance—i.e., whether cell growth is affected during the period of proliferation along, during proliferation with hyperplasia and hypertrophy, or during hypertrophy with no numerical increase in the cell population.

If the nutritional deficit occurs during the proliferation phase, the decreased rate of cell division will result in a smaller organ with fewer cells. These changes are irreversible. But if the deficit occurs during the hypertrophic phase of cell growth, the main effect will be a failure of cell enlargement. These changes are reversible (82). Chronic malnutrition leads to a symmetrical reduction in weight and length, whereas an "acute" nutritional deficit has a much greater impact on weight than on length (63).

Causes. The causes of IUGR are diverse and can be classified as maternal, placental, or fetal. Table 16.**1** lists the intrinsic and extrinsic factors that were identified by Robson and Chang (63) as causing IUGR. If there is deficient blood flow to the uterus and/or placenta, Doppler or color Doppler ultrasound is a good source of additional information (12, 23, 28, 64, 71) in the biometric diagnosis of IUGR.

Proportional Growth Retardation

Characteristics. Proportional IUGR affects the entire body and is most pronounced in the first half of the second trimester (Figs. 16.**4**, 16.**14**). Both the head and trunk parameters are too small for gestational age. Campbell (8) calls this a "low-profile" pattern of cephalic growth.

Table 16.**1**   Causes of intrauterine growth retardation (63)

Extrinsic factors	Intrinsic factors
➢ Maternal starvation, chronic malnutrition ➢ Malabsorption syndromes ➢ Excessive energy expenditure ➢ Smoking ➢ Alcohol ➢ Marihuana, cocaine, heroin ➢ Cardiac diseases ➢ Respiratory tract diseases ➢ Extreme altitude ➢ Proteinuric hypertension ➢ Sickle-cell anemia, connective-tissue diseases ➢ Renal diseases ➢ Recurrent uterine bleeding ➢ Placental vascular anomalies or tumors	➢ Chromosomal anomalies ➢ Nonchromosomal anomalies ➢ Dwarfism syndromes ➢ Fetal infections ➢ Teratogenic drugs or chemical products ➢ Ionizing radiation ➢ Constitutional factors

Causes. Proportional IUGR may be caused by fetal anomalies, chromosomal abnormalities, viral infections (rubella, cytomegalovirus), or exogenous agents (alcohol, nicotine, heroin, ionizing radiation) (Table 16.**1**). Also, the genetically small but healthy offspring of small parents may exhibit a growth pattern that falls below the fifth percentile (8, 19, 31, 59).

Further tests. Proportional IUGR detected before 20 weeks in a fetus of known gestational age should always raise suspicion of a fetal anomaly or chromosomal abnormality, and appropriate further tests (targeted imaging for fetal anomalies, chromosome analysis) should be initiated.

Chromosomal abnormalities and fetal anomalies. Up to 38% of children with chromosomal abnormalities manifest IUGR (40). Mean birth weight is reduced by 20% in children with trisomy 21 or trisomy 13 and by 38% in children with trisomy 18 (57). Triploidy is also associated with severe growth retardation of early onset (3). As for anomalies that do not occur in the setting of a chromosomal abnormality, 22% of these cases also manifest growth retardation (40).

Disproportional Growth Retardation

Characteristics. In disproportional IUGR, an initially normal period of growth is followed by a retardation of fetal growth during the third trimester. This pattern is mainly characterized by a deficiency of trunk growth with little or no retardation of head growth (Figs. 16.**5**, 16.**15**). The slowing of abdominal growth may precede that of head growth by 2–3 weeks. Campbell (8) describes this as a "late flattening" type of growth pattern.

Causes. Disproportional or asymmetrical IUGR is caused by a deficiency of uteroplacental blood flow due to maternal disease such as hypertension, gestational edema, proteinuria, and hypertension (GEPH), or diabetes mellitus (8, 16, 32) (Table 16.**1**). The growth retardation affects weight more than length. The weight loss chiefly affects the fetal internal organs (liver, lung, thymus) while sparing the brain (26).

Prognosis. Regarding the prognosis of IUGR, it is noteworthy that Fancourt et al. (21), in their follow-up examinations of small-for-date children at 4 years of age, found evidence of mental retardation only in cases where a slowing of superior growth had been noted prior to 27 weeks' gestation. Long-term studies by Low et al. (47) showed that premature SGA babies had a higher incidence of handicaps and learning deficits by 9–11 years of age than premature babies who were appropriate for gestational age (47).

Diagnosis. Various investigators have shown that only about 60% of growth-retarded fetuses can be identified by measurement of the biparietal diameter alone (43, 45, 58, 79), whereas 80% or more can be identified when a trunk parameter is added (13, 31, 43, 45, 75). This emphasizes the importance of taking both cephalic and abdominal measurements in ultrasound examinations.

Differential Diagnosis

Error in dates. The diagnosis of IUGR is problematic in cases where the first ultrasound examination is not performed until the third trimester and it is discovered that fetal growth is below the normal range (Fig. 16.**7**). This may represent true IUGR or simply an error in dates. Diagnostic problems can also arise when fetal growth parameters are within normal limits but show a definite flattening trend in subsequent examinations (Fig. 16.**6**). This may represent IUGR in a pregnancy that is actually farther along than the assigned date.

Further Tests and Treatment

Ultrasound follow-ups. If IUGR is suspected, ultrasound should be repeated after at least one week. With a shorter interval, the measurement error could be greater than the growth rate. To avoid interpersonal errors, the same examiner should perform the follow-up.

Doppler and CTG follow-ups. If ultrasound follow-ups raise suspicion of disproportional IUGR due to placental insufficiency in the third trimester, Doppler and CTG monitoring should be performed at regular intervals. If fetal growth does not rebound in response to bed rest, preferably in an inpatient setting, preterm delivery may be the best option, especially if Doppler shows additional abnormalities (0 flow, reverse flow).

Pharmacologic therapy. The maintenance and restoration of fetal growth in women treated by parenteral nutrition (62) or given oral protein and allylestrenol (39) has been reported. Renaud et al. (61) published results on the intra-amniotic instillation of amino acids to correct fetal malnutrition.

The results of low-dose maternal aspirin therapy (50–100 mg/day) for the prevention and treatment of IUGR have been controversial. While several groups of authors reported a favorable effect on IUGR (44, 74, 77), the Collaborative Low-dose Aspirin Study in Pregnancy (CLASP) published in 1994 showed no significant benefit. Carrera et al. (11) reviewed a variety of treatment strategies for IUGR. All in all, repeated doubts have been expressed as to the advisability of pharmacologic treatments for growth-retarded fetuses (33), and so far such treatments have fallen well short of expectations.

Differentiation and Quantification of IUGR

Head/Trunk Ratio

The head/trunk ratio is used to differentiate between proportional and disproportional IUGR and to quantify the severity of the growth retardation. It may be calculated as the ratio of BPD to ATD (31) or as the ratio of HC to AC (9, 16) (see Chapter 12). The head/trunk ratio is normal in proportional IUGR. It is increased in disproportional IUGR.

Confirmed dates. The gestational age must be accurately established in order to interpret the head/trunk ratio correctly. If the dates are uncertain, it is unclear whether an increased head/trunk ratio signifies disproportional IUGR in a correctly dated fetus as opposed to macrosomic head growth with a normal trunk in a younger fetus.

Uncertain dates. When dates are uncertain, additional parameters such as femur length or transverse cerebellar diameter (50, 60) should be included in the evaluation. The cerebellar diameter shows little if any change in growth retardation, however, and its importance in diagnosing IUGR is debated in the literature. Hill et al. (34, 35) found that the transverse cerebellar diameter was below the 2 SD cutoff in 60% of growth-retarded fetuses.

Isolated Retardation of Head Growth

A small head accompanied by normal trunk growth is not a result of placental insufficiency.

Microcephaly. Microcephaly is characterized by a small biparietal diameter (Fig. 16.**8**) and small head circumference but normal abdominal dimensions. The diagnosis can be confirmed by also measuring the growth of the long limb bones (37). While the head circumference is definitely too small for gestational age, the long tubular bones show growth that is appropriate for gestational age.

Spina bifida. Slightly below-normal head growth may be observed in fetuses with spina bifida (76). In fetuses that subsequently develop hydrocephalus, the biparietal diameter increases, causing the head dimensions to "rebound" into the normal range (see Chapter 23).

Dolichocephalic head shape. One danger of measuring the BPD alone is that dolichocephaly, which is common in breech-presenting fetuses (Fig. 16.**9a**), may lead to an erroneous diagnosis of IUGR. Adding the head circumference and abdominal dimensions in these cases will demonstrate normal fetal growth (Fig. 16.**9b**).

Isolated Retardation of Limb Growth

Dwarfism. Normal head growth accompanied by retarded growth of the limb bones (Fig. 16.**10**) indicates that some form of dwarfism is present. This warrants further diagnostic scrutiny.

Macrosomia, Macrocephaly

Definition. Macrosomia refers to a fetus weighing 4000 g or more at birth. Severe macrosomia denotes a birth weight of 4500 g or more. Approximately 10% of infants with a birth weight > 2500 g are macrosomic (5).

Macrocephaly is present when the fetal head dimensions are above the 95th percentile.

Prognosis. Like IUGR, macrosomia (= large for gestational age [LGA]) is associated with increased perinatal morbidity and mortality (2, 5, 30, 69). Modanlou et al. (51) found that the mortality in infants with a birth weight greater than 4500 g was twice as high as in infants of normal size. During labor, a large fetal head and trunk can cause dystocic complications. If a relative disproportion is already present, a cesarean delivery is inevitable. In some cases a cesarean section can be avoided by detecting accelerated fetal growth at an early stage and scheduling preterm induction at approximately 38 weeks.

Ultrasound diagnosis. The development of macrosomia, like that of macrocephaly, can be detected sonographically. Manual examinations, by contrast, tend to underestimate fetal size. The clinically determined symphyseal-fundal distance may be distorted due to hydramnios (69).

Macrosomic growth can be detected sonographically either by intrauterine weight estimation (22) (fetal weight > 90th percentile) or by determining the abdominal circumference (18, 29, 70). Hadlock et al.

(29) recommend using the ratio of femur length to abdominal circumference for the early detection of accelerated fetal growth. One disadvantage of weight estimation is that there is a tendency to overestimate weight due to excessive fat deposition in macrosomic fetuses (4). While fat markedly increases the abdominal girth, it is less dense than muscle tissue.

The 95th percentile is the usual cutoff point for the ultrasound diagnosis of macrosomia (49). Some authors use + 2 SD as the cutoff, and a few use the 90th percentile.

Differentiation. Macrosomia is assumed to be present when abdominal measurements yield dimensions that are above the 95th percentile. If only the head dimensions are above the 95th percentile, macrocephaly is diagnosed.

Proportional macrosomia. Macrosomic growth is described as proportional when the head and trunk dimensions are above the normal range by an equal degree. If the measurements are at or slightly above the upper limit of normal, the differential diagnosis should include a genetically large offspring of large parents (Fig. 16.**11**).

Disproportional macrosomia. If only trunk growth is accelerated, the macrosomia is described as disproportional (Figs. 16.**12**, 16.**16**). Increased abdominal growth with a relatively normal head circumference is seen in diabetic macrosomia, for example. The degree of disproportionality in these cases can be evaluated by calculating the head/trunk ratio (see Chapter 12). If only the trunk is enlarged, the head/trunk ratio will be low. With proportional macrosomia, the head/trunk ratio will be unchanged.

Macrocephaly. In macrocephaly or macrocephalic head growth due to advanced hydrocephalus (Fig. 16.**13**), both the biparietal diameter and the head circumference are too large. Because the abdominal dimensions are within normal limits, the head/trunk ratio is correspondingly high.

Causes of macrosomia. The causes of fetal macrosomia are largely unknown (Table 16.**2**). Empirical factors that can alert the physician to the development of macrosomia include the maternal birth weight (41), multiparity (41), the previous delivery of a macrosomic infant (68), maternal obesity (54), an extreme weight gain during pregnancy (72), and large parents. In some cases fetal macrosomia can be related to specific syndromes such as Wiedemann–Beckwith syndrome, Sotos syndrome, or Weaver syndrome (81). An established cause of macrosomia is maternal diabetes mellitus, although this disease is implicated in fewer than 10% of LGA cases (51).

Macrosomia in Maternal Diabetes

Pathophysiology. In diabetes mellitus, the mechanism of fetal macrosomia is a compensatory hypertrophy of the fetal islet tissue that is induced by maternal hyperglycemia. The increased fetal insulin production leads to an increased deposition of subcutaneous fat and enlargement of the internal organs (heart, liver, spleen) (hyperinsulin obesity). The size of the brain is unchanged (10, 27, 66, 69, 80).

Ultrasound findings. Ultrasound demonstrates abnormal fetal growth affecting the trunk much more than the skull (25, 30, 53), producing a disproportional macrosomic pattern with a low head/trunk ratio (30) (Fig. 16.**12**).

In occasional cases of maternal diabetes, fetuses with a deficient placental supply will develop disproportional growth retardation with abdominal dimensions that are below the fifth percentile.

In other cases of diabetic macrosomia, subcutaneous fat may be increased about the head and the trunk, creating a proportional type of

Table 16.2 Causes of fetal macrosomia

> ➢ Maternal birthweight
> ➢ Multiparity
> ➢ Prior history of macrosomia
> ➢ Maternal age > 35 years
> ➢ Maternal height > 169 cm
> ➢ Maternal obesity (initial weight > 70 kg)
> ➢ Extreme weight gain during pregnancy
> ➢ Infant delivered 7 days or more after term
> ➢ Diabetes mellitus
> ➢ Fetal syndrome (Wiedemann–Beckwith syndrome, Sotos syndrome, Weaver syndrome)

macrosomic growth. Ultrasound in these cases shows thickening of the fetal scalp with a typical double contour (38) along the skull (Fig. 16.**17**), similar to that seen in fetal hydrops or some cases of intrauterine fetal death. In fetal hydrops, however, the scalp edema is usually accompanied by ascites, hydrothorax, or pericardial effusion.

Fetal macrosomia in maternal diabetes mellitus is often associated with polyhydramnios (56). A concomitant increase in placental thickness may also be seen (65).

Glucose tolerance test. If the second screening examination already shows accelerated fetal growth with confirmed dates, an oral glucose tolerance test should be administered to assess the maternal metabolic status.

Serial examinations. Starting at 20 weeks, pregnant women with known diabetes mellitus should have an ultrasound examination every 2 weeks so that accelerated fetal growth can be promptly detected and further macrosomic development can be prevented by adjusting the insulin regimen as needed. In gestational diabetes as well, the incidence of macrosomia can be significantly reduced by the early use of insulin (15).

Congenital anomalies. Because frank diabetes mellitus is associated with an increased rate of congenital anomalies (4.5–16.8%) (2, 42, 48, 55), these patients should be carefully screened for fetal anomalies with ultrasound prior to 22 weeks. The most common malformations affect the heart, spinal column, kidneys, and inferior fetal pole (inferior regression syndrome) (2, 42, 48, 52). Given the potential for a fetal neural tube defect, a serum AFP assay is also recommended in every pregnant woman who has diabetes.

References

1. Babson, S.G., Phillips, D.S.: Growth and development of twins dissimilar in size and birth. New Engl. J. Med. 289 (1973) 937–940
2. Ballard, J.L., Holroyde, J., Tsang, R.C., Chan, G., Sutherland, J.M., Knowles, H.C.: High malformation rates and decreased mortality in infants of diabetic mothers managed after the first trimester of pregnancy (1956–1978). Amer. J. Obstet. Gynec. 148 (1984) 1111–1118
3. Benacerraf, B.R.: Intrauterine growth retardation in the first trimester associated with triploidy. J. Ultrasound Med. 7 (1988) 153–154
4. Bernstein, I.M., Catalano, P.M.: Influence of fetal fat on the ultrasound estimation of fetal weight in diabetic mothers. Obstet. Gynecol. 79 (1992) 561–563
5. Boyd, M.E., Usher, R.H., McLean, F.H.: Fetal macrosomia: Prediction, risks, proposed management. Obstet. Gynecol. 61 (1983) 715–722
6. Brandt, I.: Postnatale Entwicklung von Früh-Mangelgeborenen. Gynäkologe 8 (1975) 219–233
7. Calvert, J.P., Crean, E.E., Newcombe, R.G., Pearson, J.F.: Antenatal screening by measurement of symphysis-fundus height. Brit. med. J. 285 (1982) 846–849
8. Campbell, S.: The assessment of fetal development by diagnostic ultrasound. In: Milunsky, A.: Clinics in Perinatology, Vol. 1. Philadelphia: Saunders 1974 p. 507
9. Campbell, S., Thoms, A.: Ultrasound measurement of the fetal head to abdomen circumference ratio in the assessment of growth retardation. Brit. J. Obstet. Gynaec. 84 (1977) 165–174
10. Cardell, B.S.: The infants of diabetic mothers. J. Obstet. Gynaec. Brit. Emp. 60 (1953) 834–853
11. Carrera, J.M., Devesa, R., Mallafré, J., Lopez-Rodo, V., Ruiz, J.: Management of intrauterine growth retardation: antenatal and intrapartum strategies. In: Kurjak, A. (ed.): Textbook of Perinatal Medicine. London: Parthenon Publishing Group 1998
12. Chambers, S.E., Hoskins, P.R., Haddad, N.G., Johnstone, F.D., McDicken, W.N., Muir, B.B.: A comparison of fetal abdominal circumference measurements and Doppler ultrasound in the prediction of small-for-dates babies and fetal compromise. Brit. J. Obstet. Gynaecol. 96 (1989) 803–808
13. Chang, T.C., Robson, S.C., Boys, R.J., Spencer, J.A.D.: Prediction of the small for gestational age infant: which ultrasonic measurement is best? Obstet. Gynecol. 80 (1992) 1030–1038
14. CLASP (Collaborative Low-dose Aspirin Study in Pregnancy): CLASP: a randomised trial of low-dose aspirin for the prevention and treatment of pre-eclampsia among 9364 pregnant women. Lancet 343 (1994) 619–629
15. Coustan, D.R., Imarah, J.: Prophylactic insulin treatment of gestational diabetes reduces the incidence of macrosomia, operative delivery, and birth trauma. Amer. J. Obstet. Gynec. 150 (1984) 836–842
16. Crane, J.P., Kopta, M.M.: Prediction of intrauterine growth retardation via ultrasonographic measurement of head/abdominal circumference ratios. Obstet. Gynec. 54 (1979) 597–601
17. Deter, R.L., Harrist, R.B., Hadlock, F.P., Carpenter, R.J.: The use of ultrasound in the detection of intrauterine growth retardation. J. Clin. Ultrasound 10 (1982) 9–16
18. Deter, R.L., Hadlock, F.P.: Use of ultrasound in the detection of macrosomia: A review. J. Clin. Ultrasound 13 (1985) 519–524
19. DeVore, G., Hobbins, J.C.: Fetal growth and development: The diagnosis of intrauterine growth retardation. In: Hobbins, J.C.: Diagnostic Ultrasound in Obstetrics. New York: Churchill Livingstone 1979
20. Drillien, C.M.: Prognosis of infants of very low birth weight. Lancet I (1971) 697
21. Fancourt, R., Campbell, S., Harvey, D., Norman, A.P.: Follow-up study of small-for-dates babies. Brit. med. J. 1 (1976) 1435–1437
22. Farmer, R.M., Medearis, A.L., Hirata, G.I., Platt, L.D.: The use of a neural network for the ultrasonographic estimation of fetal weight in the macrosomic fetus. Amer. J. Obstet. Gynecol. 166 (1992) 1467–1472
23. Fok, R.Y., Pavlova, Z., Benirschke, K., Paul, R.H., Platt, L.D.: The correlation of arterial lesions with umbilical artery Doppler velocimetry in the placentas of small-for-dates pregnancies. Obstet. Gynecol. 75 (1990) 578–583
24. Frigoletto, F.D., Rothschild, S.B.: Altered fetal growth: an overview. Clin. Obstet. Gynec. 20 (1977) 915–923
25. Grandjean, H., Sarramon, M.F., Reme, J.M., Pontonnier, G.: Detection of gestational diabetes by means of ultrasonic diagnosis of excessive fetal growth. Amer. J. Obstet. Gynec. 138 (1980) 790–792
26. Gruenwald, P.: Chronic fetal distress and placental insufficiency. Biol. Neonat. 5 (1963) 215–265
27. Gruenwald, P.: Growth of the human fetus. II. Abnormal growth in twins and infants of mothers with diabetes, hypertension, or isoimmunization. Amer. J. Obstet. Gynec. 94 (1966) 1120–1132
28. Gudmundsson, S., Marsal, K.: Umbilical and uteroplacental blood flow velocity waveforms in pregnancies with fetal growth retardation. Eur. J. Obstet. Gynecol. Reprod. Biol. 27 (1988) 187–196
29. Hadlock, F.P., Harrist, R.B., Fearneyhough, T.C., Deter, R.L., Park, S.K., Rossavik, I.K.: Use of femur length/abdominal circumference ratio in detecting the macrosomic fetus. Radiology 154 (1985) 503–505
30. Hansmann, M., Hinckers, H.J.: Das große Kind. Gynäkologe 7 (1974) 81–94
31. Hansmann, M.: Ultraschallbiometrie im II. und III. Trimester der Schwangerschaft. Gynäkologe 9 (1976) 133–155
32. Hansmann, M.: Bestimmung des Gestationsalters und -gewichts und die Bedeutung für das klinische Management. In: Huch, A., Huch, R., Duc, G., Rooth, G.: Klinisches Management des kleinen Frühgeborenen. Stuttgart: Thieme 1982; S. 31–54
33. Harding, J., Owens, J., Robison, J.: Should we try to supplement the growth retarded fetus? A cautionary tale. Brit. J. Obstet. Gynaecol. 99 (1992) 707–710
34. Hill, L.M., Guzick, D., Rivello, D., Hixon, J., Peterson, C.: The transverse cerebellar diameter cannot be used to assess gestational age in the small for gestational age fetus. Obstet. Gynecol., 75 (1990) 329–333
35. Hill, L.M., Guzick, D., DiNofrio, D., Maloney, J., Merolillo, C., Nedzesky, P.: Ratios between the abdominal circumference, head circumference, or femur length and the transverse cerebellar diameter of the growth-retarded and macrosomic fetus. Amer. J. Perinatol. 11 (1994) 144–148
36. Hohenauer, L.: Studien zur intrauterinen Dystrophie. II. Folgen intrauteriner Mangelernährung beim Menschen. Eine vergleichende Studie von Zwillingspaaren mit unterschiedlichem Geburtsgewicht. Pädiatr. Pädol. 6 (1971) 17–30
37. Hohler, C.W., Quetel, T.A.: Comparison of ultrasound femur length and biparietal diameter in late pregnancy. Amer. J. Obstet. Gynec. 141 (1981) 759–760
38. Holländer, H.J.: Die Ultraschalldiagnostik während der Schwangerschaft. In: Döderlein, G., Wulf, K.H.: Klinik der Frauenheilkunde und Geburtshilfe, Bd. VI. München: Urban & Schwarzenberg 1975
39. Kaneoka, T., Taguchi, S., Shimizu, H., Shirakawa, K.: Prenatal diagnosis and treatment of intrauterine growth retardation. J. perinat. Med. 11 (1983) 204–212
40. Khoury, M.J., Erickson, J.D., Cordero, J.F., McCarthy, B.J.: Congenital malformations and intrauterine growth retardation: a population study. Pediatrics 82 (1988) 83–90
41. Klebanoff, M.A., Mills, J.L., Berendes, H.W.: Mother's birth weight as a predictor of macrosomia. Amer. J. Obstet. Gynec. 153 (1985) 253–257
42. Kucera, J.: Rate and type of congenital anomalies among offspring of diabetic women. J. reprod. Med. 7 (1971) 73–82
43. Lang, N., Bellmann, O., Hansmann, M., Nocke, W., Niesen, M.: Klinik und Diagnostik der intrauterinen Mangelentwicklung. Fortschr. Med. 95 (1977) 482–494
44. Leitich, H., Egarter, C., Husslein, P., Kaider, A., Schemper, M.: A meta-analysis of low dose aspirin for the prevention of intrauterine growth retardation. Brit. J. Obstet. Gynaecol. 104 (1997) 450–459
45. Little D., Campbell, S.: Ultrasonic evaluation of intrauterine growth retardation. Radiol. Clin. N. Amer. 20 (1982) 335–351

Continued on page 183

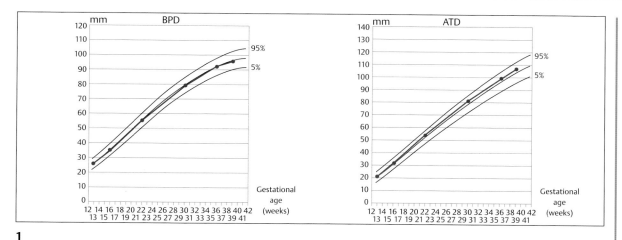

1

Normal growth and errors in dates

Fig. 16.**1**   Normal fetal growth. The BPD and ATD are at the center of the normal growth curves (the 5th, 50th, and 95th percentiles are shown) (after [49]).

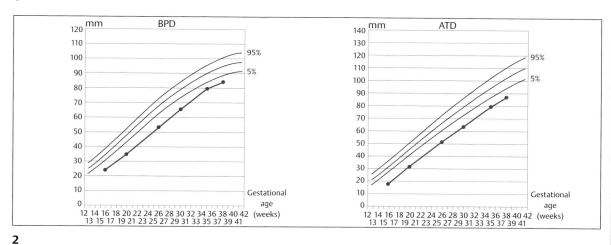

2

Fig. 16.**2**   Fetal development with a 4-week error in dates. The serial measurements indicate a normal fetal growth pattern with a consistent discrepancy relative to the assigned gestational age.

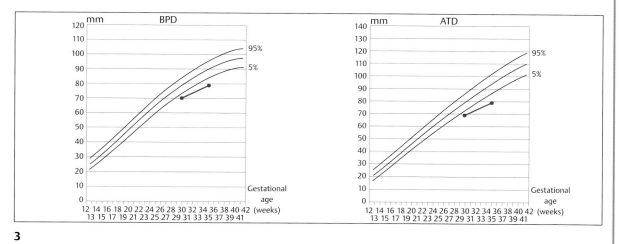

3

Fig. 16.**3**   Proportional fetal growth in a genetically small infant. The head and abdominal circumference are close to the 5th percentile.

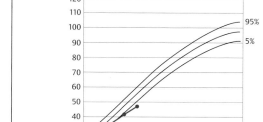

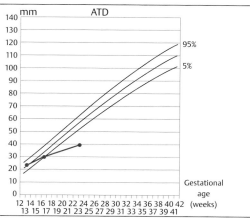

4

Various growth disturbances

Fig. 16.**4**   Severe proportional growth retardation in the second trimester in a fetus with a chromosomal abnormality (trisomy 18). The growth curve falls below the 5th percentile at an early gestational age.

Fig. 16.**5** Disproportional growth retardation due to placental insufficiency. Note the late flattening of the ATD growth curve in the third trimester. A boy weighing 1780 g with a length of 43 cm was delivered at 37 weeks.

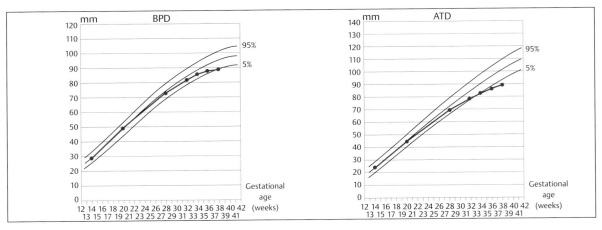

5

Fig. 16.**6** Disproportional growth retardation due to placental insufficiency, with an error in dates. Because the true gestational age was 2 weeks older, the growth curves show late flattening but the values themselves are all within normal limits.

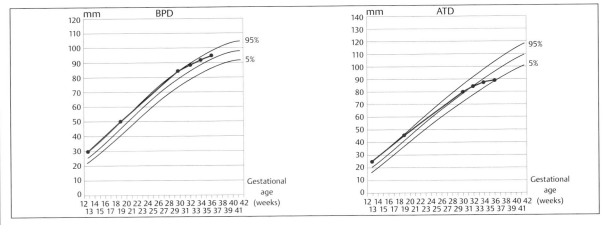

6

Fig. 16.**7** Error in dates or proportional growth retardation? Since prior sonograms are unavailable, a correct evaluation can be made only by obtaining serial scans or measuring additional growth parameters.

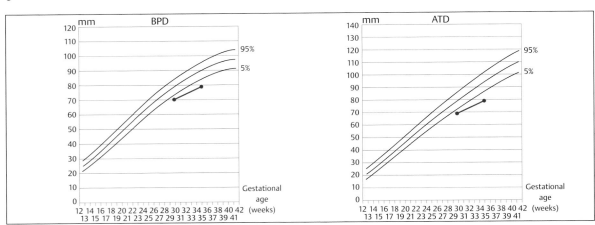

7

Fig. 16.**8** Microcephalic head development in a fetus with Seckel syndrome. The BPD lags well below the normal curve, while the abdominal diameter progresses normally. The HC and AC show a similar discrepancy.

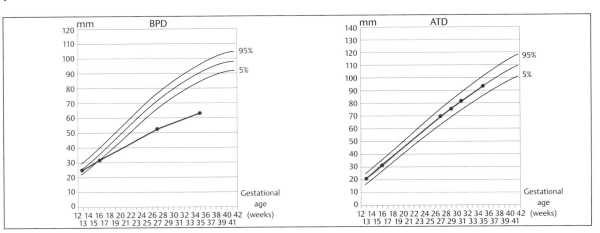

8

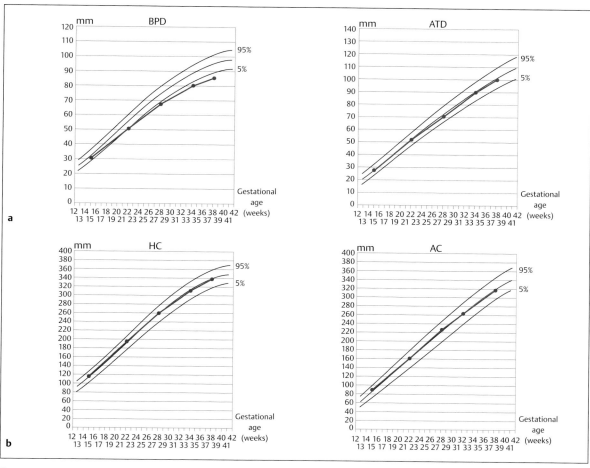

9

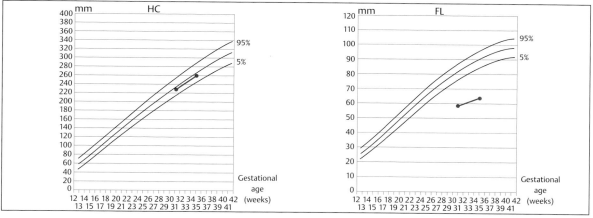

10

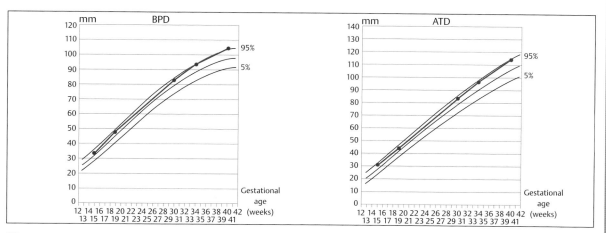

11

Fig. 16.**9** Influence of head shape.
a Dolichocephalic head shape in a breech-presenting fetus mimics growth retardation. The BPD values in the third trimester are below the fifth percentile.
b Tracking the HC instead of BPD indicates normal head development.

Fig. 16.**10** HC and femur length in dwarfism. While head circumference remains within normal limits, femur length falls well below the normal growth curve.

Fig. 16.**11** Growth of a genetically large fetus in the high-normal range. Birthweight 4090 g, length 54 cm.

Fig. 16.**12** Predominantly disproportional fetal macrosomia in poorly controlled insulin-dependent diabetes mellitus. Birthweight 4820 g (36 weeks).

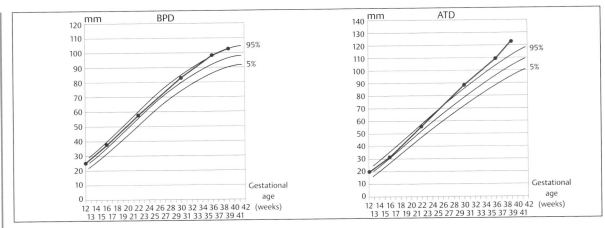

12

Fig. 16.**13** Macrocephalic development (BPD > 95th percentile) in severe hydrocephalus.

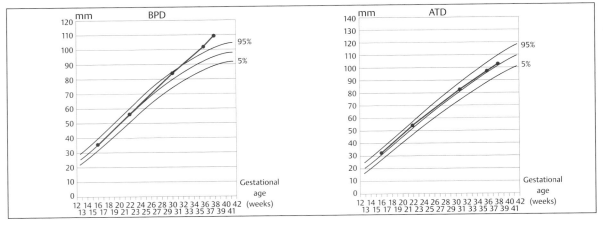

13

Fig. 16.**14** Early proportional growth retardation due to a chromosomal abnormality (trisomy 18), 21 weeks. The head and trunk are equally delayed in their growth. BPD (1) 5.0 cm, OFD (2) 5.8 cm, ATD (3) 4.8 cm, ASD (4) 5.0 cm.

Fig. 16.**15** Disproportional growth retardation secondary to a fetal infection, with hepatic calcification (32 weeks). BPD (1) 7.1 cm, OFD (2) 9.2 cm, ATD (3) 6.0 cm, ASD (4) 6.3 cm.

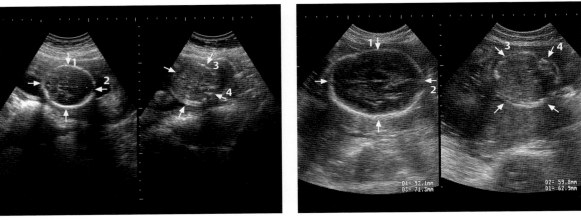

14

15

Fig. 16.**16** Fetal macrosomia in diabetes mellitus, 36 weeks. ATD 12.1 cm, ASD 11.9 cm.

Fig. 16.**17** Double contour of the skull (arrow) in proportional fetal macrosomia in a mother with poorly controlled diabetes, 34 weeks.

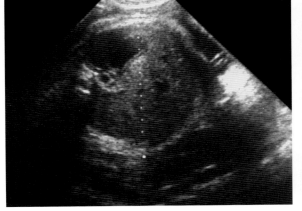

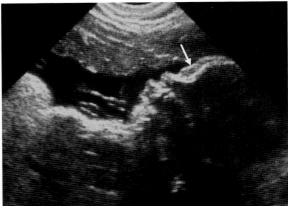

16

17

Continued from page 178

46. Low, J.A., Galbraith, R.S.: Pregnancy characteristics of IUGR. Obstet. Gynec. 44 (1974) 122–126

47. Low, J.A., Handley-Derry, M.H., Burke, S.O. et al.: Association of intrauterine growth retardation and learning deficits at age 9 to 11 years. Amer. J. Obstet. Gynecol. 167 (1992) 1499–1505

48. Malins, J.M.: Congenital malformations and fetal mortality in diabetic pregnancy. J. R. Soc. Med. 71 (1979) 205–207

49. Merz, E., Wellek, S: Das normale fetale Wachstumsprofil – ein einheitliches Modell zur Berechnung von Normkurven für die gängigen Kopf- und Abdomenparameter sowie die großen Extremitätenknochen. Ultraschall in Med. 17 (1996) 153–162

50. Meyer, W.J., Gauthier, D., Ramakrishnan, V., Sipos, J.: Ultrasonographic detection of abnormal fetal growth with the gestational age-independent, transverse cerebellar diameter/abdominal circumference ratio. Amer. J. Obstet. Gynecol. 171 (1994) 1057–1063

51. Modanlou, H.D., Dorchester, W.L., Thorosian, A., Freeman, R.K.: Macrosomia – maternal, fetal, and neonatal implications. Obstet. Gynec. 55 (1980) 420–424

52. Molsted-Petersen, L., Tygstrup, I., Pedersen, J.: Congenital malformations in newborn infants of diabetic women – correlation with maternal diabetic vascular complications. Lancet I (1964) 1124–1126

53. Ogata, E.S., Sabbagha, R., Metzger, B.E., Phelps, R.L., Depp, R., Freinkel, N.: Serial ultrasonography to assess evolving fetal macrosomia. Studies in 23 pregnant diabetic women. J. Amer. med. Ass. 243 (1980) 2405–2408

54. Parks, D.G., Ziel, H.K.: Macrosomia, a proposed indication for primary cesarean section. Obstet. and Gynec. 52 (1978) 407–409

55. Pedersen, J.F., Molsted-Pedersen, L.: Early fetal growth delay detected by ultrasound marks increased risk of congenital malformation in diabetic pregnancy. Brit. med. J. 283 (1981) 269–271

56. Peters, F.D., Roemer, V.M.: Diabetes mellitus und Schwangerschaft. Geburtsh. und Frauenheilk. 37 (1977) 557–565

57. Polani, P.E.: Chromosomal and other genetic influences on birthweight variation, in size at birth. Amsterdam: Elsevier 1974; pp. 127–159

58. Queenan, J.T., Kabarych, S.F., Cook, L.B., Anderson, G.D., Griffin, L.P.: Diagnostic ultrasound for detection of intrauterine growth retardation. Amer. J. Obstet. Gynec. 124 (1976) 865–873

59. Ramzin, M.S., Meudt, R.O., Hinselmann, M.: Prognostic significance of abnormal ultrasonographic findings during the second trimester of gestation. J. perinat. Med. 1 (1973) 60–64

60. Reece, E.A., Goldstein, I., Pilu, G., Hobbins, J.C.: Fetal cerebellar growth unaffected by intrauterine growth retardation: A new parameter for prenatal diagnosis. Amer. J. Obstet. Gynecol. 157 (1987) 632–638

61. Renaud, R., Vincendon, G., Boog, G. et al.: Injections intra-amniotiques d'acides amines dans les cas de malnutrition foetales: premiers resultats. J. Gynecol. Obstet. Biol. Reprod. 1 (1972) 231–244

62. Rivera-Alsina, M.E., Saldana, L.R., Stringer, C.A.: Fetal growth sustained by parenteral nutrition in pregnancy. Obstet. and Gynec. 64 (1984) 138–141

63. Robson, S.C., Chang, T.C.: Intrauterine growth retardation. In: Reed, G.B., Cllaireaux, A.E., Cockburn, F. (eds.): Diseases of the Fetus and Newborn. London: Chapman & Hall 1995; pp. 275–283

64. Rotmensch, S., Liberati, M., Luo, J.S. et al.: Color Doppler flow patterns and flow velocity waveforms of the intraplacental fetal circulation in growth retarded fetuses. Amer. J. Obstet. Gynecol. 171 (1994) 1257–1264

65. Schlensker, K.H.: Ultraschallplazentographie. Gynäkologe 9 (1976) 156–165

66. Schwartz, R., Susa, J.: Fetal macrosomia – animal models. Diabetes Care 3 (1980) 430–432

67. Scott, K.E., Usher, R.: Fetal malnutrition: its incidence, causes and effects. Amer. J. Obstet. Gynec. 94 (1966) 951–953

68. Stallone, L.A., Ziel, H.K.: Management of gestational diabetes. Amer. J. Obstet. Gynec. 119 (1974) 1091–1094

69. Stevenson, D.K., Hopper, A.O., Cohen, R.S., Bucalo, L.R., Kerner, J.A., Sunshine, P.: Macrosomia: Causes and consequences. J. Paediat. 100 (1982) 515–520

70. Tamura, R.K., Sabbagha, R.E., Depp, R., Dooley, S.L., Socol, M.L.: Diabetic macrosomia. Accuracy of third trimester ultrasound. Obstet. Gynecol. 67 (1986) 826–832

71. Trudinger, B.J.: Intrauterine growth retardation. In: Copell, J.A., Reed, K.L. (eds.): Doppler Ultrasound in Obstetrics and Gynecology. New York: Raven Press 1995; pp. 179–185

72. Udal, J.N., Harrison, G.G., Vaucher, Y., Walson, P.D., Morrow, G. III: Interaction of maternal and neonatal obesity. Pediatrics 62 (1978) 17–21

73. Usher, R.H., McLean, F.H.: Normal fetal growth and the significance of fetal growth retardation. In: Davis, J.A., Dobbing, J.: Scientific foundations of paediatrics. London: Heinemann 1974

74. Uzan, S., Beaufils, M., Bréart, G., Bazin, B., Capitant, C., Paris, J.: Prevention of fetal growth retardation with low-dose aspirin: findings of the EPREDA trial. Lancet 337 (1991) 1427–1431

75. Varma, T.R., Taylor, H., Bridges, C.: Ultrasonic assessment of fetal growth. Brit. J. Obstet. Gynaec. 86 (1979) 623–632

76. Wald, N., Cuckle, H., Boreham, J., Stirrat, G.: Small biparietal diameter of fetuses with spina bifida: implications for antenatal screening. Brit. J. Obstet. Gynaec. 87 (1980) 219–221

77. Wallenburg, H.C.S., Rothmans, N.: Prevention of recurrent idiopathic fetal growth retardation by low-dose aspirin and dipyridamol. Amer. J. Obstet. Gynecol. 157 (1987) 1230–1235

78. Westin, B.: Schwangerschaftsüberwachung mittels Gravidogramm. Zbl. Gynäk. 102 (1980) 257–271

79. Whetham, J.C.G., Muggah, H., Davidson, S.: Assessment of intrauterine growth retardation by diagnostic ultrasound. Amer. J. Obstet. Gynec. 125 (1976) 577–580

80. Whitelaw, A.: Subcutaneous fat in newborn infants of diabetic mothers: An indication of quality of diabetic control. Lancet I (1977) 15–18

81. Wiedemann, H.R., Grosse, F.R., Dibbern, H.: Das charakteristische Syndrom. Stuttgart: Schattauer 1982

82. Winick, M.: Fehlernährung und das Nervensystem bei Tieren und Menschen. In: Dudenhausen, J.M., Saling, E.: Perinatale Medizin IV. Stuttgart: Thieme 1973; S. 295

83. Yerushalmy, J.: Relation of birth weight, gestational age and the rate of IUGR to perinatal mortality. Clin. Obstet. Gynec. 13 (1970) 107–129

17 Immune Fetal Hydrops Due to Rhesus Incompatibility

Occurrence, Pathogenesis, and Ultrasound Features

▬ *Definition*

Immune hydrops is the most severe manifestation of fetal hemolytic disease. Fetal hemolytic anemia is caused by maternal IgG antibodies that are formed in response to fetomaternal blood group incompatibility (Rh incompatibility, Kell incompatibility, and other less common forms). Generalized immune hydrops develops when the fetal hematocrit falls below 15% (Hb < 5 g/dL) (normal hematocrit = 34–42%, normal Hb = 11.5–14.4 g/dL). As a result of the anemia, excess fluid accumulates in the subcutaneous tissues (generalized cutaneous edema), peritoneal cavity (ascites), pleural cavity (pleural effusion), and/or the pericardium (pericardial effusion). It is common to find enlargement of the fetal heart (cardiomegaly), liver, and/or spleen. Untreated, fetal hydrops due to Rh incompatibility usually leads to the death of the fetus or newborn as a result of hemolytic anemia, tissue hypoxia, and acidosis.

▬ *Incidence*

Overt prenatal fetomaternal blood group incompatibility with fetal anemia has an incidence of one in 1000 pregnancies in Central Europe (3).

The incidence of hemolytic disease with generalized fetal hydrops is closely related to prenatal care and the availability of prenatal centers experienced in the prenatal diagnosis and treatment of Rh incompatibility. In mothers who have no history of blood group incompatibility and receive appropriate prenatal care, including the intrauterine treatment of fetal anemia if required, the risk of fetal hydrops is low (2–3% of all pregnancies with fetomaternal Rh or Kell incompatibility and maternal isoantibodies) (3).

▬ *Etiology and Pathogenesis*

Sensitization. Sensitization of the maternal immune system to fetal erythrocyte antigens usually occurs during pregnancy or delivery (placental separation) as a result of fetomaternal microtransfusion(s). Despite the introduction of anti-D prophylaxis more than 30 years ago, anti-D (rhesus) incompatibility is still the most common form of fetomaternal blood group incompatibility. It occurs, for example, when Rh prophylaxis has been omitted after a delivery or has been given in an insufficient dose (macrotransfusion due to premature placental separation, which may have been partial and unnoticed). Less commonly, sensitization may occur after an early miscarriage or after a tubal or molar pregnancy. Also, intolerance reactions to "non-D antigens" (Kell, Duffy, Kidd, etc.) following sensitization in blood transfusions, etc. are becoming increasingly common (Table 17.1).

Rhesus family. Despite the many blood group antigens that can theoretically incite a fetomaternal incompatibility reaction leading to fetal hemolysis, the great majority of clinically overt cases that require a transfusion are caused by antigens of the rhesus family (especially the D antigen) and by the Kell antigen (hereafter referred to collectively as "Rh incompatibility").

Table 17.1 Fetal blood group antigens that can evoke incompatibility reactions with fetal hemolysis requiring antenatal treatment

Frequency	Blood group antigens
Common	Rhesus family: D, C, E, c, e Kell
Less common	JK^a (Kidd) Fy^a (Duffy) Kp^{a,b} K S
Rare	Do^a, Di^{a,b}, Fy^b, Hutch, Jk^b, Lu^a, M, N, s, U, Yt^a
Never	Le^{a,b}, P

Compensatory mechanisms. Frank Rh incompatibility is a condition in which maternal placental immunoglobulins (anti-D/anti-Kell IgG) destroy antigen-positive red blood cells in the fetus. Initially, the fetus compensates for the hemolytic anemia by increasing erythropoiesis in the liver and spleen (and in the bone marrow during the third trimester) and also by increasing the release of young, immature erythrocytes into the blood stream (fetal reticulocytosis). Fetal erythrocytes mostly contain hemoglobin F, which has a higher oxygen affinity than adult hemoglobin A, and the fetus also makes use of the Bohr effect (shift of the O$_2$ dissociation curve to the right with an increase in P$_{CO2}$).

Hypoxia. When the fetal hematocrit has been decreased by 50%, the anemia leads to a state of tissue hypoxia and acidosis. At this point the fetal blood flow becomes centralized to sustain vital organs such as the CNS, myocardium, kidneys, and adrenal glands, while blood flow to peripheral organs and body regions is curtailed. As the hypoxia disrupts the integrity of the endothelium, fluid is extravasated into the abdominal cavity, a generalized cutaneous edema develops, and finally fluid accumulates in the pleural and pericardial cavities, leading to a state of generalized hydrops. In severe cases of fetomaternal Rh incompatibility, fetal heart failure (myocardial damage due to hypoxia and an ineffectual attempt to compensate by increasing the cardiac output), tissue hypoxia, and acidosis lead to intrauterine fetal death within a few weeks (4).

▬ *Ultrasound Features*

Nonspecific signs. Ultrasound findings that may precede the development of fetal hydrops include a usually slight increase in the amniotic fluid volume, liver enlargement, thickening of the placenta (placental edema), and an increase in the cardiac biventricular diameter (reactive cardiomegaly).

Signs of anemia. The maximum blood flow velocity in the fetal circulation (fetal aorta, middle cerebral artery, ductus venosus) is elevated as a result of the anemia. A significant correlation with the degree of anemia is found, especially in the fetal aorta.

Severity and course. With its relatively low diagnostic accuracy, Doppler flowmetry is of questionable clinical value in evaluating the severity of fetal anemia and planning interventional therapy (2, 5, 8). Based on ultrasound findings alone, it is not possible to assess the severity of the fetal anemia before the development of hydrops or to predict the future course of the disease or the time at which fetal hydrops may occur. There are two reasons for this: (1) the "prehydropic" ultrasound changes mentioned above are present only in a small percentage of fetuses before hydrops develops, and (2) fetal hydrops can develop within a few days due to aggressive hemolysis, even if maternal antibody titers remain constant.

Full-blown hydrops. When fetal hydrops is fully established, ultrasound shows an accumulation of fluid in the subcutaneous tissues (generalized cutaneous edema) and, by definition, in at least one body cavity: the peritoneal cavity (ascites, sometimes forming a crescent between the anterior hepatic border and inner abdominal wall on transverse scans), pleural cavity (usually bilateral pleural effusion), and/or the pericardial sac (pericardial effusion). Because the fetus tries to compensate for the hemolytic anemia by increasing hematopoiesis and also by raising the cardiac output, ultrasound often shows concomitant enlargement of the liver and spleen (hepatosplenomegaly) and of the heart (cardiomegaly).

Diagnosis

■ *Differential Diagnosis*

Immune hydrops. Immune hydrops is caused by fetomaternal incompatibility in the rhesus or Kell blood group system (other blood group antigens rarely lead to fetal hydrops; Table 17.**1**) (3).

Nonimmune hydrops (see Chapter 18). Nonimmune hydrops is caused by a variety of disorders. The following list is by no means exhaustive:
- Idiopathic
- Anemia without isoimmunization (e.g., in alpha thalassemia)
- Intrauterine infections: parvovirus B19, CMV, HSV, syphilis, toxoplasmosis, etc.
- Cardiovascular: congenital defects (Ebstein anomaly, tetralogy of Fallot, AV canal, etc.), fetal tachy- or bradyarrhythmias, intracardiac tumors, fetal myocarditis or cardiomyopathy
- Pulmonary: cystic adenomatoid malformation (CAM), diaphragmatic hernia, less commonly bronchogenic cysts or sequestra, congenital hydro- or chylothorax
- Renal: prune belly syndrome, urinary tract obstruction (very rare)
- Hepatic: congenital hepatitis, biliary atresia, etc.
- Aneuploidies: trisomies, Turner syndrome, less commonly triploidy
- Twins: fetofetal transfusion syndrome (recipient)
- Cystic hygroma with or without aneuploidy
- Sacrococcygeal teratoma
- Meconium peritonitis

■ *Invasive Diagnostic Procedures*

Indirect prognostic parameters. The goal of prenatal care in Rh incompatibility is to detect and treat any fetal anemia that develops before the fetus reaches the hypoxic stage. Indirect prognostic parameters such as the course of earlier pregnancies (anemia requiring intrauterine transfusion?), paternal homo- or heterozygosity for the antigen in question (hereditary disposition), ultrasound findings (signs of hydrops?), and Doppler findings (centralization of the fetal circulation?) can be used to estimate the risk of fetal anemia. The maternal antibody titer and its progression over time are important guides for scheduling initial cordocentesis in a pregnant woman who is manifesting signs of Rh incompatibility but has no prior history of blood group isoimmunization. In later pregnancies complicated by Rh incompatibility, often the antibody titer is already elevated at the start of the pregnancy and therefore is of limited diagnostic value.

Cordocentesis

None of the indirect prognostic parameters can replace invasive testing by cordocentesis. Only cordocentesis allows for the assessment of fetal blood type, the precise evaluation of fetal anemia, and its subsequent treatment by intrauterine transfusion.

Absolute indications. The absolute indications for cordocentesis at the earliest possible time (generally 18–19 weeks, or as late as 20–21 weeks with a posterior-wall placenta or very obese patient) are listed below:

Positive history. Rh incompatibility with fetal anemia requiring a transfusion, with or without fetal hydrops, or the prior death of a fetus or newborn associated with very high maternal Rh antibody titers (high index of suspicion for death due to Rh incompatibility).

Ultrasound indication. Fetal hydrops or early hydropic changes such as cardiomegaly or an ascites crescent with a positive maternal Rh antibody test.

Serologic indication. High maternal Rh antibody titer (> 1 : 16 in second trimester, > 1 : 32 in third trimester), rapidly rising titer (suggests boosting of maternal antibody synthesis by fetomaternal microtransfusion).

Elective cordocentesis. Elective cordocentesis can be scheduled later in the pregnancy when the maternal antibody titers (checked once a week starting at 16 weeks!) are consistently between 1 : 8 and 1 : 32, ultrasound findings are normal, and there are no signs of incipient hydrops (also checked every week!) or paternal antigen heterozygosity (D or Kell antigen).

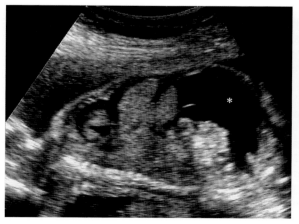

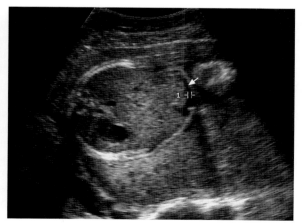

Fig. 17.**1** Fetal hydrops due to Rh incompatibility, before intravascular fetal transfusion. Massive ascites (∗).

Fig. 17.**2** The same fetus after intravascular transfusion. Residual ascites appears as a thin, hypoechoic crescent adjacent to the liver (arrow).

1

2

Preterm induction. Different considerations apply during the last 4–6 weeks before the expected delivery date. In most cases where the patient is first seen after 34 weeks and is found to have high maternal antibody titers or a history showing a high risk of fetal hemolytic anemia due to Rh incompatibility, preterm induction is preferable to cordocentesis. But in cases where fetal hydrops is detected shortly before the due date, the treatment of choice is cordocentesis with intrauterine fetal transfusion.

Technique. Cordocentesis is performed transabdominally under local anesthesia. The easiest site for cord puncture is the placental insertion of the umbilical cord. An alternative site is a free loop of umbilical cord that is easily accessible to puncture. Blood should be sampled from the umbilical vein, since puncture of the umbilical artery is associated with a higher risk of complications. When the needle has been placed in the umbilical vein under ultrasound guidance, 1–2 mL of fetal blood is withdrawn, and an immediate bedside fetal hematocrit is determined. By definition, a fetal hematocrit higher than 30% rules out anemia requiring intrauterine transfusion. In this case an additional 1–2 mL of venous blood is drawn to determine the fetal blood type, and the cordocentesis concludes as a diagnostic procedure. If the fetal hematocrit is less than 30%, an intrauterine transfusion is performed in the same sitting (see Prenatal Management) (1, 7, 9).

Chorion villus sampling and amniocentesis. In cases where the father is heterozygous for the antigen in question and there is an additional indication for karyotyping (e.g., advanced maternal age or fetal structural abnormalities) or a positive maternal history (prior pregnancy with a very aggressive Rh incompatibility), the parents should be offered early invasive testing by chorion villus sampling or amniocentesis. In these cases a gene analysis is performed by PCR directly from the DNA to determine whether the D allele is present or absent. However, the advantage of a direct gene analysis in early pregnancy (to see whether the fetus can possibly be affected by isoimmunization) should be carefully weighed against the risk of iatrogenic boosting of the immune response by the transplacental passage of red blood cells into the maternal circulation, particularly in chorion villus sampling.

Prognosis and Treatment

▬ *Prognosis, Risk of Recurrence*

Rh incompatibility has an excellent prognosis in cases of transfusion-treatable fetal anemia without hydrops (survival rate approximately 95%). Once fetal hydrops has developed, the prognosis is much less favorable (survival rates of 60–75%), especially before 24 weeks when the fetus is not yet viable.

Risk assessment. The risk posed to the fetus by maternal Rh or Kell antibodies can be estimated from the maternal history (prior pregnancies with fetal hydrops or intrauterine/neonatal death due to isoimmunization), from the maternal antibody titers and their progression over time (high or rapidly rising titers imply a high fetal risk), and from paternal homo- or heterozygosity for the blood group antigen in question: homozygosity implies a high risk, while heterozygosity implies a 50% chance that the fetus has not inherited the antigen-coding allele. B-mode ultrasound, Doppler, and cardiotocography without invasive testing (cordocentesis) are not helpful in making a prognosis, because they are only positive just before or after the onset of fetal hydrops (see Ultrasound Features).

Risk of recurrence. The risk of recurrence after a previously affected pregnancy (fetal anemia requiring transfusion) is very high when pa-

ternal antigen homozygosity is present. As a general rule of thumb, hemolytic disease takes a more severe course with each successive pregnancy. In later pregnancies, the maternal antibody titers usually start to rise earlier and reach a higher level than in previous pregnancies, and significant fetal anemia develops at an earlier stage. This means that when there has been a prior pregnancy with fetal anemia necessitating a transfusion, initial cordocentesis in subsequent pregnancies should be performed as early as possible. A transfusion setup should be ready for immediate use if needed.

If the father is heterozygous for the isoantigen in question (Rh, Kell), the recurrence risk is approximately 50%. It is still important to schedule an initial cordocentesis as early as possible to determine whether the fetuses possesses the blood group antigen in question. If it does, it will be at risk; if it does not, it will require no further evaluation (see Invasive Diagnosis).

▬ *Prenatal Management*

Rh prophylaxis. The screening examination in the first trimester of pregnancy includes determination of the maternal blood group and Rh factor. An antibody screening test (indirect Coombs test) is also performed. If no irregular blood group antibodies are found, it is recommended that Rh-D-negative women be reexamined every 2 months until term. In many countries, antenatal Rh prophylaxis is mandatory in Rh-negative women without antibodies: either a single dose of 250–300 µg administered in week 28 or 100 µg administered in weeks 28 and 34. After the delivery, Rh-negative mothers of Rh-positive newborns receive anti-D IgG Rh prophylaxis within 72 h postpartum to prevent sensitization.

Follow-ups. If the maternal serum is found to contain irregular blood group antibodies, the antibody titers and their progression over time dictate further management. Rapidly rising titers warrant an invasive procedure at an earlier stage than consistently low titers. When the titer reaches 1 : 16, the patient should be referred to a prenatal center for further evaluation and possible treatment. Starting at 16–17 weeks, ultrasound examinations are performed once a week to check for signs of fetal hydrops. Weekly serologic tests are also scheduled to track maternal antibody titers.

Cordocentesis. The initial cordocentesis is generally performed between 18 and 24 weeks (indications listed above). The setup should include facilities for intravascular fetal transfusion. If this initial sampling does not indicate fetal anemia (fetal hematocrit > 30%), additional samplings should be scheduled at approximately 4- to 6-week intervals in Rh-positive fetuses. On each of these occasions, a setup for fetal blood transfusion should be available.

Serologic tests. Serologic prognostic parameters in the fetal blood (bilirubin, free hemoglobin, reticulocytes, maternal Rh antibodies in the fetal circulation, etc.) can assist in management planning during the intervals between umbilical blood samplings. Very strict care should be taken to maintain the weekly ultrasound and serologic follow-ups, as there is no way of predicting the onset or course of fetal hydrops.

Top-up transfusion, exchange transfusion. A fetal hematocrit below 30% at cordocentesis indicates that fetal anemia is present, and transfusion should be initiated. The transfusion is performed using type O, Rh-negative, CMV- and HIV-negative, irradiated, filtered packed red blood cells with an hematocrit of approximately 75–80%. The use of packed cells can reduce both the volume and duration of the transfusion. The hematocrit is calculated after each transfusion. In nonhydropic fetuses, the desired final hematocrit is approximately 35–40%. If fetal hydrops is present (hematocrit almost always < 15%), generally a somewhat lower final hematocrit is desired for the first one or two transfusions to avoid volume overload of the fetal circulation, which is already hemodynamically unstable. A possible alternative to the classic top-up transfusion in fetal hydrops is a true exchange transfusion. This involves removing some of the fetal Rh-positive red cells before administering the Rh-negative donor red cells, resulting in less of a volume load on the fetal circulation.

Transfusion intervals. Despite the transfusion of O-negative packed red blood cells, neither fetal erythropoiesis nor maternal antibody production are halted. Moreover, the transfused red cells have an average life span of only about four weeks. From 28 to 30 days after the transfusion, therefore, the fetal hematocrit (disregarding the continued hemolysis of fetal red cells) is no higher than its initial value and may even fall below it (if the puncture has boosted maternal antibody synthesis). In cases of overt Rh incompatibility, therefore, a new intrauterine transfusion should initially be performed every 2–3 weeks. After three or four transfusions, when the fetal blood has been almost entirely replaced by the transfused Rh-negative donor red cells, the fetus can tolerate longer intervals without a drastic fall in hematocrit. Hydropic fetuses are initially transfused in smaller increments (see above) at 4- to 7-day intervals until the hydrops has been reabsorbed. They can then be placed on a standard transfusion regimen at 2- to 3-week intervals (1, 6, 7, 9).

▬ *Delivery and Postpartum Management*

As a rule, intrauterine transfusion therapy is continued until about 36 weeks' gestation, at which time labor is induced. One difference between mature neonates and preterm infants is that the blood-brain barrier in mature infants is much less permeable to bilirubin. In the fetus, bilirubin that is liberated by hemolysis crosses the placenta and is removed by the maternal circulation. Birth interrupts this transplacental bilirubin clearance, making it necessary to maintain close-interval follow-ups during the first days and weeks of life and, in some cases, to reduce bilirubin levels by phototherapy. Meanwhile, there is no longer any transfer of maternal Rh antibodies into the fetal circulation. Because the maternal isoantibodies persist in the neonate's bloodstream for up to 6 weeks, considerable additional hemolysis can occur during that period, requiring additional transfusions.

References

1. Ghidin, A., Sepulveda, W., Lockwood, C.J., Romero, R.: Complications of fetal blood sampling. Amer. J. Obstet. Gynecol. 168 (1993) 1339–1344
2. Hecher, K., Snijders, R., Campbell, S., Nicolaides, K.: Fetal venous, arterial, and intracardiac blood flows in red blood cell isoimmunization. Obstet. Gynecol. 85 (1995) 122–128
3. James, D., Smoleniec, J., Weiner, C.P.: Fetal Hydrops. In: James, D.K., Steer, P.J., Weiner, C.P., Gonik, B. (eds.): High Risk Pregnancy. Management Options. London: WB Saunders 1996; pp. 803–812
4. Nicolaides, K.H., Rodeck, C.H., Millar, D.S., Mibashan, R.S.: Fetal haematology in rhesus isoimmunization. Brit. Med. J. 290 (1985) 661–663
5. Oepkes, D., Brand, R., Vandenbussche, F.P., Meerman, R.U., Kanhai, H.H.: The use of ultrasonography and Doppler in the prediction of fetal haemolytic anaemia: a multivariate analysis. Brit. J. Obstet. Gynaecol. 101 (1994) 680–684
6. Radunovic, N., Lockwood, C.J., Alvarez, M., Plecas, D., Chitkara, U., Berkowitz, R.L.: The severely anemic and hydropic isoimmune fetus: changes in fetal hematocrit associated with intrauterine death. Obstet. Gynecol. 79 (1992) 390–393
7. Schumacher, B., Moise, K.J.: Fetal transfusion for red blood cell alloimmunization in pregnancy. Obstet. Gynecol. 88 (1996) 137–150
8. Steiner, H., Schaffer, H., Spitzer, D., Batka, M., Graf, A.H., Staudach, A:. The relationship between peak velocity in the fetal descending aorta and hematocrit in rhesus isoimmunization. Obstet. Gynecol. 85 (1995) 659–662
9. Weiner, C.P., Williamson, R.A., Wenstrom, K.D., Sipes, S.L., Grant, S.S., Widness, J.A.: Management of fetal hemolytic disease by cordocentesis. I. Prediction of fetal anemia. Amer. J. Obstet. Gynecol. 165 (1991) 546–553

18 Nonimmune Fetal Hydrops (NIHF)

Occurrence, Pathogenesis, and Ultrasound Features

▬ Definition

Fetal hydrops refers to an abnormal excess of fluid accumulation in fetal serous body cavities and soft tissues (Fig. 18.1). If there is no evidence that the hydrops has been caused by a blood group incompatibility, it is termed nonimmune fetal hydrops (NIHF).

NIHF was first described by Ballantyne in 1892 (6) and first diagnosed by E. L. Potter in 1943 (56). The condition was first imaged with ultrasound in 1967 (30). It is relatively easy to diagnose with the aid of modern, high-resolution ultrasound scanners. The extreme diversity of its causes, however, has made NIHF a particular diagnostic and therapeutic challenge.

▬ Incidence

As the incidence of immune hydrops has declined through the widespread use of Rh prophylaxis, NIHF has become the predominant form of fetal hydrops. Its incidence in large studies is between one in 2500 and one in 3500 pregnancies (33, 49).

▬ Ultrasound Features

Typical signs. The typical features of NIHF at ultrasound are: usually generalized subcutaneous edema (19), ascites, pleural effusion, pericardial effusion, and an hydropic placenta (Figs. 18.2–18.4, Table 18.1). Polyhydramnios is present in 50–75% of cases (30, 46), and oligohydramnios is occasionally seen (31). The diagnosis is established by detecting fluid collections in more than one compartment, thereby differentiating the condition from an isolated hydrothorax or ascites, pericardial effusion, cystic hygroma, or nuchal edema. Often there is no clear dividing line, however, and NIHF is on a continuum with these other conditions.

Early signs. A fluid collection that is very small or confined to one body cavity may provide an early sign of incipient fetal hydrops (26, 71). For example, initial ascites may appear as a fluid collection along the hepatic border or between loops of bowel. The development of a pleural effusion (Figs. 18.5, 18.6) or pericardial effusion (Figs. 18.7, 18.8) usually reflects severe hydrops. Isolated pericardial effusion (Fig. 18.8) has also been described as an early sign.

Generalization. The development of cutaneous edema, especially about the head (Fig. 18.3), is a sign that the hydrops is becoming generalized and often heralds the late stage of NIHF.

Heterogeneity of findings. Given the heterogeneous nature of the disease, the ultrasound signs are often atypical. For example, while ascites (Figs. 18.9, 18.10) is the most common manifestation, it may be completely absent even in severe cases. Fetal ascites as a sign of NIHF should be distinguished from isolated ascites (for the differential diagnosis of fetal ascites, see below; Fig. 18.11). In male fetuses, scrotal edema is often present as an associated feature (Fig. 18.12).

Coexisting abnormalities. An important consideration in the differential diagnosis of fetal hydrops is whether the underlying cause is a generalized fetal disease, such as infection, or a congenital anomaly such as a heart defect or diaphragmatic hernia. It is essential, therefore, to conduct a careful ultrasound search for potentially subtle anomalies. The most frequent concomitant ultrasound abnormalities in NIHF are as follows (59):
- Cystic hygroma
- Cardiac anomalies
- Multiple anomalies

The following are less common:
- Placental abnormalities
- Intrathoracic and intra-abdominal masses

Besides the assessment of fetal anatomy, an evaluation of fetal hemodynamics by echocardiography and by Doppler scanning of the arterial system and especially the venous system are essential for making a differential diagnosis, planning treatment, and offering a prognosis.

▬ Pathogenesis

Understanding the pathogenesis of fetal hydrops is the key to making an accurate differential diagnosis. In many cases, none of the following mechanisms is solely responsible for causing the hydrops; usually there is one predominant disorder that determines the prognosis and possible treatment. In many cases the hydrops cannot be related causally to a specific anomaly or disease, and it is more correct to speak of an association rather than a cause.

Fluid retention. NIHF is a late symptom of fetal diseases or anomalies that lead to fluid extravasation from the intravascular, intracellular, and interstitial compartments. The cause is an abnormal shift in the hydrostatic capillary pressure, oncotic plasma pressure, and capillary permeability (16). The set of six essential factors described by Im et al. in 1984 is helpful in acquiring a basic understanding of these mechanisms (34) (Table 18.2).

Table 18.1 Ultrasound diagnosis of nonimmune fetal hydrops (NIHF)

Cutaneous edema	Subcutaneous fluid collection > 5 mm, usually detected in head and neck region	Figs. 18.3, 18.4
Pleural effusion or hydrothorax	Usually bilateral fluid collection in the chest; visualization of the lungs, which often appear small; frequent displacement of the cardiac axis	Figs.18.5, 18.6
Pericardial effusion	Pericardial fluid collection > 2 mm	Figs. 18.7, 18.8
Ascites	Fluid collection in the abdomen, smaller amounts at the hepatic border and between bowel loops	Figs. 18.9, 18.10
Hydropic placenta	Thickened (> 5 cm), often hyperechoic placenta	
Polyhydramnios	Largest amniotic fluid pocket > 8 cm, AFI > 18	

Table 18.**2**   Pathogenesis nonimmune fetal hydrops (NIHF) (after [34])

1. **Primary myocardial heart failure or cardiac insufficiency,** caused for example by congenital heart defects, arrhythmias, or myocarditis (Figs. 18.**16**, 18.**17**).

2. **Secondary heart failure or cardiac insufficiency,** caused for example by severe anemia, AV shunts, placental tumors, or fetofetal transfusion syndrome.

3. **Reduced oncotic pressure,** caused for example by increased protein production in congenital cirrhosis or hepatitis (infections) or by increased protein loss due to a congenital nephropathy. Hypoproteinemia leading to a reduced oncotic pressure can generally be detected by the secondary capillary damage and resulting protein loss (53).

4. **Increased capillary permeability** due to severe hypoxia, infections, severe anemia, or other causes.

5. **Obstruction or disturbance of lymphatic drainage,** due to example to Turner syndrome, chylothorax, or chyloperitoneum.

6. **Obstruction of venous return,** due to example to a mass lesion such as CCAM or diaphragmatic defects

Table 18.**3**   Differential diagnosis of nonimmune fetal hydrops (NIHF)

➢ Cardiovascular causes 17–35%	➢ Infections 1.5–5.3%
➢ Chromosomal abnormalities 13.5–15.7%	➢ Pulmonary diseases 3–6%
	➢ Skeletal dysplasias 3–4%
➢ Hematologic diseases 4.2–12%	➢ Gastrointestinal causes 2–3.7%
➢ Multiple malformations (syndromes) 3–15%	➢ Urogenital causes 2.2–3%
	➢ Tumors 2.5–3%
➢ Fetofetal transfusion syndromes 3–10.3%	➢ Metabolic disorders 1%
	➢ Idiopathic cases 15.5–40%

Heart failure. Experimental studies have documented the development of NIHF in response to induced tachycardia and anemia. The cause is an increase in venous pressure caused by primary or secondary heart failure. The backward failure increases the preload in the venous limb, and the central venous pressure rises along with the pressure in the umbilical vein (35, 68). The high venous pressure leads to a rise in hydrostatic capillary pressure and, as the final sign of decompensation, generalized fetal hydrops (Figs. 18.**13**, 18.**14**). The venous pressure may fall again following successful therapy (68). Doppler scanning can demonstrate the high venous pressure by showing a decreased diastolic flow velocity in the ductus venosus and later by demonstrating pulsatile flow in the umbilical vein (23).

The elevated pressure in the atria leads to an increased secretion of atrial natriuretic peptide (ANP) and increased fetal diuresis, which may account for the polyhydramnios that is often observed.

It follows from these pathophysiologic considerations that evaluation of the fetal heart is of key importance in the differential diagnosis of NIHF. The examiner of a fetus with nonimmune hydrops should first determine whether cardiac performance is impaired and, if so, whether it might be the cause or the effect of the NIHF. This assessment will direct further differential diagnostic considerations.

Diseases Associated with NIHF

The etiology of NIHF is diverse, and reported incidence figures vary greatly from one study to the next. Table 18.**3** shows the distribution of the principal etiologies of NIHF based on a comprehensive meta-analysis by Norton (54). "Idiopathic" in this context usually means that a definitive diagnosis could not be made. The percentage of idiopathic cases has been declining in recent years owing to improved prenatal and postnatal diagnostic methods. A detailed list of possible causes is shown in Table 18.**4**.

Table 18.**4**   Anomalies and diseases associated with nonimmune fetal hydrops (NIHF), based on refs. 18, 29, 67, 69 and our own results

Cardiac causes

➢ Heart defects
➢ Left ventricular hypoplasia
➢ AV canal
➢ Transposition of the great vessels
➢ Tetralogy of Fallot
➢ Valvular atresias, dysplasias, and stenoses
➢ Ebstein anomaly
➢ Large ventricular septal defects
➢ Single ventricle
➢ Occlusion of the ductus arteriosus or foramen ovale

Arrhythmias

➢ Tachyarrhythmia
➢ Supraventricular paroxysmal tachycardia (PSVT)
➢ Atrial flutter
➢ WPW syndrome
➢ Bradyarrhythmia
➢ AV block
➢ Sick sinus

Cardiac tumors

➢ Rhabdomyomas
➢ Teratomas

Cardiomyopathy
AV shunts

➢ Sacrococcygeal teratoma
➢ Chorangioma
➢ Vein of Galen aneurysm

Heart failure

➢ Chorangioma
➢ Sacrococcygeal teratoma
➢ Vein of Galen aneurysm
➢ Fetofetal transfusion syndrome (acceptor)

Chromosomal abnormalities

➢ Monosomy X (Turner syndrome)
➢ Trisomy 21
➢ Triploidy
➢ Other trisomies (e.g., 13, 18)

Anemias

➢ α-thalassemia
➢ Parvovirus B19 infection
➢ G6PD deficiency
➢ Fetomaternal hemorrhage
➢ Fetofetal hemorrhage (donor)
➢ Fetal hemorrhages

Infections

➢ CMV
➢ Parvovirus B19
➢ Syphilis
➢ Herpes simplex type 1
➢ Coxsackievirus

Monochorionic twins

➢ Fetofetal transfusion syndrome
➢ Twin reversed arterial perfusion (TRAP)

Diseases involving the neck

➢ Cystic hygroma
➢ CHAOS (e.g., laryngeal atresia)

Thoracic diseases

➢ CCAM
➢ Diaphragmatic hernia
➢ Pulmonary sequestrum
➢ Pulmonary cysts, bronchogenic cysts
➢ Tumors: pulmonary hamartoma, pulmonary adenoma, mediastinal teratoma

Renal diseases

➢ Congenital nephrotic syndrome (Finnish type)
➢ (Prune belly syndrome)
➢ (Polycystic kidneys)

Gastrointestinal diseases

➢ Hepatic cirrhosis, fibrosis, necrosis
➢ Polycystic renal disease
➢ Hepatic hemangioma
➢ Biliary atresia
➢ Hepatitis

Metabolic disorders

➢ Gaucher disease
➢ Gangliosidosis
➢ Mucopolysaccharidosis
➢ Hurler syndrome
➢ Niemann–Pick disease

Skeletal dysplasias

➢ Achondroplasia
➢ Osteogenesis imperfecta
➢ Thanatophoric dwarfism
➢ Thoracic dystrophy
➢ Polydactyly and short rib syndrome
➢ Arthrogryposis

Neoplasias

➢ Teratomas
➢ Neuroblastomas
➢ Hemangioendotheliomas
➢ Congenital leukemia

Rare syndromes

➢ Congenital myotonic dystrophy
➢ Noonan syndrome
➢ Pterygium syndrome
➢ Yellow nail syndrome
➢ Congenital lymphangiectasis
➢ Pena–Shokeir syndrome
➢ Neu–Laxova syndrome

Placental and umbilical disorders

➢ Chorangioma
➢ Hemorrhagic endovasculitis
➢ Umbilical artery aneurysm
➢ Umbilical vein thrombosis
➢ Twisted or knotted umbilical cord

Maternal disorders

➢ Diabetes mellitus (?)
➢ Anemia
➢ Sjögren syndrome
➢ Lupus erythematosus
➢ Bourneville–Pringle disease
➢ Drugs (indomethacin, tocolytic agents, antiarrhythmic agents, etc.)

Cardiac Diseases

Primary cardiac diseases are the leading cause of nonimmune hydrops in North America and Central Europe. They can be subdivided into two groups:
- Arrhythmias without congenital heart defects
- Congenital heart defects

Often it cannot be determined whether the cardiac defect is the actual cause of the nonimmune hydrops or is just an associated anomaly. Congenital heart defects that lead to hydrops have a very poor prognosis, with a mortality rate in excess of 80% (2, 26, 50). Most of these cases involve complex structural anomalies, the premature closure of a physiologic shunt, valvular atresias and stenoses, or large septal defects. Table 18.5 shows the cardiac defects that we found to be associated with NIHF over a seven-year period. Our case material also included seven fetuses with arrhythmias and six with premature closure of the ductus arteriosus or foramen ovale.

Fetal Arrhythmias

Fetal arrhythmias have a diverse etiology (11). Both tachycardias and bradyarrhythmias can lead to a decrease in cardiac output, resulting in NIHF. Arrhythmias can often be successfully managed by the direct or transplacental administration of antiarrhythmic drugs. Some cases resolve spontaneously without treatment.

Tachyarrhythmias. These arrhythmias respond better to intrauterine therapy and have a good prognosis even when hydropic changes have already developed (1). Most cases involve supraventricular tachycardias (Figs. 18.**15**, 18.**16**). Atrial flutter is less common. Deficient atrial filling increases the cardiac preload, giving rise to NIHF.

Bradyarrhythmias. These arrhythmias are usually based on a congenital heart defect or a maternal autoimmune disease (e.g., systemic lupus erythematosus, Sjögren syndrome). The prognosis of NIHF with a severe bradyarrhythmia, such as a complete AV block, is poor (60). A complete, third-degree AV block is the result of a congenital heart defect in up to 90% of cases (20).

Table 18.**5** Nonimmune fetal hydrops (NIHF) and associated cardiac defects (based on authors' own data)

Coarctation of the aorta	n = 8
Cardiomyopathy	n = 5
Single ventricle	n = 2
Ebstein anomaly	n = 3
Tricuspid dysplasia	n = 2
Endocardial fibroelastosis	n = 1
Aortic stenosis with EFE	n = 1
Complete AV canal	n = 3
Aortic stenosis + VSD, CoA	n = 2
Heart block + I TGA	n = 1
pCFO	n = 2
DORV	n = 1
VSD	n = 2
Interruption of the aortic arch	n = 1
PT to LA fistula	n = 1
Pulmonary atresia with or without VSD	n = 3
Tricuspid atresia + VSD	n = 1
Total number of cardiac defects	n = 39

Treatment. In the treatment of fetal arrhythmias, it should be considered that the prospect for successful transplacental drug therapy is less favorable after the onset of hydrops due to impaired fetal bioavailability. This emphasizes the need for prompt and, if necessary, direct treatment of the arrhythmia.

Cardiac Tumors and Cardiomyopathy

In rare cases, nonimmune hydrops is caused by rhabdomyomas or teratomas of the fetal heart. Rhabdomyomas are very often associated with a tuberous brain sclerosis known as Bourneville–Pringle disease. Another rare cause of NIHF is intrauterine cardiomyopathy, which may have an infectious or metabolic etiology (Figs. 18.**17**, 18.**18**). Its prognosis is poor (12).

Interruption of the Fetal Circulation

Intrauterine closure of the ductus arteriosus with the subsequent development of NIHF has been documented in isolated cases (13, 38). Constriction of the ductus arteriosus may occur in response to tocolytic therapy with prostaglandin synthesis inhibitors (e.g., indomethacin). Serial ultrasound scans should be scheduled, therefore, when this type of treatment is used. Interruption of the fetal venous circulation, due for example to closure or absence of the ductus venosus, has been observed in association with NIHF.

Cardiac Volume Overload

A heterogeneous group of NIHF cases apparently result from fetal heart failure based on a chronic volume overload. These cases include fetuses with arteriovenous shunts, fetal anemia (see Anemias), or hypervolemia, like that occurring in the acceptor of a fetofetal transfusion syndrome (see Twins). Typical causes of AV shunts are sacrococcygeal teratomas, vein of Galen aneurysms, and chorangiomas. It is clear that fetal echocardiography is an essential study in the differential diagnosis of NIHF (see Management).

Chromosomal abnormalities

Turner Syndrome and Trisomy 21

Turner syndrome (monosomy X) and trisomy 21 (Fig. 18.**3**) are the aneuploidies that are most commonly associated with NIHF (10, 31, 67).

Cystic hygroma. Cystic nuchal hygroma (25) is a frequent cause of NIHF in Turner syndrome because it disrupts the connection between the lymphatic and venous systems, causing impairment of lymphatic drainage. Turner syndrome should also be suspected when chylothorax is present. When a fluid collection is found in the nuchal region, a distinction should be drawn between cystic hygroma and nuchal edema. Cystic hygromas are bilateral, septated structures that are frequently associated with Turner syndrome. By contrast, nuchal edema is probably a common early sign of incipient fetal hydrops.

Other Trisomies

Nonimmune hydrops has also been observed in other trisomies, such as 18 and 13. As in trisomy 21, the most frequent underlying cause is a cardiac defect. NIHF without a cardiac defect has also been diagnosed in sporadic cases of Down syndrome. The likely cause in these cases is a transient myeloproliferative disease, which can be diagnosed prenatally by the detection of fetal hepatosplenomegaly (28, 48).

▦ *Anemias*

Fetal anemias may develop as a result of hemoglobinopathy, chronic blood loss, or an infection, usually with parvovirus B19. The pathogenesis of NIHF may involve a chronic overload with secondary heart failure or a chronic capillary hypoxia leading to protein loss.

Alpha Thalassemia

Alpha thalassemia, inherited as an autosomal-recessive disorder, is the most frequent cause of NIHF in Southeast Asia and the Mediterranean region (4, 37, 44), with an incidence as high as 80%. The incidence in other populations is only about 10% (31, 59). Homozygous fetuses do not form alpha-globulin chains and are therefore unable to synthesize hemoglobin F, instead forming Bart hemoglobin. This abnormal hemoglobin has a very high oxygen affinity, resulting in severe, chronic tissue hypoxia (65).

Diagnosis. NIHF usually does not develop until the early third trimester, but an early diagnosis of alpha thalassemia can still be made. Parents in high-risk populations can be examined in screening tests (e.g., low MCV) and positive cases referred for DNA analysis of the fetal blood to establish the antenatal diagnosis (43). This is critically important when we consider that homozygous fetuses that develop NIHF may survive, and that the mothers of these fetuses are at greater risk for developing preeclampsia and usually suffer from microcytic anemia.

Fetal Blood Loss

Fetal blood loss can result either from fetomaternal or fetofetal transfusion. There have been few reports to date on NIHF in cases of fetomaternal transfusion (16, 66). This is because it is normal for small numbers of fetal red blood cells to enter the maternal circulation, but the passage of these cells in massive amounts usually leads to acute intrauterine distress. Prompt diagnosis (e.g., using the Kleihauer-Bethke test to detect fetal erythrocytes in the maternal blood) and intrauterine transfusion can save the affected fetus in some cases (17, 66). Apparently, bleeding within the fetus itself can also lead to severe anemia and NIHF, as illustrated by the case of intracranial hemorrhage (15).

Enzyme Defects

There have been isolated reports of glucose-6-phosphate dehydrogenase deficiency (favism), the most common pathogenic enzyme defect, occurring in association with NIHF. If the mother is a known carrier, she must avoid the ingestion of oxidative substances. Other enzymes whose deficiency can theoretically lead to intrauterine hemolysis and NIHF are glucose-phosphate isomerase, pyruvate kinase, and triphosphatisomerase.

▦ *Infections*

A number of congenital infections have been identified in association with NIHF. When generalized, these infections can lead to an intrauterine "multisystem failure" with decreased protein production due to hepatic involvement and protein loss due to capillary injury. Unfortunately, congenital infections are often indistinguishable from other diseases that can cause NIHF. But the presence of stippled or patchy echogenic areas in the fetal liver or brain and echogenic bowel loops may provide a suggestive sign.

Human Parvovirus B19 (Erythema Infectiosum)

Parvovirus B19 is a common congenital pathogen. Approximately 50% of all pregnant women are immune to parvovirus B19 infection. When an initial infection occurs, it is estimated that vertical transmission will occur in approximately one-third of cases. Fetal deaths are almost always associated with NIHF, which develops about 4–6 weeks following maternal exposure. Early manifestations have been described after just one week, however.

Pathogenesis. Fetal hydrops is attributed to anemia or heart failure secondary to myocarditis. Parvovirus B19 predominantly affects red cell precursors and can lead to bone marrow depression with severe anemia or pancytopenia (3, 31). The compensatory response consists of widespread extramedullary blood formation in other reticuloendothelial organs such as the liver and spleen, often leading to the prenatal detection of hepatosplenomegaly. The fetal bone marrow is particularly susceptible to the parvovirus between 17 and 22 weeks' gestation.

Diagnosis and treatment. If serologic tests raise suspicion of a maternal parvovirus infection, serial ultrasound examinations should be scheduled at very close intervals, for once hydrops has started to develop, the infection can be diagnosed from the fetal blood (39), and blood transfusions can be initiated with a good chance of success (64). It is unclear how vigorous the treatment regimen must be, since spontaneous remissions have been described (57). The fetal mortality rate is approximately 2.5%. Sheikh et al. (64) proposed a good diagnostic and therapeutic protocol for parvovirus infections, and we use a modified form of this protocol in our department. Treatment of the mother or fetus with hyperimmunoglobulin doses has not been recommended to date, because no specific B19 immunoglobulin is yet available. Owing to its favorable prognosis, parvovirus B19 infection is not an indication for pregnancy termination.

Cytomegalovirus

Cytomegalovirus (CMV), which belongs to the group of herpes viruses, is the most common causative organism of intrauterine infections in the western world. It is estimated that a congenital infection occurs in 20–30% of initial infections.

Symptoms. Only about 10% of infected fetuses develop symptoms such as hepatosplenomegaly with focal calcifications, microcephaly, growth retardation, oligohydramnios, cerebral calcifications, hydrocephalus, and hemolytic anemia. The development of isolated ascites or NIHF is very rare.

Prognosis. Approximately 30% of severely affected fetuses die, usually from disseminated intravascular coagulation, liver failure, or bacterial superinfection. Up to 15% of infants who appear normal at birth later develop symptoms such as hearing loss.

Diagnosis. IgM determination in the fetal blood is not reliable due to cross-reactivity. The presumptive diagnosis should be confirmed by viral culture or PCR in the amniotic fluid. Amniocentesis should be done about 6 weeks after the maternal infection but not before 20 weeks' gestation.

Toxoplasmosis and Syphilis

Congenital toxoplasmosis and syphilis infections have also been described in association with NIHF (5, 7, 46). Both infections can lead to serious complications, and both are responsive to transplacental antibiotic therapy. We therefore recommend adding maternal serum screening for toxoplasmosis in pregnancy, like the test that is already done for syphilis.

Twins

The risk of developing a serious hemodynamic overload is increased in a monochorionic twin pregnancy. Examples are fetofetal transfusion syndrome and the twin reversed arterial perfusion (TRAP) syndrome that occurs when one twin lacks a heart.

Fetofetal transfusion syndrome. Fetofetal transfusion syndrome is of particular interest with regard to NIHF, because both fetuses are at risk for developing hydrops (49, 67), although the acceptor is affected in most cases. The donor appears to be mainly affected by hypovolemia. The acceptor is chiefly affected by hypervolemia, polycythemia, and hyperalbuminemia, which can lead to secondary heart failure when of long duration (69). Ultrasound in acute cases shows the rapid development of hydrops in the acceptor. Untreated, this condition will lead to intrauterine death within a matter of hours or days.

TRAP sequence. When one twin is normal and the other is acardiac, there is a high risk that the healthy twin perfusing the placenta and the acardius (the "pump twin") will develop secondary heart failure due to the chronic overload, leading to NIHF.

Diagnosis. When a twin manifests hydrops, it should be considered that twins have an increased rate of congenital anomalies, and a very intensive ultrasound evaluation should be conducted before fetofetal transfusion is assumed to be the sole cause of the hydrops.

Diseases Involving the Neck

Besides cystic hygroma, which is among the most common ultrasound findings in nonimmune hydrops, very rare obstructions of the upper respiratory tract are also commonly associated with NIHF. This group of anomalies is known internationally by the acronym CHAOS (congenital high airway obstruction syndrome) (27). Among our own patients, we have made two antenatal diagnoses of laryngeal atresia, and both cases were associated with marked fetal hydrops (36).

Pulmonary and Other Thoracic Diseases

Hydrothorax and chylothorax. The pleural effusion in NIHF requires differentiation from an isolated hydro- or chylothorax. An obstruction of the lymphatic pathways is the most frequent cause of an isolated pleural effusion. Pronounced cases with an early onset result in unilateral or bilateral pulmonary hypoplasia. When significant chylothorax is present, especially when it is associated with a shift of the mediastinum, the fetus may develop hydrops (Figs. 18.**5**, 18.**19**, 18.**20**). Great numbers of lymphocytes are found in aspirated thoracic fluid.

Masses. Extensive thoracic masses can raise the intrathoracic pressure and obstruct the venous or lymphatic system, leading to NIHF (46). The manifestations include chylothorax, congenital cystic adenomatoid malformation (CCAM) of the lung, pulmonary sequestration (70), diaphragmatic hernia (9), and pulmonary cysts or tumors. Tumors in the thoracic region are rare. The differential diagnosis includes hamartomas, adenomas, and teratomas.

An extralobar pulmonary sequestrum can also give rise to NIHF through an interesting mechanism. The sequestrum receives its arterial supply from an abnormal vessel. If the sequestrum is drained by the pulmonary veins, a shunt develops between the systemic arteries and pulmonary veins, imposing a chronic overload on the left heart. This type of "left-to-left shunt" is not known to occur in any other anomaly.

The most frequent pulmonary cause of nonimmune fetal hydrops is CCAM (22, 58). With unilateral involvement, the prognosis is good. The prognosis worsens after the onset of hydrops, but successful intrauterine treatment has been described even after the development of NIHF

(41, 58). The prognosis depends on the type of CCAM that is present. Type III CCAM is particularly common in association with NIHF and has a poor prognosis with pulmonary and cardiac failure in the neonate.

Among our own patients, we have diagnosed 20 cases of CCAM. Seven of these fetuses developed hydrops. We observed one case of NIHF in seven fetuses with pulmonary or bronchogenic cysts and another case in four fetuses with pulmonary sequestra. Whenever CCAM is suspected, the lesion should be very carefully evaluated with ultrasound, both to determine the number and size of the cysts and also to check for subtle signs of NIHF.

Abdominal Diseases

Gastrointestinal disorders such as stenoses and atresias of the bowel, malrotation, volvulus, and meconium peritonitis usually lead to isolated ascites rather than NIHF (26, 50) and often have a better prognosis.

Hepatic Diseases

The following hepatic diseases have been described in association with NIHF (31, 33, 67):
- Cirrhosis
- Necrosis
- Polycystic liver disease
- Biliary atresia
- Hepatic hemangioma

To date we have diagnosed one case of hepatitis antenatally in a fetus with nonimmune hydrops.

Metabolic Disorders

Metabolic disorders can cause hepatomegaly leading to venous congestion. They can also lead to anemia and hypoproteinemia.

NIHF sometimes occurs in the following metabolic disorders, presumably based on the same mechanisms (45, 51, 52):
- Gaucher disease
- Gangliosidosis
- Mucopolysaccharidosis
- Hurler syndrome
- Niemann–Pick disease

In equivocal cases, a postnatal evaluation may be advised when one of these diseases is suspected, as they may be associated with a high risk of recurrence.

Renal Diseases

Renal diseases that are associated with NIHF are uncommon. Urinary ascites (Fig. 18.**11**) caused by fluid extravasation due to urinary obstruction must be differentiated from NIHF. Congenital nephrosis (Finnish type), which is inherited as an autosomal-recessive trait, can lead to hydrops as a result of excessive protein loss (24).

Skeletal Dysplasias

All severe skeletal dysplasias have been described in association with NIHF, but the pathogenic mechanism is not always clear.

In cases of skeletal dysplasia with thoracic hypoplasia (e.g., short rib–polydactyly syndrome), crowding of the thoracic organs leads to increased intrathoracic pressure during growth. The workup should include an accurate evaluation of the fetal tubular bones (length, mineralization, etc.) when NIHF is present.

Neoplasms

Teratomas. Teratomas are associated with NIHF in more than 30% of cases (18). The majority occur in the nuchal or sacrococcygeal area. When they reach a certain size and degree of vascularity, the fetal cardiac load becomes too great, resulting in heart failure with a poor prognosis (40).

Neuroblastomas. These tumors have also been described in association with NIHF. Neuroblastomas may affect the bone marrow, precipitating anemia, or tumors at certain location may compress the vena cava, promoting NIHF.

Rare Syndromes

Myotonic dystrophy. A number of very rare syndromes have been described as having causal significance in NIHF. An example is myotonic dystrophy, which has an autosomal-dominant mode of inheritance (1). Maternal symptoms can provide evidence for the presence of this disease.

There are several other diseases that tend to affect the lymphatic system:
* Noonan syndrome (8)
* Pterygium syndrome (14)
* Yellow nail syndrome
* Congenital lymphangiectasis (61)

When NIHF occurs without an identifiable cause, the parents can be screened for lymphatic abnormalities in order to detect these rare syndromes.

Placenta and Umbilical Cord

Chorangiomas. Chorangiomas of the placenta are common but usually have no pathologic significance. When their arteriovenous shunts become hemodynamically active (on reaching about 5 cm in size), they can give rise to severe fetal hydrops. The diagnosis can be established by color Doppler (29) or power Doppler imaging.

Hemorrhagic endovasculitis. In some cases of NIHF with no apparent cause, postpartum histologic examination of the placenta revealed hemorrhagic endovasculitis (55). The significance of this condition is not yet fully understood.

Umbilical cord changes. NIHF has been found to be associated with umbilical cord changes that restrict blood flow, including aneurysms, thrombosis, twisting, and knotting.

Maternal Disorders and Complications

Maternal disorders. The association of NIHF and maternal diabetes has been a subject of controversy in the literature (46, 67). Severe maternal anemias have been observed in NIHF. Reference was made above to the association of maternal autoimmune diseases such as Sjögren syndrome and systemic lupus erythematosus (SLE) with fetal arrhythmias, as well as with Bourneville–Pringle disease and metabolic diseases such as glucose-6-phosphate dehydrogenase deficiency. The history and antibody tests can furnish a presumptive diagnosis.

Pregnancy complications. The incidence of pregnancy complications such as preeclampsia, anemia, postpartum hemorrhage, and placental retention (21, 33) is known to be increased in both immune and nonimmune forms of fetal hydrops. The high complication rate appears to be closely related to the trophoblastic disturbance, polyhydramnios, and the often immature, edematous placenta.

Maternal hydrops syndrome. Several studies have shown differences between "classic" preeclampsia and that associated with hydrops (maternal anemia, low hematocrit in fetal hydrops). This has given rise to the term "maternal hydrops syndrome," known also as Ballantyne syndrome or mirror syndrome (21). When maternal GEPH-like symptoms appear in conjunction with nonimmune fetal hydrops, it is important to consider the possibility of a maternal hydrops syndrome, since serious complications such as brain edema may arise. In some cases the symptoms may be so severe that pregnancy termination is indicated on maternal grounds. In our department, we have observed one such acute case in NIHF caused by a parvovirus B19 infection at 23 weeks' gestation.

Maternal drug use. Tocolytic agents (sympathomimetics) can precipitate fetal tachyarrhythmias. Prostaglandin-synthesis inhibitors can lead to premature closure of the ductus arteriosus.

Diagnosis

Fetal hydrops is usually a late symptom of a pathological process that is caused by a serious fetal anomaly or disease or, in rare cases, by an underlying maternal disease. Often the severity of the hydrops does not correlate with the severity of the underlying disorder. Early detection and diagnosis are of critical importance in the further planning of the pregnancy and in obstetric management.

Diagnostic protocol. The diagnostic protocol is dictated by the most frequent causes of NIHF: cardiovascular disorders, chromosomal abnormalities, infectious diseases, anemias, thoracic or abdominal diseases, and monochorionic twins. Prevention or therapeutic intervention is now possible in selected cases through the recognition of individual risks. The myriad diagnostic possibilities make it necessary to follow a standard protocol (Table 18.**6**, Fig. 18.**21**). Many of the rare causes cannot be identified until after birth.

Prognosis and Treatment

Prognosis

Obstetric management and parental counseling are based on the specific diagnosis and also on gestational age. On the whole, NIHF has a guarded prognosis with a reported mortality rate ranging from 40% to 90% (33, 34, 47). When NIHF develops before 24 weeks' gestation, few fetuses survive (4% according to [26]). When it occurs after 24 weeks, almost 30% survive. In our study of fetuses with a cardiovascular etiology of NIHF, 11% survived when the hydrops was diagnosed before 24 weeks, and 35% survived when diagnosed after 24 weeks. It is evident from these figures that NIHF occurring before 24 weeks is associated with more severe anomalies and diseases. In these cases the option of pregnancy termination should be discussed with the parents. The long-term prognosis depends essentially on the underlying disease and the severity of any cardiac failure more than on the severity of the hydrops. There is also evidence that hydropic fetuses are susceptible to hypoxic brain damage (42).

In rare cases, severe maternal complications (see above) may also warrant intervention.

▬ *Treatment*

Various therapeutic options may be considered (Table 18.**7**).

Intrauterine blood transfusion. Intrauterine transfusion using directed or nondirected donor blood is the treatment of choice in anemic fetuses. We feel that human albumin should also be given to correct the primary or secondary hypoproteinemia that theoretically develops in most fetuses, although there are still no hard data to support this.

Pharmacologic therapy. If ultrasound shows evidence of fetal heart failure, direct and indirect digitalization is advised even if the fetus shows no arrhythmia. When a diagnosis has been established, specific therapy should be provided whenever possible, such as antiarrhythmic drugs for arrhythmia and antibiotics for certain infections.

Aspiration of body cavities. If significant hydrothorax develops during the first half of pregnancy with a danger of secondary pulmonary hypoplasia, it is worthwhile to attempt decompression in selected cases by intrauterine needle aspiration. Especially in the later weeks of pregnancy, however, it should be noted that the fetal lungs appear compressed at ultrasound even when they are not hypoplastic. The aspirated fluid should be tested for lymphocyte content and protein concentration to differentiate between hydrothorax and chylothorax. A hydrothorax should be aspirated shortly before delivery to facilitate postpartum ventilation. As a general rule, the needle aspiration of fetal body cavities is recommended only in rare and difficult cases, as the fluid will reaccumulate within a short time. Thus, the aspiration of body cavities is usually more diagnostic than therapeutic, consistent with the etiology of NIHF.

Fetal Ascites

It seems prudent on etiologic and prognostic grounds to distinguish isolated fetal ascites from generalized nonimmune hydrops. Any evidence of ascites should be closely followed sonographically to detect or exclude the development of hydrops at an early stage.

Differential diagnosis. Isolated ascites requires differentiation from an early manifestation of NIHF, from urinary ascites (Fig. 18.**11**), from chyloperitoneum, and from "pseudoascites."

Pseudoascites. This refers to a narrow, hypoechoic streak along the abdominal wall that is caused by the normal abdominal musculature.

Table 18.**6** Staged diagnostic evaluation of nonimmune fetal hydrops (NIHF)

I. First exclude an immunologic cause

➢ Personal and family history
➢ Indirect Coombs test, blood group with Rh antigen, antibody screen

II. Further tests of maternal venous blood to cover common differential diagnoses

➢ Hb, HCT, MCV, platelets ("small blood count")
➢ Hb electrophoresis if there is a specific suspicion of hemoglobinopathy
➢ Kleihauer–Bethke test
➢ Antibody screening for common infections (toxoplasmosis, parvovirus B19, CMV)
➢ Syphilis serology (VDLR)
➢ Maternal AFP

III. Essential imaging studies

➢ Ultrasound B-mode evaluation of the fetus, placenta, umbilical cord, and amniotic fluid volume
➢ B-mode echocardiography with cardiac biometry and evaluation of myocardial contractility (failure?). M-mode evaluation of cardiac rhythm (Fig. 18.**18**). Color and spectral Doppler evaluation of valvular function, etc. As a basic rule, the cardiac anatomy, size, rhythm, and myocardial contractility are primarily evaluated in NIHF. Echocardiography can help determine the severity of cardiac failure.
➢ Doppler examination of maternal and fetal vessels including the venous system (see also Figs. 18.**13** and 18.**14**)

Ultrasound is of greatest importance, not just in preparing for special invasive studies but also because the severity of the ultrasound findings can dictate further management before laboratory parameters such as karyotype and infectious parameters become available.

IV. Subsequent invasive fetal diagnosis

The standard workup is extended based on the preliminary findings. Since only a limited amount of fetal blood is available, the tests should be strictly prioritized. Amniocentesis and cordocentesis should be performed whenever possible. One benefit of these procedures is that they allow fast and accurate fetal karyotyping. If a chromosomal abnormality is suspected, the FISH analysis of an amniotic fluid sample is a relatively quick method for detecting a numerical chromosome anomaly.

Cordocentesis

➢ Karyotyping
➢ Hb, HCT
➢ Fetal blood type, Coombs test
➢ In suspicious cases: Hb electrophoresis
➢ Plasma albumin
➢ Antibody screening (targeted), viral PCR
➢ Targeted genetic studies

A quick hemoglobin test should be done immediately after the blood is drawn. If severe fetal anemia is detected, an intrauterine transfusion can be performed using 0 Rh-negative donor blood.

Amniocentesis

➢ In suspicious cases: viral cultures, PCR
➢ AFP

Table 18.**7** Therapeutic options for nonimmune fetal hydrops (NIHF)

General treatment options

➢ Blood transfusion
➢ Human albumin administration
➢ Digitalization

Special treatment options

➢ Antiarrhythmic drugs
➢ Antibiotics
➢ Needle aspiration of affected body cavities

Table 18.**8** Isolated fetal ascites: associated anomalies and diseases

Urogenital causes (DD: urinary ascites)

➢ Urethrovesical obstruction
➢ Prevesical obstruction
➢ Renal hypoplasia
➢ Cystic renal diseases
➢ Ovarian cysts
➢ Cloaca formation

Gastrointestinal causes

➢ Meconium peritonitis
➢ Volvulus
➢ Small bowel atresia
➢ Diaphragmatic hernia

Lebererkrankungen

➢ Hepatitis
➢ Fibrosis, necrosis
➢ Biliary atresia
➢ Tumors

Metabolic diseases

➢ Gaucher disease
➢ Gangliosidosis

Urinary ascites. Diseases that lead to a massive fluid buildup in the fetal bladder, ureters, or kidneys may cause urinary ascites as a result of transudation or rupture. Common urogenital causes of urinary ascites are listed in Table 18.**8**. The presence of fetal ascites should prompt a meticulous evaluation of the urogenital tract.

Gastrointestinal diseases. These diseases can lead to isolated ascites due to chronic inflammation of the intestinal serosa with exudation or due to obstruction of the venous and lymphatic system. The most fre-

quent cause appears to be meconium peritonitis, which may present sonographically with echogenic plaques on the peritoneum. Other frequent causes are listed in Table 18.**8**.

Hepatic diseases. Hepatic diseases that lead to obstruction of the venous system can not only lead to NIHF (see above) but can also cause isolated ascites. Various metabolic diseases have also been described in connection with ascites, but the precise cause is still unknown.

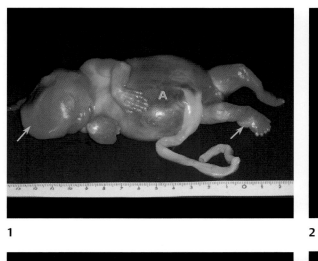

1

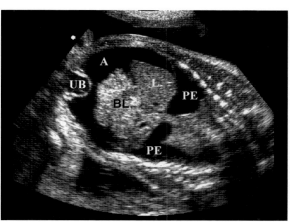

2

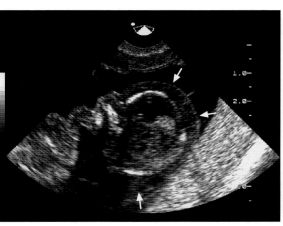

3

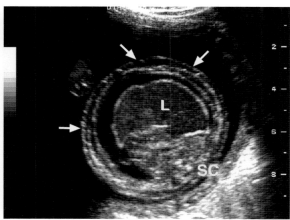

4

Clinical and ultrasound findings in NIHF

Fig. 18.**1** Generalized fetal hydrops. Photograph of a 12-week fetus with NIHF. There is marked cutaneous edema on the head and extremities (arrows). Ascites (A). Diagnosis: Turner syndrome.

Fig. 18.**2** Generalized fetal hydrops. Marked pleural effusion (PE) and ascites (A) in a fetus with severe anemia due to a parvovirus B19 infection. Abdominal organs such as the liver (L) and urinary bladder (UB) are clearly delineated by the fluid. The bowel loops (BL) appear to float freely in the ascitic fluid.

Fig. 18.**3** Cutaneous edema. Prominent cutaneous edema appears about the head in NIHF (arrows) at 13 weeks. An arteriovenous fistula was found within the liver. Diagnosis: trisomy 21.

Fig. 18.**4** Cutaneous edema. Transverse thoracic scan at the level of the liver (L) demonstrates the subcutaneous edema (arrows). Diagnosis: generalized NIHF of the acceptor twin in fetofetal transfusion syndrome. SC = spinal column.

Fig. 18.**5** Pleural effusion. Transverse thoracic scan at the four-chamber level in a fetus with bilateral pleural effusions (P). Chylothorax was identified as the cause. The lungs (L) are clearly delineated and appear compressed. Postnatally, the infant was ventilated and the effusions were drained. The chylothorax cleared without surgical intervention. SC = spinal column, H = heart.

Fig. 18.**6** Pleural effusion. Transverse thoracic scan shows bilateral pleural effusions (P) in NIHF as a result of supraventricular tachyarrhythmia. The mesentery and great vessels are defined. In response to cardioversion by maternal digitalization, a normal rhythm was reestablished and the hydrops cleared.

Fig. 18.**7** Pericardial effusion. Scan demonstrates an isolated pericardial effusion (arrows) at 24 weeks. Marked NIHF developed by 32 weeks. The infant was delivered at 34 weeks following thoracocentesis. The hydrops cleared postnatally in response to diuretic therapy. A cause could not be ascertained.

Fig. 18.**8** Pericardial effusion. Scan at the four-chamber level shows a small pericardial effusion at 16 weeks with generalized NIHF (arrows). The cause could not be determined. It is very difficult in early pregnancy to distinguish a physiologic fluid collection in the pericardium from a pathologic pericardial effusion.

Fig. 18.**9** Ascites. Transverse abdominal scan at the level of the liver (L). The bowel loops (BL) and omental bursa (arrow) appear to float within the fluid.

Fig. 18.**10** Ascites. Marked dilatation of the hepatic veins (arrows) in ascites resulting from secondary heart failure due to supraventricular tachyarrhythmia. L = liver, H = heart.

Fig. 18.**11** Urinary ascites. Scan demonstrates a small intra-abdominal fluid collection (arrows) in megacystis. The fluid consists of urine ("urinary ascites") due to transudation or bladder rupture and does not signify NIHF. UB = urinary bladder.

Fig. 18.**12** Scrotal edema. In male fetuses with generalized NIHF, it is often possible to demonstrate fluid within the scrotum (arrows).

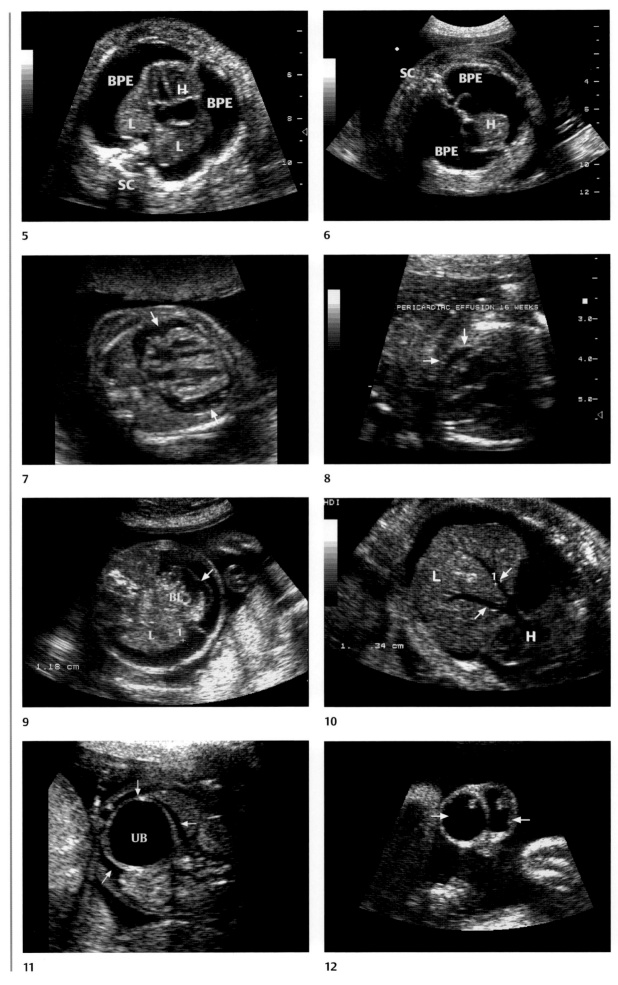

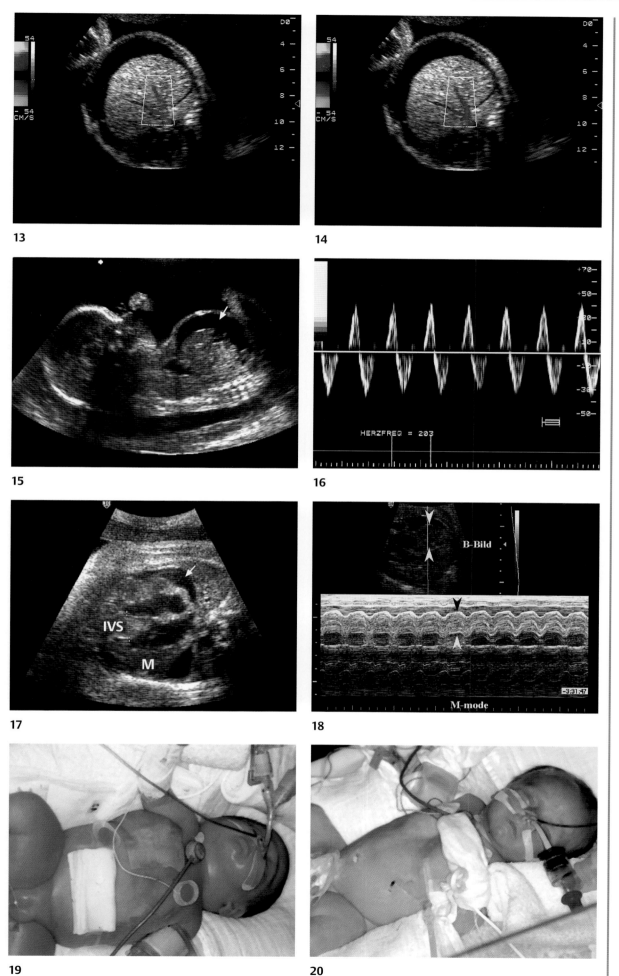

13

14

15

16

HERZFREQ = 203

17

IVS

M

18

B-Bild

M-mode

19

20

NIHF due to heart disease

Fig. 18.**13** Transverse abdominal scan at the level of the liver, demonstrating ascites.

Fig. 18.**14** Same fetus as in Fig. 18.**13**. Color Doppler can show bidirectional blood flow in the hepatic veins (retrograde red, antegrade blue) when heart failure is present (e.g., due to cardiomyopathy).

Fig. 18.**15** NIHF in a fetus with tachycardia. Longitudinal scan at 22 weeks demonstrates ascites (arrow). The cause was identified as paroxysmal supraventricular tachycardia leading to severe valvular insufficiency. The hydrops cleared in response to cardioversion by maternal digitalization.

Fig. 18.**16** NIHF in a fetus with tachycardia. Same fetus as in Fig. 18.**13**. Doppler sampling of the vena cava in supraventricular tachycardia shows a heart rate in excess of 200 bpm. The pronounced reverse flow points to heart failure as the cause of the nonimmune hydrops.

Fig. 18.**17** NIHF in fetal cardiomyopathy. Transverse thoracic scan at the four-chamber level in a fetus with NIHF (29 weeks). The heart occupies almost the entire chest cavity. The myocardium (M) and interventricular septum (IVS) are hypertrophic, and the ventricular lumina appear narrowed. This hypertrophic cardiomyopathy is presumably based on a metabolic disorder (suspected L-carnitine deficiency).

Fig. 18.**18** NIHF in fetal cardiomyopathy. Same fetus as in Fig. 18.**17**. Wall thickness (arrows) and myocardial contractility can be evaluated in the M-mode tracing. In the present case, the myocardium appears thickened and hypokinetic.

NIHF due to chylothorax

Fig. 18.**19** NIHF due to chylothorax. Immediate postpartum photograph of an infant with marked fetal hydrops due to chylothorax.

Fig. 18.**20** The same infant 6 weeks postpartum following pleural drainage and diuretic therapy. The infant was healthy enough for discharge home.

Diagnostic evaluation of NIHF

Fig. 18.**21** Flowchart for the evaluation of fetal hydrops.

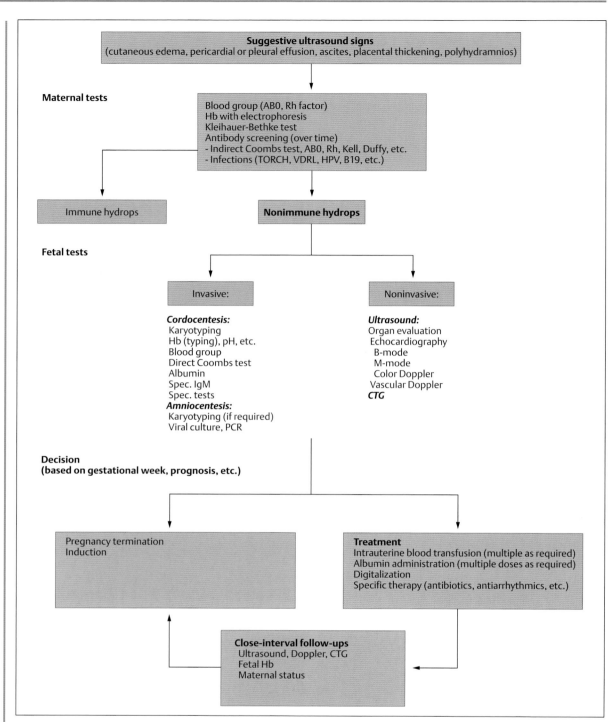

Suggestive ultrasound signs
(cutaneous edema, pericardial or pleural effusion, ascites, placental thickening, polyhydramnios)

Maternal tests

Blood group (AB0, Rh factor)
Hb with electrophoresis
Kleihauer-Bethke test
Antibody screening (over time)
- Indirect Coombs test, AB0, Rh, Kell, Duffy, etc.
- Infections (TORCH, VDRL, HPV, B19, etc.)

Immune hydrops

Nonimmune hydrops

Fetal tests

Invasive:

Cordocentesis:
Karyotyping
Hb (typing), pH, etc.
Blood group
Direct Coombs test
Albumin
Spec. IgM
Spec. tests
Amniocentesis:
Karyotyping (if required)
Viral culture, PCR

Noninvasive:

Ultrasound:
Organ evaluation
 Echocardiography
 B-mode
 M-mode
 Color Doppler
Vascular Doppler
CTG

Decision
(based on gestational week, prognosis, etc.)

Pregnancy termination
Induction

Treatment
Intrauterine blood transfusion (multiple as required)
Albumin administration (multiple doses as required)
Digitalization
Specific therapy (antibiotics, antiarrhythmics, etc.)

Close-interval follow-ups
Ultrasound, Doppler, CTG
Fetal Hb
Maternal status

21

References

1. Afifi, A.M., Bahtia, A.R., Eyal, F.: Hydrops fetalis associated with congenital myotonic dystrophy. Amer. J. Obstet. Gynecol. 166 (1992) 929–930
2. Allan, L.D., Crawford, D.C., Sheridan, R.: Aetiology of non-immune hydrops: The value of echocardiography. Brit. J. Obstet. Gynecol. 93 (1986) 223–225
3. Anand, A., Gray, E.S., Brown, T.: Human parvovirus infection in pregnancy and hydrops fetalis. New Engl. J. Med. 316 (1987) 183–186
4. Anandakumar, C., Biswas, A., Wong, Y.C. et al.: Management of non-immune hydrops: 8 years' experience. Ultrasound Obstet. Gynecol. 8 (1996) 196–200
5. Bain, A.D., Bowie, J.H., Flint, W.F.: Congenital toxoplasmosis simulating haemolytic disease of the newborn. J. Obstet. Gynecol. Br. Commonw. 63 (1956) 826–831
6. Ballantyne, J.W.: The Diseases and Deformities of the Fetus. Edinburgh: Oliver & Boyd 1892
7. Barton, J.R., Thorpe, E.M., Shaver, D.C.: Nonimmune hydrops fetalis associated with maternal infection with syphilis. Amer. J. Obstet. Gynecol. 167 (1992) 56–58
8. Bawle, E.V., Black, V.: Nonimmune hydrops fetalis in Noonan's syndrome. Amer. J. Dis. Child. 140 (1986) 758–760
9. Benacerraf, B.R., Frigoletto, F.D.: In utero treatment of a fetus with diaphragmatic hernia complicated by hydrops. Amer. J. Obstet. Gynecol. 155 (1986) 817–818
10. Bernstein, H.S., Filly, R.A., Goldberg, J.D.: Prognosis of fetuses with cystic hygroma. Prenat. Diagn. 11 (1991) 349–355
11. Bollmann, R., Chaoui, R., Schilling, H.: Pränatale Diagnostik und Management der fetalen Arrhythmien. Z. Geburtshilfe Perinatol. 192 (1988) 266–272
12. Chaoui, R., Bollmann, R., Göllner, B.: Fetal cardiomegaly: echocardiographic findings and outcome in 19 cases. Fet. Diagn. Ther. 9 (1994) 92–104
13. Chaoui, R., Hoffmann, H., Bollmann, R., Wauer, R.: Pränatale Diagnose eines vorzeitigen Verschlusses des Ductus arteriosus mit nachfolgender Entwicklung eines nichtimmunologischen Hydrops fetalis (NIHF). Geburtsh. Frauenhk. 49 (1989) 1096–1098
14. Chen, H., Immken, L, Lachman., R.: Syndrome of multiple pterygia, camptodactyly, facial anomalies, hypoplastic lungs and heart, cystic hygroma and skeletal anomalies: Delineation of a new entity and review of lethal forms of multiple pterygium syndrome. Amer. J. Med. Genet. 17 (1984) 809–826
15. Coulson, C.C., Kuller, J.A., Sweeney, W.J.: Nonimmune hydrops and hydrocephalus secondary to fetal intracranial hemorrhage. Amer. J. Perinatol. 11 (1994) 253–254
16. Fadne, H.O., Oian, P.: Transcapillary fluid balance and plasma volume regulation: a review. Obstet. Gynecol. Surv. 44 (1989) 769–773
17. Fischer, R.I., Kuhlmann, K., Grover, J.: Chronic, massive fetomaternal hemorrhage treated with repeated fetal intravascular transfusion. Amer. J. Obstet. Gynecol. 162 (1990) 203–204
18. Flake, A.W., Harrison, M.R., Adzick, N.S.: Fetal sacrococcygeal teratoma. J. Pediatr. Surg. 1 (1987) 563–565
19. Fleischer, A.C., Killam, A.P., Boehm, F.H.: Hydrops fetalis: Sonographic evaluation and clinical implications. Radiology 141 (1981) 163
20. Gembruch, U., Hansmann, M., Bald, R.: Direct intrauterine fetal treatment of tachyarrhythmia with severe hydrops fetalis by antiarrythmic drugs. Fetal Ther. 3 (1988) 210–215
21. Gough, J.D., Keeling, J.W., Castle, B.: The obstetric management of non-immunological hydrops. Brit. J. Obstet. Gynaecol. 93 (1986) 226–239
22. Graham, D., Winn, K., Dex, W.: Prenatal diagnosis of cystic adenomatoid malformation of the lung. J. Ultrasound Med. 1 (1982) 9–12
23. Gudmundsson, S., Huhta, J.C., Wood, D.C., Tulzer, G., Cohen, A.W., Weiner, S.: Venous Doppler ultrasonography in the fetus with nonimmune hydrops. Amer. J. Obstet. Gynecol. 164 (1991) 33–37
24. Hallmenn, N., Norio, R., Rapola, J.: Congenital nephrotic syndrome. Nephron 11 (1973) 101
25. Hansmann, M., Arabin, B.: Nonimmune Hydrops Fetalis. In: Chervenak, Isaacson, Campell (eds.) Ultrasound in Obstetrics and Gynecology (1993) 1027–1048
26. Hansmann, M., Gembruch, U., Bald, R.: New therapeutic aspects in nonimmune hydrops fetalis based on four hundred and two prenatally diagnosed cases. Fetal Therapy 4 (1989) 29–37
27. Hedrick, M.H., Ferro, M.M., Filly, R.A., Flake, A.W., Harrison, M.R., Adzick, N.S.: Congenital high airway obstruction syndrome (CHAOS): a potential for perinatal intervention. J. Pediatr. Surg. 29 (1994) 271–274
28. Hendricks, S., Sorensen, S., Baker, E.: Trisomy 21, fetal hydrops, and anemia: prenatal diagnosis of transient myeloproliferative disorder? Obstet. Gynecol. 82 (1993) 703–705
29. Hirata, G.I., Masaki, D.I., O'Toole, M.: Color flow mapping and doppler velocimetry in the diagnosis and management of a placental chorangioma: a case report. J. Reprod. Med. 31 (1993) 520–522
30. Hoffmann, D., Holländer, H.J., Weiser, P.: The gynecological and obstetrical importance of ultrasonic diagnosis. Gynaecologia 164 (1967) 24–36
31. Holzgreve, W., Curry, C.J.R., Golbus, M.S., Callen, P.W., Filly, R.A., Smith, J.C.: Investigation of nonimmune hydrops fetalis. Amer. J. Obstet. Gynecol. 150 (1984) 805–812
32. Holzgreve, W.: The fetus with nonimmune hydrops In: Harrison, Golbus, Filly (eds.): The unborn patient: prenatal diagnosis and treatment. W.B. Saunders Company (1991) 228–245
33. Hutchinson, A.A., Drew, J.H., Yu, V.Y.H.: Nonimmunologic hydrops fetalis: a review of 61 cases. Obstet. Gynecol. 59 (1982) 347–352
34. Im, S.S., Rizos, N., Joutsi, P., Shime, J., Benzie, R.J.: Nonimmunologic hydrops fetalis. Amer. J. Obstet. Gynecol. 148 (1984) 566–569
35. Johnson, P., Sharland, G., Allan, L.D., Tynan, M.J., Maxwell, D.: Umbilical venous pressure in nonimmune hydrops fetalis: Correlation with cardiac size. Amer. J. Obstet. Gynecol. 167 (1992) 1309–1313

36. Kalache, K.D., Tennstedt, C., Chaoui, R., Bollmann, R.: Prenatal Diagnosis of laryngeal atresia: a report of two cases. Ultrasound Obstet. Gynecol. 8 (1996) 140 (Abstract)
37. Kattamis, C., Metaxotu-Mavromati, A., Tsiarta, E.: Haemoglobin Bart's syndrome in Greece. Brit. Med. J. 281 (1980) 268–270
38. Kohler, H.G.: Premature closure of the ductus arteriosus (PCDA): a possible cause of intrauterine circulatory failure. Early Hum. Dev. 2 (1978) 15–20
39. Kovacs, B.W., Carlson, D.E., Shachbarami, B., Platt, L.D.: Prenatal Diagnosis of human parvovirus B19 in nonimmune hydrops fetalis by polymerase chain reaction. Amer. J. Obstet. Gynecol. 167 (1992) 461–466
40. Kuhlmann, R.S., Warsof, S.L., Lavy, D.L.: Fetal sacrococcygeal teratoma. Fetal Therapy 2 (1987) 95–100
41. Kuller, J.A., Yankowitz, J., Goldberg, Harrison, M.R. et al.: Outcome of antenatally diagnosed cystic adenomatoid malformations. Amer. J. Obstet. Gynecol. 167 (1992) 1038–1041
42. Laroche, J.C., Aubry, M.C., Narcy, F.: Intrauterine brain damage in nonimmune hydrops fetalis. Biol. Neonat. 61 (1992) 273–280
43. Lebo, R.V., Saiki, R.K., Swanson, K.: Prenatal diagnosis of alpha thalassemia by polymerase chain reaction and dual restriction enzyme analysis. Hum. Genet. 85 (1990) 293–299
44. Liang, S.T., Wong, V.C.W., So, W.W.K.: Homozygous alpha-thalassemia: Clinical presentation, diagnosis and management. A review of 46 cases. Brit. J. Obstet. Gynecol. 92 (1985) 680–684
45. Lissens, W., Dedobbeleer, G., Foulon, W.: Beta-glucuronidase deficiency as cause of prenatally diagnosed non-immune hydrops fetalis. Prenat. Diagn. 11 (1991) 405–410
46. Macafee, C.A., Fortune, D.W., Beischer, N.A.: Non-immunological hydrops fetalis. J. Obstet. Gynaecol. Br. Commonw. 77 (1970) 226–237
47. Machin, G.A.: Hydrops revisited: Literature review of 1414 cases published in the 1980s. Amer. J. Med. Gen. 34 (1989) 366–390
48. Macones, G.A., Johnson, A., Tilley, D., Wade, R., Wapner, R.: Fetal hepatosplenomegaly associated with transient myeloproliferative disorder in Trisomy 21. Fetal Diagn. Ther. 10 (1995) 131–133
49. Maidman, J.E., Yaeger, C., Anderson, V.: Prenatal diagnosis and management of nonimmunologic hydrops fetalis. Obstet. Gynecol. 56 (1980) 571–576
50. McCoy, M.C., Katz, V., Gould, N., Kuller, J.: Non-immune hydrops after 20 weeks' gestation: Review of 10 years' experience with suggestion for management. Obstet. Gynecol. 85 (1995) 578–582
51. Meizner, I., Levy, A., Carmi, R.: Niemann-Pick disease associated with nonimmune hydrops fetalis. Amer. J. Obstet. Gynecol. 163 (1990) 128–129
52. Nelson, J., Kenny, B., O'Hara, D.: Foamy changes of placenta cells in probable beta-glucuronidase deficiency associated with hydrops fetalis. J. Clin. Pathol. 46 (1993) 370–371
53. Nicolaides, K.: Fetoscopy in the assessment of unexplained fetal hydrops. Brit. J. Obstet. Gynaecol. 92 (1985) 671–679
54. Norton, M.E.: Nonimmune Hydrops Fetalis. Sem. Perinatol. Vol. 18 (1994) 321–332
55. Novak, P.M., Sander, C.M., Yang, S.: Report of fourteen cases of nonimmune hydrops fetalis in association with hemorrhagic endovasculitis of the placenta. Amer. J. Obstet. Gynecol. 165 (1991) 945–950
56. Potter, E.L.: Universal edema of the fetus unassociated with erythroblastosis. Amer. J. Obstet. Gynecol. 43 (1943) 130–134
57. Pryde, P.G., Nugent, C.E., Pridjian, G., Barr, M., Faix, R.: Spontaneous resolution of nonimmune hydrops fetalis secondary to human parvovirus B19 infection. Obstet. Gynecol. 79 (1992) 859–861
58. Revillon, Y., Jan, D., Platner, V.: Congenital cystic adenomatoid malformation of the lung: Prenatal management and prognosis. J. Pediatr. Surg. 28 (1993) 1009–1011
59. Santolaya, J., Alley, D., Jaffe, R., Warsof, S.: Antenatal classification of hydrops fetalis. Obstet. Gynecol. 79 (1992) 256–259
60. Schmidt, K.G., Ulmer, H.E., Silverman, N.H.: Perinatal outcome of fetal complete atrioventricular block: A multicenter experience. J. Amer. Coll. Cardiol. 17 (1991) 1360–1366
61. Scott-Emuakpor, A.B., Warren, S.T., Kapur, S.: Familial occurrence of congenital pulmonary lymphangiectasie. Amer. J. Dis. Child. 135 (1981) 532–534
62. Selm, M.V., Kanhai, H.H.H., Gravenhorst, J.B.: Maternal hydrops syndrome: a review. Obstet. Gynecol. Surv. 46 (1991) 785–788
63. Shah, Y., Hadlock, F.P.: Hydrops and Ascites. In: Nyberg, Mahony, Pretorius (eds.): Diagnostic Ultrasound of Fetal Anomalies. Mosby Year Book (1990) 563–591
64. Sheikh, A.U., Ernest, J.M., O'Shea, M.: Long term outcome in fetal hydrops from parvovirus B19 infection. Amer. J. Obstet. Gynecol. 167 (1992) 337–341
65. Thomson, M.W., McInnes, R.R., Williard, H.F. (eds.): The molecular and biochemical basis of genetic diseases. In: Thomson & Thomson: Genetics in Medicine (ed 5). Philadelphia, PA: Saunders (1991) 298
66. Thorp, J.A., Cohen, G.R., Yeast, J.D.: Nonimmune hydrops caused by massive fetomaternal hemorrhage and treated by intravascular transfusion. Amer. J. Perinatol. 9 (1992) 22–24
67. Turkel, S.B.: Conditions associated with hydrops fetalis. Clin. Perinatol. 9 (1982) 613–625
68. Weiner, C.P.: Umbilical pressure measurement in the evaluation of nonimmune hydrops fetalis. Amer. J. Obstet. Gynecol. 168 (1992) 817–823
69. Weiner, C.P., Ludomirski, A.: Diagnosis, pathophysiology, and treatment of chronic twin-to-twin transfusion syndrome. Fetal Diagn. Ther. 9 (1993) 283–290
70. Weiner, C.P., Warner, M., Pringle, K.: Antenatal diagnosis and palliative treatment of nonimmune hydrops fetalis secondary to pulmonary extralobar sequestration. Obstet. Gynecol. 68 (1996) 275–280
71. Winn, H.N., Stiller, R., Grannum, P.A.T.: Isolated fetal Aszites: Prenatal diagnosis and management. Amer. J. Perinat. 7 (1990) 370–373

19 Intrauterine Fetal Death

Causes

The causes of intrauterine fetal death may relate to the mother, the fetus, or the placenta (Tables 19.**1** and 19.**2**). According to Völker (20), who examined 487 stillbirths and the associated placentas from 13 to 41 weeks' gestation, intrauterine fetal death has a placental cause in approximately half of cases, a fetal cause in one-fourth of cases, and a combined placental and fetal cause in one-eighth of cases.

In 13.7% of cases, the cause of the intrauterine fetal death cannot be established (7).

In a review of 71 intrauterine deaths, 37 (= 52%) of the patients were primiparae, 17 had previously delivered one child, 10 had delivered two children, and 7 had delivered three or more children (21). Fifty-five percent of the patients were between 20 and 29 years of age.

Maternal causes. The maternal causes of intrauterine fetal death are as follows:
- GEPH disorders. Eschler et al. (7) found that 30% of the mothers in their series had a prior history of GEPH disorders.
- Metabolic disorders (diabetes mellitus, thyroid disease)
- Blood group incompatibility
- Intrauterine infections (cytomegalovirus, listeriosis) (11, 19)

Fetal causes. Fetal causes include major anomalies and umbilical cord complications (looping, knotting, twisting) (7, 11, 20).

Placental causes. When intrauterine fetal death is due to placental causes, 50% of cases result from chronic placental insufficiency due to delayed placental maturation, endangiitis obliterans of major villous vessels, obliterative changes, or combined placental injuries. With delayed placental maturation, placental insufficiency is usually latent despite the small placental size. It often decompensates at a late stage (perinatally) and can cause acute fetal compromise. Endangiitis obliterans of major villous vessels results in early growth retardation. In many of these cases the area of placental attachment and placental weight are below the normal-for-age percentiles. Obliterative changes in the placenta remain compensated for some time, lead to subacute placental insufficiency, and are often associated with a small, light placenta (20).

Ultrasound Detection

Absence of heart activity. Real-time ultrasound offers a fast and effective method of diagnosing intrauterine fetal death. A fetal cardiac scan can directly confirm the absence of heart activity. If it is unclear whether heart activity has ceased completely, an M-mode examination or Doppler scan will help clarify the situation. This is particularly important in delivery room emergencies where fetal monitoring is unable to distinguish fetal bradycardia from intrauterine death with fetal transmission of the maternal pulse (13).

Superior signs. If the fetus has already been dead for several days, fetal death can be diagnosed from traditional superior roentgen signs (3, 5, 6, 15) such as the "bag" sign (Fig. 19.**1**), Spalding's sign (Figs. 19.**2**, 19.**3**), the halo sign (Fig. 10.**3**), or angulation of the fetal spine (Fig. 19.**4**). The

Table 19.**1**   Causes of intrauterine fetal death in spontaneous deliveries (adapted from [20])

Placental causes	48.4%
Fetal causes	22.0%
> Fetal anomalies	10.8%
> Umbilical cord changes	2.8%
> Other fetal causesn	8.3%
Maternal causes	2.3%
Placental and maternal causes	1.0%
Placental and fetal causes	12.8%
> Placental causes and fetal anomalies	4.9%
Indeterminate	13.7%

Table 19.**2**   Placental causes of intrauterine fetal death in spontaneous deliveries (adapted from [20])

Chronic placental insufficiency	54.0%
> Delayed placental maturation	14.9%
> Endangiitis obliterans	11.8%
> Obliterative changes	5.9%
> Combinations	21.4%
Placental abruption	24.5%
Chorioamnionitis	24.5%
Chorioamnionitis and abruption	4.3%
Subclinical intervillositis	2.1%
Other causes and combinations	3.2%

thorax may also exhibit deformity (10), but this is not as conspicuous as in the head.

All of these signs provide no more than suggestive evidence that the fetus has been dead for several days. The only proof of intrauterine fetal death is ultrasound verification of the absence of heart activity.

Time of death. If the time of death is uncertain, it can be estimated by evaluating fetal growth. Due to postmortem shape distortions in the head and trunk, the lengths of the long limb bones are better for estimating the age of a dead fetus. If the fetus is affected by dwarfism or severe growth retardation, the gestational age at the time of fetal demise cannot be determined with much accuracy. It may be helpful in such cases to resort to cerebellar biometry.

Maceration. When advanced (grade II) fetal maceration has occurred, separation of the skin from the head and trunk creates bubble-like outlines in the ultrasound image (Fig. 19.**5**). Signs of maceration may not be apparent before the sixth month of pregnancy, however (11).

Determining the cause. In some cases the cause of intrauterine fetal death can be determined with ultrasound. Detectable causes include grossly visible changes in the placenta such as a large retroplacental hematoma or partial/complete placental separation (see Chapter 34), conspicuous umbilical cord changes (knotting), a severe fetal anomaly, and pronounced fetal hydrops.

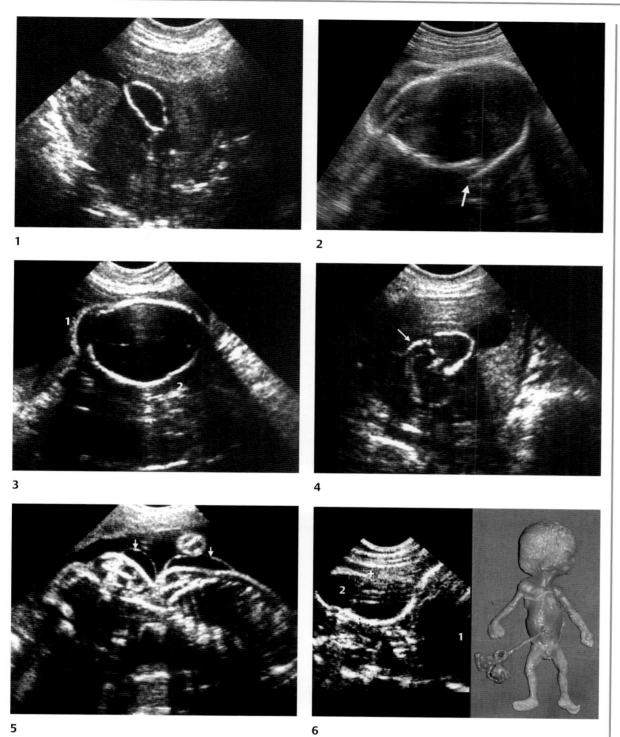

1

2

3

4

5

6

Fig. 19.**1**   Intrauterine fetal death, 16 weeks. The skull exhibits the "bag" sign of fetal death. Longitudinal scan.

Fig. 19.**2**   Intrauterine fetal death, 29 weeks. Spalding's sign (arrow), transverse scan.

Fig. 19.**3**   Intrauterine fetal death, 33 weeks. Both the halo sign (1) and Spalding's sign (2) are visible in the transverse scan.

Fig. 19.**4**   Intrauterine fetal death, 16 weeks. Note the marked angulation of the fetal spine (arrow).

Fig. 19.**5**   Intrauterine fetal death, 26 weeks. "Bubble sign" caused by separation of the skin from the head and thorax (arrows), longitudinal scan.

Fig. 19.**6**   Dead second twin in fetofetal transfusion syndrome. The first twin has a normal-appearing skull (1). The second twin has a misshapen oval skull (2). Transverse scan, 30 weeks. The photograph at right shows the corresponding fetus papyraceus after birth.

Intrauterine Fetal Death in Multiple Pregnancy

Incidence. At least one of the fetuses in a multiple pregnancy is at increased risk of intrauterine death. According to Litschgi and Stucki (14), the death of one fetus with the development of a fetus papyraceus occurs in 1.5% of all twin pregnancies. The intrauterine death of one twin is three times more common with a monochorionic placenta than with a dichorionic placenta (2).

Cause. Looping of the umbilical cord has been identified as the most frequent cause of death in monochorionic monoamniotic twins (4, 12). The main cause of death in monochorionic diamniotic twins is fetofetal transfusion syndrome (1, 9).

Further course of the pregnancy. The death of one twin during the second or third trimester does not necessarily lead to premature delivery. Litschgi and Stucki (14) found that in 6.8% of their twin pregnancies, the pregnancy continued following the intrauterine death of one twin. The interval between twin death and delivery ranged from 12 hours to 20 weeks. Feiks et al. (8) described two cases in which a period of 19 weeks and 16 weeks passed between the intrauterine death of one twin and the birth of the live twin. Among our own patients, we have had six pregnancies that continued for another 6–16 weeks following the intrauterine death of one twin due to fetofetal transfusion syndrome.

Mummification. As the pregnancy progresses, the dead twin shrivels up and is pressed flat against the uterine wall or placenta by the live, growing twin (Fig. 19.**6**), resulting in a fetus papyraceus. At birth, the mummified fetus is found in the region of the placenta or in the membranes of the surviving twin (17) (Fig. 19.**6**).

Obstetric Management and Subsequent Pregnancy

Coagulation disorder. According to Pritchard and Ratnoff (18), a maternal coagulation disorder in the form of hypofibrinogenemia does not develop before the fifth week after an intrauterine death. In the six cases that we followed for several weeks (6–16 weeks), regular coagulation tests showed no decline in maternal clotting factors. Pritchard and Ratnoff (18) recommend inducing labor when the maternal fibrinogen level falls below 150 mg/dL.

Subsequent pregnancy. Patients who have had a previous stillbirth may require close ultrasound surveillance of a subsequent pregnancy (biometry, Doppler), depending on the cause of the intrauterine fetal death. Especially in cases with a placental cause, the risk of recurrence is increased. When Monnier et al. (16) followed 62 patients who had a previous stillborn infant, they found that 8 of the women (13%) had another stillbirth in a subsequent pregnancy.

References

1. Bebbington, M.W., Wittmann, B.K.: Fetal transfusion syndrome: Antenatal factors predicting outcome. Amer. J. Obstet. Gynecol. 160 (1989) 913–915
2. Benirschke, K.: Twin placenta in perinatal mortality. N.Y. State J. Med. 61 (1961) 1499–1508
3. Borell, U., Fernström, I., Ohlson, L.: The halo sign in the living and dead fetus. Amer. J. Obstet. Gynecol. 87 (1963) 906–911
4. Colburn, D.W., Pasquale, S.A.: Monoamniotic twin pregnancy. J. reprod. Med. 27 (1982) 165–168
5. Deuel, H.: Zur Röntgendiagnose des intrauterinen Fruchttodes. Schweiz. med. Wschr. 77 (1947) 1003–1005
6. Donat, H., Heinz, W.: Beitrag zur röntgenologischen Diagnose des intrauterinen Fruchttodes. Zbl. Gynäk. 94 (1972) 402–407
7. Eschler, G., Heidegger, H., Krone, H.A.: Die Totgeburt – eine Analyse von 354 Fällen aus den Jahren 1966–1988. Geburtsh. u. Frauenheilk. 51 (1991) 293–297
8. Feiks, A., Scholler, J., Rehcek, G., Grünberger, W.: Der vorzeitig abgestorbene Mehrling – Geburtsmedizinische Implikation und Literaturübersicht. Z. Geburtsh. u. Perinat. 196 (1992) 44–46
9. Gonsoulin, W., Moise, K.J.Jr., Kirshon, B., Cotton, D.B., Wheeler, J.M., Carpenter, R.J.Jr.: Outcome of twin-twin transfusion diagnosed before 28 weeks of gestation. Obstet. Gynecol. 75(1990) 214–216
10. Gottesfeld, K.R.: The ultrasonic diagnosis of intrauterine fetal death. Amer. J. Obstet. Gynec. 108 (1970) 623–634
11. Hindemann, P.: Der intrauterine Fruchttod. In: Käser, O., Friedberg, V. (Hrsg.): Gynäkologie und Geburtshilfe Bd. II/1. Stuttgart: Thieme 1981; S. 1202
12. Holländer, H.J.: Monoamniotische Zwillinge. Z. Geburtsh. 171 (1969) 292–300
13. Hutson, J.M., Fox, H.E.: Real-time ultrasonography for the differential diagnosis of intrapartum fetal death. Amer. J. Obstet. Gynecol. 142 (1982) 1057–1059
14. Litschgi, M., Stucki, D.: Verlauf von Zwillingsschwangerschaften nach intrauterinem Fruchttod eines Föten. Z. Geburtsh. Perinat. 184 (1980) 227–230
15. Möbius, W.: Geburtshilfliche Strahlen- und Röntgendiagnostik. Berlin: Akademie Verlag 1967; S. 137
16. Monnier, J.C., Patey-Savatier, P., Dognin, C. et al.: Avenir obstetrical des femmes ayant un antécédent de mort in utero. Rev. Franc. Gyn. Obstet. 78 (1983) 781–784
17. Ottow, B.: Die Mehrlingsschwangerschaft und die Mehrlingsgeburt. In: Stoeckel, W.: Lehrbuch der Geburtshilfe. 10. Aufl. Jena: Fischer 1948; S. 254
18. Pritchard, J.A., Ratnoff, O.P.: Studies of fibrinogen and other hemostatic factors in women with intrauterine death and delayed delivery. Surg. Gynec. Obstet. 101 (1955) 467–477
19. Quinn, P.A., Butany, J., Chipman, M., Taylor, J., Hannah, W.: A prospective study of microbial infection in stillbirth and early neonatal death. Amer. J. Obstet. Gynecol. 151 (1985) 238–249
20. Völker, U.: Gewichts- und Größenvergleich von Plazenten und Feten bei intrauterinem Fruchttod. Perinatalmedizin 4 (1992) 8–16
21. Wessel, J., Lichtenegger, W., Gerold, W., Schönegg, W.: Zum Geburtsverlauf bei intrauterinem Fruchttod. Geburtsh. u. Frauenheilk. 52 (1992) 103–108

Ultrasound Examination
of Fetal Anomalies

20 General Detection of Fetal Anomalies

Basic Principles

Definition and Basic Terms

Definition of Fetal Anomalies

Deviation from normal. Fetal anomalies are defined as developmental malformations that are outside the limits of what is "normal." In the classic definition by Schwalbe (1906) (24), any deviation from the "normal range" during morphogenesis constitutes an anomaly. Minor anomalies and developmental disturbances at the microscopic, molecular, and functional levels often exist on a continuum with nonpathological normal variants.

Minor and major anomalies. In the definition established by the European Union Registry of Congenital Anomalies and Twins (EUROCAT) (5, 6), a distinction is drawn between minor and major anomalies:
"Minor anomalies" are malformations that are definitely present but are minimal and usually have no functional significance (e.g., ear tags). "Major anomalies" are defined as malformations that affect viability and/or the quality of life and require intervention.

Basic Teratologic Concepts

Teratogenic insult. Morphologic abnormalities represent only a small part of the developmental abnormalities that may affect the human embryo and fetus. As a result, teratology has long since lost the connotation of monstrous deformities that the prefix "terato" implies.

Today the term "teratogenic insults" usually refers to early injuries of any kind, including functional and regulatory disturbances that often do not become apparent until postnatal development. This has led to the widespread use of the term "congenital anomalies" and "birth defects" to describe any structural, functional, or biochemical abnormality.

Embryotoxic insult. This is a collective term for any exogenous disturbance of embryonic development ranging from reversible, curable insults to irreversible, fatal ones. Only a small percentage of these embryotoxic or fetotoxic influences are manifested by a disruption of morphogenesis and can thus be classified as "teratogenic" in the strict sense of the term.

Malformations. Malformations are morphologic defects affecting one or more organs, organ systems, or the entire body that occur during intrauterine development and are outside the normal range of variation of the species (Fig. 20.1). They are based on a primary developmental abnormality, distinguishing them from deformations and disruptions.

Anomalies. Anomalies in the strict sense refer to malformations that are on a continuum with normal variants (e.g., hypertelorism) (Fig. 20.1). But in conventional usage, the term "anomalies" is broadly applied to all birth defects.

Dysplasias. Dysplasias are defects that result from abnormalities in the organization of cells (dysplasiogenesis). By their nature, they are dynamic changes that do not reach their full extent until the cessation of body growth after puberty. This distinguishes them from malformations and anomalies, which have already become static by the completion of intrauterine growth and development.

Classification

Malformations, anomalies, and dysplasias can be classified as outlined below with regard to their time of onset, their morphogenesis, or their etiology during ontogenesis (19).

Ontogenic Classification

Individual development (ontogenesis) consists of two broad stages: (1) progenesis, in which the oocytes and sperm cells form (gametogenesis), migrate for a time, and then unite to form the zygote, and (2) cyemogenesis, consisting of the segmentation and blastocyst stage (blastogenesis), embryonic development (embryogenesis), fetal development (fetogenesis), and postfetal development.

Defects of ontogenesis can be classified as follows based on the timing of their occurrence:
- **Gametopathies:** defects that are based on abnormalities of the oocytes or sperm cells (gametes).
- **Blastopathies:** defects that are based on a developmental disturbance during blastogenesis (days 0–16 of embryonic development, or as late as day 18).
- **Embryopathies:** defects caused by developmental abnormalities that occur during embryogenesis (weeks 3–8 of embryonic development, or weeks 5–10 of gestation).
- **Fetopathies:** diseases of the fetus (9th embryonic week or later), which can lead to local or general growth disturbances or local residual defects during intrauterine or postnatal life.

Teratologic determination period. The experimentally derived law relating congenital anomalies to periods of development states that genetic defects and a variety of environmental (peristatic) factors must become active during a certain period of time in order to produce a certain pattern of injury. While we must be careful in applying experimental findings to humans, the insights that have been gained in pathologic anatomy and embryology point to the existence of a definite period in which any given anomaly can originate. Schwalbe (24) calls this the teratologic determination period. The teratologic determination point is the latest point at which a (genetic or exogenous) cause must become active in order to steer normal development in the direction of an anomaly.

Critical periods. Critical periods are periods in which there is a generally increased "accident risk" relating to a period of increased biochemical and biomorphologic activity. Critical periods should not be confused with sensitive periods, which are characterized by a particularly high sensitivity to (certain?) exogenous agents. Both periods may coincide, but they need not do so.

Organotropism. A number of exogenous teratogenic agents are organotropic, meaning that they have a certain affinity for particular developing organs. The effects of these agents are not very specific in humans, however. For example, twins with thalidomide embryopathy may each acquire a different pattern of anomalies even though they developed in the same uterus and were exposed to the same organotropic agent at the same time.

Thus, besides the timing of the exposure, the resulting anomaly depends on the nature of the teratogenic agent, the genetic background, and ecologic factors in the uterine environment. Consequently we can rarely assign particular anomalies in humans to specific teratogenic agents by referring to a timetable, and we can never pinpoint the time at which a teratogenic agent acts on the developing embryo. As a general rule, however, earlier times of exposure to environmental (peristatic) insults are associated with more severe congenital anomalies.

Morphogenetic Classification

With the tremendous advances that have been made in prenatal diagnosis, human genetics, obstetrics, pediatrics, and teratologic preventive medicine in recent years, there is a pressing need for a standard nomenclature that goes beyond pure description in order to facilitate interdisciplinary communication. The formal pathogenesis of a particular anomaly is of key importance in evaluating the importance of the condition and offering a prognosis. The following terms are used in classifying anomalies based on their pathogenesis:

- **Agenesis:** the absence of an organ or body part due to failure of appearance of the primordial organ (e.g., unilateral or bilateral renal agenesis).
- **Aplasia:** the absence of an organ or body part due to failure of development of a primordial organ, which is present only in rudimentary form (e.g., renal aplasia).
- **Atresia:** special form of aplasia marked by the absence of a normal body orifice or cavity (e.g., anal atresia, esophageal atresia).
- **Hypoplasia:** abnormal smallness of an organ or body part due to the premature cessation of growth (e.g., renal hypoplasia).
- **Stenosis:** special form of hypoplasia marked by the narrowness of an orifice, duct, or cavity (e.g., pulmonary stenosis, coarctation of the aorta).
- **Dysraphia:** an abnormal cleft due to the incomplete closure of embryonic lines of fusion (e.g., neural tube defects).
- **Vestigium:** developmental defect marked by the persistence of organs or organelles that normally regresses during intrauterine development (e.g., fistula due to persistence of the thyroglossal duct, umbilical fistula due to persistence of the omphaloenteric duct).
- **Hamartia:** local aberrant development of a tissue structure—i.e., local dysplasia. When tumor-like, the anomaly is also called a hamartoma. Hamartias are derivatives of a germ layer (e.g., cavernous hemangioma).
- **Chorista:** abnormally structured, heterotopic tissue that probably results from the displacement of differentiated tissues ("germs") into a different germ layer (e.g., heterotopic adrenal cortex). Choristas can also occur after the cessation of developmental growth (e.g., traumatic epidermal cyst).
- **Cyst:** an epithelium-lined cavity produced by excessive epithelial proliferation or the retention of substances that are normally secreted onto internal or external surfaces (e.g., renal cysts, dermoid cyst occurring as a retention cyst in a chorista, lateral cervical cyst occurring as a retention cyst in a vestigium).
- **Redundant development:** general or partial overgrowth of the organism or individual organs or the development of accessory organs or organ parts.
- **Atavism:** the reappearance of phylogenetically primitive structures (e.g., polymastia).

Multiple anomalies. Multiple anomalies can occur randomly in an individual as separate, mutually independent defects, or they may occur in certain combinations that have a common cause or interrelated pathogenesis. Additionally, there are multiple anomalies that occur together more frequently than by chance alone but whose interrelationship is not yet fully understood. The following terms are used to describe the varying patterns in which multiple anomalies can occur:

- **Field defect:** a pattern of anomalies that is based on the disturbance of a single embryonic developmental field. It is caused by a single defect that may be primary (malformation) or secondary (disruption) in nature (e.g., holoprosencephaly).
- **Sequence:** a pattern of multiple anomalies that develop as a chain reaction following a single primary or secondary disturbance (e.g., myelomeningocele sequence, Potter sequence).
- **Syndrome:** a pattern of multiple anomalies that are apparently based on a common primary or secondary disturbance in more than one developmental field (e.g., Down syndrome, Marfan syndrome, rubella syndrome).
- **Association:** two or more anomalies that occur together more frequently than by chance alone and, based on current knowledge, are not (yet) classifiable as a field defect, sequence, or syndrome (e.g., VATER association).
- **Congenital disease:** an anomaly with a conditioned pattern of progression and a tendency to become worse with aging (e.g., glycogen storage disease).

Etiologic Classification

The following terms can be used when the basic cause of an anomaly is known. Since this applies to a relatively few cases at the time of evaluation (phenotypic mapping), from a practical standpoint they cannot replace "congenital anomalies" as a collective term for birth defects.

- **Malformation:** a primary morphologic or structural abnormality in an organ, organ part, or body part based on a lack of development, redundant development, or heterotopia.
- **Disruption:** a secondary morphologic abnormality resulting from exogenous injury to a previously healthy organ, organ part, or body part.
- **Deformation:** an abnormal form, size, or position of an organ, organ part, or body part resulting from a local mechanical force in utero (e.g., in Potter sequence).

General Etiology

The cause of a congenital anomaly can be reliably determined in only a small percentage of cases. From a statistical standpoint, approximately 20% of anomalies in live-born infants are based on a defective gene, 10% are due to chromosomal abnormalities, and 10% are due mainly to exogenous injury to the conceptus. Some 60% of all congenital anomalies probably result from the interaction of adverse hereditary factors and environmental influences (Table 20.**1**).

Genetic Causes

Chromosomal abnormalities. Chromosomal aberrations can be diagnosed with relatively high confidence, as their morphologic features correspond to a particular karyotype. They almost always occur sporadically. Inheritance in the accepted sense is unusual.

Monogenic hereditary diseases. A second group consists of monogenic hereditary diseases. A familial occurrence is characteristic, and often there is a 25% or 50% risk of recurrence for first-degree relatives.

Sporadic new mutations. Problems in evaluation arise when a dominant congenital defect is so severe that it precludes reproduction. All of these cases are sporadic new mutations. A genetic etiology is indicated only by a lack of evidence for an external cause, concordance in monozygotic twins, and perhaps by the statistical dependence of new mutations on the age of the father.

Problem cases. Genetic analysis is also problematic in anomalies where no definite relationship exists between the genotype and phenotype. Many dominant genes are manifested in quantitatively and qualitatively different ways in different carriers. Their manifestation often depends largely on the overall hereditary disposition of the carrier and probably depend on environmental influences as well.

Anomalies with a multifactorial cause. The hypothesis that known or still-unknown exogenous factors also play a role in the third group of genetic defects, the multifactorial anomalies, is controversial. It is weakened by the essentially constant incidence of these anomalies in different countries and at different times.

Exogenous Causes

There is no longer any question that environmental influences can cause injuries and anomalies in both genetically normal and genetically predisposed embryos. However, the number of environmental factors that can withstand critical analysis in this regard is comparatively small.

Teratogenic agents in the strict sense. These are agents that can produce their injurious effect during embryonic development. They include high doses of ionizing radiation, cytostatic agents (e.g., aminopterin), thalidomide, rubella virus, and severe forms of maternal diabetes mellitus. Many other factors are considered suspect, but their teratogenic effects in humans have not yet been proved (e.g., oxygen lack, low-level diagnostic x-rays).

Only some effects actually produce anomalies that are teratogenic by definition (Fig. 20.**2**).

Embryopathies. Embryogenesis is essentially complete by the end of the 8th to 10th week of embryonic life, but there is no sharp dividing line between the embryonic and fetal periods. Since most embryonic cells are already differentiated by this time, so that the early daughter cells of the zygote are no longer pluripotent, a developmental disturbance that occurs during fetogenesis can no longer cause a duplication anomaly but can still cause anomalies in the individual. The earlier embryogenesis is impaired due to genetic defects or peristatic influences, the more severe the resulting abnormalities.

Although most disturbances of embryogenesis are due entirely or partly to genetic causes, the term "embryopathy" in clinical parlance is generally applied only to anomalies that have a known exogenous cause.

Alcohol and Diabetes Mellitus

Maternal alcohol abuse and diabetes mellitus consistently produce a teratogenic effect even during the fetal period. These factors, then, can cause both embryopathies and fetopathies.

Infections

Infectious agents besides the rubella virus have been identified as causing serious malformations in newborns: the Cytomegalovirus, the protozoon *Toxoplasma gondii,* the bacterium *Listeria monocytogenes,* and *Treponema pallidum.*

While early rubella infection leads to typical rubella embryopathy with Gregg syndrome (cataract formation, sensorineural hearing loss, heart defects), the other organisms generally are not harmful until the fetal period. But the resulting fetal disorders often lead to such profound developmental disturbances, especially in the brain, that they are classified along with the rubella virus as teratogenic organisms.

Radiation Embryopathy (29)

Experimental results. The teratogenic effects of ionizing radiation were observed as early as 1907, just a few years after the discovery of x-rays. The effects occurred in rabbits born to mothers that had been irradiated during early pregnancy. The animals displayed ocular anomalies that included microphthalmia, cataracts, and underdeveloped eyelids. Since then, ionizing radiation has played a large role in experimental teratology and especially in neuroteratology owing to the very high radiosensitivity of neuroblasts in the embryo. These are small, round, very metabolically active cells that still have a limited replicative capacity and transform into neurons by forming processes. The irradiation of these cells has profound effects because the destroyed cells cannot be replaced. In the rat, the first neuroblasts appear on the 7th day of embryonic development. A radiation dose of 25–40 rad on day 9 is sufficient to destroy these primitive neuroblasts. On day 12, a dose of 200–300 rad is necessary to produce the same effect. Thus, these cells become less radiosensitive as maturation proceeds.

Radiosensitivity in humans. The first neuroblasts in humans appear on the 23rd day after conception. Maximum radiosensitivity occurs between the 5th and 13th weeks of embryonic development. The human brain may remain vulnerable to extremely high radiation doses even after birth, however. Findings in survivors of the A-bomb blast in Hiroshima are consistent with findings in animal experiments and con-

Basic principles in the diagnosis of fetal anomalies

Fig. 20.1 "Normal" is only the mean of what is considered a natural range of variation in a healthy population. The manifestation of individual traits follows a gaussian distribution. Anomalies are manifestations outside the normal range that is considered typical for the species (from [19]).

Fig. 20.2 Effects of exogenous insults to the developing embryo. Only a small percentage of these insults lead to congenital anomalies, fitting the definition of teratogenic (from [19]).

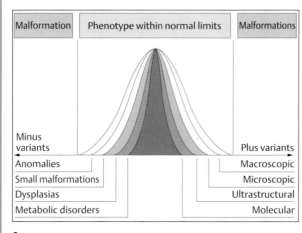

1

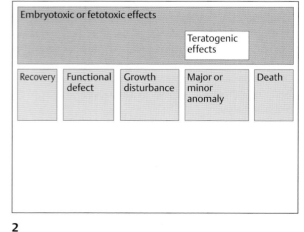

2

firm the high radiosensitivity of nerve cells between weeks 5 and 13 and the dose-dependence of the resulting injuries.

Radiation injuries. A number of radiation-induced injuries to human embryos have been known since the early days of radiography. The effects include microcephaly, mental retardation, ocular damage, growth retardation, and sporadic skeletal malformations. Many observations involved cases in which radiation exposure had occurred without knowledge of the pregnancy or of the possible harmful effects.

Radiation exposure. Experience to date indicates that maternal exposure to diagnostic x-rays of 5 rad or less does not pose a serious risk to embryofetal development.

Environmental Factors

While the number of established teratogenic agents is relatively small, there are many environmental factors that, while not causing embryopathy in the strict sense, can still compromise the growth and development of the fetus. The scale ranges from maternal enzymopathic metabolic disorders, deficiency diseases, and endocrine disorders to antifetal immune response, amniogenic or transplacental infections, and acute or chronic transplacental intoxications. Because fetal development into a mature, viable neonate occurs on a continuum, some fetal disorders take a course similar to that seen in the postnatal period. Other fetopathies display features that are specific for the fetal period.

Multifactorial Anomalies

A number of anomalies result from the interaction of several teratogenic agents. Anomalies with a multifactorial etiology include neural tube defects, limb malformations, abnormalities of sexual differentiation, and malrotation anomalies.

▬ Incidence of Fetal Anomalies

The incidence of congenital anomalies in live-born infants is between 1.3% and 4.5% (14, 27). If we add stillborn infants that weigh more than 1000 g, the incidence of congenital anomalies is two to three times higher (7, 23, 28).

Recent studies employing an active rather than passive detection system indicate that the incidence of fetal anomalies, including congenital hip dysplasia, is as high as 7.3% (20).

General Ultrasound Diagnosis of Fetal Anomalies

▬ Detection of Fetal Anomalies

The successful detection of fetal anomalies with ultrasound requires a detailed knowledge of the normal ultrasound anatomy of the fetus and a knowledge of the most common fetal anomalies and sequences so that ultrasound findings can be correctly interpreted.

Multilevel concept. Adequate experience can be gained only by the frequent observation of pathologic findings. This led Hansmann (9, 10) in 1981 to state the need for a multilevel system (proficiency levels I–III) for detecting and excluding fetal anomalies. According to this concept, every physician who performs level I ultrasound screening examinations in pregnant women (see Chapter 2) exercises a "filtering function" by noting suspicious findings and then referring the patient to a level II facility for further evaluation to confirm or exclude an anomaly. Level III centers function as the final problem solvers. However, this

three-tiered system can work only if ultrasound abnormalities are recognized during the initial screening examination. Only a few anomalies such as anencephaly or severe hydrocephalus are easy to detect even by an inexperienced examiner. In the great majority of cases, the accurate diagnosis of a fetal anomaly requires a detailed and often time-consuming ultrasound examination conducted by a highly experienced examiner using up-to-date equipment.

Favorable Periods for Detecting Fetal Anomalies, and Suggestive Ultrasound Signs

Diagnostic windows. There are two diagnostic time windows that are most favorable for detecting the suggestive signs of a fetal anomaly (Table 20.**2**). The first window is the period between 11 and 14 weeks' gestation. The second window is between 18 and 22 weeks.

The most important sign during the first window is increased nuchal translucency thickness (25) (Fig. 20.**3**). This sign not only suggests a chromosomal abnormality but is also associated with cardiac anomalies and other morphologic defects (see Chapter 2) (25, 26).

During the second time window, various suggestive signs of a fetal anomaly may be observed (Table 20.**2**). By this time the fetal organs have matured to a point where a variety of malformations can be directly visualized.

Abnormal amniotic fluid volume. The most important suggestive sign during the second and third trimesters is an abnormal amniotic fluid volume. A markedly increased amniotic fluid volume (polyhydramnios, Fig. 20.**4**), a decreased fluid volume (oligohydramnios), or the absence of amniotic fluid (anhydramnios, Fig. 20.**5**) are associated with an increased rate of fetal anomalies. There is a 7.9% (34) to 18% (11) association of fetal anomalies with polyhydramnios, and a 7% (17) to 13% (1, 21) association with oligohydramnios. Polyhydramnios is most often seen in conjunction with neural tube defects, gastrointestinal anomalies, and cardiovascular defects (30). Oligohydramnios is more suggestive of renal anomalies or urinary tract obstruction. Anhydramnios is most commonly associated with original Potter syndrome (bilateral renal agenesis).

When a decreased amniotic fluid volume is noted, rupture of the fetal membranes should be excluded before any further steps are taken.

Table 20.1 Causes of fetal anomalies (13, 19, 31)

Hereditary disease	20%
Chromosomal abnormalities	10%
Environmental insults	10%
Indeterminate or multifactorial causes	60%

Table 20.2 Ultrasound signs that suggest the presence of a fetal anomaly

First trimester

- Nuchal translucency thickness ≥ 3 mm

Second and third trimesters

- Abnormal amniotic fluid volume (polyhydramnios, oligohydramnios, anhydramnios)
- Fetal growth disturbance (early growth retardation, macrosomia)
- Disproportion of individual body parts (abnormal head/trunk ratio or head/limb ratio)
- Body surface abnormalities (defect, protrusion, abnormal head shape [lemon sign, strawberry skull])
- Abnormal internal structures (fluid, cavity, atypical four-chamber view, abnormal cerebellar shape [banana sign])
- Cardiac arrhythmias (especially bradyarrhythmia)
- Abnormal pattern of fetal movements (hypo- or hyperactivity)
- Absence of an umbilical cord artery
- Abnormal placental structure (vacuolated placenta)

Growth disturbances. In the case of growth disturbances, early IUGR as well as macrosomia may be indicative of a fetal anomaly (see Chapters 12 and 16). Ramzin et al. (22) report an 11% incidence of anomalies in fetuses showing growth retardation before 28 weeks and 17% in fetuses showing macrosomic growth. Early IUGR is especially likely to signify a chromosomal abnormality (3, 9, 15).

Disproportional growth. A disproportion between the fetal head and trunk is seen in advanced hydrocephalus, microcephaly, and severe prune belly syndrome. A disproportion between the head and limb bones is seen in the various forms of dwarfism.

Surface abnormalities. An abnormal body contour may appear as a defect (anencephaly), deformation (lemon sign, Fig. 20.**6**), or protrusion in the body surface (omphalocele, myelomeningocele, cystic hygroma).

Internal abnormalities. These may consist of fluid collections, an accessory cavity or mass, organ displacement, or an abnormal-appearing organ structure.

Depending on their location, intrafetal cystic masses may signify a gastrointestinal obstruction or urinary stasis. Organ displacement, such as dextrocardia, is seen in fetuses with a diaphragmatic hernia. Fluid collections in the fetal abdomen or thorax always indicate a serious abnormality and require prompt investigation. Remarkable organ structures, such as an abnormal-appearing four-chamber view (Fig. 20.**7**), are suspicious for an organ malformation.

Cardiac arrhythmias. Fetal cardiac arrhythmias, especially bradycardia and bradyarrhythmia (Fig. 20.**8**), warrant very close scrutiny of the heart, as it is not unusual to find an underlying heart defect as the cause.

Increased or decreased motor activity. In observing fetal movements, the examiner should watch for increased or decreased motor activity. Hectic or spasmodic movements are found in CNS defects (anencephaly), while a paucity of movements may signify a passive constraint of fetal mobility (oligohydramnios) or a true motor defect (myelomeningocele, arthrogryposis multiplex congenita).

Single umbilical artery. On observation of the umbilical cord, only one umbilical artery is seen in approximately 1% of cases (8) (Fig. 20.**9**). Careful attention should be given to this finding, for a single umbilical artery is associated with a 7% (4) to 50% (2) incidence of fetal anomalies.

Placenta. An abnormal thickness or structure of the placenta may also suggest a fetal anomaly or fetal disorder. For example, a placental thickness greater than 5 cm may signify hemolytic disease (12) while a large, vacuolated placenta may indicate triploidy (3) (Fig. 20.**10**).

■ *Exclusion of Anomalies*

Risk of recurrence. The function of prenatal ultrasound in most cases is to exclude rather than detect a fetal anomaly. This particularly applies to cases in which there is an increased risk of recurrence.

Today the availability of intensive prenatal ultrasound can relieve the fears of many parents that they will have a deformed child. In particular, it can offer hope and encouragement to couples who formerly were advised to avoid further pregnancy due to an increased familial risk for the recurrence of an anomaly.

Undetectable defects. At the same time, patients should realize that the ultrasound examination does not guarantee a healthy child. There are some defects (chromosomal defects, metabolic disorders) that even a detailed ultrasound examination either cannot detect or can only

suggest based on indirect markers. Also, it should be noted that the purpose of a screening examination is not to exclude all malformations but simply to serve as a filter for suspicious findings, which should then be referred for a more detailed investigation.

Implications of Suggestive Signs or a Detected Fetal Anomaly

If ultrasound demonstrates one of the suggestive signs listed in Table 20.**2**, this raises the possibility that a fetal anomaly is present. To confirm or exclude a fetal anomaly, the patient should be referred to a level II or level III facility for a more detailed evaluation.

If a fetal anomaly is confirmed sonographically at that facility, several options may be considered depending on the severity of the lesion (Tables 20.**3**, 20.**4**), the length of gestation, and the attitude of the parents.

Grouping fetal anomalies. Sonographically detected fetal anomalies or diseases are generally grouped according their treatability (Table 20.**3**) or the ability of the affected infant to survive (Table 20.**4**). Both classifications are closely interrelated.

■ *Anomalies and Diseases that are Incompatible with Postnatal Life*

If the detected anomaly is incompatible with life (anencephaly, thanatophoric dwarfism, original Potter syndrome), it is up to the patient to decide whether or not to terminate the pregnancy. This decision can be made without regard for gestational age. If the anomaly is not detected until the third trimester and the patient does not desire pregnancy termination, it is at least possible to avoid measures that would place an extra burden on the mother, such as prolonged tocolytic therapy or cesarean section.

■ *Fetal Anomalies and Diseases with Limited or Doubtful Postnatal Survival*

This group includes disorders in which long-term survival is doubtful (e.g., bilateral Potter I kidneys). In a broader sense, it also includes anomalies that are surgically treatable after birth but still have a dubious prognosis (e.g., severe spina bifida).

Diagnosis before reaching viability. If a fetal anomaly of uncertain outcome is detected before viability is reached (generally up to 24 weeks), it is up to the patient to decide whether pregnancy termination is an option. Preterm induction after 24 weeks is not advised, because the infant may survive and the preterm delivery would compound the infant's problems.

Table 20.**3**   Grouping of fetal anomalies and diseases by treatability

1. Anomalies that are not treatable after birth
2. Anomalies that are surgically treatable after birth but not with full curative intent
3. Anomalies that are surgically treatable after birth with full curative intent
4. Anomalies or disorders that are accessible to intrauterine treatment

Table 20.**4**   Grouping of fetal anomalies and diseases by survivability

1. Fetal anomalies and diseases that are incompatible with postnatal survival
2. Fetal anomalies and diseases with a limited, dubious, or questionable potential for postnatal survival
3. Fetal anomalies and diseases with a high likelihood of postnatal survival

Diagnosis after reaching viability. If the diagnosis is made after viability is reached and the patient desires to terminate the pregnancy, the diagnosis should be confirmed by securing a second qualified opinion on the fetal anomaly or disease, and an interdisciplinary consensus should be reached on the procedure that should be used at the institution in question. Fetocide prior to termination is an option that can be discussed with the patient or parents as a means of sparing the fetus the suffering that might result from the termination procedure (32).

Fetal Anomalies and Diseases with a High Likelihood of Postnatal Survival

This group includes anomalies and diseases that are accessible to intrauterine treatment, also anomalies that are surgically treatable after birth with curative intent.

Anomalies accessible to intrauterine treatment. The intrauterine treatment of a fetal anomaly or disease should be done at an experienced prenatal center whenever possible in order to minimize the risk to the fetus. Successful treatment also relies on interdisciplinary cooperation and effective facilities for neonatal intensive care.

Anomalies treatable after birth. With the early detection of an anomaly that normally can be treated after birth with curative intent (e.g., omphalocele), a search should be conducted for additional anomalies, and invasive diagnostic tests (amniocentesis, cordocentesis) should be applied as needed to determine the karyotype. If these tests reveal additional anomalies or a chromosomal abnormality, it is up to the patient to decide whether to terminate or continue the pregnancy. Conscientious interdisciplinary cooperation is essential for responsible, effective parental counseling in these cases.

Obstetric and neonatal management. If tests do not show significant additional anomalies, the prognosis for the newborn infant can be improved by judicious selection of the site, timing, and mode of the delivery and by planning for the care of the neonate. In particular, the risks and stresses of transporting the newborn infant can be avoided by referring the mother early to a perinatal center offering the services of a pediatric surgeon or neurosurgeon (16).

Counseling Before and After Prenatal Diagnosis

Counseling Before Prenatal Diagnosis

Necessary information. The complexity of prenatal diagnosis requires that the patient be given appropriate, ongoing counseling and information from the time of her initial visit (32). This pertains not only to targeted imaging for fetal anomalies but also to more general prenatal tests such as routine ultrasound scans. The counseling and information requirement should be appropriate for the timing of the examination and the age of the pregnancy.

Patient counseling should cover the information points listed in Table 20.**5**.

Informed consent. Informed consent is an essential prerequisite for any measure in prenatal diagnosis. The German Society for Ultrasound in Medicine (DEGUM) recommends that all pregnant patients, especially those seeking a targeted prenatal ultrasound examination, sign an information sheet that explains the goals and the limitations of prenatal diagnosis.

Counseling After Prenatal Diagnosis

Reporting the result. If a fetal anomaly is detected, it is the job of the attending and/or counseling physician to report the findings to the patient. He or she should cover all of the points listed in Table 20.**6**.

Table 20.5 Information that should be given to patients before prenatal diagnosis (after [33])

> ➤ Reason for the examination
> ➤ Goal of the examination
> ➤ Risk of the examination
> ➤ Limitations of prenatal diagnosis (disorders that cannot be detected prenatally)
> ➤ Accuracy of the result
> ➤ Nature and severity of potential or presumed disorders
> ➤ Options when an abnormality is found
> ➤ Psychological and ethical conflicts that may arise when an abnormality is found
> ➤ Possible alternatives to invasive prenatal tests

Table 20.6 Information that should be given to patients when a fetal anomaly has been detected (after [33])

> ➤ Significance of the finding
> ➤ Cause, nature, and prognosis of the detected disease or developmental abnormality
> ➤ Possible complications
> ➤ Pre- and postnatal treatment and assistance options
> ➤ Implications for obstetric management (site, time, and mode)
> ➤ Alternatives: continue or terminate the pregnancy
> ➤ Contact options for support groups and persons with similar problems
> ➤ Medical and social aid options

Counseling by a specialist. During initial counseling by the prenatal diagnostician, the patient should be offered the option of counseling by a specialist (18). This may be a neonatologist, pediatrician, geneticist, pediatric surgeon, neurosurgeon, pediatric cardiologist, pediatric neurologist, or other specialist depending on the nature of the problem. It should be noted that all subsequent counselors must rely entirely on the information that the prenatal diagnostician has provided them.

After the parents have received the necessary counseling and information, they should be given time to think before making a final decision.

References

1. Bastide, A., Manning, F., Harman, C., Lnage, I., Morrsion, I.: Ultrasound evaluation of amniotic fluid: Outcome of pregnancies with severe oligohydramnios. Amer. J. Obstet. Gynecol. 154 (1986) 895–900
2. Catanzarite, V.A., Hendricks, S.K., Maida, C., Westbrook, C., Cousins, L., Schrimmer, D.: Prenatal diagnosis of the two-vessel cord: implications for patient counseling and obstetric management. Ultrasound Obstet. Gynecol. 5 (1995) 98–105
3. Claussen, U., Hansmann, M.: Die Pipettenmethode zur schnellen Karyotypisierung bei sonographischen Verdachtskriterien für eine Chromosomenanomalie. Gynäkologe 17 (1984) 33–40
4. Csecsi, K., Kovacs, T., Hinchliffe, S.A., Papp, Z.: Incidence and associations of single umbilical artery in prenatally diagnosed malformed midtrimester fetuses: a review of 62 cases. Amer. J. Med. Genet. 43 (1992) 524–530
5. EUROCAT report: Surveillance of Congenital Anomalies 1980–1988. Eurocat Central registry, Department of Epidemiology, Catholic University of Louvain, Brussels 1991
6. EUROCAT report 6: Surveillance of Congenital Anomalies in Europe 1980–1992, Brussels: EUROCAT Central Registry, Institute of Hygiene and Epidemiology (1995)
7. Födisch, H.J., Knöpfle, G.: Patho-anatomische Teratologie. Eine aktuelle Herausforderung. Gynäkologe 17 (1984) 2–12
8. Froehlich, L.A., Fujikura, T.: Significance of a single umbilical artery. Report from the collaborative study of cerebral palsy. Amer. J. Obstet. Gynec. 94 (1966) 274–279
9. Hansmann, M.: Nachweis und Ausschluß fetaler Entwicklungsstörungen mittels Ultraschallscreening und gezielter Untersuchung – ein Mehrstufenkonzept. Ultraschall 2 (1981) 206–220
10. Hansmann, M.: Ultraschallscreening in der Schwangerschaft – Vorsicht vor übertriebenen Forderungen. Geburtsh. u. Frauenheilk. 41 (1981) 725–728
11. Hobbins, J.C., Grannum, P.A.T., Berkowitz, R.L., Silverman, R., Mahoney, M.: Ultrasound in the diagnosis of congenital anomalies. Amer. J. Obstet. Gynec. 134 (1979) 331–345
12. Holländer, H.J.: Die Ultraschalldiagnostik während der Schwangerschaft. In: Döderlein, G., Wulf, K.H.: Klinik der Frauenheilkunde und Geburtshilfe, Bd. VI. München: Urban & Schwarzenberg 1975; S. 736
13. Kalter, H., Warkany, J.: Congenital malformations. New Engl. J. Med. 308 (1983) 424–431
14. Kennedy, W.P.: Epidemiological aspects of the problem of congenital malformations. Birth Defects Orig. 3 (1967) 1
15. Kurjak, A., Kirkinen, P., Latin, V., Raijhvajn, B.: Diagnosis and assessment of fetal malformations and abnormalities. J. perinat. Med. 8 (1980) 219–235
16. Lamont, R.F., Dunlop, P.D.M., Crowley, P., Levene, M.I., Elder, M.G.: Comparative mortality and morbidity of infants transferred in utero or postnatally. J. perinat. Med. 11 (1983) 200–203

17. Mercer, L.J., Brown, L.G., Petres, R.E., Messer, R.H.: A survey of pregnancies complicated by decreased amniotic fluid. Amer. J. Obstet. Gynecol. 149 (1984) 355–361

18. Merz, E., Hackelöer, B.J., Wisser, J. et al.: Stellungnahme der Sektion Gynäkologie und Geburtshilfe der Deutschen Gesellschaft für Ultraschall in der Medizin (DEGUM), der Deutschen Gesellschaft für Pränatal- und Geburtsmedizin, der Arbeitsgemeinschaft für Ultraschalldiagnostik in der Deutschen Gesellschaft für Gynäkologie und Geburtshilfe und der Arbeitsgemeinschaft für Dopplersonographie und materno-fetale Medizin zu der im Frauenarzt 2/98 publizierten Erklärung zum Schwangerschaftsabbruch nach Pränataldiagnostik. Frauenarzt 39 (1998) 650–652

19. Müntefering, H.: Fehlbildungen. In: Riede, U.N., Wehner, H. (Hrsg.): Allgemeine und spezielle Pathologie. Stuttgart: Thieme 1986; S. 256–278

20. Queisser-Luft, A., Stopfkuchen, H., Stolz, G., Schlaefer, K., Merz, E.: Prenatal diagnosis of major malformations: Quality control of routine ultrasound examinations based on a five-year study of 20 248 newborn fetuses and infants. Prenat. Diagn. 18 (1998) 567–576

21. Rabe, D., Leucht, W., Hendrik, H.J., Boos, R., Schmidt, W.: Sonographische Beurteilung der Fruchtwassermenge. II. Oligohydramnion – Bedeutung für den Schwangerschafts- u. Geburtsverlauf. Geburtsh. u. Frauenheilk. 46 (1986) 422–426

22. Ramzin, M.S., Meudt, R.O., Hinselmann, M.J.: Prognostic significance of abnormal ultrasonic findings during the second trimester of gestation. J. perinat. Med. 1 (1973) 60–64

23. Richards, I.D.: Fetal and infant mortality associated with congenital malformations. Brit. J. prev. soc. Med. 27 (1973) 85–90

24. Schwalbe, E.: Die Morphologie der Mißbildungen des Menschen und der Tiere. 1. Teil: Allgemeine Mißbildungslehre (Teratologie). Jena: Gustav Fischer 1906

25. Snijders, R.J.M., Noble, P., Sebire, N., Souka, A., Nicolaides, K.H. for the Fetal Medicine Foundation First Trimester Screening Group. UK multicentre project on assessment of risk of trisomy 21 by maternal age and fetal nuchal-translucency thickness at 10–14 weeks of gestation. Lancet 351 (1998) 343–346

26. Souka, A.P., Nicolaides, K.H.: Diagnosis of fetal abnormalities at the 10–14-week scan. Ultrasound Obstet. Gynecol. 10 (1997) 429–442

27. Stevenson, A.C., Johnston, H.A., Stewart, M.I., Golding, D.R.: Congenital malformations: A report of a series of consecutive birth in 24 centers. Bull. WHO, Suppl. 34 (1966) 9–127

28. Stocks, P.: Incidence of congenital malformations in the region of England and Wales. Brit. J. prev. soc. Med. 24 (1970) 67–77

29. Töndury, G.: Formen der wichtigsten Embryopathien. AMI-Berichte 1 (1978) 36–42

30. Wallenburg, H.C., Wladimiroff, J.W.: The amniotic fluid. II. Polyhydramnios and oligohydramnios. J. perinat. Med. 6 (1977) 233–243

31. Wilson, J.G.: Environment and Birth Defects. New York: Academic Press 1973

32. Wissenschaftlicher Beirat der Bundesärztekammer – Bekanntmachungen: Erklärung zum Schwangerschaftsabbruch nach Pränataldiagnostik. Dtsch. Ärztebl. 95, Heft 47 (1998) A3013–3016

33. Wissenschaftlicher Beirat der Bundesärztekammer – Bekanntmachungen: Richtlinien zur pränatalen Diagnostik von Krankheiten und Krankheitsdispositionen. Dtsch. Ärztebl. 95, Heft 50 (1998) A3236–3242

34. Zamah, N.M., Gillieson, M.S., Walters, J.H., Hall, P.F.: Sonographic detection of polyhydramnios: A five-year experience. Amer. J. Obstet. Gynec. 143 (1982) 523–527

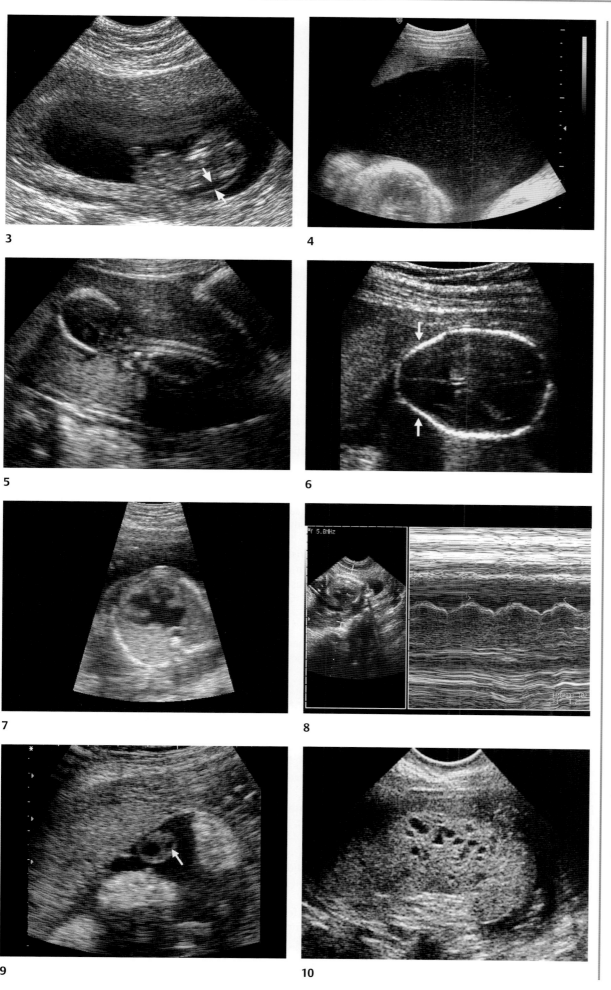

3

4

5

6

7

8

9

10

Fig. 20.**3** Increased nuchal translucency thickness (arrows, 4 mm) at 11 weeks. Karyotype: trisomy 21.

Fig. 20.**4** Massive polyhydramnios at 33 weeks.

Fig. 20.**5** Anhydramnios at 16 weeks, 5 days.

Fig. 20.**6** Lemon sign in a fetus with spina bifida and incipient hydrocephalus. The lateral indentations in the front of the skull (arrows) give the head a lemon-like shape.

Fig. 20.**7** Abnormal four-chamber view in a fetus with an AV canal (20 weeks).

Fig. 20.**8** M-mode tracing shows marked bradycardia (102 bpm) in a fetus with an AV canal (19 weeks).

Fig. 20.**9** Single umbilical cord artery at 29 weeks, 3 days. Transverse scan of the umbilical cord shows only one artery (arrow) adjacent to the large-caliber vein.

Fig. 20.**10** Vacuolated posterior-wall placenta in triploidy (18 weeks).

21 Anomalies of the Head

Neural Tube Defects

Examples of neural tube defects are anencephaly, exencephaly, encephalocele, iniencephaly, and spina bifida. Based on studies by the EUROCAT working group, the incidence of neural tube defects in Europe is 11.5 per 10,000 infants (live-born infants, still-born infants, and abortions). The incidence in Ireland and England is markedly higher, at approximately 24–38 per 10,000 infants (12).

The sections below deal with anencephaly, exencephaly, encephalocele, and iniencephaly. Spina bifida is discussed under anomalies of the spine.

■ Anencephaly

Definition. Absence of the superior vault and cerebrum. Anencephaly is the most common and severe anomaly of the central nervous system. It is also the easiest to diagnose with ultrasound.

Incidence. The reported incidence of anencephaly is one in 1000 births, with a 4 : 1 preponderance of females over males (8).

Etiology and pathogenesis. The causes are multifactorial. Various teratogenic agents such as salicylates (49) and sulfonamides (45) can produce the defect in animal models.

Embryology. The defect results from a failure of dorsal neural tube closure between the second and third weeks of embryonic development (i.e., between the fourth and fifth weeks of gestation).

Pathoanatomic features. The superior vault and cerebrum are absent. The brainstem and portions of the midbrain are present.

Ultrasound features. As early as 1979, Robinson (35) and Kurjak (25) described the reliable ultrasound diagnosis of anencephaly. The most striking feature at ultrasound is the absence of a superior vault and intracranial structures (Figs. 21.**1**–21.**6**) with large, bulging eyes marking the superior boundary of the fetus (Figs. 21.**2**, 21.**5**). The normal elliptical head shape and midline echo are not seen. When the complete body silhouette is observed (Figs. 21.**1**–21.**6**), a marked disproportion is noted between the head and trunk. Abrupt, spasmodic body movements are not uncommon.

Diagnostic problems. If the fetal head is deeply engaged in the lower pelvis, anencephaly may be missed if only the elliptical skull base can be seen. Conversely, a normal fetal head that is very low in the lower pelvis can mimic anencephaly if the superior vault is not visible in the transabdominal scan. If the entire fetal head cannot be seen despite a full maternal bladder, its superior pole can be defined by manually pressing upward on the uterus from the vagina. Usually this will bring the previously obscured upper half of the head into view. Alternatively, transvaginal scanning with an empty bladder will usually afford a complete view of the fetal head.

Time of detection. Anencephaly can be detected sonographically as early as 11 weeks' gestation (4, 37, 39). However, Bronshtein and Ornoy (4) described a case in which the head appeared normal at 9 and 11 weeks, acrania was detected at 12 weeks, and anencephaly was not diagnosed until 14 weeks. Goldstein et al. (16) published a similar case in which anencephaly was missed at 12.5 weeks.

Johnson et al. (21) reported on a multicenter study in which 53,435 single fetuses and 901 twins were screened during the initial phase of the study, and 47 cases of anencephaly were diagnosed with ultrasound. Thirty-nine of the cases were detected between 10 and 14 weeks' gestation and the other 8 between 16 and 22 weeks. Following this initial phase 20,407 fetuses were examined, and in all 16 with anencephaly, the diagnosis was made at the 10- to 14-week ultrasound scan.

Differential diagnosis. Exencephaly (1), amniotic band syndrome (15).

Associated anomalies and chromosomal defects. Polyhydramnios is present in 40–50% of cases, and oligohydramnios is occasionally detected (13). In a review of 30 anencephaly cases, Kurjak (25) found that polyhydramnios did not develop before 25 weeks. The anomaly is frequently associated with a fissure of the vertebral column (craniorachischisis). Cleft lip and palate and omphalocele can also occur as associated anomalies.

Invasive tests. Alpha-fetoprotein (AFP) levels in the amniotic fluid are elevated in more than 90% of cases (46). The amniotic fluid acetylcholinesterase (AChE) assay can detect 98% (48) to 100% (27) of fetuses with anencephaly.

Prognosis and risk of recurrence. The prognosis is grave. Live-born infants die within a few hours or days after birth. When a woman has had one previous infant with anencephaly, the risk of recurrence is approximately 4% (29). The risk following two previous affected infants is 10% (8).

Prenatal management. The severity of the condition justifies terminating the pregnancy at any stage, even in the third trimester.

■ Exencephaly

Definition. In exencephaly (acrania), all or most of the superior vault is absent while brain tissue is present.

Incidence. Exencephaly is much less common than anencephaly (7).

Etiology and pathogenesis. Animal studies have shown that certain teratogenic agents, like the antiepileptic drug valproic acid, can cause exencephaly (33, 44).

Embryology. Evidence indicates that exencephaly is a precursor stage of anencephaly (19, 52).

Pathoanatomic features. Absence of the superior vault. The brain tissue is mostly present but abnormal.

Ultrasound features. The superior vault is absent, leaving the brain tissue uncovered and exposed to the amniotic fluid (Fig. 21.**7**) (7, 19, 22,

47). Kennedy et al. (22) describe the early ultrasound detection of ex-encephaly at 10 weeks.

Differential diagnosis. Anencephaly, amniotic band syndrome.

Associated anomalies. Spina bifida, cleft lip and palate, and club foot (19).

Invasive test. The amniotic fluid AFP is markedly elevated.

Prognosis. Grave.

Prenatal management. As in anencephaly, the severity of the anomaly warrants pregnancy termination at any stage.

Cephalocele

Definition. A defect in the bony skull through which the meninges (superior meningocele) and brain substance (encephalomeningocele) may protrude (51).

Incidence. This anomaly has a reported incidence of one in 2000 live births (40). Frontoethmoid myelomeningoceles are much rarer, with an estimated incidence of one in 40,000 live births (11).

Etiology and pathogenesis. Cephalocele results from a defect of neural tube closure during the sixth week of gestation. Some cases also result from amniotic bands that become wrapped around portions of the brain (amniotic band syndrome) (6).

Pathoanatomic features. The location of the defect is midoccipital in 75% of cases, frontoethmoidal in 13%, and parietal in 12% (36). The bony defect is usually small in relation to the hernial sac (51).

Ultrasound features. Sonographically, the cephalocele appears as a sac-like protrusion at the back of the skull (Figs. 21.**8**–21.**12**). A sac that contains only meninges will appear purely cystic (Fig. 21.**8**), while a sac containing brain and meninges will also contain solid structures depending on the proportion of herniated brain (Figs. 21.**9**–21.**12**). In fetuses with a frontoethmoidal myelomeningocele (Figs. 21.**14**, 21.**15**), a hernial sac will be found between the orbits (11). A definitive diagnosis can be made only by visualizing the bony defect in addition to the hernial sac (6). If the fetal head is low in the pelvis, transvaginal scans will help to define the anomaly (Fig. 21.**12**).

Budorick et al. (5) were able to detect 24 of 26 cephaloceles antenatally. They noted amniotic fluid abnormalities in 14 of the 26 cases: 5 cases of oligohydramnios and 7 cases of polyhydramnios.

Further tests. The maternal serum AFP is frequently elevated (5) but is not always so (43). Very high AFP levels are found in the fluid aspirated from an encephalocele.

Differential diagnosis. Differentiation is required from cervical hygroma, hemangioma, teratoma, and amniotic band syndrome (Fig. 21.**11**). The latter condition should be suspected when the defect is not located at the center of the occiput. With a paucity of amniotic fluid, a loop of umbilical cord adjacent to the occiput can mimic an encephalocele (Fig. 21.**13**). Color Doppler can quickly resolve this issue by detecting blood flow (Fig. 21.**13**). A cystic frontal sac requires differentiation from a lacrimal duct cyst.

Associated anomalies. Hydrocephalus, microcephaly, spina bifida (5, 6, 17). In the study by Budorick et al. (5), additional anomalies were discovered in 17 out of 26 cases (65%). Microcephaly was ob-served in 50% of the cases. The combination of encephalocele and oligohydramnios was the most common association, occurring in 80% of cases.

Special forms. Cephaloceles may occur in isolation or as a feature of various syndromes.

Meckel–Gruber syndrome. This is perhaps the most important syndrome in which cephaloceles may occur (30) (Figs. 21.**10**, 21.**16**). Transmitted as an autosomal-recessive trait (risk of recurrence 25%), the syndrome is characterized by a combination of polycystic kidneys, cephalocele, and postaxial polydactyly. Several cases have been described sonographically (10, 26, 38).

Roberts syndrome. A frontoethmoidal myelomeningocele may be found in the setting of Roberts syndrome (tetraphocomelia syndrome), which is characterized by growth disturbance, severe limb deformities, cleft lip and palate, and other associated anomalies (11).

Prognosis. The prognosis of cephaloceles depends on the location of the defect, the amount of protruding brain tissue, and accompanying anomalies. Additional defects should always be sought at ultrasound, therefore. The concomitant presence of hydrocephalus or microcephaly generally implies a poor prognosis (6). According to Guthkelch (17), the mortality rate is 71% for infants with an encephalocele and 11% for infants with a meningocele. Meckel–Gruber syndrome is fatal.

With an isolated meningocele, almost half of affected infants develop normally following surgical repair (28). By contrast, infants with an encephalocele show significant retardation of mental development (17).

Prenatal management. When the findings are pronounced and when there are associated anomalies that are detected early before viability is reached, pregnancy termination may be considered. If the anomaly is detected late or if there is an isolated meningocele with a large hernial sac, elective cesarean delivery near term is advised to avoid potential rupture of the sac leading to meningitis (11).

Iniencephaly

Definition. Malformation characterized by encephalocele, marked dorsiflexion of the fetal head, and cervical rachischisis.

Incidence. Very rare.

Etiology and pathogenesis. The etiology is uncertain. Animal experiments have shown that the anomaly can be induced by administering certain agents such as streptonigrin (50).

Pathoanatomic features. Due to the enlarged foramen magnum and the absence of cervical vertebrae, the head assumes an extreme dorsiflexed position, and brain may herniate through a fissure in the occiput (20). Due to the extreme lordosis of the cervical spine, the face is directed upward (34) ("stargazer").

Ultrasound features. The ultrasound diagnosis is based on the detection of craniorachischisis with a short spine and marked dorsiflexion of the fetal head (Fig. 21.**17**) (32). Several cases detected prenatally have been described in the literature (3, 14, 18, 24, 31). Sherer et al. (41) described the transvaginal ultrasound diagnosis of iniencephaly at 13 weeks' gestation.

Differential diagnosis. Differentiation is required from cervical myelomeningocele and Klippel–Feil syndrome. The latter is characterized by a short and deformed cervical spine (23).

Associated anomalies. Forty-eight percent of fetuses with iniencephaly have associated anomalies (9) such as anencephaly, holoprosencephaly, polymicrogyria, vermian agenesis, hydrocephalus, cyclopia, cleft lip and palate, cardiovascular disease, diaphragmatic hernia, abdominal wall defects, situs inversus, anal atresia, polycystic kidneys, arthrogryposis multiplex congenita, club foot, and single umbilical artery (2, 9).

Invasive test. The amniotic fluid AFP is markedly elevated because of the cervical rachischisis (42).

Prognosis. The condition is fatal.

Prenatal management. The pregnancy may be terminated.

Anencephaly

Fig. 21.**1**   Anencephaly, 17 weeks. Longitudinal scan shows prominent "frog eyes" with absence of the superior vault (arrow).

Fig. 21.**2**   Postmortem view of the fetus in Fig. 21.**1**. The fetus is still enveloped by the amniotic sac.

Fig. 21.**3**   Anencephaly, 17 weeks, longitudinal scan. The spine is surmounted by an irregularly shaped "hump" in place of the normal skull.

Fig. 21.**4**   Anencephaly, 17 weeks, longitudinal scan.

Fig. 21.**5**   Anencephaly, 23 weeks. Note the absent superior vault and prominent "frog's eye" (arrow).

Fig. 21.**6**   Postmortem view of the fetus in Fig. 21.**5**.

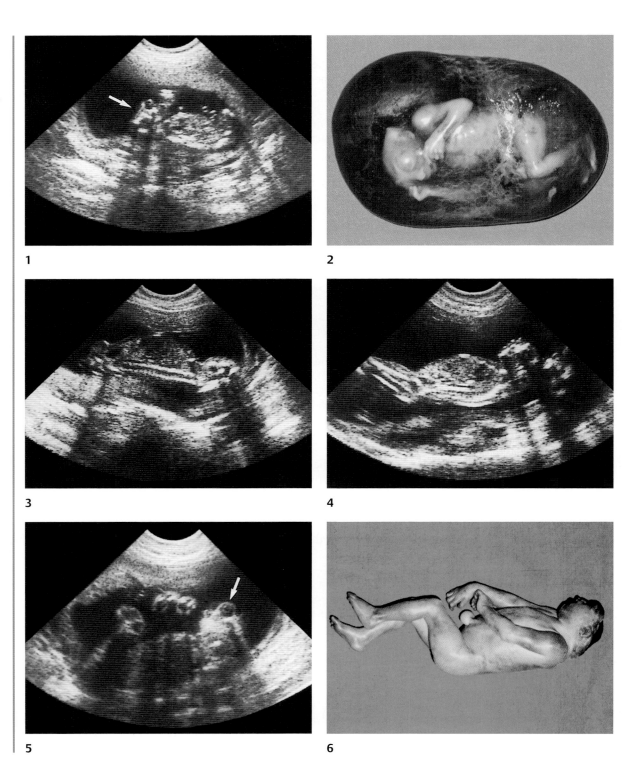

1

2

3

4

5

6

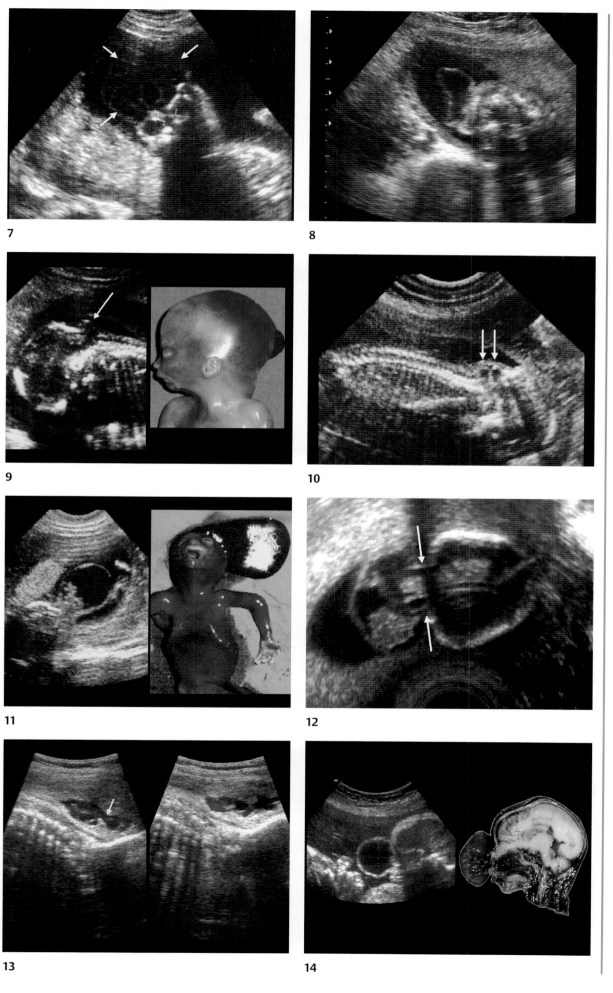

7

8

9

10

11

12

13

14

Exencephaly and cephalocele

Fig. 21.**7** Exencephaly, 19 weeks. Only brain tissue is visible above the orbits (arrows). The superior vault is absent.

Fig. 21.**8** Occipital cephalocele with a purely cystic hernial sac (meningocele) at 20 weeks. The sac was aspirated prior to ultrasound.

Fig. 21.**9** Small occipital encephalocele (1.5 cm), 22 weeks. The inset shows a postmortem view of the fetus.

Fig. 21.**10** Small double encephalocele in Meckel–Gruber syndrome (arrows) at 19 weeks.

Fig. 21.**11** Encephalocele resulting from amniotic band syndrome, 20 weeks. Transverse scan at the level of the superior defect demonstrates hyperechoic brain tissue within the cystic sac. The inset shows a postmortem view of the fetus (photo courtesy of Dr. Doetsch, Bischofsheim, Germany).

Fig. 21.**12** Encephalocele with a large central defect in the occiput (arrows) and a large amount of brain tissue in the hernial sac. Transvaginal scan, 15 weeks.

Fig. 21.**13** Left: a loop of umbilical cord behind the fetal head mimics a hypoechoic encephalocele (34 weeks, 2 days). Right: color Doppler identifies the mass as a loop of umbilical cord.

Fig. 21.**14** Left: frontoethmoidal encephalocele. Right: pathologic correlate (photo courtesy of Prof. Boll-mann, Department of Obstetrics and Gynecology, Charité Hospital, Berlin).

Fig. 21.**15**   Transverse scan of the encephalocele in Fig. 21.**14** (arrows) (photo courtesy of Prof. Bollmann, Department of Obstetrics and Gynecology, Charité Hospital, Berlin).

Fig. 21.**16**   Top left: microcephaly (BPD 5.3 cm) with a small occipital encephalocele (arrow) in Meckel–Gruber syndrome, 28 weeks. Bottom left: giant, bilateral cystic kidneys with abdominal distension (1 = left kidney, 2 = right kidney, 3 = spine). Right: corresponding postmortem view.

Iniencephaly

Fig. 21.**17**   Left: iniencephaly with extreme dorsal flexion of the head and cervical rachischisis, 28 weeks. Right: corresponding postmortem view.

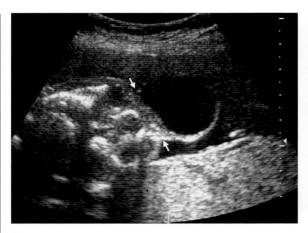

15

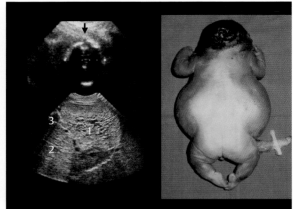

16

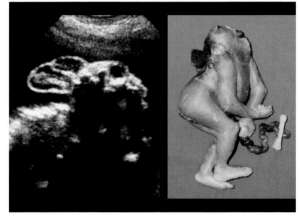

17

CNS Anomalies

Hydrocephalus

Definition. Hydrocephalus denotes the increased intracranial accumulation of cerebrospinal fluid (CSF) with expansion of the CSF spaces.

Forms.
- *Internal hydrocephalus.* Expansion of the ventricular system.
- *External hydrocephalus.* Expansion of the subarachnoid space.
- *Communicating hydrocephalus.* Internal and external hydrocephalus in which communication is maintained between the internal and external CSF spaces (132, 149).

Incidence. The reported incidence of hydrocephalus is 0.5–3 per 1000 births (38, 88).

Etiology and pathogenesis. Hydrocephalus may be caused by an obstruction of CSF flow (obstructive hydrocephalus) or the excessive production of CSF (hypersecretory hydrocephalus). The latter may be seen in association with choroid plexus papillomas (see Fig. 21.**57**).

Internal hydrocephalus. Most cases that are detectable prenatally are noncommunicating hydrocephalus in which an obstruction in the ventricular system has caused abnormal dilatation of the lateral ventricles with pressure atrophy of the brain mantle (internal hydrocephalus). The condition may be caused by infections such as cytomegalovirus and toxoplasmosis, intracranial malformations such as aqueductal stenosis (X-linked recessive inheritance), or by obstruction of the foramen of Magendie (Dandy–Walker syndrome, autosomal-recessive inheritance) (47).

Hydrocephalus ex vacuo. There are also cases in which the ventricular enlargement is not caused by an obstruction of CSF pathways but results from atrophic white matter disease (hydrocephalus ex vacuo).

Communicating hydrocephalus. In communicating hydrocephalus, the cause of the ventricular enlargement lies outside the ventricular system. An example is posthemorrhagic hydrocephalus. In some cases the etiology remains unknown.

Table 21.**1** reviews the various conditions that may underlie fetal ventricular enlargement.

Pathoanatomic features. These depend on the underlying disorder (see below).

Ultrasound features. In the early days of ultrasound, hydrocephalus could be detected only in late pregnancy by noting excessive growth of the fetal head. But with modern ultrasound equipment, it is now possible to detect hydrocephalus early in gestation, long before the skull becomes enlarged.

Severity. Severe cases can be diagnosed at a glance. Within the hemispheres, the dilated lateral ventricles appear as large, oblong, hypoechoic cystic areas that displace the brain mantle (Figs. 21.**18**, 21.**19**). Diagnosis can be difficult, however, in incipient cases (Fig. 21.**20**) or if the ventricular size varies from one examination to the next. Also, a few cases have been described in which the hydrocephalus resolved spontaneously (33, 134). Cases with borderline findings require accurate biometric analysis, taking care to avoid errors of measurement that could lead to a false-positive diagnosis (62).

Ventricular–hemispheric ratio and ventricular width. Using the ventricular–hemispheric ratio described by several authors (17, 34, 47) and

Table 21.**1** Anomalies and disorders that are associated with ventriculomegaly

Aqueductal stenosis	➢ Sporadic ➢ Postinflammatory ➢ X-linked recessive form ➢ Autosomal recessive form
CNS anomalies	➢ Dandy–Walker malformation ➢ Agenesis of corpus callosum ➢ Holoprosencephaly ➢ Porencephaly ➢ Lissencephaly
Vascular malformations	➢ Vein of Galen aneurysm ➢ Intracerebral hemorrhage
Neural tube defect	➢ Encephalocele ➢ Spina bifida ➢ Arnold–Chiari syndrome
Tumors	➢ Arachnoid cyst ➢ Neoplasms
Syndromes	➢ Apert syndrome ➢ Fragile X syndrome ➢ Roberts syndrome ➢ Smith–Lemli–Opitz syndrome
Chromosomal abnormalities	➢ Trisomy 13 ➢ Trisomy 18

the normal values for ventricular width reported by Johnson et al. (69) (see Chapter 12), abnormal enlargement of the lateral ventricles can be detected by the middle of the second trimester. However, due to the relatively large variation in normal values, especially during the second trimester, a definitive diagnosis of incipient hydrocephalus should be made only if serial scans show a marked increase in ventricular width. This presumes, of course, that the fetal head is measured at the same site on identical, nonoblique planes of section. Hansmann (60) states that the earliest manifestation of hydrocephalus is a dilatation of the frontal or occipital horns (Fig. 21.**20**). Pilu et al. (117) recommend measuring the frontal horn width, which has a normal mean value of 7.6 ± 0.6 mm regardless of gestational age. Based on the normal values derived by Johnson et al. (69), hydrocephalus is present if the lateral ventricle exceeds a width of 1.3 cm.

Third trimester. Gross enlargement of the ventricular width, often accompanied by displacement or possible undulation of the midline echo, is usually not seen before the third trimester (Figs. 21.**21**, 21.**22**). In advanced cases, rupture of the medial ventricular wall may occur (Fig. 21.**23**). Ventricular dilatation must be quite severe before superior enlargement is observed (Fig. 21.**24**).

Ultrasound misdiagnosis. A false-positive or false-negative diagnosis of hydrocephalus can occur with ultrasound, depending on the age of the pregnancy and the position of the fetal head. The hypoechoic cortex can mimic hydrocephalus (Fig. 21.**25**) (130), but the cortex is recognized by noting its position lateral to the choroid plexus. Hydrocephalus may be missed if unilateral hydrocephalus is present on the side nearer the transducer and is obscured by reverberations from the superior sutures. Similarly, suture-induced reverberations in bilateral hydrocephalus can lead to a misdiagnosis of unilateral hydrocephalus (Figs. 21.**18**, 21.**20**). If the diagnosis is uncertain, artifacts can usually be recognized by shifting the transducer and varying the scan angle. If coronal scans can be obtained, they are also helpful in clarifying equivocal findings. If insonation conditions are poor and the fetus is in a vertex presentation, transvaginal ultrasound can advance the diagnosis more quickly and easily than transabdominal scans.

Associated anomalies. Congenital hydrocephalus may occur in isolation, but it is commonly associated with a chromosomal abnormality (trisomy 13, 18) or spina bifida cystica (47). Pretorius et al. (122) found associated anomalies in 70% of hydrocephalic fetuses. They include neural tube defects, heart defects, gastrointestinal anomalies, renal anomalies, cleft lip and palate, thanatophoric dysplasia, trisomy 21, and trisomy 18 (114, 122). A syndrome should also be considered whenever hydrocephalus is found (e.g., Meckel–Gruber syndrome, Apert syndrome, Smith–Lemli–Opitz syndrome, fragile X syndrome).

Prognosis. The prognosis of hydrocephalus depends on the cause and extent of the hydrocephalus as well as on further development and the presence of associated anomalies (122).

Severity. The severity of hydrocephalus is assessed by measuring the ventricular width and the thickness of the residual brain mantle. A residual cortex less than 1 cm thick suggests a poor prognosis (146). The residual thickness of the brain mantle cannot be considered a reliable parameter, however. Conversely, a relatively thick brain mantle does not indicate a favorable prognosis because additional cerebral or other anomalies may be present that even an expert cannot detect. Asymmetrical hydrocephalus has a less favorable prognosis than symmetrical hydrocephalus.

Developmental abnormalities. In a follow-up of 40 hydrocephalus cases diagnosed antenatally, Pretorius et al. (122) found that only six children (15%) were alive after 13 months, only three of whom were normally developed. Nine of the pregnancies had been terminated. With mild ventriculomegaly (frontal horn width 10–15 mm), 9% of the infants will have a cognitive or motor delay (145).

Prenatal management. Regardless of the degree of ventricular enlargement, an effort should be made to determine the cause of the hydrocephalus.

First, a search should be made for other brain abnormalities and associated anomalies. Also, infections (toxoplasmosis, cytomegalovirus) and chromosomal abnormalities should be detected or excluded. Especially when hydrocephalus is detected early between 18 and 22 weeks, rapid karyotyping should be done by means of cordocentesis or placentocentesis. Pregnancy termination may be considered, depending on the extent of the hydrocephalus and associated anomalies.

Serial scans. If hydrocephalus does not develop until the late second or third trimester, it is recommended that serial ultrasound scans be performed at 1- to 2-week intervals. The scan intervals as well as the time and mode of delivery relate closely to the further development of the hydrocephalus. To ensure optimum perinatal management, both a pediatrician and a neurosurgeon should be consulted at an early stage with regard to further clinical management.

Timing of delivery. When moderate hydrocephalus is present, it is preferable from a neurosurgical standpoint to deliver a mature infant in order to minimize the operative risk associated with a postnatal shunting procedure. On the other hand, rapidly progressive hydrocephalus may necessitate a preterm cesarean delivery so that the infant's prognosis can be improved by a selective shunting procedure. To determine the optimum time of the delivery, Voigt (148) recommends Doppler examination of the middle cerebral artery. If normal pulsatility values are found, an expectant approach may be taken even with increasing hydrocephalus. Elevated values may be used as a criterion for electing preterm delivery. High pulsatility values in cerebral vessels signify increased intracerebral pressure and thus may indicate a cerebral perfusion deficit with impending ischemic injury.

Mode of delivery. The question of obstetric management depends on gestational age, the condition of the fetus, and the head circumference. If the head circumference is already greater than 35 cm, cesarean section is recommended to avoid obstetric complications.

Intrauterine treatment. Trials of intrauterine treatment in the form of ventriculocentesis (11) or ventriculoamniotic shunting (24, 45, 48, 71) were unable to improve the prognosis, as they treated only the ventriculomegaly and not the associated anomalies that were often present. Also, ventriculoamniotic shunting can lead to complications such as infection (12), valve malfunction (24), or shunt dislodgment (12, 71). Statistically, less than 5% of hydrocephalus cases can reasonably be expected to benefit from intrauterine shunting (48).

Intrapartum cephalocentesis is considered a destructive procedure, as it is associated with a high incidence of fetal morbidity and mortality (22). As a result, it cannot be recommended in an infant with a favorable prognosis.

Aqueductal Stenosis

Definition. Obstructive hydrocephalus due to stenosis of the sylvian aqueduct with enlargement of the lateral ventricles and third ventricle.

Special form. X-linked aqueductal stenosis (150).

Incidence. Pretorius et al. (122) found aqueductal stenosis in 17% of the 40 hydrocephalus cases that they observed.

Etiology and pathogenesis. Aqueductal stenosis can have various causes including inflammatory diseases (toxoplasmosis, cytomegalovirus, mumps, influenza [71, 141]), malformations, and genetic causes (10, 150).

Embryology. Early embryonic narrowing of the aqueduct that interconnects the third and fourth ventricles.

Pathoanatomic features. Aqueductal stenosis is marked by widening of the two lateral ventricles and the third ventricle.

Ultrasound features. Varying degrees of dilatation of the lateral ventricles and third ventricle are found, depending on the extent of the hydrocephalus (Figs. 21.**26**, 21.**27**). Hydrocephalus may be noted in the second trimester or may not appear until the third trimester, depending on whether the cause is a congenital anomaly or a postinflammatory change.

Associated anomalies. Typical flexion anomalies of the thumbs are found in fetuses with X-linked aqueductal stenosis (153).

Prognosis. The prognosis depends on the cause of the stenosis (see Hydrocephalus).

Prenatal management. See Hydrocephalus.

Communicating Hydrocephalus

Definition. Enlargement of the lateral ventricles and subarachnoid space.

Incidence. Rare antenatally.

Etiology and pathogenesis. Communicating hydrocephalus may result from an obstruction of the CSF system outside the ventricles or from the impaired reabsorption of CSF (87). The underlying cause may be a cerebral hemorrhage but is usually indeterminate.

Pathoanatomic features. Expansion of the subarachnoid space, lateral ventricles, and third and fourth ventricles.

Ultrasound features. Besides dilatation of the lateral ventricles and the third and fourth ventricles, ultrasound demonstrates expansion of the subarachnoid space lateral to the interhemispheric fissure (Figs. 21.**28**, 21.**29**) (115).

Prognosis. The prognosis appears to be more favorable than in other forms of hydrocephalus (55).

Prenatal management. See Hydrocephalus.

Hydranencephaly

Definition. Hydranencephaly is a severe congenital brain malformation in which the cerebral hemispheres are completely or almost completely absent and are replaced by a fluid-filled sac. The midbrain, basal ganglia, and cerebellum are present.

Incidence. Sporadic occurrence.

Etiology and pathogenesis. The presumed cause is a vascular occlusion involving the internal carotid arteries (98). Inflammatory processes due to toxoplasmosis have also been described as a cause (1).

Pathoanatomic features. The cerebral hemispheres are completely or almost completely absent. Rudiments may be seen in the area of the temporal or occipital cortex (57, 58).

Ultrasound features. Hydranencephaly is an extreme intracerebral fluid collection which differs from hydrocephalus in that the brain mantle is absent (Figs. 21.**30**, 21.**31**). The falx cerebri may be absent or only partially visualized (65, 139). In a coronal scan through the center of the skull, the brainstem protrudes a variable distance into the fluid-filled calvaria (Fig. 21.**31**). Lin et al. (79) reported on the early detection of hydranencephaly at 12 weeks, marked by the absence of a midline echo.

Differential diagnosis. Hydranencephaly can be difficult to distinguish sonographically from severe hydrocephalus or alobar holoprosencephaly.

Associated anomalies. There are no typical associated anomalies, nor is there an increased risk of chromosomal defects.

Prognosis. Grave.

Prenatal management. With an early diagnosis, pregnancy termination is an option. When hydranencephaly is diagnosed in the third trimester, preterm induction may be considered. If macrocephaly is also present, the head circumference can be reduced by cephalocentesis to enable a spontaneous delivery.

Holoprosencephaly

Definition. Severe brain and facial malformation.

Forms. Three forms are distinguished (40):
- *Alobar holoprosencephaly:* a single common ventricle with fusion of the thalami.
- *Semilobar holoprosencephaly:* partial separation of the ventricles and posterior cerebral hemispheres with incomplete fusion of the thalami.
- *Lobar holoprosencephaly:* normal separation of the hemispheres, lateral ventricles and thalami, with absence of the septum pellucidum.

Incidence. Approximately one in 16,000 live births (25).

Etiology and pathogenesis. The causes are diverse, and most cases are sporadic in their occurrence. The condition may occur in association with chromosomal abnormalities (usually trisomy 13) or as an autosomal-recessive disease (Meckel–Gruber syndrome). In most cases the cause is unknown (25).

Embryology. The complex cerebral developmental abnormality is based on incomplete cleavage of the prosencephalon, resulting in brain malformations in addition to various facial anomalies.

Pathoanatomic features (32).

Alobar holoprosencephaly. This form is marked by the presence of a single common ventricle. The interhemispheric fissure, corpus callosum, and third ventricle are absent, and both thalami are fused.

Semilobar holoprosencephaly. In this form a single ventricle is found in the anterior part of the skull. The cerebral hemispheres are partially separated posteriorly, and the thalami are incompletely fused.

Lobar holoprosencephaly. Lobar holoprosencephaly is the mildest form, characterized by separation of the lateral ventricles and thalami. A normal interhemispheric fissure is present, but the septum pellucidum and olfactory tract are absent.

The different forms of holoprosencephaly are shown schematically in Fig. 21.**32**.

Ultrasound features.

Alobar and semilobar forms. Both the alobar form (Fig. 21.**33**) and semilobar form (Figs. 21.**34**, 21.**35**) are characterized sonographically by a single cystic cavity between the two hemispheres in the anterior part of the skull. In contrast to hydrocephalus, scans show an absence of the midline echo (20, 51, 105, 117) and cavum septi pellucidi. A coronal scan through the head shows varying degrees of thalamic fusion, depending on the form (Fig. 21.**33**).

Lobar form. Ultrasound detection of the lobar form (67, 121) is somewhat difficult compared with the alobar and semilobar forms. Besides absence of the septum pellucidum, scans reveal a broad connection between the frontal horns and third ventricle (121). Pilu et al. (121) described a hyperechoic linear structure within the third ventricle as an additional sign (Fig. 21.**36**).

Differential diagnosis. Differentiation is required from pronounced hydrocephalus, hydranencephaly, porencephaly, or a large arachnoid cyst, depending on the extent of the findings. Table 21.**2** reviews the differential diagnosis of cystic defects according to their location.

Table 21.**2** Differential diagnosis of cystic brain structures according to the location of the cystic area

Midline defect	Asymmetrical defect
➢ Holoprosencephaly	➢ Porencephaly
➢ Agenesis of corpus callosum	➢ Choroid plexus cyst
➢ Arachnoid cyst	➢ Arachnoid cyst
➢ Vein of Galen aneurysm	➢ Unilateral hydrocephalus
➢ Dandy–Walker malformation	➢ Cystic brain tumor
	➢ Cerebral hemorrhage

Associated anomalies. DeMyer et al. (31) note that "the face predicts the brain," since a variety of facial anomalies occur in association with holoprosencephaly:
- Cyclopia (fused orbits, arrhinia with a proboscis)
- Ethmocephaly (extreme form of hypotelorism, arrhinia with a proboscis)
- Cebocephaly (hypotelorism with a proboscis-like nose)
- Midline facial cleft (see Fig. 21.71)

Any facial anomaly such as cyclopia, hypotelorism, absence of the nose, or a cleft lip and palate should be interpreted as a potential sign of holoprosencephaly.

Microcephaly (20, 31) and Meckel syndrome (68) have also been observed as associated head anomalies.

Extracranial anomalies. Extracranial anomalies (omphalocele, renal anomalies, cardiac anomalies) have also been found in the alobar and semilobar forms of holoprosencephaly. chromosomal abnormalities are often present: trisomy 13, 18, 13q, 18p and triploidy (25, 51, 105).

Prognosis. The prognosis of holoprosencephaly depends on the specific form. The alobar form is fatal. The semilobar form is compatible with life at least until childhood, and the lobar form is fully compatible with life. Both forms are associated with significant mental retardation, however (33).

Prenatal management. Fetal karyotyping is advised whenever an intracerebral cystic mass is detected at an early stage. If ultrasound reveals a severe brain malformation, pregnancy termination should be considered. If the infant is viable, further decisions will depend on the overall extent of the anomaly.

Porencephaly

Definition. Unilateral or bilateral cystic defects in the brain. The cystic areas may communicate with the ventricular system.

Incidence. Extremely rare.

Etiology and pathogenesis. It is assumed that vascular occlusion or an infectious process causes gray and white matter necrosis leading to cyst formation in the cerebral parenchyma (18, 41). Navin and Angevine (101) described porencephaly in association with a cytomegalovirus infection. Eller and Kuller (39) published a case in which porencephaly resulted from needle penetration of the fetal skull during amniocentesis. The condition is not known to have a familial occurrence.

Pathoanatomic features. Cystic areas of varying size are typically found in the region of sylvian fissure. Micropolygyria and hypoplasia/aplasia of the corpus callosum may also be present (52). In cases with unilateral cystic malacic areas, histologic examination shows signs of an inflammatory reaction or ischemia (52).

Ultrasound features. The ultrasound diagnosis of porencephaly is based on the detection of cystic areas that may be unilateral or bilateral (Fig. 21.**37**). The cysts may communicate with the ventricular system. Marked, asymmetrical ventricular dilatation with displacement of the midline echo is an important suggestive sign (19, 114).

Associated anomalies. Microcephaly.

Differential diagnosis. Arachnoid cyst, cystic brain tumor, intracerebral hemorrhage.

Prognosis. The prognosis depends on the extent of the cerebral defects. Since the condition is not treatable, the prognosis is generally poor. The defects can lead to paralysis in the newborn infant (129).

Prenatal management. Pregnancy termination is an option when porencephaly is diagnosed before viability is reached. Cases that are diagnosed later are managed the same way as hydrocephalus.

Lissencephaly

Definition. Agyria.

Incidence. Rare.

Etiology and pathogenesis. Familial cases are believed to have an autosomal-recessive mode of inheritance.

Embryology. The convolutions of the cerebral cortex fail to develop due to deficient neuronal migration (27).

Pathoanatomic features. The essential feature is an absence of cerebral gyri (27).

Ultrasound features. Prenatal diagnosis is extremely difficult in cases that do not have a positive family history. It is based on detecting an absence of cerebral gyri (Fig. 21.**38**). But gyral development is such that convolutions are not detectable with ultrasound until the third trimester (see Fig. 11.**3**), making it almost impossible to detect the anomaly at an earlier stage. It may be suggested by a familial risk (127) or by associated anomalies detected at ultrasound (Fig. 21.**38**). Motte et al. (96) described the ultrasound findings in pediatric patients as including dilatation of the occipital horns and a large, triangular appearance of the sylvian fissure. Reportedly, polyhydramnios is present in 50% of cases (109).

Associated anomalies. Hydrocephalus, microcephaly, agenesis of the corpus callosum. Associated noncerebral anomalies may include cardiac and gastrointestinal malformations, urinary tract anomalies, and limb anomalies (109).

Prognosis. Extremely poor. Infants with severe forms die during the first months of life.

Prenatal management. Since prenatal diagnosis is uncertain, management is the same as for hydrocephalus.

Arachnoid Cyst

Definition. Intracranial cystic mass arising from the arachnoid membrane.

Forms. Primary arachnoid cyst and secondary arachnoid cyst.

Incidence. Rare.

Etiology and pathogenesis (3, 23). Primary arachnoid cysts are a developmental anomaly while secondary arachnoid cysts are acquired as a result of inflammation, trauma, or intracerebral hemorrhage.

Pathoanatomic features. Most arachnoid cysts are located in the region of the sylvian fissure, interhemispheric fissure, or cisterna magna (59).

Ultrasound features. The lesion appears sonographically as a fluid-filled cyst, which may be located on the midline or at an asymmetrical site (Figs. 21.**39**, 21,**40**). As long as the cyst does not impair CSF flow, hydrocephalus does not develop.

Associated anomalies. There are no specific associated anomalies.

Differential diagnosis. Porencephaly, unilateral hydrocephalus, cystic neoplasm, holoprosencephaly, Dandy–Walker malformation, vein of Galen aneurysm, agenesis of the corpus callosum (Table 21.**2**).

Prognosis. Generally the prognosis is very good with proper neurosurgical treatment.

Prenatal management. Vaginal delivery in a perinatal center followed by neurosurgical treatment.

Agenesis of the Corpus Callosum

Definition. Absence of the corpus callosum (partial or complete aplasia).

Incidence. Rare, sporadic anomaly. The incidence in nonselected autopsy material is one in 19,000 (44).

Etiology and pathogenesis. The condition may occur sporadically or in the setting of a chromosomal abnormality (e.g., trisomy 13) (53).

Embryology. The corpus callosum is a transverse fiber tract that interconnects the cerebral hemispheres at the base of the longitudinal fissure. It is not fully developed until 18–20 weeks' gestation (54). Agenesis of the corpus callosum is based on a complete absence of the callosal fibers or their failure to cross the midline (40). It is believed to result from faulty closure of the rostral neural tube. Partial or complete aplasia may occur, depending on the time at which callosal development is inhibited.

Pathoanatomic features. Davidoff and Dyke (29) identified six characteristic features based on pneumoencephalographic studies:
- Lateralization of the lateral ventricles
- Medial angulation of the frontal horns
- Widening and elevation of the third ventricle
- Dilatation of the occipital horns
- Concave inner walls of the lateral ventricles
- Abnormal gyral development

Ultrasound features. The ultrasound detection of a corpus callosum defect (9, 54, 61, 89) is difficult and requires a very detailed examination. Given the relatively late maturation of the normal corpus callosum, a defect cannot be visualized with ultrasound until after 20 weeks' gestation. The defect can be defined by a precise midsagittal scan (Fig. 21.**41**) or coronal scan (Fig. 21.**42**). Figure 21.**43** shows diagrams of the features of corpus callosum agenesis published by Pilu et al. (120). According to Bertino et al. (9), three signs visible in the transverse scan are suspicious for corpus callosum agenesis:
- Lateralization of the lateral ventricles
- Disproportionate enlargement of the occipital horns
- Variable dilatation of the third ventricle

Associated anomalies. The agenesis may occur in isolation or in association with genetic syndromes (Aicardi syndrome, X-linked recessive) and chromosomal abnormalities (144). Among the latter, cases with trisomy 8 (9), trisomy 13 (61, 144), and trisomy 18 (136) have been observed. Bertino et al. (9) found additional malformations in 5 of 7 cases (71%) after birth. Agenesis of the corpus callosum also occurs as a feature of holoprosencephaly. According to

Parrish et al. (111), CNS malformations are present in 85% of cases and other noncerebral malformations in 62% of cases.

Differential diagnosis. Median arachnoid cyst without corpus callosum agenesis.

Prognosis. The prognosis depends on the associated anomalies. Mental development is impaired. The risk of recurrence is not significantly increased.

Prenatal management. Fetal karyotyping. Targeted imaging for additional fetal anomalies. Further management is the same as for hydrocephalus.

Vein of Galen Aneurysm

Definition. Arteriovenous malformation with dilatation of the vein of Galen, combined with an increase in blood flow.

Incidence. Rare.

Etiology and pathogenesis. Early developmental defect during the period of angioblast differentiation (108).

Pathoanatomic features. Marked dilatation of the vein of Galen caused by the union of the two internal cerebral veins. The aneurysm is located above the thalamus and drains posteriorly into the sinus rectus.

Ultrasound features. Ultrasound demonstrates a centrally located, tubular, cystic hypoechoic structure (85, 147). Doppler spectra and color Doppler scans reveal definite venous or arterial blood flow that may show turbulent characteristics (66) (Fig. 21.**44**).

Associated anomalies. There are no specific associated anomalies. However, the increased load on the heart (75) can lead to cardiomegaly, hydrops, and hepatomegaly. Polyhydramnios may also be observed.

Differential diagnosis. Differentiation is required from other centrally located cystic structures such as arachnoid cyst, agenesis of the corpus callosum, and holoprosencephaly.

Prognosis. The prognosis depends mainly on the cardiac effects. Watson et al. (151) reported on 40 cases in which a vein of Galen aneurysm was associated with congestive heart failure. Only seven of these infants survived, and two of them developed hydrocephalus.

Prenatal management. Close-interval follow-up. Vaginal delivery at term in a perinatal center.

Choroid Plexus Cyst(s)

Definition. Unilateral or bilateral cyst formation within the choroid plexus.

Incidence. Asymptomatic cysts of the choroid plexus have been found in up to 57% of autopsy material (133). Choroid plexus cysts have been detected sonographically in approximately 1% of fetuses between 16 and 24 weeks (134).

Etiology and pathogenesis. The cysts are believed to form in neuroepithelial folds within the choroid plexus (134).

Pathoanatomic features. The cysts are located within the choroid plexus. Most are smaller than 1 cm in diameter (134).

Ultrasound features. Choroid plexus cysts appear sonographically as hypoechoic, usually round structures within the choroid plexus (64, 99, 100, 135). The cysts may be unilateral or bilateral. Most cysts observed between 16 and 24 weeks are no longer detectable at 26–28 weeks (136) (Figs. 21.**45**, 21.**46**).

Associated anomalies. Various groups of authors in recent years have tried to determine whether choroid plexus cysts can serve as markers for fetal chromosomal abnormalities (13, 46, 64, 99, 100, 135). In a survey of 1806 cases published in the literature (14–38 weeks' gestation), Snijders et al. (136) found that 8% of the cases were associated with chromosomal defects, mainly trisomy 18 (121/1806 cases = 6.7%) and trisomy 21 (18/1806 cases = 1%). Other chromosomal abnormalities were much less common, accounting for 0.6% (11/1806) of the cases. The critical factor is whether the cyst is an isolated anomaly or whether other anomalies are also present. With an isolated choroid plexus cyst, the risk of a chromosomal abnormality is 1%. If additional anomalies are found, the risk is 46% (136).

Prognosis. The prognosis is generally good, provided there are no additional anomalies.

Prenatal management. When an isolated choroid plexus cyst is detected before 20 weeks, fetal karyotyping is optional if no additional ultrasound abnormalities are found. A selective search should be made for anomalies like those that may occur in trisomy 18 (cleft lip and palate, auricular deformity, myelomeningocele, heart defects, renal anomalies, limb anomalies). If an additional ultrasound abnormality is detected, the fetal chromosome set should be determined by rapid karyotyping. If the chromosome set is normal, ultrasound follow-ups are indicated.

◼ *Dandy–Walker Malformation*

Definition. Hydrocephalus, partial or complete absence of the cerebellar vermis with a posterior fossa cyst that opens directly into the fourth ventricle (28, 61).

Incidence. Approximately 10% of hydrocephalus cases.

Etiology and pathogenesis. Uncertain. Atresia of the foramina of Magendie and Luschka was originally thought to be the cause (28). But since cases have been found in which the foramina of Magendie and Luschka were not atretic (8), the syndrome is now attributed to a complex developmental abnormality involving the roof of the fourth ventricle (61, 124).

Pathology. Hydrocephalus typically affects all ventricles. Cystic dilatation of the fourth ventricle is combined with incomplete separation of the cerebellar hemispheres. The cerebellar vermis is partly or completely absent; the inferior portion is always absent (78).

Ultrasound features. Ultrasound basically shows a cystic mass in the posterior fossa and an abnormally shaped cerebellum (106, 116, 126) (Figs. 21.**47**–21.**49**). The cerebellar hemispheres are underdeveloped (30) and are splayed apart in varying degrees depending on the extent of the cerebellar defect (Figs. 21.**48**, 21.**49**). Besides a cystic mass in the posterior fossa, expansion of the lateral ventricles is also observed.

Differential diagnosis. Differentiation is required from an enlarged cisterna magna with atrophy of the cerebellar vermis and from an arachnoid cyst, but this can be very difficult to accomplish with ultrasound.

Associated anomalies. According to Murray et al. (97), Dandy–Walker malformation is associated with a variety of other disorders including syndromes (e.g., Ellis–van Creveld syndrome, Meckel–Gruber syn-

drome, Walker–Warburg syndrome), chromosomal defects (45X, triploidy, trisomy, etc.), and sporadic malformations (e.g., renal anomalies, facial hemangiomas). Dandy–Walker malformation is also observed in the setting of infectious diseases (rubella, cytomegalovirus infection), diabetes mellitus, and alcohol abuse. Ulm et al. (143) reported on the ultrasound detection of Dandy–Walker malformation at 14 weeks, associated with a chromosomal abnormality (triploidy).

Based on available evidence, it appears that associated defects are present in more than 50% of cases (61, 128). Some of these are cerebral anomalies (agyria, microgyria, agenesis of the corpus callosum) that are difficult or impossible to detect antenatally.

Prognosis. The prognosis is difficult and is generally considered unfavorable (55, 126). Russ et al. (126) report an overall mortality rate of 55%. If associated anomalies are present, the mortality rate rises to 83%.

Prenatal management. Because Dandy–Walker malformation occurs in association with chromosomal abnormalities, fetal karyotyping is indicated. When a severe form is detected before viability is reached, pregnancy termination may be considered. If the condition is detected at a later stage, ultrasound follow-ups are indicated along with early interdisciplinary consultation with a pediatrician and neurosurgeon.

◼ *Arnold–Chiari Malformation (Type II)*

Definition. A developmental defect of the cerebellum, leading secondarily to a downward protrusion of the dorsal medulla oblongata with disturbances of CSF dynamics and hydrocephalus. Myelomeningocele is also present.

Forms.
- Type I. No meningocele, first manifested at school age.
- Type II. With a meningocele.

Incidence. Pretorius et al. (122) state that 26% of fetuses with hydrocephalus have an underlying Arnold–Chiari type II malformation.

Etiology and pathogenesis. The cause is a developmental deficiency of the cerebellum marked by a downward protrusion of the dorsal part of the medulla oblongata. There is accompanying impairment of CSF circulation, with part of the cerebellum, fourth ventricle, pons, and medulla oblongata displaced into the cervical canal. Various theories on pathogenesis have been advanced (92, 132), but it is unclear which defect occurs first.

Pathoanatomic features. Besides hydrocephalus, a myelomeningocele is present in type II Arnold–Chiari malformation (16).

Ultrasound features. Bilateral hydrocephalus and a myelomeningocele are the most striking ultrasound findings (49) (Fig. 21.**50**).

Lemon sign and banana sign. Typical superior signs may also be seen in fetuses with spina bifida. One is a lemon-shaped deformation of the cranium with lateral indentation of the frontal bones ("lemon sign," Figs. 21.**50** and 21.**51**) (103, 107). Another is a banana-shaped deformation of the cerebellum ("banana sign," Fig. 21.**52**) (7, 103), which occurs when the cerebellum has been displaced into the spinal canal.

Obliteration of the cisterna magna. As it is often difficult to evaluate the cerebellum in such cases, other authors consider obliteration of the cisterna magna to be an important sign (50, 119). It is characterized by nonvisualization of the cisterna magna, which normally appears as a hypoechoic slit (Fig. 21.**53**).

Table 21.3 Grading of cerebral hemorrhage in immature newborns (after [110])

Grade	Type of hemorrhage
I	Isolated subependymal hemorrhage
II	Intraventricular hemorrhage without ventricular enlargement
III	Intraventricular hemorrhage with ventricular enlargement
IV	Intraventricular hemorrhage with bleeding into the brain parenchyma

Associated anomalies. When a sac is detected sonographically in the spinal region, attention should be given to the feet to check for signs of club foot.

Prognosis. Infants with severe forms die during the first months of life (94).

Prenatal management. Same as for hydrocephalus and myelomeningocele.

Intrauterine Cerebral Hemorrhage

Definition. Bleeding into the brain parenchyma.

Incidence. Uncertain. Based on CT studies by Burstein et al. (15), the incidence of intracranial hemorrhage is 40% in immature newborns of less than 32 weeks gestational age.

Etiology and pathogenesis. Fetal cerebral hemorrhage may be caused by hypoxic events, changes in intracranial pressure, or alloimmune thrombocytopenia (63, 95).

Pathoanatomic features. The bleeding usually occurs in the subependymal layer of the germinal matrix in the caudate nucleus, adjacent to the lateral ventricles. The bleeding may spread into the ventricles or into the brain parenchyma.

Ultrasound features. Relatively little has been published on the ultrasound diagnosis of intrauterine cerebral hemorrhage (63, 73, 82, 83, 93). Depending on its location, the intracranial hemorrhage may appear as a hyperechoic area within the brain parenchyma. If the hematoma is located within the ventricle and abuts the choroid plexus, the latter will display an exceptional size (Fig. 21.**54**). The hemorrhage may then acquire a more cystic appearance on subsequent scans. Johnson et al. (70) state that coronal and sagittal scans are best for detecting a hemorrhagic focus in newborns. In late pregnancy, however, these planes can be visualized in a vertex-presenting fetus only with transvaginal ultrasound or 3-D ultrasound. Table 21.**3** reviews the system that is used for grading cerebral hemorrhage in the immature newborn (110).

Associated anomalies. None known.

Differential diagnosis. Brain tumor.

Prognosis. The prognosis depends on the severity of the intracerebral hemorrhage. According to Fogarty et al. (43), almost 50% of fetuses with cerebral hemorrhage die in utero.

Prenatal management. Preterm induction is indicated for a mature fetus with incipient hydrocephalus.

Intracranial Tumors

Definition. Intracranial neoplasms leading to the displacement of brain structures.

Forms. Astrocytoma, ependymoma, medulloblastoma, choroid plexus papilloma, teratoma, craniopharyngioma, lipoma, and phacomatoses (2, 140).

Incidence. Rare. Approximately one-half of tumors in newborns are teratomas. Astrocytomas are the most common tumors in infancy, followed by ependymomas and medulloblastomas.

Etiology and pathogenesis. Depend on the tumor.

Pathoanatomic features. The location of the tumor may be supratentorial, infratentorial, or both (140). A choroid plexus papilloma can result in hypersecretory hydrocephalus.

Ultrasound features. Most fetal brain tumors are not diagnosed until the third trimester. Brain tumors are usually hyperechoic with a heterogeneous structure of varying echogenicity (Figs. 21.**55**–21.**57**) (26, 36, 80, 137, 152). Sites of tumor necrosis can appear as hypoechoic areas (Fig. 21.**56**). Calcifications, like those occurring in teratomas (26, 80), may cast an acoustic shadow. Different types of fetal brain tumor cannot be differentiated with ultrasound. At most, it is reasonable to assume that a tumor with a very nonhomogeneous structure is malignant. Infiltrative tumor growth often leads to the obstruction of CSF pathways and displacement of the falx cerebri. Superior enlargement may be seen in association with large, fast-growing tumors.

Associated anomalies. None.

Differential diagnosis. Arachnoid cyst, cerebral hemorrhage.

Prognosis. The prognosis is usually unfavorable. It depends critically on the type of tumor and its degree of differentiation (2). Lipomas and choroid plexus papillomas have a favorable prognosis.

Prenatal management. This depends on the size of the tumor, its growth rate, and secondary changes such as hydrocephalus or macrocephaly. Further management should be planned in consultation with a pediatrician and neurosurgeon. The infant should be delivered in a perinatal center.

Macrocephaly

Definition. The fetal head is abnormally large in relation to other, normal-for-gestational-age measurements.

Etiology and pathogenesis. Macrocephaly is not a separate disease entity but a symptom that can occur in the setting of various anomalies.
Conditions that may be associated with macrocephaly are listed in Table 21.**4**.

Ultrasound features. Macrocephaly is diagnosed at ultrasound when

Table 21.4 Conditions that are associated with macrocephaly

Bone dysplasias	➤ Achondroplasia ➤ Hypochondroplasia ➤ Thanatophoric dysplasia
Hydrocephalus	➤ Late form
Chromosomal abnormalities	➤ Tetrasomy 8p
Syndromes	➤ Bannayan–Riley–Ruvalcaba syndrome ➤ CCC (craniocerebellocardiac) syndrome ➤ Sotos syndrome

the fetal head circumference is above the 95th percentile (91) while other biometric parameters are normal for gestational age. A profile view may additionally show frontal bossing (Fig. 21.**58**) or a double superior contour signifying the increased deposition of subcutaneous fat.

Prognosis. The prognosis depends on the underlying disorder. Diseases such as thanatophoric dysplasia have a grave prognosis.

Prenatal management. This is tailored to the underlying fetal disorder. When macrocephaly is detected early, preterm induction at 38 weeks should be considered as a way to avoid cesarean delivery at term.

Cloverleaf Skull

Definition. Prominent upward bulging of the cranium with lateral bulging of the temporal regions.

Incidence. Extremely rare. Only a few cases have been described in the world literature.

Etiology and pathogenesis. Cloverleaf skull occurs in the setting of: **Holtermüller–Wiedemann syndrome** (superior deformity with severe hydrocephalus and micromelia)

Thanatophoric dysplasia (84) (see Limb Anomalies)

Guérin–Stern syndrome (form of arthrogryposis multiplex congenita with multiple flexion or extension contractures of joints and facial dysmorphia)

Cloverleaf skull is believed to be caused by defects in the differentiation and development of the superior sutures leading to synostosis (154).

Ultrasound features. The ultrasound intrauterine diagnosis of cloverleaf skull was first reported in a 1979 publication (14). Only a few cases diagnosed antenatally have been published since that time (84, 138). The most striking feature is the cloverleaf or trilobed deformity of the skull, which is best appreciated in coronal scans (Fig. 21.**59**).

Prognosis. Cases with severe hydrocephalus have a poor prognosis due to rising intracranial pressure. Cases that occur in thanatophoric dysplasia have a grave prognosis.

Prenatal management. Pregnancy termination is appropriate for cases with a grave prognosis that are diagnosed early. In cases that are detected later and show pronounced hydrocephalus, cephalocentesis may be considered to avoid a cesarean section.

Microcephaly

Definition. Abnormally small head.

Incidence. Relatively rare, with an incidence of one in 8500 births (74).

Etiology and pathogenesis. An autosomal-recessive form of microcephaly can occur in blood relatives. Other causes of microcephaly are Meckel–Gruber syndrome, Seckel syndrome, a chromosomal abnormality (trisomy 13), exposure to exogenous agents such as alcohol or cocaine (56), and infections such as cytomegalovirus (112), rubella, and toxoplasmosis.

Pathoanatomic features. Small head combined with a reduction of brain mass (microencephaly).

Ultrasound features. The ultrasound diagnosis is based on the detection of a small skull (Figs. 21.**60**, 21.**61**) (21, 77, 102). In order for the diagnosis to be made, the abnormal craniometric parameter should be too small in serial examinations, not just in a single examination (see Chapter 16).

3-SD range. Studies by Kurtz et al. (77) and Chervenak et al. (21) indicate that true microcephaly exists only when the fetal head dimensions (biparietal diameter, occipitofrontal diameter, head circumference) are below the 3-SD range.

Relative microcephaly and pseudomicrocephaly. Kurtz et al. (77) used the term "relative microcephaly" in cases where head growth is between 1 and 3 SD below the mean and "pseudomicrocephaly" in cases where the biparietal diameter only appears too small because of an unusual head shape.

Conditions. Three conditions should be met before microcephaly is diagnosed:
● The gestational age must be confirmed (ultrasound confirmation in early pregnancy).
● Fetal head size should not be evaluated by biparietal diameter (which is misleading with a dolichocephalic head shape) but by head circumference.
● The head size must be small in relation to the trunk size and the length of the limb bones.

According to Kurjak et al. (76), microcephaly should be suspected in late pregnancy when the ratio of head circumference to abdominal circumference is 1 : 2.

Transient "microcephalic" growth. Hansmann (60) observed transient "microcephalic" growth in five fetuses with spina bifida. Superior growth then "caught up" later in the pregnancy as hydrocephalus developed (see Chapter 16).

Associated anomalies. Microcephaly may be associated with a number of other anomalies, chromosomal abnormalities, and syndromes (Table 21.**5**).

Table 21.**5** Conditions that are associated with microcephaly

CNS anomalies	➢ Encephalocele ➢ Holoprosencephaly ➢ Lissencephaly
Chromosomal defects	➢ Trisomy 13 ➢ Trisomy 18 ➢ Trisomy 22 ➢ Tetrasomy 9p
Syndromes	➢ De Lange syndrome ➢ Dubowitz syndrome ➢ Lenz syndrome ➢ Meckel–Gruber syndrome ➢ Roberts syndrome ➢ Rubinstein–Taybi syndrome ➢ Seckel syndrome ➢ Smith–Lemli–Opitz syndrome ➢ Walker–Warburg syndrome
Infections	➢ Cytomegalovirus ➢ Rubella ➢ Toxoplasmosis
Exogenous agents	➢ Alcohol ➢ Cocaine
Metabolic disorders	➢ Phenylalanine embryopathy (= maternal phenylketonuria)

Differential diagnosis. Anencephaly, exencephaly.

Prognosis and risk of recurrence. The main clinical significance of this anomaly is its high association with mental retardation (86). When it occurs in Meckel–Gruber syndrome, the risk of recurrence is 25%.

Prenatal management. Fetal karyotyping should be performed whenever microcephaly is suspected. The fetus should also be scrutinized for additional anomalies.

Brachycephaly

Definition. Short skull with a markedly reduced occipitofrontal diameter.

Etiology and pathogenesis. Brachycephaly can result from craniosynostosis, with premature closure of the coronal suture leading to front-to-back shortening of the skull. Brachycephaly also occurs in various syndromes (e.g., Apert syndrome, Carpenter syndrome), in cleidocranial dysostosis, and in several chromosomal abnormalities (chromosome 3p-, chromosome 4q-, chromosome 9p-, tetrasomy 12p).

Pathoanatomic features. From an anthropologic standpoint, brachycephaly is considered to be present when the cephalic index (ratio of greatest biparietal diameter to greatest occipitofrontal diameter ? 100) is greater than 80.

Ultrasound features. Unlike the anthropologic definition used in children and adults, an ultrasound diagnosis of fetal brachycephaly is made when the cephalic index is greater than 85 (Fig. 21.**61**). In the prenatal examination of 451 fetuses with chromosomal defects, brachycephaly was found in 15% of fetuses with trisomy 21, in 28% with trisomy 18 or 13, in 10% with triploidy, and in 32% with Turner syndrome (136). However, studies by Perry et al. (113), Shah et al. (131), and our own studies (90) have shown that most fetuses with trisomy 21 still exhibit a normal cephalic index in the second trimester. Thus, a normal cephalic index cannot be taken as a criterion for a healthy infant.

Associated anomalies. Microcephaly, facial dysmorphias, polydactyly, or clavicular hypoplasia or aplasia may be found in association with brachycephaly, depending on the underlying disorder.

Prognosis. The prognosis depends mainly on any accompanying anomalies.

Prenatal management. The detection of brachycephaly should always prompt further ultrasound scrutiny in addition to fetal karyotyping.

Strawberry-Shaped Skull

Definition. Short, broad skull with narrowing of the frontal region and flattening of the occipital region.

Etiology and pathogenesis. The frontal narrowing is most likely due to hypoplasia of the face and frontal brain, and the occipital flattening to hypoplasia of the hindbrain.

Ultrasound features. Ultrasound shows a broad, brachycephalic head with a characteristic strawberry shape (Fig. 21.**62**).

Associated anomalies. In a series of 54 fetuses with a strawberry-shaped skull, Nicolaides et al. (104) found that all of them had an associated malformation. Forty-four of the 54 fetuses (81%) had a chromosomal defect (e.g., trisomy 18).

Prognosis. The prognosis depends on the associated anomalies.

Prenatal management. Finding a strawberry-shaped skull at ultrasound warrants further, detailed scrutiny of the fetus. Due to the high incidence of chromosomal defects, fetal karyotyping is always indicated.

Dolichocephaly

Definition. Elongated skull with a markedly increased occipitofrontal diameter.

Etiology and pathogenesis. Dolichocephaly may be caused by premature closure of the sagittal suture leading to an elongated head shape (scaphocephaly). It may also be a physiologic variant in a breech-presenting fetus.

Pathoanatomic features. From an anthropologic standpoint, dolichocephaly is considered to be present when the cephalic index (ratio of greatest biparietal diameter to greatest occipitofrontal diameter ? 100) is less than 75.

Ultrasound features. Besides relying on gross appearance (Fig. 21.**63**), the examiner can also calculate the cephalic index from the biparietal and occipitofrontal diameters. In prenatal ultrasound, dolichocephaly is diagnosed when the cephalic index is less than 75. It is relatively common in breech-presenting fetuses, where it is considered a physiologic finding.

Associated anomalies. The combined presence of dolichocephaly and microcephaly may occur in trisomy 10p.

Prognosis. When dolichocephaly is a physiologic variant, it has no prognostic implications.

Prenatal management. Serial scans may be indicated, depending on the fetal lie (measurement of head circumference). A chromosome analysis is unnecessary unless other sonomorphologic abnormalities are found.

Thickened Nuchal Fold

Definition. Markedly thick subcutaneous tissue layer in the nuchal area.

Incidence. A thick nuchal fold is seen in 0.06% of normal fetuses between 15 and 20 weeks (4, 5) and in 37.5% (90) to 45% (4, 5) of fetuses with Down syndrome in the second trimester. Approximately 80% of neonates with trisomy 21 were found to have excess back neck skin (123).

Ultrasound features. The skin and subcutaneous tissue at the back of the neck of a healthy fetus, called the "nuchal fold," is from 1 to 5 mm thick between 15 and 20 weeks (4). The nuchal fold is measured in a posteriorly angled transverse scan through the fetal head. It is the same plane that is used to define and measure the cerebellum (see Chapter 12, Figs. 12.**25** and 12.**26**).

Trisomy 21. Trisomy 21 should be considered whenever a thickened nuchal fold (> 5 mm) is found (4, 5, 6, 90) (Fig. 21.**64**). There are a few cases, however, in which a nuchal fold thickness > 5 mm is encountered in a chromosomally normal fetus. Benacerraf et al. (6) found a false-positive nuchal fold thickness in 0.1% of cases, Donnenfeld et al. (35) in 1.2% of cases.

Nuchal translucency. The nuchal fold should not be confused with the "nuchal translucency" at the end of the first trimester, which is caused by a fluid collection.

Prognosis. If no associated anomalies are found and the fetal chromosome set is normal, the detection of a thickened nuchal fold has no prognostic implications.

Prenatal management. The fetus should be scanned for additional anomalies, and a fetal chromosome analysis should be performed.

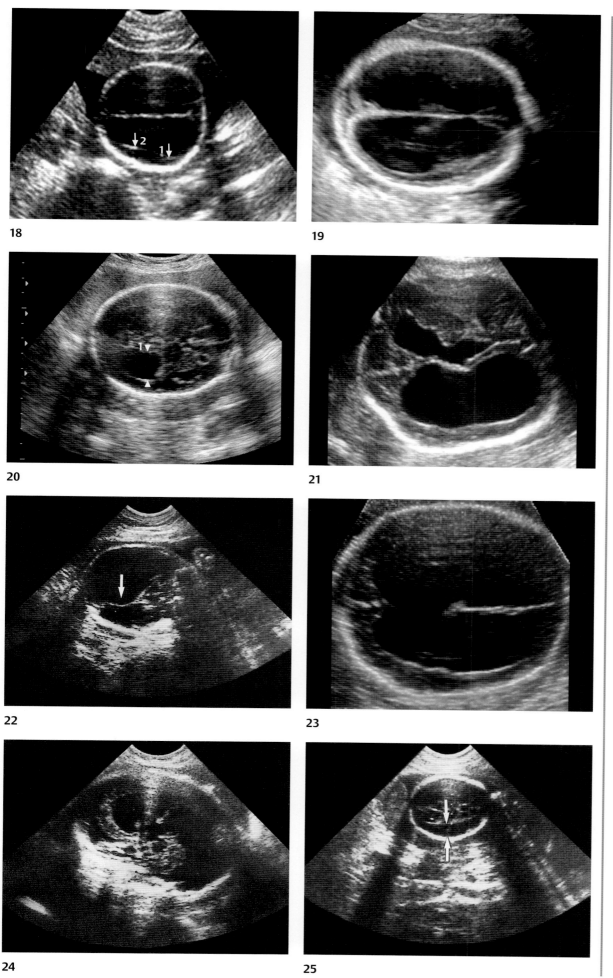

18

19

20

21

22

23

24

25

Hydrocephalus and hydranencephaly

Fig. 21.**18** Early bilateral internal hydrocephalus (19 weeks). The lateral ventricle is enlarged to 1.7 cm. Residual brain mantle thickness is 4 mm (1) and 6 mm (2). Hydrocephalus on the side near the transducer is obscured by reverberations!

Fig. 21.**19** Extensive internal hydrocephalus in a 26-week fetus (vertex presentation with the spine to the right). The lateral ventricles are enlarged to 1.7 cm. Brain mantle thickness is 4 mm.

Fig. 21.**20** Early bilateral internal hydrocephalus at 29 weeks, 3 days (vertex presentation with the spine to the right). The expansion of the lateral ventricles predominantly affects the occipital horns (19 mm).

Fig. 21.**21** Extensive, nonuniform bilateral hydrocephalus with an undulating midline echo, 31 weeks.

Fig. 21.**22** Massive, asymmetrical, predominantly left-sided internal hydrocephalus, 28 weeks. The left lateral ventricle measures 56 mm in diameter, the right lateral ventricle 16 mm. The midline echo is markedly displaced to the right (arrow). The brain mantle has been completely effaced on the left side. Coronal scan.

Fig. 21.**23** Extensive hydrocephalus with rupture of the medial ventricular wall, 34 weeks. The rupture has created a large opening between the ventricles.

Fig. 21.**24** Pronounced hydrocephalus in a sagittal scan, 29 weeks. BPD 10.7 cm.

Fig. 21.**25** Hypoechoic brain mantle on the side opposite the transducer mimics hydrocephalus (arrows). Transverse scan, 25 weeks. Vertex presentation with the spine to the right.

Fig. 21.26 Patterns of CSF circulation. a Normal pattern. b Aqueductal stenosis. The stenosis in the sylvian aqueduct (black arrows) leads to enlargement of the lateral ventricles (LaV) and third ventricle (3V). 4V = fourth ventricle, SSS = superior sagittal sinus (modified from [125]).

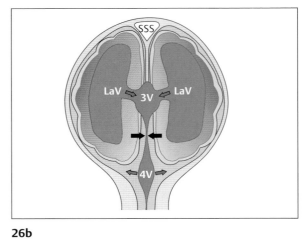

26a

26b

Fig. 21.27 Hydrocephalus due to aqueductal stenosis. There is marked frontal and occipital enlargement of the lateral ventricles. The third ventricle is also expanded (arrow). Trisomy 18, 32 weeks.

Fig. 21.28 Schematic representation of communicating hydrocephalus caused by a blockage of CSF reabsorption in the superior sagittal sinus (black arrows). The fluid buildup leads to enlargement of the lateral ventricles and expansion of the subarachnoid space (modified from [125]).

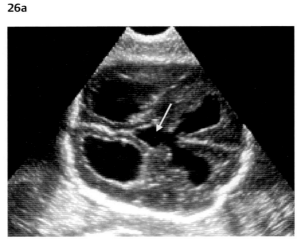

27

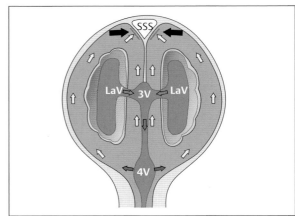

28

Fig. 21.29 Communicating hydrocephalus with dilatation of the lateral ventricles and superior sagittal sinus (arrows) at 34 weeks. Left: sagittal scan. Right: coronal scan.

Fig. 21.30 Hydranencephaly at 17 weeks, 4 days (vertex presentation with the spine to the left). The skull contains only a hypoechoic fluid collection with no visible brain structures. The midline echo is absent!

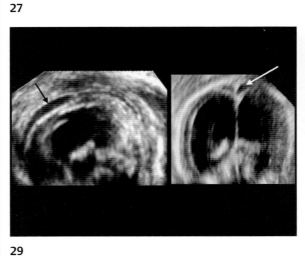

29

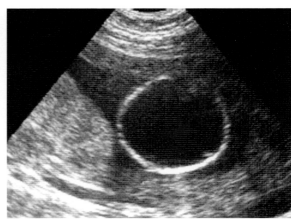

30

Fig. 21.31 Hydranencephaly, 30 weeks. The coronal scan shows a variable degree of brainstem protrusion (arrow) into the fluid-filled skull. Holoprosencephaly

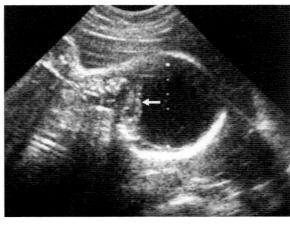

31

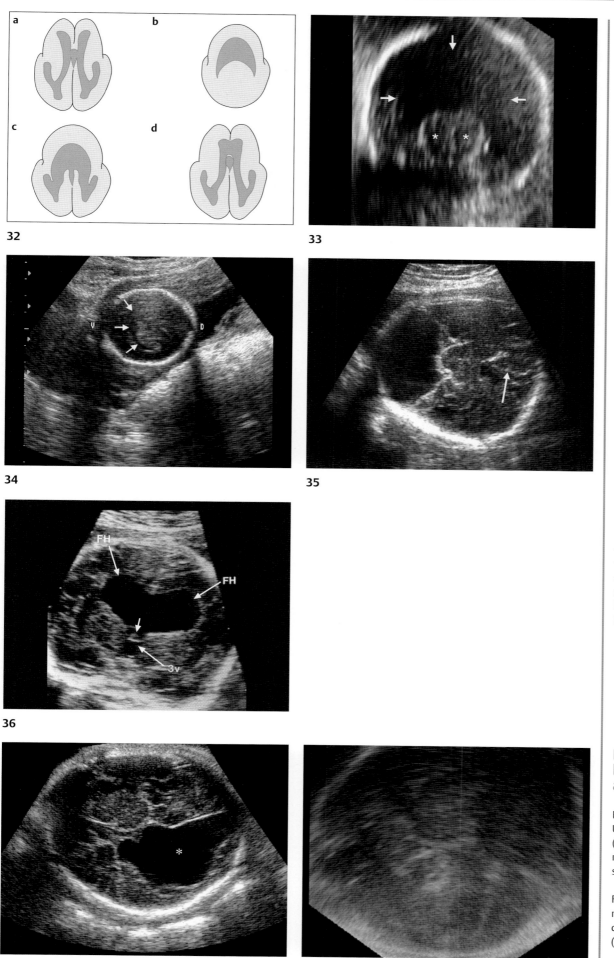

32

33

34

35

36

37

38

Fig. 21.**32**   Diagram illustrating the various forms of holoprosencephaly.
a Normal brain.
b Alobar holoprosencephaly.
c Semilobar holoprosencephaly.
d Lobar holoprosencephaly (modified from Pilu [117]).

Fig. 21.**33**   Alobar holoprosencephaly, 23 weeks. A single, dilated ventricle appears in the anterior part of the skull (arrows). The thalami (8) are fused. Oblique coronal scan.

Fig. 21.**34**   Semilobar holoprosencephaly at 21 weeks, 5 days. The lateral ventricles are normally developed anteriorly, but a common ventricle is present posteriorly (arrows). V = anterior, D = posterior (vertex presentation with the spine to the left).

Fig. 21.**35**   Semilobar holoprosencephaly, 31 weeks. The common ventricle can be seen in the anterior part of the skull. Posteriorly, the cerebral hemispheres are separated by the midline echo (arrow) (vertex presentation with the spine to the left).

Fig. 21.**36**   Lobar holoprosencephaly. Midcoronal scan through the fetal brain at 30 weeks shows absence of the septum pellucidum and fused frontal horns (FH) that communicate with the third ventricle (3v). An echogenic structure (short arrow) can be seen within the third ventricle. From Pilu et al. (121).

Porencephaly, lissencephaly, and arachnoid cysts

Fig. 21.**37**   Porencephaly, 30 weeks. Ultrasound typically shows unilateral (∗) or bilateral defects in the brain that may communicate with the ventricular system.

Fig. 21.**38**   Lissencephaly at 37 weeks, marked by an absence of gyri in the cerebral surface. Transvaginal scan (compare with Fig. 11.3).

Fig. 21.**39**   Central arachnoid cyst (39 x 38 mm), 33 weeks.

Fig. 21.**40**   Loculated arachnoid cyst located in the right posterior quadrant of the skull (45 x 36 mm), 38 weeks. Sagittal scan.

Agenesis of the corpus callosum, vein of Galen aneurysm

Fig. 21.**41**   Agenesis of the corpus callosum (arrow) with a dilated third ventricle, midsagittal scan (enlarged view). Trisomy 18, 32 weeks.

Fig. 21.**42**   Agenesis of the corpus callosum, coronal scan, 34 weeks. Above the absent corpus callosum is a markedly widened longitudinal cerebral fissure (arrows).

Fig. 21.**43 a**   Lateralization of the lateral ventricles and dilatation of the occipital horns in agenesis of the corpus callosum.
b Normal findings contrasted with the abnormalities found in agenesis of the corpus callosum. After Pilu et al. (120).

Fig. 21.**44**   Vein of Galen aneurysm, 29 weeks. Color Doppler shows definite blood flow within the central, hypoechoic tubular structure.

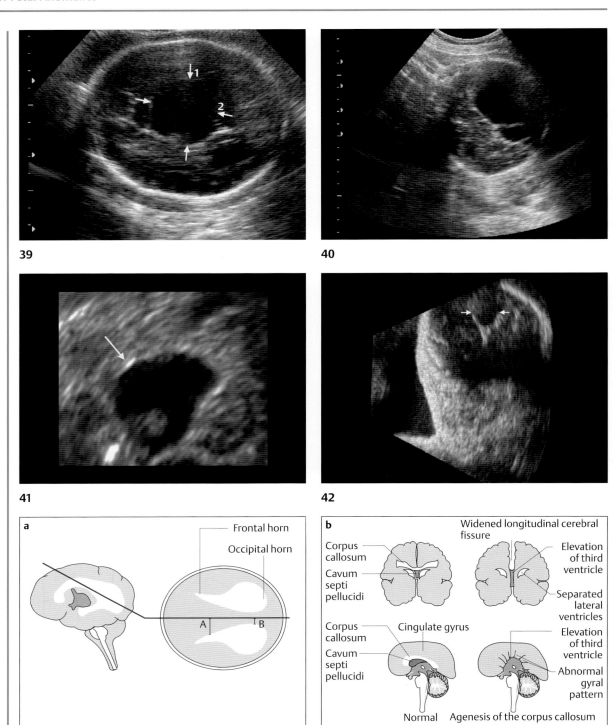

39

40

41

42

43a

43b

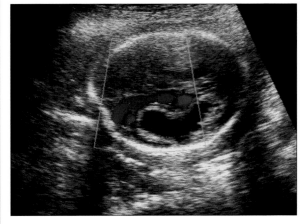

44

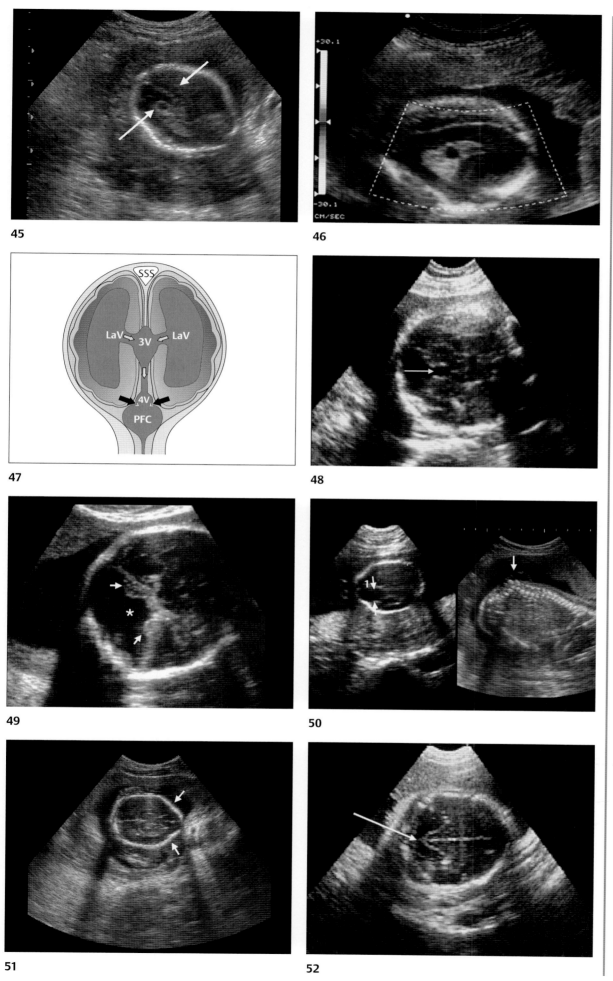

45

46

47

48

49

50

51

52

Choroid plexus cysts

Fig. 21.**45** Bilateral choroid plexus cysts (arrows), 23 weeks. Not infrequently, the cyst in the hemisphere closer to the transducer is obscured by reverberations.

Fig. 21.**46** Lateral sagittal scan of a choroid plexus cyst, 20 weeks.

Dandy–Walker malformation, Arnold–Chiari malformation

Fig. 21.**47** Diagram of a Dandy–Walker malformation. The fourth ventricle (4v) communicates with a posterior fossa cyst (PFC). The obstruction of CSF flow at the foramina of Luschka and Magendie (black arrows) leads to enlargement of the fourth ventricle, third ventricle, and lateral ventricles. SSS = superior sagittal sinus (modified from [125]).

Fig. 21.**48** Early Dandy–Walker malformation with slight enlargement of the cisterna magna and incomplete separation of the cerebellar hemispheres (arrow), 25 weeks.

Fig. 21.**49** Pronounced Dandy–Walker malformation, 33 weeks. Note the marked expansion of the cisterna magna (*) and the marked separation of the cerebellar hemispheres (arrows), which can barely be identified.

Fig. 21.**50** Arnold–Chiari type II malformation with enlarged frontal horns (arrows) and a lemon sign (image at left) with a myelomeningocele in the lumbosacral region (image at right), 23 weeks.

Fig. 21.**51** Arnold–Chiari malformation, 23 weeks. There is a conspicuous superior lemon sign, with bilateral indentation of the frontal bones (arrows).

Fig. 21.**52** Arnold–Chiari malformation, 21 weeks. Note the banana-shaped deformity of the cerebellum (arrow). The fetus is in a vertex presentation with the spine to the right.

Fig. 21.**53** Left: normal width of the cisterna magna. Right: obliteration of the cisterna magna and the lemon sign in Arnold–Chiari malformation, 22 weeks.

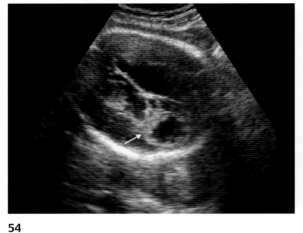

53

Cerebral hemorrhage and brain tumors

Fig. 21.**54** Pronounced, mixed hyper- and hypoechoic fetal cerebral hemorrhage (arrow) with rupture into the left ventricular system leading to ventricular dilatation, 32 weeks.

Fig. 21.**55** Mixed hyper- and hypoechoic brain tumor in the anterior part of the skull, with predominantly left-sided hydrocephalus posteriorly, 33 weeks (vertex presentation with the spine to the left). Histopathology: primitive neuroectodermal brain tumor.

54

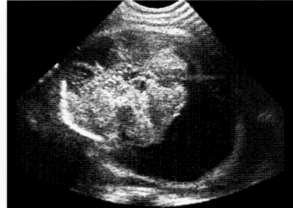

55

Fig. 21.**56** Very fast-growing brain tumor with an irregular structure, 27 weeks. The hypoechoic areas are foci of tumor necrosis. Pathology revealed a highly malignant teratoma.

Fig. 21.**57** Hypersecretory hydrocephalus associated with a choroid plexus papilloma (arrow), 31 weeks. The papilloma appears as an echogenic mass arising from the choroid plexus.

56

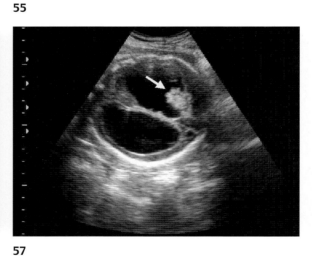

57

Macrocephaly, microcephaly, and various superior deformities

Fig. 21.**58** Macrocephaly due to severe hydrocephalus, 29 weeks. Sagittal scan. Right: postpartum appearance (infant delivered by cesarean section).

Fig. 21.**59** Cloverleaf skull in thanatophoric dysplasia, 21 weeks. Transverse scan (left) shows the irregular configuration of the superior vault. Coronal scan (right) shows the cloverleaf-shaped deformity of the skull.

58

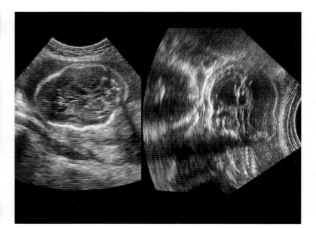

59

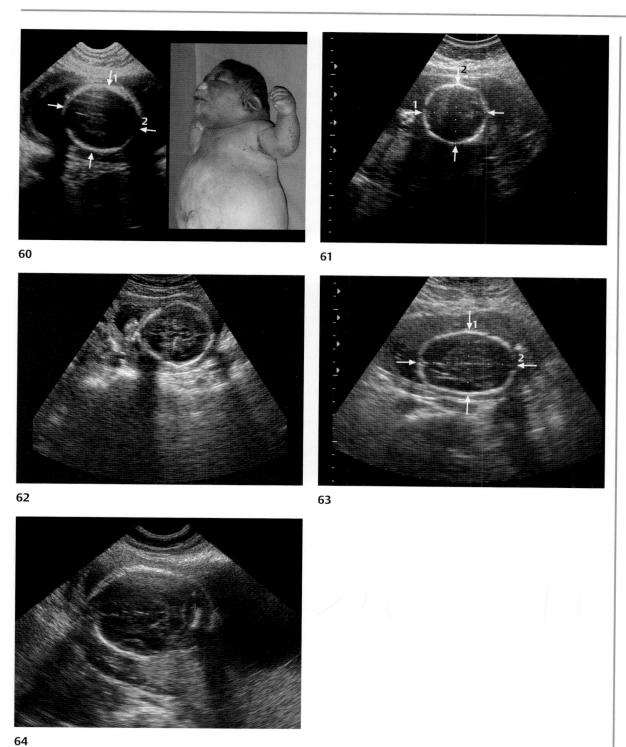

60

61

62

63

64

Fig. 21.**60**   Microcephaly (BPD [1] 5.3 cm, OFD [2] 6.0 cm) in Meckel–Gruber syndrome, 28 weeks. Right: postmortem view.

Fig. 21.**61**   Microcephaly, 23 weeks (BPD 5.2 cm [1], OFD 5.2 cm [2]).

Fig. 21.**62**   Strawberry-shaped skull, 23 weeks. The skull is narrow anteriorly and flattened posteriorly.

Fig. 21.**63**   Dolichocephaly in a breech-presenting fetus, 22 weeks. BPD 5.0 cm, OFD 7.3 cm. Cephalic index = 58.

Fig. 21.**64**   Thickened nuchal fold (arrows) (7 mm) at 19 weeks in a fetus with trisomy 21.

Facial Anomalies

▬ *Orbital Anomalies*

Hypertelorism

Definition. Increased interorbital distance.

Incidence. Rare.

Etiology and pathogenesis. Hypertelorism can occur as an isolated, sporadic anomaly, or it may occur in association with various syndromes, frontal encephaloceles, or hemangiomas (Table 21.**6**) (17).

Embryology. Normally the eyes migrate toward the facial midline during embryologic development. If this process is inhibited, hypertelorism results (18).

Pathoanatomic features. A basic distinction is drawn between *ocular and orbital hypertelorism.* Ocular hypertelorism is characterized by a broad, flat nasal root combined with a greater-than-average distance between the medial canthi of the eyes (26). Orbital hypertelorism refers to an increased distance between the medial orbital walls (31).

Ultrasound features. Orbital hypertelorism is diagnosed in the fetus by measuring the interorbital distance (= inner orbital distance) (Fig. 21.**65**). The distance between the lateral orbital walls (= outer orbital distance) can also be measured. Hypertelorism is present when the measured distance is greater than the 95th percentile (44). Chervenak et al. (8) and Donnenfeld et al. (19) reported on the prenatal diagnosis of hypertelorism in conjunction with a frontal encephalocele.

Associated anomalies. Various syndromes may be found in association with hypertelorism, as well as various chromosomal abnormalities (Table 21.**6**).

Prenatal management. Hypertelorism should prompt a detailed ultrasound search for additional fetal anomalies. Also, invasive testing is recommended to determine the fetal karyotype.

Table 21.**6**   Examples of anomalies that are associated with hypertelorism

Chromosomal abnormalities	➢ XO (Turner syndrome) ➢ Trisomy 9 ➢ Trisomy 13 ➢ Trisomy 14 ➢ Trisomy 21 ➢ Trisomy 22 ➢ Chromosome 4p syndrome ➢ Chromosome 5p syndrome ➢ Chromosome 18p syndrome
Syndromes	➢ Apert syndrome ➢ C syndrome ➢ Conradi–Huenermann syndrome ➢ Crouzon syndrome ➢ DeMyer syndrome ➢ Dubowitz syndrome ➢ Ehlers–Danlos syndrome ➢ Lange syndrome ➢ Larsen syndrome ➢ Noonan syndrome ➢ Potter syndrome ➢ Russell syndrome ➢ Secker syndrome ➢ Sotos syndrome
Hypertelorism combined with other ocular anomalies	➢ Frontal or ethmoidal encephalocele
Tumors	➢ Hemangioma

Hypotelorism

Definition. Decreased interorbital distance.

Incidence. Less common than hypertelorism.

Etiology and pathogenesis. Hypotelorism most commonly occurs in association with holoprosencephaly (12).

Embryology. It is unclear whether orbital hypotelorism results from a primary hypoplasia of the ethmoid bone or is a secondary change based on a different underlying cause (14).

Pathoanatomic features. As in hypertelorism, a distinction is made between *ocular* and *orbital hypotelorism.* Ocular hypotelorism describes a condition in which the eyes themselves are close together. Orbital hypotelorism refers to a decreased distance between the medial orbital walls (31).

Ultrasound features. The prenatal ultrasound diagnosis of orbital hypotelorism is based on the detection of a decreased interorbital distance (below the 5th percentile [44]) (Fig. 21.**66**). The outer orbital distance can also be used to diagnose hypotelorism. Pilu et al. (52) and Chervenak et al. (6) reported on the prenatal diagnosis of hypotelorism in association with holoprosencephaly.

Associated anomalies. Besides holoprosencephaly, there are several syndromes and chromosomal abnormalities that are associated with hypotelorism (Table 21.**7**).

Prenatal management. Like hypertelorism, hypotelorism should prompt a meticulous search for additional fetal anomalies, and invasive testing should be done to determine fetal karyotype.

Table 21.**7**   Examples of anomalies that are associated with hypotelorism

Chromosomal abnormalities	➢ Trisomie 13 ➢ Trisomie 21 ➢ Trisomie 18p-
CNS anomalies	➢ Holoprosencephaly ➢ Microcephaly
Syndromes	➢ Meckelsyndrome

Microphthalmos

Definition. Reduction in the size of the eye.

Incidence. Extremely rare.

Etiology and pathogenesis. Microphthalmos can occur as an isolated anomaly or in the setting of syndromes or chromosomal abnormalities. It occurs as an X-linked disorder in *microphthalmos–microcephaly syndrome* (21) and as an autosomal-dominant mandibulofacial dysmorphic syndrome in *Treacher–Collins (–Franceschetti) syndrome* (23). Exogenous factors may also have causal importance.

Pathoanatomic features. The condition may be unilateral or bilateral. The eye may be completely absent (anophthalmos). With *microphthalmos* as well as anophthalmos, there is usually retardation of orbital growth (65).

Ultrasound features. The ultrasound diagnosis is based on the detection of a small orbit whose size is below the 5th percentile for gesta-

Table 21.8 Examples of anomalies that are associated with microphthalmos

Chromosomal abnormalities	➢ Trisomy 13 ➢ Trisomy 14 mosaic ➢ Triploidy
CNS anomalies	➢ Holoprosencephaly
Syndromes	➢ Aicardi syndrome ➢ Alcoholism syndrome (37) ➢ Fraser syndrome (55) ➢ Lenz syndrome (38) ➢ Microphthalmos–microcephaly syndrome ➢ Pierre Robin syndrome ➢ Treacher–Collins syndrome

tional age (44). The eye is also small. Comparison with the opposite side is important in detecting discrepant orbital dimensions as well as abnormalities of the eye itself (Fig. 21.**67**).

Associated anomalies. Additional craniofacial, cardiac and other anomalies may be observed, depending on the underlying disorder (Table 21.**8**). Microphthalmos is combined with agenesis of the corpus callosum in *Aicardi syndrome* (20) and may coexist with limb anomalies in *Pierre Robin syndrome* (9).

Prognosis. Determined by associated anomalies.

Prenatal management. When microphthalmos is detected early, fetal karyotyping should be performed.

Synophthalmia, Cyclopia

Definition. Facial anomaly with a common orbit and two closely adjacent eyes (*synophthalmia*) or only one eye (*cyclopia*).

Incidence. Very rare.

Etiology and pathogenesis. The disorder is mainly found in association with holoprosencephaly.

Embryology. Cyclopia is characterized by deficient development of the prechordal superior segment (in front of the sella turcica), underdevelopment of the oronasal cavity, and abnormalities of the forebrain (60). Due to a severe error in the differentiation of the prosencephalon, there is partial (synophthalmia) or complete fusion (cyclopia) of the optic vesicles. If the eyes remain joined at the midline, a fleshy protuberance (proboscis) develops in place of the nose (28).

Pathoanatomic features. One or two separate, rudimentary eyes are found within the common orbit. There is concomitant arrhinia and a proboscis rooted above the orbit.

Ultrasound features. Targeting imaging of the fetal face will disclose the anomaly (40). The common orbit is best appreciated in a transverse scan through the upper half of the face (Fig. 21.**68**).

Associated anomalies. Brain malformations.

Prognosis. Because the defect is usually associated with holoprosencephaly, the prognosis is grave.

Prenatal management. Pregnancy termination is appropriate for cases that are detected early.

◼ *Nasal Anomalies*

Arrhinia

Definition. Absence of the nose.

Incidence. Very rare.

Etiology and pathogenesis. This anomaly may occur as an isolated defect, but it is usually found in association with holoprosencephaly (64).

Pathoanatomic features. Besides defects in the premaxilla, there may also be absence of the rhinencephalon (*arhinencephalia*).

Ultrasound features. Arrhinia is relatively easy to diagnose in a profile view of the fetal face (Fig. 21.**69**). If the profile cannot be defined due to an unfavorable fetal lie, the transverse scan is also diagnostic (Fig. 21.**70**).

Associated anomalies. Trisomy 13.

Prognosis. Generally unfavorable. It depends mainly on associated anomalies.

Prenatal management. Ultrasound search for additional anomalies and chromosomal analysis.

Proboscis

Definition. Snout-like protuberance on the face, usually with one opening.

Incidence. Very rare.

Etiology and pathogenesis. Occurs mainly in association with holoprosencephaly.

Pathoanatomic features. In cyclopia, the snout-like process is rooted above the rudimentary eye. In ethmocephaly it is located between the eyes, and in cebocephalia it consists of a rudimentary nose located below the eyes (Fig. 21.**71**).

Ultrasound features. The snout-like protuberance can be seen in a midsagittal scan through the fetal face, also in a coronal or transverse scan. It may appear at various levels on the face, depending on whether the fetus is cyclopic, ethmocephalic, or cebocephalic (Figs. 21.**72**, 21.**73**).

Prognosis. The prognosis is grave due to the high association with holoprosencephaly.

Prenatal management. Pregnancy termination is appropriate for cases that are detected early.

◼ *Tumors in the Facial Region*

Definition. Mass lesion in the facial region.

Incidence. Very rare.

Etiology and pathogenesis. A fetal facial mass may be a lacrimal duct cyst (16), a periorbital hemangioma, or a dermoid.

Pathoanatomic features. Lacrimal duct cysts are located inferomedial to the orbit.

Ultrasound features. The ultrasound appearance depends on whether the mass is an echogenic tumor or a purely cystic lesion (Figs. 21.**74**, 21.**75**). Doppler scanning can also be used to distinguish between a dermoid and hemangioma (43, 36).

Differential diagnosis. Frontal encephalocele.

Prognosis. Depends on the type, location, and size of the tumor.

Prenatal management. A large mass can pose an obstacle to vaginal delivery, necessitating a cesarean section.

Facial Cleft Anomalies

Cleft Lip and Palate

Definition. Cleft formation in the lip and/or maxilla and/or palate.

Forms. Lateral and median clefts.

Incidence. Clefts of the upper lip and palate are relatively common (approximately one in 1000) (29). The defect is present in 13% of all infants with congenital anomalies (25).

Etiology and pathogenesis. Abnormalities of facial development may be genetic or acquired (e.g., drug-induced). Clefts are also found in association with various syndromes (13) and chromosomal abnormalities, particularly trisomy 13 and 18.

Embryology. Given the diverse processes in which facial elevations and furrows are fused and effaced during embryonic development, there is no single, simple explanation for facial cleft anomalies. There are two basic possibilities:
1. An epithelial wall is formed but cannot be maintained (nonfusibility of the epithelium).
2. The facial processes fail to come into contact with each other (hypoplasia or faulty growth direction).
   The critical period for cleft formation is between days 36 and 42 of embryonic development (28).

Anterior and posterior clefts. According to Moore (47), anterior clefts are caused by faulty development of the primary palate based on a lack of mesenchyma in the maxillary process and premaxillary segment. Posterior clefts result from faulty development of the secondary palate—i.e., growth disturbances of the lateral palatine processes, which fail to fuse with each other.

Unilateral cleft lip. This occurs when the maxillary process fails to reach and fuse with the medial nasal process.

Bilateral cleft lip. Bilateral clefts develop in the upper lip when the maxillary processes on both sides fail to fuse with the median nasal process. The degree of cleft formation may be equal or different on both sides.

Median cleft lip. A median cleft is probably caused by a lack of mesenchyma in the central portion of the upper lip (47).

Pathoanatomic Features

Anterior clefts. These include a cleft lip with or without a cleft in the alveolar part of the maxilla. A complete anterior cleft extends through the lips and alveolus to the incisive foramen and separates the primary palate from the secondary palate.

Posterior clefts. These clefts involve the secondary (posterior) palate. They extend through the soft and hard palate to the incisive foramen and separate the secondary palate from the primary palate. The lateral defect may be unilateral or bilateral. Cleft palate may result from failure of the lateral palatine processes to fuse with each other, with the nasal septum, and/or with the posterior margin of the primary palate (47).

Ultrasound features. Cleft lip and palate can be diagnosed sonographically (3, 29, 54, 59) in a coronal or sagittal scan through the face or in a transverse scan at the level of the maxilla (Figs. 21.**76**–21.**82**). Whereas large clefts are fairly conspicuous, a small cleft is easily overlooked. Coronal and transverse scans are best for distinguishing the different types of cleft (Figs. 21.**76**–21.**79** and 21.**82**). With a small lip cleft, the coronal scan shows only a narrow defect in the upper lip (Fig. 21.**79**). A sagittal scan through the defect itself gives the impression of a perpetually open mouth (Fig. 21.**80**). When bilateral clefts are present, the tissue bridge located between the clefts appears as a protuberance in the midsagittal scan (Fig. 21.**81**).

Maxillary defect. A maxillary defect appears as a concavity in the transverse scan (Fig. 21.**82**). An isolated palatal cleft, however, can be extremely difficult to detect with ultrasound. Three-dimensional ultrasound can provide an accurate tomographic survey of cleft-lip defects (45).

Associated anomalies. Facial clefts may occur as part of a syndrome or in association with chromosomal abnormalities (Table 21.**9**). Snijders et al. (59) examined 111 fetuses with a facial cleft. The facial cleft occurred as an isolated defect in 37% of these cases, and additional anomalies were present in 63% of cases. All the fetuses with an isolated facial cleft were chromosomally normal, while 39 of the 70 cases (35%) with additional anomalies were found to have chromosomal defects. These consisted of trisomy 18 (n = 7), trisomy 13 (n = 22), unbalanced translocation between chromosomes 13 and 14 (n = 3), trisomy 21 (n = 1), trisomy 22 (n = 1), partial trisomy 4q (n = 1), deletion 21q (n = 1), deletion 4p (n = 1), inversion of chromosome 9 (n = 1), and triploidy (n = 1).

Mohr syndrome. A median cleft in the upper lip is a characteristic feature of Mohr syndrome (orofaciodigital syndrome II) (34), which is also characterized by limb malformations (syndactyly, polydactyly), growth retardation, and brain malformations.

Prognosis. The prognosis depends on whether the cleft is an isolated abnormality or whether other anomalies are present. The prognosis with a small, isolated defect is very good. Larger defects require more elaborate maxillofacial surgical procedures. The empirical recurrence risk for maxillofacial clefts depends on various factors. If both parents have congenital clefts and two siblings are affected, the recurrence risk is as high as 50% (61).

Table 21.9 Examples of anomalies that are associated with cleft lip and palate

Chromosomal abnormalities	➢ Trisomy 13 ➢ Trisomy 18 ➢ Trisomy 21 ➢ Tetrasomy 9p ➢ Chromosome 4p-
CNS anomalies	➢ Holoprosencephaly
Syndromes	➢ DeMyer syndrome (medial or bilateral cleft) ➢ Roberts syndrome (bilateral cleft) ➢ Mohr syndrome (median cleft) ➢ Smith–Lemli–Opitz syndrome (cleft palate) ➢ Amniotic band syndrome

Prenatal management. Given the high association of chromosomal defects with facial clefts, fetal karyotyping should be performed whenever a cleft is detected sonographically. If a chromosomal defect is excluded, the parents should be referred for early counseling with a geneticist and maxillofacial surgeon.

Epignathus

Definition. Epignathus is a teratoid tumor that arises from the fetal oral cavity or pharynx.

Incidence. Epignathus accounts for 2% of all congenital teratomas (24).

Etiology and pathogenesis. While epignathus was once thought to be a parasitic (asymmetric) twin malformation, current opinion attributes the tumor to the disorganized growth of pluripotent cells from Rathke's pouch (30).

Pathoanatomic features. In the strict sense, epignathus is a tumor of the upper jaw. Most of these tumors originate from the sphenoid bone or palate, however, and grow into the mouth or pharynx and occasionally into the cranium (22, 64). Histologically, the tumors contain elements of all three germ layers.

Ultrasound features. Ultrasound demonstrates a complex tumor at the front of the face. The mass may contain a mixture of hypoechoic and hyperechoic areas (7, 32, 58) (Fig. 21.**83**).

Polyhydramnios is a common associated finding, probably due to interference with fetal swallowing.

Prognosis. Although most of these tumors are benign, the prognosis tends to be unfavorable because the tumors cause airway obstruction leading to postpartum asphyxiation. The size and operability of the tumor are critical. A few cases have been described in which the infants survived with surgical intervention (5, 41, 50).

Prenatal management. Pregnancy termination is an option if the tumor is extensive and is detected early in the second trimester. Larger tumors diagnosed late in the pregnancy can obstruct delivery, necessitating a cesarean section. These cases require close interdisciplinary consultation with the pediatrician, anesthesiologist, and oromaxillary surgeon.

Macroglossia

Definition. Excessive size of the tongue.

Incidence. Rare.

Etiology and pathogenesis. Macroglossia can occur in the following settings:

Beckwith–Wiedemann syndrome (exomphalos–macroglossia–gigantism syndrome) (34)

Cornelia de Lange syndrome II (muscular hyperplasia with cerebral injury) (35)

Trisomy 21 (48)

Ultrasound features. A sagittal scan most clearly demonstrates the large tongue protruding between the upper and lower lips (Fig. 21.**84**). Measurements of the tongue circumference like those described by Achiron et al. (1) may be helpful in diagnosing macroglossia.

Trisomy 21. If a flat profile is noted in association with macroglossia, trisomy 21 should be considered (Fig. 21.**84**). Nicolaides et al. (48) examined 69 fetuses with trisomy 21 and found macroglossia in 10% of the cases observed before 28 weeks and 20% of the cases with 28 or more weeks' gestation.

Beckwith–Wiedemann syndrome. There have been reports of several cases of Beckwith–Wiedemann syndrome diagnosed prenatally with ultrasound (27, 63, 67). Detection of an accompanying abdominal wall defect suggests the correct diagnosis. Diagnostic problems arise, however, if the abdominal wall is intact (49).

Associated anomalies. Accompanying abdominal wall defects and visceromegaly are found in Beckwith–Wiedemann syndrome (67). Cornelia de Lange syndrome may additionally exhibit porencephaly.

Differential diagnosis. Bilateral cleft lip and palate with a prominent median tissue bridge.

Prognosis. The prognosis depends on the underlying disorder.

Prenatal management. Fetal chromosome analysis is recommended to detect or exclude trisomy 21.

Micrognathia, Retrognathia

Definition. Small, retruded mandible.

Incidence. Rare.

Etiology and pathogenesis. Micrognathia occurs as a feature of several syndromes (Table 21.**10**), including:
Pierre Robin syndrome (microgenia, glossoptosis, and cleft palate) (51, 53)
- *Treacher–Collins (–Franceschetti) syndrome* (autosomal-dominant mandibulofacial dysmorphic syndrome with characteristic facies) (23)
- *Smith–Lemli–Opitz syndrome II* (autosomal-recessive disease with microcephaly, typical craniofacial dysmorphias, heart defects, and pseudohermaphroditism in males) (15)
- *Kousseff syndrome* (sacral myelomeningocele, complex heart defect, craniofacial dysmorphism) (33)

Ultrasound features. The profile view demonstrates a small, receding chin (Fig. 21.**85**). Chitty et al. (10) published normal data for mandibular dimensions between 12 and 27 weeks' gestation that may permit a more objective evaluation of fetal micrognathia. Cohen et al. (11) reported on the prenatal detection of Treacher–Collins syndrome (11).

Associated anomalies. Turner and Twining (62) found an abnormal karyotype in 38% of fetuses found to have micrognathia with ultrasound (Table 21.**10**). The most common chromosomal defect is trisomy 18 (24, 48).

Table 21.**10** Anomalies that are associated with micrognathia or retrognathism

Chromosomal abnormalities	➤ Trisomy 13 ➤ Trisomy 18 ➤ Trisomy 10p
Syndromes	➤ Kousseff syndrome ➤ Nager syndrome ➤ Pierre Robin syndrome ➤ Oroacral syndrome ➤ Smith–Lemli–Opitz syndrome II ➤ Treacher–Collins syndrome

Prognosis. The prognosis depends on the underlying disorder.

Prenatal management. When micro- or retrognathia is detected sonographically, a diligent search should be made for concomitant anomalies. The fetal karyotype should also be determined.

▬ Anomalies of the Ear and Auricular Root

Definition. Malformations of the auricle and its attachment.

Etiology and pathogenesis. Auricular dysplasias are found in the setting of various syndromes (Table 21.**11**) including:

- *Treacher–Collins syndrome* (autosomal-dominant mandibulofacial dysmorphic syndrome with characteristic facies and reduction deformities of the external ear) (23)
- *Seckel syndrome* (bird-headed dwarfism with microcephaly, bird-like face with a beak-like nose, receding chin, intrauterine growth retardation, low-set dysplastic ears, clinodactyly, and club foot) (66)
- *Smith–Lemli–Opitz syndrome* (growth retardation, microcephaly, low-set ears, micrognathia, hypospadias, small penis, syndactyly of second and third toes).

Chromosomal defects. Dysplastic ears are also found in chromosomal defects such as trisomy 18 (66) (Table 21.**11**).

Embryology. The primordium of the external ear is located on the side of the neck in early development. If the lower jaw is underdeveloped, the auricle does not undergo a normal ascension and retains its "embryonic" position at the head-neck junction (28).

Table 21.**11**   Anomalies that are associated with low-set ears, auricular dysplasia, a small ear, or a preauricular tag

Low-set ears	➢ Cloverleaf skull syndrome ➢ Kousseff syndrome ➢ Smith–Lemli–Opitz syndrome ➢ Treacher–Collins syndrome
Auricular dysplasia	➢ Chromosome 9p- ➢ Trisomy 18 ➢ Seckel syndrome ➢ Smith–Lemli–Opitz syndrome type I
Small ear	➢ Trisomy 21
Preauricular tag	➢ Trisomy 10p ➢ Goldenhar syndrome

Pathoanatomic features. Auricular anomalies can assume a variety of forms. Auricular tags are most commonly located in front of the external auditory canal (47).

Ultrasound features. Low-set ears are most clearly appreciated in a longitudinal coronal scan (Fig. 21.**86**). Auricular abnormalities are best demonstrated in a tangential scan through the ear (Fig. 21.**87**). Some authors (2, 4, 39, 57) claim that a short fetal ear is also suggestive of a chromosomal abnormality. Three-dimensional ultrasound is excellent for selective visualization of the auricle, as it can provide a 3-D rendering of the auricular surface (46, 56).

Prenatal management. When ultrasound demonstrates low-set ears or auricular dysplasia, a diligent search should be made for additional anomalies, and fetal karyotyping should be performed.

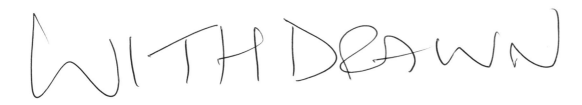

Orbital anomalies

Fig. 21.**65**   Hypertelorism with marked widening of the interorbital distance (30 mm), 32 weeks.

Fig. 21.**66**   Hypertelorism in holoprosencephaly. The interorbital distance, at 7 mm, is markedly decreased. 31 weeks.

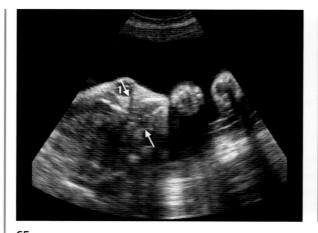

65

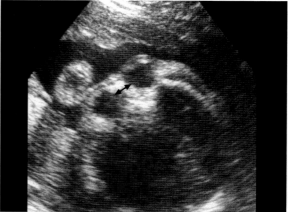

66

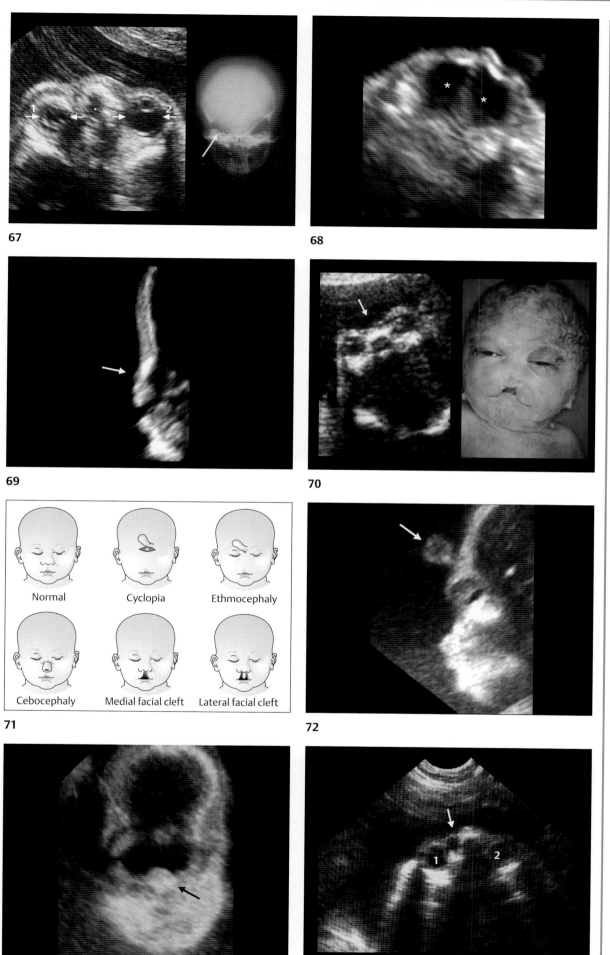

67

68

69

70

Normal   Cyclopia   Ethmocephaly

Cebocephaly   Medial facial cleft   Lateral facial cleft

71

72

73

74

Fig. 21.**67**   Right orbital hypoplasia in a breech-presenting fetus with trisomy 13. The right orbital diameter (1) is 9 mm with a small, rudimentary eye. The left orbital diameter (2) is 13 mm with a normally developed eye. 27 weeks, 6 days. The postpartum radiograph on the right demonstrates the small size of the right orbit (arrow).

Fig. 21.**68**   Synophthalmia, 26 weeks. Two adjacent, close-set eyes (*) occupy a common orbit.

Nasal anomalies and tumors of the facial region

Fig. 21.**69**   Nasal aplasia (arrow) accompanied by arrhinencephaly, 21 weeks. The midsagittal scan shows an abnormally flat profile. The nose cannot be visualized.

Fig. 21.**70**   Left: absent nose (arrow) and arrhinencephaly in a fetus with holoprosencephaly. Oblique scan, weeks. Right: postmortem view of the same fetus.

Fig. 21.**71**   Various facial abnormalities that can occur in holoprosencephaly (after [42]).

Fig. 21.**72**   Proboscis (arrow) above the rudimentary eye in cyclopia. Midsagittal scan, 25 weeks.

Fig. 21.**73**   Cebocephaly, coronal view, 26 weeks.. The snout-like process is located below the fused orbits (arrow).

Fig. 21.**74**   Cystic outpouching of the left lacrimal sac, 8 · 11 mm (arrow). Vertex presentation, 29 weeks. 1 = Left orbit, 2 = right orbit.

Fig. 21.**75** Dermoid in the area of the right cheek (54 mm in diameter). Lateral sagittal scan, 25 weeks.

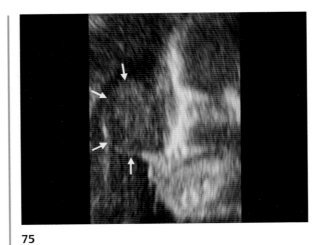

75

Cleft lip and palate

Fig. 21.**76** Left: right-sided cleft lip and palate in a coronal view. Trisomy 13, 23 weeks. Right: postmortem view of the affected fetus.

Fig. 21.**77** Left: isolated left-sided cleft lip and palate in a coronal view. Normal karyotype, 33 weeks. Right: postpartum appearance at 40 weeks.

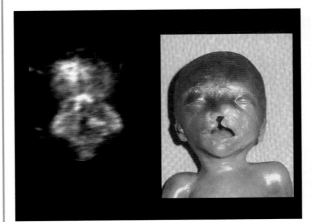

76

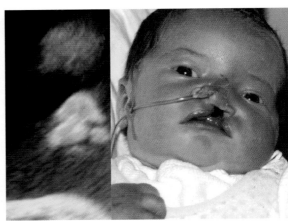

77

Fig. 21.**78** Left: bilateral cleft lip and palate in a coronal view. Trisomy 18, 22 weeks. Right: corresponding postmortem view.

Fig. 21.**79** Small cleft in the lip and maxilla (arrow), 36 weeks.

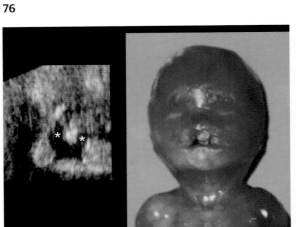

78

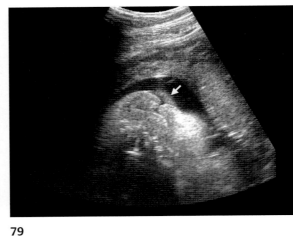

79

Fig. 21.**80** Left: large median cleft in a profile view. Partial tetrasomy 9, 30 weeks. A striking feature is the open mouth, which does not close even when observed for a prolonged period. Right: corresponding postmortem view.

Fig. 21.**81** Left: bilateral clefts in a profile view, 22 weeks. The knob of tissue between the two clefts appears as a protuberance below the nose (arrow). Right: corresponding postmortem view.

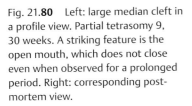

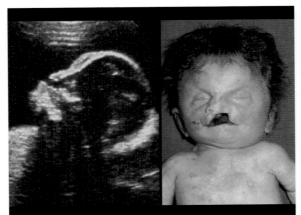

80

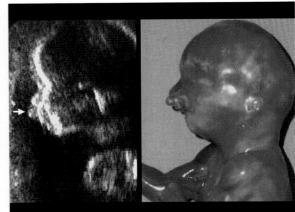

81

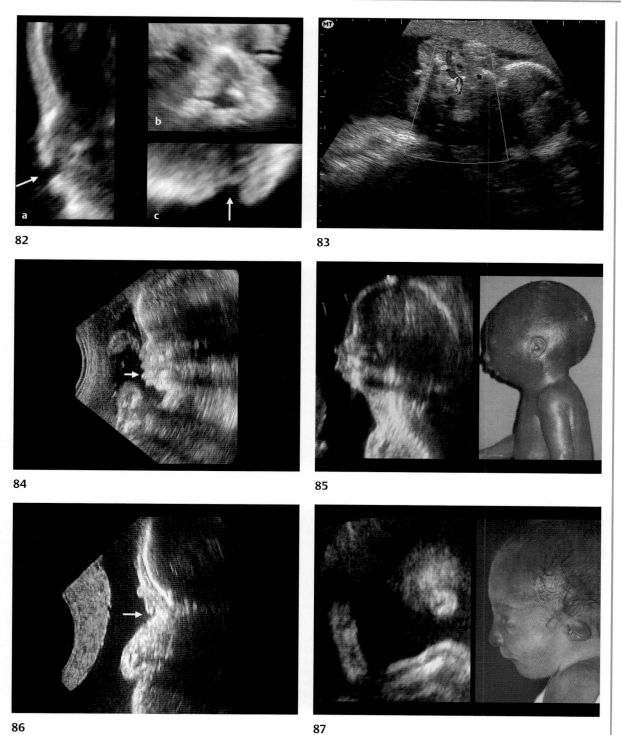

82

83

84

85

86

87

Fig. 21.**82**   Median cleft in a fetus with holoprosencephaly, 29 weeks.
a Profile view (arrow).
b Coronal view.
c Transverse scan. The cleft appears in this plane as a concave defect (arrow).

Fig. 21.**83**   Epignathus in lateral view, 22 weeks. Color Doppler defines the tumor's vascular supply.

Fig. 21.**84**   Macroglossia (arrow) in a 30-week fetus with trisomy 21. The profile view shows a flat face and open mouth with a large, protruding tongue.

Fig. 21.**85**   Micro- and retrognathia in trisomy 18. Profile view, 23 weeks. Right: corresponding postmortem view.

Auricular anomalies

Fig. 21.**86**   Low-set ear in Pena–Shokeir syndrome, 28 weeks. The lower part of the left earlobe almost touches the shoulder (arrow).

Fig. 21.**87**   Dysplastic auricle in trisomy 18. Tangential scan, 33 weeks. Right: corresponding postmortem view.

References

Neural Tube Defects

1. Achiron, R., Malinger, G., Tadmor, O. et al.: Exencephaly and anencephaly: a distinct anomaly or an embryologic precursor: in utero study by transvaginal sonography. Israel. J. Obstet. Gynecol. 1 (1990) 60–63
2. Aleksic, S., Budzilovich, G., Greco, M.A., Feigin, I., Epstein, F., Pearson, J.: Iniencephaly: Neuropathologic study. Clin. Neuropathol. 2 (1983) 55–61
3. Boos, R., Rabe, D., Schmidt, W.: Pränatale Diagnose eines schweren Neuralrohrdefektes bei negativen biochemischen Befunden. Z. Geburtsh. Perinat. 188 (1984) 244–247
4. Bronshtein, M., Ornoy, A.: Acrania: anencephaly resulting from secondary degeneration of a closed neural tube: two cases in the same family. J. Clin. Ultrasound, 19 (1991) 230–234
5. Budorick, N.E., Pretorius, D.H., MacGahan, J.P., Grafe, M.R., James, H.E., Slivka, J.: Cephalocele detection in utero: sonographic and clinical features. Ultrasound Obstet. Gynecol. 5 (1995) 77–85
6. Chervenak, F.A., Isaacson, G., Mahoney, M.J., Berkowitz, R.L., Tortora, M., Hobbins, J.C.: Diagnosis and management of fetal cephalocele. Obstet. Gynecol. 64 (1984) 86–91
7. Cox, G.G., Rosenthall, S.J., Holsapple, J.W.: Exencephaly: Sonographic findings and radiologic-pathologic correlation. Radiology 155 (1985) 755–756
8. Cunningham, M.E., Walls, W.I.: Ultrasound in the evaluation of anencephaly. Radiology 118 (1976) 165–167
9. David, T.J., Nixon, A.: Congenital malformations associated with anencephaly and iniencephaly. J. Med. Genet. 13 (1976) 263–265
10. Degenhardt, F., Mühlhaus, K.: Pränatale Diagnostik eines Meckel-Syndroms bei einer vorbelasteten Familie. Ultraschall 6 (1985) 226–228
11. Donnenfeld, A.E., Hughes, H., Weiner, S.: Prenatal diagnosis and perinatal management of frontoethmoidal meningoencephalocele. Amer J. Perinatology 5 (1988) 51–53
12. EUROCAT Working Group. Prevalence of neural tube defects in 20 regions of Europe and the impact of prenatal diagnosis, 1980–1986. J. Epidemiol. Community Health 45 (1991) 52–58
13. Fiske, C.E., Filly, R.A.: Ultrasound evaluation of the normal and abnormal fetal neural axis. Radiol. Clin. N. Amer. 20 (1982) 285–296
14. Foderaro, A.E., Abu-Yosef, M.M., Benda, J.A., Williamson, R.A., Smith, W.L.: Antenatal diagnosis of iniencephaly. J. Clin. Ultrasound 15 (1988) 550–554
15. Goldstein, R.B., Filly, R.A.: Prenatal diagnosis of anencephaly: Spectrum of sonographic appearances and distinction from the amniotic band syndrome. Amer. J. Roentgenol. 151 (1988) 547–550
16. Goldstein, R.B., Filly, R.A., Callen, P.W.: Sonography of anencephaly: pitfalls in early diagnosis. J. Clin. Ultrasound 17 (1989) 397–402
17. Guthkelch, A.N.: Occipital cranium bifidum. Arch. Dis. Child 45 (1970) 104–109
18. Hackelöer, B.J., Nitschke, S.: Frühdiagnose des Anencephalus und Iniencephalus durch Ultraschall. Geburtsh. u. Frauenheilk. 35 (1975) 866–871
19. Hendricks, S.K., Cyr, D.R., Nyberg, D.A., Raabe, R., Mack, L.A.: Exencephaly – Clinical and ultrasonic correlation to anencephaly. Obstet. Gynecol. 72 (1988) 898–901
20. Howkins, J., Lawrie, R.S.: Inienzephalus. J. Obstet. Gynaec. Brit. Emp. 46 (1939) 25–31
21. Johnson, S.P., Sebire, N.J., Snijders, R.J.M., Tunkei, S., Nicolaides, K.H.: Ultrasound screening for anencephaly at 10–14 weeks of gestation. Ultrasound Obstet. Gynecol. 9 (1997) 14–16
22. Kennedy, K.A., Flick, K.J., Thurmond, A.S.: First-trimester diagnosis of exencephaly. Amer. J. Obstet. Gynecol. 162 (1990) 461–463
23. Klippel, M., Feil, A.: Un cas d'absence des verèbres cervicales. Nouv. Iconogr. Salpêtrière 25 (1912) 223–250
24. Kossoff, G., Garrett, W.J., Radovanovich, G.: Grey scale echography in obstetrics and gynaecology. Aust. Radiol. 18 (1974) 62–111
25. Kurjak, A.: Direct ultrasonic diagnosis of fetal malformations and abnormalities. In: Murken, J.D., Stengel-Rutkowski, S., Schwinger, E.: Prenatal Diagnosis. Stuttgart: Enke 1979; p. 175
26. Leucht, W., Heyes, H., Müller, E., Schmidt, W.: Das Meckel-Syndrom. Seine Bedeutung für die pränatale Diagnostik und für den Frauenarzt. Geburtsh. u. Frauenheilk. 41 (1981) 765–768
27. Loft, A.G., Hogdall, E., Larsen, S.O., Norgaard-Pedersen, B.: A comparison of amniotic fluid alpha-fetoprotein and acetylcholinesterase in the prenatal diagnosis of open neural tube defects and anterior abdominal wall defects. Prenat. Diagn. 13 (1993) 93–109
28. Lorber, J., Schofield, J.K.: The prognosis of occipital encephalocele. Z. Kinderchir. Grenzgeb. 28 (1979) 347–351
29. Masterson, J.G.: Empiric risk, genetic counseling and preventive measures in anencephaly. Acta genet. (Basel) 12 (1962) 219–229
30. Mecke, S., Passarge, E.: Encephalocele, polycystic kidneys, and polydactyly as an autosomal recessive trait simulating certain other disorders. The Meckel syndrome. Ann. Genet. 14 (1971) 97–103
31. Meizner, I., Bar-Ziv, J.: Preantal ultrasonic diagnosis of a rare case of iniencephaly apertus. J. Clin. Ultrasound 15 (1987) 200–203
32. Mórocz, I., Szeifert, G.T., Molnár, P., Tóth, J., Csécsei, Papp, Z.: Prenatal diagnosis and pathoanatomy of iniencephaly. Clin. Genetics 30 (1986) 81–86
33. Nau, H., Hauck, R.S., Ehlers, K.: Valproic acid-induced neural tube defects in mouse and human: aspects of chirality, alternative drug development, pharmacokinetics and possible mechanisms. Pharmacol. Toxicol. 69 (1991) 310–321
34. Patt, V., Niesen, M.: Dystokie durch fetale Mißbildungen und Anomalien des mütterlichen Genitale. Gynäkologe 7 (1974) 106–115
35. Robinson, H.P.: The role of ultrasound in the prenatal diagnosis of neural tube defects. In: Murken, J.D., Stengel-Rutkowski, S., Schwinger, E.: Prenatal Diagnosis. Stuttgart: Enke 1979; p. 179
36. Robinson, H.P., Hood, V.D., Adam, A.H., Gibson, A.A., Ferguson-Smith, M.A.: Diagnostic ultrasound: Early detection of fetal neural tube defects. Obstet. Gynec. 56 (1980) 705–710
37. Rottem, S., Bronshtein, M., Thaler, I., Brandes, J. M.: First trimester transvaginal sonographic diagnosis of fetal anomalies. Lancet 1 (1989) 444–445
38. Schmidt, W., von Host, T., Schröder, T., Kubli, F.: Pränatale Diagnose des Meckel-Gruber-Syndroms durch Ultraschall. Z. Geburtsh. Perinat. 185 (1981) 67–71
39. Schmidt, W., Kubli, F.: Early diagnosis of severe congenital malformations by ultrasonography. J. Perinat. Med. 10 (1982) 233–241
40. Schulman, K.: Encephalocele. In: Bergsma, D., Alan, R.: Birth Defects Compendium. 2nd ed. Liss 1979; p. 390
41. Sherer, D.M., Hearn-Stebbins, B., Harvey, W., Metlay, L.A., Abramowicz, J.S.: Endovaginal sonographic diagnosis of iniencephaly apertus and craniorachischisis at 13 weeks' menstrual age. J. Clin. Ultrasound 21 (1993) 124–127
42. Shoham, Z., Caspi, B., Chemke, J., Dgani, R., Lancet, M.: Iniencephaly: prenatal ultrasonographic diagnosis – case report. J. Perinat. Med. 16 (1988) 139–143
43. Simpson, D.A., David, D.J., White, J.: Cephaloceles: Treatment, outcome, and antenatal diagnosis. Neurosurgery 15 (1984) 14–21
44. Sonoda, T., Ohdo, S, Ohba, K., Okishima, T., Hayakawa, K.: Teratogenic effects of sodium valproate in the Jcl: ICR mouse fetus. Acta Paediatr. Jpn. 32 (1990) 502–507
45. Tuchmann-Duplessis, H., Mercier-Parot, L.: Sur l'action teratogene d'un sulfamide hypoglycemiant, etude experimentale chez la ratte. J. Physiol. 51 (1959) 65–83
46. U. K. Collaborative study on alpha-1-fetoprotein in relation to neural tube defects. Lancet I (1977) 1323–1332
47. Vergani, P., Ghidini, A., Sirtori, M., Roncaglia, N.: Antenatal diagnosis of fetal acrania. J. Ultrasound Med. 6 (1987) 715–717
48. Wald, N., Cuckle, H., Nanchahal, K.: Amniotic fluid acetylcholinesterase measurement in the prenatal diagnosis of open neural tube defects. Second report of the Collaborative Acetylcholinesterase Study. Prenat. Diagn. 9 (1989) 813–829
49. Warkany, J., Takacs, E.: Experimental production of congenital malformations in rats by salicylate poisoning. Amer. J. Pathol. 35 (1959) 315–331
50. Warkany, J., Takacs, E.: Congenital malformations in rats from streptonigrin. Arch. Pathol. 79 (1965) 65–79
51. Warkany, J.: Congenital Malformations. Year Book Medical Publishers, Chicago 1971; p. 414
52. Wilkins-Haug, L., Freedman, W.: Progression of exencephaly to anencephaly in the human fetus – an ultrasound perspective. Prenat. Diagn. 11 (1991) 227–233

CNS Anomalies

1. Altshuler, G.: Toxoplasmosis as a cause of hydranencephaly. Amer. J. Dis. Child. 125 (1973) 251–252
2. Alvord, E.C., Jr., Shaw, C.M.: Neoplasmas of the nervous system. In: Ducket, S.: Pediatric Neuropathology. Baltimore: Williams and Wilkins 1995; pp. 640–718
3. Anderson, F., Landing, B:. Cerebral arachnoid cysts in infants. J. Pediatr. 69 (1966) 88–96
4. Benacerraf, B.R., Barss, V.A., Laboda, L.A.: A sonographic sign for the detection in the second trimester of the fetus with Down syndrome. Amer. J. Obstet. Gynecol. 151 (1985) 1078–1079
5. Benacerraf, B.R., Gelman, R., Frigoletto, F.D.: Sonographic identification of second trimester fetuses with Down's syndrome. New Engl. J. Med. 317 (1987) 1371–1376
6. Benacerraf, B.R., Frigoletto, F.D.Jr.: Soft tissue nuchal fold in the second-trimester fetus: Standards for normal measurements compared with those in Down syndrome. Amer. J. Obstet. Gynecol. 157 (1987) 1146–1149
7. Benacerraf, B.R., Stryker, J., Frigoletto, F.D.Jr.: Abnormal US appearance of the cerebellum (banana sign): indirect sign of spina bifida. Radiology 171 (1989) 151–153
8. Benda, C.E.: The Dandy-Walker syndrome or the socalled atresia of the foramen Magendie. J. Neuropathol. Exp. Neurol. 13 (1954) 14–29
9. Bertino, R.E., Nyberg, D.A., Cyr, D.R., Mack, L.A.: Prenatal diagnosis of agenesis of the corpus callosum. J. Ultrasound Med. 7 (1988) 251–260
10. Bickers, D.S., Adams, R.D.: Hereditary stenosis of the aqueduct of Sylvius as a cause of congenital hydrocephalus. Brain 72 (1949) 246–262
11. Birnholz, J.C., Frigoletto, F.D.: Antenatal treatment of hydrocephalus. New Engl. J. Med. 304 (1981) 1021–1023
12. Bland, R.S., Nelson, L.H., Meis, P.J., Weaver, R.L., Abramson, J.S.: Gonococcal ventriculitis associated with ventruculoamniotic shunt placement. Amer. J. Obstet. Gynecol. 147 (1983) 781–784
13. Bollmann, R., Chaoui, R, Zienert, A., Körner, H.: Plexus chorioideus-Zysten im II. Trimenon – ein Hinweiszeichen für eine Trisomie 18. Zentralbl. Gynäkol. 114 (1992) 171–174
14. Brahman, S., Jenna, R., Wittenauer, H.J.: Sonographic in utero appearance of Kleeblattschädel syndrome. J. Clin. Ultrasound 7 (1979) 481–484
15. Burstein, J., Papile, L., Burstein, R.: Intraventricular hemorrhage and hydrocephalus in premature newborns: A prospective study with CT. Amer. J. Roentgenol. 132 (1979) 631–635
16. Cameron, A.H.: Arnold-Chiari and other neuro-anatomical malformations associated with spina bifida. J. Path. Bact. 73 (1957) 195–211
17. Campbell, S.: Early prenatal diagnosis of fetal abnormality by ultrasound B-scanning. In: Murken, J.D., Rutkowski, S., Schwinger, E.: Prenatal Diagnosis. Stuttgart: Enke 1979; S. 183
18. Cantu, R.C., LeMay, M.: Porencephaly caused by intracerebral hemorrhage. Radiology 88 (1967) 526–530
19. Chervenak, F.A., Berkowitz, R.L., Romero, R. et al.: The diagnosis of fetal hydrocephalus. Amer. J. Obstet. Gynecol. 147 (1983) 703–716

20. Chervenak, F.A., Isaacson, G., Mahoney, M.J., Tortora, M., Mesologites, T., Hobbins, J.: The obstetric significance of holoprosencephaly. Obstet. Gynecol. 63 (1984) 115–121
21. Chervenak, F.A., Jeanty, P., Cantraine, F. et al.: The diagnosis of fetal microcephaly. Amer. J. Obstet. Gynec. 149 (1984) 512–517
22. Chervenak, F.A., McCullough, L.B.: Ethical challenges in prenatal medicine: the intrapartum management of pregnancy complicated by fetal hydrocephalus with macrocephaly. Semin. Perinatol. 1 (1987) 232–239
23. Chuang, S., Harwood-Nash, D.: Tumors and cysts. Neuroradiology 28 (1986) 436–475
24. Clewell, M.H., Johnson, M.L., Meier, P.R. et al.: A surgical approach to the treatment of fetal hydrocephalus. New. Engl. J. Med. 306 (1982) 1320–1325
25. Cohen, M.M.: An update on the holoprosencephalic disorders. J. Pediat. 101 (1982) 865–869
26. Crade, M.: Ultrasonic demonstration in utero of an intracranial teratoma. JAMA 247 (1982) 1173
27. Dambska, M., Wisniewski, K., Sher, J.H.: Lissencephaly: Two distinct clinico-pathologic types. Brain Dev. 5 (1983) 302–310
28. Dandy, W.E.: The diagnosis and treatment of hydrocephalus due to occlusion of the foramina of Magendie and Luschka. Surg. Gynecol. Obstet. 32 (1921) 112–124
29. Davidoff, L.M., Dyke, C.G.: Agenesis of the corpus callosum: Its diagnosis by encephalography. AJR 32 (1934) 1–10
30. Dempsey, P.J., Koch, H.: In utero diagnosis of the Dandy-Walker syndrome: Differentiation from extra-axial posterior fossa cyst. J. clin. Ultrasound 9 (1981) 403–405
31. DeMyer, W., Zeman, W., Palmer, C.: The face predicts the brain: Diagnostic significance of median facial anomalies for holoprosencephaly (arhinencephaly). Pediatrics 34 (1964) 256–263
32. DeMyer, W: Classification of cerebral malformations. Birth Defects 7 (1971) 78–93
33. DeMyer, W.: Holoprosencephaly (cyclopia-arhinencephaly). In: Vinken, P.J., Bruyn, G.W. (eds.): Handbook of Clinical Neurology. Vol. 30. Amsterdam: Elsevier/North Holland Biomedical Press 1977; pp. 431–478
34. Denkhaus, H., Winsberg, F.: Ultrasonic measurement of the fetal ventricular system. Radiology 131 (1979) 781–787
35. Donnenfeld, A.E., Carlson, D.E., Palomaki, G.E., Librizzi, R.J., Weiner, S., Platt, L.: Prospective multicenter study of second-trimester nuchal skinfold thickness in unaffected and Down syndrome pregnancies. Obstet. Gynecol. 84 (1994) 844–847
36. Doren, M., Tercanli, S., Gulotta, F., Holzgreve, W.: Prenatal diagnosis of highly undifferentiated brain tumour: a case report and review of the literature. Prenat. Diagn. 17 (1997) 967–971
37. Dreazen, E., Tessler, F., Sarti, D., Crandall, B.F.: Spontaneous resolution of fetal hydrocephalus. J. Ultrasound Med. 8 (1989) 155–157
38. Edwards, J.H.: Congenital malformations of the nervous system in Scotland. Brit. J. prev. soc. Med. 12 (1958) 115–130
39. Eller, K.M., Kuller, J.A.: Porencephaly secondary to fetal trauma during amniocentesis. Obstet. Gynecol. 85 (1995) 865–867
40. Encha-Razavi, F.: Fetal neuropathology. In: Duckett, S.: Pediatric neuropathology. Baltimore: Williams & Wilkins 1995 108–122
41. Evrard, P., Kadhim, H.J., de Saint-Georges, P., Gadisseau, J.F.: Abnormal development and destructive processes of the human brain during the second half of gestation. In: Evrard, P., Minkowski, A. (eds.): Developmental Neurobiology. Nestlé Nutrition Workshop Series Vol. 12. New York: Vevey/Raven Press 1989; pp.153–176
42. Findlay, J.W.: The choroid plexuses of the lateral ventricles of the brain, their histology, normal and pathological (in relation specially to insanity). Brain 22 (1899) 161
43. Fogarty, K., Cohen, H.L., Haller, J.O.: Sonography of fetal intracranial hemorrhage: Unusual causes and a review of the literature. J. Clin. Ultrasound 17 (1989) 366–370
44. Freytag, E., Lindenberg, R: Neuropathic findings in patients of a hospital for the mentally deficient. A survey of 359 cases. Hopkins Med. J. 121 (1967) 379–392
45. Frigoletto, F.D.jr., Birnholz, J.C., Greene, M.F.: Antenatal treatment of hydrocephalus by ventriculoamniotic shunting. J. Amer. med. Ass. (1982) 2496–2497
46. Gabrielli, S., Reece, A.R., Pilu, G. et al.: The significance of prenatally diagnosed choroid plexus cysts. Amer. J. Obstet. Gynecol. 160 (1989) 1207–1210
47. Garrett, W.J.: Ultrasound in discerning normal fetal anatomy. In: Hobbins, J.C.: Diagnostic Ultrasound in Obstetrics. New York: Churchill Livingstone 1979; p. 57
48. Golbus, M.S., Holzgreve, W., Harrison, M.R.: Intrauterine Direktbehandlung des Feten. Gynäkologe 17 (1984) 62–71
49. Goldhofer, W., Merz, E., Ackermann, R., Al-Hami, S.: Pränatale Ultraschallbefunde bei der Arnold-Chiarischen Missbildung. Z. Geburtsh. Perinat. 189 (1985) 42–44
50. Goldstein, R.B., Podrasky, A.E., Filly, R.A., Callen, P.W.: Effacement of the fetal cisterna magna in association with myelomeningocele. Radiology 172 (1989) 409–413
51. Green, M.F., Benacerraf, B.R., Frigoletto, F.D.jr.: Reliable criteria for the prenatal diagnosis of alobar holoprosencephaly. Amer. J. Obstet. Gynecol. 156 (1987) 687–689
52. Gross, H., Jellinger, K.: Morphologische Aspekte cerebraler Mißbildungen. Wien. Z. Nervenheilk. 27 (1969) 9–37
53. Grouchy de, J., Turleau, C.: Atlas des maladies chromosomiques. Deuxième édition. Paris, Expansion Scietnifique Francaise (1982)
54. Guibert-Tranier, F., Piton, J., Billerey, J., Caillé, J.M.: Agenesis of the corpus callosum. J. Neuroradiology 9 (1982) 135–160
55. Guthkelch, A.N., Riley, N.A.: Influence of aetiology on prognosis in surgically treated infantile hydrocephalus. Arch. Dis. Child. 44 (1969) 29–35
56. Hadeed, A.J., Siegel, S.R.: Maternal cocaine use during pregnancy: effect on the newborn infant. Pediatrics 84 (1989) 205–210
57. Halsey, J.H., Allen, N., Chamberlin, H.R.: Hydranencephaly. In: Vinken, P.J., Bruyn, G.W. (eds.): Handbook of Clinical Neurology. Vol. 30. Amsterdam: Elsevier/North Holland Biomedical Press 1977; 661–680
58. Hamby, W.B., Krauss, R.F., Beswick, W.F.: Hydranencephaly: Clinical diagnosis. Presentation of 7 cases. Pediatrics 6 (1950) 371–383
59. Hanieh, A., Simpson, D.A., North, J.B.: Arachnoid cyst: A ctitical survey of 41 cases. Childs Nerv. Syst. 4 (1988) 92–96
60. Hansmann, M.: Nachweis und Ausschluß fetaler Entwicklungsstörungen mittels Ultraschallscreening und gezielter Untersuchung – ein Mehrstufenkonzept. Ultraschall 2 (1981) 206–220
61. Hart, M.N., Malamud, N., Ellis, W.G.: The Dandy-Walker syndrome: A clinicopathological study bases on 28 cases. Neurology 22 (1972) 771–780
62. Heiserman, J., Filly, R.A., Goldstein, R.B.: Effect of measurement errors on sonographic evaluation of ventriculomegaly. J. Ultrasound Med. 4 1991) 121–124
63. Herman, J.H., Jumbelic, M., Ancona, R., Kickler, T.S.: In utero cerebral hemorrhage in alloimmune thrombocytopenia. Amer. J. Pediatr. Hematol. Oncol. 8 (1986) 312–317
64. Hertzberg, B.S., Kay, H.H., Bowie, J.D.: Fetal choroid plexus lesions. Relationship of antenatal sonographic appearance to clinical outcome. J. Ultrasound Med. 8 (1989) 77–82
65. Hidalgo, H., Bowie, J., Rosenberg, E.R., Ram, P.C., Ford, K., Lipsit, E.: In utero sonographic diagnosis of fetal cerebral anomalies. Amer. J. Roentgenol. 139 (1982) 143–148
66. Hirsch, J.H., Cyr, D., Eberhardt, H., Zunkel, D.: Ultrasonographic diagnosis of an aneurysm of the vein of Galen in utero by duplex scanning. J. Ultrasound Med. 2 (1983) 231–233
67. Hofman-Tretin, J.C., Horoupian, D.S., Koenisberg, M., Schnur, M.J., Liena, J.F.: Lobar holoprosencephaly with hydrocephalus: antenatal demonstration and differential diagnosis. J. Ultrasound Med. 5 (1986) 691–697
68. Hsia, Y.E., Bratu, M., Herbordt, A.: Genetics of the Meckel syndrome (dysencephalia splanchnocystica). Pediatrics 48 (1971) 237–247
69. Johnson, M.L., Dunne, M.G., Mack, L.A., Rashbaum, C.L.: Evaluation of fetal intracranial anatomy by static and real-time ultrasound. J. Clin. Ultrasound 8 (1980) 311–318
70. Johnson, M.L., Rumack, C.M., Mannes, E.J., Appareti, K.E.: Detecting of neonatal intracranial hemorrhage utilizing real-time and static ultrasound. J. Clin. Ultrasound 9 (1981) 427–433
71. Johnson, M.L., Pretorius, D., Clewell, W.H., Meier, P.R., Manchester, D.: Fetal hydrocephalus. Diagnosis and management. Semin. Perinat. 7 (1983) 83–89
72. Johnson, R.T., Johnson, K.P., Edmonds,C.J.: Virus-induced hydrocephalus: Development of aqueductal stenosis in hamsters after mumps infection. Science 157 (1967) 1066–1067
73. Kim, M., Elyaderani, M.K.: Sonographic diagnosis of cerebroventricular hemorrhage in utero. Radiology 142 (1982) 479–480
74. Koch, G.: Genetics of microcephaly in man. Acta. Genet. med. (Roma) 8 (1959) 75–86
75. Koh, A., Grundy, H.: Fetal heart rate tracing with congenital aneurysm of the great vein of Galen. Amer. J. Perinatol. 5 (1988) 98–100
76. Kurjak, A., Kirkinen, P., Latin, V., Raijhvajn, B.: Diagnosis and assessment of fetal malformations and abnormalities. J. perinat. Med. 8 (1980) 219–235
77. Kurtz, A.B., Wapner, R.J., Rubin, C.S., Cole-Beuglet, C., Ross, R.D., Goldberg, B.B.: Ultrasound criteria for in utero diagnosis of microcephaly. J. clin. Ultrasound 8 (1980) 11–16
78. Lemire, R.J., Loeser, J.D., Leech, R.W., Alvord, E.C.: Normal and abnormal development of the human nervous system. New York: Harper & Row 1975
79. Lin, Y., Chang, F., Liu, C.: Antenatal detection of hydranencephaly at 12 weeks' menstrual age. J. Clin. Ultrasound 20 (1992) 62–64
80. Lipman, S.R, Pretorius, D., Rumack, C., Manco-Johnson, M.L.: Fetal intracranial teratoma: US diagnosis of three cases and a review of the literature. Radiology 157 (1985) 491–494
81. Lockwood, C.J., Ghidini, A., Aggarwal, R., Hobbins, J.: Antenatal diagnosis of partial agenesis of the corpus callosum: a benign cause of ventriculomegaly. Amer. J. Obstet. Gynecol. 159 (1988) 184–186
82. Lustig-Gillman, I., Young, B.K., Silverman, F. et al.: Fetal intraventricular hemorrhage: Sonographic diagnosis and clinical implications. J. Clin. Ultrasound 11 (1983) 277–280
83. MacGahan, J.P, Haesslein, H.C, Meyers, M., Ford, K.B.: Sonographic recognition of in utero intraventricular hemorrhage. AJR 142 (1984) 171–173
84. Mahony, B.S., Filly, R.A., Callen, P.W., Golbus, M.S.: Thanatophoric dwarfism with the cloverleaf skull: A specific antenatal diagnosis. J. Ultraosund Med. 4 (1985) 151–154
85. Mao, K., Adams, J.: Antenatal diagnosis of intracranial arteriovenous fistula by ultrasonography. Case report. Brit. J. Obstet. Gynaecol. 90 (1983) 872–873
86. Martin, H.: Microcephaly and mental retardation. Amer. J. Dis. Child 119 (1970) 128–131
87. McComb, J.G.: Recent research into the nature of cerebrospinal fluid formation and absorption. J. Neurosurg. 59 (1983) 369–383
88. McIntosh, R., Merritt, K.K., Richards, M.R., Samuels, M.H., Bellows, M.T.: The incidence of congenital malformations: a study of 5.964 pregnancies. Pediatrics 14 (1954) 505–521
89. Meizner, I., Barki, Y., Hertzanu, Y.: Prenatal sonographic diagnosis of agenesis of corpus callosum. J. Clin. Ultrasound 15 (1987) 262–264
90. Merz, E.: Hinweisende Diagnostik durch Ultraschalluntersuchung. In: Dudenhausen, J.W. (Hrsg.): Down-Syndrom: Früherkennung und therapeutische Hilfen. Frankfurt: Umwelt & Medizin 1992; S. 24–30
91. Merz, E., Wellek, S.: Das normale fetale Wachstumsprofil – ein einheitliches Modell zur Berechnung von Normkurven für die gängigen Kopf- und Abdomenparameter sowie die großen Extremitätenknochen. Ultraschall in Med. 17 (1996) 153–162
92. Milhorat, T.H.: Hydrocephalus and the cerebrospinal fluid. Baltimore: Williams & Wilkins (1972) 97–102
93. Mintz, M.C., Arger, P.H., Coleman, B.G.: In utero sonographic diagnosis of intracerebral hemorrhage. J. Ultrasound Med. 4 (1985) 375–376
94. Montserrat, J.M., Picado, C., Austi-Vidal, A.: Arnold-Chiari malformation and paralysis of the diaphragm. Respiration 53 (1992) 128–131
95. Morales, W., Stroup, M.: Intracranial hemorrhage in utero due to isoimmune neonatal thrombocytopenia. Obstet. Gynecol. 65 (1985) 20S–21S
96. Motte, J., Gomes, H., Morville, P., Cymbalista, M.: Sonographic diagnosis of lissencephaly. Pediatr. Radiol. 17 (1987) 362–364

97. Murray, J., Johnson, J., Bird, T.: Dandy-Walker malformation: Etiologic heterogenity and empiric recurrence risks. Clin. Genet. 28 (1985) 272–283
98. Myers, R.E.: Brain pathology following fetal vascular occlusion: An experimental study. Invest. Ophthalmol. 8 (1969) 41–50
99. Nadel, A.S., Bromley, B.S., Frigoletto, F.D.jr., Estroff, J.A., Benacerraf, B.R.: Isolated choroid plexus cysts in the second-trimester fetus: is amniocentesis really indicated? Radiology 185 (1992) 545–548
100. Nava, S., Godmilow, L., Reeser, S., Ludominky, A., Donnenfeld, A.E.: Significance of sonographically detected second trimester choroid plexus cysts: a series of 211 cases and a review of the literature. Ultrasound Obstet. Gynecol. 4 (1994) 448–451
101. Navin, J.J., Angevine, J.M.: Congenital cytomegalic inclusion disease with porencephaly. Neurology (Minneap.) 18 (1968) 470–472
102. Nguyen, T.H., Pescia, G., Deonna, T. et al.: Early prenatal diagnosis of genetic microcephaly. Prenat. Diagn. 5 (1985) 345–347
103. Nicolaides, K.H., Campbell, S., Gabbe, S.G.: Ultrasound screening for spina bifida: cranial and cerebellar signs. Lancet 2 (1986) 72–74
104. Nicolaides, K.H., Salvesen, D., Snijders, R.J.M., Gosden, C.M.: Strawberry shaped skull: associated malformations and chromosomal defects. Fetal Diagn. Ther. 7 (1992) 132–197
105. Nyberg, D.A., Mack, L.A., Bronstein, A., Hirsch, J., Pagon, R.A.: Holoprosencephaly: prenatal sonographic diagnosis. Amer. J. Roentgenol. 49 (1987) 1050–1058
106. Nyberg, D.A., Xyr, D.R., Mack, L., Fitzsimmons, J., Hickok, D., Mahony, B.S.: The Dandy-Walker malformation. Prenatal sonographic diagnosis and its clinical significance. J. Ultrasound Med. 7 (1988) 65–71
107. Nyberg, D.A., Mack, L.A., Hirsch, J., Mahony, J.S.: Abnormalities of fetal cranial contour in sonographic detection of spina bifida: Evaluation of the "lemon" sign. Radiology 167 (1988) 387–392
108. Olivecrona, H., Ladenheim, J.: Congenital arterioveneous aneurysmas of the carotid and vertebral arterial systems. Berlin: Springer 1957
109. Opitz, J.M.: Lissencephaly syndrome. In: Bergsma, D. (ed.): Birth Defects Compendium, 2 ed., New York: Alan R. Liss 1979; p. 658
110. Papile, L., Burstein, J., Burstein, R., Kofer, H.: Incidence and evolution of subependymal and intraventricular hemorrhage. A study of infants with birth weight less than 1500 grams. J. Pediatr. 92 (1978) 529–534
111. Parrish, M., Roessmann, U., Levinsohn, M.: Agenesis of the corpus callosum: A study of the frequency of associated malformations. Ann. Neurol. 6 (1979) 349–354
112. Perlman, J.M., Argyle, C.: Lethal cytomegalovirus infection in preterm infants: clinical, radiological, and neuropathological findings. Ann. Neurol. 31 (1992) 64–68
113. Perry, T.B., Benzie, R.J., Cassar, N.: Fetal cephalometry by ultrasound as a screening procedure for the prenatal detection of Down syndrome. Brit. J. Obstet. Gynaecol. 91 (1984) 138–143
114. Pilu, G., Rizzo, N., Orsini, L.F., Bovicelli, L.: Antenatal detection of fetal cerebral anomalies. Ultrasound Med. Biol. 12 (1986) 319–326
115. Pilu, G., DePalma, L., Romero, R., Bovicelli, L, Hobbins, J.C.: The fetal subarachnoid cisterns: An ultrasound study. With report of a case of communicating hydrocephalus. J. Ultrasound Med. 5 (1986) 365–372
116. Pilu, G., Romero, R., De Palma, L. et al.: Antenatal diagnosis and obstetrical management of Dandy-Walker syndrome. J. Reprod. Med. 31 (1986) 1017–1022
117. Pilu, G., Romero, R., Rizzo, N., Jeanty, P., Bovicelli, L., Hobbins, J.C.: Criteria for the prenatal diagnosis of holoprosencephaly. Amer. J. Perinatol. 4 (1987) 41–49
118. Pilu, G.L., Reece, E.A., Goldstein, I.: Sonographic evaluation of the normal developmental anatomy of the fetal cerebral ventricles: II. The atria. Obstet. Gynecol. 73 (1988) 250–257
119. Pilu, G., Romero, R., Reece, A., Goldstein, I., Hobbins, J.C., Bovicelli, L.: Subnormal cerebellum in fetuses with spina bifida. Amer. J. Obstet. Gynecol. 158 (1988) 1052–1056
120. Pilu, G., Sandri, F., Perolo, A. et al.: Sonography of fetal agenesis of the corpus callosum: a survey of 35 cases. Ultrasound Obstet. Gynecol. 3 (1993) 318–329
121. Pilu, G., Arnbrosetto, P., Sandri, T. et al.: Intraventricular fused fornices: a specific sign of fetal lobar holoprosencephaly. Ultrasound Obstet. Gynecol. 4 (1994) 65–67
122. Pretorius, D.H., Davis, K., Manco-Johnson, M.L., Manchester, D., Meier, P.R., Clewell, W.H.: Clinical course of fetal hydrocephalus: 40 cases. Amer. J. Roentgenol. 144 (1985) 827–831
123. Rex, A.P., Preuss, M.: A diagnostic index for Down syndrome. J. Pediatr. 100 (1982) 903–906
124. Roesmann, U.: Congenital malformations. In: Duckett, S.: Pediatric neuropathology. Baltimore: Williams & Wilkins 1995; pp. 123–148
125. Romero, R., Pilu, G., Jeanty, P., Ghidini, A., Hobbins, J.C.: Prenatal diagnosis of congenital anomalies. Norwalk: Appleton & Lange 1988
126. Russ, P.D., Pretorius, D.H., Johnson, M.J.: Dandy-Walker-syndrome: a review of fifteen cases evaluated by prenatal sonography. Amer. J. Obstet. Gynecol. 161 (1989) 401–406
127. Saltzman, D.H., Krauss, C.M., Goldman, J.M., Benacerraf, B.R.: Prenatal diagnosis of lissencephaly. Prenat. Diagn. 11 (1991) 139–143
128. Sawaya, R., McLaurin, R.L.: Dandy-Walker syndrome: Clinical analysis of 23 cases. J. Neurosurg. 55 (1981) 89–98
129. Scher, M.S., Belfar, H., Martin, J., Painer, M.J.: Destructive brain lesions of presumed fetal onset: antepartum causes of cerebral palsy. Pediatrics 88 (1991) 898–906
130. Schoenecker, S.A., Pretorius, D.H., Manco-Johnson, M.L.: Artifacts seen commonly on ultrasonography of the fetal cranium. J. Reprod. Med. 30 (1985) 541–544
131. Shah, Y.G., Eckl, C.J., Stinson, S.K., Woods, J.R.: Biparietal diameter/femur length ratio, cephalic index, and femur length measurements: not reliable screening techniques for Down syndrome. Obstet. Gynecol. 75 (1990) 186–188
132. Shaw, C.M., Alvord, E.C.jr.: Hydrocephalus. In: Duckett, S.: Pediatric neuropathology. Baltimore: Williams & Wilkins 1995; pp. 149–211
133. Shuangshoti, S., Netsky, M.G.: Neuroepithelial (colloid) cysts of the nervous system: Further observations on pathogenesis, location, incidence and histochemistry. Neurology 16 (1966) 887
134. Shuangshoti, S., Netsky, M.G.: Histogenesis of choroid plexus in man. Amer. J. Anat. 118 (1966) 283–316
135. Snijders, R.J.M., Shawwa, L., Nicolaides, K.H.: Fetal choroid plexus cysts and trisomy 18: assessment of risk based on ultrasound findings and maternal age. Prenatal Diagn. 14 (1994) 1119–1127
136. Snijders, R.J.M., Farrias, M., von Kaisenberg, C., Nicolaides, K.H.: Fetal abnormalities. In: Snijders, R.J.M., Nicolaides, K.H.(eds.): Ultrasound markers for fetal chromosomal defects. New York: The Parthenon Publishing Group 1996; pp. 1–62
137. Snyder, J.R., Lustig-Gillman, I., Milio, L. et al.: Antenatal ultrasound diagnosis of an intracranial neoplasm (craniopharyngioma). J. Clin. Ultrasound 14 (1986) 304–306
138. Stamm, E.R., Pretorius, D.H., Rumack, C.M., Manco-Johnson, M.L.: Kleeblattschadel anomaly: In utero sonographic appearance. J. Ultrasound Med. 6 (1987) 319–324
139. Strauss, S., Bouzouki, M., Goldfarb, H., Uppal, V., Costales, F.: Antenatal ultrasound diagnosis of an unusual case of hydranencephaly. J. clin. Ultrasound 12 (1984) 420–422
140. Takaku, A., Kodama, N., Ohara, H. et al.: Brain tumor in newborn babies. Child's Brain 4 (1973) 365–375
141. Timmons, G.D., Johnson, K.P.: Aqueductual stenosis and hydrocephalus after mumps encephalitis. New Engl. J. Med. 283 (1970) 1505–1507
142. Toi, A.: Spontaneous resolution of fetal ventriculomegaly in a diabetic patient. J. Ultrasound Med. 6 (1987) 37–39
143. Ulm, B., Ulm, M.R., Deutinger, J., Bernaschek, G.: Dandy-Walker malformation diagnosed before 21 weeks of gestation: associated malformations and chromosomal abnormalities. Ultrasound Obstet. Gynecol. 10 (1997)167–170
144. Vergani, P., Ghidini, A., Strobelt, N. et al.: Prognostic indicators in the prenatal diagnosis of agenesis of corpus callosum. Amer. J. Obstet. Gynecol. 170 (1994) 753–758
145. Vergani, P., Locatelli, A., Strobelt, N. et al.: Clinical outcome of mild ventriculomegaly. Amer. J. Obstet. Gynecol. 178 (1998) 18–22
146. Vintzileos, A.M., Ingardia, C.J., Nochimson, D.J.: Congenital hydrocephalus: A review and protocol for perinatal management. Obstet. Gynecol. 62 (1983) 539–549
147. Vintzileos, A.M., Eisenfeld, L.I., Campbell, W.A., Herson, V.C., DiLeo, P.E., Chameides, L.: Prenatal ultrasonic diagnosis of arteriovenous malformation of the vein of Galen. Amer. J. Perinatol. 3 (1986) 209–211
148. Voigt, H.J.: Diagnostisch-therapeutisches Konzept bei Hydrozephalus. Gynäkologe 28 (1995) 346–355
149. Voth, D., Schwarz, M.: Hydrozephalus im Kindesalter. In: Hopf, H.C., Deuschl, G., Diener, H.C., Reichmann, H. (Hrsg.): Neurologie in Klinik und Praxis, Band 2. Stuttgart: Thieme 1997
150. Warren, M.C., Lu, A.T., Ziering, W.H.: Sex-linked hydrocephalus with aqueductal stenosis. J. Pediatr. 63 (1963) 1104–1110
151. Watson, D., Smith, R., Brann, A.: Ateriovenous malformation of the vein of Galen. Amer. J. Dis. Child 130 (1976) 520–525
152. Weber, G., Macchiella, D., Bahlmann, F., Merz, E.: Pränatale Diagnose intrakranieller Hirntumoren. Ultraschall Klin. Prax. 6 (1991) 92–95
153. Willems, P.J., Brouwer, O.F., Dijkstra, I., Wilmink, J.: X-linked hydrocephalus. Amer. J. Med. Genet. 27 (1987) 921–928
154. Witt, P.D., Hardesty, R.A., Zuppan, C., Rouse, G., Hasso, A.N., Boyne, P.: Fetal kleeblattschadel cranium: morphologic, radiographic, and histologic analysis. Cleft Palate Craniofac. J. 29 (1992) 363–368

Facial Anomalies

1. Achiron, R., Ben-Arie, A., Gabbay, U., Mashiach, S., Rotstein, Z., Lipitz, S.: Development of the fetal tongue between 14 and 26 weeks of gestation: in utero ultrasonographic measurements. Ultrasound Obstet. Gynecol. 9 (1997) 39–41
2. Awwad, J.T., Azar, G.B., Karam, K.S., Nicolaides, K.H.: Ear length: a potential sonographic marker for Down syndrome. Int. J. Gynecol. Obstet. 44 (1994) 233–238
3. Babcook, C.J., McGahan, J.P.: Axial ultrasound imaging of the fetal maxilla for accurate characterization of facial clefts. J. Ultrasound Med. 16 (1997) 619–625
4. Birnholz, J.C., Farell, E.E.: Fetal ear length. Pediatrics 81 (1988) 555–558
5. Catalano, P.J., Urken, M.L., Alvarez, M. et al.: New approach to the management of airway obstruction in "high risk" neonates. Head Neck Surg. 118 (1992) 306–309
6. Chervenak, F.A., Berkowitz, R.L., Romero, R. et al.: The diagnosis of fetal hydrocephalus. Amer. J. Obstet. Gynecol. 147 (1983) 703–716
7. Chervenak, F.A., Tortora, M., Moya, F.R. et al.: Antenatal sonographic diagnosis of epignathus. J. Ultrasound Med. 3 (1984) 235–237
8. Chervenak, F.A., Isaacson, G., Rosenberg, J.C., Kardon, N.B.: Antenatal diagnosis of frontal cephalocele in a fetus with atelosteogenesis. J. Ultrasound Med. 5 (1986) 111–113
9. Chitayat, D., Meunier, C.M., Hodkonson, K.A., Azouz, M.E.: Robinson sequence with facial and digital anomalies in two half-brothers by the same mother. Amer. J. Med. Genet. 40 (1991) 167–172
10. Chitty, L.S., Campbell, S., Altman, D.G.: Measurement of the fetal mandible: feasibility and construction of a centile chart. Prenat. Diagn. 13 (1993) 749–756
11. Cohen, J., Ghezzi, G., Goncalves, L., Fuentes, J.D., Paulyson, K.J., Sherer, D.M.: Prenatal sonographic diagnosis of Treacher Collins syndrome: a case report and review of the literature. Amer. J. Perinatol. 12 (1995) 416–419
12. Cohen, M.M.jr., Jirasek, J.E., Guzman, R.T., Gorlin, R.J., Peterson, M.Q.: Holoprosencephaly and facial dysmorphia: Nosology, etiology and pathogenesis. Birth Defects 7 (1971) 125–135
13. Cohen, M.M.jr.: Syndromes with cleft lip and cleft palate. Cleft Palate J. 15 (1978) 306–328
14. Currarino, G., Silverman, F.N.: Orbital hypotelorism, arhinencephaly trigonocephaly. Radiology 74 (1960) 206–217
15. Curry, C.J., Carey, J.C., Holland, J.S. et al.: Smith-Lemli-Opitz-syndrome II: Multiple congenital anomalies wtih male pseudohermaphroditism and frequent early lethality. Amer. J. Med. Genet. 26 (1987) 45–57

16. Davis, W.K., Mahony, B.S., Carroll, B.A., Bowie, J.D.: Antenatal sonographic detection of benign dacrocystoceles (lacrimal duct cysts). J. Ultrasound Med. 6 (1987) 641–645
17. DeMyer, W.: Median facial malformations and their implications for brain malformations. Birth Defects 11 (1975) 155–181
18. DeMyer, W.: Orbital hypertelorism. In: Vinken, P.J., Bruyn, G.W. (eds.): Handbook of Clinical Neurology. Vol. 30. Amsterdam: Elsevier/North Holland Biomedical Press 1977; pp. 235–255
19. Donnenfeld, A.E., Hughes, H., Weiner, S.: Prenatal diagnosis and perinatal management of frontoethmoidal meningoencephalocele. Amer. J. Perinatol. 5 (1988) 51–53
20. Donnenfeld, A.E., Packer, R.J., Zackai, E.H., Chee, C.M., Sellinger, B., Emanuel, B.S.: Clinical, cytogenetic, and pedigree findings in 18 cases of Aicardi syndrome. Amer. J. Med. Genet. 32 (1989) 461–467
21. Duker, J.S., Weiss, J.S., Siber, M., Bieber, F.R., Albert, D.M.: Ocular findings in a new heritable syndrome of brain, eye, and urogenital abnormalities. Amer. J. Ophthalmol. 99 (1985) 51–55
22. Ehrich, W.E.: Teratoid parasites of the mouth. Amer. J. Orthodont. 31 (1945) 650–659
23. Franceschetti, A., Klein, D.: The mandibulo-facial dysostosis. A new hereditary syndrome. Acta ophtal. Kbl. 27 (1949) 143–224
24. Gilman, P.A.: Epidemiology of human teratomas. In: Damjarov, I., Knowles, B.B., Solter, D. (eds.): The human teratomas. Experimental and clinical biology. Clifton, New Jersey: Humana Press 1985; pp. 94–105
25. Gorlin, R.J., Cervenka, J., Pruzansky, S.: Facial clefting and its syndromes. Birth Defects Orig. Artic. Ser. 7 (1971) 3–49
26. Greig, D.: Hypertelorism: A hitherto undifferentiated congenital cranio-facial deformity. Edinburgh Med. J. 31 (1924) 560–593
27. Harker, C.P., Winter, T. 3rd, Mack, L.: Prenatal diagnosis of Beckwith-Wiedemann syndrome. Amer. J. Roentgenol. 168 (1997) 520–522
28. Hinrichsen, K.V.: Gesichtsentwicklung. In: Hinrichsen, K.V. (Hrsg.): Humanembryologie. Berlin: Springer 1993; S. 650–692
29. Houze, de l'Aulnoit, D., Ellart, D., Furby, F., Ghazi, D., Brabant, G., Delcroix, M.: Diagnostic echographique antenatal des fentes labiales et labio-palatines. A propos de 10 observations. J. Gynecol. Obstet. Biolo. Reprod. Paris 20 (1991) 325–331
30. Isaacs, H. jr.: Tumors of the fetus and the newborn. Philadelphia: Saunders 1997
31. Judisch, G.F., Kraft, S.P., Bartley, J.A., Jacoby, C.G.: Orbital hypotelorism. An isolated autosomal dominant trait. Arch. Ophthalmol. 102 (1984) 995–997
32. Kang, K.W., Hissong, S.L., Langer, A.: Prenatal ultrasonic diagnosis of epignathus. J. clin. Ultrasound 6 (1978) 330–331
33. Kousseff, B.G.: Sacral meningocele with conotruncal heart defects: a possible autosomal recessive trait. Pediatrics 74 (1984) 395–398
34. Kunze, J., Wiedemann, H.R.: Das Wiedemann-Beckwith-Syndrom. Ergeb. Inn. Med. Kinderheilk. 61 (1993) 303–338
35. Lange, C.: Congenital hypertrophy of the muscles, extra-pyramidal motor disturbances and mental deficiency. Amer. J. Dis. Child. 48 (1934) 243
36. Lasser, D., Preis, O., Dor, N. et al.: Antenatal diagnosis of giant cystic cavernous hemangioma by Doppler velocimetry. Obstet. Gynecol. 72 (1988) 476–477
37. Lemoine, P., Harousseau, H., Boteyru, J.P., Menuet, J.C.: Les enfants de parents alcooliques; anomalies observées. Apropos de 127 cas. Quest. Med. 25 (1968) 477
38. Lenz, W.: Rezessiv-geschlechtsgebundene Mikrophthalmie mit multiplen Fehlbildungen. Kinderheilk. 77 (1955) 384–390
39. Lettieri, L., Rodis, J.F., Vintzileos, A.M., Feeney, L., Ciarleglio, L., Craffey, A.: Ear length in second-trimester aneuploid fetuses. Obstet. Gynecol. 81 (1993) 57–60
40. Lev-Gur, M., Maklad, N.F., Patel, S.: Ultrasonic findings in fetal cyclopia. A case report. J. Reprod. Med. 28 (1983) 554–557
41. Levine, A.B., Alvarez, M., Wedgewood, J. et al.: Contemporary management of a potentially lethal fetal anomaly: a successful perinatal approach to epignathus. Obstet. Gynecol. 76 (1990) 962–966
42. Mahoney, B.S., Hegge, F.N.: The face and the neck. In: Nyberg, D.A., Mahony, B.S., Pretorius, D.H. (eds.): Diagnostic ultrasound of fetal anomalies. St. Louis: Mosby Year Book 1990; S. 212

43. Meizner, I., Bar-Ziv, J., Holcberg, G. et al.: In utero prenatal diagnosis of fetal facial tumor-hemangioma. J. Clin. Ultrasound 13 (1985) 435–437
44. Merz, E., Wellek, S., Püttmann, S., Bahlmann, F., Weber, G.: Orbitadurchmesser, innerer und äußerer Orbitaabstand. Ein Wachstumsmodell für die fetalen Orbitamaße. Ultraschall in Med. 16 (1995) 12–17
45. Merz, E., Weber, G., Bahlmann, F., Miric-Tesanic, D.: Application of transvaginal and abdominal three-dimensional ultrasound for the detection or exclusion of malformations of the fetal face. Ultrasound Obstet. Gynecol. 9 (1997) 237–243
46. Merz, E., Bahlmann, F., Weber, G., Miric-Tesanic, D.: Fetal malformations: Assessment by three-dimensional ultrasound in the surface mode. In: Merz, E. (ed.): 3-D ultrasound in Obstetrics and Gynecology. Philadelphia: Lippincott, William and Wilkins 1998
47. Moore, K.L.: Embryologie. Stuttgart: Schattauer 1985
48. Nicolaides, K.H., Salvesen, D.R., Snijders, R.J.M., Gosden, C.M.: Fetal facial defects: associated malformations and chromosomal abnormalities. Fetal Diagn. Ther. 8 (1993) 1–9
49. Nowotny, T., Bollmann, R., Pfeifer, L., Windt, W.: Beckwith-Wiedemann syndrome: difficulties with prenatal diagnosis. Fetal Diagn. Ther. 9 (1994) 256–260
50. Oliveira-Filho, A.G., Carvalho, M.H., Bustorff-Silva, J.M., Sbragia-Neto, L., Miyabara, S., Oliveira, E.R.: Epignathus: report of a case with successful outcome. J. Pediatr. Surg. 33 (1998) 520–521
51. Pilu, G., Romero, R., Reece, E.A., Jeanty, P., Hobbins, J.C.: The prenatal diagnosis of Robin anomalad. Amer. J. Obstet. Gynecol. 154 (1986) 630–632
52. Pilu, G., Romero, R., Rizzo, N., Jeanty, P., Bovicelli, L., Hobbins, J.C.: Criteria for the prenatal diagnosis of holoprosencephaly. Amer. J. Perinatol. 4 (1987) 41–49
53. Robin, P.: Glossoptosis due to atresia and hypotrophy of the mandible. Amer. J. Dis. Child 48 (1934) 541
54. Savoldelli, G., Schmid, W., Schinzel, A.: Prenatal diagnosis of cleft lip and palate by ultrasound. Prenat. Diagn. 2 (1982) 313–317
55. Schauer, G.M., Dunn, L.K., Godmilow, L., Eagle, R.C.jr., Knisely, A.S.: Prenatal diagnosis of Fraser syndrome at 18.5 weeks gestation, with autopsy findings at 19 weeks. Amer. J. Med. Genet. 37 (1990) 583–591
56. Shi, J.C., Shyu, M.K., Lee, C.N., Wu, C.H., Lin, G.J., Hsieh, F.J.: Antenatal depiction of the ear with three-dimensional ultrasonography. Obstet. Gynecol. 91 (1998) 500–505
57. Shimidzu, T., Salvador, L., Hughes-Benzie, R., Dawson, L., Nimrod, C., Allanson, J.: The role of reduced ear size in the prenatal detection of chromosomal abnormalities. Prenat. Diagn. 17 (1997) 545–549
58. Smith, N.M., Chambers, S.E., Billson, V.R., Laing, I., West, C.P., Bell, J.E.: Oral teratoma (epignathus) with intracranial extension: a report of two cases. Prenat. Diagn. 13 (1993) 945–952
59. Snijders, R.J.M., Sebire, N.J., Psara, N., Souka, A., Nicolaides, K.H.: Prevalence of fetal facial cleft at different stages of pregnancy. Ultrasound Obstet. Gynecol. 6 (1995) 327–329
60. Starck, D.: Embryologie. Stuttgart: Thieme 1975
61. Tolarova, M.: Empirical recurrence rsik for genetical counseling of clefts. Acta Chri. Plast (Praha) 14 (1972) 204–235
62. Turner, G.M., Twining, P.: The facial profile in the diagnosis of fetal abnormalities. Clin. Radiol. 47 (1993) 389–395
63. Viljoen, D.L., Jaquire, Z., Woods, D.L.: Prenatal diagnosis in autosomal dominant Beckwith-Wiedemann syndrome. Prenat. Diagn. 11 (1991) 167–175
64. Warkany, J.: Congenital Malformations. Year Book Medical Publishers Inc., Chicago 1971; p. 414
65. Wessely, K.: Beiträge zu den Wachstumsbeziehungen zwischen dem Augapfel und seinen Nebenorganen. Arch. Ophthal. 105 (1921) 491–501
66. Wiedemann, H.R., Grosse, F.R., Dibbern, H.: Das charakteristische Syndrom. Stuttgart: Schattauer 1982; 60–61
67. Whisson, C.C., Wyte, A., Ziesing, P.: Beckwith-Wiedemann syndrome: antenatal diagnosis. Australas. Radiol. 38 (1994) 130–131

22 Anomalies of the Neck

Significance. Numerous reports from the literature have proven that the prompt prenatal diagnosis of soft-tissue anomalies in the fetal neck region can significantly affect the postnatal outcome. A number of morphologic abnormalities can interfere with normal functional processes (breathing, swallowing), jeopardizing the survival of the fetus or neonate (Tables 22.1, 22.2). Thus, evaluation of the fetal neck region should be included in every obstetric ultrasound examination.

Neoplasms

▄ *Cystic Hygroma*

Definition. Cystic hygroma is an anomaly of the lymphatic system that appears sonographically as a thin-walled, uni- or multiloculated cystic mass. Approximately 80% are located on the posterolateral aspect of the fetal neck. Other common sites of occurrence are the axilla, mediastinum, and anterior chest wall.

Incidence. Cystic hygroma occurs in 0.3–2% of fetuses (2, 33). The incidence depends, however, on the population examined and on gestational age.

Etiology and pathogenesis. Two types are distinguished based on the period in which they develop: an early form (8–29 weeks) and a late form (after 30 weeks or postnatally). The early form is most likely caused by anomalous development of the thoracic duct. The etiology of the late form is unknown. Development of the lymphatic system is completed by the end of 8 weeks. Normally, lymph is drained via the thoracic duct from the lymphatic sacs to the junction of the subclavian and internal jugular veins. When communication with the venous system is obstructed, the lymphatic sacs undergo a cystic dilatation (10, 38).

Ultrasound features. The lymphatic cysts appear as thin-walled cystic structures, devoid of internal echoes, located in the fetal neck region (Fig. 22.1). A typical feature is the "nuchal ligament," which appears as a dorsal cord on transverse scans (Figs. 22.2, 22.3). If the connection between the venous and lymphatic systems is reestablished, the cysts regress and resolve. Webbing of the neck may occur as a residual condition due to stretching of the skin. If the obstruction persists, the cysts may reach monstrous proportions. Giant cysts that completely fill the amniotic cavity are easily mistaken for amniotic fluid and overlooked (Figs. 22.3, 22.4). If the lymph cysts persist, it is common for peripheral lymphedema or nonimmune hydrops to develop over time, resulting in intrauterine fetal death. Differentiation is required from cervical meningocele, myelomeningocele, and hemangioma.

Associated anomalies. Cystic hygromas are associated with chromosomal abnormalities in 50–80% of cases (2, 3, 8, 27, 33). The most common chromosome defect, accounting for 65% of cases, is monosomy XO (Turner syndrome). Other possible anomalies are trisomy 18, 21, 22, 8, and structural chromosomal anomalies. In fetuses with a normal karyotype, cystic hygroma of the neck may be a cardinal feature of various nongenetic syndromes including Noonan syndrome (Turner-like syndrome), Roberts syndrome, fetal alcohol syndrome, and fatal multiple pterygium syndrome (10, 21). Cystic hygroma coexists with a congenital heart defect in up to 90% of cases, principally coarctation of the aorta and conotruncal anomalies (22).

Table 22.1 Ultrasound features of fetal neck masses, which may or may not have functional significance

Tumor	Incidence	Ultrasound features, echo texture	Typical sign	Prognosis
Anterior neck region				
➤ Goiter	Rare	Solid	Bilobed shape	Good
➤ Thyroglossal duct cysts	Common	Cystic	–	Good
Anterolateral neck region				
➤ Teratoma	Rare	Mixed solid/cystic	Well circumscribed with calcifications	Uncertain
➤ Neuroblastoma	Rare	Solid	Calcifications	Poor
➤ Hemangioma	Common	Cystic	Poorly demarcated, rarely exhibits flow	Uncertain
Lateral neck region				
➤ Branchiogenic cysts	Common	Cystic	–	Good

Table 22.2 Ultrasound features of anomalies that may affect functional processes in the fetal neck region

Anomaly	Incidence	Ultrasound features, indirect signs	Direct signs	Prognosis
Esophageal atresia	Common	➤ Gastric bubble small or not visualized ➤ Polyhydramnion	Rhythmic filling and emptying of a lateral neck cyst during fetal swallowing	Good
Laryngeal atresia	Rare	CHAO syndrome: ➤ Large, echogenic lungs ➤ Dilated trachea ➤ Hydrops	No detectable flow in the trachea during fetal breathing movements	Poor

Prognosis. Generally unfavorable. Generalized fetal hydrops often develops secondarily, and intrauterine fetal death is a common outcome.

Prenatal management. An invasive procedure for karyotyping is absolutely indicated. If the karyotype is normal, further ultrasound examinations are recommended along with fetal echocardiography. If an isolated hygroma is suspected and the pregnancy is continued, an elective cesarean section near term may be considered to prevent obstetric complications. The late form of cystic hygroma may enlarge rapidly and warrants close-interval follow-up (12). Delivery should take place in a perinatal center, since compression of the upper airways can lead to postnatal complications.

Goiter

Definition. Enlargement of the fetal thyroid gland.

Incidence. Rare.

Etiology and pathogenesis. A goiter can develop in association with fetal hypo- or hyperthyroidism.

Fetal hyperthyroidism. Maternal hyperthyroidism is present in 0.2% of pregnancies (6). The most frequent cause of maternal hyperthyroidism is the presence of circulating thyroid-stimulating autoantibodies (thyroid-stimulating immunoglobulin, TSI). These substances can cross the placental barrier, in 2–12% of cases inducing fetal hyperthyroidism with the formation of a goiter (37). Hyperstimulation of the fetal thyroid continues may occur even after normalization after the maternal thyroid status.

Fetal hypothyroidism. Fetal hypothyroidism, on the other hand, is extremely rare. It has three main causes:
1. The treatment of maternal hyperthyroidism with thyrostatic agents or iodine-containing drugs. These agents can cross the placenta and suppress fetal thyroid function (23).
2. Circulating maternal antibodies that are directed against the thyroid gland (thyrotropin-binding inhibitory immunoglobulin, TBII).
3. A primary disorder of fetal thyroid metabolism.

Pathoanatomic features. Fetal hyperthyroidism and hypothyroidism are both characterized by massive enlargement of the fetal thyroid gland.

Ultrasound features. The enlarged thyroid gland appears sonographically as a bilobed structure, usually hyperechoic, located on the anterior aspect of the neck (Fig. 22.**5**). It often causes hyperextension of the fetal head (Fig. 22.**6**). The enlarged thyroid may interfere with fetal swallowing, leading to polyhydramnios. The common carotid artery is often displaced posteriorly. Compression of the upper respiratory tract has not been described.

Further tests. The most reliable way to distinguish between fetal hypo- and hyperthyroidism is to determine the fetal thyroid hormone status (T_3, T_4, TSH, TSI, TBII) in a fetal blood sample obtained by cordocentesis. Standard values for these hormones have been established (32). Determination of thyroid hormone levels in the amniotic fluid is controversial, however (14). The detection of increased blood flow in the fetal goiter is considered an uncertain sign of hyperthyroidism. Surprisingly, we found increased blood flow in a case of fetal hypothyroidism using power Doppler imaging (Fig. 22.**7**).

Associated anomalies. Not described.

Prognosis. Fetal goiter generally has a good prognosis when pharmacologic treatment is initiated without delay. If fetal hypothyroidism goes untreated, there is a risk of severe physical and mental retardation. Hyperthyroidism can lead to tachycardia with secondary fetal hydrops and to premature bone maturation or craniosynostosis.

Prenatal management. Cordocentesis is indicated to determine the fetal thyroid hormone status (T_3, T_4, TSH, TSI, TBII). Serial fetal blood tests are necessary to evaluate prenatal response to therapy.

Teratomas

Definition. Germ-cell tumors of the fetal neck region.

Incidence. Teratomas are relatively rare congenital tumors (1 in 40,000 live births). Only 5% of teratomas occur in the fetal neck region (15, 30, 31). Generally a distinction is drawn between "true" cervical teratomas and those that originate in the oropharynx or nasopharynx (epignathus).

Etiology and pathogenesis. Unknown.

Ultrasound features. Cervical teratomas most commonly occur in the anterolateral neck region (Figs. 22.**8**, 22.**9**). They appear sonographically as well-circumscribed masses with a mixed solid/cystic structure. Calcifications with associated acoustic shadows and clumps of echogenic material are characteristic signs (36). Polyhydramnios often develops when the tumor compresses the esophagus and interferes with fetal swallowing. Cardiac compression can lead to fetal hydrops.

Associated anomalies. Teratomas usually occur in isolation. In a series of seven cases (two craniocervical and five sacrococcygeal teratomas), we were unable to find any accompanying anomalies (1).

Prognosis. Postnatal survival depends on rapid intubation. Levine et al. (20) described a cesarean delivery in which a life-saving tracheostomy was performed with the placenta still in place. The teratoma was successfully removed several hours later. Most teratomas are benign (15), but the benign or malignant nature of the tumor does not correlate with its ultrasound appearance. Ultimately, postnatal histologic examination is the only accurate tool for benign-malignant differentiation. Once an airway has been established, most cervical teratomas are well demarcated from the surrounding tissue and can be easily removed with an acceptable cosmetic and functional result (19).

Prenatal management. Large cervical teratomas can cause dystocic complications due to the extended position of the head. A cesarean delivery is preferable in these cases. Antenatal needle aspiration of the cystic components to reduce the tumor volume is strictly contraindicated due to the risk of hemorrhage.

Hemangiomas

Definition. Hemangiomas are defined as an abnormal, reversible proliferation of endothelial cells.

Incidence. Hemangiomas are the most common congenital lesion of the craniocervical region (29).

Etiology and pathogenesis. Unknown.

Ultrasound features. Cervical hemangioma appears sonographically as a cystic/solid mass located on the anterolateral aspect of the neck (Fig. 22.**10**). Its echo texture usually resembles that of the placenta. Contrary to former beliefs, an arteriovenous venous plexus is rarely visualized. Typically, the mass is poorly demarcated from the surrounding tissue. It may be extremely large and may extend to the thoracic region (Fig. 22.**11**). Fetal hydrops due to cardiac decompensation is a frequent development (4). Most hemangiomas are exophytic and rarely cause compression of adjacent organs.

Associated anomalies. Hemangiomas are not known to be associated with other anomalies or chromosomal defects.

Prognosis. Hemangiomas show an initial period of rapid growth (proliferation phase), followed by gradual spontaneous regression over a period of 5–8 years (regression phase) (29). Surgical intervention is sometimes warranted for a fast-growing tumor or impending functional compromise. Serious iatrogenic complications are not unusual following surgery (bleeding, sepsis, necrosis). The development of noninvasive treatment methods (cortisol, interferon) could improve the survival prospects of affected fetuses in the future (28).

Prenatal management. A cesarean delivery near term is the preferred course of action due to the risk of vascular rupture. As with teratomas, antenatal aspiration of the cystic components to reduce the tumor volume is strictly contraindicated due to the risk of hemorrhage.

▨ Thyroglossal Duct Cysts and Branchiogenic Cysts

Definitions.

Thyroglossal duct cysts. These are among the most common cervical cystic lesions of childhood (25). They may develop anywhere along the thyroglossal duct from the foramen cecum to the thyroid gland.

Lateral branchiogenic neck cysts. These cysts are remnants of the cervical sinus, second branchial cleft, or second pharyngeal pouch. Often they are first noticed in adulthood, when they appear as a slowly increasing, usually painless swelling in the neck region.

Incidence. Rare.

Etiology and pathogenesis. Unknown.

Ultrasound features. Thyroglossal duct cysts appear as echo-free masses located in the anterior midline of the neck. A branchiogenic cyst usually appears as an isolated anechoic structure located in the anterolateral neck region just below the sternocleidomastoid muscle (Fig. 22.**12**).

Associated anomalies. Not described.

Prognosis. Only postnatal examination can establish the origin of the cyst and differentiate it from other cystic anomalies.

▨ Malignant Tumors

Definition. Malignant tumors in fetuses include lymphadenopathies along with cervical tumors and neuroblastomas that have metastasized from a different fetal primary tumor. Sarcomas (5) and melanomas (7) are rare.

Incidence. Rarely described prenatally.

Cervical Neuroblastoma

Ultrasound features. Cervical neuroblastoma appears sonographically as a solid, hyperechoic mass located in the lateral part of the neck. Like teratomas, the tumor may contain calcifications with associated acoustic shadows. The two tumors are distinguishable, however. Ter-

atomas contain cystic components and are usually located in the anterior part of the neck.

The primary tumor, fetal neuroblastoma, can be identified as a predominantly cystic mass at the level of the adrenal gland (11). The catecholamines synthesized by a fetal neuroblastoma can cross the placenta and cause dramatic maternal symptoms such as tachycardia, hypertension, vomiting, and sweating.

Prognosis. Very poor.

Functional Impairment

▨ Esophageal Atresia

Incidence. Esophageal atresia is a relatively common anomaly, with an incidence of approximately one in 3000–3500 live births.

Pathoanatomic features. The various forms of esophageal atresia can be classified into six types, as described by Vogt (35) (Fig. 22.**13**).

Ultrasound features. Ordinarily the collapsed upper portion of the esophagus cannot be visualized with ultrasound in the fetus.

Indirect signs. The prenatal suspicion of esophageal atresia is based mainly on two indirect signs: the presence of polyhydramnios and a small or nonvisualized fetal gastric bubble.

Atresia without a fistula. When atresia occurs without a proximal tracheo-esophageal fistula (Vogt types II and IIIb), the presumptive diagnosis can sometimes be confirmed by careful examination of the fetal neck region. The examiner can define the esophagus by moving the transducer slightly posteriorly from the coronal plane that simultaneously defines the pharynx, larynx, and trachea. The rhythmic filling and emptying of the blindly ending proximal esophageal pouch can be observed during fetal swallowing movements (Fig. 22.**14**). The abnormally dilated esophagus can also be visualized in a transverse scan at the level of the thyroid gland (Fig. 22.**15**).

Swallowing movements. If esophageal atresia is suspected prenatally, one of the first diagnostic measures should be a detailed evaluation of the fetal neck. The examiner should wait for fetal swallowing movements in order to detect any abnormalities. Atresia is confirmed by observing alternate filling and emptying of the proximal blind esophageal pouch (9, 17, 26, 34).

Associated anomalies. Associated anomalies are fairly common in fetuses with esophageal atresia (50%) and should be excluded (39). The cardiovascular system is most frequently affected, followed by the gastrointestinal tract. Chromosomal abnormalities, especially trisomy 21, should also be excluded. The VACTERL syndrome refers to an association of vertebral body defects (V), anorectal anomalies (A), cardiac anomalies (C), tracheo-esophageal fistula (T), esophageal atresia (E), renal anomalies (R), and limb malformations (L).

Prognosis. The prognosis of esophageal atresia has improved substantially in recent years owing to advances in surgical techniques. It depends mainly on the severity of associated anomalies and only secondarily on the level of the esophageal atresia.

Prenatal management. The goal is spontaneous delivery near term at a perinatal center.

Laryngeal Atresia

Definition. Malformation involving complete closure of the upper fetal respiratory tract.

Incidence. Extremely rare.

Etiology and pathogenesis. Unknown.

Pathoanatomic features. When the upper respiratory tract is atretic, lung fluid cannot escape through the airway. This fluid buildup leads to a well-defined clinical entity with the acronym CHAOS (congenital high airway obstruction syndrome) (13).

Ultrasound features. The ultrasound signs are characteristic:
- Bilateral enlargement of the lungs
- Dilatation of the trachea
- Ascites and/or hydrops secondary to cardiac compression

The presence of these signs should prompt a detailed examination of the fetal neck region. It is normal to see the larynx opening and closing during fetal breathing movements. With laryngeal atresia, a coronal or sagittal scan of the upper respiratory tract shows a closed, stenotic larynx that does not open and close with breathing movements (Figs. 22.**16**–22.**18**). The trachea is extremely dilated (16) and shows no evidence of fluid flow (18).

Associated anomalies. Fraser syndrome.

Prognosis. Newborns with the congenital high airway obstruction syndrome (CHAOS) have very little chance of survival. The prognosis is extremely poor.

Prenatal management. When the anomaly is detected early, termination of the pregnancy should be considered. If the parents refuse this option, preparations should be made for a tracheostomy at the time of delivery. The infant has a chance of survival only if the stenosis is relieved by an "EXIT operation" before the cord is clamped (24).

Conclusion

The fetal neck region is complex and best evaluated using the most modern ultrasound technology. It is not normally done as part of the routine examination.

However, particularly close attention should be given to the fetal neck region when one or more of the suggestive signs in Table 22.3 are noted. Further management should then be performed at a specialized center.

Table 22.**3**   Suggestive signs of a disturbance or anomaly in the neck region

➤ Polyhydramnios
➤ Hyperextension of the fetal head
➤ Stomach small or not visualized
➤ Ascites and/or hydrops

References

1. Bloechle, M., Bollmann, R., Ziener, A. et al.: Fetale Teratome – Diagnostik und Management. Zbl. Gynäkol. 114 (1992) 175–180
2. Bronshtein, M., Bar-Hava, I., Blumenfeld, I., Bejar, J., Toder, V., Blumenfeld, Z.: The difference between septated and nonseptated nuchal cystic hygroma in the early second trimester. Obstet. Gynecol. 81 (1993) 683–687
3. Brumfield, C.G., Wenstrom, K.D., Davis, R.O., Owen, J., Cosper, P.: Second-trimester cystic hygroma: prognosis of septated and nonseptated lesions. Obstet. Gynecol. 88 (1996) 979–982
4. Bulas, D.I., Johnson, D., Allen, J.F. et al.: Fetal Hemangioma. Sonographic and color flow finding. J. Ultrasound Med. 11 (1992) 499–501
5. Bulic, M., Urbanke, A., Ciglar, S., Dominis, M.: Bösartiger Tumor (Sarkom) am Hals eines Fetus, durch Ultraschall während der Gravidität festgestellt. Zbl. Gynäkol. 97 (1975) 747–753
6. Burrow, G.N.: The management of thyreotoxicosis in pregnancy. New Engl. J. Med. 313 (1985) 562–565
7. Campbell, W.A., Storlazzi, E., Vintzileos, A.M., Wu, A., Schneiderman, H., Nochimson, D.J.: Fetal malignant melanoma: Ultrasound presentation and review of the literature. Obstet. Gynecol. 70 (1987) 434–439
8. Chervenak, F.A., Isaacson, G., Blakemore, K.J. et al.: Fetal cystic hygroma. Cause and natural history. New Engl. J. Med. 309 (1983) 822–825
9. Eyheremendy, E., Pfister, M.: Antenatal real-time diagnosis of esophageal atresias. J. Clin. Ultrasound 11 (1983) 395–397
10. Fryns, J.P., Vandenberghe, K., Moerman, P., van den Berghe, H.: Cystic hygroma and multiple pterygium syndrome. Ann. Genet. 27 (1984) 252–253
11. Gadwood, K.A., Reynes, C.J.: Prenatal sonography of metastatic neuroblastoma. J. Clin. Ultrasound 11 (1983) 512–515
12. Gonzales, R., Sommer, F.G., Taylor, K.J.: Prenatal Diagnosis of fetal cystic hygroma. Rev. Interam. Radiol. 5 (1980) 121
13. Hedrick, M.H., Ferro, M.M., Filly, R.A., Flake, A.W., Harrison, M.R., Adzick, N.S.: Congenital high airway obstruction syndrome (CHAOS): a potential for perinatal intervention. J. Pediatr. Surg. 29 (1994) 271–274
14. Hollingsworth, D.R., Alexander, N.M.: Amniotic fluid concentration of iodothyronine and thyrotropin do not reliably predict fetal thyroid status in pregnancy complicated by maternal thyroid disorders or anencephaly. J. Clin. Endocrin. Metab. 57 (1983) 349–355
15. Jordan, R.B., Gauderer, M.W.: Cervical teratomas: An analysis, literature review and proposed classification. J. Pediatr. Surg. 23 (1988) 583–591
16. Kalache, K.D., Franz, M.F., Chaoui, R., Bollmann, R.: Ultrasound measurements of the diameter of the fetal trachea, larynx and pharynx throughout gestation and applicability to prenatal diagnosis of obstructive anomalies of the upper respiratory-digestive tract. Prenat. Diag. 19 (1999) 211–218
17. Kalache, K.D., Chaoui, R., Bollmann, R.: The „upper neck pouch": a prenatal sonographic sign for congenital esophageal atresia. Ultrasound Obst. Gynecol. 11 (1998) 138–140
18. Kalache, K.D., Chaoui, R., Tennstedt, C., Bollmann, R.: Prenatal diagnosis of laryngeal atresia in two cases with Congenital High Airway obstruction Syndrome (CHAOS). Prenat. Diag. 17 (1997) 577–581
19. Kerner, B., Flaum, E., Matwews, H. et al.: Cervical teratoma: Prenatal diagnosis and long-term follow-up. Prenat. Diag. 8 (1998) 51–59
20. Levine, A.B., Alvarez, M., Wedgwood, J., Berkowitz, R.L., Holzman, I.: Contemporary management of a potentially lethal anomaly: A successfull perinatal approach to epignathus. Obstet. Gynecol. 76 (1990) 962–966
21. Moerman, P., Fryns, J.P., Cornelis, A., Bergmans, G., Vandenberghe, K., Lauweryns, J.M.: Pathogenesis of the lethal multiple pterygium syndrome. Amer. J. Med. Genet. 35 (1990) 415–421
22. Miyabara, S., Sugihara, H., Maehara, N. et al.: Significance of cardiovascular malformations in cystic hygroma: a new interpretation of the pathogenesis. Amer. J. Med. Genet. 34 (1989) 489–501
23. Nicolini, U., Venegoni, E., Acaia, B., Cortelazzi, D., Beck-Peccoz, P.: Prenatal treatment of fetal hypothyroidism: is there more than one option? Prenat. Diag. 16 (1996) 443–448
24. Richards, D.S., Yancey, M.K., Duff, P., Stieg, F.H.: The perinatal management of severe laryngeal stenosis. Obstet. Gynecol. 80 (1992) 537–540
25. Santiago, W., Ryback, L.P., Bass, R.M.: Thyreoglossal duct cyst of the tongue. J. Otolaryngol. 14 (1985) 261–264
26. Satoh, S., Takashima, T., Takeuchi, H., Koyanagi, T., Nakano, H.: Antenatal sonographic detection of the proximal esophageal segment: specific evidence for congenital esophageal atresia. J. Clin. Ultrasound 23 (1995) 419–423
27. Schwanitz, G., Zerres, K., Gembruch, U., Bald, R., Hansmann, M.: Rate of chromosomal aberrations in prenatally detected hydrops fetalis and hygroma colli. Hum. Genet. 84 (1989) 81–82
28. Soumeck, B., Adams, G.L., Shapiro, R.S.: Treatment of head and neck hemangiomas with recombinant interferon alpha 2B. Ann. Otol. Rhinol. Laryngol. 105 (1996) 201–205
29. Stal, S., Hamilton, S., Spira, M.: Haemangioma, Lymphangioma and vascular malformations of the head and neck. Otolaryngol. Clin. North Amer. 19 (1986) 769–796
30. Tapper, D., Lack, E.E.: Teratomas in infancy and childhood. A 54-years experience at the Childrens Hospital Medical center. Ann. Surg. 13 (1983) 1079–1084
31. Teal, L.N., Augtuaco, T.L., Jimenez, J.F., Quirk, J.G.: Fetal teratomas: antenatal diagnosis and clinical management. J. Clin. Ultrasound 16 (1988) 329–336
32. Thorpe-Beeston, J.G., Nicolaides, K.H., McGregor, A.M.: Fetal thyroid function. Thyroid 2 (1992) 207–217
33. Trauffer, P.M.L., Anderson, C.E., Johnson, A., Heeger, S., Morgan, P., Wapner, R.J.: The natural history of euploid pregnancies with first-trimester cystic hygromas. Amer. J. Obstet. Gynecol. 170 (1994) 1279–1284
34. Vijayaraghavan, S.B.: Antenatal diagnosis of esophageal atresia with tracheoesophageal fistula. J. Ultrasound Med. 15 (1996) 417–419

35. Vogt, E.C.: Congenital esophageal atresia. Amer. J. Roentgenol. 22 (1929) 463
36. Weber, G., Macchiella, D., Bahlmann, F., Merz, E.: Pränatale Diagnose fetaler Teratome. Ultraschall in Med. 14 (1993) 187–192
37. Wenstrom, K.D., Weiner, C.P., Williamson, R.A., Grant, S.S.: Prenatal diagnosis of fetal hyperthyroidism using funipuncture. Obstet. Gynecol. 76 (1990) 513–517
38. Zadvinskis, D.P., Benson, M.T., Kerr, H.H. et al.: Congenital malformations of the cervicothoracic lymphatic system: embryology and pathogenesis. Radiographics 12 (1992) 1175–1189
39. Zienert, A., Chaoui, R., Bollmann, R.: Die Trachealatresie – eine besondere Assoziation bei Ösophagusatresie und Hydramnion. Ultraschall Med. 12 (1991) 22–24

Neoplasms

Fig. 22.**1**   Cystic hygroma. Transverse scan through the neck of a 15-week fetus. The lymph cysts (∗) appear as thin-walled, cystic masses with no internal echoes, located at the back and sides of the fetal neck. Ha = hands, VB = vertebral body.

Fig. 22.**2**   Cystic hygroma. Transverse scan of the posterior head and neck of the fetus in Fig. 22.**1**. The "nuchal ligament," a typical feature of cystic hygroma, is visible (arrows).

Fig. 22.**3**   Extensive cystic hygroma (XO karyotype) and oligohydramnios, 20 weeks. Transverse scan at the level of the fetal neck (1) in a breech-presenting fetus. The large, hypoechoic lymph cysts (2) may be mistaken for amniotic fluid pockets. The "nuchal ligament" (arrow) may be misinterpreted as an amniotic cord (observation by Prof. Merz).

Fig. 22.**4**   Extensive cystic hygroma, 20 weeks. Postmortem view of the fetus in Fig. 22.**3** (observation by Prof. Merz).

Fig. 22.**5**   Fetal goiter. Transverse scan through the neck at the level of the thyroid gland in a 23-week fetus with hypothyroidism. The enlarged thyroid gland appears as a bilobed, echogenic structure (arrow) in the anterior part of the neck.

Fig. 22.**6**   Fetal goiter. Sagittal scan through the neck of the fetus in Fig. 22.**5**. The trachea (small arrows) is displaced posteriorly by the goiter (large arrows).

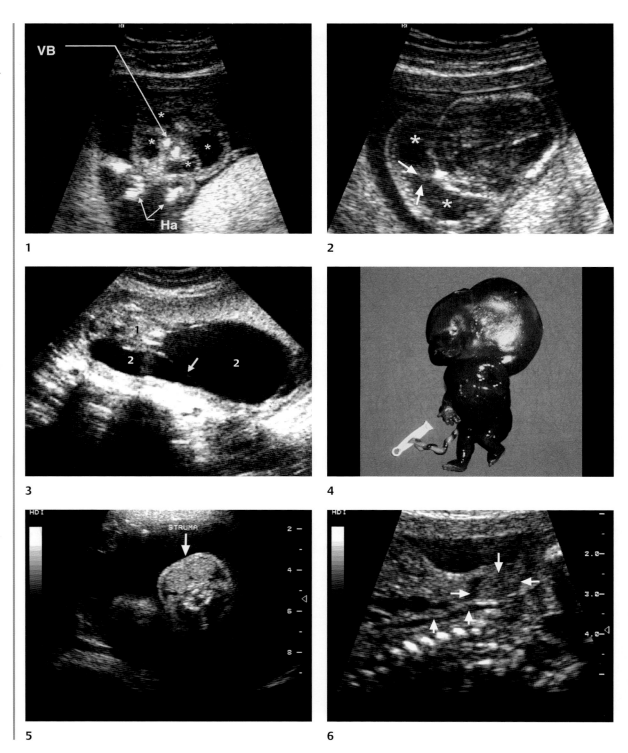

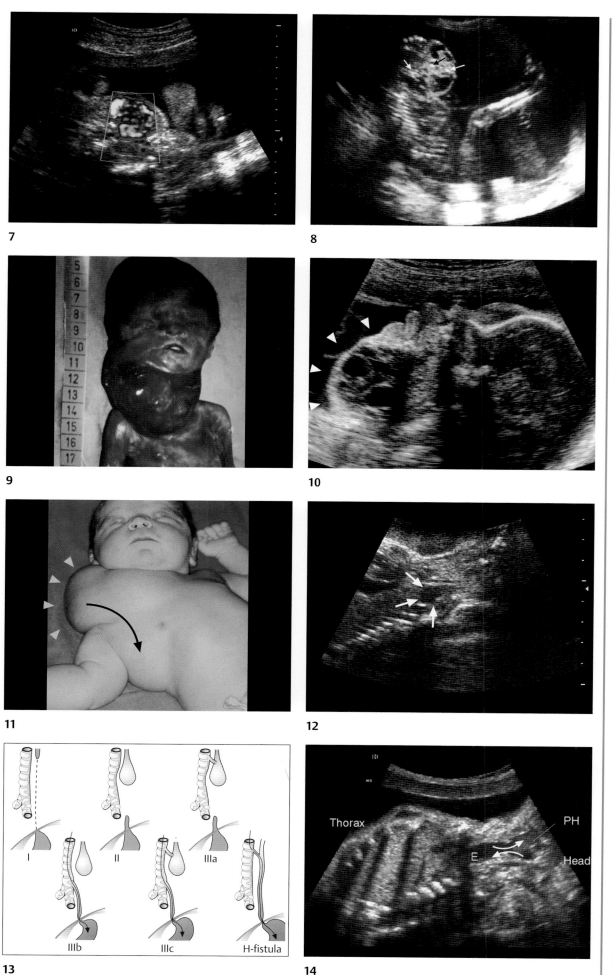

7

8

9

10

11

12

13

14

Fig. 22.**7**   Fetal goiter. Transverse scan through the neck at the level of the thyroid gland. Same fetus as in Figs. 22.**5** and 22.**6** (23 weeks). Power color Doppler demonstrates hypervascularity of the goiter.

Fig. 22.**8**   Fetal cervical teratoma. A well-circumscribed, mixed solid/cystic, echogenic anterior neck mass is demonstrated in a 21-week fetus. The echogenic calcifications (arrows) are a typical feature of teratomas.

Fig. 22.**9**   Fetal cervical teratoma, 21 weeks. Postmortem view of the fetus in Fig. 22.**8**.

Fig. 22.**10**   Fetal cervical hemangioma. Sagittal scan of a fetus at 27 weeks. The tumor appears as a poorly circumscribed, mixed solid/cystic anterior neck mass (arrows).

Fig. 22.**11**   Postnatal view of the fetus in Fig. 22.10. A huge cervical hemangioma extends into the right upper quadrant of the chest.

Fig. 22.**12**   Branchiogenic cyst. Sagittal scan through the neck of a 27-week fetus demonstrates an isolated, smooth-walled cyst (arrows). The "teardrop" shape is typical of a laterally situated branchiogenic cyst.

Functional impairment

Fig. 22.**13**   The Vogt classification of esophageal atresia (35) (from Richter and Ernst: Radiologische Anatomie des Neugeborenen, 1990). Type IIIb (blindly ending esophagus with a distal tracheo-esophageal fistula) is the most common form. Antenatal dilatation of the upper blind pouch has been observed only in types II and IIIb.

Fig. 22.**14**   Esophageal atresia. Coronal scan through the neck of a 27-week fetus with Vogt type II esophageal atresia (the transducer was moved a few millimeters posteriorly). During fetal swallowing movements, rhythmic filling and emptying of the blindly terminating proximal esophagus (E) are observed during fetal swallowing. PH = pharynx. From Kalache et al. 1998 (17).

Fig. 22.**15**   Esophageal atresia. Transverse scan through the neck at the level of the thyroid gland, same fetus as in Fig. 22.**14**. Note the proximally dilated esophagus (arrows) lateral to the trachea (TR). From Kalache et al. 1998 (17).

Fig. 22.**16**   Laryngeal atresia. The closed, stenotic larynx (SL) prevents the normal drainage of lung fluid. Dilatation of the trachea (TR) occurred in this case despite the presence of a tracheo-esophageal fistula (arrow). It occurred because an associated complete duodenal atresia led to fluid stasis in the upper gastrointestinal tract (compare with Fig. 22.**13**). E = esophagus, Ao = aorta. From Kalache et al. 1997 (18).

Fig. 22.**17**   Diagram of the case shown in Fig. 22.**16**. Laryngeal atresia was combined with esophageal atresia and duodenal atresia.

Fig. 22.**18**   Laryngeal atresia. Pathology specimen from the case in Figs. 22.**16** and 22.**17**, demonstrating the cartilaginous laryngeal closure. From Kalache et al. 1998 (18).

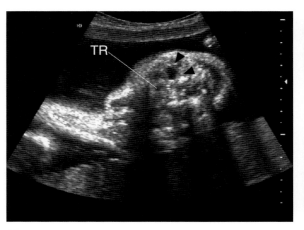

15

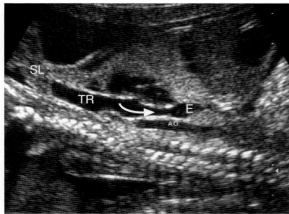

16

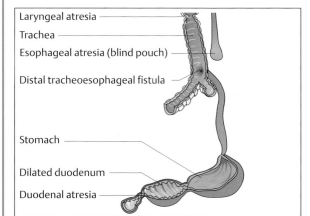

17

18

23 Spina Bifida

Occurrence, Pathogenesis, and Ultrasound Features

Definition

Spina bifida is a combined developmental defect involving the spinal canal and its contents and characterized by partial or complete absence of the vertebral arches. Several forms are distinguished according to the involvement of the spinal cord, meninges, and skin (14):
Complete spina bifida (rachischisis)
Partial spina bifida
- Myelocele
- Spina bifida cystica (meningocele, myelomeningocele)

Open and closed forms. Partial spina bifida may be open or closed, depending on whether the defect is covered by skin (14).

Anterior and posterior forms. Spina bifida is classified as anterior or posterior, depending on whether the defect involves the anterior or posterior surface of the bony spinal canal (39).

Incidence

Posterior defects of neural tube closure are among the most common fetal anomalies. Spina bifida aperta (open spinal defect) is particularly important in prenatal diagnosis, and its incidence varies markedly among different countries. Its average reported incidence is 0.17% of all live births in Germany (18) but is considerably higher in Great Britain, with an incidence of 0.5% (24). Most of these cases involve posterior defects; anterior spina bifida is very rare.

Etiology and Pathogenesis

Spina bifida is believed to result from a primary failure of closure of the posterior vertebral arches involving one or more spinal segments (14, 54).

Endogenous and exogenous factors. Animal studies have shown that neural tube defects are ultimately based on the inadequate expression of certain pattern control genes such as the Hox-1.6 gene. In humans, this could be caused by endogenous factors (gene deletion), exogenous teratogenic agents such as valproinic acid and carbamazepine (48), or a vitamin deficiency (46).

Embryology

Araphias and dysraphias. The primary failure of neural tube closure is believed to occur before the end of the sixth week of embryonic development (56). The failure of posterior vertebral arch fusion is variable in its degree, and accordingly the defect may involve only a few vertebral segments or the entire spinal column. Forms in which the neural groove remains open are called araphias. These are distinguished from dysraphias, in which a neural tube has formed but there is defective closure along the posterior raphe (14). Araphias have an earlier teratologic determination period than dysraphias (14).

The lesion most commonly occurs in the lumbosacral area (almost 80% of cases). It occurs occasionally in the cervical spine and is least common in the thoracic spine (14, 50).

Pathoanatomic Features (39)

Spina bifida occulta. This is the mildest form of spina bifida, in which there is no protrusion of the spinal cord or meninges. The skin covering the bony spinal canal defect shows changes such as increased local hair growth, pigmentation changes, angioma formation, and dimpling (14) (Fig. 23.**1a**).

Spina bifida aperta. The occult form contrasts with spina bifida aperta (myelocele and spina bifida cystica), which is an open spinal defect.
A *myelocele* refers to open spina bifida with an exposed neural plate (Fig. 23.**1b**).
Spina bifida cystica is characterized by the protrusion of meninges (meningocele) (27) (Fig. 23.**1c**) or of the spinal cord and meninges (myelomeningocele) (40) (Fig. 23.**1d**). Pure meningoceles account for only about 10% of open spinal defects; the rest are myelomeningoceles (50).

Complete rachischisis. This very rare condition is the most severe of the cleft anomalies. The spinal cord forms a flat, elongated, dark red plaque (area medullovasculosa) located within the open vertebral groove.

Ultrasound Features

Clefts in the spinal canal are among the defects that require great care and experience in their ultrasound detection. In contrast to anencephaly, the majority of spinal defects are still overlooked in routine prenatal screening examinations. According to a 1993 survey published by Carstens and Niethard (9), only 27% of a total of 488 myeloceles were detected prior to delivery cases, and 83% were detected between 30 and 40 weeks.

AFP and AChE tests. Given the poor detection rate with ultrasound, the maternal serum alpha-fetoprotein (AFP) continues to be the preferred screening test for fetal spinal defects (13, 30, 53). Elevated maternal serum acetylcholinesterase (AChE) levels can also provide evidence of spina bifida when detected in early pregnancy (2).

Dating the pregnancy. Once an elevated serum AFP has been found, ultrasound can be used to selectively examine the fetus for a spinal defect. Ultrasound dating can also be used at this time to screen out cases in which the false assumption of a younger gestational age created the impression of elevated AFP levels. If the AFP levels are found to be within normal limits after the gestational age has been adjusted, and if targeted imaging shows no evidence of spina bifida, it is unnecessary to proceed with amniocentesis in these patients.

Amniocentesis. If the serum AFP is elevated or if there is a positive family history of spina bifida despite normal ultrasound findings, amniocentesis should be performed to determine the AFP level and CNS-specific acetylcholinesterase (3, 51). The patient may also be referred to a prenatal diagnostic center for targeted imaging.

Essential points. Targeted ultrasound imaging can resolve three essential points:

- In most cases the defect in the spinal column can be directly visualized with ultrasound (6, 7, 8, 17, 44, 45). The size and location of the defect have prognostic implications.
- If the elevated AFP level is caused by a different anomaly, such as omphalocele or gastroschisis (35), the causal defect can be specifically defined.
- Skin-covered spinal defects can also be detected, especially in high-risk cases (19, 25). These defects are not disclosed by biochemical tests when they are associated with normal serum and amniotic fluid AFP levels (31, 32).

Favorable period. According to Campbell (7), the most favorable period for ultrasound evaluation of the fetal spine is between 16 and 20 weeks' gestation, for at this time the spine can be visualized in its entire length. With transvaginal ultrasound, a detailed evaluation of the spine can be performed as early as 10 weeks if the fetus is in a favorable position.

Scan planes. To ensure the reliable detection or exclusion of a spinal defect, the fetal spine should be scrutinized in sagittal and coronal views as well as in transverse planes. A spinal defect cannot be excluded with high confidence until a complete series of transverse scans demonstrate the ossification centers of all the vertebral segments, and no defect in the body surface is visible on sagittal examination.

Amniotic fluid volume and breech presentation. A decreased amniotic fluid volume can make it much more difficult to detect spina bifida. In these cases the fetal spine usually lies against the uterine wall, obscuring the spinal defect. But even with a normal amniotic fluid volume, a lumbosacral defect can be difficult to appreciate if the fetus is in a breech presentation with the rump deeply engaged in the lower pelvis. If the transabdominal findings are equivocal, transvaginal scanning should additionally be performed.

Ultrasound Forms

Spina Bifida Occulta

In this form, ultrasound shows only a circumscribed expansion of the spinal canal with no visible defect in the body surface (28) (Figs. 21.**1a**, 23.**2**).

Spina Bifida Aperta

The ultrasound appearance of this condition varies depending on the location and nature of the defect (spinal defect with or without a cystic swelling).

Differentiation. It can be difficult or impossible to distinguish between a myelocele and myelomeningocele when the cystic sac lies relatively flat against the spinal defect. The same applies to differentiating a meningocele from a myelomeningocele. For example, the ultrasound appearance may be that of a meningocele, but postpartum histologic examination of the cystic sac may reveal spinal cord tissue in the herniated sac, identifying the lesion as a myelomeningocele.

Myelocele, Open Spinal Canal

Scan planes. Spinal clefts that are not associated with a definite cystic sac are easily missed on ultrasound examination. Figure 23.**3** illustrates the importance of scanning the spine in various planes and at various angles.

Oblique sagittal scan. An oblique scan may cut the ossification centers of the individual vertebrae at an angle which makes it appear that the spinal column is intact. There may be only a slight irregularity at the lumbosacral level suggesting the presence of a defect (Fig. 23.**3a**).

Midsagittal scan. On a precise midsagittal scan through the dorsoanterior fetus, the defect in the lumbosacral area is plainly defined (Fig. 23.**3b**). The advantage of a precise midsagittal scan is that it can demonstrate both the bony spinal defect and the body surface defect in the same image. It should be noted, however, that spina bifida is still easily missed even in a dorsoanterior fetus if the defect is very shallow (Figs. 23.**4**, 23.**5**) or if it consists of a small, pore-like opening at the sacral level (Fig. 23.**6**).

Coronal scan. If the fetus is lying on its side, a longitudinal coronal scan will demonstrate the spinal defect as a variable-sized fusiform expansion of the spinal canal (Fig. 23.**7**).

"Pseudodefect." If the lesion is a circumscribed defect in the lumbar region and the fetus is lying on its side, the acoustic shadow cast by the near iliac wing can obscure the spinal defect. Also, the shadow from the iliac wing can occasionally mimic spina bifida in a healthy fetus (Fig. 23.**8**). This "pseudodefect" is recognized by noting that it equals the exact width of the iliac wing shadow and that it does not appear in sagittal or transverse views of the spine.

Transverse scan. On an axial scan through a spinal defect, the spinal canal does not form a complete ring but is interrupted posteriorly by a V- or U-shaped opening (7) (Figs. 23.**9**, 23.**10**).

Rachischisis

Complete rachischisis is an extreme form of spina bifida in which most of the spinal canal is disrupted by a fusiform opening (Fig. 23.**11**). In craniorachischisis, which occurs in some cases of anencephaly, a longitudinal coronal scan shows triangular expansion of the spinal canal at the craniocervical junction (Fig. 23.**12**).

Spina Bifida Cystica

Meningocele. A meningocele is a small, sac-like, fluid-filled protrusion posterior to the spinal defect (Fig. 23.**13**). Despite the absence of echoes in the hernial sac, a meningocele cannot be confidently distinguished from a myelomeningocele with ultrasound because peripheral spinal cord fibers may be present that cannot be detected sonographically.

Myelomeningocele. In a myelomeningocele, ultrasound may show punctate to cord-like echogenic structures within the cystic sac, depending on the scan plane and the size of the sac (Figs. 23.**14**–23.**20**). A flat myelomeningocele cannot be distinguished sonographically from a myelocele, because the cystic sac may closely overlie the defect (Figs. 23.**15**, 23.**16**).

Arnold–Chiari type II malformation. The detection of a myelomeningocele always warrants a meticulous examination of the fetal head (lateral ventricles, cerebellum) to detect or exclude an Arnold–Chiari type II malformation (Fig. 23.**21**). This condition is a syndrome characterized by defective development of the cerebellum with downward extension of the dorsal medulla oblongata, hydrocephalus, and a myelomeningocele (4, 47) (see Chapter 21).

Diagnosis

Ultrasound Signs that Suggest Spina Bifida

Superior biometry. When the growth pattern of fetuses with spina bifida is evaluated with ultrasound, head growth is found to be decreased while trunk growth progresses normally. Wald et al. (54), in a study of 20 fetuses with spina bifida in the second trimester, found that the superior biparietal diameter was an average of 16% smaller than in normal controls. Hansmann (17) also noted a transient period of microcephalic growth in serial observations of five fetuses with spina bifida. As term approaches, growth of the fetal head accelerates due to the development of hydrocephalus. Figure 23.**22** shows an example of this "rebound growth" in one of our own cases. A relative decrease in head growth should be diagnosed only if the abdominal circumference and femur length show a concomitant growth pattern that is normal for gestational age.

Lemon sign and banana sign. Besides a small biparietal diameter and hydrocephalus, two other head parameters provide important suggestive signs of a spinal defect (Table 23.**1**). These are the lemon sign (36, 37), referring to a lemon-shaped deformity of the head due to anterolateral collapse of the frontal bones (see Figs. 21.**50** and 21.**51**), and the banana sign (1, 36), referring to a banana-shaped cerebellum that has been displaced into the spinal canal (see Fig. 21.**52**).

The lemon sign has proved to be a particularly sensitive marker of spina bifida during the second trimester. In a retrospective study, Nicolaides et al. (36) found that this sign could be detected in all 54 spina bifida cases before 24 weeks' gestation. However, a similar type of superior deformation is found in 1% of healthy fetuses (5, 37).

The banana sign is more difficult to recognize. Pilu et al. (42) found a decreased cerebellar diameter in 19 fetuses with spina bifida. In another 7 fetuses, they were unable to define the cerebellum with ultrasound. This has led several authors to use obliteration of the cisterna magna as a suggestive sign of spina bifida, rather than the banana sign (15, 42).

Foot deformities. In addition to the superior deformities listed in Table 23.**1**, fetuses with spina bifida also manifest foot deformities such as pes equinovarus and impaired leg movements.

Angulation of the spine. Angulation of the fetal spine (Fig. 23.**13**) also warrants a complete and detailed examination of the spinal column.

Despite the suggestive signs described above and despite a targeted search by an experienced examiner (7, 17, 44), the ultrasound detection of spina bifida may be unsuccessful. Usually this is due to poor imaging conditions or an unfavorable fetal position.

Associated Anomalies

Vintzileos et al. (52) observed hydrocephalus in 80% of fetuses with spina bifida. Other possible associated anomalies include heart defects, cleft lip and palate, abdominal wall defects, and limb malformations (21, 43). Spinal defects located at higher levels are more commonly associated with nonneural anomalies than spinal defects at lower levels (21). Defects unrelated to the neural tube are found in 14.5% of spina bifida cases (49).

Rachischisis is almost invariably combined with other anomalies such as cranioschisis, anencephaly, or an abdominal cleft (39).

Chromosomal abnormalities. In a study of CNS anomalies, Nyberg et al. (38) found a chromosomal defect in 8% of fetuses with hydrocephalus and spina bifida and in 33% of fetuses with spina bifida alone. The most common chromosomal abnormality found in association with neural tube defects is trisomy 18 (20).

Table 23.1 Ultrasound abnormalities that suggest spina bifida

Head abnormalities	➢ Enlargement of the lateral ventricles ➢ Head growth at lower limit of normal ➢ Altered head shape (lemon sign) ➢ Altered cerebellar shape (banana sign) ➢ Decreased cerebellar diameter (12, 42) ➢ Obliteration of the cisterna magna
Other spinal abnormalities	➢ Angulation of the fetal spine
Abnormalities of the legs or feet	➢ Pes equinovarus ➢ Absence of leg movements

Differential Diagnosis

Sacrococcygeal teratoma and lipoma. When a cystic structure is found in the lumbosacral area, conditions to be considered other than spina bifida cystica include a cystic sacrococcygeal teratoma (closed spinal column!) and a lumbosacral lipoma (41). If the cystic structure is located in the thoracic area and a spinal defect has been excluded, the lesion is presumed to be a lipoma (Figs. 23.**23**, 23.**24**).

Other Tests

If ultrasound findings are equivocal, amniocentesis should be performed to determine the AFP and acetylcholinesterase (AChE) levels in the amniotic fluid.

Prognosis and Prenatal Management

Prognosis

The prognosis of spina bifida depends on several factors including the level, nature, and size of the defect. Possible associated anomalies also play a significant role.

Paralysis. Whereas spina bifida occulta is innocuous, myelomeningoceles are usually associated with flaccid paralysis. Lesions above the L3 vertebral body can cause total paraplegia, depending on their extent, while lesions at or below the level of the L4 vertebral body typically cause motor paralysis of the legs, bladder paralysis, and anorectal paralysis. Lesions at or below S3 mainly cause impairment of bladder and bowel emptying (39) (Table 23.**2**).

Impaired leg function. If a complete absence of fetal leg motion is noted sonographically for a prolonged period despite an adequate amniotic fluid volume, it is reasonable to assume that a motor dysfunction is present. A concomitant foot deformity should increase the index of suspicion. On the other hand, the detection of leg movements in a fe-

Table 23.2 Clinical manifestations of dysraphic myelodysplasias (39)

1. Lesions above L3	Complete paraplegia
2. Lesions at or below L4	Loss of hip extensors and knee flexors, total foot paralysis, bladder and bowel incontinence
3. Lesions at or below S1	Weakness of hip extensors and knee flexors, loss of foot flexors, weak pronation and supination of the foot, loss of toe spreaders, bladder and anorectal paralysis
4. Lesions at or below S3	No motor deficits, but likely bladder and anorectal paralysis

tus with spina bifida is not necessarily a good prognostic sign, because paralysis of the lower extremities has been found postnatally in infants that actively moved their legs while still in utero (7, 28).

Level of the defect. The precise level of the defect is not always easy to determine with two-dimensional ultrasound. For example, Kollias et al. (22) reported on cases in which the actual lesion was underestimated with ultrasound (it appeared lower than it really was) as well as cases in which the lesion was overestimated (appearing higher than it actually was). Three-dimensional ultrasound may yield better results in the future, as it permits an accurate tomographic survey of spinal defects (29).

Risk of Recurrence

If a patient has previously had an infant with spina bifida (or anencephaly), the risk of recurrence is approximately 4% (26).

Prenatal Management

When spina bifida is detected before viability is reached, pregnancy termination may be considered depending on the size and level of the defect and the presence of accompanying anomalies (10). If the parents want to continue the pregnancy, the fetal karyotype should be determined to exclude a chromosomal abnormality such as trisomy 18 (55).

Interdisciplinary management. Optimum interdisciplinary management is important in ensuring optimum care of the newborn infant, especially in fetuses with a large spina bifida cystica. An elective cesarean delivery (10) can be planned to avoid rupturing the sac, and preparations can be made for immediate pediatric care and subsequent neurosurgical treatment of the newborn.

Gressens et al. (16) published the follow-up results of 137 spina bifida cases in 1998.

Prospective Management

Folic acid. Various prospective studies (11, 33, 34) have documented the efficacy of folic acid supplementation in preventing neural tube defects in groups with a genetic and/or geographic risk. A risk reduction of up to 72% could be achieved, depending on the study. For this reason, it is recommended that women who have already had a child with a neural tube defect take a daily dose of 4 mg of folic acid prior to conception and during the first 3 months of their pregnancy.

References

1. Benacerraf, B.R., Stryker, J., Figoletto, J.D.jr.: Abnormal US appearance of the cerebellum (banana sign): indirect sign of spina bifida. Radiology 171 (1989) 151–153
2. Brennand, D.M., Jehanli, A.M., Wood, P.J., Smith, J.L.: Raised levels of maternal serum secretory acetylcholinesterase may be indicative of fetal neural tube defects in early pregnancy. Acta Obstet. Gynecol. Scand. 77 (1998) 8–13
3. Brock, D.J., Hayward, C.: Gel electrophoresis of amniotic fluid acetylcholinesterase as an aid to the prenatal diagnosis of fetal defects. Clin. chim. Acta 108 (1980) 135–141
4. Cameron, A.H.: Arnold-Chiari and other neuro-anatomical malformations associated with spina bifida. J. Path. Bact. 73 (1957) 195–211
5. Campbell, J., Gilbert, W.M., Nicolaides, K.H., Campbell, S.: Ultrasound screening for spina bifida: cranial and cerebellar signs in a high-risk population. Obstet. Gynecol. 70 (1987) 247–250
6. Campbell, S., Pryse-Davies, J., Coltart, T.M., Seller, M.J., Singer, J.D.: Ultrasound in the diagnosis of spina bifida. Lancet 1 (1975) 1065–1068
7. Campbell, S.: Early prenatal diagnosis of neural tube defects by ultrasound. Clin. Obstet. Gynec. 20 (1977) 351–359
8. Campbell, S.: Early prenatal diagnosis of fetal abnormality by ultrasound B-scanning. In: Murken, J.D., Stengel-Rutkowski, S., Schwinger, E.: Prenatal Diagnosis. Stuttgart: Enke 1979; p. 183
9. Carstens, C., Niethard, F.U.: Der gegenwärtige Stand der pränatalen Diagnostik einer Myelomeningozele: Ergebnisse einer Fragenbogenaktion. Geburtsh. Frauenheilkd. 53 (1993) 182–185
10. Chervenak, F.A., Duncan, C., Ment, L.R., Tortora, M., McClure, M., Hobbins, J.C.: Perinatal management of meningomyelocele. Obstet. Gynecol. 63 (1984) 376–380
11. Czeizel, A.E., Dudas, I.: Prevention of the first occurrence of neural tube defects by periconceptional vitamin supplementation. New Engl. J. Med. 327 (1992) 1832–1835
12. De Courcy-Wheeler, R.H., Pomeranz, M.M., Wald, N.J., Nicolaides, K.H.: Small fetal transverse cerebellar diameter: a screening test for spina bifida. Brit. J. Obstet. Gynaecol. 101 (1994) 904–905
13. Fuhrmann, W.: Die Alpha-Fetoproteinbestimmung in der pränatalen Diagnostik und Vorsorge. Diagn. Intensivther. 6 (1983) 1–7
14. Gerlach, J., Jensen, H.P.: Mißbildungen des Rückenmarks – B. Verschlußstörungen. In: Handbuch der Neurochirurgie, Band VII/I., Springer 1967, S. 308 ff
15. Goldstein, R.B., Podrasky, A.E., Filly, R.A., Callen, P.W.: Effacement of the fetal cisterna magna in association with myelomeningocele. Radiology 172 (1989) 409–413
16. Gressens, P., Collin, P., Lebarbier, P. et al.: Le diagnostic prenatal et le devenir des patients atteints de spina bifida. Arch. Pediatr. 5 (1998) 1004–1008
17. Hansmann, M.: Nachweis und Ausschluß fetaler Entwicklungsstörungen mittels Ultraschallscreening und gezielter Untersuchung – ein Mehrstufenkonzept. Ultraschall 2 (1981) 206–220
18. Harnack von, G.A., Kirsten, B.: Meningo- und Myelomeningocele. Nachuntersuchungen über 103 Kinder, die 1946–1956 behandelt wurden. Dtsch. med. Wschr. 83 (1958) 2122–2126
19. Hood, V.D., Robinson, H.P.: Diagnosis of closed neural tube defects by ultrasound in the second trimester of pregnancy. Brit. med. J. 2 (1978) 931
20. Hume, R.F.jr., Drugan, A., Reichler, A. et al.: Aneuploidy among prenatally detected neural tube defects. Amer. J. Med. Genet. 61 (1996) 171–173
21. Kalien, B., Robert, E., Harris, J.: Associated malformations in infants and fetuses with upper or lower neural tube defects. Teratology 57 (1998) 56–63
22. Kollias, S.S., Goldstein, R.B., Cogen, P.H., Filly, R.A.: Prenatally detected myelomeningoceles: sonographic accuracy in estimation of the spinal level. Radiology 185 (1992) 109–112
23. Kries von, R., Lenard, H.G.: Anmerkung zur Prävention von Neuralrohrdefekten (NRD) durch Folsäure. Monatsschr. Kinderheilk. 142 (1994) 705–711
24. Lawrence, K.M., David, P.A.: The incidence of major central nervous system malformations in South Wales. Arch. Dis. Childh. 38 (1963) 98
25. Leucht, W., Müller, E., Heyes, H., Töllner, U., Jonatha, W.: Probleme bei der pränatalen Diagnose von Neuralrohrdefekten. Z. Geburtsh. Perinat. 183 (1979) 434–437
26. Masterson, J.G.: Empiric risk, genetic counseling and preventive measures in anencephaly. Acta genet. (Basel) 12 (1962) 219–229
27. McComb, J.G.: Spinal meningoceles. In: Albright, L., Pollack, I., Adelson, D. (eds.): Principles and practice of pediatric neurosurgery. New York: Thieme 1999; pp. 271–289
28. Merz, E.: Prenatal diagnosis of neural tube defects by ultrasound. In: Voth, D., Glees, P.: Spina bifida – Neural Tube Defects. In collaboration with L. Lorber. Berlin: de Gruyter 1986; p. 159
29. Merz, E., Bahlmann, F., Weber, G.: Volume scanning in the evaluation of fetal malformations: A new dimension in prenatal diagnosis. Ultrasound Obstet. Gynecol. 5 (1995) 222–227
30. Milunsky, A., Alpert, E.: The value of alpha-fetoprotein in prenatal diagnosis of neural tube defects. J. Pediat. 84 (1974) 889–893
31. Milunsky, A., Alpert, E.: Prenatal diagnosis of neural tube defects. I. Problems and pitfalls: analysis of 2495 cases using the alphafetoprotein assay. Obstet. Gynec. 48 (1976) 1–5
32. Milunsky, A., Alpert, E.: Pranatal diagnosis of neural tube defects. II. Analysis of false positive and false negative alpha-fetoprotein results. Obstet. Gynec. 48 (1976) 6–12
33. Milunsky, A., Jick, H., Jick, S.S. et al.: Multivitamin/folic acid supplementation in early pregnancy reduces the prevalence of neural tube defects. JAMA 262 (1989) 2847–2852
34. MRC Vitamin Study Research Group: Prevention of neural tube defects: results of medical research council vitamin study. Lancet 338 (1991) 131–137
35. Mühlhaus, K., Weitzel, H.K., Schneider, J.: Pränatale Diagnostik von Neuralrohr- und Bauchwanddefekten im II. Trimenon. Geburtsh. u. Frauenheilk. 45 (1985) 98–100
36. Nicolaides, K.H., Campbell, S., Gabbe, S.G.: Ultrasound screening for spina bifida: cranial and cerebellar signs. Lancet 2 (1986) 72–74

37. Nyberg, D.A., Mack, L.A., Hirsch, J., Mahony, J.S.: Abnormalities of fetal cranial contour in sonographic detection of spina bifida: Evaluation of the „lemon" sign. Radiology 167 (1988) 387–392
38. Nyberg, D.A., Shepard, T., Mack, L.A., Hirsch, J., Luthy, D., Fitzsimmons, J.: Significance of a single umbilical artery in fetuses with central nervous system malformations. J. Ultrasound Med. 9 (1988) 265–273
39. Pache, H.D.: Die Dysrhaphien des Rückenmarks. In: Opitz, H., Schmid, F. (Hrsg.): Handbuch der Kinderheilkunde, VIII/1. Berlin: Springer 1969; S. 169
40. Park, T.S.: Myelomeningocele. Mahony, J.S.: Abnormalities of fetal cranial contour in sonographic detection of spina bifida: Evaluation of the „lemon" sign. Radiology 167 (1988) 291–320
41. Pierre-Kahn, A., Zerah, M., Renier, D. et al.: Congenital lumbosacral lipomas. Childs Nerv. Syst. 13 (1997) 298–334
42. Pilu, G., Romero, R., Reece, A., Goldstein, I., Hobbins, J.C., Bovicelli, L.: Subnormal cerebellum in fetuses with spina bifida. Amer. J. Obstet. Gynecol. 158 (1988) 1052–1056
43. Record, R.G., McKeown, T.: Congenital malformations of the central nervous system. II. Brit. J. soc. Med. 4 (1950) 26
44. Robinson, H.P.: The role of ultrasound in the prenatal diagnosis of neural tube defects. In: Murken, J.D., Stengel-Rutkowski, S., Schwinger, E.: Prenatal Diagnosis. Stuttgart: Enke 1979; p. 179
45. Robinson, H.P., Hood, V.A., Adam, A.H., Gibson, A.A.M., Ferguson-Smith, M.A.: Diagnostic ultrasound: Early detection of fetal neural tube defects. Obstet. and Gynec. 56 (1980) 705–710
46. Schlote, W., Riede, U.N., Wiestler, O.D.: Nervensystem. In: Riede, U.N., Schaefer, H.E.: Allgemeine und spezielle Pathologie. Stuttgart: Thieme 1995; S. 1021–1094

47. Shaw, C.M., Alvord, E.C.jr.: Hydrocephalus. In: Duckett, S.: Pediatric neuropathology. Baltimore: Williams & Wilkins 1995; pp. 149–211
48. Shurtleff, D.B., Lemire, R.J.: Epidemiology, etiologic factors, and prenatal diagnosis of open spinal dysraphism. Neurosurg. Clin. N. Amer. 6 (1995) 183–193
49. Simpson, J.L., Mills, J., Rhoads, G.G., Cunningham, G.C., Conley, M.R., Hoffman, H.J.: Genetic heterogeneity in neural tube defects. Ann. Genet. 34 (1991) 279–286
50. Stauffer, U.G.: Mißbildungen im Bereich der Wirbelsäule. In: Rickham, P.P., Soper, R.T., Stauffer, U.G.: Kinderchirurgie. Stuttgart: Thieme 1975; S. 115
51. U.K. Collaborative acethylcholinesterase study. Amniotic fluid acetylcholinesterase electrophoresis as a secondary test in the diagnosis of anencephaly and open spina bifida in early pregnancy. Lancet 2 (1981) 321–324
52. Vintzileos, A.M., Ingardia, C.J., Nochimson, D.J.: Congenital hydrocephalus: A review and protocol for perinatal management. Obstet. and Gynec. 62 (1983) 539–549
53. Wald, N.J., Cuckle, H., Brock, J.H., Peto, R., Polani, P.E., Woodford, F.P.: Maternal serum-alpha-fetoprotein measurement in antenatal screening for anencephaly and spina bifida in early pregnancy. Report of U.K. collaborative study on alpha-fetoprotein in relation to neural-tube defects. Lancet 1 (1977) 1323–1332
54. Wald, N., Cuckle, H., Boreham, J., Stirrat, G.: Small biparietal diameter of fetuses with spina bifida: implications for antenatal screening. Brit. J. Obstet. Gynaec. 87 (1980) 219–221
55. Warkany, J., Passarge, E., Smith, L.B.: Congenital malformations in autosomal trisomy syndromes. Amer. J. Dis. Child. 112 (1966) 502–517
56. Warkany, J.: Congenital Malformations: Spina bifida. Year Book Medical Publishers Inc., Chicago 1971; p. 272

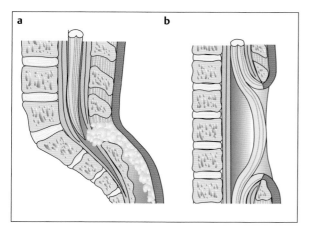

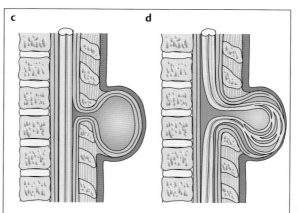

Fig. 23.**1** Schematic representation of spinal dysraphias (modified from [46]).
a Spina bifida occulta with a lipoma.
b Myelocele.
c Meningocele.
d Myelomeningocele.

Spina bifida occulta

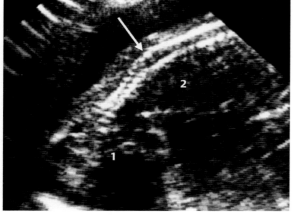

Fig. 23.**2** Spina bifida occulta in the thoracic region (arrow) of a breech-presenting fetus, 22 weeks. Ultrasound shows only a slight fusiform expansion of the spinal canal. The body surface itself is intact. 1 = Head, 2 = trunk.

Spina bifida aperta and myelocele

Fig. 23.3 Spina bifida (myelocele) in the lumbosacral region (arrows), 26 weeks.
a The spinal column appears closed in this oblique longitudinal scan.
b With a precise midsagittal scan of the dorsoanterior fetus, the defect is clearly defined by the break in the surface contour.

Fig. 23.4 Lumbosacral spina bifida, 22 weeks. A shallow defect (arrows mark its upper and lower boundaries) is easily overlooked.

Fig. 23.5 Postmortem view of the fetus in Fig. 23.4.

Fig. 23.6 Left: spina bifida at the sacral level, consisting only of a pore-like opening (arrow), 22 weeks. Karyotype: trisomy 18. Right: postmortem view.

Fig. 23.7 Left: lumbar spina bifida, 20 weeks. Karyotype: trisomy 18. In a longitudinal coronal scan through the spinal column, the defect is obscured by shadowing from the upper iliac wing (arrow). The spinal canal itself is widened at this level, however. Right: postmortem view.

Fig. 23.8 Longitudinal coronal scan of a normal fetal spine, 20 weeks. The acoustic shadow from the iliac wing near the transducer mimics spina bifida in the underlying spinal segment (arrow). The "pseudodefect" equals the exact width of the acoustic shadow.

Fig. 23.9 Transverse scan of spina bifida, 25 weeks. Note the V-shaped posterior opening in the spinal canal (arrow).

Fig. 23.10 Transverse scan of spina bifida, 25 weeks. This case shows a more U-shaped posterior opening (arrow).

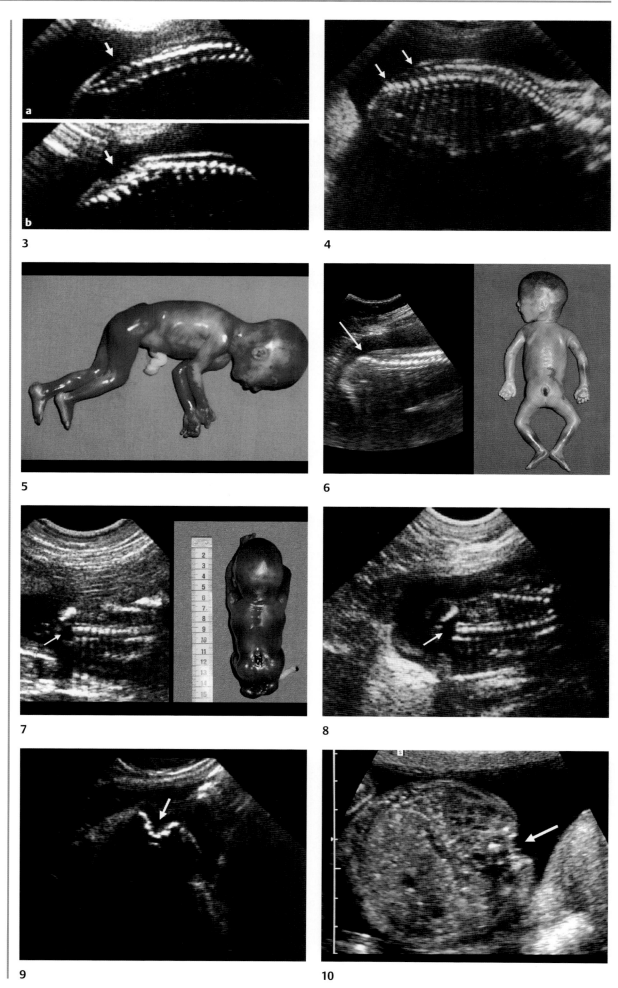

3

4

5

6

7

8

9

10

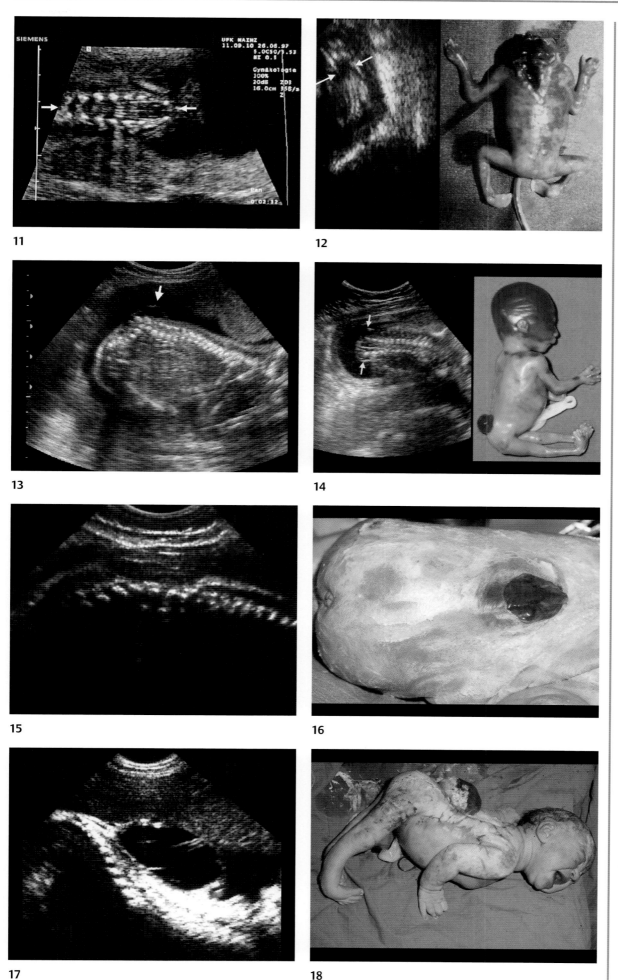

11

12

13

14

15

16

17

18

Rachischisis

Fig. 23.**11** Complete rachischisis, 25 weeks. A fusiform defect extends the full length of spinal canal (arrows), which is open posteriorly. Longitudinal coronal scan in a breech-presenting fetus (2nd position).

Fig. 23.**12** Left: craniorachischisis in an anencephalic fetus, 13 weeks. Longitudinal coronal scan through the spinal column shows a triangular defect at the craniocervical junction. Right: postmortem appearance.

Spina bifida cystica

Fig. 23.**13** Small meningocele in the lumbar area (arrow) with concomitant angulation of the spine, 23 weeks. The sac itself appears echo-free.

Fig. 23.**14** Small myelomeningocele in the lumbosacral area (arrows). Vertex presentation with the spine to the right, 21 weeks. The photograph at right shows the protruding sac along with an extension contracture of the legs and clubbed feet.

Fig. 23.**15** Thoracic spina bifida with a flat myelomeningocele. Vertex presentation, 36 weeks. The defect appears as a concave depression in the longitudinal sagittal scan. When the sac is flat as in this case, ultrasound cannot distinguish between a myelocele and myelomeningocele.

Fig. 23.**16** Postpartum view of the fetus in Fig. 23.**15**.

Fig. 23.**17** Large lumbar myelomeningocele, 37 weeks. Nerve fibers running peripherally from the spinal canal can be seen within the sac. Longitudinal sagittal scan, vertex presentation.

Fig. 23.**18** Postpartum view of the fetus in Fig. 23.**17**.

Fig. 23.**19** Transverse scan of a large, skin-covered myelomeningocele (7.6 x 5.0 x 8.1 cm). Fetus is in a vertex presentation with the spine to the right. Several nerve fibers runs from the open spinal canal to the periphery of the cystic sac.

Fig. 23.**20** Postpartum view of the fetus in Fig. 23.**19** (cesarean delivery).

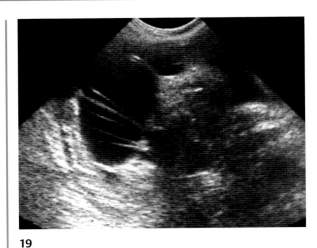
19

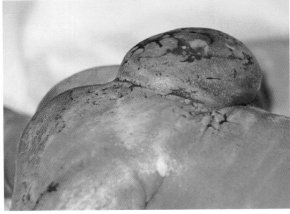
20

Fig. 23.**21** Left: Arnold–Chiari malformation (19 weeks) with a myelomeningocele at the thoracolumbar junction (single arrow on the right) and concomitant displacement of the cerebellum into the cervical canal (2 arrows on the left). Right: post-mortem view.

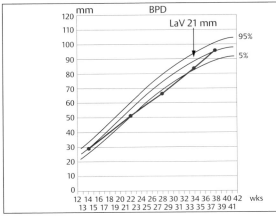
21

Fig. 23.**22** Head and trunk growth in a vertex-presenting fetus with spina bifida. While the abdominal transverse diameter (ATD) stays within normal limits, the biparietal diameter (BPD) falls below the 5th percentile starting at 22 weeks ("pseudomicrocephaly"). The growth of the head "rebounds" some weeks later (arrow) due to the development of hydrocephalus (lateral ventricle (LaV) = 2.1 cm), causing the BPD to return to the normal range. Differentiation from lipoma

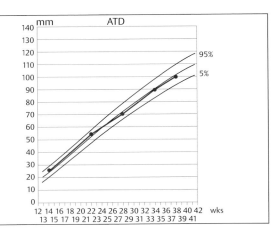
22

Fig. 23.**23** Hypoechoic, cystic-appearing mass at the cervicothoracic junction (3.8 x 1.5 x 3.4 cm) with no apparent defect in the spinal column. Breech presentation, 36 weeks. Histopathology: lipoma.

Fig. 23.**24** Postpartum view of the fetus in Fig. 23.**23**. The lipoma is well covered by skin, and the infant itself displays normal motor function.

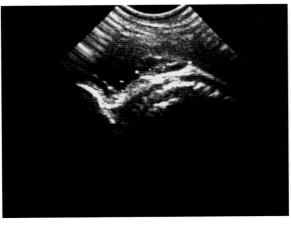
23

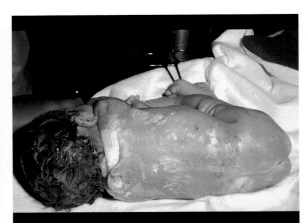
24

24 Thoracic Anomalies

Pulmonary Hypoplasia

Definition. Deficient lung development with a reduction in lung size due to a decreased size and number of acini.

Incidence. 1.4% of all live births (38).

Etiology and pathogenesis. Normal lung development depends on various factors, including an adequate intrathoracic space, normal fetal breathing movements, sufficient pressure in the trachea, and a normal fluid balance (54). The lung fluid is of key importance in this regard. Animal studies have shown that the continuous removal of this fluid leads to pulmonary hypoplasia (4).

Various factors can lead to pulmonary hypoplasia: prolonged rupture of the membranes, skeletal dysplasias with a narrow thorax, renal anomalies with pronounced oligohydramnios, diaphragmatic hernia, and severe hydrothorax (16, 50, 53, 55, 61, 80) (Table 24.1).

Embryology. Impairment of lung development usually occurs after 16 weeks' gestation, at a stage when development of the bronchial tree is nearly complete. If the disturbance occurs before 16 weeks, bronchial malformations are also observed.

Pathoanatomic features. The pathoanatomic diagnosis is based on a low ratio of lung weight to body weight and on the detection of a low radial alveolar count (RAC) (6).

Ultrasound features. Pronounced pulmonary hypoplasia in the setting of a skeletal dysplasia is easily recognized on ultrasonograms by the narrow, often bell-shaped fetal chest (Fig. 24.1). In less pronounced cases, both thoracic and pulmonary measurements may have to be obtained for the intrauterine diagnosis of pulmonary hypoplasia (24, 36, 50, 54, 55, 61, 63, 72, 80) (Fig. 24.2). These measurements should be taken on a consistent, well-defined plane (see Chapter 12) (49) to avoid the large variations that would otherwise occur between measurements.

Oblique lung diameter. In a prospective study of 32 fetuses with pulmonary hypoplasia, Merz et al. (50) found that the oblique lung diameter (LD) was the most effective diagnostic criterion, regardless of the underlying disorder. The lung diameter was below the 5th percentile in all 32 cases (=100%) (Fig. 24.3).

Table 24.1 Possible causes of pulmonary hypoplasia

Pronounced oligohydramnios	➢ Renal anomaly (Potter sequence, bilateral cystic renal malformation) ➢ Prolonged rupture of the membranes (> 8 weeks)
Narrow thorax	➢ Skeletal dysplasias
Intrathoracic mass	➢ Hydrothorax, chylothorax ➢ Diaphragmatic hernia ➢ Cystic adenomatoid lung malformation ➢ Cardiomegaly
Syndromes	➢ Pena–Shokeir syndrome
Chromosomal abnormalities	➢ Trisomy 13, 18, 21

Thoracic measurements. Pulmonary hypoplasia could be diagnosed in just 53.1% of cases using the thoracic transverse diameter (TTD < 5%) at the level of the cardiac valve plane (50). It could be diagnosed in 46.8% of cases using the thoracic sagittal diameter (TSD < 5%) and 78.1% of cases using the ratio of lung diameter to thoracic circumference (LD : TC) (< 5%). Perhaps the use of three-dimensional ultrasound to measure lung volumes (41, 59) will increase the level of diagnostic confidence.

Associated anomalies. Because pulmonary hypoplasia usually occurs in the setting of an underlying disorder (Table 24.1), it should prompt a careful search for additional anomalies that occur in association with those disorders.

Prognosis. The mortality rate associated with the detection of pulmonary hypoplasia is very high (80–100%), regardless of the underlying fetal disorder (50, 55, 75). With borderline lung dimensions in the range of the 5th percentile, the prognosis depends critically on the underlying disorder.

Prenatal management. When fetal pulmonary hypoplasia is diagnosed, further management depends mainly on the nature of the underlying disorder and on gestational age. If a large pleural effusion is present, it may be drained in an effort to forestall the development of pulmonary hypoplasia (64). In cases with pronounced oligohydramnios, serial amnioinfusions may be tried as a preventive measure. A chromosomal abnormality should be excluded first, however.

Hydrothorax, Chylothorax

Definition. Unilateral or bilateral effusions within the pleural cavity.

Incidence. The estimated incidence of chylothorax is one in 10,000 births (35).

Etiology and pathogenesis.

Hydrothorax. Hydrothorax may be an isolated condition, or it may occur in association with infections, immune or nonimmune fetal hydrops, fetal heart failure due to tachyarrhythmia, or in the setting of chromosomal abnormalities (XO, trisomy 21). It is usually bilateral.

Chylothorax. Chylothorax may be caused by a malformation of the thoracic duct or an obstruction of lymphatic pathways. Most cases are unilateral and usually affect the right side. Bilateral chylothorax has also been described (20).

Ultrasound features. Fluid collections in the chest are easily detected with ultrasound (40, 43, 47, 62). An incipient fluid collection in the pleural fissures appears as a crescent-shaped hypoechoic area between the lung and bony thorax (Fig. 24.4). As the hydro-/chylothorax increases, the pleural cavity increasingly fills with a hypoechoic fluid (Figs. 24.5–24.7, 24.13), causing marked compression of the lung tissue. Large, unilateral fluid collections cause a mediastinal shift and cardiac compression.

Differential diagnosis, further tests. Hydrothorax and chylothorax are not distinguished prenatally by their color. Needle aspiration in both conditions yields a clear, yellowish fluid. Hydrothorax and chylothorax are distinguished by determining the lymphocyte content of the aspirated fluid, as the fluid in chylothorax contains abundant lymphocytes. Chylomicrons are not detected in chylothorax until the newborn infant has begun to feed. Fluid aspirated at that time will show a typical milky turbidity.

Associated anomalies. Congenital chylothorax may occur in association with a chromosomal abnormality (trisomy 21) (79, 84) as well as anomalies of the blood vessels or lymphatics (67, 83). It is usually associated with polyhydramnios (40).

Prognosis. In cases that have an early onset and a pronounced intrathoracic fluid collection with a prolonged elevation of the intrathoracic pressure, pulmonary hypoplasia may develop (16, 50). If the fetus has a disorder that can be treated prenatally (e.g., tachyarrhythmia), the hydrothorax may resolve completely after the underlying disorder has been corrected. The spontaneous remission of pleural effusion has also been described in isolated cases (42).

Prenatal management. The detection of a pleural effusion always warrants further tests, including the diagnosis or exclusion of infection. The fetal karyotype should also be determined in cases where viability has not been reached.

Thoracocentesis just before delivery. Fluid collections in the thoracic cavity usually lead to acute respiratory distress in the neonate, depending on their location and extent. In the past, this often led to neonatal deaths resulting from deficient aeration of the lungs. This can be prevented by passing a needle into both pleural cavities under ultrasound guidance just before the infant is delivered (by cesarean section) and aspirating the fluid (34, 57). This will permit effective lung aeration in the newborn infant.

Thoracoamniotic shunt. To prevent the development of pulmonary hypoplasia caused by an extensive, early effusion, Rodeck et al. (64) recommended the intrauterine placement of a thoracoamniotic shunt. A single, early drainage of the pleural effusion is unlikely to be of benefit, as the fluid reaccumulates within a short time. Serial aspirations are a more promising alternative.

Due to the necessity of fetal therapy and the potential for neonatal complications, the infant should be delivered at a perinatal center.

Congenital Cystic Adenomatoid Lung Malformation

Definition. Congenital cystic adenomatoid malformation (CCAM) is a unilateral, hamartomatous dysplasia of the lung.

Incidence. Rare.

Pathoanatomic features. CCAM is characterized histologically by an overgrowth of ductule- and bronchiolus-like structures (71). Stocker (73) described three pathologic types:
- Type I with cysts > 2 cm in diameter
- Type II with cysts < 1 cm in diameter
- A predominantly solid type with microcysts (Type III) (Fig. 24.**8**)

Ultrasound features. Consistent with the pathoanatomic changes, ultrasound may demonstrate the macrocystic type I malformation (Fig. 24.**9**), the microcystic type II (Figs. 24.**10** and 24.**11**), or the predominantly solid type III (Fig. 24.**12**) (18, 21, 29, 37, 44, 46, 52, 58).

The affected lung is markedly enlarged in all three types, causing a mediastinal shift to the opposite side. Normal lung areas are compressed, promoting the development of pulmonary hypoplasia. Compression of the heart and inferior vena cava can compromise venous return, leading to the development of fetal hydrops.

Differential diagnosis. Isolated bronchogenic cyst, pulmonary sequestration (Fig. 24.**13**).

Associated anomalies. Possible associated abnormalities include fetal hydrops, cardiac and skeletal malformations, Potter syndrome, and gastrointestinal atresias. These anomalies occur predominantly in type II CCAM and are less common in type I. Associated anomalies are consistently absent in type III (56, 81).

Polyhydramnios. Hypersecretion by the affected lung and hyporesorption by the hypoplastic lung, along with compression of the esophagus, may account for the polyhydramnios that is often found in CCAM (81). Reports on the frequency of polyhydramnios range from 30% (51) to 80% (56) of cases.

Prognosis. The prognosis depends on the histologic type.

Type I. This is the most common form of CCAM and has the best prognosis of the three types, with a survival rate of 69% (73).

Type II and type III. Both of these types have a poor prognosis. Stocker (73) reported a mortality rate of 100% for both types. The deaths in type II cases were due mainly to severe accompanying anomalies (56).

Other factors. The prognosis is also influenced by the development of fetal hydrops, the severity of pulmonary hypoplasia on the opposite side, and the timing of diagnosis and early surgical intervention (2, 23).

Prenatal management. When an extensive type II or type III malformation is detected before viability is reached, pregnancy termination should be considered because of the poor prognosis (pulmonary and cardiac insufficiency in the newborn). If the anomaly is detected later and if the findings are type I, the patient should be referred to a perinatal center for scheduling the delivery and providing optimum neonatal care.

Bronchogenic Cysts

Definition. Bronchogenic cysts are isolated cysts occurring within the thorax.

Incidence. Rare.

Etiology and pathogenesis. The cysts are believed to result from faulty arborization of the bronchial tree.

Pathoanatomic features. The cysts, lined with bronchial epithelium, are of variable size and can occur at various sites. They are filled with fluid and may be aerated after birth if they communicate with the bronchial system (39).

Ultrasound features. A bronchogenic cyst appears sonographically (5, 46, 69) as an isolated, hypoechoic, smoothly marginated structure in the lung region (Fig. 24.**14**). Bronchogenic cysts usually occur in the area of the mediastinum and are less common within the lung parenchyma (26).

Differential diagnosis. The first condition to be considered in the differential diagnosis (Fig. 24.**13**) is a diaphragmatic hernia, which is characterized by intrathoracic fluid-filled stomach or bowel. Differentiation is also required from CCAM and intrathoracic teratoma.

Associated anomalies. Rare (22). Bronchogenic cysts may coexist with other anomalies that originate from the same embryonic structures, including anomalies of the spinal column, trachea, esophagus, or lung.

Prognosis. When sufficiently large, these cysts can cause a mediastinal shift or obstruction of the bronchial tree.

Prenatal management. Serial examinations are recommended to detect any changes in the size of the cyst. The infant should be delivered in a perinatal center due to the potential need for neonatal surgery.

Pulmonary Sequestration

Definition. Pulmonary sequestration (not to be confused with a sequestrum = a demarcated area of necrotic tissue!) is defined as a congenital developmental anomaly in which a portion of the lung is separated from the bronchial tree in the rest of the lung and receives its blood supply directly from the aorta or its side branches (12). Two types of pulmonary sequestration are distinguished:
- Intralobar
- Extralobar

Incidence. Rare. The extralobar type is three times more common in males than females (15).

Etiology and pathogenesis. Two different theories have been proposed: the traction theory and the excess theory.

Traction theory. This theory postulates an error in the development of the pulmonary artery, with a persistence of anomalous arterial connections that exert downward traction on the area of lung tissue that they supply. This theory is most useful for explaining abdominal pulmonary sequestration.

Excess theory. This theory postulates a hamartomatous surplus of lung tissue. It is mainly supported by the fact that other associated anomalies such as diaphragmatic gaps and hernias, heart defects, etc. are frequently present and that the sequestration is sometimes connected to the stomach or esophagus by a bridge of tissue (12).

Embryology. Pulmonary sequestration is a type of bronchopulmonary foregut malformation, a class of anomalies that originate from the primitive foregut and involve the respiratory and gastrointestinal tract. With an intralobar sequestration, the lung and pulmonary sequestration are surrounded by a common pleura because the accessory lung area formed before the pleura. In the extralobar type, the pulmonary sequestration has its own pleura because the accessory lung area formed after the pleura (13, 66).

Pathoanatomic features. An *intralobar sequestration* is located within an otherwise normal pulmonary lobe. Usually it is drained by a pulmonary vein. An *extralobar sequestration* is separate from the rest of the lung and has its own pleura. It is usually drained by extrapulmonary veins (superior or inferior vena cava, azygos or hemiazygos vein, intercostal veins) (12). The sequestration has a firm, rubbery consistency.

Ultrasound features. An extralobar sequestration appears sonographically as an isolated, echogenic, intrathoracic structure (Figs. 24.**13**, 24.**15**) (37, 45, 46, 65, 76). Color Doppler can demonstrate the separate vascular supply of the sequestration.

Differential diagnosis. CCAM, renal tumor, neuronal tumor, pulmonary hamartoma (46).

Associated anomalies. Associated anomalies may involve organs that are also derived from the foregut: tracheo-esophageal fistula, esophageal diverticulum, esophageal cyst, bronchogenic cyst. Other possible anomalies include diaphragmatic hernia, skeletal dysplasias, heart defects, renal anomalies, hydrocephalus, and nonimmune fetal hydrops (68, 74, 76).

Prognosis. The prognosis is uncertain. It depends on the extent of the sequestration and any accompanying anomalies. Associated anomalies suggest an unfavorable prognosis and high mortality rate (68).

Prenatal management. The delivery (vaginal) should take place in a perinatal center with facilities for neonatal intensive care. After birth, treatment consists of operative removal of the sequestered lung area.

Diaphragmatic Hernia

Definition. Unilateral or bilateral diaphragmatic defect allowing abdominal viscera to herniate into the chest.

Incidence. Relatively common: one in 2500 live births (7).

Etiology and pathogenesis. Deficient closure of the pleuroperitoneal duct.

Pathoanatomic features. The hernia is posterolateral in 90% of cases (30). Abdominal organs herniate into the chest cavity through the diaphragmatic defect, which is usually large and occurs on the left side in 75% of cases (17). The herniated abdominal contents displace and compress the thoracic organs (Fig. 24.**13**).

Ultrasound features. Prenatal ultrasound diagnosis (9, 48) is based on the detection of fluid-filled stomach or bowel within the thoracic cavity (Figs. 24.**16**–24.**19**). A longitudinal scan of the dorsoposterior fetus may show a defect in the diaphragmatic contour in proximity to the spine (Fig. 24.**16**). With a large, left-sided diaphragmatic defect allowing a portion of the liver to herniate into the chest, a transverse scan through the thorax may show displacement of the heart toward the right side (Fig. 24.**17**) (48). With a right-sided defect (Fig. 24.**19**), the right lobe of the liver usually herniates into the chest cavity, displacing the heart toward the left side.

Associated anomalies. Congenital diaphragmatic hernia may be isolated or may coexist with other defects such as hydrocephalus, spina bifida, meningocele, heart defects, omphalocele, or a renal anomaly (9, 82). Chromosomal defects, mainly trisomy 18, are found in 18% of cases. The prevalence of chromosomal abnormalities is just 2% with an isolated diaphragmatic hernia but rises to 34% when additional anomalies are present (70). Polyhydramnios is also observed in some cases (33, 48).

Prognosis. The prognosis of a diaphragmatic hernia depends on the size of the defect, the presence of accompanying anomalies, and early prenatal diagnosis.

Heart failure. A prolonged elevation of the intrathoracic pressure with compression of the heart and lung can lead to cardiac failure with the development of ascites (37) and to severe pulmonary hypoplasia (60). The latter is responsible for respiratory insufficiency and death in newborns. The mortality rates reported in the literature mostly range from 60% to 80% (1, 3, 10, 19, 77). In a prospective study published by Harrison et al. (31), the mortality rate of isolated diaphragmatic hernias that had been diagnosed before 24 weeks and subsequently referred for optimum interdisciplinary management was 58%. When associated anomalies such as pulmonary hypoplasia are also detected prenatally, the mortality rate rises to 100% (8).

Sequelae. Infants who survive have a high incidence of gastroesophageal reflux, swallowing difficulties, and bronchopulmonary dysplasia (11).

Diaphragmatic hernia is not associated with an increased risk of recurrence.

Prenatal management. Especially when the condition is detected early, the delivery can take place in a perinatal center and specific preparations made for repair of the defect by a pediatric surgeon.

▬ *Pentalogy of Cantrell*

Definition. The pentalogy of Cantrell is characterized by the following five features:
- Ectopia cordis
- Omphalocele
- Anterior diaphragmatic defect
- Defect in the lower sternum
- Defect in the pericardium (14)

Incidence. Rare.

Pathogenesis and embryology. A defect forms in the anterior thoracic or abdominal wall and in the diaphragm due to faulty development and differentiation of the lateral mesodermal plates between days 14 and 18 of embryonic development.

Pathoanatomic features. The abdominal wall defect is a supraumbilical defect that may present as an omphalocele, gastroschisis, or simple rectus diastasis. Ectopia cordis is accompanied by various heart defects: atrial septal defects, ventricular septal defects, tetralogy of Fallot, and pulmonary stenosis.

Ultrasound features. Besides a prominent omphalocele, ultrasound reveals a dystopic position of the heart. The heart may be partially or completely outside the chest (Figs. 24.**20**, 24.**21**). In one case we were able to detect the anomaly as early as 12 weeks, 5 days with transvaginal ultrasound (Fig. 24.**22**). If the cardiac topography is uncertain, adjunctive studies such as M-mode scanning, color Doppler, or power Doppler can clarify the situation.

Associated anomalies. Spinal deformities, craniofacial anomalies, ascites, and chromosomal abnormalities (trisomy 13, 18, and Turner syndrome) have been reported (25, 78).

Differential diagnosis. Isolated ectopia cordis, amniotic band syndrome.

Prognosis. Pronounced forms have a very poor prognosis (28, 85).

Prenatal management. In pronounced forms and cases diagnosed before viability is reached, pregnancy termination should be considered because of the poor prognosis. Due to the potential for a chromosomal defect, fetal karyotyping is always recommended. In milder cases or cases diagnosed later in the pregnancy, the infant should be delivered in a perinatal center with facilities for pediatric and cardiac surgery.

Pulmonary hypoplasia

Fig. 24.**1**   Fetus with a markedly narrow, bell-shaped thorax and pulmonary hypoplasia (1). Underlying disease: thanatophoric dysplasia, 23 weeks. Note the marked stepoff (arrows) at the junction of the thorax with the abdomen (2).

Fig. 24.**2**   Pulmonary hypoplasia in osteogenesis imperfecta, 29 weeks. Left: thoracic biometry: transverse diameter of the bony thorax (1) is 36 mm, lung diameter (2) is 8 mm. Right: abdominal biometry: abdominal transverse diameter (3) is 57 mm.

Fig. 24.**3**   Bony thoracic circumference (TC) and oblique lung diameter (LD) in 32 fetuses with pulmonary hypoplasia and various underlying disorders.
∗ = Skeletal dysplasia, □ = renal agenesis, ● = diaphragmatic hernia, ◆ = hydrothorax, ▲ = other disorders.

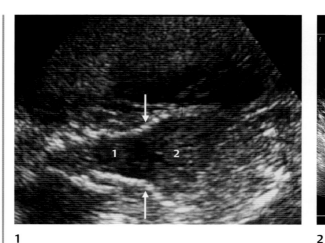

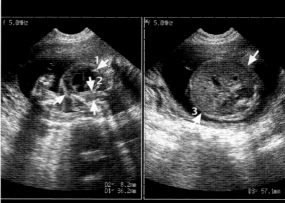

1

2

3

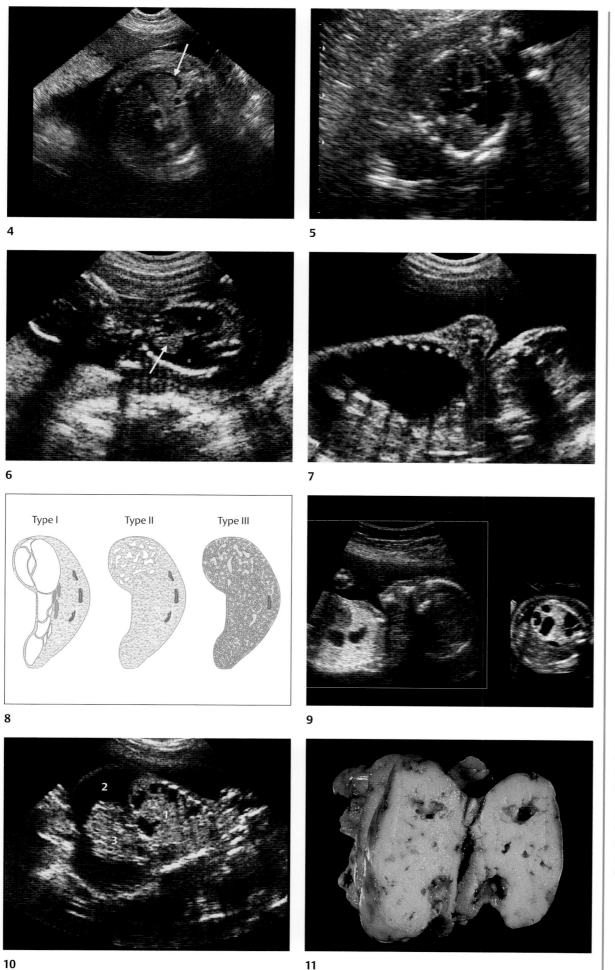

4

5

6

7

8

Type I Type II Type III

9

10

11

Hydrothorax, chylothorax

Fig. 24.**4**   Incipient bilateral hydrothorax, 36 weeks, transverse scan (vertex presentation with the spine to the left). A thin, hypoechoic fluid crescent (arrow) is visible behind the right lung. The opposite side is obscured by shadowing from the spine.

Fig. 24.**5**   Unilateral right-sided chylothorax, 21 weeks, transverse scan (vertex presentation with the spine to the right).

Fig. 24.**6**   Bilateral hydrothorax (∗) in Turner syndrome, 19 weeks, longitudinal scan (breech presentation). The lung appears as a small, triangular, echogenic structure (arrow).

Fig. 24.**7**   Massive chylothorax filling the entire left pleural cavity at 26 weeks, 4 days.

CCAM

Fig. 24.**8**   Classification of congenital cystic adenomatoid lung malformation, after Stocker (73).

Fig. 24.**9**   Type I CCAM, 24 weeks. Left: longitudinal scan in a vertex presentation. Right: transverse scan. On both images, the hyperechoic lung is seen to contain cysts larger than 2 cm.

Fig. 24.**10**   Type II CCAM at 24 weeks, vertex presentation. The lung (1) contains peripheral cysts up to 1 cm in diameter. 2 = Ascites, 3 = bowel.

Fig. 24.**11**   Gross pathology specimen from the fetus in Fig. 24.10 (photo courtesy of Prof. Müntefering, Department of Pediatric Pathology, University of Mainz, Germany).

Fig. 24.**12**　Type III CCAM of the left lung, 21 weeks, vertex presentation. Note the conspicuous hyperechoic structure of the affected lung. Large cysts are absent.

Fig. 24.**13**　Schematic representation of various fetal lung findings. Modified from Hilpert and Pretorius (32).
a　Normal findings.
b　Hydrothorax.

c　CCAM.
d　Extralobar sequestration.
e　Diaphragmatic hernia, displacing the heart (H) toward the right side. The stomach (St) and bowel (B) have herniated into the chest.
f　Bronchogenic cyst (adjacent to the mediastinum).

Bronchogenic cyst, pulmonary sequestration

Fig. 24.**14**　Bronchogenic cyst, 27 weeks. Isolated, solitary intrathoracic cystic mass (observation by Prof. Bernaschek, Vienna).

Fig. 24.**15**　Pulmonary sequestration, 25 weeks. The sequestered lung area (arrows) is more echogenic than the rest of the lung (observation by Prof. Bernaschek, Vienna).

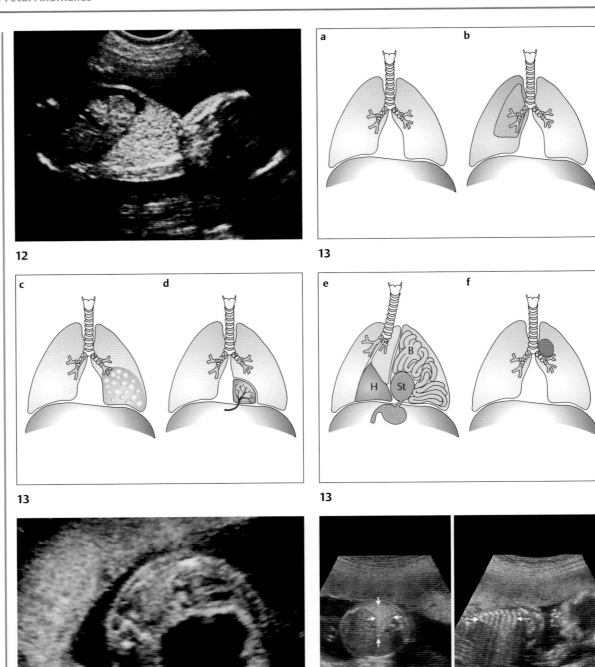

12

13

13

13

14

15

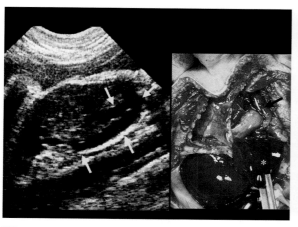

16

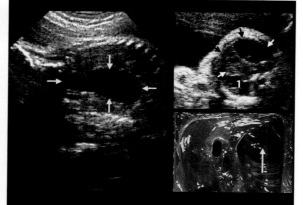

17

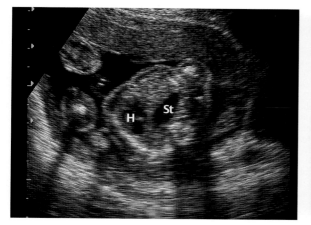

18

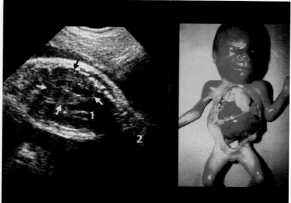

19

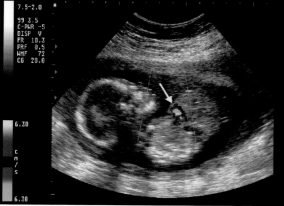

20

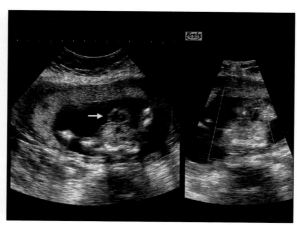

21

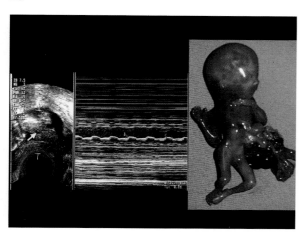

22

Diaphragmatic hernia

Fig. 24.**16**   Left: diaphragmatic hernia, 33 weeks. Longitudinal scan, vertex presentation. Posteriorly, the fluid-filled bowel (arrows) appears as a tubular structure passing from the abdomen into the chest and back again. Right: corresponding pathoanatomic view showing the large, left-sided diaphragmatic defect through which stomach, bowel (arrow), spleen, pancreas, and left hepatic lobe (∗) have herniated into the left chest cavity (photo courtesy of Dr. Röhrig, Department of Pediatric Pathology, University of Mainz, Germany).

Fig. 24.**17**   Large, left-sided diaphragmatic hernia, 32 weeks. The stomach and liver have herniated into the chest cavity (arrows), and the heart (1) is displaced toward the right side (dextrocardia). Breech presentation, 1st position. Left: longitudinal scan. Upper Right: transverse scan. Lower Right: pathoanatomic view showing the large, left-sided diaphragmatic defect (photo courtesy of Prof. Müntefering, Department of Pediatric Pathology, University of Mainz, Germany).

Fig. 24.**18**   Left-sided diaphragmatic hernia with dextrocardia at 23 weeks, 2 days. Transverse scan, breech presentation, 1st position. H = heart, St = stomach.

Fig. 24.**19**   Left: right-sided diaphragmatic hernia, 30 weeks. Longitudinal scan, vertex presentation. To the right of the heart, the right lobe of the liver has herniated into the chest cavity along with a fluid-filled loop of bowel (arrows). 1 = Right hemithorax, 2 = head. Right: corresponding pathoanatomic view showing the large, right-sided diaphragmatic defect (photo courtesy of Prof. Müntefering, Department of Pediatric Pathology, University of Mainz).

Pentalogy of Cantrell

Fig. 24.**20**   Pentalogy of Cantrell with omphalocele and partial ectopia cordis (arrow) at 19 weeks, 3 days. Breech presentation.

Fig. 24.**21**   Left: pentalogy of Cantrell with complete ectopia cordis (arrow), transverse scan. Right: power Doppler image of the heart.

Fig. 24.**22**   Left: pentalogy of Cantrell with omphalocele and partial ectopia cordis (arrow) at 12 weeks, 5 days. Breech presentation, 2nd position. Transvaginal M-mode tracing of the dystopic heart. Right: postmortem view.

References

1. Adzick, N.S., Harrison, M.R., Glick, P.L., Nakayama, D.K., Manning, F.A., Lorimier de, A.: Diaphragmatic hernia in the fetus: prenatal diagnosis and outcome in 94 cases. J. Pediatr. Surg. 20 (1985) 357–361
2. Adzick, N.S., Harrison, M.R., Glick, P.L. et al.: Fetal cystic adenomatoid malformation: prenatal diagnosis and natural history. J. Pediatr. Surg. 20 (1985) 483–488
3. Adzick, N.S., Vacanti, J.P., Lillehei, C.W., O'Rourke, P.P., Crone, R.K., Wilson, J.M.: Fetal diaphragmatic hernia: ultrasound diagnosis and clinical outcome in 38 cases. J. Pediatr. Surg. 24 (1989) 654–658
4. Alcorn, D., Adamson, T.M., Lambert, T.F., Maloney, J.E., Ritchie, B.C., Robinson, P.M.: Effects of chronic tracheal ligation and drainage in the fetal lamb. J. Anat. 123 (1977) 649–660
5. Asher, J.B., Sabbagha, R.E., Tamura, R.K., Luck, S., Gerbie, A.B.: Fetal pulmonary cyst: Intrauterine diagnosis and management. Amer. J. Obstet. Gynec. 151 (1985) 97–98
6. Askenazi, S.S., Pearlman, M.: Pulmonary hypoplasia: lung weight and radial alveolar count as criteria of diagnosis. Arch. Dis. Child. 54 (1979) 614–618
7. Askin, F.B.: Diaphragm-congenital anomalies. In: Kissane, J.M.: Pathology of Infancy and Childhood. St. Louis: Mosby 1975; p. 560
8. Bahlmann, F., Merz, E., Hallermann, C., Stopfkuchen, H., Krämer, W., Hofmann, M.: Congenital diagphragmatic hernia: ultrasonic measurement of fetal lungs to predict pulmonary hypoplasia. Ultrasound Obstet. Gynecol. 14 (1999) 1–7
9. Bell, M.J., Ternberg, J.L.: Antenatal diagnosis of diaphragmatic hernia. Pediatrics 60 (1977) 738–740
10. Benacerraf, B.R., Adzick, N.S.: Fetal diaphragmatic hernia: ultrasound diagnosis and clinical outcome in 19 cases. Amer. J. Obstet. Gynecol. 156 (1987) 573–576
11. Bernbaum, J., Schwartz, I., Gerdes, M., D'Agostini, J., Coburn, C., Polin, R.: Survivors of extracorporal membrane oxygenation at 1 year of age: the relationship of primary diagnosis with health and neurodevelopmental sequelae. Pediatrics 96 (1995) 907–913
12. Böhm, N.: Kinderpathologie. Stuttgart: Schattauer 1984
13. Boiskin, I., Brunner, J.S., Jeanty, P.: Extralobar intrathoracic sequestration of the lung. Fetus 2 (1991) 74–85
14. Cantrell, J.R., Haller, J.A., Ravitch, M.M.: A syndrome of congenital defects involving the abdominal wall, sternum, diaphragm, pericardium and heart. Surg. Gynecol. Obstet. 107 (1958) 602–614
15. Carter, R.: Pulmonary sequestration. Ann. Thorac. Surg. 7 (1969) 68–88
16. Castillo, R.A., Devoe, L.D., Falls, G., Holzmann, G.B., Hadi, H.A., Fadel, H.E.: Pleural effusions and pulmonary hypoplasia. Amer. J. Obstet. Gynecol. 1547 (1987) 1252–1255
17. David, T.J., Illingworth, C.A.: Diaphragmatic hernia in the southwest of England. J. Med. Genet. 13 (1976) 253–262
18. Diwan, R.V., Brennan, J.N., Philipson, E.H., Jain, S., Bellon, E.M.: Ultrasonic prenatal diagnosis of type III congenital cystic adenomatoid malformation of lung. J. clin. Ultrasound 11 (1983) 218–221
19. Dommergues, M., Louis-Sylvestre, C., Mandelbrot, L. et al.: Congenital diaphragmatic hernia: can prenatal ultrasonography predict outcome? Amer. J. Obstet. Gynecol. 74 (1996) 1377–1381
20. Doolittle, W.M., Ohmart, D., Egan, E.A.: Congenital bilateral pleural effusions: A cause for respiratory failure in the newborn. Amer. J. Dis. Child. 125 (1973) 435–437
21. Dumez, Y., Mandelbrot, L., Radunovic, N. et al.: Prenatal management of congenital cystic adenomatoid malformation of the lung. J. Pediatr. Surg. 28 (1993) 36–41
22. DuMontier, C., Graviss, E.R., Silberstein, M.J., McAlister, W.H.: Bronchogenic cysts in children. Clin. Radiol. 36 (1985) 431–436
23. Fine, C., Adzick, N.S, Doubilet, P.M.: Decreasing size of a congenital cystic adenomatoid malformation in utero. J. Ultrasound Med. 7 (1988) 405–408
24. Fong, K., Ohlsson, A., Zalev, A.: Fetal thoracic circumference: A prospective cross-sectional study with real-time ultrasound. Amer. J. Obstet. Gynecol. 158 (1988) 1154–1160
25. Fox, J.E., Gloster, E.S., Mirchandani, R.: Trisomy 18 with Cantrell pentalogy in a stillborn infant. Amer. J. Med. Genet. 31 (1988) 391–394
26. Fraser, R.G., Pare, J.A.P.: Pulmonary abnormalities of developmental origin. In: Pare, P.D., Fraser, R.S., Bernereux, G.P. (eds): Diagnosis of Diseases of the Chest. 3rd ed. Philadelphia: Saunders 1989; pp. 695–773
27. Geary, M.P., Chitty, L.S., Morrison, J.J., Wright, V., Pierro, A., Rodeck, C.H.: Perinatal outcome and prognostic factors in prenatally diagnosed congenital diaphragmatic hernia. Ultrasound Obstet. Gynecol. 12 (1998) 107–111
28. Ghidini, A., Sirtori, M., Romero, R., Hobbins, J.C.: Prenatal diagnosis of pentalogy of Cantrell. J. Ultrasound Med. 7 (1988) 567–572
29. Glaves, J., Baker, J.L.: Spontaneous resolution of maternal hydramnios in congenital cystic adenomatoid malformation of the lung. Antenatal ultrasound features. Case report. Brit. J. Obstet. Gynaecol. 90 (1983) 1065–1068
30. Gross, R.E.: The Surgery of Infancy and Childhood. Philadelphia: Saunders 1953; p. 428
31. Harrison, M.R., Adzick, N.S., Estes, J.M., Howell, L.J.: A prospective study of the outcome for fetuses with diaphragmatic hernia. J. Amer. Med. Assoc. 271 (1994) 82–84
32. Hilpert, P.L., Pretorius, D.: The Thorax. In: Nyberg, D.A, Mahony, B.S., Pretorius, D.H. (eds.): Diagnostic Ultrasound of Fetal Anomalies. St. Louis: Mosby Year-Book 1990; pp. 262–299
33. Hobbins, J.C., Grannum, P.A.T., Berkowitz, R.L., Silverman, R., Mahoney, M.J.: Ultrasound in the diagnosis of congenital anomalies. Amer. J. Obstet. Gynec. 134 (1979) 331–345
34. Holländer, H.J.: Die Ultraschalldiagnostik in der Schwangerschaft. München: Urban & Schwarzenberg 1984; S. 149
35. John, E.: Pleural effusion in the newborn. Med. J. Aust. 1 (1974) 102–103
36. Johnson, A., Callan, N.A., Bhutani, V.K., Colmorgen, G.H., Weiner, S., Bolognese, R.J.: Ultrasonic ratio of fetal thoracic to abdominal circumference: an association with fetal pulmonary hypoplasia. Amer. J. Obstet. Gynecol. 157 (1987) 764–769
37. Knochel, J.Q., Lee, T.G., Melendez, M.G., Henderson, S.C.: Fetal anomalies involving the thorax and abdomen. Radiol. Clin. N. Amer. 20 (1982) 297–310
38. Knox, W.F., Barson, A.J.: Pulmonary hypoplasia in a regional perinatal unit. Early Hum. Dev. 14 (1986) 1433–1442
39. Landing, B.H.: Anomalies of the respiratory tract. In: Nelson, E.D. (ed.): Pediatrics clinics of North America, Symposium on respiratory disorders. Philadelphia: Saunders 1957; pp. 73–102
40. Lange, I.R., Manning, F.A.: Antenatal diagnosis of congenital pleural effusions. Amer. J. Obstet. Gynec. 140 (1981) 839–840
41. Lee, A., Kratochwil, A., Stümpflen, I., Deutinger, J., Bernaschek, G.: Fetal lung volume determination by three-dimensional ultrasonography. Amer. J. Obstet. Gynecol. 175 (1996) 588–592
42. Lien, J.M., Colmorgen, G.H., Gebret, J.F., Evantash, A.B.: Spontaneous resolution of fetal pleural effusion diagnosed during the second trimester. JCU 18 (1990) 54–56
43. Linder, R., Grumbrecht, C., Stosiek, U., Maier, W.A., Wolkewitz, W.U.: Behandlung des pränatal diagnostizierten fetalen Chylothorax. Geburtsh. u. Frauenheilk. 42 (1982) 720–722
44. Macchiella, D., Merz, E.: Pränatale Diagnose der adenomatoiden Lungendysplasie Typ II. Geburtsh. u. Frauenheilk. 50 (1990) 495–498
45. Mariona, F., McAlpin, G., Zador, I., Phillipart, A., Jafri, S.Z.: Sonographic detection of fetal extrathoracic pulmonary sequestration. J. Clin. Ultrasound 5 (1986) 283–285
46. Mayden, K.L., Tortora, M., Chervenak, F.A., Hobbins, J.C.: The antenatal sonographic detection of lung masses. Amer. J. Obstet. Gyn. 148 (1984) 349–351
47. Meizner, I., Carmi, R., Bar-Ziv, J.: Congenital chylothorax – Prenatal ultrasonic diagnosis and successful post partum management. Prenat. Diagn. 6 (1986) 217–221
48. Merz, E., Goldhofer, W., Friese, K., Rörig, R.: Intrauteriner Nachweis der dorsolateralen Zwerchfellhernie mittels Ultraschall. Geburtsh. u. Frauenheilk. 47 (1987) 54–56
49. Merz, E., Wellek, S., Bahlmann, F., Weber, G.: Sonographische Normkurven des fetalen knöchernen Thorax und der fetalen Lunge. Geburtsh. u. Frauenheilk. 55 (1995) 77–82
50. Merz, E., Miric-Tesanic, D., Bahlmann, F., Weber, G., Hallermann, C.: Prenatal sonographic chest and lung measurements for predicting severe pulmonary hypoplasia. Prenat. Diagn. 19 (1999) 614–619
51. Miller, H.K., Sieber, W.K., Yunis, E.J.: Congenital adenomatoid malformation of the lung. Pathol. Annual Part 1, 15 (1980) 387–402
52. Morcos, S.F., Lobb, M.O.: The antenatal diagnosis by ultrasonography of type III congenital cystic adenomatoid malformation of the lung. Case report. Brit. J. Obstet. Gynaecol. 93 (1986) 1002–1005
53. Nicolini, U., Fisk, N.M., Rodeck, C.H., Talbert, D.G., Wigglesworth, J.S.: Low amniotic pressure in oligohydramnios – is this the cause of pulmonary hypoplasia? Amer. J. Obstet. Gynecol. 161 (1989) 1098–1101
54. Nimrod, C., Davies, D., Iwanicki, S., Harder, J., Persaud, D., Nicholson, S.: Ultrasound prediction of pulmonary hypoplasia. Obstet. Gynecol. 68 (1986) 495–498
55. Nimrod, C., Nicholson, S., Davies, D., Harder, J., Dodd, G., Sauve, R.: Pulmonary hypoplasia testing in clinical obstetrics. Amer. J. Obstet. Gynecol. 158 (1988) 277–280
56. Östör, A.G., Fortune, D.W.: Congenital cystic adenomatoid malformation of lung. Amer. J. clin. Path. 70 (1978) 595–604
57. Petres, R.E., Redwine, J.P., Cruikshank, J.P.: Congenital bilateral chylothorax. J. Amer. med. Ass. 248 (1982) 1360–1361
58. Pezzuti, R.T., Isler, R.J.: Antenatal ultrasound detection of cystic adenomatoid malformation of lung: Report of a case and review of the recent literature. J. clin. Ultrasound 11 (1983) 342–346
59. Pöhls, U.G., Rempen, A.: Fetal lung volumentry by three-dimensional ultrasound. Ultrasound Obstet. Gynecol. 11 (1998) 6–12
60. Potter, E.L.: Diaphragmatic and abdominal hernias: In: Pathology of the Fetus and Infant: Year Book Medical Publishers, Chicago 1962; p. 370
61. Quinlan, R.W., Cruz, A.C., Huddleston, J.F.: Sonographic detection of fetal urinary tract anomalies. Obstet. Gynecol. 67 (1986) 558–565
62. Rempen, A., Dame, W., Jorch, G., Pfefferkorn, J.: Pränatale Diagnostik und Therapie des Hydro-/Chylothorax mit Hydrops fetalis. Z. Geburtsh. u. Perinat. 188 (1984) 90–93
63. Roberts, A.B., Mitchell, J.M.: Direct ultrasonographic measurements of fetal lung length in normal pregnancies and pregnancies complicated by prolonged rupture of membranes. Amer. J. Obstet Gynecol. 163 (1990) 1560–1566
64. Rodeck, C.H., Fisk, N.M., Fraser, D.I., Nicolini, U.: Long-term in utero drainage of fetal hydrothorax. New Engl. J. Med. 319 (1988) 1135–1138
65. Romero, R., Chervenak, F.A., Kotzen, J., Berkowitz, R.L., Hobbins, J.C.: Antenatal sonographic findings of extralobular pulmonary sequestration. J. Ultrasound Med. 1 (1982) 131–132
66. Sade, R.M., Clouse, M., Ellis, F.H.jr.: The spectrum of pulmonary sequestration. Ann. Thorac. Surg. 18 (1974) 644–658
67. Samuel, N., Sirotta, L., Bar-Ziv, J., Dicker, D., Feldberg, D., Goldman, J.A.: The ultrasonic appearance of common pulmonary vein atresia in utero. J. Ultrasound Med. 7 (1988) 25–28
68. Savic, B., Birtel, F.J., Tholen, W., Funke, H.D., Knoche, R.: Lung sequestration: report of seven cases and review of 540 published cases. Thorax 34 (1979) 96–101
69. Schramm, T., Brusis, E.: Ultrasonographische Diagnostik einer fetalen Lungenzyste. Geburtsh. u. Frauenheilk. 46 (1986) 118–120
70. Snijders, R.J.M., Farrias, M., von Kaisenberg, C., Nicolaides, K.H.: Fetal abnormalities. In: Snijders, R.J.M., Nicolaides, K.H. (eds.): Ultrasound markers for fetal chromosomal defects. New York: Parthenon Publ. 1996; pp. 1–62
71. Spencer, H.: Pathology of the lungs. Oxford: Pergamon 1977; 976 ff
72. Songster, G.S., Gray, D.L., Crane, J.P.: Prenatal prediction of lethal pulmonary hypoplasia using ultrasonic fetal chest circumference. Obstet. Gynecol. 73 (1989) 261–266
73. Stocker, J.T., Madewell, J.E., Drake, R.M.: Congenital cystic adenomatoid malformation of the lung. Classification and morphologic spectrum. Hum. Path. 8 (1977) 155–171
74. Stocker, J.T., Kagan-Hallet, K.: Extralobular pulmonary sequestration. Analysis of 15 cases. Amer. J. Clin. Pathol. 72 (1979) 917–925
75. Swischuk, L.E., Richardson, C.J., Nichols, M.M., Ingman, M.J.: Primary pulmonary hypoplasia in the neonate. J. Pediatr. 95 (1979) 573–577

76. Thomas, C.S., Leopold, G.R., Hilton, S., Key, T., Coen, R., Lynch, F.: Fetal hydrops associated with extralobular pulmonary sequestration. J. Ultrasound Med. 5 (1986) 668–671
77. Tibboel, D., Bos, A.P., Hazebroeck, W.J., Lachmann, B., Molenaar, J.C.: Changing concepts in the treatment of congenital diaphragmatic hernia. Klin. Paediatr. 205 (1993) 67–70
78. Toyama, W.M.: Combined congential defects of the anterior abdominal wall, sternum diaphragm, pericardium and heart: A case report and review of the syndrome. Pediatrics 50 (1972) 778–792
79. Van Aerde, J., Campbell, A.N., Smyth, J.A., Lloyd, D., Bryan, M.H.: Spontaneous chylothorax in newborns. Amer. J. Dis. Child. 138 (1984) 961–964
80. Vintzileos, A.M., Campbell, W.A., Rodis, J.F., Nochimson, D.J., Pinette, M.G., Petrikovsky, B.M.: Comparison of six different ultrasonographic methods for predicting lethal fetal pulmonary hypoplasia. Amer. J. Obstet. Gynecol. 161 (1989) 606–612
81. Vogel, M.: Mißbildungen und Anomalien der Lunge. In: Doerr, W., Seifert, G., Uehlinger, E. (Hrsg.): Spezielle pathologische Anatomie. Pathologie der Lunge. Bd. 16/1. Berlin: Springer 1970; S. 157
82. Warkany, J.: Congenital diaphragmatic hernias. In: Congenital Malformations. Year Book Medical Publishers, Chicago 1971; S. 751
83. Wilson, R.H.J., Duncan, A., Hume, R., Bain, A.D.: Prenatal pleural effusion associated with congenital pulmonary lymphangiectasia. Prenat. Diagn. 5 (1985) 73–76
84. Yoss, B.S., Lipsitz, P.J.: Chylothorax in two mongoloid infants. Clin. Genet. 12 (1977) 357–360
85. Zachariou, Z., Daum, R., Roth, H., Benz, G.: Cantrell's syndrome. Z. Kinderchir. 42 (1987) 255–259

25 Anomalies and Diseases of the Fetal Heart

Epidemiology and Indications for Fetal Echocardiography

▬ Epidemiologic Aspects

It is generally known that approximately 15–20% of pregnancies in the second trimester end in spontaneous abortion and that some of these pregnancies are associated with anomalies, particularly involving the heart. Thus, the prenatal examiner will encounter a higher rate of heart defects in second-trimester fetuses than in newborns, for which the incidence of heart defects is five in 1000 births (12).

Perinatal mortality. Even with the improved treatment options that are now available, every fifth child with a congenital heart defect dies during the first year of life (Table 25.**5**). The mortality rate correlates closely with the severity of the heart defect and its early clinical manifestations. Approximately 40% of infants who are symptomatic during the first week of life die before one year of age, compared with just 5% of infants who do not become symptomatic until after 12 weeks of life (20). It is reasonable to assume that the first group includes heart defects that can be readily detected by fetal echocardiography. By diagnosing these conditions prenatally, it may be possible to reduce perinatal morbidity and mortality.

▬ Fetal Echocardiography: Who, Whom, When, and How?

Who?

The main question is how to detect fetal heart disease most effectively. In Germany, approximately 800,000 pregnant women undergo ultrasound screening examinations each year. In most cases the obstetrician is still the primary examiner who evaluates the overall anatomy of the fetus, including cardiac anatomy (22). It is only by intensive training that examiner experience can be increased, improving the detection rate of cardiac anomalies in the 20-week screening at a secondary center. In fetal echocardiography, the examiner should work closely with a pediatric cardiologist (21). When a cardiac abnormality is detected, this specialist can be called in to help make a precise diagnosis and assess the prognosis.

Whom?

Low-risk and high-risk groups. It is important in prenatal ultrasound to distinguish between groups that have a low risk or a high risk for congenital heart disease. While the risk of finding a heart defect in the low-risk group is less than 0.5%, it is approximately 10% (!) in the high-risk group. For this reason, cases that are at high risk for congenital heart disease should be referred directly to an examiner who is experienced in fetal echocardiography.

Indications for fetal echocardiography. The indications for fetal echocardiography are listed in Table 25.**2**. Although recurrence in cases with a positive history is rare (caution: hypoplastic left heart!), fetal echocardiography is still of major value in providing reassurance and relieving parental concerns. The cases that offer the highest "yield" of heart defects consist of ultrasound indications such as an abnormal four-chamber view at screening, the presence of extracardiac anomalies, nonimmune fetal hydrops, and AV block (11).

Improved screening. Since congenital heart defects usually have multifactorial causes, the majority are not found in the high-risk group. Consequently, detection rates can be increased only by improving the screening process (22). Recent studies have shown that increased nuchal translucency thickness in early pregnancy not only suggests a chromosomal abnormality but also suggests the presence of a heart

Table 25.1   Abbreviations used in the text, tables, and figures

Ao	=	Aorta
AoV	=	Aortic valve
AS	=	Aortic stenosis
ASD I	=	Atrial septal defect type I = incomplete AV canal
ASD II	=	Atrial septal defect type II
AV block III°	=	Third degree atrioventricular block
AVSD	=	AV canal = atrioventricular canal or septal defect
CCHB	=	Congenital complete heart block (= third degree AV block)
CMP	=	Cardiomyopathy
CoA	=	Coarctation of the aorta
D-TGA	=	Complete transposition of the great arteries
DA	=	Ductus arteriosus
DAP	=	Ductus arteriosus persistens (persistent ductus arteriosus)
DOLV	=	Double-outlet left ventricle
DORV	=	Double-outlet right ventricle
EFE	=	Endocardial fibroelastosis
FO	=	Foramen ovale
Heterotaxia	=	left and right isomerism, polysplenia and asplenia syndrome
HLHS	=	Hypoplastic left heart syndrome
IAS	=	Interatrial septum
IUGR	=	Intrauterine growth retardation
IVS	=	Interventricular septum
L-TGA	=	Corrected transposition of the great arteries
LA	=	Left atrium
LV	=	Left ventricle
LVOT	=	Left ventricular outflow tract
MV	=	Mitral valve
PA/IVS	=	Pulmonary atresia with intact ventricular septum
PAPVR	=	Partial anomalous pulmonary venous return
PLSVC	=	Persistent left superior vena cava
PS	=	Pulmonary stenosis
PSVT	=	Paroxysmal supraventricular tachycardia
PT	=	Pulmonary trunk
PV	=	Pulmonary valve
RA	=	Right atrium
RV	=	Right ventricle
RVOT	=	Right ventricular outflow tract
Sp	=	Spinal column
SVES	=	Supraventricular extrasystole
TA	=	Tricuspid atresia
TAC	=	Truncus arteriosus (communis)
TAPVR	=	Total anomalous pulmonary venous return
TGA	=	Transposition of great arteries
TOF	=	Tetralogy of Fallot
TV	=	Tricuspid valve
VCI	=	Inferior vena cava
VCS	=	Superior vena cava
VSD	=	Ventricular septal defect

defect. According to a 1999 study, this feature has a sensitivity of 60% in the detection of congenital heart defects (26).

When?

The optimum time to perform a screening examination is the period from 20 to 22 weeks. The period of 16–18 weeks was preferred in the past, but recent findings indicate that 20–22 weeks is better because at that time the fetal cardiac structures can be defined more clearly with screening ultrasound in more than 90% of cases (30). A 5.0-MHz transducer should be used for adequate resolution.

How?

Systematic examination. It is important to explore the somewhat difficult path from noting a cardiac abnormality to making a diagnosis. Only by following a systematic approach (see Chapter 11) can the examiner identify specific fetal cardiac structures, describe any abnormalities that are found, and make a presumptive diagnosis. In most cases this can be done without the use of color Doppler. Color imaging can then be used to define the details of the abnormality.

From symptom to diagnosis. This section of the chapter, presented below, covers the most important suggestive signs in the systematic analysis of fetal heart structures. It is intended to help the reader recognize what is normal and formulate a differential diagnosis for any abnormalities that are found.

Specific cardiac anomalies and diseases. In this part of the chapter, specific heart defects are described and placed in diagnostic groups so that when a fetal heart defect is suspected, the examiner can look up the typical B-mode and color Doppler findings and use them in formulating a differential diagnosis. The tables divide the principal heart defects into right-sided (Table 25.**9**) and left-sided defects (Table 25.**10**). Major vascular anomalies, septal defects, malrotation anomalies, and fetal arrhythmias are reviewed in Tables 25.**11**–25.**19**.

Abbreviations. The abbreviations used in the text and tables are explained in Table 25.**1**.

Prognosis of Cardiac Anomalies

Relatively little attention is given to the prognosis of congenital heart defects in this chapter, because every case must be considered individually. The neonatal data available in the literature often indicate much better prognoses than are found in cases that are detected prenatally. This is mainly because there is a tendency to detect more severe anomalies prenatally and because the association with extracardiac anomalies is higher in cases diagnosed prenatally than postnatally (50% versus 28%). Reference data from the Baltimore-Washington Infant Study (20) on survival rates and associations with extracardiac anomalies are presented in Tables 25.**3**–25.**5**.

Table 25.**2** Indications for fetal echocardiography

Positive history
➢ Family history:
• Congenital heart defects
• Other malformations or syndromes commonly associated with heart defects
➢ Exposure to various insults during pregnancy:
• Chemical substances (e.g., antiepileptic drugs, lithium, alcohol)
• Maternal diseases (e.g., diabetes mellitus, phenylketonuria)
• Infections (e.g., rubella, cytomegalovirus, coxsackie)
• High doses of ionizing radiation

Detection of fetal abnormalities
➢ Ultrasound suspicion of a heart defect (e.g., suspicious four-chamber view)
➢ Cardiovascular symptoms:
• Arrhythmias
• Nonimmune hydrops (NIHF)
• Early increase in nuchal translucency thickness or cystic hygroma
➢ Early (before 32 weeks) and/or more symmetrical growth retardation
➢ Anomalies commonly associated with heart defects:
• Abnormal cardiac position
• CNS anomalies (hydrocephalus, microcephalus, agenesis of the corpus callosum, encephalocele)
• Mediastinum (esophageal atresia, diaphragmatic hernia)
• Gastrointestinal tract (duodenal atresia, visceral transposition)
• Abdominal wall (omphalocele, ectopia cordis)
• Kidneys (renal dysplasia)
• Syndromes associated with cardiac defects
• Single umbilical artery
➢ Detected chromosomal abnormality (e.g., Turner syndrome)
➢ Twin pregnancies:
• Monozygotic twins
• Conjoined twins

Invasive test for karyotyping has been omitted due to:
➢ High risk based on advanced maternal age
➢ Suspicious biochemical parameters in maternal blood (AFP, HCG, uE3)
➢ Familial risks

Table 25.**3** Percentage distribution of heart defects in 4390 infants (Baltimore–Washington Infant Study 1981–1989) (adapted from [20])

Diagnostic group	%	Diagnostic group	%
VSD	32.1	CMP	1.9
PS	9.0	PA/IVS	1.7
ASD II	7.7	Peripheral PS	1.5
AVSD	7.4	TAPVD	1.4
TOF	6.8	TAC	1.2
D-TGA	4.7	L-TGA	1.1
CoA	4.6	Ebstein anomaly	1.0
HLHS	3.8	TA	0.7
AS	2.9	Interruption of the aortic arch	0.7
DAP	2.4	Other "left-sided" defects	0.6
Heterotaxia	2.3	Double inlet ventricle	0.4
DORV	2.0	Other "right-sided" defects	0.2
Bicuspid aortic valve	1.9	Cor triatriatum	0.1

From Symptom to Diagnosis

The systematic examiner will conduct a step-by-step analysis of the individual cardiac structures, as described under "Cardiac Examination" in Chapter 11. An accurate diagnosis can be made, however, only if an abnormal finding is correctly interpreted and proper consideration is given to associated findings and differential diagnoses.

Systematic interpretation of abnormal findings. Since this chapter deals with the typical features of specific heart defects, Tables 25.**6**–25.**12** are designed to make it easier to get from an abnormal finding to an initial working diagnosis. Possible abnormalities are presented in the same order that is followed when conducting a systematic examination.

Table 25.**4**   Distribution of the association of noncardiac anomalies by diagnostic groups (Baltimore–Washington Infant Study 1981–1989) (adapted from [20])

Diagnostic group	n	Association with syndromes, major organ anomalies and deformations (%)
L-TGA	47	32
Heterotaxia	99	80
D-TGA	208	11
TAC	51	37
DORV	86	40
TOF	297	35
Double inlet ventricle	18	11
AVSD	326	80
TAPVD	60	23
TA	32	12
PA/IVS	73	10
Cor triatriatum	5	0
HLHS	167	17
Interruption of aortic arch	31	48
Ebstein anomaly	43	23
PS	395	13
AS	128	19
CoA	203	26
Bicuspid aortic valve	84	21
Peripheral PS	65	35
VSD	1411	18
ASD II	340	30
DAP	104	32
CMP	82	37
Other	35	74
All cases	4390	28

Table 25.**5**   Survival rates of congenital heart defects: survivors with and without surgical treatment during the first year of life; n = 4390 infants (Baltimore–Washington Infant Study 1981–1989) (adapted from [20])

Diagnostic group	Survivors with and without surgery (%)
L-TGA	64
Heterotaxia	48
D-TGA	72
TAC	35
DORV	56
TOF	78
Double inlet ventricle	61
AVSD	71
TAPVD	60
TA	69
PA/IVS	57
Cor triatriatum	25
HLHS	15
Interruption of aortic arch	35
Ebstein anomaly	70
PS	98
AS	82
CoA	82
Bicuspid aortic valve	95
Peripheral PS	92
VSD	95
ASD II	94
DAP	94
CMP	77
Other	91
All cases	82

Table 25.**6**   Principal findings in the fetal upper abdomen

Normal	Suspicious
Stomach on left side, filled	➢ Stomach small or not visualized: esophageal atresia, diaphragmatic defect, or stomach on right side ➢ Stomach on right side or centered: rotation anomaly such as isomerism (situs ambiguus) or situs inversus abdominalis ➢ Stomach in chest cavity: diaphragmatic hernia
Liver on right side	➢ Liver on left side or centered: rotation anomalies Liver protruding: omphalocele
Aorta on left side	➢ Aorta on right side or centered: rotation anomalies or heart defects with right-sided aortic arch
Inferior vena cava	➢ No confluence of inferior vena cava and hepatic veins: azygos continuation in left isomerism ➢ Inferior vena cava and aorta on the same side: right isomerism ➢ Inferior vena cava dilated: severe heart failure or severe hypoxia in IUGR

Table 25.**7**   Differential diagnosis of suspected abnormalities of cardiac position

Normal	Suspicious
➢ Two-thirds of the heart is in the left hemithorax ➢ Cardiac axis points to the left	➢ Heart is partially or completely outside the chest: ectopia cordis ➢ Heart is shifted to the right, with its apex toward the left: dextroposition of the heart (diaphragmatic defect, intrathoracic mass, unilateral agenesis of the right lung, unilateral pleural effusion) ➢ Heart is shifted far to the left within the chest: levocardia due to an intrathoracic mass on the right side (right-sided diaphragmatic defect, right lung cysts, etc.) or due to abdominal displacements, as in gastroschisis ➢ Heart on the left, stomach on the right: situs inversus with levocardia ➢ Heart on the midline: mesocardia ➢ Mirror-image inversion of the heart: mirror dextrocardia in situs inversus; right ventricle is anterior ➢ Heart is rotated toward the right: cardiac dextroversion; the left ventricle is anterior

Table 25.**8**   Differential diagnosis of suspected abnormalities of cardiac position

Normal	Suspicious
Heart occupies approximately one-third of the chest cavity (see curves for cardiac dimensions)	➢ Pseudocardiomegaly: normal heart in intrauterine growth retardation (CT ratio abnormal with a normal cardiac width or area) ➢ Extreme cardiomegaly: dilated cardiomyopathy (all chambers dilated and hypokinetic), Ebstein anomaly or tricuspid valve dysplasia (marked dilatation of right atrium) ➢ Large heart due to a cardiac defect, usually with tricuspid insufficiency; defect may be AV canal, pulmonary atresia, pulmonary stenosis, etc. ➢ Volume overload (see under Tricuspid Insufficiency)

Table 25.**9**   Differential diagnosis of principal right-heart findings in the four-chamber view

Normal	Suspicious
➢ Lumen of right ventricle (RV) is slightly shorter than that of the left ventricle ➢ RV shows trabeculation ➢ Moderator band is visualized ➢ Normal contractility	➢ Suspicious ➢ Low insertion of the tricuspid valve in the RV, right atrium is strongly dilated: Ebstein anomaly (often with cardiomegaly due to severe tricuspid insufficiency) ➢ Tricuspid valve has normal insertion but dysplastic leaflets, right atrium is strongly dilated: tricuspid valve dysplasia (often with cardiomegaly due to severe tricuspid insufficiency) ➢ Right atrium is visualized but RV is not visualized, single ventricle is perfused from the left atrium: tricuspid atresia with a single ventricle ➢ RV is very small with an echogenic wall, tricuspid valve shows ineffective movements, hypertrophic myocardium with interventricular septum shifted slightly to the left: pulmonary atresia with an intact septum (PA/IVS) ("hypoplastic right heart") ➢ RV is very small, tricuspid valve is not defined, but a VSD is present: tricuspid valve atresia with VSD ➢ Lumen of RV is small with hypertrophic myocardium and hypokinesia: severe pulmonary stenosis ➢ RV is extremely dilated with a very thin wall: Uhl anomaly (prenatal cases extremely rare)

Table 25.10 Differential diagnosis of principal left-heart findings in the four-chamber view

Normal	Suspicious
➤ Lumen of left ventricle (LV) is slightly longer than that of the RV ➤ Normal contractility	➤ LV is not visualized and left atrium is difficult to define, only one ventricle is perfused from the right atrium: mitral atresia and aortic atresia in HLHS ➤ LV lumen is visible but extremely small with an echogenic wall, mitral valve shows ineffectual movements, myocardium frequently hypertrophic: aortic atresia with mitral valve dysplasia in HLHS ➤ LV is very small, small mitral valve, presence of VSD: mitral valve atresia with VSD ➤ LV is dilated with hypokinetic wall and often with echogenic myocardium: endocardial fibroelastosis due to critical aortic stenosis ➤ LV is considerably smaller than RV, but its contractility is preserved (sometimes with VSD): coarctation of the aorta, hypoplasia of the aortic arch, tubular hypoplasia or interruption of the aortic arch ➤ LV is dilated, left atrium is extremely dilated: isolated aortic atresia with patent (but incompetent) mitral valve

Table 25.11 Differential diagnosis of an overriding aorta

Normal	Suspicious
➤ Aorta and septum present continuity	➤ Aorta is overriding, pulmonary artery is patent with a normal caliber: malalignment VSD ➤ Aorta is overriding, pulmonary artery is narrow with patent (separate) valve: tetralogy of Fallot ➤ Aorta is overriding, pulmonary artery is narrow and difficult to define, atretic pulmonary valve: pulmonary atresia with VSD (formerly: extreme tetralogy of Fallot) ➤ Pulmonary arteries arise from the aorta: truncus arteriosus ➤ Aorta arises mostly (> 50%) from the RV, with variable interrelationship of the vessels (normal or with D or L malposition): double-outlet right ventricle

Table 25.12 Differential diagnosis of tricuspid insufficiency

Slight tricuspid valve regurgitation	➤ Normal due to immaturity of fetal lung (often with pulmonary valve regurgitation) or to myocardial immaturity
Heart defects with primary dysplasia of the tricuspid valve, heart defects with "optional" tricuspid insufficiency	➤ Ebstein anomaly ➤ Tricuspid valve dysplasia ➤ AV canal ➤ Hypoplastic left heart ➤ Mitral atresia with DORV ➤ Coarctation of the aorta
Heart defects and diseases with right ventricular obstruction	➤ Pulmonary atresia ➤ Pulmonary stenosis ➤ Constriction of ductus arteriosus (moderate to severe tricuspid insufficiency)
Volume overload (frequent tricuspid insufficiency with mitral insufficiency)	➤ Fetal anemia: Rh isoimmunization, parvovirus ➤ Peripheral arteriovenous fistula: veins of Galen, sacrococcygeal teratoma, chorangioma ➤ Acceptor in twin–twin transfusion syndrome ➤ Cardiac recirculation defect ➤ Severe arrhythmia: tachycardia, bradycardia
Myocardial dysfunction (frequent tricuspid insufficiency with mitral insufficiency)	➤ Myocarditis: infection, connective tissue disease ➤ Cardiomyopathy: dilated CMP, following a severe arrhythmia or volume overload ➤ Myocardial damage due to hypoxia: severe IUGR with abnormal Doppler findings in the periphery

Specific Cardiac Anomalies and Diseases

▬ *Tricuspid Atresia (TA)*

Definition. In this anomaly, the normal connection between the right atrium and right ventricle is absent. If there is an accompanying ventricular septal defect (VSD), a right (hypoplastic) ventricle can be identified (TA with VSD) (Fig. 25.**1**). Otherwise the heart has only a single (left) ventricle. TA is divided into two types according to the position of the great vessels:

- Type I: ventriculoarterial concordance (70% of cases)
- Type II: discordance (30% of cases)

In turn, types I and II are each subdivided into a patent, stenotic, and atretic form depending on the morphology of the pulmonary valve (18).

Incidence. TA occurs in 0.7% of all live births with a congenital heart defect.

Associated anomalies and chromosomal abnormalities. Besides the cardiac anomalies associated with the different types, TA is frequently accompanied by an atrial septal defect. Typical extracardiac anomalies are not known and are rather uncommon. It is most important to exclude malrotation anomalies (left and right isomerism).

Ultrasound Diagnosis

B-mode image. The four-chamber view shows an absent or hypoplastic right ventricle. Only the AV valve on the left side (mitral valve) opens during diastole, connecting the left atrium to the ventricle. If the right ventricle has a demonstrable lumen, then a VSD (of variable size) can always be detected (Fig. 25.**2**). By defining the great vessels (e.g., in a short-axis view), the examiner can distinguish normal vascular origins from a malposition of the great vessels. When pulmonary atresia is present, a hypoplastic pulmonary trunk is often found.

Color and spectral Doppler. Color Doppler (Fig. 25.**3**) confirms an absence of blood flow from the right atrium to the "right" ventricle. Blood flows from the right atrium through the foramen ovale to the left atrium, from which it enters the left ventricle during diastole (Fig. 25.**3**). If a VSD is also present, the unidirectional left-to-right shunt can be optimally visualized with color Doppler (Fig. 25.**4**). In evaluations of the great vessels, color Doppler also helps differentiate the aorta and pulmonary trunk, and it can help in defining a right ventricular obstruction (see above). Color flow can demonstrate antegrade perfusion through the open pulmonary valve or retrograde perfusion through the ductus arteriosus in pulmonary atresia.

Differential diagnosis. When a single ventricle is found, other anomalies with a univentricular heart should be considered. With a hypoplastic right ventricle, the differential diagnosis should include pulmonary atresia with an intact ventricular septum and severe pulmonary stenosis. If isomerism is found (see below), it can be difficult to make a precise differential diagnosis (mitral valve atresia with VSD?).

Intrauterine course and prognosis. Tricuspid atresia can lead to intrauterine heart failure. For this reason, pregnancies that are carried to term should be examined at regular intervals, giving particular attention to the single AV valve (mitral valve) to look for signs of valvular insufficiency. Doppler examinations of the hepatic veins, vena cava, and

Tricuspid atresia

Fig. 25.**1**   Diagram of tricuspid atresia with a VSD (modified from [30]).

Fig. 25.**2**   Apical four-chamber view of tricuspid atresia with VSD, 25 weeks. The atretic tricuspid valve appears as an echogenic tissue band, and the lumen of the right ventricle (RV) is hypoplastic, as it receives flow only from the left ventricle (LV) through the VSD (left-to-right shunt) (compare with Figs. 25.**3** and 25.**4**). The small right ventricle shows good contractility.

Fig. 25.**3**   TA + VSD (compare with Figs. 25.**1** and 25.**2**). Color Doppler demonstrates how blood flows from the left atrium (LA) through the LV (red) and VSD (blue) to the RV.

Fig. 25.**4**   Doppler spectrum recorded over the ventricular septal defect in a fetus with TA + VSD (compare with Figs. 25.**1**–25.**3**). Because the tricuspid valve is atretic, blood enters the right ventricle only through the VSD in late diastole, creating a unidirectional left-to-right shunt.

Pulmonary atresia

Fig. 25.**5**   Hypoplasia of the right ventricle in pulmonary atresia with an intact ventricular septum (PA/IVS). The lumen of the right ventricle is hypoplastic compared with the left ventricle, its wall is hypertrophic, and the ventricle appears hypokinetic in the real-time image. The tricuspid valve is dysplastic. Visualization of the pulmonary trunk would confirm the diagnosis of pulmonary atresia.

Fig. 25.**6**   Pulmonary atresia, 25 weeks. Tangential view of the aortic arch (blue) and pulmonary trunk in a longitudinal scan. While blood normally flows in the same direction through both vessels (encoded in blue), pulmonary atresia leads to retrograde perfusion of the pulmonary trunk through the patent ductus arteriosus (DA) (encoded in red).

Fig. 25.**7**   In a 35-week fetus with pulmonary atresia, the right and left pulmonary arteries (Rpa, Lpa) and pulmonary trunk (PT) are hypoplastic. By contrast, the ascending aorta (Aoa) appears dilated. Aod = descending aorta.

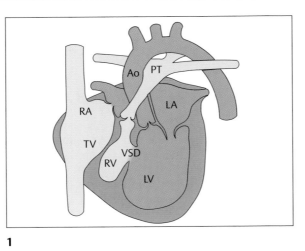

1

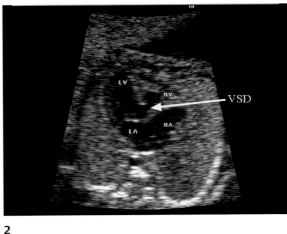

2

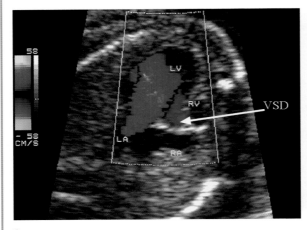

3

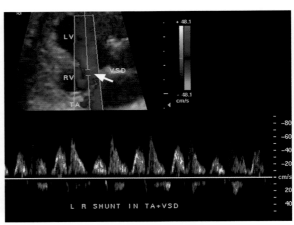

4

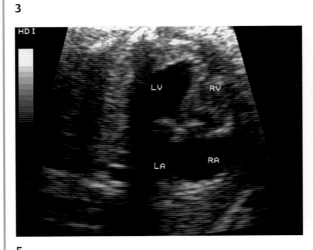

5

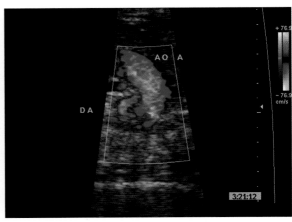

6

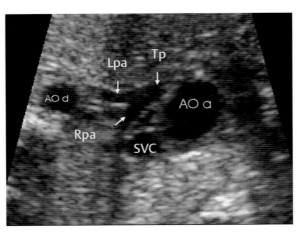

7

ductus venosus (24, 26) are also helpful in assessing an atrial volume overload.

Pulmonary Atresia with an Intact Ventricular Septum (PA/IVS)

Definition. This term includes various defects in which the pulmonary valve is atretic and the interventricular septum is intact. Pulmonary atresia also occurs in several complex cardiac anomalies (double-outlet right ventricle [DORV], "extreme" tetralogy of Fallot). Atresia of the pulmonary valve leads to hypoplasia of the right ventricle with pronounced myocardial hypertrophy and secondary dysplasia of the tricuspid valve (Fig. 25.**5**). There are also less common forms marked by a normal-size or even enlarged right ventricle with a dysplastic tricuspid valve. Today, this latter group is increasingly classified as a form of primary tricuspid dysplasia (see below).

Incidence. PA/IVS occurs in approximately 1–2% of all live births with a congenital heart defect.

Associated anomalies and chromosomal abnormalities. Extracardiac anomalies are somewhat rare in PA/IVS. An atrial septal defect is often present as an associated cardiac anomaly. Also, connections are occasionally found between the lumen of the right ventricle and the coronary vessels (ventriculocoronary fistulae), which we have been able to detect in utero (14). The presence of these connections is a poor prognostic sign.

Ultrasound Diagnosis

B-mode image. The four-chamber view demonstrates hypoplasia, myocardial hypertrophy, and hypokinesia of the right ventricle. Not infrequently, slight endocardial fibrosis is noted in the form of an echogenic rim, and the right ventricle bulges to the left. The motion of the tricuspid valve appears restricted. The pulmonary trunk is underdeveloped compared with the aorta (Fig. 25.**7**) (pulmonary trunk biometry or Ao/PT ratio; see Chapter 12), and typical opening movements of the pulmonary valve are not observed. The origins of the pulmonary arteries should be visible, but the arteries themselves are often hypoplastic (Fig. 25.**7**).

Color and spectral Doppler. In the four-chamber view, flow through the tricuspid valve in diastole is absent or greatly diminished, depending on the degree of right ventricular hypoplasia. Regurgitation through the tricuspid valve may be noted during systole. Evaluation of the pulmonary trunk demonstrates retrograde flow through the ductus arteriosus (Fig. 25.**6**). Color Doppler can also detect any ventriculocoronary fistulae that are present. In fetuses with other forms of pulmonary atresia, such as PA with a VSD or in cases of DORV, the examiner should consider that atypical pulmonary arteries may arise directly from the aorta. This type of pattern can be detected only with color Doppler.

Differential diagnosis. With hypoplasia of the right ventricle, differentiation is first required from tricuspid atresia with a VSD (see above). Since the hypoplasia may be mild, the differential diagnosis should also include pulmonary stenosis (Doppler scanning of the pulmonary artery). Hypokinesia of the ventricle should also raise the possibility of cardiomyopathies or hemodynamic changes (e.g., acceptor in twin–twin transfusion). It should be noted that a less experienced examiner may confuse the sides and mistake the finding for a hypoplastic left heart syndrome. Finally, PA/IVS requires differentiation from pulmonary atresia with a VSD. In the latter condition, it is rare to find an extremely small, hypokinetic right ventricle.

Intrauterine course and prognosis. Intrauterine follow-up examinations are done mainly for the early recognition of heart failure, giving particular attention to retrograde flow in the systemic veins. It is also important to follow the development of the right ventricular lumen, for if the chamber is well developed, chances are good that a catheter procedure can be performed in the neonatal period to open up the valves.

Ductus arteriosus. Since cyanosis occurs in the early neonatal period as the ductus arteriosus begins to close, it is important to assess the size, course, and perfusion of the ductus arteriosus when PA/IVS is present. The pediatric cardiologist may need this information if neonatal stent insertion into the ductus is planned or if prostaglandin therapy is required. Under no circumstances should indomethacin be administered during the pregnancy to inhibit labor.

Tricuspid Dysplasia, Ebstein Anomaly

Definition. Both of these tricuspid valve anomalies have clinical and hemodynamic features that often cause them to be erroneously grouped together as "Ebstein anomaly." In tricuspid dysplasia, the valve is markedly thickened and flaccid but has a normal site of insertion (Fig. 25.**8**). In Ebstein anomaly, however, the valve inserts considerably lower in the right ventricle and has decreased mobility (Fig. 25.**11**). A common feature of the both anomalies is that the dysplastic valve is usually incompetent (Figs. 25.**9**–25.**11**), often leading to dilatation of the right atrium and fetal cardiomegaly.

Incidence. These rare anomalies occur in 1% of all live births with a congenital heart defect.

Associated anomalies and chromosomal abnormalities. Associated cardiac anomalies include right ventricular outflow tract obstruction (pulmonary stenosis or atresia), which occurs in 30% of fetuses with Ebstein anomaly and in 80% with tricuspid dysplasia. Extracardiac anomalies are somewhat rare, but several authors have observed associated skeletal deformities and chromosomal abnormalities (e.g., trisomy 13). Fetal hydrops may develop as a complication of cardiomegaly, and the chronically elevated intrathoracic pressure in pronounced cases can lead to pulmonary hypoplasia. Diagnosis is aided in these cases by determining the CTA ratio (ratio of cardiac and thoracic areas) (9). A value > 0.6 is strongly suspicious for pulmonary hypoplasia (10).

Ultrasound Diagnosis

B-mode image. In both anomalies, the four-chamber view demonstrates cardiomegaly and dilatation of the right atrium. As a result, these anomalies are relatively easy to detect at ultrasound screening. On subsequent planes, particular attention should be given to the right ventricular outflow tract, the opening movements of the pulmonary valve, and the caliber of the pulmonary trunk.

Color and spectral Doppler. Color Doppler can vividly demonstrate the incompetence of the tricuspid valve. Color flow is also helpful in assessing the perfusion of the pulmonary trunk to detect right ventricular obstruction. Doppler is of limited value, however, in correctly identifying a RVOT obstruction in cases with severe tricuspid insufficiency (10). Even if the pulmonary valve appears closed in the B-mode image and color Doppler shows only retrograde flow through the pulmonary trunk, the pulmonary valve may still be "open" since the incompetent tricuspid valve allows blood to reflux into the atrium during systole, and no pressure is generated to open the pulmonary valve, simulating atresia (10). The detection of pulmonary insufficiency is evidence for an open pulmonary valve.

Tricuspid dysplasia

Fig. 25.**8** Tricuspid valve dysplasia with extreme cardiomegaly, 32 weeks. Left: the tricuspid valve (TV) is at the correct location (differential diagnosis: Ebstein anomaly), but it is thickened and dysplastic (right arrow). The severe tricuspid insufficiency has led to cardiomegaly. Right: spectral features of severe tricuspid insufficiency, with a peak velocity of 3 m/s.

Fig. 25.**9** In a color Doppler view of the fetus in Fig. 25.**8**, the severe valvular insufficiency produces retrograde flow with a mosaic pattern. The newborn infant was also found to have pulmonary hypoplasia and died on the 2nd day of life.

Fig. 25.**10** Same fetus as in Figs. 15.**8** and 15.**9**. Color Doppler M-mode image shows the diastolic and systolic perfusion of the valve, indicating holosystolic tricuspid insufficiency.

Fig. 25.**11** Color Doppler view of an Ebstein anomaly, 32 weeks. In this condition the tricuspid valve insertion is lower in the right ventricle (long arrow) compared with the mitral valve insertion (two short arrows). Color Doppler indicates severe tricuspid insufficiency (turbulent flow with a mosaic pattern).

Pulmonary stenosis

Fig. 25.**12** Isolated pulmonary stenosis, 31 weeks. In a longitudinal scan over the pulmonary trunk, color Doppler indicates turbulence over the pulmonary valve.

Fig. 25.**13** Isolated pulmonary stenosis as in Fig. 25.**12**. CW Doppler shows peak velocities as high as 3.5 m/s!

Hypoplastic left heart syndrome

Fig. 25.**14** Diagram of HLHS with aortic atresia and mitral valve dysplasia. In this case the left ventricle is demonstrable and hypoplastic (after [30]).

Fig. 25.**15** Specimen of a fetal heart with left ventricular hypoplasia following pregnancy termination at 19 weeks. Note the hypoplastic ascending aorta (Ao).

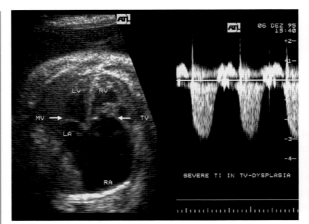

8

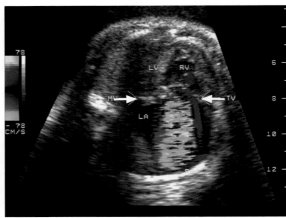

9

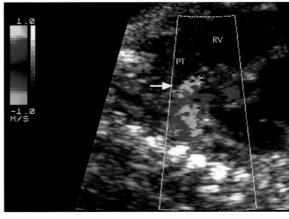

10

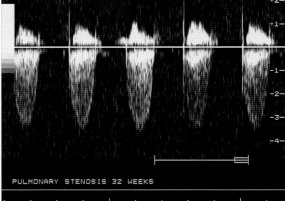

11

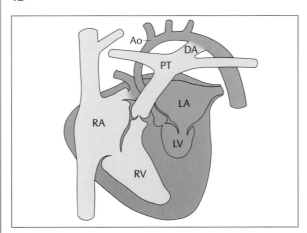

12

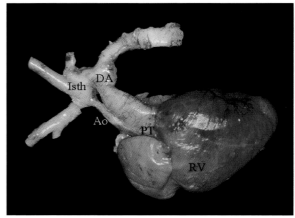

13

14

15

Differential diagnosis. Table 25.**8** lists the numerous conditions that should be considered in the differential diagnosis of cardiomegaly. The differential diagnosis of tricuspid insufficiency is also extensive, ranging from functional and hemodynamic disturbances to complex cardiac anomalies (Table 25.**12**). A logical, systematic approach is needed to make an accurate differential diagnosis, and subsequent follow-ups during the pregnancy often permit an accurate diagnosis to be made.

Intrauterine course and prognosis. These heart defects tend to take an unfavorable course. Serial examinations during pregnancy are done mainly for the purpose of detecting progression of tricuspid insufficiency. The examiner should also assess the quality of blood flow into the venous system (hepatic veins, ductus venosus, and inferior vena cava). The development of NIHF implies a considerably worse prognosis, with intrauterine fetal death occurring in more than 50% of cases (10).

Pulmonary Stenosis

Definition. Pulmonary stenosis refers to a narrowing of the right ventricular outflow tract in the area of the pulmonary valve. The stenosis is classified by its location as follows:
- Valvular (isolated)
- Subvalvular (infundibular and subinfundibular)
- Supravalvular

This section deals mainly with isolated valvular pulmonary stenosis.

Incidence. Pulmonary stenosis is the second most common heart defect after VSD, occurring in 9% of all live births with a congenital heart defect.

Associated Anomalies and Chromosomal abnormalities

Extracardiac anomalies. These are somewhat rare, occurring in just 12% of cases (20). As part of a genetic syndrome, pulmonary stenosis is a common feature of Noonan syndrome. It is rarely associated with chromosomal abnormalities, although invasive testing is recommended.

Intracardiac anomalies. Pulmonary stenosis is frequently isolated, but it also occurs as an associated cardiac anomaly as in ASD II or anomalous pulmonary venous return. It is also commonly found as part of a complex cardiac anomaly, especially in association with VSD and conotruncal anomalies (e.g., tetralogy of Fallot, DORV, transposition of the great arteries).

Ultrasound Diagnosis

B-mode image. Isolated pulmonary stenosis is rarely diagnosed prenatally with B-mode ultrasound and is difficult to detect. For this reason, pulmonary stenosis is a rare finding in prenatal examinations (6). The four-chamber view can detect only pronounced cases in which the right ventricle is already hypokinetic or third-trimester cases in which right ventricular hypertrophy or tricuspid insufficiency has caused visible dilatation of the right atrium. Proximal dilatation of the pulmonary trunk and a rigid, dome-like opening movement of the pulmonary valve can be important suggestive signs. At screening, however, pulmonary stenosis is usually detected only by the routine use of color Doppler, which can demonstrate the turbulence associated with the stenosis.

Color and spectral Doppler. Color Doppler can demonstrate tricuspid insufficiency in the four-chamber view, but usually this is seen most clearly during the third trimester. In some cases the insufficiency may be so pronounced that the resulting dilatation of the right atrium prompts immediate referral for a fetal echocardiographic examination.

Pulmonary stenosis is then diagnosed by detecting turbulent antegrade flow at the poststenotic level, evidenced by a typical mosaic pattern over the pulmonary valve (Fig. 25.**12**). Spectral Doppler (CW Doppler) can record peak flow velocities in excess of 2 m/s (Fig. 25.**13**).

Differential diagnosis. Isolated forms are not difficult to diagnose with the aid of color Doppler. In our experience, pulmonary stenosis can be difficult to distinguish from pulmonary atresia in cases with severe tricuspid insufficiency and cardiac dilatation (10, 28).

Intrauterine course and prognosis. Pulmonary stenosis is a valvular-obstruction type of heart defect that can develop in utero. Even if the heart appears normal during the second trimester, pulmonary stenosis may be present by the end of the pregnancy. Once pulmonary stenosis has developed, the fetal condition may deteriorate. Sharland et al. (28) investigated the natural history of severe tricuspid insufficiency and cardiomegaly in fetuses. They noted several cases in which pulmonary stenosis in the second trimester had progressed to pulmonary atresia by the end of gestation.

Surveillance. The surveillance of fetuses with pulmonary stenosis includes monitoring the pressure gradient of the stenotic valve along with the detection and possible documentation of increasing tricuspid insufficiency. The examiner should also check for retrograde flow in the systemic veins. When we see a deterioration of these findings, we induce labor no later than 36 weeks' gestation and perform a balloon valvuloplasty on the infant. If the right ventricle appears to be functioning normally, it is safe to take an expectant approach. The prognosis of isolated pulmonary stenosis is very good.

Hypoplastic Left Heart Syndrome (HLHS)

Definition. This is a group of heart defects in which the left ventricle may be nonvisualized or extremely hypoplastic as a result of aortic atresia and mitral valve atresia, dysplasia, or stenosis (Fig. 25.**14**).

Incidence. HLHS is present in 4% of all live-born infants with a congenital heart defect.

Associated anomalies and chromosomal abnormalities. Associated extracardiac anomalies are usually absent. Approximately 10% of fetuses with HLHS have an associated chromosomal abnormality, usually in the form of trisomy 13, trisomy 18, or Turner syndrome.

Ultrasound Diagnosis

B-mode image. HLHS is detectable by B-mode screening. In severe forms, the four-chamber view is already abnormal during the second trimester. The lumen of the left ventricle may be extremely small or nonvisualized (Fig. 25.**16**). The aorta is often extremely hypoplastic, and its origin and course are often difficult to define in the five-chamber view (Fig. 25.**15**). There is compensatory dilatation of the right ventricle and pulmonary trunk.

Color and spectral Doppler. Absent or greatly reduced diastolic filling of the left ventricle is quickly evident in the color flow image (Fig. 25.**17**). The pattern of unilateral perfusion through the right ventricular inflow tract is highly characteristic. Due to the increased perfusion of the right ventricle, a small amount of regurgitation may occur through the tricuspid valve. Another feature of HLHS is retrograde perfusion of the brachiocephalic arteries and coronary arteries through the pulmonary trunk and ductus arteriosus via the aortic isthmus. Color Doppler can demonstrate this retrograde flow in the aortic arch and ascending aorta, directed toward the aortic valve (Fig. 25.**18**).

Differential diagnosis. Differentiation is required from other forms of left ventricular obstruction. If the left ventricle shows good contractility, coarctation of the aorta should not be mistaken for HLHS, as it has a much more favorable prognosis.

Intrauterine course and prognosis. In recent theories on the pathogenesis of heart defects, several anomalies such as aortic stenosis, HLHS, and coarctation of the aorta are placed in the category of heart defects "with impaired intracardiac blood flow." This means that the cardiac defect does not already exist in the embryo in its definitive form, such as an AV canal with a septal defect. Instead, the impairment of intracardiac blood flow leads to decreased perfusion of the left ventricular inflow and outflow tracts, especially in the area of the foramen ovale. In other words, the intrauterine circulatory system, with its natural protective mechanisms, witnesses the increasing "evolution" of this type of obstruction as term approaches. Allan et al. (2) described one fetus in which the left ventricle was still well developed at 20 weeks' gestation, but scans at term revealed a severe form of HLHS. Many other authors have published similar observations. As a result, some cases of HLHS are not detected during the second trimester because the screening four-chamber view still appears normal at this stage of gestation.

Aortic Stenosis

Definition. In aortic stenosis, the narrowing may affect the aortic valve itself (valvular form, approximately 80%) or it may be located below the valve (approximately 15%) or above it (approximately 5%). Two types of aortic stenosis should be distinguished because of their different prognoses:

- "Simple" aortic stenosis
- "Critical" aortic stenosis

The latter is a severe form that causes severe prenatal changes in the wall of the left ventricle, described pathologically as endocardial fibroelastosis (Fig. 25.**19**).

Incidence. Aortic stenosis occurs in 3% of live births with a congenital heart defect.

Associated anomalies and chromosomal abnormalities. Associated extracardiac anomalies are somewhat rare in aortic stenosis. A critical type of stenosis can lead to intrauterine heart failure, and therefore this lesion should be considered when NIHF is present. A chromosome analysis should be performed.

Ultrasound Diagnosis

B-mode image. Mild forms of *"simple" aortic stenosis* are very difficult to diagnose prenatally. Left ventricular hypertrophy or dilatation does not develop until the third trimester, if at all. The attentive examiner may be able to recognize a mild form by the restricted opening movements of the valve (dome-like bulge) and by poststenotic dilatation of the ascending aorta. The mild forms are easier to detect when color Doppler is used.

With a *"critical" aortic stenosis*, the B-mode four-chamber view often shows a dilated left ventricle with a densely echogenic wall due to (incipient) endocardial fibroelastosis (Fig. 25.**19**). Besides ventricular dilatation and rounding of the cardiac apex, hypokinesia of the ventricle is a typical finding. The aortic root appears normal or narrowed in the five-chamber view and often shows poststenotic dilatation.

Color and spectral Doppler. *"Simple" aortic stenosis* can be detected with color Doppler. Turbulent, antegrade blood flow with a mosaic pattern is clearly apparent in the five-chamber view (Fig. 25.**20**). Doppler spectral measurement of peak flow velocities (using pulsed-wave or continuous-wave Doppler) shows values higher than 2 m/s (Fig. 25.**21**).

With a *"critical" aortic stenosis,* turbulent antegrade flow can be detected over the aortic valve. The turbulence may be less pronounced if severe endocardial fibroelastosis is present. With the increased pressure in the left ventricle, it is common to detect mitral insufficiency in systole, possibly with a left-to-right shunt through the foramen ovale. Retrograde perfusion of the aortic arch is observed in severe cases.

Differential diagnosis. The differential diagnosis of a dilated left ventricle should include dilatative cardiomyopathy, which is distinguished by the fact that it involves all the cardiac chambers. Also, a small aortic valve, with or without associated turbulence, may result from a left ventricular obstruction with involvement of the aortic arch. Aortic stenosis may be associated with hypoplasia of the aortic arch, especially when there is a coexisting VSD (Table 25.**10**).

Intrauterine course and prognosis. In an interesting retrospective analysis, Sharland et al. (29) studied the data from 30 fetuses with a critical aortic stenosis and left ventricular dysfunction. One of their most important observations was that the aortic valve in five cases was definitely open (and stenotic) prenatally but was found to be atretic several weeks later at autopsy. The authors also described five cases with an initially dilated left ventricle that subsequently developed into a hypoplastic left heart syndrome.

Intrauterine development. The authors underscore this observation, which supports the intrauterine development of valvular obstructions. Thus a critical stenosis or hypoplastic left heart may be associated with a normal-appearing four-chamber view at 18 weeks, causing it to be missed at screening. Moreover, a reliable prognosis cannot be offered when left ventricular dysfunction is detected, because the subsequent intrauterine course cannot be predicted.

Serial scans. For this reason, serial examinations should be conducted when this defect is present so that the subsequent development of endocardial fibroelastosis or NIHF can be recognized.

Aortic Arch Anomalies

Definition. Aortic arch anomalies basically consist of the following malformations:

- Interruption of the aortic arch
- Tubular hypoplasia of the aortic arch
- Tubular coarctation of the aorta
- "Simple" coarctation of the aorta (Fig. 25.**22**) involving the segment opposite the opening of the ductus arteriosus into the descending aorta ("juxtaductal" form) (13)

Incidence. Coarctation of the aorta occurs in approximately 5% of all live births with congenital heart disease, interruption of the aortic arch in 0.7%.

Associated Anomalies and Chromosomal Abnormalities

Intracardiac anomalies. These mainly include ventricular septal defect, AV canal, double-outlet right ventricle, and a dysplastic aortic valve. It is also very likely that these anomalies have an important pathogenetic role: By equalizing the pressure between the left and right sides of the fetal circulation, these defects give rise to a "chronic" underperfusion of the aortic isthmus, inhibiting its development. This is supported by the fact that defects with greater aortic perfusion, such as tetralogy of Fallot (TOF) and truncus arteriosus communis (TAC), are almost never associated with coarctation of the aorta.

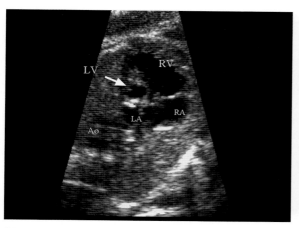

16

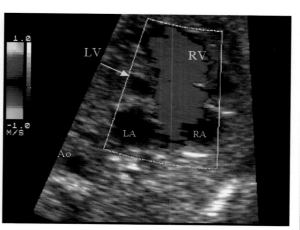

17

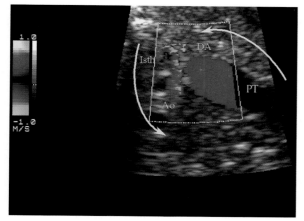

18

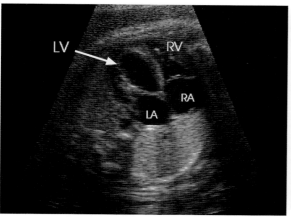

19

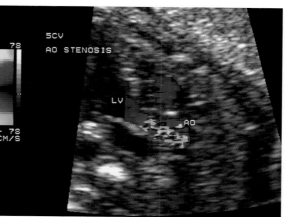

20

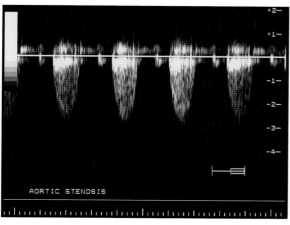

21

Fig. 25.**16** Hypoplastic left heart syndrome, 28 weeks. Apical four-chamber B-mode image shows a hypoplastic left ventricle (arrow). Hypokinesia of the left ventricle is evident in the real-time image.

Fig. 25.**17** Color Doppler confirms the finding in Fig. 25.**16** by showing unidirectional perfusion through the right ventricular inflow tract.

Fig. 25.**18** Color Doppler view of the great vessels in HLHS. Often the aortic arch cannot be seen in the B-mode image, but color Doppler clearly demonstrates retrograde flow through the isthmic portion of the aorta toward the ascending aorta.

Aortic stenosis

Fig. 25.**19** Endocardial fibroelastosis in the apical four-chamber view, 31 weeks. The left ventricle (LV) is dilated, its wall is densely echogenic ("porcelain-like"), and its contractility is extremely diminished. Critical aortic stenosis is present.

Fig. 25.**20** Valvular aortic stenosis, 26 weeks. Color Doppler in the apical five-chamber view shows typical turbulence (mosaic pattern) over the aortic valve.

Fig. 25.**21** Valvular aortic stenosis in CW Doppler, 26 weeks. Continuous-wave Doppler is used to prevent aliasing at the high flow velocities. Vmax is approximately 280 cm/s.

Extracardiac anomalies. Coarctation of the aorta is accompanied by extracardiac anomalies in 26% of cases and by interruption of the aortic arch in 50% of cases. The rate is much higher in prenatal studies, due largely to the fact that most cases are detected based on the presence of extracardiac anomalies. Typical anomalies include those whose embryonic development coincides with the timing and location of aortic arch development, such as upper gastrointestinal tract anomalies (esophageal atresia, diaphragmatic defect).

With an interruption of the aortic arch, the group of velocardiac anomalies should be considered (DiGeorge syndrome, Sphrintzen syndrome, etc.), and chromosome analysis should include a specific search for a deletion on chromosome 22 (CATCH 22: *c*ardiac defects, *a*bnormal facies, *t*hymic hypoplasia, *c*left palate, *h*ypocalcemia) using the fluorescence in-situ hybridization (FISH) technique.

Ultrasound Diagnosis

B-mode image. A simple coarctation of the aorta is very difficult to diagnose prenatally (1, 13). Other aortic arch anomalies such as tubular hypoplasia, aortic arch hypoplasia, and interruption of the aortic arch can be detected prenatally, but many of these cases are still difficult to diagnose (25). Visualization of the aortic arch in longitudinal section is of minor importance in prenatal diagnosis. Primary attention should be given to disproportion between the left and right ventricles and between the aortic arch and pulmonary trunk (Fig. 25.**24**) (1, 25). The "small" left ventricle shows normal contractility in these cases – an important sign in the prenatal differentiation of left ventricular hypoplasia (Fig. 25.**23**, Table 25.**10**). Even in a healthy fetus, however, scanning in the third trimester will show a discrepancy between the left and right ventricles, making it more difficult to distinguish between normal and abnormal.

Color and spectral Doppler. Spectral and color Doppler have contributed relatively little to the prenatal diagnosis of coarctation of the aorta. Although the lesion is a "stenosis," turbulence is not observed in the area of the coarctation. Allan et al. (1) found that fetuses with coarctation of the aorta had a low flow volume across the aortic valve and twice as much flow through the tricuspid valve as through the mitral valve. In cases with pronounced findings, such as a coexisting VSD or aortic stenosis, color Doppler may demonstrate retrograde perfusion in the aortic isthmus.

Differential diagnosis. Although several ultrasound signs have been described for coarctation of the aorta, all authors note that the signs are unreliable and stress the possibility of false-positive and false-negative findings (25). The differential diagnosis should include a normal heart, therefore. In some cases even an experienced examiner cannot diagnose the lesion with confidence. HLHS should also be considered when a small left ventricle is found, but that condition is distinguished by a hypoplastic ventricle and a nonpatent aortic valve (Table 25.**10**).

Intrauterine course and prognosis. The main purpose of serial scans is to observe the development of the aortic arch from the aortic valve to the termination of the ductus arteriosus. In cases that are detected early, the discrepancy between the right and left ventricles (RV/LV) and between the pulmonary trunk and ascending aorta (25) (see curves in Chapter 12) during the course of the pregnancy can serve as important parameters in evaluating progression.

Atrial Septal Defect (ASD)

Definition. A defect in the atrial septum is seldom mentioned in prenatal studies, because it can rarely be diagnosed antenatally. Four types of defect are distinguished:
- A sinus venosus defect
- An ostium secundum defect (ASD II)
- A septum primum defect
- A common atrium

Incidence. ASD II occurs as an isolated anomaly in approximately 7–8% of all live births with a congenital heart defect.

Associated anomalies and chromosomal abnormalities. ASD II does occur in isolation but is more often part of a complex cardiac anomaly (TGA, PS, Fallot, TAPVD, PLSVC, etc.). It is also found in association with extracardiac anomalies (right and left isomerism, Holt–Oram syndrome) and chromosomal abnormalities.

Ultrasound Diagnosis

B-mode image. An atrial septal defect is very difficult to diagnose prenatally. ASD I (Fig. 25.**25**) and a common atrium can be diagnosed by an experienced examiner, however, whereas a sinus venosus defect and ASD II usually go undetected.

Color Doppler. Color Doppler is less important than B-mode in evaluating these defects. But if a large ASD II is suspected, it can be confirmed with color Doppler, which demonstrates a left-to-right shunt in addition to the physiologic right-to-left shunt. With a septum primum defect, the examiner can use color flow to confirm his suspicion. Color Doppler will show any communication that exists between the right atrium and left ventricle or between the left atrium and right ventricle.

Differential diagnosis. Differential diagnosis rarely presents a problem with these defects. In fetuses who have a persistent left superior vena cava (PLSVC), that vessel usually opens into a dilated coronary sulcus. When viewed in a plane slightly inferior to the four-chamber view, the site where the vena cava enters the coronary sulcus may be mistaken for an ASD. The septum primum and secundum can be visualized, however, in a plane slightly superior to the four-chamber view.

Intrauterine course and prognosis. ASD is considered to have a very good prognosis when it is not associated with other cardiac or extracardiac anomalies. When present, these anomalies usually take precedence over septal defects. Invasive testing is strongly indicated in cases with ASD I and II to exclude a chromosomal abnormality.

Ventricular Septal Defect (VSD)

Definition. Two types are distinguished by their location:
- Defect in the membranous part of the interventricular septum (80% of VSDs)
- Defect in the muscular part of the septum (20%)

Incidence. VSD is the most common heart defect, occurring in 30% of live births with a congenital heart defect.

Associated Anomalies and Chromosomal Abnormalities

Complex defects. VSD often occurs in isolation but may also be part of numerous complex cardiac defects that involve the ventricles and great vessels (Table 25.**13**), including tricuspid atresia, mitral atresia, pulmonary atresia, tetralogy of Fallot, DORV, TAC, TGA, tubular hypoplasia of the aortic arch, and interruption of the aortic arch. Thus whenever a VSD is detected prenatally, the patient should be referred for a detailed fetal cardiac scan that includes a precise evaluation of the great vessels.

Extracardiac anomalies. VSD also occurs in association with a number of extracardiac anomalies and in the setting of syndromes. An isolated VSD detected prenatally may be a sign of a chromosomal abnormality such as trisomy 21, 18, or 13 (4). The likelihood of aneuploidy increases significantly when extracardiac anomalies or abnormalities are present.

Ultrasound Diagnosis

B-mode image. Because VSDs vary in size, their accessibility to prenatal diagnosis also varies. They are most reliably detected by scanning from different directions in multiple contiguous planes. Even with optimum examination conditions, however, a VSD cannot be excluded with complete confidence. Whereas larger VSDs can be recognized in the B-mode image as early as 13 weeks' gestation, small muscular defects may be missed and may not be detected until the third trimester, aided if necessary by color Doppler imaging (Fig. 25.**26**).

But most defects are located in the membranous, subaortic portion of the interventricular septum and are best visualized in the five-chamber view (Fig. 25.**27**). So even if the four-chamber view appears normal, a large membranous VSD may still be present.

Color and spectral Doppler. Large VSDs (> 5–6 mm) can quickly be detected in the B-mode image. Color Doppler is mainly of value in the detection or confirmation of small VSDs (< 2 mm) (Fig. 25.**28**). Although VSDs are easier to detect in lateral views, is not uncommon for the shunt flow across small defects to produce high flow velocities and turbulence that can also be seen in an apical view (i.e., at a less favorable angle) (Fig. 25.**26**). While postnatal scans indicate a unidirectional left-to-right shunt that follows the pressure gradient, prenatal scans of an isolated defect show a bidirectional shunt (Fig. 25.**26**). This shunt is directed from right to left in systole and early diastole and is reversed thereafter. But in fetuses with a complex cardiac anomaly causing obstruction of the inflow or outflow tract, a predominantly unidirectional shunt is found. A left-to-right shunt is seen with obstruction of the left ventricular outflow tract, tricuspid atresia, and DORV. A right-to-left shunt is seen with mitral atresia, pulmonary atresia, and pulmonary stenosis.

With a membranous VSD, color Doppler can also demonstrate the shunt flow across the septal defect. This is best accomplished in the five-chamber or short-axis view.

Power Doppler imaging. Our own recent studies suggest that power Doppler imaging may one day be useful in the detection of small muscular VSDs. The problem of optimum equipment settings remains to be solved.

Differential diagnosis. A VSD as small as 2 mm in diameter can be detected with B-mode ultrasound using high-resolution equipment.

Dropout effects. Dropout effects in an apical cardiac scan can mimic a VSD. Typically this occurs up to 20 weeks' gestation or when insonation conditions are poor. The examiner can confirm or refute his presumptive diagnosis by obtaining a lateral view in which the sound waves are directed perpendicular to the septum. The inlet and trabecular portions of the septum can be evaluated in the four-chamber view. The potential for false-positive findings was noted above.

AV canal. Differentiation is mainly required from AV canal, which should be considered whenever a VSD is found.

Table 25.**13** Cardiac anomalies that may be associated with a ventricular septal defect

➢ Tricuspid atresia
➢ Mitral atresia
➢ Pulmonary atresia
➢ Tetralogy of Fallot
➢ DORV
➢ TAC
➢ TGA
➢ Tubular hypoplasia of the aortic arch
➢ Interruption of the aortic arch

Incomplete diagnosis. The main problem in the prenatal diagnosis of VSD is making an incomplete diagnosis that misses associated cardiac anomalies (e.g., involving the great vessels). Tubular hypoplasia or interruption of the aortic arch is often associated with a VSD and can be detected only by specific evaluation of the aortic arch (see above). Another problem is the difficulty of detecting and describing malpositions of the great vessels (ventriculoarterial discordance).

Intrauterine course and prognosis. Small VSDs may close spontaneously in prenatal or postnatal life and usually have a good prognosis when they are not associated with other cardiac or extracardiac anomalies. Larger VSDs can be occluded with a "shield" in an interventional procedure or operatively repaired. Surgery should be done promptly, before the pulmonary vessels have been damaged by the postnatal left-to-right shunt.

■ *Atrioventricular Septal Defect (AVSD, AV Canal)*

Definition. These defects involve a combination of atrial and ventricular septal defects. They are divided into two forms:
- Incomplete AV septal defect (ASD I)
- Complete AV septal defect (CAVSD, AV canal)

Incidence. An AV canal occurs in 7.4% of all live births with a congenital heart defect.

Associated Anomalies and Chromosomal Abnormalities

Extracardiac anomalies. An AV canal is usually associated with extracardiac anomalies, which should always be excluded when this defect is found. Most are chromosomal abnormalities such as Down syndrome, which occurs in at least 50% of all cases (4). Also, an AV canal is often found in association with an abnormal cardiac position such as left- or right-sided isomerism. These forms, however, are very rarely associated with Down syndrome or other chromosomal abnormalities.

Intracardiac anomalies. These may occur in any cardiac structures. At the atrial level, the septum secundum may be affected in addition to the septum primum, and a common atrium may be present in extreme cases. At the ventricular level, hypoplasia of the left ventricle is sometimes found (this form, too, is rarely associated with Down syndrome). The following anomalies may involve the great vessels: tetralogy of Fallot, DORV, pulmonary atresia or stenosis, TGA, and TAC or coarctation of the aorta, especially in cases with isomerism. The AV canal may be combined with cardiac arrhythmias (especially AV block) due to possible anatomic impairment of the impulse conduction system (23).

Ultrasound Diagnosis

B-mode image. ASD I is considerably more difficult to diagnose than a complete AV canal. It should be considered whenever a defect is noted

Aortic arch anomalies

Fig. 25.22   Coarctation of the aorta.

Fig. 25.23   Coarctation of the aorta in the four-chamber view, 21 weeks. The scan shows a small left ventricle with normal contractility. This is an important suggestive sign of coarctation.

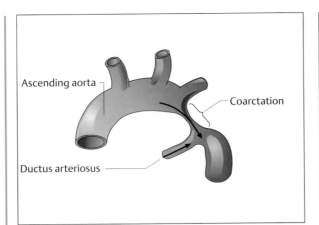

22

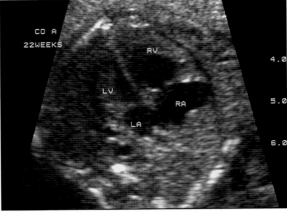

23

Fig. 25.24   Tubular hypoplasia of the aortic arch (plane 5). Besides the normally developed pulmonary trunk (PT) and ductus arteriosus (DA), the scan gives a tangential view of the hypoplastic aortic arch.

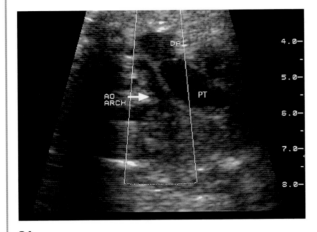

24

Septal defects

Fig. 25.25   Atrial septal defect (arrow) in the septum primum area of a fetus with mitral valve atresia and a hypoplastic left ventricle, 33 weeks.

Fig. 25.26   Ventricular septal defect (VSD), 33 weeks. Color Doppler reveals a bidirectional shunt in the central, muscular part of the interventricular septum. The VSD was not visible in the B-mode image and could be diagnosed only by visualizing the shunt with color Doppler.

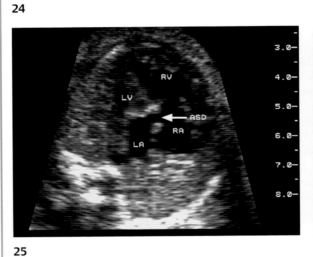

25

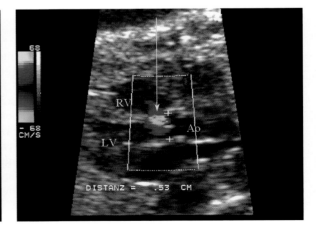

26

Fig. 25.27   Small, membranous VSD in a lateral five-chamber view, 28 weeks. Often these VSDs are clearly defined only at the subaortic level. The aorta appears in continuity with the interventricular septum and is not "overriding" (compare with Fig. 25.33).

Fig. 25.28   Color Doppler view of the VSD in Fig. 25.27. The right-to-left shunt confirms the finding.

27

28

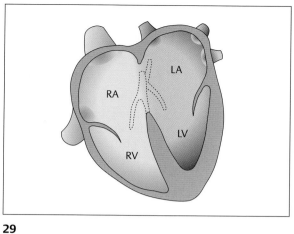

29

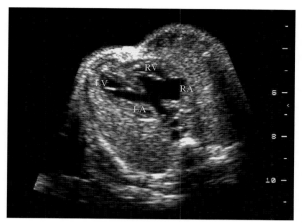

30

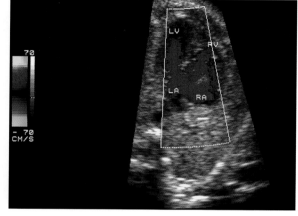

31

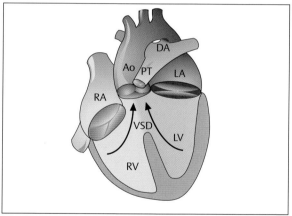

32

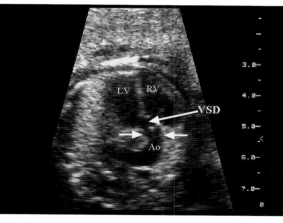

33

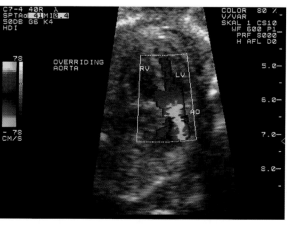

34

Fig. 25.**29** Diagram of a complete atrioventricular septal defect ("AV canal"). The dotted outlines indicate the missing structures (modified from [31]).

Fig. 25.**30** Complete AV canal, 31 weeks. The complete absence of the endocardial cushion is evident in the four-chamber view. A combined ventricular and atrial septal defect with only two AV valve leaflets are characteristic. In more than 50% of cases, an AV canal is associated with Down syndrome (as was the case with this fetus).

Fig. 25.**31** Complete AV canal at 33 weeks, with mixing of blood from both inflow tracts via the atrial and ventricular septal defects during diastole. Note the typical "H" configuration.

Tetralogy of Fallot

Fig. 25.**32** The tetralogy of Fallot is characterized by four abnormalities: ventricular septal defect (VSD), overriding aorta, pulmonary stenosis, and right ventricular hypertrophy. Only the first two of these signs can be detected prenatally (modified from [31]).

Fig. 25.**33** Tetralogy of Fallot, 31 weeks. The dilated, overriding aorta (short arrows) is visible above the ventricular septal defect (long arrow) in the apical five-chamber view. Right ventricular enlargement can rarely be detected prenatally.

Fig. 25.**34** Tetralogy of Fallot, apical five-chamber view, 31 weeks. During systole, blood flows from the left and right ventricles across the VSD and then through the aortic valve into the ascending aorta. Note the typical "Y" pattern in the color Doppler image.

in the portion of the atrial septum near the AV valves (septum primum) in the four-chamber view (Fig. 25.**25**).

A large *complete AV canal* is most conspicuous in the four-chamber view during diastole when the valve is open. The central portion of the heart appears "punched out" (Fig. 25.**29**). During systole, the atrial and ventricular septal defects can be seen above and below the closed AV valves (Figs. 25.**30**, 25.**44**). An AV canal can be diagnosed as early as the late first trimester, as it is already fully developed in the embryo. Color Doppler is a tremendous aid to prenatal diagnosis.

Since an AV canal may also occur in *isomerism,* the detection of the defect warrants a segmental analysis of the upper abdomen (Figs. 25.**43**, 25.**44**), especially when there is a coexisting heart block.

Color Doppler. Color Doppler in the four-chamber view shows a lack of separation between the right and left ventricular inflow tracts in diastole, producing a typical "H" configuration (Fig. 25.**31**). With color flow, blood can be seen mixing in the area of the septum primum defect, the dysplastic AV valves, and the ventricular septal defect. Also, incompetence of the dysplastic AV valve is often evident during systole, and color flow is needed to evaluate the degree of the valvular insufficiency. It may be severe enough to produce fetal heart failure with ascites.

Differential diagnosis. Questions of differential diagnosis mainly arise in distinguishing between a complete and incomplete AV canal. Differentiation is also required from a simple VSD. A hypoplastic left heart or single ventricle may sometimes be confused with an AV canal, particularly due to the moderator band in the right ventricle.

When color Doppler is used, increasing the color gain scale can simulate the atrioventricular mixing of blood (false-positive finding). This can be clarified by scrutinizing the B-mode image and by adding a lateral view of the heart.

Intrauterine course and prognosis. NIHF may develop as a result of valvular insufficiency. Cardiac biometry, valvular insufficiency, and Doppler ultrasound findings in the venous vessels should be evaluated on serial scans. The prognosis of AV canal depends critically on associated extracardiac anomalies.

Tetralogy of Fallot

Definition. Tetralogy of Fallot (TOF, Fig. 25.**32**) is defined by the presence of four abnormalities:
- A large ventricular septal defect (VSD)
- An overriding aorta ("dextroposition" of the aorta)
- Infundibular pulmonary stenosis
- Right ventricular hypertrophy (a secondary condition)

Incidence. TOF occurs in approximately 6–7% of all live births with congenital heart disease.

Associated Anomalies and Chromosomal Abnormalities

Extracardiac anomalies. TOF, as a conotruncal anomaly, has a relatively high association with extracardiac anomalies (approximately 30–50% of cases) (5). Chromosomal abnormalities are found in 10–25% of cases (4). Associated gastrointestinal anomalies are particularly common. Cleft anomalies and associations with syndromes (e.g., VACTERL association) are also common.

Intracardiac anomalies. Associations with intracardiac anomalies often alter the classification of the disorder. For example, if an associated AV canal is present, the anomaly is classified as an atrioventricular septal defect. Another anomaly that has an extremely rare association with TOF is the absence of the pulmonary valve (absent pulmonary valve

syndrome), characterized by massive dilatation and insufficiency of the pulmonary trunk. Agenesis of the ductus arteriosus is usually present and contributes to the pathogenesis of the condition.

Ultrasound Diagnosis

B-mode image. Only two of the four abnormalities that characterize TOF—the VSD and overriding aorta—can definitely be detected in the fetus. Pulmonary stenosis usually results from underperfusion of the valve and "develops" during intrauterine and postnatal life. Right ventricular hypertrophy develops as a secondary response to the increased workload on the right ventricle. Generally hypertrophy is diagnosed postnatally, but a few cases are detected in late pregnancy.

The VSD is sometimes detectable in the four-chamber view and is always detectable in the five-chamber view, preferably using a lateral scan direction (see above). A presumptive diagnosis of TOF can be made in the five-chamber view by demonstrating the *overriding aorta* (Fig. 25.**33**) above the VSD. The aorta typically shows marked dilatation, which can be confirmed by biometry (16). The diagnosis is completed by evaluating the *pulmonary trunk,* which typically shows a smaller caliber than the aorta. An overriding aorta raises several diagnostic possibilities (Table 25.**11**), the most common being the tetralogy of Fallot.

Color and spectral Doppler. Color Doppler is of key importance in the diagnosis and differential diagnosis of TOF. The VSD is clearly visualized with color Doppler, and the typical overriding aorta is displayed in the five-chamber view. Since the ascending aorta receives simultaneous flow from both ventricles, a characteristic "Y" configuration is seen in the apical five-chamber view (Fig. 25.**34**). In the next plane, the perfusion of the pulmonary trunk is evaluated as an aid to differential diagnosis. Pulmonary atresia with VSD or truncus arteriosus can be recognized in this view. Differentiation from a double-outlet right ventricle is still difficult in many cases, even when color Doppler is used.

Differential diagnosis. The five-chamber view is first used to distinguish a simple VSD from an overriding aorta or a double-outlet right ventricle, where the aorta emerges mainly from the right ventricle. When an overriding aorta is found, it can sometimes be difficult to differentiate among the various forms (Table 25.**11**). B-mode biometry and Doppler evaluation of the pulmonary trunk are necessary in order to distinguish a VSD in the setting of TOF from pulmonary atresia with VSD, truncus arteriosus, and absent pulmonary valve syndrome.

Intrauterine course and prognosis. When a tetralogy of Fallot is diagnosed, the intrauterine follow-up focuses on the development of the pulmonary trunk, which will dictate the strategy for neonatal care. Heart failure with fetal hydrops is unlikely to develop in the setting of TOF, but it is possible, especially if the pulmonary valve is absent. Allan and Sharland (5) analyzed the prognoses of 23 fetuses with TOF and found a mortality rate of 75% in the 16 pregnancies that were continued. Thus, on detecting a heart defect with an otherwise "good" prognosis, the examiner should first exclude extracardiac anomalies, especially chromosomal defects.

Double-Outlet Right Ventricle (DORV)

Definition. In this anomaly the aorta and pulmonary trunk both arise from the right ventricle (Fig. 25.**35**). Usually these trunks are parallel to each other, forming an L or D type of malposition. The morphologic forms of DORV are correspondingly diverse.

Incidence. This anomaly occurs in 2% of live births with a congenital heart defect.

Associated Anomalies and Chromosomal abnormalities

Intracardiac anomalies. DORV is often associated with anomalies at the AV level such as AV canal or mitral atresia. Possible anomalies of the great vessels include coarctation of the aorta and pulmonary stenosis or atresia. The VSD in DORV may be very large, creating the appearance of a single ventricle.

Extracardiac anomalies. Associated extracardiac anomalies consist mainly of malrotation anomalies (polysplenia or asplenia syndrome); gastrointestinal tract anomalies such as esophageal atresia, diaphragmatic defect, and omphalocele; and facial malformations (DiGeorge syndrome, Charge syndrome, etc.). DORV is also found in fetuses with chromosomal abnormalities (e.g., trisomy 18) and in the fetuses of diabetic women (11, 19).

Ultrasound Diagnosis

B-mode image. Because of its diverse morphology, DORV does not have a "typical" ultrasound appearance. The four-chamber view may be abnormal in fetuses with a large VSD, a single ventricle, or coexisting mitral valve atresia (Fig. 25.**25**) (small left ventricle!). But a precise evaluation of the great vessels is necessary in order to make a presumptive diagnosis (Fig. 25.**36**). Often there is a conspicuous malposition of the great vessels with a discrepancy in the calibers of the aorta and pulmonary trunk. Occasionally, a tetralogy of Fallot is diagnosed in the initial examination and the diagnosis is revised later. Since DORV may occur in the setting of a heterotaxic syndrome (right or left isomerism), the segmental evaluation of cardiac anatomy is always advised.

Color and spectral Doppler. Usually there is a large VSD that can be visualized with color Doppler. With concomitant mitral atresia, the absence of flow between the left atrium and small left ventricle can be directly visualized, and the VSD displays a right-to-left shunt. Not infrequently, a relative tricuspid insufficiency is present due to the volume overload.

In many cases the origin of the two great vessels from the right ventricle is defined more easily and clearly with color Doppler (Fig. 25.**37**) than with B-mode ultrasound, supporting the presumptive diagnosis. Often, color Doppler can also more easily define the parallel course of the two great arteries in cases where a malposition is present. Especially when vascular anatomy is uncertain, color Doppler can help to differentiate the two vessels by defining the bifurcation of the two pulmonary arteries or the origin of the vascular trunks.

Differential diagnosis. Differential diagnosis can be quite difficult in fetuses with DORV, depending on the findings and the experience of the examiner. But a distinction should be made between "true" difficulties and "academic" problems. The true difficulties consist mainly of determining whether the great vessels are in an L or D relationship to each other and whether the hypoplastic vessel is the aorta or pulmonary trunk. The "academic" problems mainly involve questions of nomenclature and determining whether the anomaly is a tetralogy of Fallot, pulmonary atresia with a VSD, or a form of DORV. The small left ventricle can mimic HLHS, especially when mitral atresia is present. If there is suspicion of L-TGA or D-TGA with a VSD, it is important to exclude a DORV or DOLV.

Intrauterine course and prognosis. Intrauterine follow-up should focus on signs of AV valvular insufficiency so that heart failure can be detected without delay. Checking the hepatic veins for retrograde perfusion is particularly helpful in this respect. The association of this complex heart defect with other anomalies (including chromosomal abnormalities) helps explain the high intrauterine fetal death rate of 60% that we have documented in our own cases. If pulmonary stenosis or atresia is present, indomethacin should not be used during the pregnancy to inhibit labor.

Complete Transposition of the Great Arteries

Definition. In this anomaly (dextro-transposition of the great arteries, D-TGA), the aorta arises from the right ventricle and the pulmonary trunk from the left ventricle (ventriculoarterial discordance), with otherwise normal connections between the atria and ventricles (atrioventricular concordance) (Fig. 25.**41b**).

Incidence. D-TGA is a relatively frequent cardiac anomaly, occurring in approximately 5–7% of all live births with a congenital heart defect.

Associated anomalies and chromosomal abnormalities. Associated intracardiac anomalies are common. Pulmonary stenosis or a ventricular or atrial septal defect is present in 25% of cases.

Associated extracardiac anomalies are somewhat rare, occurring in less than 10% of cases. Trisomies and other chromosomal defects are very rare in D-TGA (4).

Ultrasound Diagnosis

B-mode image. D-TGA cannot be detected in the B-mode four-chamber view. Its detection requires a systematic evaluation of the origin and course of the two great vessels. The four-chamber view appears normal except in cases with a VSD. D-TGA may also be missed in the five-chamber view. The condition is diagnosed by attempting to define the vessel arising from the right ventricle, for that vessel (the aorta) does not cross the other vessel (pulmonary trunk) in the normal way but runs parallel and to the right of it (hence the "D" prefix). Defining the parallel course of both vessels in one plane, along with their valves, is characteristic of D-TGA (Fig. 25.**38**). Examiners who prefer the short-axis plane will find the aorta located anterior to the pulmonary trunk (Fig. 25.**40**) and will not see the typical "circle and sausage" sign.

Color and spectral Doppler. Color Doppler is mainly helpful in quickly defining the parallel course of both vessels (Fig. 25.**39**) and quickly distinguishing between the aorta and pulmonary trunk. Once the diagnosis has been established, color Doppler can help to exclude possible associated cardiac anomalies such as VSD and pulmonary stenosis.

Intrauterine course and prognosis. In most cases D-TGA has no clinical manifestations and first becomes symptomatic postnatally with the reversal of the circulation. In cases where pulmonary stenosis or a VSD is present, attention should be given to the prenatal course. It is also advisable to check for constriction of the foramen ovale during the final weeks of pregnancy, as this could necessitate an acute neonatal intervention (Rashkind balloon atrioseptostomy).

Corrected Transposition of the Great Arteries

Definition. In the "corrected" form of TGA (levo-transposition of the great arteries, L-TGA), the ventriculoarterial discordance is accompanied by atrioventricular discordance. The right atrium is connected to the morphologic left ventricle, which gives rise to the pulmonary trunk. The left atrium is connected to the morphologic right ventricle, which gives rise to the aorta (Fig. 25.**41c**). Although the vessels are anatomically transposed, there is no resulting circulatory impairment in this "corrected" form of the anomaly.

Incidence. L-TGA occurs in 1% of all live births with a congenital heart defect.

Associated anomalies and chromosomal abnormalities. This anomaly is often associated with a third-degree AV block (23). Also, an L malposition of the great vessels with ventriculoarterial discordance is not an uncommon finding in a heterotaxia syndrome or other complex cardiac anomalies (tricuspid atresia, double-outlet right ventricle, single ventricle, etc.). Extracardiac anomalies and chromosomal abnormalities are rare in "classic" L-TGA.

Ultrasound Diagnosis

B-mode image. Aside from cases associated with a third-degree AV block, an "isolated" L-TGA can be diagnosed only by a highly experienced examiner. Even in the four-chamber view, the experienced examiner can recognize that the morphologic left ventricle is on the right side while the right ventricle, with its moderator band and trabeculation, is on the left side. The origin of the great vessels appears suspicious at once, for when the transducer is tilted toward the five-chamber plane, the pulmonary trunk is seen emerging from the ventricle on the right side (the anatomic left ventricle). In the next plane, the aorta is found to be located anterior and to the left of the pulmonary trunk (hence the "L" prefix). The two vessels are parallel to each other. The inability to obtain a typical short-axis view supports the diagnosis.

Color and spectral Doppler. Although L-TGA can be diagnosed in the B-mode image, the use of color flow can confirm the diagnosis. It can differentiate the vessels more clearly and reveal additional defects such as VSD or pulmonary stenosis.

Differential diagnosis. Differentiation from D-TGA can be difficult. Complex defects with an L malposition of the great vessels can be difficult to distinguish from a D malposition.

Intrauterine course and prognosis. Most cases of L-TGA that are detected prenatally are a form of isomerism and/or are associated with a third-degree AV block. Both conditions have a high incidence of intrauterine fetal death. In follow-up, therefore, particular attention should be given to the development of fetal hydrops, which is a poor prognostic sign (23). If hydrops is not present and no significant intracardiac anomalies are found, the prognosis is very good. Some infants will not even require treatment by a pediatric cardiologist in the neonatal period.

▬ Truncus Arteriosus

Definition. In this anomaly a common arterial trunk arises from the base of the heart and gives rise to the systemic (aorta), pulmonary, and coronary arteries (Fig. 25.**42**). Several types are recognized. The classification of Collett and Edwards (15), which identifies four types (I–IV) according to the origin of the pulmonary arteries, is commonly used.

Incidence. Truncus arteriosus occurs in approximately 1–1.5% of all live births with a congenital heart defect.

Associated anomalies and chromosomal abnormalities. Possible associated cardiac anomalies include mitral atresia, aortic arch anomalies, and almost complete absence of the interventricular septum, creating a single ventricle. Truncus arteriosus is more common in the offspring of diabetic women (19). Extracardiac anomalies are found in 30% of cases, often in connection with a syndrome such as DiGeorge syndrome (molecular genetics!) or with midline defects. When a truncus arteriosus is found, therefore, a standard chromosome analysis is not enough and should be supplemented by a search for rare molecular genetic anomalies (CATCH 22) using the FISH technique.

Ultrasound Diagnosis

B-mode image. Truncus arteriosus can be diagnosed in the B-mode image by defining the origin of the great vessels (planes 2 and 3), but this is difficult. Either the VSD or possible associated anomalies are the dominant findings in the four-chamber view. In the five-chamber view, the dilated arterial trunk (first thought to be the aorta) is clearly seen overriding the defect in the ventricular septum (8). A careful search for the pulmonary trunk in plane III or IV will suggest the more common diagnosis of pulmonary atresia with a VSD. But the patient examiner will be able to define the root of a small-caliber pulmonary trunk arising from the truncus arteriosus (in type I). This finding is confirmed with color Doppler.

Color and spectral Doppler. Color Doppler is of major value in this anomaly. Initially the findings resemble those seen in the tetralogy of Fallot ("Y" configuration, see above). But color Doppler in type I cases can demonstrate the origin of the pulmonary trunk from the truncus along with antegrade flow. In the five-chamber view, it is common to observe turbulence over the truncal valve, and valvular insufficiency may already be evident in utero.

Differential diagnosis. Differentiation is mainly required from defects with an overriding aorta such as the tetralogy of Fallot, pulmonary atresia with a VSD, and double-outlet right ventricle with pulmonary atresia (Table 25.**11**).

Intrauterine course and prognosis. Because the valve of the arterial trunk is dysplastic and often shows regurgitant flow, the fetus should be watched for early signs of heart failure during follow-up.

▬ Isomerism, Situs Inversus (Heterotaxia Syndromes)

Definition. This group includes the following conditions:
- Partial situs inversus
- Complete situs inversus
- Left isomerism (formerly known as polysplenia syndrome) (32, 33)
- Right isomerism (formerly known as asplenia syndrome) (32, 33)

A common feature of these anomalies is a tendency to find a symmetrical arrangement of the asymmetrically formed organs—i.e., a mirror-image arrangement of structures between the two sides of the chest and abdomen.

Incidence. A malrotation anomaly is present in approximately 4% of all live-born infants with a congenital heart defect.

Associated cardiac and extracardiac anomalies. By definition, isomerism denotes the presence of multiple associated cardiac and extracardiac (e.g., visceral) malformations (Tables 25.**14**, 25.**15**). In fetuses with heterotaxia (right and left isomerism), an association with aneuploidy is very rare (4). Malrotation anomalies have occasionally been found in children with trisomy 13. Some forms are thought to have an autosomal-recessive mode of inheritance (25% recurrence risk), and therefore an aggregation of malrotation anomalies is found in marriages between relatives. Malrotation anomalies are also more common in the fetuses of diabetic mothers.

Ultrasound Diagnosis

B-mode image. A malrotation anomaly is usually easy to detect, for a systematic analysis will quickly disclose the commonly associated anomalous positions of the heart and stomach (Tables 25.**6**, 25.**7**). The

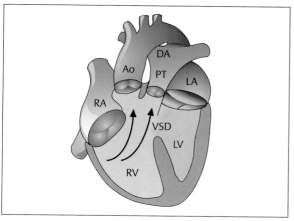

35

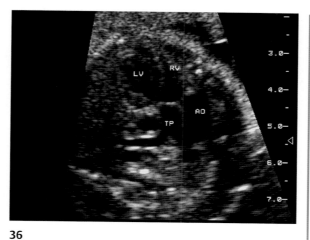

36

Double-outlet right ventricle

Fig. 25.**35** With a double-outlet right ventricle, both the aorta and pulmonary trunk arise from the right ventricle. The relative positions of the vessels are highly variable (modified from [31]).

Fig. 25.**36** Double-outlet right ventricle (DORV), 26 weeks. The apical view shows both the pulmonary trunk and aorta arising from the right ventricle and running parallel to each other.

Fig. 25.**37** Double-outlet right ventricle (DORV). Color Doppler shows the parallel origins of both vessels from the right ventricle.

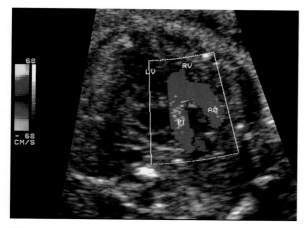

37

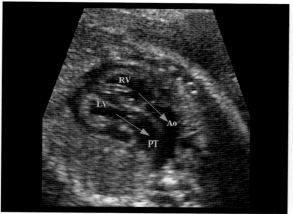

38

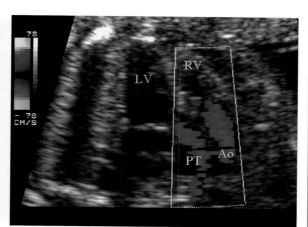

39

Transposition of the great arteries

Fig. 25.**38** Complete transposition of the great arteries (D-TGA), 25 weeks. When the ventriculoarterial connection is evaluated in a lateral scan, both vessels show a typical parallel course ("double-barreled" pattern). The aorta arises from the right ventricle and the pulmonary trunk from the left ventricle. Both semilunar valves are visualized in one plane.

Fig. 25.**39** Complete transposition of the great arteries (D-TGA), 25 weeks. Color Doppler demonstrates the typical parallel pattern of the two great vessels.

Fig. 25.**40** Origin of the pulmonary arteries in a fetus with D-TGA, 25 weeks. The standard short-axis view cannot be obtained, and the aorta is anterior to the pulmonary trunk. Rpa = right pulmonary artery, Lpa = left pulmonary artery.

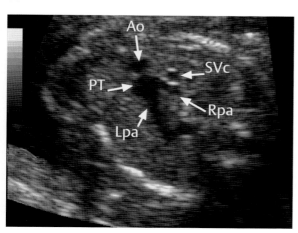

40

Fig. 25.**41** Schematic representation of D-TGA and L-TGA.

a Diagram of a normal fetal heart (patent ductus arteriosus). There are normal connections between the right and left atria and the right and left ventricles, which in turn have normal connections with the pulmonary trunk (PT) and the aorta. "Normal," then, refers to a situation of atrioventricular (AV) and ventriculoarterial concordance. The right-sided anatomic structures of the heart are shown in blue, the left-sided structures in red.

b In D-TGA, the atria connect normally with their ventricles but the great vessels arise from the wrong ventricles (the aorta from the RV, the pulmonary trunk from the LV). This creates a situation of AV concordance and ventriculoarterial discordance.

c In L-TGA, the right atrium connects to the LV and the left atrium to the RV. As in the D form, the LV is connected to the pulmonary trunk and the RV to the aorta. This creates a situation of AV and ventriculoarterial discordance. The aorta and pulmonary trunk are parallel to each other (adapted and modified from [30]).

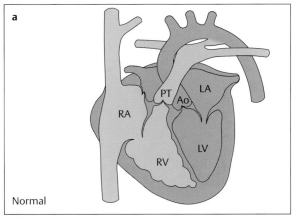

41 a

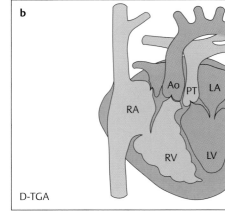

41 b

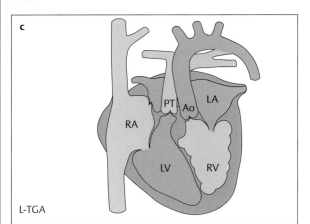

41 c

Truncus arteriosus

Fig. 25.**42** Diagram of truncus arteriosus (type I). A large vascular trunk (TAC = truncus arteriosus communis) overrides the VSD. The aorta and pulmonary trunk arise from the common trunk.

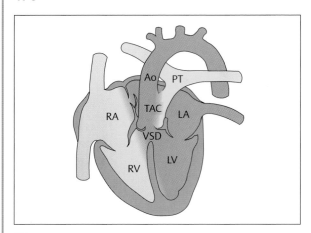

42

Heterotaxia syndromes

Fig. 25.**43** Heterotaxia syndrome. The stomach (ST) is located on the right side of the upper abdomen in this fetus. The aorta is to the left of the spine. Just to the right of the spine (not anterolateral), the inferior vena cava persists as the azygos vein (AZ). The findings are consistent with a polysplenia syndrome (left isomerism).

Fig. 25.**44** Four-chamber view of the fetus in Fig. 25.**43** demonstrates a complete AV canal (curved arrows). The aorta is visible behind the heart on the left side, and to the right is the dilated azygos vein (see also Fig. 25.**45**).

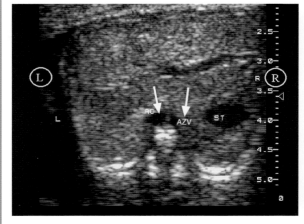

43

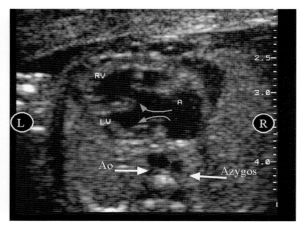

44

presence of bradycardia (AV block) may also be a sign of left isomerism.

A scan of the upper abdomen showing the course of the hepatic veins and inferior vena cava is the most important B-mode tool for diagnosing a malrotation anomaly.

- **In situs solitus,** the aorta is to the left of the spine and the inferior vena cava (IVC) is to the right of the spine.
- In **situs inversus,** there is a mirror-image arrangement of both vessels.
- In **right isomerism** (asplenia), the aorta and IVC are always on the same side, and the IVC is usually anterior to the aorta.
- In **left isomerism** (polysplenia), the hepatic IVC is frequently absent. Venous blood from the periphery flows through the azygos vein (azygos continuation) or hemiazygos vein on the right or left side of the spine (Figs. 25.**43**, 25.**44**) behind the aorta and enters the superior vena cava, which is on the left or right side (Fig. 25.**45**), or flows directly into the atrium. Often the hepatic veins open directly into the right atrium.

Although these findings are not consistently present in all heterotaxia syndromes or malrotation anomalies, they are still the most reliable suggestive signs in echocardiography. On moving to the next planes, the examiner should adhere strictly to a segmental analysis, for as Tables 25.**14** and 25.**15** indicate, there is no typical heart defect in this group. The precise differentiation of a heart defect in isomerism continues to be one of the greatest challenges in fetal echocardiography.

Color and spectral Doppler. Color Doppler is of major importance in assessing the vascular anatomy of the heart. If the IVC is not visualized, color Doppler can demonstrate a persistent azygos vein running parallel to the aorta to its site of termination (Fig. 25.**45**). The hepatic veins and their connection can also be clearly defined as well as the pulmonary veins. When a malposition is present, color Doppler makes it easier to distinguish the aorta and pulmonary trunk and diagnose stenoses and atresias.

Differential diagnosis. A false-positive diagnosis of situs inversus is most often due to faulty placement of the transducer or confusion of the sides in breech- and vertex-presenting fetuses. Also, the detection of an abnormal organ position should always prompt consideration of an intrathoracic mass (diaphragmatic defect, unilateral pulmonary atresia, lung cysts, etc.) (Tables 25.**6**, 25.**7**).

It can be difficult to distinguish partial situs inversus (Fig. 25.**46**) or complete situs inversus from isomerism, but this distinction is important owing to the better prognosis of situs inversus. The anomalous venoatrial connection is the key feature in differentiating these conditions. Differentiating between the forms of isomerism is described above.

Intrauterine course and prognosis. The course is variable, depending on the nature of the anomaly. With complete situs inversus, no adverse hemodynamic effects can be detected prenatally or postnatally. By contrast, left isomerism with a complex cardiac anomaly and AV block may be associated with fetal hydrops and intrauterine death. A detailed analysis is of major importance, therefore, and venous Doppler ultrasound can be a very helpful tool for prenatal surveillance.

Table 25.14 Most common findings in right isomerism (adapted from [32])

Right isomerism (asplenia)	
Association with a heart defect	Almost 100%
Stomach	Left, right, or central
Liver	Often central, asymmetrical
Aorta and inferior vena cava	Usually on the same side (left or right)
Dextrocardia	40%
Anomalous pulmonary venous return	Almost 100%
Bilateral superior vena cava	Almost 100%
AV canal	85%
Single ventricle	50%
TGA	60%
Pulmonary stenosis or atresia	70%

Table 25.15 Most common findings in left isomerism (adapted from [32])

Left isomerism (asplenia)	
Association with AV block (bradycardia)	Frequent
Interruption of inferior vena cava and persistence as azygos (or hemiazygos) vein	70%
Azygos (or hemiazygos) vein dilated	Posterior to the aorta
Aorta	Centrally locatede
Stomach and liver	Left or right
ASD	35%
AV canal	43%
TGA, DORV	20%
Dextrocardia	35%
Bilateral superior vena cavae	50%

Anomalies of Systemic and Pulmonary Venous Return

Total and Partial Anomalous Pulmonary Venous Return

Definition. Total or partial anomalous pulmonary venous return (TAPVR or PAPVR) is present when all or some of the pulmonary veins drain into the right atrium or into the venae cavae that enter the right atrium.

Incidence. These anomalies occur in approximately 1.5% of all live births with a congenital heart defect.

Associated anomalies and chromosomal abnormalities. The anomaly may be isolated but is more commonly associated with right or left isomerism (approximately 100% in asplenia syndrome, 70% in polysplenia syndrome). Also, it is common to find TAPVR associated with atrial septal defects or an AV canal. Other associated cardiac anomalies include pulmonary vein stenoses. Extracardiac anomalies mainly involve the lung and gastrointestinal tract.

Ultrasound Diagnosis

B-mode image. Prenatal diagnosis is extremely difficult in the absence of associated cardiac anomalies. Possible suggestive signs include a left atrium that is somewhat smaller than the right atrium or the presence of a persistent left superior vena cava (Figs. 25.**47**, 25.**48**). There are cases where the pulmonary veins are clearly defined in the standard four-chamber view (Fig. 25.**49**), but color Doppler is generally more rewarding than the B-mode scan.

Color and spectral Doppler. Often the pulmonary veins are plainly defined with color Doppler at a low velocity setting (low PRF), and different types of anomalous drainage patterns can be identified. This requires an examiner who is very experienced in the Doppler interrogation of slow flows and the interpretation of subtle findings. It is hoped that these anomalies can be detected by the consistent, systematic visualization of the pulmonary veins with color Doppler (17).

Differential diagnosis. The pulmonary arteries and veins close to the atria are apt to be confused in the B-mode image, and so the diagnosis should rely on color Doppler. When the right pulmonary veins are evaluated on an oblique plane, they are easily confused with the hepatic veins. In cases of isomerism, moreover, anatomic orientation is often very complicated, making it difficult to identify and evaluate the pulmonary veins.

Intrauterine course and prognosis. The emphasis in follow-up is on associated cardiac anomalies. There has been no experience with isolated forms of fetal TAPVR. But since the fetal pulmonary circulation as a whole does not affect hemodynamics, there should be no circulatory compromise during the prenatal period.

Persistent Left Superior Vena Cava (PLSVC)

Definition. This condition, known also as left superior vena cava (LSVC), is the most common venous anomaly. It results from a failure of obliteration of the left cardinal vein. The vessel is located anterior to the aortic arch, often running in front of the ductus arteriosus on the left side (Fig. 25.**48**). It usually bypasses the left atrium (Fig. 25.**47**), opens into the coronary sinus from below, and drains directly into the right atrium. In rare cases it opens directly into the left atrium, and in approximately 20% of cases the right superior vena cava is not present.
Associated anomalies. PLSVC may be associated with other cardiac anomalies (e.g., heterotaxia syndromes or anomalous pulmonary venous return), but its occurrence as an isolated anomaly is not uncommon.

Ultrasound diagnosis. PLSVC is relatively easy to diagnose in fetal echocardiography (when it is considered) by demonstrating a venous vessel on the left side wall of the left atrium in the four-chamber view (Fig. 25.**47**) or by demonstrating a "fourth" vessel with venous flow adjacent to the ductus arteriosus in the three-vessel view (plane V) (Fig. 25.**48**). Not infrequently, the right atrium appears slightly broader than the left atrium in the four-chamber view.

▬ *Cardiomyopathies*

Definition. This group includes a number of heart diseases whose common feature is an impairment of myocardial contractility.

Etiology and pathogenesis. Cardiomyopathies have a broad etiologic spectrum ranging from infectious diseases to congenital metabolic storage diseases. In most cases, however, the cause is not discovered and the cardiomyopathy is described as "idiopathic."

Forms. It is not uncommon in prenatal diagnosis to find decreased myocardial contractility in association with fetal hydrops (immune or nonimmune). This *secondary cardiomyopathy* can aggravate the severity of the hydrops as a result of cardiac failure. These cases require dif-

ferentiation from the primary idiopathic forms, which may present either as *hypertrophic* or *dilatative cardiomyopathy.* In the hypertrophic form, the myocardium is thickened and has a very narrow lumen. But in the dilatative form, the heart appears "stretched out" and remains compensated until a relatively late stage. Dilatative cardiomyopathy is usually manifested by cardiomegaly.

Prognosis. In our experience, both forms have an unfavorable prognosis. In cases that have a known cause such as arrhythmia, volume overload (e.g., acceptor in fetofetal transfusion syndrome), pressure overload (e.g., constriction of the ductus arteriosus, IUGR), or diabetes mellitus, the prognosis is determined chiefly by the primary disease.

▬ *Cardiac Tumors*

On the whole, cardiac tumors very rarely occur as congenital anomalies. The majority are benign and consist of rhabdomyomas (60% of cases) or teratomas (20%). Cardiac rhabdomyomas may be multiple (Fig. 25.**50**), often affect the interventricular septum, and sometimes undergo spontaneous remission. They may be detected incidentally in the fetus, but often there are associated supraventricular extrasystoles or nonimmune hydrops due to circulatory obstruction by the tumor.

Associated anomalies and chromosomal abnormalities. Although most cardiac tumors occur in isolation, rhabdomyoma is an exception: 50–90% of these tumors are a symptom of tuberous sclerosis (Bourneville–Pringle disease), which is associated with mental retardation and seizures. This disease is usually inherited as an autosomal-dominant trait, but it also has a high spontaneous mutation rate. Thus, genetic family counseling is indicated whenever a cardiac tumor is detected prenatally, and the fetus should be examined sonographically for CNS abnormalities (dilatation of cerebral ventricles) and renal tumors.

Fetal Arrhythmias

Incidence and significance. Arrhythmias are among the most common "cardiologic" symptoms in fetuses, with an incidence between 0.2% and 2%. Transient fetal arrhythmias are also a common finding (10%) in pregnancies that are evaluated by auscultation, CTG, or ultrasound. As a result, fetal arrhythmias are one of the most frequent indications for fetal echocardiographic evaluation. Except in fetuses with a heart block, arrhythmias are rarely associated with cardiac anomalies (< 5% of cases).

Cause, course, and prognosis. Cardiac arrhythmias are a nonhomogeneous group that can vary greatly in their cause, course, and prognosis, and so a differentiated approach is recommended. An accurate diagnostic workup is essential, relying particularly on prenatal M-mode and Doppler examination (only the QRS complex can be recorded in the fetal ECG).

Special Aspects in the Analysis of Fetal Arrhythmias

The examiner who evaluates a fetus with an arrhythmia should keep in mind several aspects that distinguish fetal from postnatal arrhythmias:
- **Immaturity.** The development of the heart, like that of other fetal organs, is not yet completed at birth. The physiologic immaturity of the impulse formation and conduction system in the fetal heart may be manifested by arrhythmias. Most of these arrhythmias are caused by ectopic stimuli in the atria or ventricles, which are registered as extrasystoles.

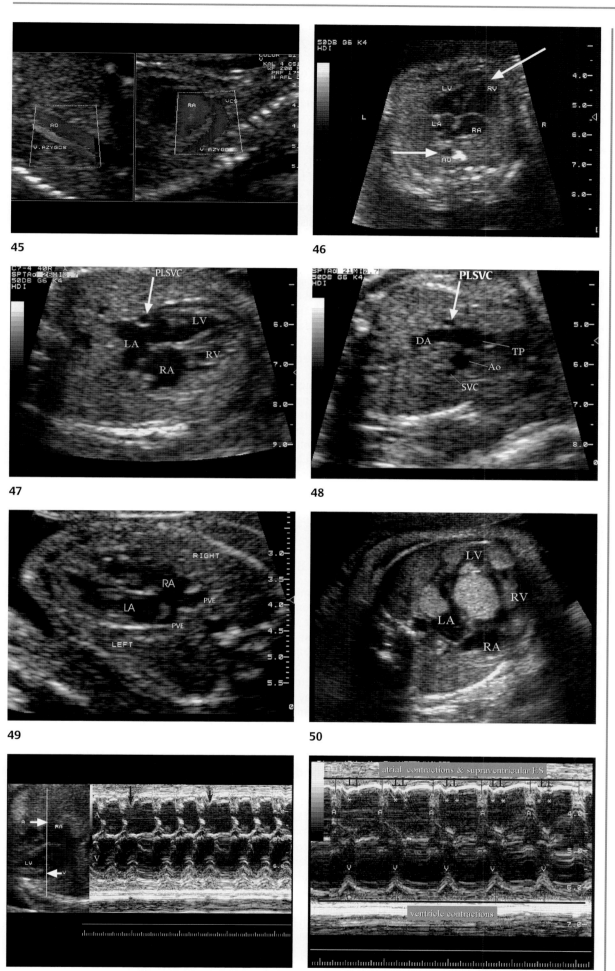

45

46

47

48

49

50

51

52

Fig. 25.**45** Same fetus as in Figs. 25.**43** and 25.**44**. Left: Color Doppler shows the aorta and azygos vein side-by-side in the longitudinal scan. Right: Another longitudinal scan shows the termination of the azygos vein at the superior vena cava.

Fig. 25.**46** Dextrocardia. In this fetus the descending aorta is found to the left of the spine (lower arrow) but the cardiac apex points to the right (upper arrow). Only about one-third of the heart is located in the left hemithorax.

Anomalies of systemic and pulmonary venous return

Fig. 25.**47** Persistent left superior vena cava (PLSVC) in the four-chamber view. The vessel appears in transverse section directly adjacent to the left atrium.

Fig. 25.**48** Same fetus as in Fig. 25.**47**. The persistent vessel is seen more clearly in the "three-vessel view" (plane 5), appearing as a fourth vessel to the left of the pulmonary trunk. Aorta and (right) superior vena cava (SVC).

Fig. 25.**49** Termination of the pulmonary veins at the right atrium in total anomalous pulmonary venous return. Associated right isomerism was detected initially.

Cardiac tumors

Fig. 25.**50** Multiple echogenic cardiac tumors (rhabdomyomas). Tuberous sclerosis should be considered when this type of lesion is found.

Fetal arrhythmias

Fig. 25.**51** Supraventricular extrasystole. The M-mode cursor is positioned in the four-chamber view so that it passes through a ventricle (below), the interventricular septum, and an atrium (above). The M-mode tracing shows two supraventricular extrasystoles in the atrium (arrows), which are not conducted to the ventricle.

Fig. 25.**52** Blocked extrasystoles, 23 weeks. The M-mode cursor is aligned across the right ventricle (below) and right atrium (above). The extrasystoles from the atrium reach the impulse conduction system of the ventricle while it is still refractory, and so only the next atrial beat is conducted.

- **Structural anomalies.** When evaluating a fetal arrhythmia, the examiner should always consider that a structural anomaly in the heart may be the underlying cause. This means that fetal echocardiography should be performed without delay.
- **Vagal dominance.** It is not unusual to find transient bradycardia, especially in the second trimester, as a manifestation of vagal dominance. Every examiner is familiar with episodes (e.g., at about 20 weeks) in which the fetal heartbeat stops briefly during the ultrasound examination and then slowly resumes a few seconds later.
- **Short circuits.** Connective-tissue development in the atrioventricular (AV) plane is not yet complete in the fetus, and this can cause ventricular contractions to be initiated via "short circuits" between the atria and ventricles. In some cases, for example, a supraventricular extrasystole can trigger circuitous excitations via these accessory pathways (or even through the AV node itself). This reentry mechanism in the fetus can trigger paroxysmal tachycardia, which when sustained can lead to cardiac failure.
- **Maternal factors.** It should be kept in mind that the fetus is a "patient within a patient." When seeking the cause of a fetal arrhythmia, therefore, the examiner should also look for maternal factors that could adversely affect the fetal heart rhythm. For example, maternal diseases such as systematic lupus erythematosus, diabetes mellitus, hyperthyroidism, as well as smoking, alcohol consumption, and the use of (cardioactive) drugs can provoke fetal cardiac arrhythmias.

Differential Diagnosis of Fetal Arrhythmias as a Basis for Optimum Management

Before deciding whether a detected fetal arrhythmia should be treated, the examiner should first exclude a structural heart defect using B-mode ultrasound and then accurately classify the arrhythmia using the M-mode technique (7). In this technique the M-mode cursor is positioned under B-mode guidance to produce a simultaneous tracing of heart activity as a function of time. The cursor should be placed so that it passes through an atrium and a ventricle (or across a semilunar valve). This makes it possible to analyze atrioventricular (AV) conduction and determine whether it is impaired (AV block). The high temporal resolution in the M-mode tracing also allows precise measurement of the heart rate, as the examiner cannot distinguish between paroxysmal tachycardia and atrial flutter by using B-mode alone. Modern color-encoded M-mode echocardiography is useful both for classifying the arrhythmia and analyzing its hemodynamic effects.

Three groups. Fetal arrhythmias are divided into three groups based on practical criteria:
- The large group of extrasystoles (85% of all arrhythmias): the supraventricular and ventricular forms with a basal heart rate in the normal range.
- The group of sustained bradycardias (incidence 5–10%), in which the basal heart rate is lower than 100 bpm.
- The group of sustained tachycardias (incidence 10%), in which the basal heart rate is higher than 190 bpm.

▬ Extrasystoles

Incidence and etiology. Extrasystoles are by far the most common type of fetal arrhythmia, with an incidence between 80% and 90%. Most extrasystoles are supraventricular (Fig. 25.**51**). Ventricular extrasystoles are much less common. Extrasystoles are usually attributed to the immaturity of the impulse formation and conduction system in the fetal heart. This immaturity also makes the heart susceptible to exogenous agents (including beta mimetic drugs). Sinus arrhythmias are also observed in association with fetal movements (including hiccups). Although extrasystoles are an innocuous finding, a morphologic cause is detectable in 1–2% of cases.

Prognosis. This type of arrhythmia has a very good prognosis (except for cases with a heart defect). The condition resolves spontaneously in most fetuses, and in most other cases it ceases during the initial weeks after birth.

In 1–2% of cases, however, this harmless arrhythmia can progress to sustained paroxysmal tachycardia, most likely through a reentry mechanism (58). This poses a danger of cardiac decompensation with the development of NIHF. For this reason, fetuses with extrasystoles should be examined at regular intervals. Prenatal treatment is unnecessary owing to the good prognosis, and follow-ups can be conducted on an ambulatory basis.

▬ Bradyarrhythmias

Three principal subgroups are distinguished antenatally:
- Blocked atrial extrasystoles
- Sinus bradycardia
- Congenital heart block (second or third degree AV block)

Blocked Atrial Extrasystoles

When, following a normal excitation pattern, an atrial extrasystole reaches an AV node that is still in a refractory state, the impulse will not be transmitted to the ventricles, and ventricular systole will not occur until the arrival of the next normal impulse (Fig. 25.**52**). When these extrasystoles alternate with sinus beats, the heart appears to be contracting in a bradycardiac rhythm. Although this arrhythmia is perceived as bradycardia on auscultation, it is actually a type of extrasystole from an electrophysiologic standpoint. In any case, it is a rare condition that usually resolves spontaneously, has a good prognosis, and requires maternal (transplacental) digitalis therapy only when it persists.

Sinus Bradycardia

The most common form is a transient, harmless bradycardia that occurs in the second trimester as an expression of vagal dominance. Sinus bradycardia very rarely occurs as a persistent, sustained bradycardia, which is usually a preterminal event caused by fetal hypoxia. This category would include intrapartum bradycardias that necessitate a cesarean delivery. Sinus bradycardia has also occasionally been found in fetuses with heterotaxia syndromes (e.g., polysplenia). Transient sinus bradycardia may be induced by compression of the skull or umbilical cord. Not infrequently, we have found low basal fetal heart rates of 90–110 bpm in women who are heavy smokers.

Complete Congenital Heart Block (CCHB, Second- or Third-Degree AV Block)

Definition. In fetuses with a third-degree heart block, the atria beat at a normal rate (120–160 bpm) while the ventricles beat at their own (bradycardiac) rate with no evidence of AV conduction (Fig. 25.**53**). In the much less common second-degree heart block, an impulse is conducted to the ventricles at every other atrial contraction (which occur at equal intervals) (Fig. 25.**54**). These forms often progress to a third-degree heart block.

Association with heart defects. Among the arrhythmias, AV blocks have the highest association with heart defects, which are present in up to 40% (!) of cases (7). Most of these defects consist of morphologic abnormalities at the AV level, particularly AV canal, AV discordance with corrected TGA, and heterotaxia syndrome (e.g., polysplenia syndrome).

Association with maternal connective-tissue diseases. If a structural heart defect is not found in the B-mode image, an immediate search should be made for a maternal connective-tissue disease. The most frequent of these disorders are systemic lupus erythematosus (SLE) and Sjögren syndrome, in which anti-Ro or anti-La antibodies (also called anti-SS-A or anti-SS-B antibodies) can be detected in the maternal serum (7). Etiologically, it has been found that these IgG autoantibodies are able to cross the placenta, enter the fetal circulation, and bind to the impulse conduction system at the AV level. There they incite a nonspecific inflammation that heals with fibrous tissue transformation, creating an irreversible break within the conduction system. It is interesting that the pregnant women are often (still) asymptomatic at this stage, so that the detection of fetal CCHB and maternal antibodies leads to the diagnosis of SLE.

Prognosis. The prognosis of CCHB depends on its etiology. Fetuses with a cardiac malformation are prone to intrauterine cardiac decompensation with the development of NIHF leading to the death of the fetus or neonate. By contrast, fetuses with CCHB based on maternal SLE have a good prognosis unless the fetus develops nonimmune hydrops due to the connective-tissue disease.

Treatment. There is disagreement whether CCHB is accessible to prenatal medical treatment with orciprenaline or other beta-mimetic drugs. A major consideration is whether it is desirable to increase the ventricular rate. In cases with a maternal connective-tissue disease, we have had good results with serial plasmapheresis and corticosteroid therapy.

▬ Tachyarrhythmias

Three principal subgroups are distinguished:
- Sinus tachycardia
- Paroxysmal supraventricular tachycardia
- Atrial flutter
  Ventricular tachycardia is extremely rare.

Sinus Tachycardia

With a basal heart rate in the range of 180 to 205 bpm, a CTG with good variability can still be recorded.

Etiology. Sinus tachycardia can occur in response to exogenous factors such as tocolytic therapy with beta mimetics, infection (fever, chorioamnionitis!), and hyperthyroidism. Persistent accelerations are occasionally seen in the CTG of a particularly active fetus.

Treatment. Causal treatment can produce remission, but follow-ups are still necessary to watch for potential complications or a recurrence. Antiarrhythmic therapy is not indicated in these cases, and the arrhythmia itself has a favorable prognosis.

Paroxysmal Supraventricular Tachycardia

Etiology and pathogenesis. Paroxysmal supraventricular tachycardia (heart rate 210–300 bpm) is usually caused by a reentry mechanism in which extrasystoles, usually of supraventricular origin, set up circuitous, repetitive excitations via accessory conduction pathways or through the AV node itself. Since the heart responds to the fastest pacemaker, the reentrant impulses cause it to beat at a very rapid rate, typically between 220 and 260 bpm. Often the examiner notices a sudden onset of the reentry tachycardia, and in some cases it may cease spontaneously. M-mode ultrasound can clearly document this type of arrhythmia and differentiate it from other forms (Fig. 25.**55**).

Prognosis. Paroxysmal supraventricular tachycardia poses a significant hazard to the fetus, because if it persists, it can lead to heart failure with the development of nonimmune hydrops. In a number of cases, however, the tachycardia is not detected until the fetus is being evaluated for nonimmune hydrops. It is believed that heart failure will not develop if the tachycardia is interrupted by periods with a normal heart rate, even if these periods are of only a few minutes" duration.

Treatment. These fetuses are considered to be at very high risk, and there is an urgent need for treatment. Intrauterine therapy aimed at pharmacologic cardioversion and the clearing of fluid collections should be instituted without delay. Since earlier treatment means a better chance of success, these fetuses should be referred at once to the nearest prenatal center that is experienced in this area. The prognosis in such cases is very good, with less than a 10% mortality rate. Today, fetal tachycardia belongs to the diseases that can be treated antenatally with considerable success.

To interrupt the reentry circuit, the antiarrhythmic drug should suppress the formation of extrasystoles, delay AV conduction, and prolong the refractory period of the AV node. The prenatal drug of choice is digoxin, which also improves myocardial contractility owing to its positive inotropic effect.

Second-line drugs include a number of antiarrhythmic agents, most notably verapamil and flecainide (e.g., in NIHF) (3). Further details on the treatment of fetal arrhythmias can be found in the specialized literature (3, 7) (Fig. 25.**57**) (see also Chapter 47).

Atrial Flutter

Etiology and pathogenesis. Atrial flutter (> 300 bpm) is much less common than the other tachyarrhythmias. It is caused by a reentry circuit at the atrial level. An atrial rate of 400–480 bpm is often found in association with a 2 : 1 to 4 : 1 AV block, and so the ventricular rate may be 200–240 bpm or less (Fig. 25.**56**). Atrial flutter is indistinguishable from paroxysmal supraventricular tachycardia (PSVT) in the B-mode image, and so M-mode is used to count the rates of the atria and ventricles and evaluate AV conduction.

Prognosis and treatment. Like PSVT, atrial flutter can lead to nonimmune hydrops culminating in fetal death. In the absence of a complex cardiac anomaly, fetal therapy should be instituted without delay. With few exceptions, the treatment is the same as for PSVT (see above).

▬ Conclusions

In closing, it should be emphasized that a knowledge of the basic pathophysiology of fetal arrhythmias and the optimum use of ultrasound in the setting of fetal echocardiography are essential for making a precise diagnosis and differential diagnosis. The appropriate management is decided only after the arrhythmia has been classified. Recommended approaches to the management of fetal arrhythmias are reviewed in Tables 25.**16**–25.**19**. The indications for treatment and the details of therapy should be decided on an individual basis. Ultimately, the lack of fetal response to many otherwise effective cardiac drugs emphasizes the need to develop new drugs that are tailored specifically to the fetal heart.

Table 25.**16**   Steps to follow when a fetal arrhythmia has been diagnosed

> ➤ Check fetal anatomy
> ➤ Exclude a cardiac anomaly
> ➤ Exclude NIHF
> ➤ Use M-mode to diagnose and classify the arrhythmia
> ➤ Exclude maternal disease, drug use, and other exogenous factors
> ➤ Refer to a specialized center

Table 25.**17**   Management of irregular cardiac arrhythmias

> ➤ Supraventricular or ventricular extrasystole?
> ➤ Exclude cardiac anomalies (including foramen ovale prolapse)
> ➤ Discontinue caffeine, nicotine, alcohol, and "cardiac drugs"
> ➤ Check weekly for potential complications of tachycardia (reentry!)

Table 25.**18**   Management of bradyarrhythmias

Use M-mode to evaluate atrioventricular conduction

Management after diagnosis
> ➤ Sinus bradycardia
>   • Intermittent? Vagal dominance, immaturity
>   • Persistent? Possible hypoxia? Doppler, CTG, induction of labor?
> ➤ Blocked atrial extrasystoles (see Table 25.17)
>   • Transplacental digoxin therapy rarely necessary
> ➤ Complete congenital heart block (third-degree heart block)
>   • Exclude cardiac anomaly!!! (isomerism with AV discordance, AV canal, etc.)
>   • Maternal connective tissue disease? (anti-Ro antibodies?)

Check weekly for signs of nonimmune hydrops (= poor prognosis)

May consider prophylactic beta-mimetic agent, corticosteroids

Table 25.**19**   Management of tachyarrhythmias

> ➤ Classify the tachycardia using M-mode
> ➤ Hospitalize the patient
> ➤ Exclude NIHF
>
> ➤ Sinus tachycardia? Identify and treat the cause (maternal or fetal)
>
> ➤ Paroxysmal supraventricular tachycardia or atrial flutter
>   (with or without AV block)
>   • Check indication for intrauterine therapy
>   • Consult with pediatric cardiologist and neonatologist
>   • Induce lung maturity
>   • Select drug therapy. First choice: digoxin. If no response, add a medication (see Chapter 47)
>   • Select mode of therapy: transplacental; with NIHF, direct therapy + plasma assay (rarely indicated today)

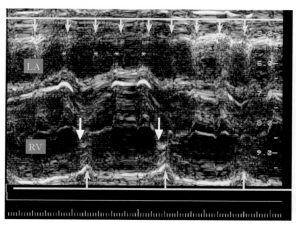

53

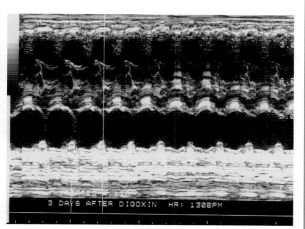

AV BLOCK II IN ANTI RO AB

54

Fig. 25.**53** Congenital complete heart block. In a third-degree atrioventricular heart block, the atria and ventricles beat independently of one another. The M-mode cursor is placed across a ventricle (below) and an atrium (above). The atria (A) show a rate of 130 bpm, while the ventricles (V) have a rate of only 60 bpm. The mother in this case had a previously undiagnosed case of visceral lupus erythematosus (detection of anti-Ro antibodies).

Fig. 25.**54** Second-degree congenital heart block. While the left atrium (LA) shows regular contractions, one ventricular contraction is skipped after every second atrial beat.

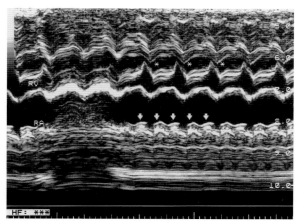

PSVT

55 a

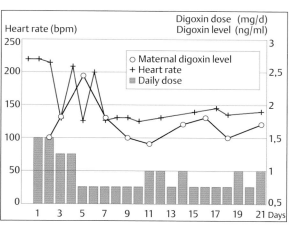

3 DAYS AFTER DIGOXIN   HR: 130BPM

55 b

Fig. 25.**55** Paroxysmal supraventricular tachycardia (PSVT), 30 weeks.

a M-mode cursor across atrium (below) and ventricle. The atria and ventricles in this fetus are beating at a rate of 222/min. Before hydrops developed, this fetus was quickly treated with maternally administered digoxin.

b M-mode tracing three days later demonstrates cardioversion with a rate of 113/min.

56

57

Fig. 25.**56** Atrial flutter with a 2:1 block, 30 weeks. This case was referred for persistent tachycardia. Only M-mode (ventricle above, atrium below) can classify the tachycardia as an atrial flutter with a 2:1 block. The atria are beating at a rate of 460/min (RA and arrows), the ventricles at a rate of 230/min (RV and *). Cardioversion was achieved by means of direct intrauterine digoxin therapy.

Fig. 25.**57** Example of the intrauterine treatment of paroxysmal supraventricular tachycardia, 27 weeks. Days since the start of treatment are shown on the abscissa. Heart rate in beats per minute (bpm) is shown on the left ordinate, and the digoxin levels (ng/mL) and daily digoxin dose (mg/d) are shown on the right ordinate (from [23]).

References

1. Allan, L.D., Chita, S.K., Anderson, R.H., Fagg, N., Crawford, D.C., Tynan, M.J.: Coarctation of the aorta in prenatal life: an echocardiographic, anatomical, and functional study. Brit. Heart J. 59 (1988) 356–360
2. Allan, L.D., Sharland, G.K., Tynan, M.J.: The natural history of the hypoplastic left heart syndrome. Int. J. Cardiol. 25 (1989) 341–343
3. Allan, L.D., Chita, S.K., Sharland, G.K., Maxwell, D., Priestley, K.: Flecainide in the treatment of fetal tachycardias. Brit. Heart J. 65 (1991) 46–48
4. Allan, L.D., Sharland, G.K., Chita, S.K., Lockhart, S., Maxwell, D.J.: Chromosomal anomalies in fetal congenital heart disease. Ultrasound Obstet. Gynecol. 1 (1991) 8–11
5. Allan, L.D., Sharland, G.K.: Prognosis in fetal tetralogy of Fallot. Pediatr. Cardiol. 13 (1992) 1–4
6. Allan, L.D., Sharland, G.K., Milburn, A. et al.: Prospective diagnosis of 1006 consecutive cases of congenital heart disease in the fetus. J. Amer. Coll. Cardiol. 23 (1994) 1452–1458
7. Chaoui, R., Bollmann, R., Hoffmann, H., Göldner, B.: Fetale Echokardiographie: Teil III. Die fetalen Arrhythmien. Zentbl. Gynäkol. 113 (1991) 1335–1350
8. Chaoui, R., Bollmann, R., Zienert, A., Weichold, K., Göldner, B., Semmler, K.: Pränatale Diagnose eines Truncus arteriosus communis (Typ I) bei einer diabetischen Schwangerschaft. Zentbl. Gynäkol. 114 (1992) 198–200
9. Chaoui, R., Heling, K.S., Bollmann, R.: Sonographische Messungen am fetalen Herzen in der Vierkammerblick-Ebene. Geburtsh. Frauenheilk. 54 (1994) 92–97
10. Chaoui, R., Bollmann, R., Göldner, B., Heling, K.S., Tennstedt, C.: Fetal cardiomegaly: echocardiographic findings and outcome in 19 cases. Fetal Diagn. Ther. 92 (1994) 92–104
11. Chaoui, R., Kalache, K., Heling, K.S. et al.: Einsatzmöglichkeiten der fetalen Echokardiographie. In: Schmidt, W. (Hrsg.): Jahrbuch der Gynäkologie und Geburtshilfe 1995/1996. Zülpich: Biermann 1995; S. 51–72
12. Chaoui, R., Gembruch, U.: Zur Epidemiologie der kongenitalen Herzfehler beim Feten und Neugeborenen. Gynäkologe 30 (1997) 165–169
13. Chaoui, R., Tennstedt, C., Göldner, B., Heling, K.S., Awwadeh, H., Bollmann, R.: Pränatale Diagnostik von Herzfehlbildungen mit linksventrikulärer Ausflußtraktobstruktion. Gynäkologe 30 (1997) 240–248
14. Chaoui, R., Tennstedt, C., Göldner, B., Bollmann, R.: Prenatal diagnosis of ventriculo-coronary communications in a second trimester fetus using transvaginal and transabdominal Color-Doppler-sonography. Ultrasound Obstet. Gynecol. 9 (1997) 194–197
15. Collett, R.W., Edwards, J.E.: Persistent truncus arteriosus: a classification according to anatomic types. Surg. Clin. North Amer. 29 (1949) 1245–1255
16. DeVore, G.R., Siassi, B., Platt, L.D.: Fetal echocardiography. VIII. Aortic root dilatation – a marker for tetralogy of Fallot. Amer. J. Obstet. Gynecol. 159 (1988) 129–136
17. DiSessa, T.G., Emerson, D.S., Felker, R.E., Brown, D.L., Cartier, M.S., Becker, J.A.: Anomalous systemic and pulmonary venous pathways diagnosed in utero by ultrasound. J. Ultrasound Med. 9 (1990) 311–317
18. Edwards, J.E., Burchell, H.B.: Congenital tricuspid atresia: a classification. Med. Clin. North Amer. 33 (1947) 1177–1196
19. Ferencz, C., Rubin, J.D., McCarter, R.J., Clark, E.: Maternal diabetes and cardiovascular malformations: Predominance of double outlet right ventricle and truncus arteriosus. Teratology 41 (1990) 319–326
20. Ferencz, C., Rubin, J.D., Loffredo, C.A., Magee, C.A.: Epidemiology of congenital heart disease. The Baltimore-Washington Infant Study 1981–1989. Perspectives in pediatric cardiology. vol. 4. Mount Kisco: Futura Publishing Company 1993
21. Fermont, L., De Geeter, B., Aubry, M.C.: A close collaboration between obstetricians and pediatric cardiologists allows antenatal detection of severe cardiac malformations by two-dimensional echocardiography. In: Doyle, E.F. et al. (eds.): Pediatric cardiology: Proceedings of the Second World Congress. New York (1985), Springer (1985)
22. Fermont, L., Kachaner, J., Sidi, D.: Detection of congenital heart disease: Who and why to screen a population. In: Chervenak, F.A., Isaacson, G.C., Campbell, S. (eds.): Ultrasound in obstetrics and gynecology. Boston: Little, Brown 1993; pp. 1115–1122
23. Gembruch, U., Hansmann, M., Redel, D.A., Bald, R., Knöpfle, G.: Fetal complete heart block: Antenatal diagnosis, significance and management. Eur. J. Obstet. Gynecol. Reprod. Biol. 31 (1989) 9–22
24. Hecher, K.: Was sagen venöse Blutflußkurven über die Funktion des fetalen Herzens aus. Gynäkologe 30 (1997) 222–229
25. Hornberger, L.K., Weintraub, R.G., Pesonen, E. et al.: Echocardiographic study of the morphology and growth of the aortic arch in the human fetus – Observations related to the prenatal diagnosis of coarctation. Circulation 86 (1992) 741–747
26. Hyett, J., Perdu, M., Sharland, G., Snijders, R., Nicolaides, K.: Using fetal nuchal translucency to screen for major congenital cardiac defects at 10–14 weeks of gestation: population based cohort study. BMJ 318 (1999) 81–85
27. Kanzaki, T., Chiba, Y.: Evaluation of the preload condition of the fetus by inferior vena caval blood flow pattern. Fetal Diagn. Ther. 5 (1990) 168–174
28. Sharland, G., Chita, S., Allan, L.: Tricuspid valve dysplasia and displacement in intrauterine life. J. Amer. Coll. Cardiol. 17 (1991) 944–949
29. Sharland, G.K., Chita, S.K., Fagg, N.L. et al.: Left ventricular dysfunction in the fetus: relation to aortic valve anomalies and endocardial fibroelastosis. Brit. Heart J. 66 (1991) 419–424
30. Schumacher, G., Bühlmeyer, K. (Hrsg.): Diagnostik angeborener Herzfehler. Erlangen: Perimed 1989
31. Soto, B., Kassner, G., Baxley, W. (Hrsg.): Imaging of cardiac disorders. New York: Gower Medical Publishing 1992
32. Van Mierop, L.H.S., Gessner, I.H., Schiebler, G.L.: Asplenia and polysplenia syndrome. Birth Defects 8 (1972) 36
33. Van Praagh, R.: The segmental approach to diagnosis in congenital heart disease. Birth Defects 8 (1972) 4–23

26 Anomalies of the Gastrointestinal Tract and Anterior Abdominal Wall

Atresias

▬ *Esophageal Atresia*

Definition. Esophageal atresia is an anomalous closure of the esophagus that may or may not be associated with a tracheoesophageal fistula. Esophageal atresia is divided into four types in the classification of Vogt (137) (Table 26.**1**, see also Fig. 22.**13**).

Incidence. Reports on the incidence of esophageal atresia range between one in 1500 (116) and one in 5000 (51) live births.

Embryology. Esophageal atresia is based on an error in the differentiation of the primitive foregut into the esophagus, trachea, and lung. The disturbance occurs between the fourth and sixth weeks of gestation. Faulty development of the tracheoesophageal septum leads to various forms of esophageal atresia with or without a tracheoesophageal fistula (13).

Pathoanatomic features. A low tracheoesophageal fistula is present in approximately 90% of all cases (129).

Ultrasound features. Diagnosis is difficult with prenatal ultrasound. Polyhydramnios and nonvisualization of the fetal stomach (30, 45, 46) are helpful suggestive signs (Fig. 26.**1**). The detection of a fluid-filled gastric bubble does not exclude the anomaly, however, since fluid can enter the stomach through the low tracheoesophageal fistula that is usually present.

Small stomach and polyhydramnios. A consistently small fetal stomach combined with polyhydramnios is still considered an important suggestive sign of esophageal atresia (79, 96, 127). But since the stomach is not always visualized even in a healthy fetus, serial scans should be obtained.

Upper neck pouch sign. In a few cases, esophageal atresia can be directly visualized by demonstrating a dilated, fluid-filled proximal esophageal pouch: the "upper neck pouch sign" (30) (see Chapter 22). The reported ultrasound detection rate of esophageal atresia ranges from 12.2% (4) to 42% (127).

Differential diagnosis. Empty stomach in a normal fetus.

Associated Anomalies

Polyhydramnios. While polyhydramnios is considered typical of esophageal atresia, it is not a sensitive marker because usually it does not appear until after 24 weeks' gestation (96) and also occurs in numerous other disorders.

Table 26.1   Vogt classification of esophageal atresia (137)

Type	Features
I	Complete atresia without a fistula
II	Segmental atresia without a fistula
III	Segmental atresia with a tracheoesophageal fistula
IV	Tracheoesophageal fistula without atresia ("H fistula")

In 64% of cases (28), esophageal atresia is associated with other anomalies of the gastrointestinal tract, heart, urogenital tract, skeletal system, and CNS (28, 35, 108). Consequently, associated anomalies should be looked for whenever esophageal atresia is suspected.

VACTERL syndrome. Esophageal atresia also occurs as a feature of the VACTERL syndrome (acronym for vertebral defects, anal atresia, cardiac anomalies, tracheoesophageal fistula with esophageal atresia, renal dysplasia, and limb anomalies) (5).

Chromosomal abnormality. Some fetuses with esophageal atresia are found to have an abnormal karyotype (trisomy 18) (86, 110, 127). McKenna et al. (79) found an abnormal karyotype in 38% of fetuses with a nonvisualized stomach and in 4% with a small stomach.

Invasive testing. A chromosomal abnormality should be excluded by amniocentesis or cordocentesis, depending on gestational age.

Prognosis. The prognosis of esophageal atresia is influenced by several factors, most notably the presence of associated anomalies as well as the birth weight (28, 35, 96, 127). The survival rate, ranging from 17% (79) to 97% (126), depends critically on accompanying anomalies and on birth weight.

Prenatal management. In cases with marked polyhydramnios, decompression amniocentesis can be performed to relieve the patient's abdominal discomfort. Spontaneous delivery is preferred and should take place in a perinatal center.

▬ *Intestinal Atresias*

Definition. Congenital closure of a bowel segment.

Incidence. According to Ravitch and Barton (99), the incidence of intestinal atresias is one in 2710 live births.

Etiology. Various etiologic mechanisms are possible, depending on the location of the atresia.

Ultrasound features. Obstructions of the intestinal tract usually do not become evident until after 20 weeks' gestation. They appear sonographically as unusual intra-abdominal cystic masses that are located at various sites, depending on the level of the atresia (Figs. 26.**2**–26.**8**). The development of polyhydramnios also depends on the level of the closure.

Duodenal Atresia

Definition. Congenital closure of the duodenum.

Incidence. Duodenal atresia has a reported incidence of one in 10,000 live births (32).

Embryology. The condition results from a failure of recanalization of the duodenum during early embryonic development (130).

Pathoanatomic features. A total of three types are distinguished:
- Type I: membranous atresia
- Type II: blindly terminating bowel loops interconnected by a fibrous band
- Type III: complete separation of the bowel loops

Membranous atresia is the most common form. Approximately 20–30% of fetuses with duodenal atresia have an annular pancreas (32, 101), in which the pancreas grows around the duodenum and compresses it, eventually occluding the bowel lumen. The cause is anomalous rotation of the duodenum with fusion of the ventral and dorsal pancreatic rudiments.

Ultrasound features. The ultrasound hallmark of duodenal atresia is the "double bubble sign" (44, 45, 52, 74, 84) (Fig. 26.**2a**). This consists of two adjacent, fluid-filled cavities in the upper abdomen: a lateral and usually somewhat larger cavity representing the dilated stomach, and a medial cavity representing the distended proximal duodenum between the pylorus and the stenosis. Since this finding can be mimicked by a scan that cuts two separate portions of a curved stomach (45), duodenal atresia should be suspected only if dual cavities are noted on two planes (longitudinal and transverse) and continue to appear on repeat scans. When the fetal bladder is full, a total of three intra-abdominal cystic areas may be seen in the longitudinal scan (Fig. 26.**3**). Duodenal atresia is accompanied by polyhydramnios in 53% of cases (107).

Differential diagnosis. Differentiation is required from a full stomach and from intra-abdominal cysts: hepatic (63), choledochal (22), renal, ovarian, and peritoneal. Bilateral hydronephrosis can have a similar appearance (Fig. 26.**2b**), but the cystic cavities have a more posterior location in the fetal cross section. Some cases of apparent duodenal atresia may actually be a functional phenomenon caused by intestinal peristalsis (145). Hence, duodenal atresia should be diagnosed only if the same finding is noted on subsequent scans.

Associated anomalies. More than half of fetuses with duodenal atresia have associated cardiac, renal, musculoskeletal, or CNS anomalies (107, 144). Atwell and Klidjian (2) found associated vertebral anomalies in 37% of cases. Trisomy 21 is present in 30–43% of all cases (32, 44, 86, 88, 133).

Invasive testing. Whenever the double bubble sign is found, amniocentesis is indicated for chromosome analysis.

Prognosis. Infants with duodenal atresia have a reported survival rate of 91% (143) to 95% (107). Overall mortality is more closely related to associated anomalies than to birth weight (143). When duodenal atresia is combined with esophageal atresia, the mortality rate is high, exceeding 60% (126).

Prenatal management. Since polyhydramnios is often present, there is a 43% incidence of premature delivery (54). To prevent this, serial amniocentesis should be performed when significant polyhydramnios is present. The goal is a vaginal delivery at a perinatal center that offers the services of a pediatric surgeon.

Jejunal and Ileal Atresia

Definition. Complete distal closure of the small-bowel lumen at the level of the jejunum or ileum.

Incidence. Approximately one in 6000. Most cases are jejunal atresia (40).

Embryology and pathogenesis. Besides incomplete revacuolization during intestinal development, atresias of the jejunum, ileum, and colon may be secondary conditions due to postembolic or postthrombotic ischemia, volvulus, or intussusception (13, 107, 133).

Pathoanatomic features. Different pathomorphologic types of atresia are encountered, analogous to the types of duodenal atresia.

Ultrasound features. Ileal and jejunal atresias (31, 138) usually appear as multiple cystic areas within the fetal abdomen (Figs. 26.**4**–26.**6**). These areas may change their shape during prolonged observation as a result of peristalsis. Most cases are not diagnosed until the third trimester.

Differential diagnosis. When ultrasound raises suspicion of a distal bowel atresia, the differential diagnosis should include other cystic malformations that may arise from the various adjacent organs in the intra- or retroperitoneal space:
- A mesenteric cyst (62)
- Renal cysts or hydronephrosis
- An ovarian cyst (128)
- A cystic sacrococcygeal teratoma with retroperitoneal extension (37)
- A nonobstructive dilatation of the small bowel is found in congenital chloride diarrhea (66) and may also be seen in a preterminal fetus.

Associated anomalies. Associated anomalies are much less common in jejunal atresia (15%) than in duodenal atresia (133). They mainly involve the gastrointestinal tract (73). Trisomy 21 is found in 1% of cases (107). Ileal and jejunal atresias may be associated with polyhydramnios, but this need not occur if there is adequate bowel length available for reabsorbing the swallowed amniotic fluid (71). The more distal the site of the atresia, the less likely it is that polyhydramnios will be present. Polyhydramnios was found in 32% of cases with proximal jejunal atresia versus 17% of cases with distal ileal atresia (73).

Invasive testing. Although an associated chromosomal abnormality is extremely rare, a chromosome analysis should be considered in cases with an early diagnosis of ileal or jejunal atresia.

Prognosis. As with duodenal atresia, the prognosis of distal small-bowel atresias also depends on the birth weight, associated anomalies, and any complications that arise. In rare cases, intrauterine rupture of the bowel may occur leading to meconium peritonitis (11, 114) and a much lower survival rate. An overall mortality rate of 80% was reported for children with meconium ileus in 1966 (23).

Prenatal management. Because ileal and jejunal atresia are surgically correctible conditions, intrauterine diagnosis can provide a sound basis for peripartum management. If a distal small-bowel obstruction does lead to bowel perforation and meconium peritonitis, this usually necessitates an early delivery.

Colonic Atresia

Definition. Colonic atresia is a congenital closure of the large bowel.

Incidence. Colonic atresia is rare (14). It is believed to have an incidence of one in 10,000 to one in 20,000 live births (55).

Etiology and pathogenesis. The defect is believed to result from deficient blood flow and inflammatory changes (92).

Hirschsprung disease. Hirschsprung disease (congenital megacolon) is based on the deficient migration of parasympathetic neuroblasts into the bowel during the 9th to 12th weeks of embryonic development. Depending on the time at which this defect occurs, it results in a terminal colonic segment of variable length in which there is no modu-

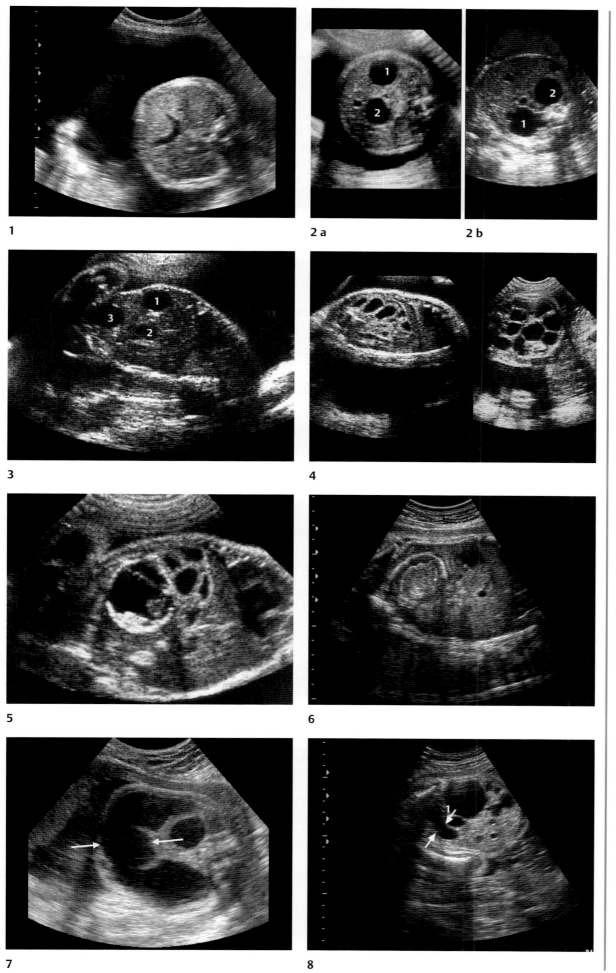

1

2 a   2 b

3   4

5   6

7   8

Atresias

Fig. 26.1 Esophageal atresia, 29 weeks, vertex presentation with the spine to the left. Note the polyhydramnios and nonvisualization of the fetal stomach.

Fig. 26.2 Duodenal atresia.
a Transverse scan through the fetal abdomen at 28 weeks shows the double bubble sign of duodenal atresia. Breech presentation, 1st position. 1 = Stomach, 2 = duodenum.
b Bilateral hydronephrosis, 27 weeks, vertex presentation with the spine to the left. 1 = Left renal pelvis, 2 = right renal pelvis.

Fig. 26.3 Duodenal atresia, 27 weeks, longitudinal scan, vertex presentation. The stomach (1) and duodenum (2) appear as two adjacent cystic structures within the fetal abdomen (double bubble sign). The urinary bladder (3) appears as a third cystic structure in the lower abdomen.

Fig. 26.4 Conspicuous, fluid-filled small bowel loops in jejunal atresia, 36 weeks. Left: longitudinal scan of the fetus in a vertex presentation; Right: transverse scan, vertex presentation with the spine to the right. Polyhydramnios is present.

Fig. 26.5 Ileal atresia with volvulus, vertex presentation, 34 weeks. In addition to several small bowel loops, the longitudinal scan shows a large cystic mass with an echogenic rim. The amniotic fluid volume is normal.

Fig. 26.6 Ileal atresia with volvulus, vertex presentation, 29 weeks, longitudinal scan. The small bowel shows a whorled configuration due to distal volvulus. There is no evidence of polyhydramnios.

Fig. 26.7 Massive dilatation of the large bowel in Hirschsprung disease (diameter = 25 mm) at 35 weeks. Transverse scan, vertex presentation with the spine to the left.

Fig. 26.8 Anal atresia with a dilated rectum (arrows) (diameter = 12 mm) and a multicystic left kidney in VACTERL syndrome. Longitudinal scan at 27 weeks.

lating effect of the intramural parasympathetic plexus on the extramural plexus (105). The predominance of extramural parasympathetic outflow in the aganglionic segment induces a sustained contraction of the annular muscle (= functional stenosis), causing a two-to three-fold dilatation of the prestenotic bowel segment.

Pathoanatomic features. Massive distension of the prestenotic colon segment develops as a secondary change. Morphologically, the disease produces an aganglionic colon segment that may be grossly normal or constricted and is histologically devoid of ganglion cells in the submucous and myenteric plexus (105). In more than 90% of cases, the aganglionic segment extends only to the rectum and distal sigmoid.

Ultrasound features. Marked dilatation of the large bowel is noted within the fetal abdomen (Fig. 26.**7**). Wrobleski and Wesselhoeft described the prenatal ultrasound diagnosis of Hirschsprung disease in 1979 (141).

Differential diagnosis. The dilated colon loops cannot be further differentiated with ultrasound. Dilated, fluid-filled bowel segments are occasionally found even in healthy fetuses, especially during the third trimester (see Chapter 11). As early as 1981, Skovbo and Smith-Jensen (122) described how fluid-filled bowel loops could mimic the ultrasound appearance of gastrointestinal atresia.

Associated anomalies. These are rare and involve other disorders of the gastrointestinal tract. An association with trisomy 21 has been described in Hirschsprung disease (9).

Invasive testing. Karyotyping is recommended to exclude a fetal chromosomal abnormality.

Prognosis. Isolated colonic atresia has a good prognosis, as it is curable by resection of the atretic bowel segment.

Prenatal management. Serial scans should be obtained during the pregnancy to detect any complications that arise. Arrangements should be made for delivery at a perinatal center where a pediatric surgeon is in attendance.

Anal Atresia

Definition. Congenital closure of the anus.

Incidence. One in 2000 to one in 3000 births (81).

Embryology. The condition results from a failure of perforation of the embryonic anal membrane (106).

Pathoanatomic features. The pathoanatomic findings are variable, ranging from simple membranous closure of the anus to a complex cloacal malformation. The rectum may terminate above (40%), level with (15%) or below (40%) the pelvic floor. In the latter cases, the rectum often forms a fistula with the urinary bladder, urethra, or vagina (106).

Ultrasound features. Enlarged, fluid-filled loops of large bowel are found in some fetuses with anal atresia (6) (Fig. 26.**8**). Others have normal-appearing colon loops. Among our own patients, we have had a total of five cases in which we could see no abnormal dilatation of the large bowel. Thus, ultrasound cannot exclude anal atresia with complete confidence.

The ultrasound detection of calcified, hyperechoic, intraluminal meconium is considered another suggestive sign of anorectal atresia (119).

Differential diagnosis. The differential diagnosis includes ovarian cyst, mesenteric cyst, and ureteral dilatation.

Associated anomalies. Anal atresia is commonly associated with other anomalies, often involving the urogenital tract. The presence of a markedly dilated rectum should suggest the possibility of a VACTERL syndrome (Fig. 26.**8**), which is characterized by vertebral anomalies; anal atresia; cardiovascular, tracheoesophageal, and renal anomalies; and limb malformations.

Anal atresia is not usually associated with polyhydramnios, since an adequate length of bowel is available for the absorption of swallowed amniotic fluid (3). But if the anal atresia is one feature of a VACTERL syndrome with esophageal atresia, polyhydramnios may develop.

Other noninvasive tests. Van Rijn et al. (135) found significantly lower serum AFP levels in fetuses with anal atresia than in fetuses with a higher-level obstruction.

Invasive testing. Fetal karyotyping is optional.

Prenatal management. Serial scans should be performed whenever a dilated rectum is found. The infant should be delivered in a perinatal center.

Meconium-Related Diseases

Meconium Ileus

Definition. Meconium ileus refers to an obstruction of the distal small bowel by inspissated meconium.

Incidence. One in 1500 to one in 2000 live births (124).

Etiology and pathogenesis. The most frequent cause of meconium ileus is cystic fibrosis (mucoviscidosis). This autosomal-recessive disorder of the exocrine system, marked by the overproduction of a viscous mucus, is based on a defect in the chloride ion-transporting anion canal. In the bowel, the functional disturbance of the intestinal glandular epithelium leads to the secretion of a very viscous intestinal mucus.

Ultrasound features. Ultrasound in meconium ileus typically shows a dilated ileum with dense internal echoes (29). During the third trimester, meconium ileus may produce increased bowel echogenicity with acoustic shadowing, but there may be no detectable bowel dilation (7) (Fig. 26.**9**).

Differential diagnosis. Echogenic intra-abdominal calcifications are also found in viral infections. A hyperechoic bowel is also seen in trisomy 21 (Fig. 26.**10**). Yaron et al. (142) observed a viral infection (cytomegalovirus, herpes simplex virus, varicella zoster virus, parvovirus B12) in 6.3% of 79 midtrimester fetuses with a hyperechoic bowel, and they found a chromosomal abnormality in 6.3% of the cases. Echogenic meconium may occur as a normal, isolated finding during the third trimester, but it may also be seen in association with meconium ileus, meconium peritonitis, and anorectal anomalies (91).

Associated anomalies. None.

Invasive testing. Cystic fibrosis is confirmed or excluded by chorionic villus sampling with DNA analysis.

Prognosis. Approximately half of fetuses with meconium ileus develop other gastrointestinal complications such as volvulus, bowel perforation, and meconium peritonitis. The overall mortality rate in newborns is high. The cause of death is almost always a severe pulmonary complication.

Prenatal management. If a bowel rupture has not occurred, there is no reason to induce labor. A fetal chromosome analysis should be considered to exclude a chromosomal abnormality.

■ *Meconium Peritonitis*

Definition. A sterile inflammation of the peritoneum following bowel perforation with the extravasation of meconium.

Incidence. One in 35,000 live births (33).

Etiology and pathogenesis. Local vascular insufficiency develops in the bowel wall as a result of small-bowel obstruction, volvulus, intussusception, or mesenteric arterial thrombosis. This leads to necrosis and perforation of the bowel wall, allowing meconium to extravasate into the peritoneal cavity. This causes a severe chemical irritation and inflammation of the peritoneum. It is believed that the stimulation of peritoneal macrophages by the meconium incites a massive inflammatory reaction (65).

Pathoanatomic features. The intrauterine perforation usually occurs in the small bowel (ileum) (47) but may involve the colon (114).

Ultrasound features. The ultrasound findings depend on the underlying disorder, the gestational age, the size of the defect, and the time elapsed since the bowel rupture. A decreased luminal diameter is usually seen following the perforation of dilated bowel loops (47, 102). Ascites and intra-abdominal densities or calcifications (acoustic shadows!) have been described as characteristic ultrasound signs (11, 82, 114) (Fig. 26.**11**). The volume of the ascites presumably depends on the amount of meconium that has been extravasated and the intensity of the peritoneal inflammatory response. If the bowel perforation has been present for several days, thickened bowel loops may be found within the abdomen in addition to echogenic calcifications.

Schild et al. (113) described meconium peritonitis in fetuses with a parvovirus B19 infection.

Differential diagnosis. The differential diagnosis includes ascites in nonimmune fetal hydrops, urinary ascites, meconium ileus, and viral infection.

Calcifications. Calcifications are found in the setting of TORCH infections (toxoplasmosis, other infections, rubella, cytomegalovirus, and herpes simplex virus) but also occur as isolated normal findings that may have no clinical significance (49).

Invasive testing. Percutaneous aspiration of the ascites yields a brownish-yellow fluid (Fig. 26.**11**).

Prognosis. The prognosis depends on the underlying disorder, gestational age, and the duration of the meconium peritonitis. The reported mortality rate was still 80% in 1966 (23). Today it ranges between 40% (65) and 62% (124).

Prenatal management. In the case of a mature fetus with suspected meconium peritonitis, delivery should be induced. If the fetus is still immature, cesarean delivery is preferred following the stimulation of lung maturation with cortisone.

Situs Inversus

Definition. Situs inversus is the term for a partial or complete mirror-image transposition of the viscera. Situs inversus is a typical feature of *Kartagener syndrome*, marked by a triad of bronchiectasis, situs inversus, and sinusitis (57).

Etiology and pathogenesis. Situs inversus is believed to result from an absence of ciliary motion on the embryonic epithelial cells. These cells are responsible for producing the normal rotation and bilateral symmetry of the internal organs (104).

Ultrasound features. Besides an abnormal location of the stomach on the right side (Fig. 26.**12**), the heart also may be found on the contralateral side.

Prenatal management. A meticulous search should be made for additional anomalies.

Ventral Abdominal Wall Defects

Ventral wall defects occur along median lines of embryonic fusion.

Types. Four main types of ventral wall defect are distinguished:
● Omphalocele
● Umbilical hernia
● Gastroschisis
● Eventration

All four types are based on a different causal mechanism. Additionally, there are disorders in which the abdominal wall defect represents one part of a complex anomaly.

■ *Omphalocele and Umbilical Hernia*

Definition. Ventral abdominal wall defect with a midgut hernial sac containing abdominal viscera.

Incidence. Omphalocele is the most common ventral wall defect, with an incidence of one in 2280 to one in 10,000 births (58).

Embryology

Omphalocele. Omphalocele occurs during the third week of embryonic development. It results from primary deficient closure of the ventral abdominal wall, marked by a failure of formation of the umbilical ring (24). The hernial sac contains liver and bowel (hepatomphalos).

Umbilical hernia. Umbilical hernia resembles omphalocele but occurs somewhat later in embryonic development, after the umbilical ring has already formed. It results from an incomplete reduction of the bowel from the physiologic umbilical hernia (60). The defect is smaller than in omphalocele and contains only bowel.

Pathoanatomic features. Both omphalocele and umbilical hernia present as an extracorporeal sac.

Ultrasound features. Both conditions are hereafter referred to as omphalocele, because they both have a hernial sac and differ sonographically only by their size and contents.

Meconium-related disorders

Fig. 26.**9** Ascites and hyperechoic bowel with partial shadowing in meconium ileus at 28 weeks. Transverse scan, vertex presentation with the spine to the right. Note the dense acoustic shadow behind the spinal column.

Fig. 26.**10** Conspicuous, hyperechoic bowel (arrow) in trisomy 21 at 15 weeks. Breech presentation.

Fig. 26.**11** Meconium peritonitis secondary to bowel rupture in the ileal region at 29 weeks. Transverse scan, vertex presentation with the spine to the left. Note the echogenic bowel and marked ascites with fine internal echoes. Because of the ruptured bowel, needle aspiration of the ascites yielded a dark brown fluid (syringe at left).

Situs inversus

Fig. 26.**12** Situs inversus at 19 weeks, 2 days. Vertex presentation with the spine to the left. Left: longitudinal scan. Right: transverse abdominal scan demonstrating the stomach on the right side. r = right, l = left.

Omphalocele and umbilical hernia

Fig. 26.**13** Transvaginal transverse scan of a physiologic umbilical hernia at 9 weeks, 3 days (not an omphalocele!).

Fig. 26.**14** Small, relatively flat omphalocele (arrows) in a transverse scan at 21 weeks, 4 days. Vertex presentation with the spine to the left.

Fig. 26.**15** Prominent omphalocele (arrows) 4.6 cm in diameter at 23 weeks. Longitudinal scan, breech presentation.

Fig. 26.**16** Same fetus delivered by cesarean section at 37 weeks. The sac diameter now measures 8 cm.

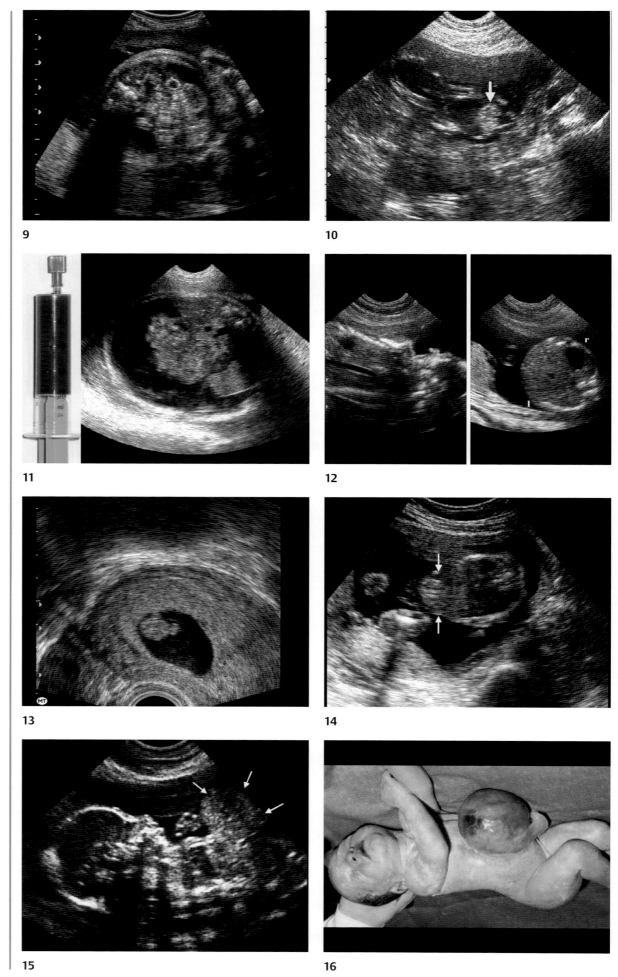

9

10

11

12

13

14

15

16

Hernial sac. Both longitudinal and transverse ultrasound scans show a hernial sac located in front of the abdominal wall and connected to the abdomen by a base of variable width (Figs. 26.**14**–26.**18**) (17, 72, 87, 97, 112). Depending on the size of the defect, the sac may contain only bowel loops or it may contain stomach and liver. The sac may closely envelop the visceral contents or it may contain copious fluid that separates the sac from the extruded viscera. In some cases the cystic sac may be accompanied by a demonstrable umbilical cyst (Fig. 26.**18**). From a biometric standpoint, the fetus with omphalocele has an abdominal diameter or circumference that is too small in relation to the superior biparietal diameter.

Physiologic umbilical hernia. Several authors have described the early ultrasound diagnosis of omphalocele between 10 and 14 weeks' gestation (10, 46, 49, 89, 115, 136). It should be noted, however, that the physiologic umbilical hernia is still present up to 12 weeks' gestation and may be misinterpreted as an omphalocele (Fig. 26.**13**). Serial scans should be obtained in equivocal cases.

Differential diagnosis. Gastroschisis, umbilical cyst.

Associated anomalies. From 45% (70) to 60% (140) of live-born infants have associated anomalies. In cases detected antenatally, Rabe et al. (97) found that 77% had associated anomalies (neural tube defects, skeletal malformations, cardiovascular anomalies, gastrointestinal anomalies). A chromosomal abnormality was present in 35% of all cases. In a screening study for chromosomal abnormalities, Snijders et al. (123) discovered an abnormal karyotype in 11 of 18 fetuses with omphalocele (= 61%): nine with trisomy 18, one with trisomy 13, and one with triploidy. Thus, trisomy 18 was the most common chromosomal defect. Fetuses with omphalocele are not at increased risk for trisomy 21 (131).

Noninvasive testing. Elevated maternal serum AFP levels are found in a high percentage of omphalocele cases. Palomaki et al. (90) were able to detect 78% of omphalocele cases based on elevated maternal serum AFP levels in the second trimester.

Invasive testing. A chromosome analysis should always be performed due to the high incidence of chromosomal abnormalities.

Prognosis. The prognosis of omphalocele depends on the size of the defect and on associated anomalies. The larger the defect, the more challenging it can be to repair the abdominal wall after birth. Also, pulmonary problems are not uncommon in these infants. Mayer et al. (78) reported a mortality rate of 34%.

Prenatal Management

Pregnancy termination. Various factors will influence the decision whether to consider pregnancy termination in cases where an omphalocele is detected in a previable fetus. These factors include the size of the defect, the detection of associated anomalies, and the result of the chromosome analysis.

Mode of delivery. From an obstetric standpoint, large omphaloceles can pose an obstacle to delivery. The recommended mode of delivery in these cases is cesarean, especially when the liver has herniated into the sac. Cesarean delivery avoids the risk of hernial sac rupture and infection, and timing the delivery allows for optimum postnatal management by a pediatric surgeon. With only a small omphalocele, a vaginal delivery may be considered in consultation with the pediatric surgeon. The preferred mode of delivery is a controversial topic in the literature. Lewis et al. (68) and Snipes et al. (121) could see no benefit of cesarean section over vaginal delivery in fetuses with uncomplicated abdominal wall defects.

Conditions that are Combined with Omphalocele

Beckwith–Wiedemann Syndrome

In addition to omphalocele, ultrasound in these cases shows accelerated growth of the fetal abdomen (values still below the 90th percentile) and polyhydramnios (98, 139). Also, a scan of the facial profile may demonstrate an enlarged tongue.

Pentalogy of Cantrell

Omphalocele is also found in the pentalogy of Cantrell, which is marked by a combination of omphalocele, diaphragmatic hernia, sternal defect, ectopia cordis, and heart defects.

OEIS Complex (Omphalocele, Exstrophy, Imperforate Anus, Spinal Defects)

Definition. The OEIS complex is an association of various anomalies:
- Omphalocele
- Bladder exstrophy
- Anal atresia
- Spinal defects

Incidence. OEIS complex has a reported incidence of one in 200,000 to one in 400,000 pregnancies (67).

Embryology. Because this complex occurs in monozygotic twins and is also characterized by various anomalies, it is presumably based on an early disturbance of blastogenesis (43, 67).

Ultrasound features. To date, only a few cases have been detected with prenatal ultrasound (43, 56). A presumptive diagnosis of OEIS complex can be made when an omphalocele and a spinal abnormality are detected sonographically but the fetal bladder cannot be clearly visualized (Fig. 26.**19**).

▬ *Gastroschisis*

Definition. Gastroschisis is an open, sporadically occurring abdominal wall defect with extruded loops of bowel.

Incidence. Gastroschisis is much less common than omphalocele, with an incidence of one in 30,000 births (103).

Embryology and pathogenesis. Gastroschisis develops between the fifth and sixth weeks of embryonic development. Instead of the physiologic umbilical hernia with bowel extruded into the umbilical cord, a rupture forms in the ventral abdominal wall adjacent to the umbilical cord insertion, allowing the free extrusion of bowel loops (120). The rupture is attributed to a premature obliteration of the right umbilical vein, creating a weak spot in the abdominal wall (120).

Pathoanatomic features. Gastroschisis differs from omphalocele and umbilical hernia in that the extruded viscera are not covered by a hernial sac. The defect is located to the right of the umbilical cord insertion.

Ultrasound features. Since there is no hernial sac, the bowel loops extruded from the paraumbilical defect on the right side of the abdomen float freely in the amniotic fluid (10, 39, 45, 97) (Figs. 26.**20**–26.**25**). The condition can be diagnosed by the end of the first trimester with transvaginal ultrasound (20, 41, 64).

Floating bowel loops. The eviscerated, fluid-filled bowel loops are clearly visible during late pregnancy. The extruded viscera usually consist of duodenum, jejunum, ileum, and portions of the colon (146). If the defect is small and only a few bowel loops have been extruded, the lesion may be mistaken for tangled loops of umbilical cord. These doubts are quickly resolved by color Doppler imaging (Fig. 26.**23**). A fetal limb placed over the abdominal wall can obscure a small defect.

Abdominal diameter too small. In cases where bowel and liver have been extruded through a large ventral wall defect, the abdominal diameter will be too small for gestational age, as in the case of omphalocele (Figs. 26.**25**, 26.**26**). Because of the small abdominal diameter, the fetal weight will appear to be too low in 43% of cases (100). In reality, a reduced birth weight is found in only 23% (100) to 36% (48) of newborns with gastroschisis.

Gastroschisis is indistinguishable from a ruptured omphalocele with ultrasound unless the hernial sac or abdominal wall defect can be identified directly adjacent to the normal umbilical cord insertion.

Differential diagnosis. Ruptured omphalocele, tangled loops of umbilical cord.

Associated anomalies. In contrast to omphalocele, only 5% of fetuses with gastroschisis have associated anomalies (70). These almost always involve the gastrointestinal tract in the form of intestinal anomalies such as nonrotation or malrotation (60, 146), which do not have true pathologic significance (146). Chromosomal abnormalities are rarely observed. Only one of 33 fetuses with gastroschisis in our series was found to have trisomy 21 (3).

Noninvasive testing. Maternal serum AFP levels are markedly elevated in pregnancies associated with gastroschisis (3, 90). Using a cutoff of 2 multiples of the median, Palomaki et al. (90) were able to detect 99% of gastroschisis cases based on elevated serum AFP levels.

Invasive testing. Because gastroschisis has an extremely low association with chromosomal abnormalities, an invasive procedure for fetal karyotyping is more of an option than a necessity. It may be prudent, however, if there is suspicion of a ruptured omphalocele or if the findings are equivocal.

Prognosis. The mortality rate associated with gastroschisis, at 10% (42) to 12.7% (78), is considerably lower than that of omphalocele except in cases where the liver is partially or completely outside the body (50% mortality rate) (Figs. 26.**25**, 26.**26**). Based on the impressive therapeutic results achieved with primary abdominal wall closure in 84% of cases (42) and the very low association with other anomalies, the early diagnosis of gastroschisis no longer appears to warrant pregnancy termination from a pediatric surgical standpoint (146). Prenatal diagnosis and delivery at a perinatal center provide the most effective basis for the successful surgical treatment of gastroschisis (42).

Prenatal Management

Mode of delivery. Both vaginal delivery (1, 58, 68, 121) and cesarean section (10, 97, 121) may be considered. The preferred mode of delivery is controversial. While some groups of authors found that cesarean section did not improve the perinatal outcome in uncomplicated gastroschisis (1, 68, 121), Sakala et al. (109) did a comparative study showing that elective cesarean section was associated with a lower rate of sepsis, a shorter hospital stay, and a shortened period of parenteral nutrition. Cesarean section is preferred over vaginal delivery in fetuses with a large defect. One reason for this is that cesarean section simplifies perinatal management.

Timing of delivery. The recommended time of delivery from a surgical standpoint is 37 weeks. After that time, the volume of the bowel increases markedly, making it more difficult to achieve primary abdominal closure.

▬ *Eventration*

Definition. An extensive abdominal wall defect with the protrusion of abdominal viscera. Eventration is found in connection with an absent umbilical cord (body stalk anomaly) and the amniotic band sequence.

Incidence. Complete eventration is a very rare event. Among our own patients, we have seen an abdominal wall defect of this magnitude in only 4 cases over a 20-year period. Two of these cases involved an absent/short umbilical cord sequence, and two involved an amniotic band sequence.

Embryology and pathogenesis. It may be that the absent umbilical cord sequence and the amniotic band sequence are both caused by an early amniotic rupture, since both anomalies are frequently combined (12).

Ultrasound features. The ultrasound hallmark is absence of the abdominal wall. The abdominal viscera may be covered by an amnioperitoneal sleeve or exposed to the amniotic fluid, depending on the cause of the defect.

Prognosis. Grave.

Prenatal management. Because of the grave prognosis, pregnancy termination is justified at any stage of gestation.

Body Stalk Anomaly (Limb/Body Wall Defect, Absent Umbilical Cord Sequence)

Definition. An anomalous sequence characterized by a large abdominal wall defect, a rudimentary umbilical cord, and fetal kyphoscoliosis.

Incidence. One in 14,000 births.

Embryology and pathogenesis. Body stalk anomaly occurs during the third week of embryonic development as part of a complex malformation sequence. The normal folding of the embryo away from the yolk sac is impaired, and the umbilical cord does not develop normally from the connecting stalk (12).

Pathoanatomic features. The abdominal viscera are enclosed within a short amnioperitoneal sleeve that connects the fetus to the placenta (Fig. 26.**27**). The umbilical vessels are only a few centimeters long and run along the wall of the amnioperitoneal sleeve. One umbilical artery is frequently absent (12).

Ultrasound features. The ultrasound hallmarks are a large ventral wall defect, a short or poorly defined umbilical cord, and severe kyphoscoliosis (Figs. 26.**28**, 26.**29**) (19, 21, 36, 53, 125). In one multicenter study covering 10–14 weeks' gestation, a body stalk anomaly was found in 14 of 106,727 fetuses examined. Increased nuchal translucency was noted in 71% of these cases (21).

Differential diagnosis. Amniotic band sequence, large omphalocele, pronounced gastroschisis.

Prognosis. Grave.

Prenatal management. Because of the grave prognosis, pregnancy termination is justified at any stage.

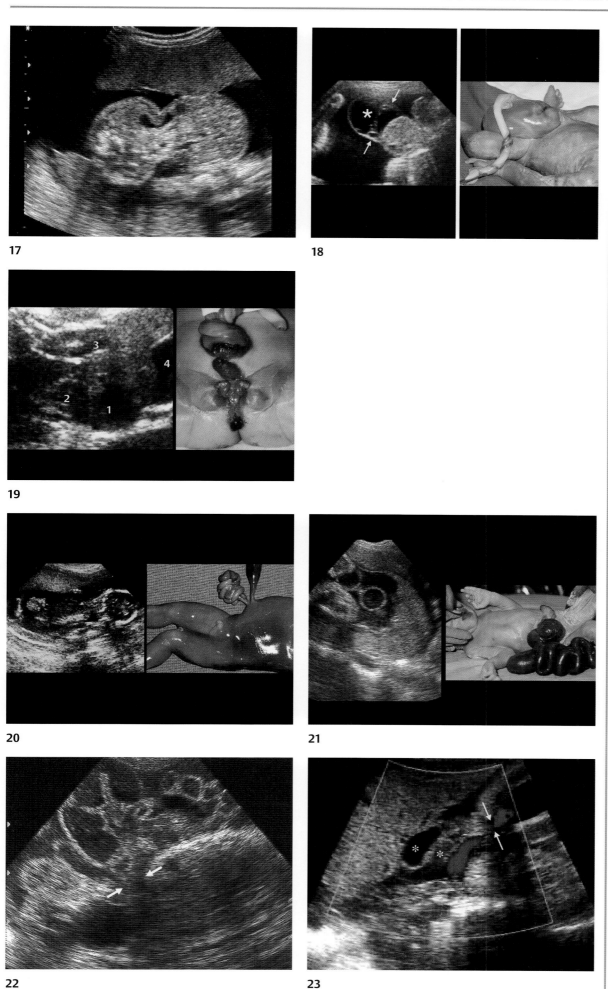

17

18

19

20

21

22

23

Fig. 26.**17**   Large omphalocele containing bowel loops and liver, transverse scan at 27 weeks. Vertex presentation with the spine to the left. The hypoechoic stomach is visible on the left side. Half of the stomach is still inside the abdomen and half is within the hernial sac. Since the liver has also herniated into the sac, the measured abdominal diameter is too small.

Fig. 26.**18**   Left: omphalocele with a large cystic sac (8.6 · 5.2 · 5.7 cm) (arrows) and an accompanying umbilical cyst (∗). Longitudinal coronal scan at 33 weeks. Right: postnatal appearance.

Fig. 26.**19**   OEIS complex with omphalocele and bladder exstrophy at 40 weeks. Left: longitudinal scan, vertex presentation. 1 = Small omphalocele, 2 = bladder region with absence of definite bladder filling, 3 = kidney in longitudinal section, 4 = heart. Right: postnatal appearance.

Gastroschisis

Fig. 26.**20**   Gastroschisis, 17 weeks. Left: longitudinal scan, vertex presentation with the spine to the right. Bowel loops have been extruded through a abdominal defect on the rig
ht side of the fetus, adjacent to the umbilical cord insertion. Right: appearance of the aborted fetus.

Fig. 26.**21**   Gastroschisis, 35 weeks. Left: two adjacent bowel loops, imaged in cross section, resemble "eyeglasses" floating in the amniotic fluid. Right: appearance after cesarean delivery.

Fig. 26.**22**   Extensive gastroschisis (arrows = abdominal wall defect) with abundant fluid-filled bowel loops floating freely in the amniotic fluid. Longitudinal scan, vertex presentation, 33 weeks.

Fig. 26.**23**   Small gastroschisis with hernial opening to the right of the umbilical vein (arrows). Transverse abdominal scan at 35 weeks, vertex presentation with the spine to the left. Without color Doppler, the extruded bowel loops (∗) could be mistaken for umbilical cord.

Fig. 26.**24** Gastroschisis with a mass of bowel loops floating in the amniotic fluid (∗), 35 weeks. The fluid-filled bowel loops have a ring-like appearance in cross section.

Fig. 26.**25** Large gastroschisis with the evisceration of bowel, stomach, and liver (∗). A hernial sac cannot be identified. The arrows indicate the defect in the ventral trunk (arrows). Longitudinal scan, vertex presentation, 31 weeks.

Fig. 26.**26** Pronounced gastroschisis with the extrusion of liver, spleen, and stomach. Postpartum view of the fetus in Fig. 26.**25**.

Eventration

Fig. 26.**27** Diagram of the gross pathoanatomy seen in body stalk anomaly. Green: amnioperitoneal sleeve. Red: chorionic plate (from [13]).

Fig. 26.**28** Eventration in body stalk anomaly, 18 weeks, longitudinal scan, breech presentation. The anterior abdominal wall is not clearly delineated. In its place, an amniotic sac with a web (arrow) is found between the placenta (∗) and the fetus. Marked oligohydramnios.

Fig. 26.**29** Eventration in body stalk anomaly, 18 weeks. Postmortem appearance of the fetus in Fig. 26.**28**. The amniotic sac between the fetus and placenta was opened.

Fig. 26.**30** Eventration in amniotic band sequence, 21 weeks. Transverse scan of a dorsoanterior fetus. Several arched bowel loops (arrows) are seen in place of a normal, well-defined ventral abdominal wall.

Fig. 26.**31** Extensive eventration with a concomitant defect in the anterior chest wall in amniotic band sequence, 21 weeks. Postmortem appearance of the fetus in Fig. 26.**30**. Arrows = amniotic bands.

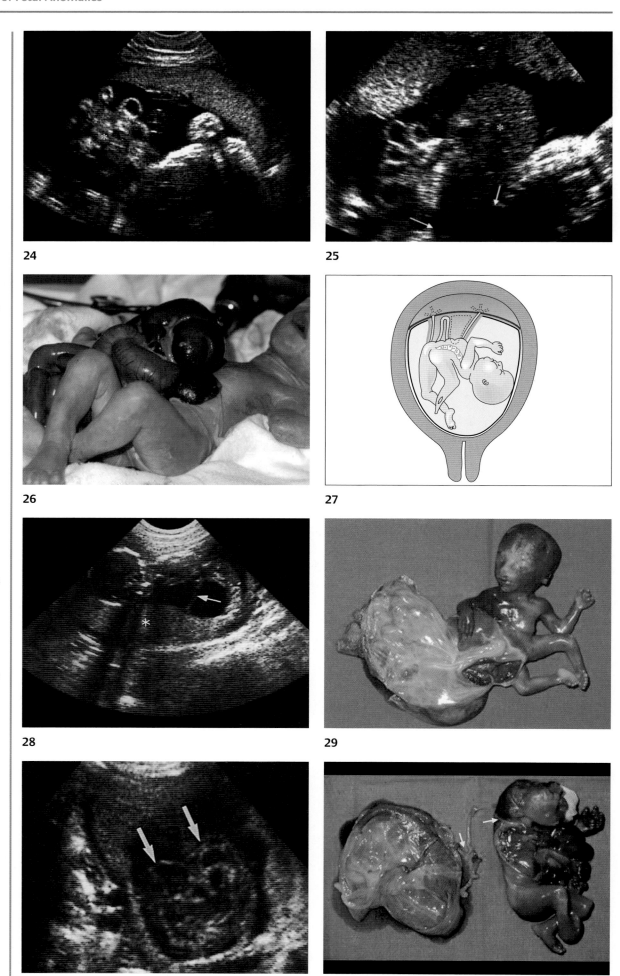

24

25

26

27

28

29

30

31

Amniotic Band Sequence (Amniotic Rupture Sequence, ADAM Complex = Amniotic Deformity, Adhesions, Mutilations)

Definition. The formation of amniotic bands that cause severe ectodermal disruption.

Incidence. Approximately one in 10,000 newborns.

Etiology and pathogenesis. According to Torpin (132), this condition is based on an early amnion rupture, producing amniotic bands that can wrap around fetal parts, causing severe ectodermal defects.

Pathoanatomic features. The spectrum of morphologic changes is extremely variable. Broad fibrous strands or patchy adhesions can produce severe craniofacial defects, large abdominal wall defects, and constrictions or amputations of the extremities (75, 117).

Ultrasound features. In the two cases with a severe abdominal wall defect that we have observed, the main feature was absence of the anterior abdominal wall. In its place were bowel loops floating freely in the amniotic fluid. In one of these cases the anterior thoracic wall was also ill-defined due to the presence of an extensive chest wall defect (80) (Figs. 26.**30**, 26.**31**). This case also showed very severe scoliotic deformity of the spine, with 180° of lateral angulation. In both cases diagnosis was hampered by a paucity of amniotic fluid.

In cases with a large ventral wall defect and the evisceration of bowel and liver, possibly accompanied by thoracoschisis, an amniotic band sequence should be considered even if the bands themselves are not visible because of oligohydramnios (75).

Differential diagnosis. Body stalk anomaly, large omphalocele, pronounced gastroschisis.

Prognosis. The prognosis of this condition is quite variable and depends on the size of the defect. With a large defect involving the head or trunk, the prognosis is grave.

Prenatal management. If there is an extensive defect involving the head or abdomen and the condition is diagnosed before 24 weeks' gestation, pregnancy termination should be discussed with the parents since an anomaly of that magnitude is not compatible with life.

Ultrasound Abnormalities of the Liver, Gallbladder, and Spleen

Hepatic Calcifications

Besides the intra-abdominal calcifications that are seen in meconium peritonitis, calcific foci are also occasionally found in the fetal liver. When Bronshtein and Blazer (15) examined 24,600 pregnancies between 14 and 26 weeks' gestation, they found one or more calcifications within the fetal liver in one out of 1750 pregnancies.

Etiology and pathogenesis. Hepatic calcifications can have various causes including viral infections (TORCH complex) (111) and ischemic hepatic necrosis (85). Bronshtein and Blazer (15) found that trisomy 18 was present in 2 of 14 cases. In a large percentage of fetuses with intrahepatic calcifications, the cause is unknown. If an infection or chromosome disorder can be ruled out, it is very likely that the ultrasound abnormality has no clinical importance (15, 49).

Ultrasound features. Intra- and perihepatic calcifications appear as round, elliptical, or flat hyperechoic areas that contrast sharply with the normal hepatic structure (Fig. 26.**32**).

Prenatal management. An infection (TORCH serology) should be excluded whenever an hepatic calcification is detected. This finding should also prompt a thorough ultrasound search for fetal anomalies. The parents may also be offered an invasive procedure for fetal karyotyping.

Hepatomegaly, Splenomegaly

Etiology and pathogenesis. Intrauterine enlargement of the liver and/or spleen can have various causes including fetal infections such as toxoplasmosis, cytomegalovirus infection, syphilis, and rubella. Other potential causes are hemolytic anemias (e.g., homozygous beta-thalassemia) and hypothyroidism (27). Hepatosplenomegaly also occurs in the setting of syndromes (Beckwith–Wiedemann syndrome, Zellweger syndrome) (139).

Ultrasound features. The liver appears markedly enlarged in its craniocaudal dimension. Concomitant ascites may also be present (Fig. 26.**33**).

Hepatic Tumors

Hepatic tumors are an extremely rare finding in fetuses. The following types have been described:
- Cysts of the liver and spleen (69, 93)
- Hepatic hemangiomas (18, 83, 94, 118)
- Mesenchymal hamartomas (34, 50, 77)
- Adenomas (76)
- Hepatoblastomas (134)

Hepatic cysts. These appear as intrahepatic hypoechoic round lesions with smooth margins. Differentiation is required from choledochal cysts, which are found in the area of the common bile duct.

Hepatic hemangiomas. Hemangiomas have been described as hyperechoic, hypoechoic, or mixed tumors. Calcifications may also be seen. The tumors range from a few millimeters to several centimeters in size. If larger vessels are present, blood flow can be detected with pulsed Doppler (38) and color Doppler (Fig. 26.**34**).

Mesenchymal hamartomas. These may appear sonographically as irregular cysts, sometimes very large, or as predominantly solid tumors.

Adenomas. Adenomas appear as hyperechoic tumors within the liver (76).

Hepatoblastomas. These are the most common malignant tumors of the liver during the neonatal period (16). They show a densely echogenic structure with conspicuous vascularity. The rich blood supply of the tumor is well demonstrated by color Doppler.

Prenatal management. When an hepatic tumor has been detected with ultrasound, close-interval follow-up should be maintained to monitor tumor growth. Large hepatic hemangiomas with arteriovenous shunts can lead to fetal heart failure. The mode and timing of the delivery depend on the size of the tumor. If the tumor remains small on follow-up scans, there should be no obstacle to a vaginal delivery at term. But if the tumor exhibits marked growth, a cesarean delivery may be required.

Abnormalities of the liver, gallbladder, and spleen

Fig. 26.**32** Abnormal calcification in the anterior part of the liver (arrow) in a fetus with 4 weeks' growth retardation. The fetus had a prior viral infection. 32 weeks, 6 days.

Fig. 26.**33** Hepatomegaly (arrows) and ascites in cytomegalovirus infection. Longitudinal scan, 37 weeks, vertex presentation. The length of the liver (7.8 cm) is markedly increased.

Fig. 26.**34** Very well-perfused, hypoechoic tumor in the right lobe of the liver (hemangioma). Power Doppler image at 33 weeks, 2 days.

Fig. 26.**35** Transverse scan of a choledochal cyst at 40 weeks.

Fig. 26.**36** Gallstone (2 x 1 mm) (arrow) at 18 weeks. Transverse scan, vertex presentation with the spine to the left.

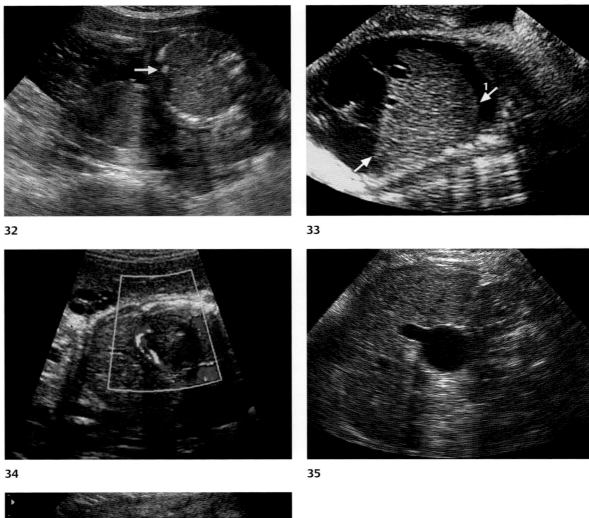

32

33

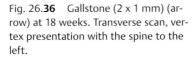

34

35

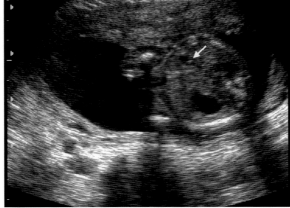

36

Choledochal Cyst

This lesion consists of a cystic outpouching in the area of the common bile duct. The hypoechoic cyst is found in direct proximity to the gallbladder (26) (Fig. 26.**35**). The differential diagnosis includes hepatic cyst, mesenteric cyst, and renal cystic disease. When the prenatal diagnosis is known, pediatric surgery can be performed in the neonate to prevent hepatic damage.

Gallstones

A few authors have been able to detect fetal gallstones in utero (8, 59). They appear sonographically as densely echogenic structures inside the gallbladder (Fig. 26.**36**). The cause of fetal gallstones is unclear. Hemolytic and nonhemolytic diseases have been discussed (8).

Kiserud et al. (59) reported finding echogenic material within the fetal gallbladder in 6 cases between 28 and 42 anomalies, and chromosomal aberrations were also observed (1 case with trisomy 21, one case with translocation 10;11).

References

1. Adra, A.M., Landy, H.J., Nahmias, J., Gomez-Marin, O.: The fetus with gastroschisis: Impact of route of delivery and prenatal ultrasonography. Amer. J. Obstet. Gynecol. 174 (1996) 540–546
2. Atwell, J.D., Klidjian, A.M.: Vertebral anomalies and duodenal atresia. J. Pediatr. Surg. 17 (1982) 237–240
3. Bahlmann, F., Merz, E., Weber, G., Macchiella, D.: Prenatal diagnosis and management of gastroschisis and omphalocele. Pediatr. Surg. Int. 11 (1996) 67–71
4. Baronciani, D., Scaglia, C., Corchia, C., Torcetta, F., Mastroiacovo, P.: Ultrasonography in pregnancy and fetal abnormalities: Screening or diagnostic tests? IPIMC 1986–1990 register data. Prenat. Diagn. 15 (1995) 1101–1108
5. Baumann, W., Greinacher, I., Emmrich, P., Spranger, J.: Vater- oder Vacterl-Syndrom. Klin. Pädiat. 188 (1976) 328–337
6. Bean, W.J., Calonje, M.A., Aprill, C.N., Geshner, J.: Anal atresia: A prenatal ultrasound diagnosis. J. clin. Ultrasound 6 (1978) 111–112
7. Benacerraf, B., Chaudhury, A.K.: Echogenic fetal bowel in the third trimester associated with meconium ileus secondary to cystic fibrosis. A case report. J. Reprod. Med. 34 (1989) 299–300
8. Beretsky, I., Lanken, D.H.: Diagnosis of fetal cholelithiasis using real-time high-resolution imaging employing digital detection. J. Ultrasound Med. 2 (1983) 381–383
9. Bergsma, D.: Birth Defects Compendium. New York: Alan R. Liss 1979
10. Bernaschek, S., Schaller, A.: Die pränatale Differenzialdiagnostik der Bauch- und Nabelschnurbrüche. Z. Geburtsh. Perinat. 189 (1985) 259–264
11. Blumenthal, D.H., Rushovich, A.M., Williams, R.K., Rochester, D.: Prenatal sonographic findings of meconium peritonitis with pathologic correlation. J. clin. Ultrasound 10 (1982) 350–352
12. Böhm, N.: Das Fehlende-Nabelschnur-Syndrom – eine typische Mißbildungs-Sequenz. Verh. dtsch. Ges. Path. 66 (1982) 436–439
13. Böhm, N.: Kinderpathologie. Stuttgart: Schattauer 1984; S. 190
14. Boles, E.T.Jr., Vassy, L.E., Ralston, M.: Atresia of the colon. J. Pediat. Surg. 11 (1976) 69–75
15. Bronshtein, M., Blazer, S.: Prenatal diagnosis of liver calcifications. Obstet. Gynecol. 86 (1995) 739–743
16. Brunelle, F., Chaumont, P.: Hepatic tumors in children: Ultrasonic differentiation of malignant from benign lesions. Radiology 150 (1984) 695–699
17. Campbell, S., Rodeck, C., Thoms, A., Little, D., Roberts, A.: Early diagnosis of exomphalos. Lancet I (1978) 1098–1099
18. Chung, W.M.: Antenatal detection of hepatic cyst. J. Clin. Ultrasound 14 (1986) 217–219
19. Craven, C.M., Carey, J.C., Ward, K.: Umbilical cord agenesis in limb body wall defect. Amer. J. Med. Genet. 71 (1997) 97–105
20. Cullen, M.T., Green, J., Whetham, J., Salfia, C., Gabrielli, S., Hobbins, J.C.: Transvaginal ultrasonographic detection of congenital anomalies in the first trimester. Amer. J. Obstet. Gynecol. 163 (1990) 466–476
21. Daskalakis, G., Debire, N.J., Jurkovic, D., Snijders, R., Nicolaides, K.H.: Body stalk anomaly at 10–14 weeks of gestation. Ultrasound Obstet. Gynecol. 10 (1997) 416–418
22. Dewbury, K.C., Aluwihare, A.P.R., Birch, S.J., Freeman, N.V.: Prenatal ultrasound demonstration of a choledochal cyst. Brit. J. Radiol. 53 (1980) 906–907
23. Donnison, A.B., Shwachman, H., Gross, R.E.: A review of 164 children with meconium ileus seen at the Children's Hospital Medical Center Boston. Pediatrics 37 (1966) 833–850
24. Duhamel, D.: Embryology of exomphalos and allied malformations. Arch. Dis. Child. 38 (1963) 142–147
25. Dunne, M.G., Johnson, M.L.: The ultrasonic demonstration of fetal abnormalities in utero. J. Reprod. Med. 23 (1979) 195–206
26. Eirad, H., Mayden, K.L., Ahart, S.: Prenatal ultrasound diagnosis of choledochal cyst. J. Ultrasound Med. 4 (1985) 553–555
27. Eliezer, S., Ester, F., Ehud, W., Henryk, Z.: Fetal splenomegaly, ultrasound diagnosis of cytomegalovirus infection: a case report. J. Clin. Ultrasound 12 (1984) 520–521
28. Engum, S.A., Grosfeld, J.L., West, K.W., Rescorla, F.J., Scherer, L.R. 3rd: Analysis of morbidity and mortality in 227 cases of esophageal atresia and/or tracheoesophageal fistula over two decades. Arch. Surg. 130 (1995) 502–508
29. Estroff, J.A., Parad, R.B., Benacerraf, B.R.: Prevalence of cystic fibrosis in fetuses with dilated bowel. Radiology. 183 (1992) 677–680
30. Eyheremendy, E., Pfister, M.: Antenatal real-time diagnosis of esophageal atresias. J. clin. Ultrasound 11 (1983) 395–397
31. Fletman, D., McQuown, D., Kanchanapoom, V., Gyepes, M.T.: „Apple peel" atresia of the small bowel: Prenatal diagnosis of the obstruction by ultrasound. Pediat. Radiol. 9 (1980) 118–119
32. Fonkalsrud, E.W., de Lorimier, A.A., Hays, D.M.: Congenital atresia and stenosis of the duodenum. A review compiled from the members of the surgical section of the American Academy of Pediatrics. Pediatrics 43 (1969) 79–83
33. Foster, M.A., Nyberg, D.A., Mahony, B.S., Mack, L.A., Marks, W.M., Rabe, R.D.: Meconium peritonitis: Prenatal sonographic findings and clinical significance. Radiology 165 (1987) 661–665
34. Foucar, E., Williamson, R.A., Yiu-Chiu, V.: Mesenchymal hamartoma of the liver identified by fetal sonography. Amer. J. Roentgenol. 140 (1983) 970–972
35. German, J.C., Mahour, G.H, Wooley, M.M.: Esophageal atresia and associated anomalies. J. Pediat. Surg. 11 (1976) 299–306
36. Goldhofer, W., Merz, E.: Das Syndrom der fehlenden Nabelschnur im Ultraschall. Z. Geburtsh. Perinat. 189 (1985) 241–243
37. Goldhofer, W., Merz, E., Bauer, H., Koltai, I.L.: Pränatale sonographische Diagnose eines zystischen Steißbeinteratoms mit retroperitonealer Ausbreitung. Geburtsh. u. Frauenheilk. 46 (1986) 121–123
38. Gonen, R., Fong, K., Chiasson, D.A.: Prenatal sonographic diagnosis of hepatic hemangioendothelioma with secondary nonimmune hydrops fetalis. Obstet. Gynecol. 73 (1989) 485–487
39. Grossman, M., Fischermann, E.A., German, J.: Sonographic findings in gastroschisis. J. clin. Ultrasound 6 (1978) 175–176
40. Guttman, F.M., Braun, P., Garance, P.H. et al.: Multiple atresias and a new syndrome of hereditary multiple atresias involving the gastrointestinal tract from stomach to rectum. J. Pediatr. Surg. 8 (1973) 633–640
41. Guzman, E.P.: Early prenatal diagnosis of gastroschisis with transvaginal sonography. Amer. J. Obstet. Gynecol. 162 (1990) 1253–1254
42. Haddock, G., Davis, C.F., Raine, P.A.: Gastroschisis in the decade of prenatal diagnosis: 1983–1993. Eur. J. Pediatr. Surg. 6 (1996) 18–22
43. Haldar, A., Sharma, A.K., Phadke, S.R., Jain, A., Agarwal, S.S.: OEIS complex with craniofacial anomalies – defect of blastogenesis? Amer. J. Med. Genet. 53 (1994) 21–23
44. Hancock, B.J., Wiseman, N.E.: Congenital duodenal obstruction: the impact of an antenatal diagnosis. J. Pediatr. Surg. 24 (1989) 1027–1031
45. Hansmann, M.: Nachweis und Ausschluß fetaler Entwicklungsstörungen mittels Ultraschallscreening und gezielter Untersuchung – ein Mehrstufenkonzept. Ultraschall 2 (1981) 206–220
46. Hansmann, M., Gembruch, U.: Gezielte sonographische Ausschlußdiagnostik fetaler Fehlbildungen in Risikogruppen. Gynäkologe 17 (1984) 19–32
47. Hatzmann, W., Dieckgießer, U., Dieckgießer, A.: Ultrasonografische Dignose eines fetalen Ascites mit Polyhydramnion infolge partieller Dünndarmatresie und sekundärer Darmwandperforation. Ultraschall 5 (1984) 144–147
48. Heydanus, R., Raats, A.M., Tibboel, D., Lost, F.J. Wladimiroff, J.W.: Prenatal diagnosis of fetal abdominal wall defects: a retrospective analysis of 44 cases. Prenat. Diagn. 16 (1996) 411–417
49. Hill, L.H.: Sonographic detection of fetal gastrointestinal anomalies. Ultrasound Quarterly 6 (1988) 35–67
50. Hirata, G.I., Matsunaga, M.L., Medearis, A.L.: Ultrasonographic diagnosis of a fetal abdominal mass: a case of a mesenchymal liver hamartoma and a review of the literature. Prenat. Diagn. 10 (1990) 507–512
51. Ingalls, T.H., Prindle, R.A.: Esophageal atresia with tracheoesophageal fistula: epidemiologic and teratologic implications. New Engl. J. Med. 240 (1949) 987–995
52. Jassani, M.N., Gauderer, M.W.L., Fanaroff, A.A., Fletcher, B., Merkatz, I.R.: A perinatal approach to the diagnosis and management of gastrointestinal malformations. Obstet. Gynecol. 59 (1982) 33–39
53. Jauniaux, E., Vyas, S., Finlayson, C., Moscoso, G., Driver, M., Campbell, S.: Early sonographic diagnosis of body stalk anomaly. Prenat. Diagn. 10 (1990) 127–132
54. Jolleys, A.: An examination of the birthweigths of babies with some abnormalities of the alimentary tract. J. Pediatr. Surg. 16 (1981) 160–163
55. Joppich, I., Kellnar, S.: Chirurgie der Atresien des Gastrointestinaltraktes. Chirurg 67 (1996) 576–583
56. Kant, S.G., Bartelings, M.M., Kibbelaar, R.E., van Haeringen, A.: Severe cardiac defect in a patient with the OEIS complex. Clin. Dysmorphol. 6 (1997) 371–374
57. Kartagener, M.: Zur Frage der Bronchiektasen. Familiäres Vorkommen von Bronchiektasen. Beitr. Klin. Tbk. 84 (1933) 73
58. Kirk, E.P., Wah, R.M.: Obstetric management of the fetus with omphalocele or gastroschisis: A review and report of one hundred twelve cases. Amer. J. Obstet. Gynec. 146 (1983) 512–518
59. Kiserud, T., Gjelland, K., Bogno, H., Waardal, M., Reigstad, H., Rosendahl, K.: Echogenic material in the fetal gallbladder and fetal disease. Ultrasound Obstet. Gynecol. 10 (1997) 103–106
60. Klein, M.D., Kosloske, A.M., Hertzler, J.H.: Congenital defects of the abdominal wall. A review of the experience in New Mexico. J. Amer. med. Ass. 245 (1981) 1643–1646
61. Klingensmith, W.C. III, Ragan-Cioffi, D.T.: Fetal gallstones. Radiology 167 (1988) 143–144
62. Kossoff, G., Garrett, W.J., Radovanovich, R.: Grey scale echography in obstetrics and gynecology. Aust. Radiol. 18 (1974) 62–111
63. Kurjak, A., Kirkinen, P., Latin, V., Rajhvajn, B.: Diagnosis and assessment of fetal malformations and abnormalities by ultrasound. J. perinat. Med. 8 (1980) 219–235
64. Kushnir, O., Izquierdo, L., Vigil, D., Curet, L.B.: Early transvaginal diagnosis of gastroschisis. J. Clin. Ultrasound 18 (1990) 194–197

65. Lally, K.P., Mehall, J.R., Xue, H., Thompson, J.: Meconium stimulates a pro-inflammatory response in peritoneal macrophages: implications for meconium peritonitis. J. Pediatr. Surg. 34 (1999) 214–217
66. Langer, J.C., Winthrop, A.L., Burrows, R.F., Issenman, R.M., Caco, C.C.: False diagnosis of intestinal obstruction in a fetus with congenital chloride diarrhea. J. Pediatr. Surg. 26 (1991) 1282–1284
67. Lee, D.H., Cottrell, J.R., Sanders, R.C., Meyers, C.M., Wulfsberg, E.A., Sun, C.C.: OEIS complex (omphalocele – exstrophy – imperforate anus – spinal defects) in monozygotic twins. Amer. J. Med. Genet. 84 (1999) 29–33
68. Lewis, D.F., Towers, C.V., Garite, T.J., Jackson, D.N., Nageotte, M.P., Major, C.A.: Fetal gastroschisis and omphalocele: is cesarean section the best mode of delivery? Amer. J. Obstet. Gynecol. 163 (1990) 773–775
69. Lichman, J.P., Miller, E.I.: Prenatal ultrasonic diagnosis of splenic cyst. J. Ultrasound Med. 7 (1988) 637–638
70. Lindham, S.: Teratogenetic aspects of abdominal wall defects. Z. Kinderchir. 38 (1983) 211–216
71. Lloyd, J.R., Clathworthy H.W.Jr.: Hydramnios as an aid to the early diagnosis of congenital obstructions of the alimentary tract. A study of the maternal and fetal factors. Pediatrics 21 (1958) 903–909
72. Lomas, F., Stanford-Bell, M., Tymus, A.: Prenatal ultrasound in the diagnosis and management of fetal exomphalos. Case reports. Brit. J. Obstet. Gynaec. 86 (1979) 581–584
73. Lorimier de, A.A., Fonkalsrud, E.W., Hays, D.M.: Congenital atresia and stenosis of the jejunum and ileum. Surgery 65 (1969) 819–827
74. Loveday, B.J., Barr, J.A., Aitken, J.: The intra-uterine demonstration of duodenal atresia by ultrasound. Brit. J. Radiol. 48 81975) 1031–1032
75. Mahony, B.S., Filly, R.A., Callen, P.W., Golbus, M.S.: The amniotic band syndrome: Antenatal sonographic diagnosis and potential pitfalls. Amer. J. Obstet. Gynec. 152 (1985) 63–68
76. Marks, F., Thomas, P., Lustig, I.: In utero sonographic description of a fetal adenoma. J. Ultrasound Med. 9 (1990) 119–122
77. Mason, B.A., Hodges, W., Goodman, J.R.: Antenatal sonographic detection of a rare solid hepatic mesenchymal hamartoma. Matern. Fetal Med. 1 (1992) 134–136
78. Mayer, T., Black, R., Matlak, M., Johnson, D.: Gastroschisis and omphalocele – an eight-year review. Ann. Surg. 192 (1980) 783–787
79. McKenna, K.M., Goldstein, R.B., Stringer, M.D.: Small or absent fetal stomach: prognostic significance. Radiology 197 (1995) 729–733
80. Merz, E., Gerlach, R., Hofmann, G., Goldhofer, W.: Das Amnionbänder-Syndrom im Ultraschall. Geburtsh. u. Frauenheilk. 44 (1984) 576–578
81. Moore, K.L., Persaud, T.V.N.: Embryologie. Stuttgart: Schattauer 1996; S. 275–308
82. Moslinger, D., Chalubinski, K., Radner, M. et al.: Meconium peritonitis: intrauterine follow-up – postnatal outcome. Wien. Klin. Wochenschr. 107 (1995) 141–145
83. Nakamoto, S.K., Dreilinger, A., Dattel, B., Mattrey, R.F., Key, T.C.: The sonographic appearance of hepatic hemangioma in utero. J. Ultrasound Med. 2 (1983) 239–241
84. Nelson, L.H., Clark, C.E., Fishburne, J.I., Urban, R.B., Penry, M.F.: Value of serial sonography in the in utero detection of duodenal atresia. Obstet. and Gynec. 59 (1982) 657–660
85. Nguyen, D.L., Leonard, J.C.: Ischemic hepatic necrosis: A cause of fetal liver calcification. AJR 147 (1986) 596–597
86. Nicolaides, K.H., Snijders, R.J.M., Cheng, H.H., Gosden, C.: Fetal gastrointestinal and abdominal wall defects: associated malformations and chromosomal anomlies. Fetal Diagn. Ther. 7 (1992) 102–115
87. Niesen, M., Hansmann, M.: Omphalozele, präpartale Ultraschalldiagnostik und Konsequenzen. Gynäkologe 12 (1979) 80–83
88. Nixon, H.H., Tawes, R.: Etiology and treatment of small intestinal atresias: Analysis of a series of 127 jejunoileal atresia and comparison with 62 duodenal atresia. Surgery 69 (1971) 41–51
89. Pagliano, M., Mossetti, M., Ragno, P.: Echographic diagnosis of omphalocele in the first trimester of pregnancy. J. Clin. Ultrasound 18 (1990) 658–660
90. Palomaki, G.E., Hill, L.E., Knight, G.J., Haddow, J.E., Carpenter, M.: Second-trimester maternal serum alpha-fetoprotein levels in pregnancies associated with gastroschisis and omphalocele. Obstet. Gynecol. 71 (1988) 906–909
91. Paulson, E.K., Hertzberg, B.S.: Hyperechoic meconium in the third trimester fetus: an uncommon normal variant. J. Ultrasound Med. 10 (1991) 677–680
92. Peck, D.A., Lynn, U.B., Harris, C.E.: Congenital atresia and stenosis of the colon. Arch. Surg. 87 (1963) 428–439
93. Petrovic, O., Haller, H., Rukavina, B.: Prenatal diagnosis of a large liver cavernous hemangioma associated with polyhydramnios. Prenat. Diagn. 12 (1992) 70–71
94. Platt, L.D., DeVore, G.R., Benner, P., Siassi, B., Ralls, P.W., Mikity, V.G.: Antenatal diagnosis of a fetal liver mass. J. Ultrasound Med. 2 (1983) 521–522
95. Prenzlau, P., Bayer, H., Schulte, R.: Möglichkeit und Grenzen der Ultraschalldiagnostik bei der antenatalen Erkennung von Mißbildungen. Zbl. Gynäkol. 99 (1977) 45–51
96. Pretorius, D.H., Drose, J.A., Dennis, M.A., Machester, D.K., Manco-Johnson, M.L.: Tracheoesophageal fistula in utero. J. Ultrasound Med. 6 (1987) 509–513
97. Rabe, D., Hendrik, H.J., Leucht, W., Roth, H., Walter, Ch., Schmidt, W.: Ventrale Bauchwanddefekte – antenatale Diagnose, Schwangerschaftsverlauf und postpartale Therapie. Geburtsh. u. Frauenheilk. 45 (1985) 176–182
98. Ranzini, A.C., Day-Salvatore, D., Turner, T., Smulian, J.C., Vintzileos, A.M.: Intrauterine growth and ultrasound findings in fetuses with Beckwith-Wiedemann syndrome. Obstet. Gynecol. 89 (1997) 538–542
99. Ravitch, M.M., Barton, B.A.: The need for pediatric surgeons as determined by the volume of work and the mode of delivery of surgical care. Surgery 76 (1974) 754–763
100. Raynor, B.D., Richards, D.: Growth retardation in fetuses with gastroschisis. J. Ultrasound Med. 16 (1997) 13–16
101. Reid, I.S.: The pattern of intrinsic duodenal obstruction. Aust. N. Z. J. Surg. 42 (1973) 349–352
102. Rempen, A., Kaesemann, H., Feige, A., Fiedler, K.: Sonografische Pränataldiagnostik und klinische Konsequenzen bei Dünndarmobstruktionen. Z. Geburtsh. Perinat. 190 (1986) 73–82
103. Rickham, P.P., Johnston, J.H.: Neonatal Surgery. London: Appleton-Century-Corfts (Division of Meredith Pub.) 1969; p. 257
104. Riede, U.N., Schaefer, H.E., Rohrbach, R., Müller, H.J.: Störungen der zellulären und extrazellulären Organisation. In: Riede, U.N., Schaefer, H.E. (Hrsg.): Allgemeine und spezielle Pathologie. Stuttgart: Thieme 1995; 7–76
105. Riede, U.N., Schaefer, H.E.: Dickdarm. In: Riede, U.N., Schaefer, H.E. (Hrsg.): Allgemeine und spezielle Pathologie. Stuttgart: Thieme 1995; S. 718–734
106. Riede, U.N.: Analregion. In: Riede, U.N., Schaefer, H.E. (Hrsg.): Allgemeine und spezielle Pathologie. Stuttgart: Thieme 1995; S. 735–737
107. Robertson, F.M., Crombleholme, T.M., Paidas, M., Harris, B.H.: Prenatal diagnosis and management of gastrointestinal anomalies. Semin. Perinat. 18 (1994) 182–195
108. Rokitansky, M.D., Kolankaya, M.D., Bichler, M.D., Mayr, J., Menardi, G.: Analysis of 309 cases of esophageal atresia for associated congenital malformations. Amer. J. Perinat. 11 (1994) 123–128
109. Sakala, E.P., Erhard, L.N., White, J.J.: Elective cesarean section improves outcomes of neonates with gastroschisis. Amer. J. Obstet. Gynecol. 169 (1993) 1050–1053
110. Satoh, S., Takashima, T., Takeuchi, H., Koyanagi, T., Nakano, H.: Antenatal sonographic detection of the proximal esophageal segment: specific evidence for congenital esophageal atresia. J. Clin. Ultrasound 23 (1995) 419–423
111. Schackelford, G.D., Kirks, D.R.: Neonatal hepatic calcification secondary to transplacental infection. Radiology 122 (1977) 753–757
112. Schaffer, R.M., Barone, C., Friedman, A.: The ultrasonographic spectrum of fetal omphalocele. J. Ultrasound Med. 2 (1983) 219–222
113. Schild, R.L., Plath, H., Thomas, P., Schulte-Wissermann, H., Eis-Hubinger, A.M., Hansmann, M.: Fetal parvovirus B19 infection and meconium peritonitis. Fetal Diagn. Ther. 13 (1998) 15–18
114. Schlensker, K.H., Günther, H., Bolte, A.: Pränatale Diagnose einer fetalen Mekoniumperitonitis, Therapie und Verlauf. Mit einem Beitrag zur Differentialdiagnose des fetalen Ascites. Geburtsh. u. Frauenheilk. 44 (1984) 435–440
115. Schmidt, W., Gabelmann, J., Garoff, L., Kubli, F.: Ultrasonographische Diagnose einer Omphalocele im ersten Schwangerschaftsdrittel. Geburtsh. u. Frauenheilk. 41 (1981) 562–565
116. Scott, J.S., Wilson, J.K.: Hydramnios as an early sign of esophageal atresia. Lancet 1957/II, 569–572
117. Seeds, J.W., Cefalo, R.C., Herbert, W.N.P.: Amniotic band syndrome. Amer. J. Obstet. Gynecol. 144 (1982) 243–248
118. Sepulveda, W.H., Donetch, G., Guiliano, A.: Prenatal sonographic diagnosis of fetal hepatic hemangioma. Eur. J. Obstet. Gynecol. Reprod. Biol. 48 (1993) 73–76
119. Shalev, E., Weiner, E., Zuzherman, H.: Prenatal ultrasound diagnosis of intestinal calcification with imperforate anus. Acta Obstet. Gynecol. Scand. 62 (1983) 95–96
120. Shaw, A.: The myth of gastroschisis. J. pediat. Surg. 10 (1975) 235–244
121. Sipes, S.L., Weiner, C.P., Sipes, D.R. 2nd, Grant, S.S., Williamson, R.A.: Gastroschisis and omphalocele: does either antenatal diagnosis or route of delivery make a difference in perinatal outcome? Obstet. Gynecol. 76 (1990) 195–199
122. Skovbo, P., Smith-Jensen, S.: Hyperdistended fluid-filled bowel loops mimicking gastrointestinal atresia. J. clin. Ultrasound 9 (1981) 463–465
123. Snijders, R.J.M., Sbire, N.J., Souka, A., Santiago, C., Nicolaides, K.H.: Fetal exomphalos and chromosomal defects: relationship to maternal age and gestation. Ultrasound Obstet. Gynecol. 6 (1995) 250–255
124. Soong, J.H., Hsieh, C.C., Chiu, T.H. et al.: Meconium peritonitis – antenatal diagnosis by ultrasound. Chang Keng I Hsueh. 15 (1992) 155–160
125. Souka, A.P., Nicolaides, K.H.: Diagnosis of fetal abnormalities at the 10-14-week scan. Ultrasound Obstet. Gynecol. 10 (1997) 429–442
126. Spitz, L., Kiely, E.M., Morecroft, J.A., Drake, D.P.: Oesophageal atresia: at risk group for the 1990's. J. Pediatr. Surg. 29 (1994) 723–725
127. Stringer, M.D., McKeena, K.M., Goldstein, R., Filly, R.A., Adzick, N.S., Harrison, M.R.: Prenatal diagnosis of esophageal atresia. J. Pediatr. Surg. 30 (1995) 1258–1263
128. Suita, S., Ikeda, K., Koyanagi, T., Nakano, H.: Neonatal ovarian cyst diagnosed antenatally: Report of two cases. J. clin. Ultrasound 12 (1984) 517–519
129. Swenson, O., Lipman, R., Fischer, J.H., Deluca, F.G.: Repair and complications of esophageal atresia and tracho-esophageal fistula. New Engl. J. Med. 267 (1962) 960–963
130. Tandler, J.: Zur Entwicklungsgeschichte des menschlichen Duodenums in frühen Embryonalstadien. Gegenbaurs morph. Jb. 29 (1900) 187
131. Torfs, C.P., Honore, L.H., Curry, C.J.: Is there an association of Down syndrome and omphalocele? Amer. J. Med. Genet. 73 (1997) 400–403
132. Torpin, R.: Amniochorionic mesoblastic fibrous strings and amniotic bands. Amer. J. Obstet. Gynec. 91 (1965) 65–75
133. Touloukian, R.J.: Intestinal atresia. Clin. Perinat. 5 (1978) 3–18
134. Van der Bor, M., Verwey, R.A., Van Pel, R.: Acute polyhydramnios associated with fetal hepatoblastoma. Eur. J. Obstet. Gynecol. Reprod. Biol. 20 (1985) 65–69
135. Van Rijn, M., Christaens, G.C., Hagenaars, A.M., Visser, G.H.: Maternal serum alpha-fetoprotein in fetal anal atresia and other gastrointestinal obstructions. Prenat. Diagn. 18 (1998) 914–921
136. Van Zalen-Sprock, R.M., van Vugt, J.M.G., van Geijn, H.P.: First trimester sonography of physiological midgut herniation and early diagnosis of omphalocele. Prenat. Diagn. 17 (1997) 511–518
137. Vogt, E.C.: Congenital esophageal atresia. Amer. J. Roentgenol. 22 (1929) 463
138. Voigt, H.J., Hümmer, H.P., Böwing, B.: Pränatale Ultraschalldiagnose einer Jejunalatresie. Z. Geburtsh. Perinat. 189 (1985) 144–146
139. Weinstein, L., Anderson, C.: In-utero diagnosis of Beckwith-Wiedemann syndrome by ultrasound. Radiology 134 (1980) 474
140. Willital, G.H., Belin, R.P., Linke, R.: Die chirurgische Bedeutung von Korrelationspathologika des gastrointestinalen Systems bei Omphalozelen und Gastroschisis. Z. Kinderchir. 11 (1972) 426–432
141. Wrobleski, D., Wesselhoeft, C.: Ultrasonic diagnosis of prenatal intestinal obstruction. J. pediat. Surg. 14 (1979) 598–600
142. Yaron, Y., Hassan, S., Geva, E., Kupferminc, M.J., Yavetz, H., Evans, M.I.: Evaluation of fetal echogenic bowel in the second trimester. Fetal. Diagn. Ther. 14 (1999) 176–180

143. Young, D.G., Wilkinson, A.W.: Mortality in duodenal obstruction. Lancet 1966/ II, 18–20
144. Young, D.G., Wilkinson, A.W.: Abnormalities associated with neonatal duodenal obstruction. Surgery 63 (1968) 832–836
145. Zimmer, E.Z., Bronshtein, M.: Early diagnosis of duodenal atresia and possible sonographic pitfalls. Prenat. Diagn. 16 (1996) 564–566
146. Zimmermann, H.J., Dziuba, M., Mühlhaus, K.: Zum Problem der pränatalen Diagnose: Gastroschisis – Kinderchirurgische Überlegungen und Bericht über 13 Fälle. Z. Geburtsh. Perinat. 189 (1985) 188–191

27 Anomalies and Diseases of the Kidneys and Urinary Tract

Embryology of the Kidneys

The kidneys in the embryo develop from the nephrogenic ridge, which is a mesodermal derivative. Renal development consists of three partially overlapping stages: the pronephros, mesonephros, and metanephros. Each of these organs succeeds the other in a superior-to-inferior progression. The first two stages regress during fetal development but are important inductors for the formation of the third stage. The ureteral bud, which is derived from the wolffian duct, grows toward the metanephros and induces the differentiation of the nephrogenic blastema to the renal parenchyma.

Pronephros. The pronephros forms at the end of the third week of conceptual age in the cervical region, developing from the superior portions of the nephrogenic ridge. It regresses again in just the fifth week. It consists of several tubules and vesicles. The mesonephric duct (wolffian duct) develops caudally from the pronephros and communicates with the cloaca by the end of the fourth week.

Mesonephros. The mesonephros is formed in the thoracic and lumbar part of the mesoderm. By the sixth week, it has developed into an elongated organ on each side. It already contains glomeruli and tubules, which empty into the wolffian duct. By the end of the eighth week, the structures of the mesonephros almost completely degenerate in a superior-to-inferior direction.

Metanephros and ureteral bud. As the mesonephros regresses, the metanephros, or permanent kidney, develops inferior to it from the intermediate mesoderm (called also the metanephrogenic blastema) starting in the fifth week of gestation. Meanwhile, the ureteral bud forms in the inferior part of the wolffian duct starting in the fourth week. The ureteral bud grows dorsally and penetrates the metanephrogenic blastema. The interaction of both components induces the formation of nephrons from the metanephrogenic blastema. In a parallel process, the ureteral bud undergoes repeated branching to form the renal pelvis, calices, papillary ducts, collecting tubules, and connecting tubules.

Interaction. It is clear that the interaction between the metanephrogenic blastema and the ureteral bud is an important foundation for normal renal development. Any disturbance of this interaction leads to renal abnormalities of varying extent, depending on the timing of the disturbance. The earlier it occurs, the more serious the renal anomaly (Fig. 27.**1**).

Incidence of Anomalies and Associated Anomalies

Incidence and associated anomalies. The incidence of urinary tract anomalies is 1.8% in the first trimester, 0.65% in the second and third trimesters, 0.3–1.0% at birth, and 0.3% in adults (11, 37, 60, 62). Fetal ovarian cysts are rare and comprise only 1% of all tumors in newborns (18). Up to 40% of anomalies detected antenatally involve the urogenital system. Twelve percent of these cases have an associated chromosomal abnormality, with a 30-fold increase in the risk for other organ malformations. Renal abnormalities are responsible for 4% of perinatal deaths due to congenital anomalies (1, 40, 71).

Ultrasound Survey

Most urogenital anomalies can be detected in an ultrasound survey of the fetus, appearing as fluid-filled spaces within the fetal abdomen. Absent or deficient fetal urine production or an obstruction located in the excretory portion of the urinary tract leads to oligo- or anhydramnios. A fetal ovarian cyst or uterine anomaly, on the other hand, is associated with a normal amniotic fluid volume.

Checklist. Malformations of the fetal kidneys and urinary tract are detected in general ultrasound screening and in selected patients with an increased recurrence risk. Holzgreve (47) presents the following checklist for the ultrasound detection or exclusion of fetal urinary tract anomalies:

Determine the amniotic fluid volume.
- Whenever oligohydramnios is detected, a urinary tract anomaly should be strongly suspected after premature rupture of the membranes and extreme early growth retardation have been excluded (Fig. 27.**2**).
- Check for distension of the renal pelvis and ureters.
- Some authors diagnose renal pelvic dilatation when the renal pelvis is larger than 5 mm. Others use a cutoff of 10 mm. Since even a mild dilatation of 6–9 mm is associated with an increased incidence of chromosomal abnormalities and associated anomalies, special vigilance is called for in the overall ultrasound evaluation of the fetus. With a negative study, the fetus should be reexamined in two weeks (Fig. 27.**3**).
- If dilatation is found, determine its extent and location. Check for ascites or a urinoma after any decompressive measures have been carried out.
- Detect or exclude renal cysts (Fig. 27.**4**).
- The size, outlines, and echogenicity of the kidneys should be determined.
- Define the fetal bladder and check for distension. Nonvisualization of the bladder with a normal amniotic fluid volume suggests bladder exstrophy (Fig. 27.**5**).
- If a urogenital anomaly is found, carefully inspect the fetus for associated anomalies, including those that may be syndromic. The parents should be offered chromosome testing (Fig. 27.**6**).

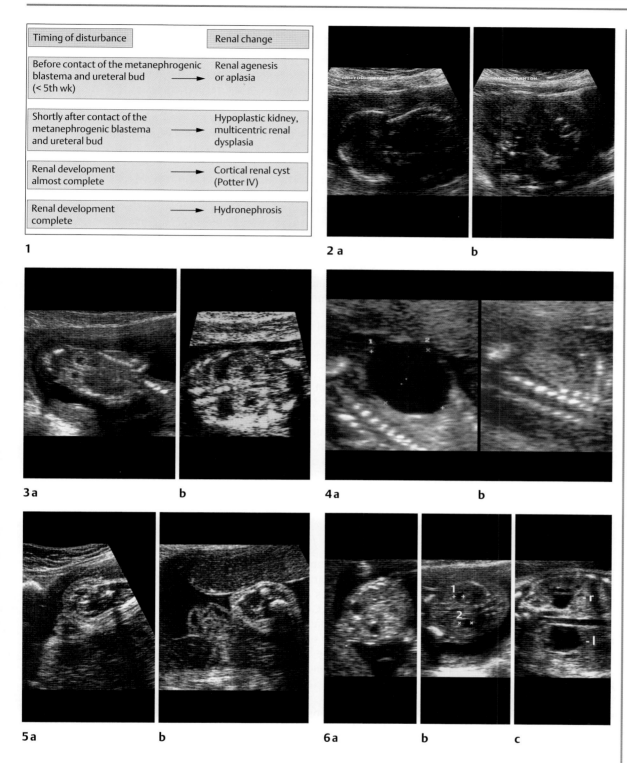

Timing of disturbance	Renal change
Before contact of the metanephrogenic blastema and ureteral bud (< 5th wk)	→ Renal agenesis or aplasia
Shortly after contact of the metanephrogenic blastema and ureteral bud	→ Hypoplastic kidney, multicentric renal dysplasia
Renal development almost complete	→ Cortical renal cyst (Potter IV)
Renal development complete	→ Hydronephrosis

1

2 a   **b**

3 a   **b**

4 a   **b**

5 a   **b**

6 a   **b**   **c**

Embryology of the kidneys

Fig. 27.**1**   Renal changes versus the timing of the disturbance in the interaction between the metanephrogenic blastema and ureteral bud (after 100).

Ultrasound checklist

Fig. 27.**2**   Anhydramnios in bilateral renal agenesis (19 weeks, 3 days).
a Longitudinal scan.
b Transverse scan. The scan quality is poor due to the paucity of amniotic fluid.

Fig. 27.**3**   Renal pelvic dilatation.
a Fetal kidneys with renal pelvic dilatation. Normal amniotic fluid volume, normal development during the rest of the pregnancy (14 weeks, 4 days).
b Hyperechoic renal parenchyma and incipient renal dysplasia in a fetus with renal pelvic dilatation and megalocystis (17 weeks, 1 day).

Fig. 27.**4**   Cystic renal disease.
a Unilateral cystic kidney.
b Corresponding adrenal gland (14 weeks, 5 days).

Fig. 27.**5**   Absence of the urinary bladder.
a Female genitalia, normal amniotic fluid volume, no visible bladder filling (35 weeks, 2 days).
b Gastroschisis. Bowel loops are visible anterior to the vulva. Bladder exstrophy appears as a solid structure.

Fig. 27.**6**   Renal changes and associated anomalies.
a Bilateral renal pelvic dilatation with a defect in the spinal column (12 weeks, 4 days).
b Bilateral renal pelvic dilatation with an extensive diaphragmatic hernia and trisomy 13 (12 weeks, 4 days).
c Bilateral hydronephrosis with a normal amniotic fluid volume. Subpelvic stenosis with no additional anomalies (25 weeks, 4 days).

Diseases of the Kidneys

▬ *Renal Agenesis, Renal Aplasia (Classic Potter Sequence)*

Definition. Since both anomalies (renal agenesis and aplasia) are similar from a diagnostic and prognostic standpoint in prenatal life, they will be discussed under the same heading.

Renal agenesis. This refers to complete absence of the kidney.

Renal aplasia. This denotes the presence of ureters and rudimentary renal tissue.

Original Potter syndrome or Potter sequence. This term applies to the bilateral occurrence of both disorders, where the underlying renal anomalies are accompanied by typical abnormalities of fetal development such as pulmonary hypoplasia, facial dysmorphias, and limb deformities (26, 84).

Incidence. Bilateral renal agenesis has a reported incidence of 0.1–0.3 per 1000 births (review in 84). Unilateral renal agenesis is considerably more common, with a frequency of two in 1000 births (92), and usually it does not have the sequelae of bilateral agenesis.

Embryology, etiology and pathogenesis. Since the development of the kidney through the pronephros, mesonephros, and metanephros stages and the budding of the ureters from the wolffian duct are critical factors in the development of the kidneys and ureters, problems at these early developmental stages can lead to renal agenesis or aplasia.

Isolated renal agenesis generally occurs sporadically and is rarely the expression of a heritable disorder. By contrast, bilateral renal agenesis can occur as part of a syndrome and may reflect a chromosome disorder (family marker syndrome, 4p syndrome), an autosomal-recessive disorder (Fraser syndrome, cerebro-oculofacioskeletal syndrome, acro-renal-mandibular syndrome), or an autosomal-dominant disorder (branchio-oto-renal syndrome) (84). Moreover, preexisting diabetes mellitus has been discussed as a possible cause of renal agenesis (59).

Pathoanatomic findings, associated anomalies. Based on the early occurrence of severe oligohydramnios or anhydramnios, the affected fetuses develop pulmonary hypoplasia, characterized by a reduction of the alveoli and airways. The lung weight may be reduced by more than 50%. The decreased amniotic fluid volume leads to limb anomalies with joint deformities in the hands and feet, joint contractures, hip dislocation, and bowing of the tubular bones. There are also a typical facial appearance with low-set ears, a flat nose, micrognathia, epicanthal folds, and a crease below the lower lids (84, 100).

There may be other associated anomalies besides the typical changes that define Potter syndrome. Forty percent of cases have muscular or skeletal anomalies (radial or fibular aplasia, finger anomalies, vertebral anomalies, facial cleft, diaphragmatic hernia), 19% have gastrointestinal anomalies (malrotation, omphalocele, duodenal or anal atresia, tracheoesophageal fistula), 14% have cardiovascular anomalies (tetralogy of Fallot, septal defects, hypoplastic left ventricle, univentricular heart, dextrocardia, transposition of the great vessels, cardiac valve defects), and 11% have CNS abnormalities (hydrocephalus, microcephaly, cele formation, holoprosencephaly) (97). Unilateral renal agenesis is commonly associated with anomalies of unilateral organs that are also of meso- or paramesonephric origin. In boys, this can lead to an absent or undescended testis or anomalies of the seminiferous structures. Girls may have anomalies of the ovaries, fallopian tubes, uterus, and vagina (5).

Ultrasound Abnormalities, Differential Diagnosis

Decreased amniotic fluid. Pregnancies with bilateral fetal renal agenesis or aplasia are generally marked by the development of oligohydramnios or anhydramnios in the second trimester. The amniotic fluid volume may be normal during the first trimester, because most amniotic fluid at that time is produced by the fetal membranes, and it is not until the 16th week that it consists mainly of fetal urine (92). The decrease in amniotic fluid may be less dramatic in fetuses with an accompanying anomaly that hampers the circulation of amniotic fluid (e.g., esophageal atresia or cerebral malformation) (58).

Nonvisualization of the kidneys. An important ultrasound sign that distinguishes renal agenesis from other renal anomalies with impaired renal function is nonvisualization of the fetal kidneys. Normally, the kidneys can be consistently visualized with high-resolution ultrasound by the 12th week of gestation (84). Confusion may occur in cases where the adrenal glands are not compressed by normally growing kidneys and cannot assume their normal discoid shape. As a result, the adrenals may appear enlarged and may be mistaken for kidneys. The absence of a renal pelvis serves to differentiate the adrenal gland from the kidney, however. The diagnosis of renal agenesis is aided by color Doppler imaging, which can confirm absence of the renal arteries.

Nonvisualization of the bladder. Another important ultrasound feature is nonvisualization of the fetal bladder. This requires serial ultrasound examinations, however. With an initial absence of bladder filling, it is normal to find urine transport into the bladder about 30 minutes later. An interval of at least two hours is advised, however, to make a definitive evaluation of bladder dynamics (96). The maternal administration of furosemide (20–60 mg i.v.) to stimulate fetal urine production (98) is no longer practiced today, because furosemide has difficulty crossing the placental barrier and there is a potential for false-negative results (84).

Amnioinfusion. Sodium chloride or a 5% glucose solution can be infused into the amniotic cavity to obtain better ultrasound delineation of the fetal organs. This also aids in the detection of possible accompanying anomalies and any signs of pulmonary hypoplasia. A dye can be added (Indigo Carmine Blue, indigotindisulfonate sodium 0.8% solution, Taylor Pharmaceuticals) to exclude rupture of the fetal membranes. In case of severe oligohydramnios, amnioinfusion is a helpful tool to diagnose bilateral renal agenesis (Fig. 27.**7**).

The ultrasound features of bilateral renal agenesis or aplasia are summarized in Table 27.**1**.

Prognosis. The prognosis of bilateral renal agenesis or aplasia is grave. In 24–38% of cases the fetus dies while still in utero. The remaining infants die within a few days after birth from the effects of pulmonary hypoplasia (5, 84). Almost half of affected infants are growth-retarded.

Unilateral cases, on the other hand, have a favorable prognosis. The healthy kidney enlarges slightly and assumes the function of both organs. There may still be associated anomalies of the internal genital organs on the ipsilateral side, such as a double uterus, uterine hypoplasia, and atresia of the fallopian tube or epididymis. Generally these changes cannot be diagnosed until after birth or in later life.

Table 27.**1** Ultrasound features of bilateral renal agenesis or aplasia

> ➢ Oligohydramnios or anhydramnios developing in the second trimester
> ➢ Nonvisualization of the fetal bladder, even after amnioinfusion
> ➢ Nonvisualization of the fetal kidneys (do not confuse with enlarged adrenals!)
> ➢ Nonvisualization of the renal arteries
> ➢ Signs of pulmonary hypoplasia (champagne-cork thorax, small lungs)
> ➢ Limb deformity

Recurrence risk. The risk of having another child with renal agenesis in a subsequent pregnancy is 3–4%. This rate may be higher when one parent has unilateral renal agenesis. It should be noted that when bilateral fetal renal agenesis is detected, the risk of unilateral renal agenesis in a first-degree relative is 13%. This climbs to 30% in two affected pregnancies (85).

Prenatal management. Given the grave prognosis of confirmed bilateral renal agenesis or aplasia, pregnancy termination should be considered, regardless of the trimester. The decision on continuing or terminating the pregnancy lies with the parents. In confirmed cases of bilateral renal agenesis or aplasia, the priority concern in obstetric management is the safety of the mother. Cesarean section should not be performed in these cases for a fetal indication. Due to the risk of unilateral renal agenesis in first-degree relatives, these individuals should be scheduled for an ultrasound examination. Chromosome testing is indicated only in fetuses with syndromes.

Cystic Renal Diseases

Classification. Cystic diseases of the kidneys are the most frequent congenital renal anomalies. They are a heterogenous group of disorders whose common feature is a renal cystic abnormality that is highly variable in its extent. The best known and most widely used classification at present is that of Osathanondh and Potter (75). Classifying cystic renal changes into four categories (Potter types I–IV), this system is based entirely on morphologic criteria and does not cover all known variants of cystic renal changes. Newer classifications, like those proposed by Risdon (82), Bernstein (5), Gleason (32), Spence (88), and Zerres (100), take genetic and clinical aspects into account besides pathomorphologic features. Below we shall review fetal cystic renal diseases that are relevant to prenatal diagnosis based on an up-to-date, generally accepted classification that can accommodate the classic Potter types of multicystic kidneys (Table 27.**2**).

Autosomal-Recessive Polycystic Kidney Disease (ARPKD)

Definition. Autosomal-recessive polycystic kidney disease (ARPKD) corresponds to infantile polycystic kidney disease (IPKD) or Potter type I cystic kidney. ARPKD has become the preferred term based on the mode of inheritance of the disease and its possible clinical variability. The term "sponge kidney" was formerly used due to the pathologic appearance of the organ.

Incidence. ARPKD is a somewhat rare anomaly, with an incidence between one in 6000 and one in 40,000 births (5, 99).

Embryology, etiology and pathogenesis. ARPKD is an autosomal-recessive disease with high penetrance. The defect is located on the short arm of chromosome 6 (5, 46). Pathogenetically, the development of the renal collecting tubules is impaired while the remaining portions of the nephron and pelvicaliceal system develop normally.

Pathoanatomic findings, associated anomalies. ARPKD is characterized by a bilateral, symmetrical enlargement of the kidneys, which are diffusely permeated by multiple radially arranged cysts 1–2 mm in size. This gives the kidney a typical sponge-like appearance. The small cysts

Table 27.**2**   Classification of cystic renal diseases (after 31, 100)

> Autosomal-recessive polycystic kidney disease (ARPKD)
> Autosomal-dominant polycystic nephropathy (ADPKD)
> Multicystic dysplastic kidneys
> Obstructive multicystic kidneys
> Polycystic kidneys in syndromes

represent dilated, hyperplastic collecting tubules (75). The absolute number of nephrons is unchanged, but their function is impaired.

Hepatic changes. The cystic renal malformation is consistently accompanied by an intrahepatic biliary anomaly consisting of biliary dysgenesis with hepatic fibrosis. The absence of these hepatic changes rules out ARPKD (100). There are forms of the disease in which the renal changes are relatively minor and the prognosis is determined by subsequent, progressive liver problems in childhood or adulthood (5). Otherwise there are no associations with other congenital malformations or chromosomal abnormalities (5, 84).

Ultrasound features, differential diagnosis. Given the phenotypic variability of the disease, the prenatal findings are highly variable (Fig. 27.**8**, Table 27.**3**). Some affected fetuses display only subtle abnormalities, and others show none at all. It is common, however, to find oligohydramnios or anhydramnios in the early second trimester, comparable to the findings in bilateral renal agenesis. Both kidneys appear enlarged at ultrasound, and the renal parenchyma shows increased echogenicity. Generally the kidneys have a sponge-like appearance because of their diffuse permeation by small cysts. Because renal function is impaired, bladder filling is not observed. Anhydramnios combined with enlarged, hyperechoic kidneys and nonvisualization of the bladder are considered pathognomonic for ARPKD (Fig. 27.**9**). The hepatic changes described above usually cannot be visualized with ultrasound. In cases that show early onset of severe oligohydramnios or anhydramnios, there may be ultrasound signs of pulmonary hypoplasia such as a "champagne-cork" thorax and small lungs.

Amnioinfusion. Ultrasound visualization of the fetal organs can sometimes be improved by infusing a dye solution into the amniotic cavity. Generally this can distinguish ARPKD from other causes of early oligohydramnios such as fetal renal agenesis, premature rupture of the membranes, or severe placental insufficiency. Differentiation from multicystic dysplasia can be difficult.

The ultrasound features of autosomal-recessive polycystic kidney disease are summarized in Table 27.**3**.

Table 27.**3**   Ultrasound features of autosomal-recessive polycystic kidney disease (ARPKD)

> Oligohydramnios or anhydramnios developing in the second trimester
> Nonvisualization of the fetal bladder, even after amnioinfusion
> Both kidneys enlarged and hyperechoic with diffuse small cysts ("sponge kidney")
> Signs of pulmonary hypoplasia (champagne-cork thorax, small lungs)
> Limb deformity

Prognosis. The phenotypic changes in ARPKD are variable. In approximately 90% of cases ARPKD leads to intrauterine fetal death, or neonatal death results from respiratory insufficiency due to pulmonary hypoplasia (31, 100). As mentioned above, there are forms of ARPKD in which the renal changes are less severe and the postpartum course is dictated by hepatic changes. The prenatal ultrasound findings will be less pronounced in these cases than in the classic form of ARPKD. In other rare cases, the patient may have chronic renal failure in adulthood but exhibit no signs of liver dysfunction (100).

Recurrence risk. Given the autosomal-recessive mode of inheritance, the recurrence risk in a couple with an affected child is 25%.

Prenatal management. The pediatric prognosis depends mainly on the signs and risks of pulmonary hypoplasia. In cases with a grave prognosis comparable to that in renal agenesis, pregnancy termination may be considered at any stage of pregnancy. This decision rests with the parents. In late pregnancy the kidneys may become large enough to

Renal agenesis

Fig. 27.**7** Bilateral renal agenesis at 24 weeks, 6 days.

a Anhydramnios. Renal contours are not visualized due to poor imaging conditions.

b Presumed amniotic fluid pockets contain only loops of umbilical cord.

c Amnioinfusion with 200 mL of 5% glucose solution.

d Five minutes after amnioinfusion, the fetal stomach is seen in the left side of the abdomen.

e Vena cava and aorta at the renal level, with no visible branch vessels.

f Aorta at the level of the renal beds. Renal arteries are not visualized. The enlarged adrenals appear as diffuse echoes at the renal level (arrows).

Cystic renal diseases

Fig. 27.**8** Potter I microcystic renal degeneration, ARPKD (16 weeks).

Fig. 27.**9** Potter I juvenile cystic kidneys, ARPKD.

a Anhydramnios. Longitudinal scan at 37 weeks, 3 days.

b Transverse scan of renal vascular supply.

c Longitudinal scan through a juvenile cystic kidney. Multiple small cysts are defined, but the caliceal system is not visualized.

Fig. 27.**10** Adult cystic kidney, ADPKD.

a Unilateral adult cystic kidney (ADP-KD) with a normal contralateral kidney (38 weeks, 0 days).

b Ulceration hydronephrosis with renal dysplasia. The contralateral kidney appears to be displaced (32 weeks, 5 days).

c Slightly enlarged contralateral kidney with mild renal pelvic dilatation (32 weeks, 5 days).

Fig. 27.**11** Left: bilateral multicystic kidneys. Right: corresponding specimen photograph (Prof. Müntefering, Department of Pediatric Pathology, University of Mainz).

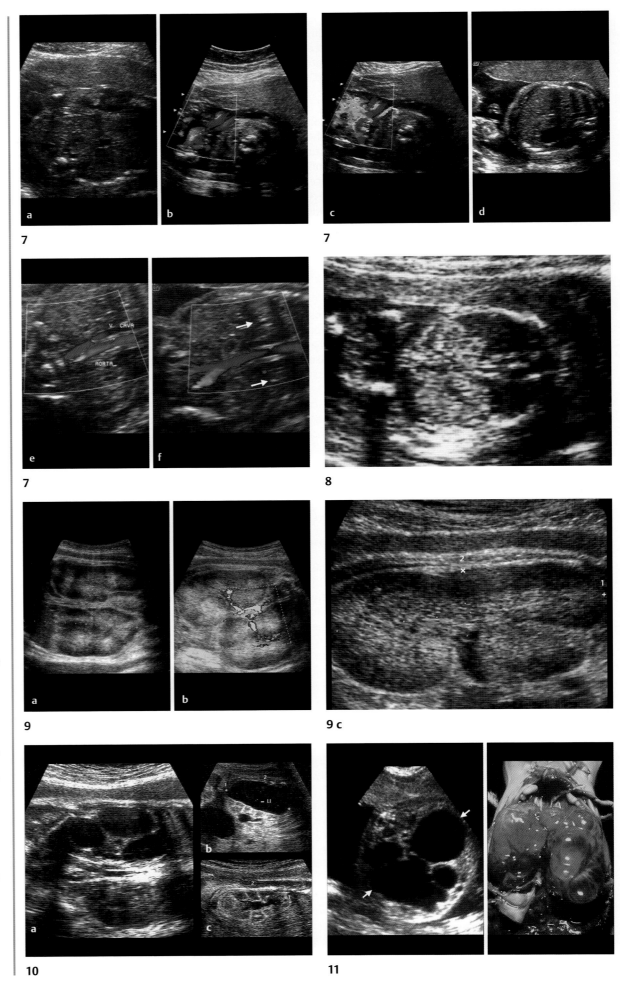

cause obstetric complications. If the fetal prognosis is deemed hopeless, the safety of the mother should be the prime concern, and a cesarean section should not be done for the purpose of fetal salvage. Given the etiology of the disease, the parents should be offered genetic counseling. Couples with a prior history of an affected child can also be offered invasive testing by chorionic biopsy in early pregnancy (101).

Autosomal-Dominant Polycystic Kidney Disease (ADPKD)

Definition. ADPKD is the new term for the disease formerly known as adult polycystic kidney disease or Potter type III cystic kidney.

Incidence. With an incidence of one in 200 to one in 1000 in the overall population, ADPKD is considerably more common than the autosomal-recessive form (5). This makes it one of the most common hereditary diseases in general. It is also one of the major causes of chronic renal failure in humans.

Embryology, etiology and pathogenesis. ADPKD has an autosomal-dominant mode of inheritance. Its phenotypic variability includes the fact that clinically significant compromise of renal function can occur at any stage of life. Usually it does not appear until adulthood, and in some patients the functional impairment has no significant effects (13).

Approximately 95% of patients have a genetic mutation on the short arm of chromosome 16. Another mutation has been identified on chromosome 4 (5, 31).

The development of ADPKD appears to result from abnormal branching of the ureteral bud (84) leading to cyst formation in the duct system. Because these abnormalities are localized, they result in kidneys with a combination of cystic changes and normal renal parenchyma.

Pathoanatomic findings, associated anomalies. Cystic changes may be detectable before symptoms appear and are often identified in children and fetuses. The lesions consist of cysts of varying size affecting both glomerular and tubular structures in the kidney. The cysts range in size from a few millimeters to several centimeters (31). Cysts are usually found in other organs as well, particularly the liver (50% of cases), pancreas (5–10%), and spleen (5), and cerebral aneurysms are found in up to 40% of cases (100).

Ultrasound features. Since approximately 95% of cases have prenatal renal enlargement, antenatal ultrasound can often provide at least a presumptive diagnosis of ADPKD (31). Besides renal enlargement and increased echogenicity of the renal parenchyma, one or more cysts may be detectable in the fetus. The changes may be unilateral or bilateral and are generally discovered during the second half of pregnancy (Fig. 27.**10**, Table 27.**4**). Because significant compromise of renal function does not occur until later life, the amniotic fluid volume is usually normal. Whenever ADPKD is suspected, both parents should definitely be scheduled for a renal ultrasound examination. Since normal renal ultrasound in persons over 20 years of age makes it unlikely that ADPKD is present, this examination can confirm or refute the presumptive diagnosis.

Prognosis. As a general rule, ADPKD does not become symptomatic until 30–50 years of age, at which time the patient develops impaired renal function. The degree of function impairment is variable. In 50% of cases, terminal renal failure develops before 60 years of age (31). Renal function impairment is rare in children and newborns but may still occur (84, 100). The extrarenal manifestations are usually asymptomatic, but the cerebral aneurysms mentioned above may rupture in later life. Based on the autosomal-dominant mode of inheritance, the risk of a couple with one carrier having an affected child is 50%.

Prenatal management. Since ADPKD causes no renal function impairment or does so only in adult life and may be treatable, the discovery of this disease is not an indication for pregnancy termination. It should, however, prompt comprehensive counseling that may include a pediatrician or nephrologist, and psychotherapeutic counseling should be offered. A prenatal investigation in the form of molecular genetic testing by chorion villus sampling or amniotic fluid analysis is an option and may be indicated for affected couples.

Multicystic Dysplastic Kidneys

Definition. Multicystic dysplastic kidneys, known also as dysplastic kidneys, correspond to Potter type II multicystic renal disease. In Potter type IIA, the kidneys are normal sized or enlarged. In Potter type IIB, the kidneys are reduced in size.

Incidence. This condition occurs in approximately one in 1000 births (99). The bilateral form has a reported incidence of one in 10,000.

Embryology, etiology and pathogenesis. Multicystic dysplastic kidneys occur sporadically (79). A familial incidence is uncommon. A significant number of cases are associated with complex malformation syndromes or chromosomal abnormalities (100).

The pathogenesis is based on an abnormal interaction between the ureteral bud and the metanephrogenic blastema in early embryonic development. As a result of this, normal nephrons cannot form. Because this developmental stage lasts for several weeks starting in week 6, the extent of the anomaly can vary considerably.

Pathoanatomic findings, associated anomalies. Generally one kidney is affected, and bilateral involvement is rare. The changes may affect the entire kidney or only segments of it. Histologic examination reveals primitive duct cysts and abnormal differentiation of the metanephrogenic blastema (100). Cartilaginous foci and other dysplastic tissue types may also be detected. In 90% of cases there are obstructive changes in the ureter, which may appear dilated. With a unilateral dysplastic kidney, the opposite kidney also exhibits changes in approximately 40% of cases (6). Usually these are relatively mild anomalies such as malrotation of the kidney or distension of the ureter or renal pelvis. Rarely, however, contralateral renal agenesis can occur.

Besides other renal changes, both unilateral and bilateral renal dysplasia may be associated with other congenital anomalies. These include abnormalities of the CNS (e.g., hydrocephalus), gastrointestinal tract and heart as well as cleft anomalies of the spine. Multicystic dysplastic kidneys also occur in association with various syndromes (Table 27.**6**) and chromosomal abnormalities. When both kidneys are affected, a first-degree relative will be found to have a renal anomaly (usually unilateral renal agenesis) in approximately 10% of cases, showing that hereditary forms can occur (5, 100).

Table 27.**4** Ultrasound features of autosomal-dominant polycystic kidney disease (ADPKD)

> Enlargement of both kidneys
> Visualization of individual renal cysts of varying size
> Normal bladder filling and amniotic fluid volume
> Parent with cystic renal change

Table 27.**5** Ultrasound features of multicystic dysplastic kidneys

> Complete or segmental involvement, usually unilateral
> Kidneys enlarged with multiple, pleomorphic, noncommunicating cysts (Potter IIA)
> Small kidneys (Potter IIB)
> Nonvisualization of renal pelvis
> Nonvisualization of fetal bladder and oligohydramnios/anhydramnios with bilateral involvement

Ultrasound features, differential diagnosis. The variability of renal dysplasia leads to a variety of ultrasound appearances. One or both kidneys may be affected. In Potter type IIA renal dysplasia, the kidney is enlarged and permeated completely or segmentally by pleomorphic, noncommunicating cysts of various sizes (Fig. 27.**11**, Table 27.**5**). The kidney loses its reniform shape. The fact that the cysts are noncommunicating is important in differentiating this condition from hydronephrosis, in which the cystic cavities communicate with one another. Dysplastic kidneys assume a cluster-of-grapes appearance. Generally the renal pelvis is not visualized. In Potter type IIB dysplasia, the kidneys are hypoplastic, and cystic transformation is often not apparent. This form requires differentiation from renal agenesis with enlarged adrenal glands. With unilateral renal dysplasia, the contralateral side appears normal. Bladder filling is seen, and the amniotic fluid volume is normal or slightly decreased. In bilateral cases, on the other hand, the bladder is not visualized, and oligohydramnios or anhydramnios begins to develop in the second trimester.

Prognosis. The prognosis depends on whether the changes are unilateral or bilateral and on the extent of the renal changes. Ultimately the prognosis is determined by how much renal function remains. Bilateral involvement with inadequate renal function leads to a Potter sequence comparable to bilateral renal agenesis, and the prognosis is grave. By contrast, unilateral or segmental involvement is associated with normal intrauterine urine production and an unremarkable postpartum course. With passage of time, the patient may develop symptoms such as recurrent urinary tract infections or hypertension. Most affected children are managed conservatively. Nephrectomy should be reserved for a very select group of patients (5).

Recurrence risk. For a child with oligohydramnios syndrome and renal dysplasia, the recurrence risk is approximately 5%. The risk increases if a parental renal anomaly is found (100).

Prenatal management. In cases with bilateral renal involvement and the development of oligohydramnios or anhydramnios, pregnancy termination should be considered as in cases of bilateral renal agenesis. If the parents want to continue the pregnancy or if the condition is detected very late, a cesarean section for fetal salvage should be avoided due to the poor prognosis for fetal survival. If unilateral involvement is detected before viability is reached, chromosomal abnormalities should be excluded. Given the association with other congenital anomalies and syndromes, detailed scanning should be performed to check for fetal anomalies. Unilateral involvement suggests a favorable prognosis, and ordinary obstetric management is indicated. The parents and siblings may also have a renal anomaly and should be scheduled for ultrasound.

Obstructive Multicystic Kidneys (Potter IV)

Pathogenesis. Multicystic renal anomalies result from a mechanical blockage affecting the excretory portion of the urinary tract. Cysts develop in the renal cortex as the nephrons continue to produce urine against the pressure in the urinary drainage tract. The parenchymal destruction predominantly affects the renal cortex (Fig. 27.**12**).

Ultrasound features. The ultrasound features of the resulting dysplasia consist of increased echogenicity in the renal cortex and subsequent cyst formation. The course and prognosis are typical of obstructive uropathies.

Polycystic Kidneys in Syndromes

Polycystic renal changes are often part of a congenital syndrome. It is very common to find dysplastic renal changes of variable degree in syndromes, with or without cystic changes. Whenever renal abnormalities are detected in a fetus, it is essential to conduct a detailed examination of the other organ systems. Table 27.**6** lists some of the genetically determined syndromes that are frequently associated with cystic renal anomalies. Since many of these conditions are hereditary, genetic counseling should be offered and a genetic evaluation, including prenatal testing, should be considered. Cystic renal diseases or other renal anomalies may also be found in association with chromosomal abnormalities, which may affect almost all chromosome pairs (90). For example, 15–30% of fetuses with trisomy 13 or 18 are found to have renal anomalies, usually of subtle degree, besides the typical changes described elsewhere.

Table 27.**6** Congenital syndromes that are frequently associated with cystic renal anomalies (adapted from 31, 100)

Syndrome	Incidence (1 : births)	Mode of inheritance (locus of mutation)	Principal findings
Meckel–Gruber syndrome	1 : 9000	Autosomal-recessive (chromosome 17)	Renal cysts, encephalocele, hydrocephalus, polydactyly, hepatic cysts; grave prognosis
Tuberous sclerosis	1 : 7000	Autosomal-dominant (chromosome 16) (variable expression)	Renal cysts or angiomyolipomas, cerebral glial nodules, oligophrenia, rhabdomyomas in the heart
von Hippel–Lindau syndrome	< 1 : 45,000	autosomal dominant (chromosome 3) (variable expression)	Cysts or tumors of the kidneys and pancreas, cerebral and retinal hemangioblastomas; clinical manifestations appear at 20—40 years of age
Branchio-oto-renal dysplasia	1 : 40,000	autosomal dominant (chromosome 8) (variable expression)	Renal cysts, cleft lip and palate, preauricular fistula, deafness
Short Rib–polydactyly syndrome		Autosomal-recessive	Various renal anomalies, limb shortening, heart defects, small thorax; poor prognosis
Orofaciodigital syndrome I	1 : 80,000	X-linked dominant (variable expression)	Cleft lip and palate, cleft tongue, frenular hyperplasia, syndactyly, type III-like renal cysts (often lethal in boys)
Jeune syndrome		Autosomal-recessive (variable expression)	Narrow thorax, short limbs, hypoplastic pelvis, type II kidneys
Roberts syndrome		Autosomal-recessive	Tetraphocomelia, cleft lip and palate, facial dysmorphism, growth retardation, microcephaly, renal cysts
Zellweger syndrome	1 : 100,000	Autosomal-recessive	High forehead, hepatomegaly, renal anomalies, psychomotor retardation

▬ *Obstructive Urinary Tract Anomalies*

Definition. Obstructive fetal urinary tract anomalies are manifested by the distension of various portions of the fetal urinary tract: the renal pelvis, ureters, and bladder. The stenosis may cause a partial or complete blockage of fetal urinary drainage, depending on its location and degree. The critical anatomic sites are the junction of the renal pelvis with the ureters (ureteropelvic junction), the insertion of the ureters into the bladder (ureterovesical junction), and the fetal urethra (obstruction of the bladder outlet). If a fetal bladder obstruction is severe enough to cause a substantial rise in pressure, the entire urinary tract will become dilated due to reflux from the ureteral orifices into the renal pelves.

Incidence. Obstructive uropathies are relatively frequent, occurring in 0.3–1% of births (1, 37, 60, 62). Only a small number of these anomalies warrant surgical intervention (urinary diversion from the bladder or renal pelves).

Embryology, normal ultrasound appearance. Both the fetal bladder and kidneys can be demonstrated by transvaginal scanning between 11 and 12 weeks' gestation. Absence of the bladder should be suspected if it cannot be visualized in repeated scans performed at 15 weeks. The renal cortex and medulla can be differentiated by 18 weeks. The growth of the kidneys parallels overall fetal growth and can be compared with established norms up to 20 years of age (36, 53). Until the second trimester of pregnancy, the amniotic fluid volume is controlled mainly by secretions from the amniotic cavity, umbilical cord, and fetal skin. Starting at 14 weeks, homeostasis of the amniotic fluid volume is increasingly determined by fetal urine production.

The genital tubercle can be defined as early as the first trimester (23). A prominent genital tubercle should not be mistaken for male genitalia, however. Occasionally it is visible in female fetuses prior to 14 weeks. The urethra in male fetuses can be identified at 28 weeks or later.

Pathoanatomic Findings

Renal dysplasia. In cases of obstructive uropathy without associated anomalies, fetal renal function depends on whether the condition is associated with renal dysplasia. It is still uncertain whether renal dysplasia is caused by elevated pressure in the urinary tract or by a parallel, pathophysiologic embryonic process that is independent of urinary tract pressure. If the latter hypothesis is correct, it would eliminate the rationale for intrauterine shunt procedures for urinary obstruction, because they are almost always done at 14 weeks, after renal dysplasia has already developed. Experiments in sheep fetuses have shown, however, that relieving an iatrogenic obstruction created during the first half of pregnancy can prevent renal failure in later pregnancy (76).

Complete outflow obstruction. In most cases of obstructive uropathy with a total outflow obstruction, terminal renal failure develops during the second trimester. This results in oligohydramnios or anhydramnios, since the amniotic fluid volume in the second and third trimesters is determined chiefly by fetal urination into the amniotic fluid. Compression of the fetus by the uterine musculature prevents expansion of the fetal thorax, leading to pulmonary hypoplasia that usually causes neonatal death. Intrauterine fetal death due to umbilical cord compression and anomalies such as Potter sequence result from the deficient amniotic fluid.

Prognosis. Oligohydramnios occurring after 24 weeks' gestation is not necessarily associated with pulmonary hypoplasia, but there may be a terminal renal function deficit as a result of dysplasia. If normal fetal urine parameters are found, the prognosis is favorable. If the obstruc-

tion is accompanied by a normal or decreased amniotic fluid volume, the prognosis is still good if fetal urine parameters are within normal limits. But if the urine values are abnormal, the infant will be born with elevated serum creatinine levels. These levels can be lowered by relieving the obstruction in the postpartum period. No long-term data are available on the progression of renal function in these children.

Most children with urinary tract dilatation during fetal life will survive and have normal kidney function. This particularly applies to unilateral obstructions with a normal contralateral kidney. The most important prognostic sign is an adequate amniotic fluid volume. Fluid pockets 2 cm in size located at two opposing sites in the amniotic cavity are considered to represent an adequate fluid volume. In cases of bilateral obstruction with a normal amniotic fluid volume, fetal urinalysis should be performed only if the renal parenchyma appears markedly hyperechoic. The location of the obstruction has a low prognostic significance.

Sites of Obstructive Urinary Tract Anomalies

Subpelvic ureteral obstruction. Subpelvic ureteral obstruction is the most common fetal urinary tract anomaly (27). It is rarely associated with a duplication anomaly or aberrant renal vessels.

Megaureter. A megaureter results from a lesion or dysfunction at the ureterovesical junction.

Ureterocele. A ureterocele is a cystic expansion of the terminal portion of the ureter at the bladder leading to ureteral dilatation. Often there is concomitant duplication of the ureters and kidneys.

Obstruction of the fetal urethra. This usually leads to megacystis with hypertrophy of the bladder musculature and reflux into the renal pelves. The hydronephrosis may be associated with renal dysplasia. The most frequent cause of bladder distension is a valve created by a mucosal fold in the posterior wall of the urethra. Urethral atresia is less common and leads to fetal anuria and intrauterine fetal death in the second trimester.

Vesicourethral reflux. Vesicourethral reflux is occasionally observed prenatally in late pregnancy and has no immediate impact on renal function. A prenatal diagnosis should, however, prompt observation of the child and the avoidance of urinary tract infections, with a potential need for early surgery.

Cloacal malformation. This results from deficient development of the urogenital sinus. In females it is associated with vesicovaginal and urethrovaginal fistulas, and affected males often have anorectal fistulas.

Prune belly syndrome. Prune belly syndrome is a combination of several defects: absence of the abdominal wall muscles, a grossly distended bladder, renal dysplasia, and in males absence of the prostate and cryptorchidism (68). The syndrome is rare (one in 50,000 births), and 97% of affected fetuses are male. Obstruction of the urethra leads to megacystis and bilateral megaureters (Fig. 27.**13**). Affected female fetuses have associated genital anomalies: vaginal atresia, rectovaginal or rectovesical fistula, and bicornuate uterus. The absence of the abdominal wall muscles leads to wrinkling of the skin (especially after bladder drainage), which gives the syndrome its name. Often the condition is not distinguishable prenatally from a urethral valve. As in any uropathy, the prognosis depends on the function of the remaining intact renal tissue.

Urachal cyst. A urachal cyst develops when the portion of the urachus between the bladder and abdominal wall remains patent. It appears as an echogenic structure extending into the umbilical cord insertion and

Fig. 27.**12** Obstructive multicystic kidneys at 32 weeks.
a Left cystic kidney: internal echoes, loss of corticomedullary differentiation.
b Right hydronephrosis with a cyst at the apical pole.
c Hyperechoic structure of the renal parenchyma following needle aspiration. Bilateral renal dysplasia.

Obstructive urinary tract anomalies

Fig. 27.**13** Left: prune belly syndrome with massive dilatation of the bladder. Breech presentation at 15 weeks, 5 days (observation by Prof. Merz, Frankfurt). Right: corresponding specimen photograph.

Fig. 27.**14** Sacrococcygeal teratoma as an associated anomaly.
a Renal pelvic obstruction and dysplastic degeneration associated with an intra- and extra-abdominal sacrococcygeal teratoma. The extra-abdominal component is shown (21 weeks, 4 days).
b Renal dysplasia and intra-abdominal component of a sacrococcygeal teratoma (21 weeks, 4 days).

Fig. 27.**15** Ultrasound findings associated with a chromosomal abnormality.
a Increased nuchal transparency (3.1 mm) at 11 weeks, 6 days.
b Megacystis, hyperechoic structure above the bladder.
c Megacystic, hyperechoic structure in the colon region, trisomy 18.

Fig. 27.**16** Urethral valve, megaureter, mild renal pelvic dilatation. The kidney is normally differentiated into a cortex and medulla, signifying a good prognosis (37 weeks, 6 days).

Fig. 27.**17** Megacystis at 15 weeks, 4 days.
a Megacystis with suspicion of a urethral valve/urethral dysplasia. Note the bottleneck narrowing toward the urethra.
b Color Doppler shows an umbilical artery on both sides of the enlarged bladder.

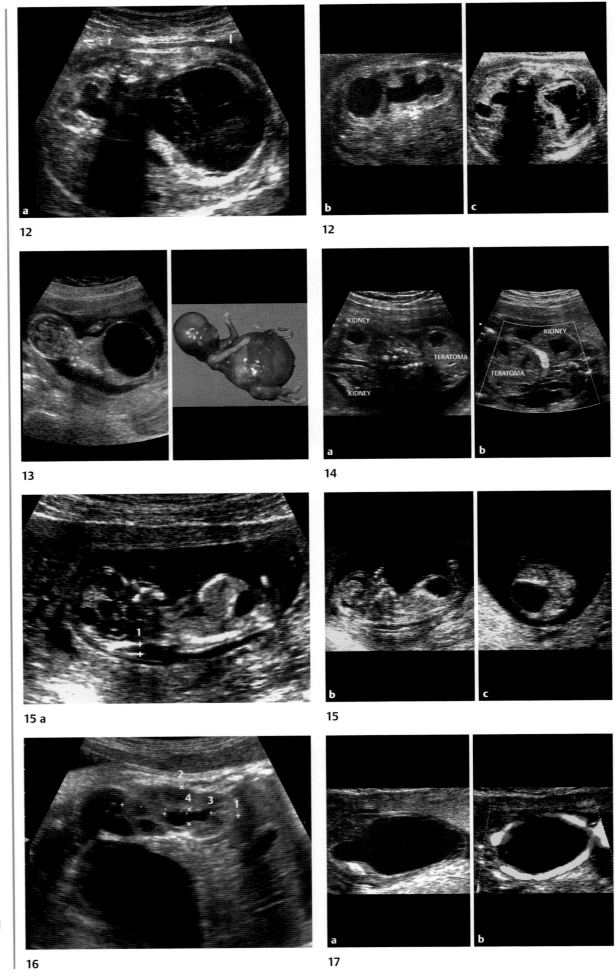

may persist in newborns as a vesicocutaneous fistula. The cyst itself has no pathologic significance and usually disappears as the pregnancy progresses.

Associated Anomalies, Chromosomal abnormalities

The ultrasound detection of urinary stasis is a spot diagnosis. Obstructions are commonly associated with anomalies outside the urinary tract (Fig. 27.**14**), making it imperative that the fetus be very carefully examined (34, 72).

Bladder exstrophy. With a normal amniotic fluid volume and nonvisualization of the fetal bladder in serial examinations, a presumptive diagnosis of bladder exstrophy may be made. In some cases it can be directly visualized (Fig. 27.**4**) (2).

Persistent cloaca, anal and rectal atresia. Other associated anomalies are difficult to diagnose even with a normal amniotic fluid volume, because they display subtle features and are not detectable until the third trimester. This pertains to the various forms of cloacal persistence (86), anal atresia, and rectal atresia. Usually a prognosis for postpartum reconstruction cannot be made. In all cases the parents should be referred to an experienced pediatric surgeon and urologist.

Megacystis–microcolon–hypoperistalsis syndrome. This rare syndrome is difficult to distinguish from prune belly syndrome, but a presumptive diagnosis can be made when a dilated urinary bladder is found in association with distended bowel loops. Usually it cannot be distinguished from dilated ureteral loops, although this distinction would be important given the poor prognosis in cases where bowel function is absent (65).

Chromosomal abnormalities. Chromosomal abnormalities are reportedly present in 12% of fetuses with renal anomalies (34). This includes fetuses with associated anomalies. With an isolated urinary tract obstruction such as a urethral valve, there is little risk that an abnormal karyotype is present. Nevertheless, the parents should still be offered karyotyping, as in any prenatal anomaly, so that an accurate prognosis can be made (Fig. 27.**15**). A normal karyotype is important in postnatal operative planning and in motivating the parents to continue the pregnancy. With mild bilateral dilatation of the renal pelves, which is found in 2% of cases at 20 weeks, the possible need for karyotyping may be discussed. With isolated bilateral pyelectasis, the risk is increased by a factor of 1.2–6 (21, 87, 93, 95). But if pyelectasis is combined with even a mild associated anomaly, the risk of aneuploidy is increased 10- to 20-fold (3, 17). Although the data are not yet conclusive in our opinion, we feel that a risk assessment based on maternal age, absent nuchal translucency, and a low-risk maternal serum screen cannot be combined with the marker of mild pyelectasis, because it has not been proven that the markers affect risk independently of one another.

Ultrasound Features of Uropathy

Renal pelvic dilatation. There is no generally accepted definition and grading system for renal pelvic dilatation in the fetus. Using anatomic criteria, we could define pyelectasis as pelvic dilatation that does not involve the calices (Fig. 26.**16**), whereas hydronephrosis includes dilatation of the calices. In the classification of Grignon (38), grade I represents a normal fetus, grade II is dilatation < 1.5 cm, and grades III and IV represent hydronephrosis. This grading system has not become widely adopted because it has no definite clinical implications.

In the literature, pyelectasis is defined as an anteroposterior renal pelvic diameter of 4–6 mm in the second trimester and 8–10 mm in the third trimester, measured in a transverse abdominal scan (21). These measurements have very little clinical significance. A spot check

during pregnancy can exclude any increase in pyelectasis. Only an anteroposterior diameter > 1.0 cm would warrant postnatal follow-up.

Hydronephrosis. In simple terms, hydronephrosis is defined as enlargement of the renal pelvis to more than 1.5 cm in its anteroposterior dimension (38). The renal calices are only slightly dilated in mild hydronephrosis (grade III), but in grade IV cases the renal contours are rounded and there are cystic areas that communicate with the renal pelvis. Unlike renal cysts, these areas are not discrete lesions but communicate with one another. With even greater distension (grade V), the calices can no longer be distinguished from the renal pelvic outline, and the renal parenchyma is thinned to a few millimeters. The thin cortex in itself does not mean that renal function is poor, however. If the cortex and medulla can still be differentiated and there are no cysts, it is reasonable to assume that renal function is good. The ultrasound evaluation of hydronephrotic kidneys is inferior to biochemical analysis, however (49, 69).

Dilated ureter. Only a dilated ureter can be identified as a cystic mass between the kidney and bladder; a normal ureter cannot be visualized with ultrasound. If the renal pelvis is dilated and peristalsis can be seen, a megaureter is present. A distended bladder indicates vesicourethral reflux (12).

Dilated fetal bladder. A dilated fetal bladder should empty during a 20-minute ultrasound examination. If this does not occur, it should be assumed that a urethral obstruction is present. Color Doppler can be used to distinguish the urinary bladder from a cystic structure located within the fetal abdomen. The bladder is flanked by the two umbilical arteries. A narrow outpouching of the bladder in the area of the symphysis signifies a urethral valve (Fig. 27.**17**). If the obstruction has been present for some time, the bladder musculature may thicken to more than 3 mm. Bladder diverticula appear as small protrusions. The presence of bladder dilatation and male fetal genitalia make it likely that a urethral valve is present, although that lesion is indistinguishable from urethral atresia. With vesicourethral reflux, the bladder and lower portions of the ureters are distended while the renal pelves are unchanged. Complex urogenital anomalies should be excluded whenever a urinary tract obstruction is found. They are more common in female fetuses (Fig. 27.**18**). Attempting to drain a distended fetal bladder with a percutaneous needle can trigger urinary ascites (Fig. 27.**19**). Spontaneous rupture of the bladder wall and ureteral rupture with urinoma formation can also occur.

Table 27.**7** reviews the ultrasound features of obstructive uropathy and their prognostic significance.

Table 27.**7** Ultrasound features of obstructive uropathy, with prognostic implications

> - Amniotic fluid volume normal or reduced (oligohydramnios or anhydramnios < 24 weeks: poor prognosis; amniotic fluid pockets at 2 sites = 2 cm after 24 weeks: good prognosis)
> - Variable dilation of pelvicaliceal system, ureters, and bladder: prognosis depends on site and degree of obstruction
> - Loss of corticomedullary differentiation: poor prognosis
> - Cysts in renal parenchyma indicating cystic renal dysplasia: poor prognosis
> - Hyperechoicity of renal parenchyma: poor prognosis

Prognosis

Surgical options. The ultrasound detection of obstructive uropathy is a spot diagnosis. To determine the exact site of the lesion and assess the prognosis, it is necessary to know the specific course of the disease and the surgical options. Once the diagnosis has been established, it is helpful to call in a urologist experienced in pediatric urology. An isolated uropathy can be surgically corrected with a good prognosis, provided renal function is not impaired.

Prune belly syndrome. The prognosis of prune belly syndrome is uncertain and depends on renal function after birth. Rarely the disease affects consanguine male siblings, with an associated risk of recurrence. The severity of the syndrome varies, and hence the prognosis is also variable. There is a 20% incidence of stillbirth or death during the first 2 months of life, with only 50% of children surviving the first 2 years. Mental development proceeds normally. The reported incidence is one in 20,000 to one in 40,000 births, and the prenatal incidence is presumably higher. Intrauterine urinary diversion is not appropriate for this complex anomaly. The life expectancy of surviving infants can be improved by hemodialysis and renal transplantation. The parents should be given detailed information on the condition. Pregnancy termination may be considered in some cases.

Main ultrasound parameters. The most important ultrasound parameters for determining the prognosis of obstructive uropathy are the amniotic fluid volume and the presence of cysts in the renal parenchyma. Oligohydramnios prior to 24 weeks is almost always associated with renal dysplasia and pulmonary hypoplasia and is incompatible with survival (19). Renal cysts in obstructive uropathy can be seen as early as 20 weeks, but they may appear later in the pregnancy, making it difficult to predict renal dysplasia with much accuracy (63).

Prenatal Management

Invasive tests. The management and prognosis of isolated fetal obstructive uropathy depend upon intrauterine renal function.

Ultrasound and urine analysis. In most cases of obstructive uropathy, the prognosis can be determined from ultrasound parameters with reasonable confidence. In cases where pregnancy termination or intrauterine therapy is being considered, fetal renal function should be assessed by urinalysis. This test is based on the ability of the renal tubules to reabsorb various components of the glomerular filtrate. Fetal urinalysis is not based on the same excretory products that are used in postnatal urinalysis, which are regulated by the maternal kidneys. Normal values for fetal urine have been determined in fetuses that were without uropathy prior to pregnancy termination (74). The most important parameters are sodium, potassium, calcium, phosphate, glucose, and β_2-microglobulin. When the prognostic importance of these parameters was determined in a study of fetuses over 20 weeks, a good correlation was found between a renal function deficit and a poor prognosis (20). The value of the test before 20 weeks has not been well established. Electrolyte values for sodium > 100 mEq/L, chlorine > 90 mEq/L, and osmolarity > 210 mOsm/L indicate an unfavorable prognosis (19, 22, 55). Some authors believe that ultrasound parameters are good predictors of perinatal mortality due to obstructive uropathy alone, while fetal urinalysis can provide information on postnatal morbidity (69).

Oligohydramnios in the second and third trimesters. When oligohydramnios occurs in the second and third trimesters due to fetal urinary tract obstruction after an initially normal amniotic fluid volume, and ultrasound reveals structural abnormalities in the renal parenchyma (lack of corticomedullary differentiation, hyperechoic renal tissue, cysts in the renal cortex, Potter IV signs), analysis of the fetal urine can support suspicion of renal failure by showing elevated urinary levels of sodium and β_2-microglobulin (Fig. 27.**20**). If oligohydramnios occurs in the third trimester with a normal-appearing renal parenchyma and borderline urine values, options include early delivery, intrauterine shunting, or an expectant approach allowing physiologic onset of labor.

Renal function in the first 2 years of life. The problem with studies of biochemical parameters in the fetal urine is that, while these parameters yield good information on the prognosis for survival, they tell us little about subsequent renal function due to a lack of long-term data. To gain interim information on fetal and postnatal renal function, Muller et al. (70) investigated various urinary compounds in 70 fetuses with obstructive uropathy. They assumed that a serum creatinine less than or equal to 50 ?mol/L at age 1–2 years indicated satisfactory renal function, and that fetuses with those values would not develop renal failure in later life. They found that urinary sodium and β_2-microglobulin levels above the 95th percentile in fetuses correlated with elevated serum creatinine levels during childhood (1–2 years of age), indicating that renal failure would probably develop in later life. When findings are borderline, sequential samples should be analyzed (56).

Invasive intrauterine therapy. The German Society for Pediatric Urology rejects any therapeutic intervention based on the data that have been published to date on intrauterine therapy.

Vesicoamniotic shunts. Ultrasound-guided vesicoamniotic shunts have been used in the treatment of obstructive uropathy since 1984 (4, 35, 83). This procedure sprang from the simple notion that bypassing the obstruction could decompress the kidneys and prevent dysplasia while providing sufficient amniotic fluid for lung maturation. This assumption was based on experimental studies in fetal sheep (33, 43, 44). So far, however, there is no evidence to prove that shunting is of significant general benefit in human fetuses with obstructive uropathy (15, 28, 66).

Methods. Transvesical fetoscopy for the elimination of urethral valves by electrocautery and laser treatment has not proven successful (24, 80). In theory, the fetal bladder can be fenestrated with a fetoscope and laser or entered through an open surgical approach. A less invasive method, and also the most popular option, is a vesicoamniotic shunt using a double pigtail catheter (74). Complications include catheter displacement or clogging and urinary ascites. Early obstructions may resolve spontaneously. There have been other cases (including the authors') in which the diagnostic aspiration of megacystis has relieved the obstruction, allowing the pregnancy to continue normally. In our opinion, vesicoamniotic shunting cannot be offered as a general therapeutic option for obstructive uropathy (Table 27.**8**). There are some situations, however, in which it is likely that the fetus will survive (mild oligohydramnios, normal fetal urinary sodium levels) but there is still a risk to subsequent renal function as indicated by hyperechoic parenchyma and a mild elevation of β_2-microglobulin. In these cases shunting can be discussed with the parents as an experimental option. The parents should also understand the potential complications of the procedure (rupture of the fetal membranes, premature labor, chorioamnionitis).

Table 27.8 Intrauterine therapy of obstructive uropathy in the recent literature

Author and year	Ultrasound exclusion of renal dysgenesis	Fetal urinalysis, adequate function	Benefit in selected cases	General
Freedman AL 1997 (29)	+	+	(+)	–
Lewis KM et al. 1998 (61)	+	+	(+)	–
Szaflik K et al. 1998 (89)	+	+	+	–
Bonsib SM 1998 (8)	+	+	(+)	–
Johnson MP et al. 1999 (57)	+	+	(+)	–
Freedman AL et al. 1999 (30)	+	+	–	–
Makino Y 2000 (64)	+	+	(+)	–
Irwin BH et al. 2000 (50)	+	+	–	–

Benefit: – No benefit   (+) Limited benefit   + Definite benefit

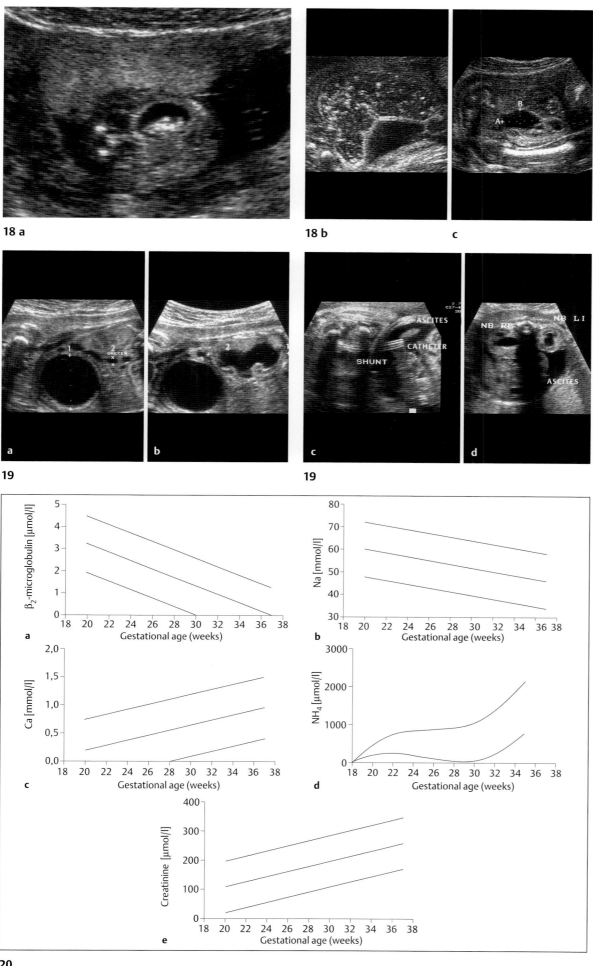

18 a

18 b   **c**

19   **19**

a   **b**   **c**   **d**

Fig. 27.**18** VACTERL syndrome: an association of anomalies of the spinal column, rectum, trachea, esophagus, limbs, heart, and kidneys.
a Cyst with solid contents in the colon area, normal amniotic fluid volume (16 weeks, 5 days).
b Megacolon, cystic area in the abdomen (24 weeks, 5 days).
c Anhydramnios, deformed urinary bladder, and urachal cyst (24 weeks, 5 days).

Fig. 27.**19** Megacystis and renal pelvic dilatation due to a urethral valve.
a Oligohydramnios, megacystis (1), and urethral obstruction (2) (29 weeks, 3 days).
b Renal pelvic dilatation, calices are still defined (29 weeks, 3 days).
c Development of urinary ascites following shunt insertion (30 weeks, 3 days).
d Moderate decompression of the renal pelvis after shunt insertion.

Fig. 27.**20** Reference curves for parameters of fetal urinalysis. Regression curves for the 5th, 50th, and 95th percentiles (modified from 70).
a β_2-microglobulin.
b Sodium.
c Calcium.
d Ammonia.
e Creatinine.

20

Fig. 27.**21** Management of obstructive uropathy.

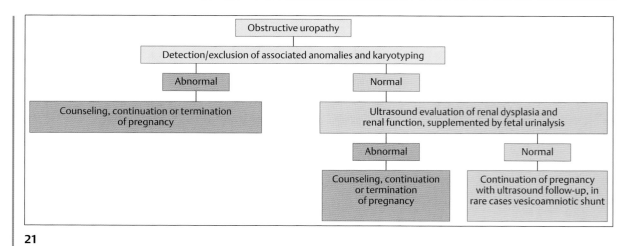

21

Tumors

Fig. 27.**22** Wilms' tumor.
a Retroperitoneal mass below the left kidney (31 weeks, 0 days).
b Wilms' tumor (31 weeks, 0 days).

Fig. 27.**23** Solid mass in the right kidney, 5.6 x 4.2 x 5.1 cm. Color Doppler shows neovascularization. Histology: mesoblastic nephroma (30 weeks, 3 days) (observation by Prof. Merz, Frankfurt am Main).

22 **23**

Fig. 27.**24** Differential diagnosis of a hemorrhagic mass.
a Cystic/solid mass superior to the kidneys, causing renal deformation. 1 = Bladder, 2 = kidney, 3 = mass.
b Normal left kidney. The mass results from bleeding into the right adrenal gland. Infarction of the right kidney has occurred.

Fig. 27.**25** Right-sided adrenal adenoma (arrow), 35 x 31 mm (37 weeks, 6 days) (observation by Prof. Merz, Frankfurt).

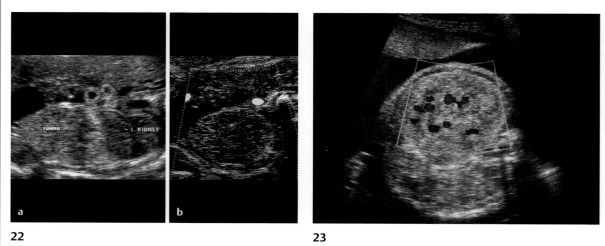

24 **25**

Prenatal care and obstetric management. In cases of obstructive uropathy with multiple anomalies and terminal renal failure, most parents will request pregnancy termination. It is possible to continue the pregnancy, even with a grave prognosis, as there is no increased maternal threat from a pregnancy-specific disease. Cesarean section for a fetal indication should be avoided, however. Fetuses with obstructive uropathy and a good likelihood of survival should receive normal antenatal surveillance and appropriate perinatal care. Early delivery is indicated only in selected cases where it is thought that renal damage can be avoided. Preterm delivery with risk of pulmonary problems should be weighed against the questionable benefit (Fig. 27.**21**).

Renal and Adrenal Tumors

Congenital renal and adrenal tumors are rare. When present, they often appear prenatally as solid, cystic, or mixed solid/cystic masses. The differential diagnosis consists mainly of neuroblastoma, Wilms tumor, and mesoblastic nephroma. Clear-cell sarcomas and rhabdoid tumors of the kidney are extremely rare lesions that often metastasize early and have a poor prognosis. Fetal abdominal masses can also result from duplications of the digestive tract, teratomas, subdiaphragmatic pulmonary sequestra, and cysts of the pancreas, biliary tract, ovaries, and mesentery (94). The differential diagnosis of intra-abdominal masses is reviewed in Table 27.**9**.

Wilms Tumor and Congenital Mesoblastic Nephroma

Definition. Wilms tumors, also called nephroblastomas, are malignant embryonic mixed tumors of the kidney. Congenital mesoblastic nephroma (synonymous with fetal renal hamartoma), on the other hand, is generally a benign renal tumor.

Incidence. Congenital Wilms tumor occurs in approximately 0.1% of all births (48) and accounts for 0.8–3% of all Wilms tumors (41, 48). The majority of renal neoplasms detected prenatally and formerly identified as Wilms tumors are actually congenital mesoblastic nephromas. In two studies, 67–90% of congenital renal tumors were found to be of this type.

Embryology, etiology and pathogenesis. Molecular genetic studies indicate that both tumor types have a different pathogenesis (90). Wilms tumors result from an abnormal proliferation of metanephrogenic blastema, whereas congenital mesoblastic nephromas are apparently derived from undifferentiated nephrogenic mesenchyme. This type of tumor rarely metastasizes and is classified as essentially benign.

In cytogenic and molecular genetic studies of children with Wilms tumors, a small percentage of patients were found to have a deletion on chromosome 11 or a mutation of the WT1 and WT2 genes on chromosome 11 (52, 77). Most of these children had bilateral tumors or a coexisting syndrome.

Pathoanatomic findings, associated anomalies. Renal tumors are unilateral in 95% of cases. Wilms tumor is a solid, invasive tumor with an exophytic or endophytic growth pattern that can completely permeate the renal parenchyma. It may consist of blastomatous, epithelia, and stromal components. Intrauterine metastasis can occur. Fourteen percent of affected fetuses have a coexisting anomaly, usually involving the genitourinary system (e.g., hypospadias, renal dysplasia, duplicated ureters, cryptorchidism) (9). Wilms tumor may also be associated with various syndromes leading to gigantism, especially Beckwith–Wiedemann syndrome and isolated hemihypertrophy. Other syndromic associations are less common (Perlmann, Sotos, Simpson/Golabi/Behmel) (14).

Like Wilms tumors, congenital mesoblastic nephromas invade the renal parenchyma and renal pelvis with no distinct line of demarca-

tion. The renal capsule usually remains intact. The tumor surface resembles that of a myoma. Histologically, congenital mesoblastic nephroma consists of a web-like arrangement of spindle-shaped aggregates of fibroblasts and myofibroblasts (90). Rarely, this tumor is associated with syndromes such as hemihypertrophy and Beckwith–Wiedemann syndrome (52).

Ultrasound features. Both tumor types appear sonographically as a solid mass. It should be noted that solid tumors in the renal area are sometimes difficult to distinguish from the kidney itself because of their similar echogenicities (Figs. 27.**22**, 27.**23**). Often, however, the normal renal structure is completely destroyed by the tumor. Wilms tumor and mesoblastic nephroma cannot be distinguished from each other antenatally. Hydramnios is a common associated finding (81). Signs of hydrops and congestive heart failure have also been reported in association with mesoblastic nephroma (91). Since both tumors are associated with syndromes, their detection should prompt a detailed ultrasound evaluation of the fetus.

Prognosis. It should be emphasized that most renal tumors diagnosed prenatally are congenital mesoblastic nephromas, and therefore benign. These tumors rarely metastasize, and surgical removal is curative in most cases. Wilms tumors are also considered to have a favorable prognosis. The cure rate for Wilms tumors of all types and stages is approximately 85–90% (16, 41).

Risk. Based on the familial incidence of Wilms tumors, a unilateral tumor in one parent is associated with a 5% chance of occurrence in the offspring, and bilateral disease is associated with a 32% chance. In couples with an affected child, the recurrence risk in subsequent offspring is less than 1% with a unilateral tumor and 1–2% with bilateral tumors (7, 10).

Prenatal management. Because fetal ultrasound cannot provide a tissue diagnosis and many of these tumors are benign, the prenatal detection of a solid renal mass generally is not an indication for early delivery to allow for prompt tumor treatment (41). Some tumors can reach a considerable size, and cesarean section may be appropriate in these cases to avoid dystocic complications.

Congenital Adrenal Neuroblastoma

Definition. Neuroblastoma is a malignant tumor of the autonomic nervous system, composed of neuroectodermal cells. It usually develops from stem cells of the sympathetic nervous system. The most common sites of occurrence are the adrenal glands and sympathetic trunk, and so the majority of these tumors are retroperitoneal (45).

Incidence. Neuroblastomas are the most common congenital and neonatal tumors, accounting for 14–50% (52). More than half of all abdominal malignancies in newborns are neuroblastomas (51). The reported overall incidence of these tumors is approximately one in 10,000 live births (25).

Embryology, etiology and pathogenesis. The adrenal cortex develops from mesenchymal cells of the coelomic epithelium, while the adrenal medulla is of neuroectodermal origin. Neuroblastomas result from the anomalous maturation of neuroblastic cells. There have been isolated reports of neuroblastomas occurring in siblings and twins, and a familial predisposition is believed to exist in approximately 20% of cases (84).

Location and metastasis. More than half of all neuroblastomas are located in the abdominal cavity. Less common sites are the mediastinum, neck, and brain (45, 52, 94). The most characteristic finding, therefore,

Table 27.**9** Differential diagnosis of abdominal masses in newborns (adapted from 78, 94)

> Renal diseases
  • Hydronephrosis
  • Cystic or dysplastic renal disease
  • Ectopic or fused kidneys

> Renal tumors
  • Wilms' tumor
  • Mesoblastic nephroma

> Renovascular thrombosis

> Adrenal diseases
  • Neuroblastoma
  • Hemorrhage
  • Adenoma

> Hepatic tumors

> Teratomas

> Duplications of the digestive tract

> Subdiaphragmatic pulmonary sequestra

> Cysts of the pancreas or biliary tract

> Ovarian cysts

> Mesenteric cysts

is an intra-abdominal mass, usually an adrenal tumor ranging from a few millimeters to several centimeters in size. Most adrenal neuroblastomas are unilateral. Occasionally, hepatomegaly is present as a signal that extensive metastasis has already occurred. The tumor may also seed to the bone marrow and skin and in rare cases to the placenta (52, 84). A special lesion is the stage IV-S neuroblastoma, in which the primary tumor is absent or very small and has already metastasized to the liver, bone marrow, and/or skin. The overall rate of metastasis at birth is approximately 50%.

Complications. Fetal hydrops can develop in some cases. Comparable to a hemolytic disease, this condition is characterized by anemia, hepatosplenomegaly, jaundice, and increased numbers of erythrocyte precursors in the peripheral blood. Epidemiologic studies do not show an increased risk for associated anomalies (54, 67).

Because 75–90% of neuroblastomas secrete catecholamines, which pass through the placenta into the maternal circulation, the mother may exhibit sympathotonic symptoms such as nausea, vomiting, headache, or arterial hypertension (84). When these symptoms are combined with the ultrasound detection or a fetal mass, a neuroblastoma should be suspected.

Ultrasound features, differential diagnosis. The ultrasound features of congenital neuroblastomas are diverse (45, 84). Most tumors are located in the abdomen, usually on the superior pole of the kidney, but a smaller number occur in the lung or brain (45). Prenatal ultrasound may demonstrate the tumor as a cystic, solid, or cystic/solid mass. Intratumoral calcifications may be seen. Generally this tumor is not distinguishable antenatally from other adrenal processes such as intra-adrenal hemorrhage (Fig. 27.**24**) and adrenal adenoma (Fig. 27.**25**). Often it is even difficult to localize a mass to the adrenal gland or kidney with prenatal ultrasound. As a result, a congenital adrenal neuroblastoma cannot be differentiated from the intra-abdominal masses in Table 27.**9** with complete confidence. Cordocentesis can be helpful in distinguishing a nephroblastoma from a neuroblastoma. The levels of neuron-specific enolase (NSE) in the cord blood are elevated with neuroblastoma but not with nephroblastoma.

Occasionally, attention is directed toward these tumors by the presence of other ultrasound abnormalities such as fetal hydrops, hydramnios, or calcified masses in the liver signifying hepatic metastasis.

Prognosis. The postnatal prognosis depends chiefly on age and tumor stage. Newborns and infants have a better prognosis than older children. If distant metastasis (stage I–III lesion) has not occurred, a cure can be achieved in up to 100% of cases. Even with distant metastasis, 50% of cases are curable, and this figure rises to 80% when stage IV-S disease is present (39). The treatment for localized disease is surgical removal. More advanced forms will require adjuvant radiotherapy and/or chemotherapy (94). Spontaneous regression has been described for some cases, especially those with IV-S neuroblastomas, but the predictability and frequency of these cases are unknown (42).

Prenatal management. If there is prenatal suspicion of neuroblastoma, serial examinations should be performed to check for signs of possible metastasis. If significant tumor enlargement is noted, early delivery should be considered. With fetal hydrops or marked hepatic enlargement, cesarean section may be indicated to avoid dystocic complications (84).

References

1. Barakat, A.Y., Butler, M.G., Cobb, C.G., Coursey, J.W., Shah, D.: Reliability of ultrasound in the prenatal diagnosis of urinary tract abnormalities. Pediat. Nephrol. 5 (1991) 12–14
2. Barth, R., Filly, R., Sontheimer, F.: Prenatal sonographic findings in bladder exstrophy. J. Ultrasound Med. 9 (1990) 359–361
3. Benacerraf, B.R., Nadel, A., Bromley, B.: Identification of second trimester fetuses with autosomal trisomy by use of a sonographic scooting index. Radiology 193 (1994) 135–140
4. Berkowitz, R., Glickmann, M., Smith, G. et al.: Fetal urinary tract obstruction: what is the role of surgical intervention in utero? Amer. J. Obstet. Gynecol. 144 (1982) 367
5. Bernstein, J., Risdon, R.A., Gilbert-Barnes, E.: Renal System. In: Gilbert-Barnes, E. (ed.): Potter's Pathology of the fetus and infant. Vol. 2. Mosby 1997; pp. 863–919
6. Bloom, D.A., Brosman, S.: The multicystic kidney. J. Urol. 120 (1978) 211–216
7. Bonaiti-Pellie, C., Chompret, A., Tournade, M.F. et al.: Genetics and epidemiology of Wilms' tumor: The French Wilms' tumor study. Med. Pediatr. Oncol. 20 (1992) 284–291
8. Bonsib, S.M. Fetal obstructive uropathy without renal dysplasia: a study of the renal findings in 13 cases presenting with megacystis. J. Urol. 160 (1998) 2166–2170
9. Breslow, N.E., Beckwith, J.B.: Epidemiological features of Wilms' tumor: Results of the National Wilms' Tumor Study. J. Natl. Cancer Inst. 62 (1982) 429–435
10. Brodeur, G.M.: Genetic and cytogenetic aspects of Wilms' tumor. In: Pochedly, C., Baum, E.S. (eds): Wilms' Tumor: Clinical and Biological Manifestation. New York: Elsevier 1984; pp. 125–145
11. Bronshtein, M., Yoffe, N., Brandes, J.M., Blumfeld, Z.: First and early second trimester-diagnosis of fetal urinary tract anomalies using transvaginal sonography. Prenat. Diagn. 10 (1990) 653–666
12. Caione, P., Patricolo, M., Lais, A., Capitanucci, M.L., Capozza, N., Ferro, F.: Role of prenatal diagnosis in the treatment of congenital obstructive megaureter in a solitary kidney. Fetal Diagn. Ther. 11 (1996) 205–209
13. Cam, G., Simon, P., Ang, K.S.: Prevalence of symptomatic forms of adult polycystic kidney disease. Kidney Int. 37 (1990) 247 (abstract)
14. Clericuzio, C.L.: A comprehensive and critical assessment of overgrowth and overgrowth syndrom. Adv. Hum. Genet. 18 (1989) 181–185
15. Coplen, D.E., Hare, J.Y., Zderic, S.A., Canning, D.A., Snyder, H.M., Duckett, J.W.: 10-year experience with prenatal intervention for hydronephrosis. J. Urol. 156 (1996) 1142–1145
16. Corn, B.W., Goldwein, J., Evans, I., Dángio, G.J.: Outcomes in low-risk babies treated with half-dose chemotherapy according to the third National Wilms Tumor Study. J. Clin. Oncol. 10 (1992) 1305–1309
17. Corteville, J.E., Dicke, J.M., Crane, P.: Fetal pyelectasis and Down Syndrom: is genetic amniocentesis warranted? Obstet. Gynecol. 79 (1992) 770–772
18. Costin, M.E., Kennedy, R.I.J.: Ovarian cysts in newborn. Amer. J. Roentgenol. 116 (1972) 664–672
19. Crombleholme, T.M., Harrison, M.R., Golbus, M.S. et al.: Fetal intervention in obstructive uropathy: prognostic indicators and efficacy of intervention. Amer. J. Obstet. Gynecol. 162 (1990) 1239–1244
20. Daikha Dahmane, F., Dommergues, M., Muller, F. et al.: Development of human fetal kidney in obstructive uropathy: correlations with ultrasonography and urine biochemistry. Kid. Int. 52 (1977) 21–32
21. Dremsek, P.A., Ginde, K., Voith, P. et al.: Renal pyelectasis in fetuses and neonates: diagnostic value of renal pelvis diameter in pre- and postnatal sonographic screening. Amer. J. Roentgenol. 168 (1997) 1017–1019
22. Elder, J.S., O'Grady, P., Ashmead, G. et al.: Evaluation of fetal renal function: unreliability of fetal urinary electrolytes. J. Urol. 144 (1990) 574
23. Emerson, D.S., Felker, R.E., Brown, D.L.: The sagittal sign – an early second trimester sonographic indicator of fetal gender. J. Ultrasound Med. 8 (1989) 293–297
24. Estes, J.M., MacGillivray, T.E., Hedrick, M.H., Adzick, N.S., Harrison, M.R.: Fetoskopic surgery for the treatment of congenital anomalies. J. Pediatr. Surg. 27 (1992) 950–954
25. Estroff, J.A., Shamberger, R.C., Diller, L., Benacerraf, B.R.: Neuroblastoma. The Fetus 1 (1991) 1–6
26. Fantal, A.G., Shepard, R.H.: Potter syndrome: nonrenal features induced by oligohydramnion. Amer. J. Dis. Child 129 (1976) 1346–1351
27. Flake, A., Harrison, M., Sauer, L., Adzick, S., deLorenier, A.: Uteropelvic junction obstruction in the fetus. J. Ped. Surg. 21 (1986) 1058–1063
28. Freedmann, A.L., Bukowski, T.P., Smith, C.A., Evans, M.I., Johnson, M.P., Gonzales, R.: Fetal therapy for obstructive uropathy: diagnosis specific outcomes. Urology 156 (1996) 720–723
29. Freedmann, A.L., Bukowski, T.P., Smith, C.A. et al.: Use of urinary beta-2-microglobulin to predict severe renal damage in fetal obstructive uropathy. Fetal Diagn. Ther. 12 (1997) 1–6
30. Freedmann, A.L., Johnson, M.P., Smith, C.A., Gonzales, R., Evans, M.I.: Long-term outcome in children after antenatal intervention for obstructive uropathies. Lancet 354 (1999) 374–377
31. Friedmann, W., Vogel, M., Dimer, J.S., Luttkus, A., Büscher, U., Dudenhausen, J.W.: Perinatal differential diagnosis of polycystic kidney disease and urinary tract obstruction: anatomic pathologic, ultrasonographic and genetic findings. Eur. J. Obstet. Gynecol. Reprod. Biol. 89 (2000) 127–133
32. Gleason, D.G., McAlister, W.H., Kissane, J.: Cystic diseases of the kidney in children. Amer. J. Roentgenol. 100 (1967) 135–141
33. Glick, P.L., Harrison, M.R., Noall, R.A., Villa, R.L.: Corrections of congenital hydronephrosis in utero III. Early mid-trimester urethral obstruction produces renal dyspharia. J. Pediatr. Surg. 18 (1983) 681–687
34. Gocci, G., Magnani, C., Morini, M.S. et al.: Urinary tract anomalies (UTA) and associated malformations: data of the Emilia-Romagna registry. Eur. J. Epidemiol. 12 (1996) 493–497
35. Golbus, M., Harrison, M., Filly, R. et al.: In utero management of urinary tract obstruction. Amer. J. Obstet. Gynecol. 142 (1982) 383
36. Grancurn, R., Bracken, M., Silverman, R., Hobbins, J.: Assessment of fetal kidney size in normal gestation by comparison of ratio of kidney circumference to abdominal circumference. Amer. J. Obstet. Gynecol. 136 (1980) 249–254
37. Greig, J.D., Raine, P.A.M., Young, D.G. et al.: Value of antenatal diagnosis of abnormalities of the urinary tract. Brit. Med. J. 298 (1989) 1417–1419
38. Grignon, A., Filion, R., Filatrault, D. et al.: Urinary tract dilatation in utero: classification and clinical applications. Radiology 160 (1986) 645–647
39. Grosfeld, J.L., Rescoria, F.J., West, K.W.: Neuroblastoma in the first year of life: Clinical and biologic factors influencing outcome. Semin. Pediatr. Surg. 2 (1993) 37–42
40. Gunn, T.R., Mora, J.D., Pease, P.: Outcome after antenatal diagnosis of upper urinary tract dilatation by ultrasonography. Arch. Dis. Childh. 63 (1988) 1240–1243
41. Gutjahr, P.: Konnatale Wilmstumoren sind meist (benigne) mesoblastische Nephrome – Bedeutung des pränatal nachgewiesenen soliden Nierentumors. Geburtsh. u. Frauenheilk. 51 (1991) 124–126
42. Haas, D., Ablin, A.R., Miller, C.: Complete pathologic maturation and regression of stage IVS neuroblastoma without treatment. Cancer 62 (1988) 818–824
43. Harrison, M., Nakayama, D., Noall, R., deLorimer, A.: Correction of congenital hydronephrosis in utero II. Decompression reverses the effects of obstruction on the fetal lung and urinary tract. J. Ped. Surg. 17 (1982) 965–974
44. Harrison, M., Ross, N., Noall, R., Lorimer, A.: Correction of congenital hydronephrosis in utero I. The model: fetal urethral obstruction produces hydronephrosis and pulmonary hypoplasia in fetal lamb. J. Ped. Surg. 18 (1983) 247–256
45. Heling, K.S., Bollmann, R., Chaoui, R., Tennstedt, C., Kirchmair, F.: Eine isolierte fetale Nierenzyste als Zeichen für ein kongenitales Neuroblastom. Geburts. u. Frauenheilk. 55 (1995) 347–350
46. Hildebrandt, F., Weber, M., Brandis, M.: Molekulare Genetik von Nierenerkrankungen. Dtsch. Ärztebl. 93 (1996) 308–313
47. Holzgreve, W., Miny, P., Evans, M.: Genitourinary malformations. In: High risk pregnancy, management options. Philadelphia: W.B. Saunders 1996; pp. 901–918
48. Hrabovsky, E.E., Othersen, H.B., de Lorimier, A.: Wilms' tumor in neonate. A report from the national Wilms' Tumor Study. J. Pediatr. Surg. 21 (1987) 385–387
49. Hutton, K.A., Thomas, D.F., Davies, B.W.: Prenatally detected posterior urethral values: qualitative assessment of second trimester scand and prediction of outcome. J. Urol. 158 (1997) 1022–1025
50. Irwin, B.H., Vane D.W.: Complications of intrauterine intervention for treatment of fetal obstructive uropathy. Urology-Online 55 (2000) 774
51. Isaacs, H.: Perinatal (congenital and neonatal) neoplasmas: A report of 110 cases. Pediatr. Pathol. 3 (1985) 165–216
52. Isaacs, H.: Tumors. In: Gilbert-Barness, E. (ed.): Potter's Pathology of the Fetus and the Infant. Vol. 2. St. Louis: Mosby 1997; pp. 1242–1339
53. Jeanty, P., Dramaix-Wilmet, M., Elkazea, N., Hubimont, C., Regemorter, V.: Measurement of fetal kidney growth on ultrasound. Radiology 144 (1982) 159–162
54. Johnson, C.C., Spitz, M.R.: Neuroblastoma: Case control analysis of birth characteristics. J. Natl. Cancer Inst. 74 (1985) 789–796
55. Johnson, M.P., Bukowski, T.P., Reitelman, C. et al.: In utero surgical treatment of fetal obstructive uropathy: a new comprehensive approach to identify appropriate candidates for vesicoamniotic shunt therapy. Amer. J. Obstet. Gynecol. 170 (1994) 1770
56. Johnson, M.P., Corsi, P., Bradfield, W. et al.: Sequential urinanalysis improves evaluation of fetal renal function in obstructive uropathy. Amer. J. Obstet. Gynecol. 173 (1995) 59–65
57. Johnson, M.P., Freedman, A.L.: Fetal uropathy. Curr. Opin. Obstet. Gynecol. 11 (1999) 185–194
58. Krous, H.F., Harper, H.F., Perlman, M.: Congenital cystic adenomatoid malformation in bilateral renal agensis. Arch. Pathol. Lab. Med. 104 (1980) 368–371
59. Kucera, J.: Rate and type of congenital anomalies among offspring of diabetic women. J. Reprod. Med. 7 (1971) 61
60. Leck, I., Record, R.G., Mckeon, T., Edward, J.H.: The incidence of malformation in Birmingham, England, 1950–1959. Teratology 1 (1968) 263–280
61. Lewis, K.M., Pinckert, T.L., Cain, M.P., Ghidini, A.: Complications of intrauterine placement of a vesicoamniotic shunt. Obstet. Gynecol. 91 (1998) 825–827
62. Livera, L.N., Brookfield, D.S.K., Egginton, J.A., Hawnaur, J.N.: Antenatal ultrasonography to defeat fetal renal abnormalities: A prospective screening programme. Brit. Med. J. 298 (1989) 1421–1423
63. Mahony, B.S., Filly, R.A., Callen, P.W.: Fetal renal dysplasia: sonographic evaluation. Radiology 152 (1984) 143–146
64. Makino, Y., Kobayashi, H., Kyono, K., Oschima, K., Kawarabayashi, T.: Clinical results of fetal obstructive uropathy treated by vesicoamniotic shunting. Urology 55 (2000) 118–122
65. Mandell, J., Blyth, B.R., Peters, C.A., Retik, A.B., Estroff, J.A., Banacerraf, B.R.: Structural genitourinary defects defeeted in utero. Radiology 178 (1991) 193–196
66. Manning, F.A., Harrison, M.R., Rodeck, C.: Catheter shunts for fetal hydronephrosis and hydrocephalus. Report of the international fetal surgery registry. New Engl. J. Med. 315 (1986) 336–340
67. Miller, R.W.: Relation between cancer and congenital defects in man. New Engl. J. Med. 275 (1966) 87–93
68. Moerman, P., Fryus, J.P., Godderis, P., Laweryus, J.: Pathogenesis of the prune belly syndrome; a functional urethral obstruction causes by prostatic hypoplasia. Pediatrics 73 (1984) 470–475
69. Muller, F., Dommergues, M., Mandelbrot, L., Aubry, M.E., Nihoul-Fekete, C., Dumez, Y.: Fetal urinary biochemistry predicts postnatal renal function in children with bilateral obstructive uropathies. Obstet. Gynecol. 82 (1993) 813–820
70. Muller, F., Dommergues, M., Bussiers, L. et al.: Development of human renal function: reference intervalls for 10 biochemical markers in fetal urine. Clin. Chem. 42 (1996) 1855–1860
71. Nakamura, Y., Hosohawa, Y., Yano, H. et al.: Primary cause of perinatal death: an autopsy study of 1000 cases in Japanese infants. Hum. Pathol. 13 (1982) 54–61
72. Nicolaides, K.H., Cheng, H.H., Abbas, A., Snijders, R.J.M., Gosden, C.: Fetal renal defects: associated malformations and chromosomal defects. Fetal Diagn. Ther. 7 (1992) 1–11
73. Nicolini, U., Rodeck, C., Fisk, N.: Shunt treatment for fetal obstructive uropathy. Lancet 2 (1987) 1338–1339

74. Nicolini, U., Fisk, N.M., Rodeck, C.H., Beacham, J.: Fetal urine biochemistry: an index of renal maturation and dysfunction. Brit. J. Obstet. Gynecol. 99 (1992) 46–50
75. Osathanondh, V., Potter, E.L.: Pathogenesis of polycystic kidneys. Historical survey. Arch. Pathol. 77 (1964) 459–465
76. Peters, C.A., Carr, M.C., Lais, A., Retik, A.B., Mandell, J.: The response of the fetal kidney to obstruction. J. Urol. 148 (1992) 503–509
77. Petruzzi, M.J., Green, D.M.: Wilms' Tumor. Pediatr. Clin. North Amer. 44 (1997) 939–952
78. Pinto, E., Guignard, J.P.: Renal masses in the neonate. Biol. Neonate 68 (1995) 175–184
79. Potter, E.L.: Type II cystic kidney: Early ampullary inhibition. In: Normal and Abnormal Development of the Kindney. Chicago, Year Book 1972; pp. 154–181
80. Quintero, R., Hume, R., Smith, C. et al.: Percutaneous fetal cystoscopy and endoscopic fulguration of posterior urethral valves. Amer. J. Obstet. Gynecol. 172 (1995) 206–209
81. Rempen, A., Kirchner, T., Frauendienst-Egger, G., Hoechst, B.: Congenital mesoblastic nephroma. Fetus 2 (1992) 7535
82. Risdon, R.A.: Development, developmental defects, and cystic diseases of the kidney. In: Heptinstall, R.H. (ed.): Pathology of the kidney. Vol 1. Boston: Little-Brown 1992; pp. 93–118
83. Rodeck, C., Nicolaides, K.: Ultrasound guided invasive procedures in obstetrics. Clin. Obstet. Gynecol. 10 (1983) 515
84. Romero, R., Pilu, G., Jeanty, P., Ghidini, A., Hobbins, J.: The Urinary Tract and Adrenal Glands. In: Romero, R., Pilu, G., Jeanty, P., Ghidini, A., Hobbins, J. (eds.): Prenatal Diagnosis of Congenital Anomalies. Norwalk: Appeleton & Lange 1988; pp. 255–307
85. Roodhooft, A.M., Birnholz, J.C., Holmes, L.B.: Familial nature of congenital absence and severe dysgenesis of both kidneys. New Engl. J. Med. 310 (1984) 1341–1343
86. Smith, D.P., Felker, R.E., Noe, H.N., Emerson, D.S., Mercer, B.: Prenatal diagnosis of genital anomalies. Urology 47 (1996) 114–117
87. Snijders, R.J.M., Sebire, N.J., Faria, M., Patel, F., Nicolaides, K.H.: Fetal mild hydronephrosis and chromosomal defects: relation to maternal age and gestation. Fetal Diagn. Ther. 10 (1995) 349–355
88. Spence, H.M., Singleton, R.: Cysts and cystic disorders of the kidney: types, diagnosis, treatment. Urol. Surv. 22 (1972) 131–137

89. Szaflik, K., Kozarzewski, M., Adamczewski, D.: Fetal bladder catheterization in severe obstructive uropathy before the 24th week of pregnancy. Fetal Diagn. Ther. 13 (1998) 133–135
90. Thorner, P., Bernstein, J., Landing, B.H.: Kidneys and lower urinary tract. In: Reed, G.B., Claireaux, A.E., Cockburn, J. (eds.): Diseases of the Fetus and Newborn. Vol 1. London: Chapman & Hall Medical 1995; pp. 609–661
91. Tsuchida, Y., Shimizu, K., Hata, J.: Renin production in congenital mesoblastic nephroma in comparison with that in Wilms' Tumor. Pediatr. Pathol. 13 (1993) 155–161
92. Tutschek, B., Rodeck, C.H.: Diagnostisch-therapeutisches Konzept bei Fehlbildungen der Nieren und der ableitenden Harnwege. Gynäkologe 28 (1995) 356–367
93. Vintzileos, A.M., Campbell, W.A., Guzman, E.R. et al.: Second-trimester ultrasound markers for detection of trisomy 21: which markers are the best? Obstet. Gynecol. 89 (1997) 941–944
94. Weitzman, S., Grant, R.: Neonatal Oncology: Diagnostic and Therapeutic Dilemmas. Sem. Perinat. 21 (1997) 102–111
95. Wickström, E.A., Thangaveln, M., Parilla, B.V., Tamura, R.K., Sabbagha, R.E.: A prospective study of the association between isolated fetal pyelectasis and chromosomal abnormality. Obstet. Gynecol. 88 (1996) 379–382
96. Wilhelm, C.: Urogenitaltrakt, Fruchtwasser. In: Sohn, C., Holzgreve, W. (Hrsg.): Ultraschall in Gynäkologie und Geburtshilfe. Stuttgart: Thieme 1995; S. 282–304
97. Wilson, R.D., Baird, P.A.: Renal agenesis in British Columbia. Amer. J. Med. Genet. 21 (1985) 153–159
98. Wladimiroff, J.W.: Effect of furosemid on fetal urine production. Brit. J. Obstet. Gynaecol. 82 (1975) 221–226
99. Zerres, K.: Genetics of cystic kidney diseases. Pediatr. Nephrol. 1 (1987) 397–404
100. Zerres, K., Waldherr, R.: Zystische Nierenerkrankungen – Klassifikation und neue Aspekte. Dtsch. Ärztebl. 87 (1990) 2356–2362
101. Zerres, K., Mucher, G., Becker, J. et al.: Prenatal diagnosis of autosomal recessive polycystic kidney disease (ARPKD): molecular genetics, clinical experience, and fetal morphology. Amer. J. Med. Genet. 76 (1998) 137–144

28 Genital Anomalies

Publications on the fetal genitalia deal primarily with the accurate prediction of fetal sex (3, 5, 8, 20). Aside from ovarian cysts and testicular hydrocele, anomalies of the genitalia are not commonly diagnosed in the fetus (7, 21). The ultrasound detection of these anomalies requires optimum visualization of the fetal genital region.

Genital Anomalies in the Male Fetus

▬ Testicular Hydrocele

Definition. A collection of serous fluid within the scrotum.

Incidence. Common in cases of nonimmune fetal hydrops.

Etiology and pathogenesis. Testicular hydrocele is found in the setting of a cardiac anomaly or fetal hydrops.

Pathoanatomic findings. The fluid collection is located in the tunica vaginalis of the testicle.

Ultrasound features. Ultrasound shows a distended scrotum filled with hypoechoic fluid in which the testes, if fully descended, appear as solid, elliptical, echogenic structures (6, 16) (Figs. 28.**1**, 28.**2**). Testicular descent occurs between 28 and 34 weeks' gestation (4). If testes are not found in the scrotum after 34 weeks, it should be assumed that *cryptorchidism* is present.

Prenatal management. Testicular hydrocele has no obstetric implications when seen as an isolated finding. If it occurs in the setting of another disease, further management depends on the underlying disease.

▬ Micropenis

Definition. Extremely small penis.

Incidence. Very rare.

Etiology and pathogenesis. A micropenis can occur in the setting of certain syndromes. Examples are the short rib–polydactyly syndrome (25) and Pallister–Hall syndrome (9).

Ultrasound features. The penis is markedly small in relation to the scrotum (Fig. 28.**3**).

Differential diagnosis. Differentiation from a small penis in a healthy child is difficult. The differential diagnosis should include clitoral hypertrophy in a female fetus with very large labia.

Associated anomalies. Other abnormalities may be found in syndromic cases. These consist of delayed bone growth and polydactyly in short rib–polydactyly syndrome. The associated anomalies in Pallister–Hall syndrome are intrauterine growth retardation, facial dysmorphias, auricular dysplasia, postaxial polydactyly, and cardiac anomalies.

Prognosis. The prognosis depends on the underlying disease.

Hermaphroditism

Definition. In true hermaphroditism, both ovarian and testicular tissue are present in the same fetus.

Incidence. Rare.

Etiology and pathogenesis. Poorly understood.

Pathoanatomic findings. The external genitalia range from purely male to purely female. Prader (24) classified intersex genitalia into five main types.

Ultrasound features. A genital anomaly should be suspected if a specific sex cannot be identified at ultrasound. The external genitalia may feature both male and female components (Fig. 28.**4**).

Differential diagnosis. The ultrasound detection of ambiguous gender provides no specific information on the underlying disorder. The differential diagnosis includes pseudohermaphroditism, adrenogenital syndrome, and other conditions such as camptomelic dysplasia (14).

Associated anomalies. When ambiguous gender occurs in the setting of a camptomelic syndrome (9), there may be accompanying abnormalities such as facial dysplasia (depressed nasal bridge, micrognathia, cleft palate) and bowing of the tibiae.

Prognosis. Children with camptomelic dysplasia usually die while in utero or shortly after birth.

Prenatal management. The ultrasound detection of abnormal external genitalia does not affect prenatal management when noted as an isolated finding.

Genital Anomalies in the Female Fetus

▬ Ovarian Cyst

Definition. Solitary, sharply circumscribed cyst of the ovary, typically unilateral.

Incidence. Most frequent intra-abdominal cystic mass in fetuses.

Pathoanatomic findings. Follicular cysts are the most common. Cystic teratomas are rare.

Ultrasound Features

Simple ovarian cysts. These lesions appear sonographically as sharply circumscribed cystic masses in the lower to midabdomen (2, 13, 17). They may be anechoic or may contain scattered internal echoes (Figs. 28.**5**–28.**7**).

Hemorrhagic ovarian cysts. Hemorrhagic cysts contain both streaks and clumps of echogenic densities (Figs. 28.**8**, 28.**9**). The hemorrhage may result from *ovarian torsion* (11, 15, 22), which has an overall reported incidence of 36% (17).

Differential diagnosis. An ovarian cyst cannot be confidently distinguished from a mesenteric cyst in female fetuses. Differentiation from an ectopic, hydronephrotic kidney can be difficult but is possible when the kidney is accurately defined in all three planes.

Associated anomalies. None.

Invasive tests. If the findings are equivocal and the mass is seen to enlarge, needle aspiration may be considered. A high estradiol level in the cystic fluid confirms the diagnosis of an ovarian cyst.

Prognosis. Ovarian cysts usually have a good prognosis. Spontaneous regression will even occur in some cases. Ovarian torsion is a poor prognostic sign. Unless corrected by an interventional procedure, it will lead to loss of the adnexa.

Prenatal management. When an ovarian cyst is detected, serial scans should be obtained to check for cyst enlargement that could lead to ovarian torsion or pulmonary compression (1, 2, 11). If there is extreme cyst enlargement causing the displacement of other organs, aspiration of the cyst contents should be considered. If ovarian torsion is suspected, Mas et al. (19) recommend cesarean section so that the newborn can be referred to a pediatric surgeon without delay. A small, simple ovarian cyst does not affect the mode of delivery.

▬ Clitoral Hypertrophy

Definition. Marked enlargement of the clitoris.

Incidence. Rare.

Etiology and pathogenesis. Clitoral hypertrophy can occur in the setting of adrenogenital syndrome (12, 18), Roberts syndrome (pseudothalidomide syndrome) (18, 26), and trisomy 18 (18).

Adrenogenital syndrome. In adrenogenital syndrome (AGS), a deficiency of various adrenocortical enzymes necessary for cortisol and aldosterone synthesis leads to an increase in androgen synthesis. The enzyme defects (21-hydroxylase, 11β-hydroxylase, 3β-hydroxysteroid dehydrogenase) result in the prenatal virilization of female fetuses

(12). The intersex anomaly of the external genitalia varies in degree, depending on the severity of the enzyme defect. All three forms are transmitted by autosomal-recessive inheritance.

Roberts syndrome. Roberts syndrome also has an autosomal-recessive mode of inheritance.

Pathoanatomic findings. It can be difficult to distinguish between a normal-size clitoris and one that is abnormally enlarged. Ethnic differences should also be taken into account when evaluating clitoral length (23).

Ultrasound features. The clitoris appears markedly enlarged in relation to the labia majora, especially in a coronal scan (Fig. 28.**10**).

Differential diagnosis. Small penis.

Associated Anomalies

Roberts syndrome. Roberts syndrome is associated with other major anomalies such as tetraphocomelia, facial dysplasia with bilateral cleft lip and palate, retrognathia, microphthalmia, and microcephaly.
Trisomy 18. In this syndrome, growth retardation is combined with characteristic facial dysmorphias, auricular dysplasia, cardiac anomalies, CNS anomalies, diaphragmatic hernia, and polydactyly.

Invasive tests. A 21-hydroxylase deficiency can be diagnosed prenatally by determining 17-hydroxyprogesterone in the amniotic fluid or by the HLA typing of cultured amniotic cells or chorionic villi. An 11?-hydroxylase deficiency can be diagnosed by performing a steroid assay (11-deoxycortisol, tetrahydro-11-deoxycortisol) in the amniotic fluid. If there is a known p450c11 mutation, a molecular genetic analysis of chorionic villi or amniotic cells can also be used for prenatal diagnosis.

Invasive testing should always include a determination of fetal karyotype to exclude trisomy 18.

Prognosis. The prognosis depends on the underlying disease. In fetuses with AGS, subsequent treatment will depend on the severity of the malformation of the female external genitalia. Approximately 50% of fetuses with Roberts syndrome are stillborn, or the infants die during the first weeks of life (26). The detection of trisomy 18 implies a grave prognosis.

Prenatal management. The ultrasound detection of abnormal female external genitalia has little or no effect on prenatal management when noted as an isolated finding.

When a 21-hydroxylase deficiency is detected in a female fetus, masculinization can be prevented by the prompt maternal administration of dexamethasone.

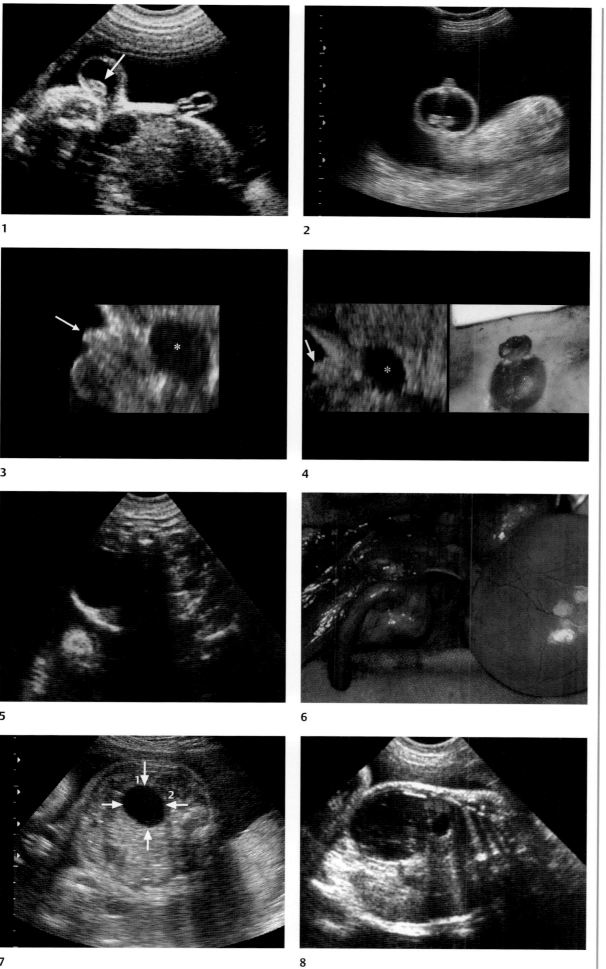

1

2

3

4

5

6

7

8

Genital anomalies in the male fetus

Fig. 28.1 Isolated testicular hydrocele with a normally descended testis (arrow). Longitudinal scan at 32 weeks.

Fig. 28.2 Marked bilateral testicular hydrocele in NIHF. Both descended testes are visible as small echogenic structures. Transverse scan through the scrotum at 31 weeks.

Fig. 28.3 Minipenis (arrow) in a fetus with short rib–polydactyly syndrome. Midsagittal scan at 34 weeks. (∗) = Urinary bladder

Hermaphroditism

Fig. 28.4 Left: intersex genitals with a clitoris (arrow) and scrotum (hermaphroditism) in camptomelic dysplasia. Midsagittal scan at 31 weeks. (∗) = Urinary bladder. Right: postpartum appearance.

Genital anomalies in the female fetus

Fig. 28.5 Hypoechoic right ovarian cyst (5.6 · 4.8 · 4.5 cm). Transverse scan in a 35-week fetus in a vertex presentation. The normal-size kidneys are visible on each side of the spinal column.

Fig. 28.6 Intraoperative appearance of the ovarian cyst in Fig. 28.**5** (photo courtesy of Dr. Koltai, Department of Pediatric Surgery, Mainz University Hospital, Mainz, Germany).

Fig. 28.7 Small, hypoechoic right ovarian cyst (2.8 · 2.6 · 2.6 cm) with faint internal echoes (arrows). Transverse scan at 31 weeks, vertex presentation with the spine to the left.

Fig. 28.8 Large, hemorrhagic ovarian cyst with a dense internal echo pattern (diameter 4.5 cm). Longitudinal scan at 35 weeks.

Fig. 28.**9** Hemorrhagic ovarian cyst (diameter 4 cm) with dense internal echoes (arrows) at 34 weeks. Located below the stomach, the cyst mimics a solid, left-sided intra-abdominal tumor.

Fig. 28.**10** Chromosome in AGS, 34 weeks.

a On a coronal scan through the external genitalia, the clitoris (arrow) appears markedly enlarged in relation to the labia majora.

b Transverse scan through the genitalia at the level of the enlarged clitoris.

c Transverse scan through the genitalia at the level of the labia majora.

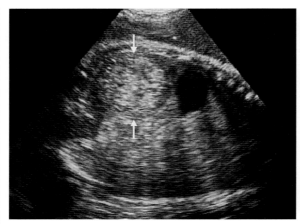

9

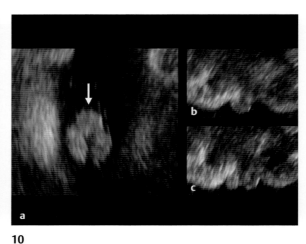

10

References

1. Ahmed, S.: Neonatal and childhood ovarian cyst. J. Pediat. Surg. 6 (1971) 702–708
2. Avni, E.F., Godart, S., Israel, C., Schmitz, C.: Ovarian torsion cyst presenting as a wandering tumor in a newborn: antenatal diagnosis and postnatal assessment. Pediat. Radiol. 13 (1983) 169–171
3. Benoit, B.: Early fetal gender determination. Ultrasound Obstet. Gynecol. 13 (1999) 299–300
4. Birnholz, J.C.: Determination of fetal sex. New Eng. J. Med. 309 (1983) 942–944
5. Bronshtein, M., Rottem, S., Yoffe, N., Blumenfeld, Z., Brandes, J.M.: Early determination of fetal sex using transvaginal sonography: techniques and pitfalls. J. Clin. Ultrasound 18 (1990) 302–306
6. Conrad, A.R., Rao, S.A.: Ultrasound diagnosis of fetal hydrocele. Radiology 127 (1978) 232
7. Cooper, C., Mahony, B.S., Bowie, J.D., Pope, I.I.: Prenatal ultrasound diagnosis of ambiguous genitalia. J. Ultrasound Med. 4 (1985) 433–436
8. Efrat, Z., Akinfenwa, O.O., Nicolaides, K.H.: First-trimester determination of fetal gender by ultrasound. Ultrasound Obstet. Gynecol. 13 (1999) 305–307
9. Finnigan, D.P., Clarren, S.K., Haas, J.E.: Extending the Pallister-Hall syndrome to include other central nervous system malformations. Amer. J. Med. Genet. 40 (1991) 395–400
10. Garel, L., Filiatrault, D., Brandt, M. et al.: Antenatal diagnosis of ovarian cysts: natural history and therapeutic implications. Pediatr. Radiol. 21 (1991) 182–184
11. Hafner, E., Rosen, A., Schuchter, K., Geissler, W.: Stieldrehung einer fetalen Ovarialzyste. Geburtsh. u. Frauenheilk. 58 (1998) 152–154
12. Heinrich, U., Gerhard, I. In: Runnebaum, B., Rabe, T. (Hrsg.): Gynäkologische Endokrinologie. Berlin: Springer 1987; S. 239–276
13. Holzgreve, W., Edel, G., Gerlach, B., Miny, P.: Differenzialdiagnose und Management fetaler Ovarialzysten – Erfahrungen bei 9 Fällen. Arch. Gynecol. Obstet. 245 (1989) 135–138
14. Houston, C.S., Opitz, J.M., Spranger, J.W. et al.: The campomelic syndrome. Amer. J. Med. Genet. 15 (1982) 3–28
15. Katz, V.L., McCoy, M.C. Kuller, J.A., Hansen, W.F., Watson, W.J.: Fetal ovarian torsion appearing as a solid abdominal mass. J. Perinatol. 16 (1996) 302–304
16. Köhler, C., Schuhmacher, G., Meierhofer, J.N., Peter, B.: Pränatale Ultraschalldiagnostik eines schweren Herzvitiums. Geburtsh. u. Frauenheilk. 41 (1981) 36–41
17. Kühl, G., Heep, J., Paulski, H.J., Schütze, U.: Die pränatale ultrasonografische Diagnose von Ovarialzysten und deren Häufigkeit bei Neugeborenen. Z. Kinderchir. 39 (1984) 344–346
18. Leiber, B., Olbrich, G.: Die klinischen Syndrome. Syndrome, Sequenzen und Symptomenkomplexe. München: Urban & Fischer 1996
19. Mas, M., Fontes, J., Salcedo, J.: Ultrasonographic diagnosis of twisted fetal ovarial cyst in utero. Int. J. Gynaecol. Obstet. 52 (1996) 185–186
20. Meagher, S., Davison, G.: Early second-trimester determination of fetal gender by ultrasound. Ultrasound Obstet. Gynecol. 8 (1996) 322–324
21. Merz, E., Miric-Tesanic, D., Bahlmann, F., Sedlaczek, H.: Prenatal diagnosis of fetal ambiguous gender using three-dimensional sonography. Ultrasound Obstet. Gynecol. 13 (1999) 217–219
22. Nussbaum, A.R., Sanders, R.C., Beantor, R.M., Hartman, D.S., Dudgeon, D.L., Parmley, T.H.: Neonatal ovarian cysts: sonographic-pathologic correlation. Radiology 168 (1988) 817–821
23. Philip, M., De Boer, C., Pilpel, D., Karplus, M., Sofer, S.: Clitoral and penile sizes of full term newborns in two different ethnic groups. J. Pediatr. Endocrinol. Metab. 9 (1996) 175–179
24. Prader, A.: Genitalbefund beim Pseudohermaphroditismus femininus des kongenitalen adrenogenitalen Syndroms: Morphologie, Häufigkeit, Entwicklung und Vererbung der verschiedenen Genitalformen. Helv. Paediatr. Acta 9 (1954) 231–248
25. Spranger, J., Maroteaux, P.: The lethal osteochondrodysplasias. Adv. Hum. Genet. 19 (1990) 1–103
26. Wiedemann, H.R., Grosse, F.R., Dibbern, H.: Das charakteristische Syndrom. Stuttgart: Schattauer 1982

29 Sacrococcygeal Teratoma

Definition. Teratomas are dysontogenic germ-cell tumors that contain elements derived from all three germ layers. As a result, they contain various epithelial, mesenchymal, and neural tissue components. The contents may include organoid structures and even fully differentiated organ segments such as bowel wall, pancreatic tissue, bronchial structures, and bony structures.

"Sacrococcygeal teratoma" is often used as a collective term for all germ-cell tumors located in the sacrococcygeal region.

Classification of teratomas. Teratomas can be classified as follows, regardless of their location:
- Mature teratomas
- Immature teratomas
- Teratomas with malignant transformation

Teratomas with malignant transformation are rare. They differ from other malignant teratomas in that "conventional" malignancies such as squamous-cell carcinoma, adenocarcinoma, and sarcoma can develop in them through the secondary transformation of mature, preexisting structures. These secondary tumors then dictate the course and prognosis (8). The size and location of the teratoma may have a greater bearing on treatment strategy than tumor histology.

In the American Academy of Pediatrics Surgical Survey (AAPSS) classification (1), sacrococcygeal teratomas are classified into four types based on their location (Table 29.1, Fig. 29.1).

Location and frequency. Teratomas are the most frequent group of tumors occurring in newborns (2). The most common sites of occurrence in infants and children are, in descending order of frequency, the sacrococcygeal region (Fig. 29.1), the ovaries, the testes, and the retroperitoneum (14).

Although sacrococcygeal teratoma is rare in absolute terms (one in 38,500 live births), it is the most frequent large tumor in neonates and the most common germ-cell tumor in children. Girls predominate over boys by a ratio of 3–4 : 1. In terms of location, 47% of the tumors are completely postsacral, 35% are predominantly postsacral, 9% are predominantly presacral, and 10% are completely presacral.

Biologic behavior. Eighty percent of sacrococcygeal tumors are teratomas, and one-fifth of these are of the immature type. The remaining 20% are malignant, in which case the malignant component is usually a yolk sac tumor (8). Sacrococcygeal teratomas are usually benign during the first months of life. After 12 months of age, however, 62% are malignant. Malignant transformation is more common in boys than girls and more common in presacral than postsacral tumors (8).

Embryology. Teratomas always form during early embryonic development, regardless of when they produce clinical manifestations.

Etiology and pathogenesis. Teratomas belong to the category of germ-cell tumors, whose etiology is poorly understood. The histogenesis of

these tumors was debated for many years. The debate centered on whether these neoplasms were derived from primordial gametes or from embryonic tissue (4). Today it is agreed that all germ-cell tumors, including teratomas, originate from immature (primordial) germ cells.

Several arguments support this "unitarian" or holistic histogenesis for germ-cell tumors:
- The frequent occurrence of different tumor types within the same lesion
- The occurrence of histologically similar tumors at extragonadal sites
- The similar histologies of these tumor types in male and female gonads and at extragonadal sites
- The cytogenetic detection of an isochromosome on the short arm of the chromosome 12 (i (12p)) with greater-than-average frequency (7)

Ultrasound Diagnosis

Nonhomogeneous echo structure. A characteristic ultrasound finding is a jumbled array of cystic and solid areas, with the solid areas often showing a nonhomogeneous echo structure and possible echogenic calcifications (13) (Figs. 29.2–29.8). The cystic structures have irregular boundaries and represent morphologic cavities with different epithelial structures (3).

The nonhomogeneous echo pattern in the solid elements is caused by the presence of tissues of varying density such as cartilage, bone, liver, and brain tissue (6).

Fetal hydrops. The differentiation of solid and cystic tumor components based on their ultrasound features can be important in predicting intrauterine growth, since predominantly cystic tumors (Figs. 29.5–29.8) have little effect on intrauterine growth whereas large, solid tumors can lead to fetal hydrops with intrauterine demise (10).

The cause of fetal hydrops is chronic anemia secondary to tumoral hemorrhage, fluid transudation in the tumor, and arteriovenous shunting across the tumor. These arteriovenous shunts can greatly increase the venous return to the fetal heart, initially causing an increased output from both ventricles and increased flow in the aorta and placenta. Eventually the volume overload on the fetal heart leads to decompensation with fetal hydrops and placentomegaly. Doppler scanning can demonstrate the arteriovenous shunts within the tumor as well as the waveform changes in affected vascular segments. Overall, approximately 25% of fetuses with sacrococcygeal teratoma develop fetal hydrops. Polyhydramnios develops in 70% of cases as a result of the changes described above (11).

Size, location, and biologic behavior. Besides defining tumor morphology, ultrasound is particularly important in evaluating the size and location of the tumors, since pediatric mortality from sacrococcygeal teratomas correlates with an increase in tumor size (9). There are no definite ultrasound signs of immature or malignant tumor components, and so there is no correlation between ultrasound findings and the biologic behavior of teratomas (12).

Secondary signs. Secondary signs that suggest the presence of a sacrococcygeal teratoma in the ultrasound examination include possible bladder displacement by the tumor and possible ureteral obstruction leading to hydronephrosis or renal dysplasia.

Table 29.1 Classification of sacrococcygeal teratomas (1)

Type 1	Predominantly external with a minimal presacral component
Type 2	Predominantly external with a significant intrapelvic component
Type 3	Predominantly internal with intra-abdominal extension
Type 4	Completely internal with no external component

Differential diagnosis. The differential diagnosis of sacrococcygeal teratomas depends largely on the solid or cystic structure of the neoplasm. Other, predominantly solid tumors in the sacrococcygeal region are lipomas, neurogenic tumors, rhabdomyosarcomas, hemangiomas, and malignant melanomas. A predominantly cystic tumor mainly requires differentiation from myelomeningocele. The latter lesion is associated with a bony defect in the spinal column, whereas a sacrococcygeal teratoma is not (Fig. 29.**5**).

Invasive tests. The determination of N-acetylcholinesterase and AFP in the amniotic fluid cannot reliably differentiate cystic tumors from myelomeningocele, because both parameters may be elevated with a sacrococcygeal teratoma.

It may be helpful to aspirate the tumor for cytologic analysis. If cells from two or three germ layers are identified in the aspirate, this establishes the diagnosis of sacrococcygeal teratoma (10).

Associated anomalies. Sacrococcygeal teratomas are associated with other anomalies in 18% of cases. Most of these anomalies involve the musculoskeletal system (5).

Prognosis and treatment. Except for malignancies, the prognosis of sacrococcygeal teratoma depends mainly on the location and size of the tumor. Also, purely cystic sacrococcygeal teratomas generally have a better prognosis than predominantly solid tumors, which are usually more vascular and are more commonly associated with fetal hydrops.

Mature teratomas. The prognosis following the complete removal of a mature teratoma is excellent. This applies to all sites of occurrence of mature teratomas in young patients.

Immature teratomas. These tumors rarely metastasize, but they have a strong tendency for locoregional recurrence after incomplete removal. A correlation exists between the degree of immaturity and tumor prognosis. The survival rate is much poorer with grade II or higher teratomas than with grade 0–1 tumors.

Prenatal Management

Timing of delivery. If ultrasound reveals a fast-growing tumor or if there are poor associated prognostic signs such as fetal heart failure, fetal hydrops or polyhydramnios, it can be difficult to weigh the risks of prematurity, which can compound the difficulty of surgical resection, against the risk of intrauterine fetal death. Lung maturation therapy should be instituted without delay. Maternal digitalization is indicated in selected cases for hemodynamic stabilization of the fetus.

Mode of delivery. Fetuses with an external sacrococcygeal teratoma should be delivered by cesarean section to avoid dystocic complications and tumor hemorrhage.

Surgical treatment. After the baby has been delivered, the goal of the pediatric surgeon is to remove the tumor completely. This may necessitate reconstruction of the pelvic floor. Due to the risk of malignant transformation of residual tumor tissue, the coccyx should be resected with the tumor. The infant should be delivered at a perinatal center that allows for teamwork among the obstetrician, pediatrician, and pediatric surgeon.

References

1. Altman, R.P., Randolph, J.G., Lilly, J.R.: Sacrococcygeal teratoma: American Academy of Pediatrics Surgical Survey – 1973, vol. 9. Philadelphia: Grune a. Stratton 1994; pp. 389–398
2. Barson, A.J.: Congenital neoplasia: The society's experience. Arch. Dis. Child. 53 (1978) 436
3. Chervenak, F.A., Isaacson, G., Touloukian, R., Tortura, M., Berkowitz, I., Hobbins, C.: Diagnosis and Management of fetal teratomas. Obstet. Gynecol. 66 (1983) 666–671
4. Damjanov, I., Solter, D.: Experimental teratome. Curr. Topics. Pathol. 59 (1994) 69–130
5. Ein, S.H., Adeyemi, S.D., Mancer, K.: Benign sacrococcygeal teratoma in infants and children: A 25 year review. Ann. Surg. 191 (1980) 382–384
6. Goldhofer, W., Merz, E., Bauer, H., Koltai, L.: Pränatale sonographische Diagnose eines zystischen Steißbeinteratomes mit retroperitonealer Ausbreitung. Geburtsh. u. Frauenheilk. 46 (1986) 121–123
7. Harms, D., Schmidt, D.: Solide Tumoren des Kindes- und Adoleszentenalters. Keimzelltumoren. In: Remmele, W. (Hrsg.): Pathologie, Bd. 4. Berlin: Springer 1997; S. 539–542
8. Harms, D., Schmidt, D.: Solide Tumoren des Kindes- und Adoleszentenalters. Teratome. In: Remmele, W. (Hrsg.): Pathologie, Bd. 4. Berlin: Springer 1997; S. 542–545
9. Holzgreve, W.: Sonographic demonstration of fetal sacrococcygeal teratoma. Prenat. Diagn. 5 (1985) 245–257
10. Kainer, F., Winter, R., Hofmann, H.M., Karpf, E.F.: Das sacrococcygeale Teratom. Pränatale Diagnose und Prognose. Zbl. Gynäkol. 112 (10) (1990) 609–616
11. Nyberg, D.A., Mach, L.A.: The spine and neural tube defects. In: Nyberg, D.A., Mahony, B.S., Pretorius, D.H. (eds.): Diagnostic ultrasound of fetal anomalies: Text and Atlas. St. Louis: Mosby Year 1990; S. 146–202
12. Sheth, S., Nussbaum, A.R., Sanders, R.C., Hampe, U.K., Davidson, A.J.: Prenatal diagnosis of sacrococcygeal teratoma: sonographic pathologic correlation. Radiology 169 (1988) 131–136
13. Weber, G., Macchiella, D., Bahlmann, F., Merz, E.: Pränatale Diagnose fetaler Teratome. Ultraschall in Med. 14 (1993) 187–192
14. Wodley, M.M., Ginsburg, S., Dicensa, S., Snyder W.H.Jr.: Teratomas in infancy and childhood. A review of the clinical experience at the children's hospital of Los Angeles. Kinderchir. 4 (1967) 283–307

Sacrococcygeal teratoma

Fig. 29.**1**   American Academy of Pediatrics Surgical Survey classification of sacrococcygeal teratomas (modified from 1) (see also Table 29.**1**).

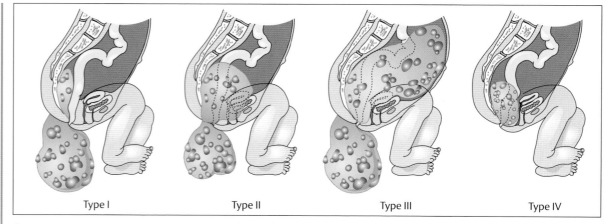

Type I   Type II   Type III   Type IV

1

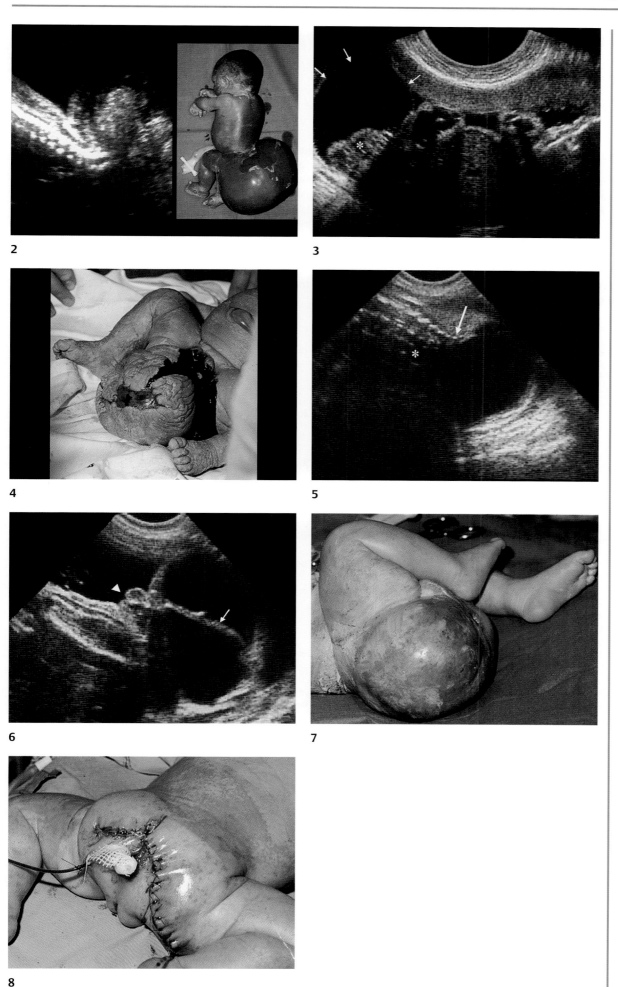

2

3

4

5

6

7

8

Fig. 29.**2** Left: Predominantly solid, immature sacrococcygeal teratoma (12 · 10 · 15 cm) appears as an exophytic mass on the coccyx of a breech-presenting fetus at 27 weeks. Right: Actual appearance. Intrauterine fetal death occurred at 28 weeks (1700 g!).

Fig. 29.**3** Mixed cystic/solid sacrococcygeal teratoma (10.5 · 13 · 12 cm) at 32 weeks. General longitudinal scan of a fetus in the vertex presentation (140°). Cystic sac (arrows). Solid portion of sacrococcygeal teratoma (∗).

Fig. 29.**4** Appearance of sacrococcygeal teratoma in a newborn (same case as in Fig. 29.**3**).

Fig. 29.**5** Purely cystic sacrococcygeal teratoma with partial retroperitoneal extension (∗). Overall size 12 · 10 cm. Occipitoanterior breech presentation, longitudinal scan at 36 weeks. The lower part of the spinal column is closed (arrow).

Fig. 29.**6** Same cystic teratoma as in Fig. 29.**5**. Transverse scan from the superior aspect. A septum (arrow) is visible within the predominantly right-sided sacrococcygeal teratoma. Female genitalia (arrowhead).

Fig. 29.**7** Female newborn with a loculated cystic sacrococcygeal teratoma. Clinical appearance of the case in Figs. 29.**5** and 29.**6**.

Fig. 29.**8** Postoperative appearance of the infant in Figs. 29.**5**–29.**7** (photo courtesy of Dr. Koltai, Department of Pediatric Surgery, Mainz University Hospital, Mainz, Germany).

30 Anomalies of the Extremities

Forms, Causes, and Ultrasound Visualization

Anomalies of the extremities occur in approximately 2.2% of all newborns (120). There may be general abnormalities of bone and cartilage growth, or the changes may be confined to individual bones or limb segments.

Genetic defects. Various forms of osteochondrodysplasia occur as hereditary, familial disorders. The mode of inheritance is usually recessive but is dominant in some conditions (Table 30.1). Anomalies that are confined to specific bones or limb segments can also result from a genetic defect.

Exogenous agents. We have known since the thalidomide tragedy (76) that exogenous agents can have causal importance in congenital limb anomalies. Besides thalidomide, exposure to various other compounds such as ethyl alcohol and diphenylhydantoin can produce limb malformations (115).

Amniotic band syndrome. Another cause of partial limb defects is the amniotic band syndrome, in which bands in the amniotic fluid become entangled around part of the limb in an early stage of development, leading to peromelia.

Table 30.**1** International classification of osteochondrodysplasias, partial listing (adapted from Spranger [140])

Group	Diseases	Mode of inheritance, comments	Group	Diseases	Mode of inheritance, comments
Achondroplasia group	Achondroplasia	AD	Acromelias and acromesomelic dysplasias	Acromicric dysplasia	AR
	Hypochondroplasia	AD		Brachydactylies A—E	AD
	Thanatophoric dysplasia I + II	AD, L		Pseudohypoparathyroidismb	AD
Spondylodysplastic dysplasia group	Platyspondylic dysplasias	AR, L		Acromesomelic dysplasia	AR
	Achondrogenesis IA	AR, L	Dysplasias with prominent membranous bone involvement	Cleidocranial dysplasia	AD
Metatrophic dysplasia group	Fibrochondrogenesis	AR, L		Osteodysplasia	AD
	Schneckenbecken dysplasia	AR, L	Bowing group	Camptomelic dysplasia	AD
	Metatrophic dysplasiab	AD	Dysplasias and congenital dislocations	Larsen syndrome	Het
Short rib–polydactyly groupa	I Saldino–Noonan	AR, L		Desbuquois syndrome	AR
	II Majewski	AR, L	Dysostosis multiplex group	Mucopolysaccharidoses	Het
	III Verma–Naumoff	AR, L		Oligosaccharidoses	Het
	IV Beemer–Langer	AR, L	Osteodysplastic slender bone group	Type I osteodysplastic dysplasia	
	Asphyxiating thoracic dysplasia	AR, OL		Type II osteodysplastic dysplasia	
	Ellis–van Creveld syndrome	AR	Dysplasias with decreased bone density	Osteogenesis imperfecta I—IV	AR
Atelosteogenesis–omodysplasia group	Atelosteogenesis I	L		Type II	L
	Omodysplasia I	AD		Osteoporosis–pseudoglioma	AD
	Omodysplasia II	AR		Geroderma osteodysplastica	AR
	Otopalatodigital syndrome II	L		Idiopathic osteoporosis	
	Atelosteogenesis II	XR, L	Mineralization defectsa	Hypophosphatasia, early form	ARA
	De la Chapelle dysplasia	AR, L		Severe form	L
Diastrophic dysplasia group	Diastrophic dysplasia	AR		Hypophosphatasia, late form	D
	Achondrogenesis IB	AR, L	Osteosclerosis without modification of bone shape	Osteopetrosisb	Het
	Atelosteogenesis II	AR, L		Osteopetrosis + renal acidosis	AR
Dyssegmental dysplasia group	Silverman–Handmaker type	AR, L		Pyknodysostosis	AR
	Rolland–Desbuquois type	AR, L	Osteosclerosis with diaphyseal dysplasia	Camurati–Engelmann syndrome	AD
Type II collagenopathiesa	Achondrogenesis II	AD, L		Craniodiaphysial dysplasia	AR?
	Hypochondrogenesis	AD, L	Osteosclerosis with metaphyseal dysplasia	Pyle disease	AR
	Kniest dysplasia	AD		Craniometaphyseal dysplasiab	Het
	Congenital spondyloepiphyseal dysplasia	AD		Frontometaphysial dysplasia	XR
	Stickler dysplasiab	AD		Dysosteosclerosisb	Het
Type XI collagenopathies	Stickler dysplasiab	AD	Severe neonatal osteosclerosis	Numerous individual forms with smooth or fragmented bone formation	Het, L
	Otospondylomegaepiphyseal dysplasia	AD			
Multiple epiphyseal dysplasia group	Pseudoachondroplasia	AD	Dysplasias with disorganized tissue development	Dysplasia epiphysealis hemimelica	
	Multiple epiphyseal dysplasia	AD		Fibrous dysplasia	AD
Chondrodysplasia punctata group	Rhizomelic type	AR, SL		Fibrodysplasia ossificans progressiva	AD
	Conradi–Hünermann type	XD	Osteolysesa	Carpotarsal form	Het
	Brachytelephalangial type	XR		François syndrome	AR
Mesomelic dysplasiasa	Dyschondrosteosis	AD		Winchester syndrome	AR
	Robinow typeb	Het		Torg syndrome	AD
				Hajdu–Cheney syndrome	AR
				Mandibuloacral syndrome	

aGroups shown to have a uniform pathogenesis. bVarious forms.
AD = autosomal-dominant, AR = autosomal-rezessive, XD = X-linked dominant, XR = X-linked recessive, Het = genetically heterogeneous, L = fatal, OL = often fatal, SL = semifatal

Oligohydramnios. Abnormal positioning or constraint of the fetal limbs can occur in cases of prolonged oligohydramnios or in conditions such as arthrogryposis multiplex congenita. A familial incidence has been documented in some cases.

Targeted search and screening. Since the individual fetal limbs and especially the ossified shafts of the long bones can be defined with ultrasound by 12 weeks' gestation (98, 100, 121), targeted imaging for fetal limb anomalies can be performed as early as the second trimester. This is particularly important in cases that are at risk by family history. But in ordinary screening examinations as well, conspicuous anomalies such as a micromelic growth pattern can be detected if measurements of the fetal limb bones are routinely included in the examination protocol.

Of course, the accurate detection, differentiation, and confident exclusion of fetal limb anomalies require an experienced examiner. It is not uncommon to find ossification defects that cannot be definitely classified, even by radiographic examination in the neonatal period, and can ultimately be diagnosed only by following their progression over time.

Osteochondrodysplasias (Skeletal Dysplasias)

Frequency

As the Italian multicenter study of 1978–1981 showed, the incidence of skeletal dysplasias is approximately one in 4100 newborns, including stillbirths (13). The following anomalies were most commonly found:
- Thanatophoric dysplasia
- Achondroplasia
- Achondrogenesis
- Osteogenesis imperfecta

The results were similar in the prenatal multicenter study published by Goncalves et al. (42), except that osteogenesis imperfecta was found with somewhat greater frequency (Fig. 30.**1**). Data from a population-based registry of congenital anomalies (144) confirm that the four anomalies listed above are the most prevalent skeletal dysplasias.

Ultrasound Differentiation of Skeletal Anomalies

The ultrasound detection and differentiation of skeletal and limb anomalies requires a careful, general ultrasound evaluation of the fetus (especially the head, spinal column, bony thorax, and limbs) in addition to accurate biometry, especially of the long tubular bones.

Femur–foot length comparison. If bone length cannot be accurately interpreted due to uncertain dates, it can be helpful to compare the lengths of the femur and foot. Because the femur and foot have similar antenatal lengths, at least during the second trimester, a femur that is considerably shorter than the foot is always suspicious for skeletal dysplasia (Fig. 30.**2**).

Patterns of limb shortening. The following patterns of limb shortening, or dwarfism, may be observed with ultrasound:
- *Micromelia* (proximal and distal long bones are equally shortened)
- *Rhizomelia* (proximal long bones are shortened)
- *Mesomelia* (distal long bones are shortened) (Table 30.**2**, Fig. 30.**3**).

Besides the growth patterns of the extremity bones, various others parameters can be used for the prenatal differentiation of the various forms of limb shortening (Tables 30.**3** and 30.**4**, Figs. 30.**4** and 30.**5**).

Table 30.**2**   Patterns of limb shortening

Rhizomelia	Shortening of the proximal long bones (femur, humerus)
Mesomelia	Shortening of the distal long bones (tibia, fibula, radius, ulna)
Acromelia	Shortening of the distal segments (hands, feet)
Micromelia	Shortening of the proximal and distal long bones

Table 30.**3**   Parameters for the differentiation of skeletal anomalies

Skelettabschnitt	Parameter
Limb bones	➤ Bone length ➤ Pattern of bone shortening (rhizomelia, mesomelia, micromelia) ➤ Absence or hypoplasia of a bone (e.g., radial or fibular aplasia) ➤ Abnormal bone structure (diaphysis, metaphysis) ➤ Degree of bowing ➤ Detection of bone fractures
Head	➤ Head size (macrocephaly) ➤ Abnormal head shape (cloverleaf) ➤ Ossification of calvaria ➤ Deformable calvaria ➤ Hypertelorism ➤ Abnormal facial profile (flat profile, frontal bossing, depressed nasal bridge, cleft lip and palate, retrognathia)
Spinal column	➤ Abnormal curvature ➤ Hypomineralization
Clavicle	➤ Aplasia, hypoplasia
Scapula	➤ Aplasia, hypoplasia
Thorax	➤ Thoracic shape (champagne-cork thorax, bell-shaped) ➤ Hypoplasia of bony thorax ➤ Pulmonary hypoplasia ➤ Cardiac anomaly
Pelvic bones	➤ Absent or delayed ossification
Hands	➤ Polydactyly
Feet	➤ Pes equinovarus
Movement pattern	➤ Decreased motor activity

▬ *Fatal Skeletal Dysplasias*

An essential goal of prenatal diagnosis is the early detection or exclusion of fatal forms of skeletal dysplasia (Table 30.**5**)—i.e., anomalies that cause the death of the fetus or neonate.

Incidence. The incidence of fatal osteochondrodysplasias is approximately one in 19,000 live births (21).

Pathoanatomic findings. This group of dysplasias is characterized by short limb bones, a narrow thorax, and hypoplastic lungs.

Ultrasound features. The prenatal ultrasound diagnosis is based on short limb bones and a narrow thorax in relation to the abdomen, causing the head and torso to resemble a "champagne cork" when viewed in longitudinal section (49) (Fig. 30.**5**). In transverse scans, the two thoracic diameters are markedly smaller than the abdominal diameter, and the lungs appear small (Fig. 30.**6**).

In recent years, prenatal ultrasound has been able to detect various skeletal dysplasias both in high-risk cases and in screening examinations (71, 89, 92). In some of these cases, the dysplasias could be diagnosed earlier than 24 weeks.

Fig. 30.**1** Frequency distribution of 132 skeletal dysplasias detected prenatally. Data based on an international multicenter study published by Goncalves and Jeanty 1994 (42).

Ultrasound differentiation

Fig. 30.**2** Marked growth discrepancy between the foot (1) (38 mm) and femur (2) (19 mm) in thanatophoric dysplasia, 23 weeks (foot–femur length ratio = 2!).

Fig. 30.**3** Patterns of limb shortening.

a Rhizomelia: short femoral shaft (23 mm) with normal lengths of the tibia (31 mm) and fibula (30 mm), 21 weeks.

b Mesomelia: the shafts of the distal arm bones are short [radius (1) = 20 mm and ulna (2) = 21 mm] with a normal humeral length (34 mm), 22 weeks.

c Acromelia: short fingers, 30 weeks.

d Micromelia: proximal and distal bones are equally shortened; here: tibia (2) 12 mm, fibula (1) 11 mm, femur 15 mm, 20 weeks.

Fig. 30.**4** Ultrasound abnormalities of the long tubular bones.

a Abnormally short femoral shaft (30 mm) in osteochondrodysplasia (chondrodysplasia punctata, rhizomelic type) at 25 weeks, 4 days.

b Abnormal bowing of the femoral shaft (26 mm) in camptomelic dysplasia, 23 weeks.

c Expansion and hyperechoicity of the metaphysis and epiphysis (arrow) with a very short humerus (34 mm) (short rib–polydactyly syndrome), 32 weeks.

d Deficient ossification at the center of the bone in hypophosphatasia.

e Stepoff caused by a midshaft fracture of the femur (osteogenesis imperfecta), 23 weeks.

f Marked angulation and deficient ossification of the tibia following a fracture (osteogenesis imperfecta).

Fig. 30.**5** Skeletal deformities in osteochondrodysplasias.

a Frontal bossing in thanatophoric dysplasia, 23 weeks.

b Marked bulging of the calvaria in thanatophoric dysplasia with a cloverleaf skull, 21 weeks.

c Very narrow thorax (arrows) with a large head and normal-size abdomen (champagne-cork phenomenon) in osteogenesis imperfecta, 23 weeks.

d Heptadactyly in short rib–polydactyly syndrome, 22 weeks.

e Club foot in arthrogryposis multiplex congenita, 35 weeks.

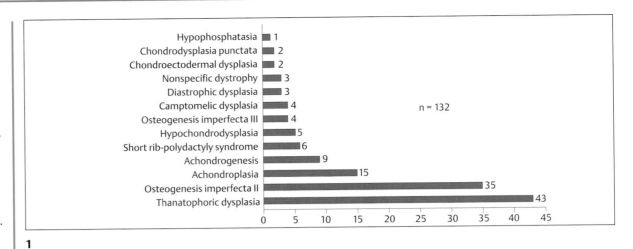

1

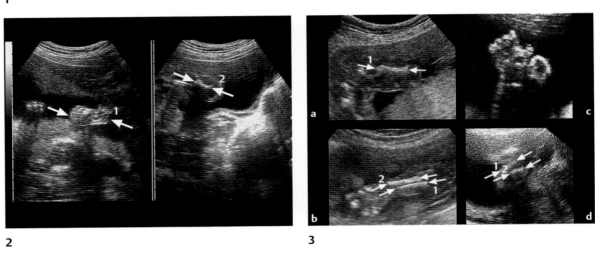

2

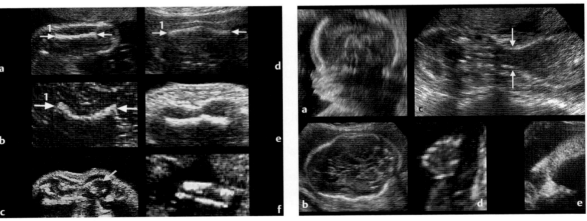

3

4

5

The "most common" fatal forms of osteochondrodysplasia will be discussed below.

Hypophosphatasia

Definition. Disease characterized by severe, rickets-like defects in skeletal mineralization, vitamin-D resistant.

Forms. Hypophosphatasia (= Rathbun syndrome) (116) has four forms that are distinguished by their severity and the age at which the changes are manifested (74):

- Prenatal form (congenital fatal hypophosphatasia)
- Early infantile form
- Infantile-juvenile form
- Adult form

Table 30.**4** Differential diagnosis of ultrasound limb and bone abnormalities

Ultrasound finding	Possible diagnoses
Micromelia	Achondrogenesis Thanatophoric dysplasia Short rib–polydactyly syndrome Diastrophic dysplasia
Rhizomelia	Thanatophoric dysplasia Chondrodysplasia punctata, rhizomelic type Diastrophic dysplasia Cardiofaciomelic dysplasia Congenital short femur
Mesomelia	Mesomelic dysplasia Cardiofaciomelic dysplasia
Normal bone length	Cleidocranial dysplasia Arthrogryposis multiplex congenita Larsen syndrome Craniosynostoses
Abnormal metaphysis	Metatrophic dysplasia Short rib–polydactyly syndrome type III Kniest syndrome Diastrophic dysplasia Fibrochondrogenesis
Abnormal bowing of a bone	Thanatophoric dysplasia Osteogenesis imperfecta Hypophosphatasia Camptomelic dysplasia
Bone fractures	Osteogenesis imperfecta Hypophosphatasia Achondrogenesis IA (Houston–Harris type)
Radial aplasia or hypoplasia	Roberts syndrome Vater association
Fibular aplasia or hypoplasia	Camptomelic dysplasia Mesomelic dysplasia, Langer type and Reinhart type Atelosteogenesis
Acromesomelia	Ellis–van Creveld syndrome
Polydactyly of the hand	Short rib–polydactyly syndrome Vater association Smith–Lemli–Opitz syndrome
Polydactyly of the foot Abducted ("hitchhiker") thumbs	Short rib–polydactyly syndrome Diastrophic dysplasia
Syndactyly	Cranioectodermal dysplasia
Pes equinovarus (clubfoot)	Osteogenesis imperfecta Chondrodysplasia punctata Diastrophic dysplasia Metatrophic dysplasia Arthrogryposis multiplex congenita Camptomelic dysplasia Pena–Shokeir syndrome Atelosteogenesis
Macrocephaly	Thanatophoric dysplasia Achondroplasia
Cloverleaf skull	Thanatophoric dysplasia with cloverleaf skull
Microcephaly	Smith–Lemli–Opitz syndrome Meckel–Gruber syndrome Seckel syndrome Roberts syndrome

Ultrasound finding	Possible diagnoses
Hypomineralization of the calvaria	Osteogenesis imperfecta type II Hypophosphatasia
Deformable skull	Osteogenesis imperfecta type II Hypophosphatasia
Frontal bossing of the skull	Thanatophoric dysplasia
Flat facial profile	Weissenbacher–Zweymüller syndrome
Hypertelorism	Weissenbacher–Zweymüller syndrome
Depressed nasal bridge	Thanatophoric dysplasia Achondrogenesis Achondroplasia Osteogenesis imperfecta type II Camptomelic dysplasia Chondrodysplasia punctata Larsen syndrome Atelosteogenesis
Cleft lip and palate	Diastrophic dysplasia Larsen syndrome Short rib–polydactyly syndrome Camptomelic dysplasia Roberts syndrome Weissenbacher–Zweymüller syndrome Camptomelic dysplasia Weissenbacher–Zweymüller syndrome
Retro- or micrognathia	Metaphyseal chondrodysplasia, Murk–Hansen type Mesomelic dysplasia, Langer type Atelosteogenesis
Deficient ossification of the vertebral bodies	Dyssegmental dysplasia Atelosteogenesis
Scoliosis	Diastrophic dysplasia Chondrodysplasia punctata, X-linked dominant form
Clavicular aplasia or hypoplasia	Cleidocranial dysostosis
Scapular hypoplasia	Camptomelic syndrome
Hypoplasia of bony thorax	Thanatophoric dysplasia Achondrogenesis Homozygous achondroplasia Osteogenesis imperfecta Asphyxiating thoracic dysplasia Short rib–polydactyly syndrome Chondroectodermal dysplasia Camptomelic dysplasia Hypophosphatasia Fibrochondrogenesis Atelosteogenesis
Cardiac anomalies	Chondroectodermal dysplasia Short rib–polydactyly syndrome type I/II Cardiofaciomelic dysplasia Smith–Lemli–Opitz syndrome type I
Absent or delayed ossification of the ischium and pubis	Achondrogenesis
Decreased motor activity	Arthrogryposis multiplex congenita Pena–Shokeir syndrome Atelosteogenesis

Fig. 30.5 Fatal forms of osteochondrodysplasia (adapted from 139)

1	**Hypophosphatasia and morphologically similar disorders**
1.1	Hypophosphatasia
2	**Chondrodysplasia punctata and similar disorders**
2.1	Rhizomelic chondrodysplasia punctata
2.2	Fatal chondrodysplasia punctata, x-linked dominant
2.3	Greenberg dysplasia
2.4	Stippled diaphyseal dysplasia
3	**Achondrogenesis and similar disorders**
3.1	Achondrogenesis IA (Houston–Harris)
3.2	Achondrogenesis IB (Fraccaro)
3.3	Achondrogenesis II (Langer–Saldino)
3.4	Hypochondrogenesis
4	**Thanatophoric dysplasia and similar disorders**
4.1	Thanatophoric dysplasia type 1
4.2	Thanatophoric dysplasia type 2
4.3	Homozygous achondroplasia
4.4	Fatal achondroplasia
4.5	Glasgow variant
5	**Platyspondylitic fatal chondrodysplasias**
5.1	Platyspondylitic chondrodysplasia, Torrance type
5.2	Platyspondylitic chondrodysplasia, San Diego type
5.3	Platyspondylitic chondrodysplasia, Luton type
5.4	Platyspondylitic chondrodysplasia, Shiraz type
5.5	Opsismodysplasia
6	**Short rib–polydactyly syndromes**
6.1	Short rib–polydactyly syndrome type I (Saldino–Noonan)
6.2	Short rib–polydactyly syndrome type II (Verma–Naumoff)
6.3	Short rib–polydactyly syndrome type II (Le Marec)
6.4	Short rib–polydactyly syndrome type IV (Yang)
6.5	Asphyxiating thoracic dysplasia (Jeune)
6.6	Short rib–polydactyly syndrome type VI (Majewski)
6.7	Short rib–polydactyly syndrome type VII (Beemer)
7	**Fatal metatrophic dysplasia and similar disorders**
7.1	Fatal metatrophic dysplasia (hyperchondrogenesis)
7.2	Fibrochondrogenesis
7.3	Schneckenbecken dysplasia
8	**Kniest-like disorders**
8.1	Dyssegmental dysplasia, Silverman type
8.2	Dyssegmental dysplasia, Rolland–Desbuquois type
8.3	Blomstrand chondrodysplasia
9	**Fatal osteochondrodysplasias with predominantly diaphyseal abnormalities**
9.1	Camptomelic syndrome
9.2	Stüve–Wiedemann syndrome
9.3	Boomerang dysplasia
9.4	Atelosteogenesis
9.5	De la Chapelle dysplasia
9.6	McAlister dysplasia
9.7	Pseudodiastrophic dysplasia
10	**Osteogenesis imperfecta and similar disorders**
10.1	Osteogenesis imperfecta IIA
10.2	Osteogenesis imperfecta IIB
10.3	Osteogenesis imperfecta IIC
10.4	Astley–Kendall dysplasia
11	**Fatal diseases with fragile bones**
11.1	Fetal hypokinesia
11.2	Fatal osteochondrodysplasia with fragile bones

The prenatal form, known also as the "malignant" form, is the most unfavorable.

Incidence. The reported incidence is one in 100,000 (34).

Etiology and pathogenesis. There is a severe decrease in alkaline phosphatase activity with an essentially normal serum phosphate level.
The mode of inheritance is autosomal-recessive.

Pathoanatomic findings. Based on the severe disturbance of mineralization and ossification, osteolytic defects are distributed throughout the skeleton. Fractures and pseudofractures also occur. The calvaria is "membranous" due to deficient ossification.

Ultrasound features. The ultrasound diagnosis (23, 73, 151, 159) is based on the detection of abnormal bone growth and decreased superior ossification. The shafts of the limb bones exhibit marked shortening and bowing with decreased echogenicity (Fig. 30.**7**). Fractures may also be seen. Because of the decreased calvarial density, the brain structures show a remarkably distinct echo pattern (Fig. 30.**8**). Laughlin and Lee (73) describe a prominent falx cerebri. The amniotic fluid volume is increased.

Further tests. The alkaline phosphatase activity in the amniotic fluid can be determined by amniocentesis and culturing the amniotic fluid cells (104). Alkaline phosphatase activity can also be determined in the fetal blood following cordocentesis (104).

Differential diagnosis. Osteogenesis imperfecta II, Jeune syndrome.

Prognosis. In the prenatal fatal form of hypophosphatasia, the infants are either stillborn or die within a short time after birth.

Clinical management. Given the fatal outcome of the prenatal form, pregnancy termination is justified at any stage of gestation.

Chondrodysplasia Punctata, Rhizomelic Type

Definition. A dysplastic syndrome in which dwarfism is manifested prenatally. It is associated with facial abnormalities and stippled calcifications in the epiphyses.

Forms. Two major forms are distinguished in the group of chondrodysplasia punctata syndromes:
- Fatal, rhizomelic form
- Nonfatal form, known also as Conradi–Hünermann disease

Incidence. Rare. Only 36 cases were described as of 1971 (157).

Etiology and pathogenesis. The disease is transmitted as an autosomal-recessive trait (135).

Pathoanatomic findings. There is a disproportionate rhizomelic dwarfism with predominant shortening of the femora and humeri. This is accompanied by multiple joint contractures. The face is flat, and the nasal bridge is broad and depressed. Microcephaly is usually present and is associated with significant psychomotor retardation. Radiographs show grossly shortened proximal limb bones with metaphyseal flaring and epiphyseal stippling in the humerus and femur.

Associated anomalies. Ichthyosiform skin changes are not uncommon. Unilateral or bilateral cataracts are present in approximately two-thirds of cases.

Prognosis. Affected infants are either stillborn or die shortly after birth (37, 51).

Ultrasound features (111, 119). Ultrasound demonstrates rhizomelic dwarfism with marked shortening of the humerus and femur (Fig. 30.**9**). Cephalometry may indicate microcephalic growth. Because of the flexion contractures, restricted motion is noted in various joints.

Differential diagnosis. Differentiation is required from other forms of rhizomelic dysplasia. The stippled epiphyseal calcifications seen on radiographs are not specific for chondrodysplasia punctata and also occur in trisomy 18, trisomy 21, Smith–Lemli–Opitz syndrome, and warfarin embryopathy (53).

Other tests. Chorion villus sampling can detect the disease as early as the first trimester (56).

Clinical management. When the fatal rhizomelic form is diagnosed, pregnancy termination may be considered due to the extremely poor prognosis.

Achondrogenesis

Definition. Severe skeletal dysplasia with extreme micromelia, macrocephaly, and short trunk.

Forms. For many years, only two forms of achondrogenesis were distinguished: type I (Parenti–Fraccaro) and type II (Langer–Saldino) (136). According to Whitley and Gorlin (156), a total of four types are recognized today. Spranger and Maroteaux (139) subdivide type I into the subtypes IA (Houston–Harris) and IB (Fraccaro) (Table 30.**5**).

Incidence. Approximately one in 43,000 births (13).

Pathoanatomic Findings

Types IA and IB. These disproportionate forms of dwarfism involve an extreme micromelia that affects both the proximal and distal limb segments. Other features are macrocephaly with a round face and short nose, a very short trunk with a protuberant abdomen (and possible hydrops), and a short neck (33, 132, 136).

Type IA. Radiographs in type IA show decreased ossification of the calvaria, almost no ossification of the vertebral bodies, thin ribs that may contain multiple fractures, and short, crescent-shaped ilia. The femora are greatly shortened and may be bowed (139).

Type IB. This type resembles IA but differs in the absence of rib fractures and slightly better ossification of the vertebral bodies. The femora exhibit a triangular shape (139).

Type II. The overall changes in this type are somewhat less pronounced than in IA and Ibd (139). The fetuses attain a body length of 27–36 cm and a weight of 1000–2800 g. They are hydropic and have short limbs. The forehead is more prominent and the nose slightly longer than in type I cases. Radiographs show better ossification of the calvaria than in achondrogenesis type I, but the vertebral bodies show very poor ossification. The scapulae are small and irregular. The ribs show a horizontal orientation. The long bones of the extremities are shortened and have deeply cupped metaphyses.

Types III and IV. These are generally less pronounced than the other types, with considerably longer femora (156).

Etiology and pathogenesis. Types I and II have an autosomal-recessive inheritance (21). Type I affects both enchondral and membranous bone, while type II affects only enchondral bone. Type II is caused by a defect in the biosynthesis of type II collagen (59).

Ultrasound features. The fatal forms of achondrogenesis can be diagnosed sonographically (4, 41, 44, 49, 132, 154) by noting the extreme micromelia that affects all the long bones of the extremities (Fig. 30.**10**) and is already detectable early in the second trimester. Ultrasound also reveals macrocephaly with a flat face, a narrow thorax, and a poorly ossified spinal column. There may also be decreased density of the calvaria, fetal hydrops, and polyhydramnios (4, 44, 49).

Soothill et al. (133) were able to detect achondrogenesis type II at only 12 weeks' gestation by transvaginal scanning.

Differential diagnosis. In principle, it is possible to distinguish among the various forms of achondrogenesis in the second trimester based on the differentiating ultrasound features noted above. Ultimately, however, this differentiation relies on postnatal x-ray examination. If the micromelia is slightly less pronounced, *hypochondrogenesis* may be a more accurate diagnosis (Fig. 30.**11**).

Prognosis. Affected infants are either stillborn or die within a few hours after birth.

Clinical management. Because of the fatal outcome, pregnancy termination is justified at any gestational age.

Thanatophoric Dysplasia

Definition. Fatal skeletal dysplasia with a large skull, a narrow thorax of normal length, and pronounced rhizomelic dwarfism.

Forms. Two forms of thanatophoric dysplasia are distinguished:
- Thanatophoric dysplasia type 1
- Thanatophoric dysplasia type 2 (139)

Type 2 is very similar to type 1 but is associated with a cloverleaf skull.

Incidence. In 1971, Thompson and Parmley (148) estimated the incidence of thanatophoric dysplasia at one in 100,000 births. But if we take into account the data from the Italian multicenter study (13), thanatophoric dysplasia appears to be the second most common form of dwarfism, with an incidence of approximately one in 17,000. In the 1994 prenatal multicenter study published by Goncalves and Jeanty (42), thanatophoric dysplasia was also found to be the second most common form of prenatally detectable osteochondrodysplasia.

Etiology and pathogenesis. The cause is uncertain. The disease is based upon a very severe defect of enchondral ossification. Males predominate by about a 2 : 1 ratio (109). Chromosomal studies have revealed a normal karyotype (68, 72). Most cases to date appear to have occurred sporadically (109, 136). However, some cases of familial recurrence have been described (15, 43), prompting speculation on an autosomal-dominant inheritance (125). The autosomal-recessive mode of inheritance suggested by some authors (15, 67) has not been confirmed.

Pathoanatomic Findings

Thanatophoric dysplasia type 1. The typical thanatophoric dwarf has a large cranium (head circumference up to 40 cm at term) with a prominent forehead and saddle nose. The thorax is markedly narrow in relation to the frequently protuberant abdomen (hypoplastic lungs). The trunk length is normal. The limbs are very short, and there is redundant subcutaneous fat. The overall length of the thanatophoric dwarf ranges from 36 to 47 cm at birth (83, 136). The large tubular bones are short and bowed with a "telephone receiver" shape, and the metaphyses are flared (21, 136). The ribs are short, and the vertebral bodies are flattened. The ilia are short and broad.

Thanatophoric dysplasia type 2. This type is distinguished by the additional presence of a *cloverleaf skull* (11, 17, 141, 153). The cloverleaf deformity of the skull is caused by premature closure of the coronal and lambdoid sutures. The cloverleaf skull itself is a nonspecific feature. It may occur as an isolated defect or may coexist with ankyloses, syndactylies, or various skeletal dysplasias.

Other differences from type 1: the limb bones are slightly thinner and are not bowed, the ribs are not as thin, the vertebral bodies are not as flat, and the scapulae and pelvic bones show more uniform contours (139).

Associated anomalies. Several anomalies have been described in association with thanatophoric dysplasia: hydrocephalus (in type 1), cardiac anomalies, and renal anomalies.

Ultrasound features. Prenatal ultrasound diagnosis is based on the following criteria (27, 40, 72, 95, 126): stubby limbs with very short, bowed long tubular bones (Fig. 30.**12**); a very narrow thorax that tapers superiorly to a conical shape and contrasts sharply with the protuberant abdomen ("champagne cork" phenomenon) (49) (Figs. 30.**6**, 30.**13**); and macrocephaly with frontal bossing and a depressed nasal bridge (Fig. 30.**13**). Polyhydramnios is present in most cases (148). The long bones of the extremities are already so grossly shortened in the second trimester that a diagnosis can be made before 20 weeks' gestation (Fig. 30.**14**).

In type 2, a cloverleaf skull is noted in addition to the shortened limb bones (11, 81) (Fig. 30.**15**).

Differential diagnosis. Thanatophoric dysplasia may be confused with all the other fatal forms of osteochondrodysplasia that are associated with a very narrow thorax.

Prognosis. Affected infants are either stillborn or die shortly after birth from cardiorespiratory failure secondary to pulmonary hypoplasia (109, 136).

Clinical management. Given the fatal outcome of the prenatal form, pregnancy termination is justified even in older fetuses.

In fetuses that have been carried to term, macrocephaly can cause dystocic complications. In view of the grave prognosis, early delivery is advised to spare the mother the needless risk of a cesarean section.

Short Rib–Polydactyly Syndromes

Definition. The short rib–polydactyly syndromes are a group of fatal osteochondrodysplasias characterized by a narrow thorax, brachymelia, and polydactyly. Various organ malformations may also be found. One confusing aspect of this group is that there are also forms without polydactyly.

Forms. Short rib–polydactyly syndrome is currently classified into seven different forms, as described by Spranger and Maroteaux (139):
1. Short rib–polydactyly syndrome type I (Saldino–Noonan)
2. Short rib–polydactyly syndrome type II (Verma–Naumoff)
3. Short rib–polydactyly syndrome type III (Le Marec)
4. Short rib–polydactyly syndrome type IV (Yang)
5. Asphyxiating thoracic dystrophy (Jeune)
6. Short rib–polydactyly syndrome type VI (Majewski)
7. Short rib–polydactyly syndrome type VII (Beemer)

Below we shall describe several of these syndromes in greater detail. Information on the other, extremely rare forms can be found in the specialized literature (74, 139).

Short Rib–Polydactyly Syndrome Type I (Saldino–Noonan)

Incidence. Rare.

Etiology and pathogenesis. Autosomal-recessive disorder with no chromosomal abnormalities.

Pathoanatomic findings (118, 139). Besides pronounced brachymelia and postaxial polydactyly of the hands and feet, affected fetuses have a very narrow thorax with pulmonary hypoplasia. The body length ranges from 33 to 34 cm at 36–37 weeks. The nasal root is depressed. Radiographs demonstrate short ribs and hypoplasia of the scapulae and pelvic bones. The long bones of the extremities have a band-like shape with pointed ends.

Associated anomalies. The following anomalies are found in association with this syndrome: cardiac anomalies (transposition), renal anomalies (aplasia, hypoplasia, polycystic kidneys), and gastrointestinal anomalies (esophageal atresia, malrotation, absent gallbladder, hepatic cysts, anal atresia). Other possible anomalies include cleft lip and palate and genital malformations.

Short Rib–Polydactyly Syndrome Type II (Verma–Naumoff)

Incidence. More common than type I.

Etiology and pathogenesis. An autosomal-recessive inheritance is assumed. The disease appears to be more common in male than female newborns (129).

Pathoanatomic findings. On the whole, ossification if more advanced than in type I. The long bones of the extremities have frayed ends that resemble an opened banana peel (139). Polydactyly is absent in some cases. Affected infants are often hydropic at birth.

Associated anomalies. The same organ malformations are observed as in type I.

Asphyxiating Thoracic Dystrophy (Jeune)

Incidence. Between one in 100,000 and one in 130,000 (105).

Etiology and pathogenesis. Autosomal-recessive inheritance.

Pathoanatomic findings. A very narrow thorax is combined with a short sternum, short ribs, and hypoplastic iliac wings (63, 78). The bones are shortened but show normal contours. Polydactyly may be present.

Associated anomalies. Infants with a pronounced form are hydropic and have relatively short limb bones. In contrast to other short rib–polydactyly syndromes, there are no lip or palatal clefts and no urogenital anomalies.

Prognosis. Pronounced cases are stillborn or die within a few days. Less severe forms survive the neonatal period.

Short Rib–Polydactyly Syndrome Type VI (Majewski)

Incidence. As of 1987, at least 10 cases in eight families had been described (139).

Etiology and pathogenesis. Autosomal-recessive inheritance.
Pathoanatomic findings (82, 137). The thorax is very narrow with short ribs. The long bones of the extremities are well developed except for the tibia, which is very short and has a characteristic rounded, oval proximal end. Polysyndactyly may occur.

Associated anomalies. Infants with a pronounced form are hydropic. The head is large with a depressed nasal bridge, cleft lip and palate, and micrognathia. Other associated anomalies are the same as in the other short rib–polydactyly syndromes. Polyhydramnios may occur.
Prognosis. Pronounced cases are stillborn or die within a few days. Less severe forms survive the neonatal period.

Ultrasound Diagnosis, Differential Diagnosis, and Clinical Management of the Short Rib–Polydactyly Syndromes

Ultrasound features. Among the various forms of short rib–polydactyly syndrome, there are isolated cases that can be diagnosed prenatally, especially in patients who have a risk of recurrence (24, 38, 64, 78, 93, 94, 149, 158, 162).

Besides micromelia (Figs. 30.**16**, 30.**17**), the most prominent features of this group of osteochondrodysplasias are pronounced thoracic and pulmonary hypoplasia (Fig. 30.**18**) and polydactyly of the hand and/or foot (Fig. 30.**5**). The latter is not always found, however. The ribs are short. Both of the scapulae and the pelvic bones may show poor ossification. In scrutinizing the organs, particular attention should be given to the face, heart, kidneys, and intestinal tract.

Either polyhydramnios (type VI) or oligohydramnios (type I) may be observed, depending on the presenting form.

Differential diagnosis. It is difficult to distinguish among the various types of short rib–polydactyly syndrome, even in the neonatal period. Prenatally, differentiation is required from all other osteochondrodysplasias that are associated with a small thorax. The same applies to Ellis–van Creveld syndrome (Table 30.**6**).

Prognosis. Grave. If the infant is not stillborn, it will soon die from respiratory failure due to pulmonary hypoplasia.

Clinical management. Because of the grave prognosis, pregnancy termination may be considered at any gestational age.

Camptomelic Syndrome

Definition. Mesomelic dysplasia with symmetrical bowing and shortening of the lower extremities. Camptomelic syndrome belongs to the group of fatal osteochondrodysplasias with predominant diaphyseal involvement (Table 30.**5**).

The syndrome was recognized as a separate entity in 1970 by Spranger et al. (134) and in 1971 by Maroteaux et al. (84).

Incidence. Rare. Houston (60) published a review of 97 cases in 1982.

Etiology and pathogenesis. Occurrence is usually sporadic. It may be an autosomal-recessive or heterogeneous congenital disorder. It is believed to result from damage to the cartilage model in the bony shaft of the femur and tibia and also the bones of the pelvic girdle, scapulae, and thoracic spine (108).

Pathoanatomic Findings

Extremities. This mesomelic form of dwarfism is characterized by severe, predominantly mesomelic limb curvatures plus fibular hypoplasia or aplasia. The lower legs are bowed forward, and the feet show a fixed club foot deformity. The infants are 43 cm long at birth.

Head. The head is relatively large and dolichocephalic. Auricular malformations are present. Facial abnormalities include a depressed nasal bridge, hypertelorism, a long philtrum, cleft palate, and micrognathia.

Trunk and genitalia. The trunk is short, the thorax is narrow, and the scapulae are hypoplastic. There is a distinctive disturbance of genital development ranging from hypospadias to pseudogynecotropia (female external genitalia with an XY chromosome pattern) (139).

Associated anomalies. Arhinencephaly, cardiac anomalies, hydronephrosis, tracheal dysplasia, craniosynostosis, hydrocephalus, cerebral dysplasias, and genital anomalies.

Prognosis. Some babies are stillborn. Most die during the first weeks of life.

Ultrasound features. Ultrasound abnormalities (35, 55) can be recognized during the first half of the second trimester. Besides shortening of the long limb bones, there is marked bowing of the femur (Fig. 30.**19**) and especially of the tibia and fibula (Fig. 30.**19**). The fibula may be absent. The feet are clubbed. The thorax is abnormally narrow.

Attention should also be given to the genitalia, since camptomelic syndrome has an association with genital anomalies (Fig. 28.**4**).

Polyhydramnios is frequently present.

Differential diagnosis. Differentiation is required from all other fatal skeletal dysplasias with the bowing of bones (Stüve–Wiedemann dysplasia [146], boomerang dysplasia [147], atelosteogenesis [86], De la Chapelle dysplasia [22], McAlister dysplasia [88]).

Osteogenesis Imperfecta Type II

Definition. Heterogeneous condition characterized by disproportionate dwarfism and multiple fractures of the long bones of the extremities.

Incidence. Approximately one in 54,000 births (13).

Forms. According to Sillence et al. (128), four different types are distinguished. Type II is the most severe and is not compatible with life. This type is further divided into various subgroups (Table 30.**5**).

Etiology and pathogenesis. This condition may have an autosomal-recessive mode of inheritance or may result from a new dominant mutation (87, 127, 136, 138). According to Byers et al. (12), the disease is caused by dominant mutations of genes that code type I collagen.

Pathoanatomic findings. The main features of osteogenesis imperfecta are shortened and deformed limbs with multiple bone fractures. Rib fractures can also occur (85, 136). The head is large and shows deficient ossification of the calvaria.

Table 30.1 Differentiation of short rib–polydactyly syndromes from Ellis–van Creveld syndrome

Parameter	Short rib–polydactyly syndromes				Ellis-van-Creveld-syndrome
	Typ I	Typ II	Jeune	Typ VI	
Bone shortening					
- Proximal	++	++	–	++	±
- Distal	++	++	+	++	+++
Metaphyseal dysplasia	++	++	+	–	–
Bone shape	Bandlike with pointed ends	Banana peel, torpedo	Tibia very short		
Polydactyly	++	±	± (20%)	+++	+++
Metacarpal fusion	–	–	±	+	+++
Degree of thoracic dysplasia	++	++	++	++	+
Rib shortening	++	++	++	++	+
Cleft lip and palate	+	+	–	+	–
Cardiac anomalies	++	+	–	++	++ (50%)
Renal anomaly	+	+	–	+	±
Genital anomaly	+	+	–	+++	+
Anal atresia	+	+	–	–	–

Ultrasound features. There have been numerous reports on the intrauterine diagnosis of this disease (2, 6, 9, 18, 26, 97, 102, 127, 142, 158, 160). It can be detected prior to 24 weeks, not just in patients with a familial risk but also in screening examinations of patients with a negative history (97).

Fractures. Ultrasound demonstrates marked shortening of the long tubular bones, which are found to contain isolated fractures (Figs. 30.**20**, 30.**21**). These fractures may lead to angulation of the bone segments (Fig. 30.**20**) or of the entire limb (Fig. 30.**22**). Fetal movements are restricted (26).

Membranous calvaria. Another abnormal finding is a thin, poorly ossified calvaria (26, 97, 102, 160). As a result, the skull is easily deformed by external pressure ("membranous" calvaria) (Fig. 30.**23**) and brain structures appear unusually distinct. Milsom et al. (102) were also able to demonstrate a narrow thorax with multiple rib fractures.

It should be assumed that a fatal form of osteogenesis imperfecta is present when the above changes are already detectable in the second trimester.

Differential diagnosis. Hypophosphatasia, achondrogenesis IA.

Prognosis. Infants with osteogenesis imperfecta type II are usually stillborn or survive for only a short time (85).

Spranger et al. (138) published a prognostic scoring system for osteogenesis imperfecta in 1982. A score of 2.7 or higher was associated with an 88% mortality rate.

The recurrence risk of congenital osteogenesis imperfecta is approximately 25% (160) or less (87, 138).

Clinical management. With early intrauterine detection of osteogenesis imperfecta, pregnancy termination should be considered. If the abnormalities are mild (e.g., an isolated fracture) and are not detected until the third trimester, it is unlikely that a fatal form is present. These cases should be managed by elective cesarean section to prevent additional fractures, which might occur in a spontaneous delivery.

Differential Diagnosis of Fatal Forms of Dwarfism

The principal differential diagnostic criteria for fatal osteochondrodysplasias are listed in Table 30.7.

Narrow thorax. It is noteworthy that all fatal forms of dwarfism feature a narrow thorax (Figs. 30.**5**, 30.**6**), which explains the development of pulmonary hypoplasia. If ultrasound thoracometry indicates that the thorax is markedly narrow for gestational age and in relation to other body parameters, this should be interpreted as a poor prognostic sign.

▬ *Nonfatal Skeletal Dysplasias*

Heterozygous Achondroplasia

Definition. Generalized skeletal dysplasia with disproportionate rhizomelic dwarfism, lumbosacral lordosis, and a large head.

Incidence. With an incidence of approximately one in 27,000 births (13), this condition is among the most common skeletal dysplasias.

Etiology and pathogenesis. The disease can be transmitted as an autosomal-dominant trait. In over 80% of cases, however, it occurs as a new mutation (124).

Enchondral ossification processes are greatly delayed due to absence of the zone of chondroblast proliferation.

Pathoanatomic findings. A characteristic finding is disproportionate growth retardation (birth length 38–47 cm) (74) with a large head and depressed nasal bridge. The trunk is of normal length, and the limbs show rhizomelic micromelia. Radiographs demonstrate short, stout bones with marked flaring of the metaphyses (136). The abdomen is protuberant due to lumbosacral lordosis. Genital development is normal.

Associated anomalies. Hydrocephalus may be observed in some cases.

Ultrasound features. A prenatal ultrasound diagnosis (30, 70, 122) usually cannot be made before 24 weeks' gestation.

Femoral shortening. Filly et al. (30) were able to detect a marked reduction of femoral growth no earlier than the late second trimester or early third trimester in three heterozygous achondroplastic dwarfs. Similarly, in the seven cases described by Kurtz et al. (70), none showed definite femoral shortening in the early second trimester. In five cases seen by the author, only one fetus showed marked femoral shortening as early as 22 weeks. In the other fetuses, flattening of the growth curve was not apparent until 26 weeks (Figs. 30.**14**, 30.**24**). In the case described by Schlotter and Pfeiffer (122), the humerus showed a more pronounced growth lag than the femur at the end of the second trimester.

Differential diagnosis. Thanatophoric dysplasia, chondrodysplasia punctata of the Conradi–Hünermann type, hypochondrodysplasia, pseudoachondroplasia.

Prognosis. The prognosis depends on the particular form of the disease.

Heterozygous achondroplasia. This form is compatible with life (74). Most children show normal intellectual development, but in some cases severe cerebral dysplasia with hydrocephalus is observed (74).

Homozygous achondroplasia. In cases where both patients have the disease, the affected infant usually dies from respiratory problems during the first 3 months.

Clinical management. Spontaneous delivery is desirable if the head circumference is not markedly enlarged. If macrocephaly is present, there should be little hesitation in recommending a cesarean delivery.

If the patient herself suffers from heterozygous achondroplasia, an elective cesarean section is indicated on maternal grounds due to the anatomic constraints to a vaginal delivery.

Table 30.7 Criteria for differentiating fatal fetal osteochondrodysplasias

Skeletal region	Osteogenesis imperfecta II	Achondrogenesis	Homozygous achondroplasia	Thanatophoric dysplasia	Camptomelic dysplasia
Skull	Compressible	Macrocephaly	Depressed nasal bridge	Saddle nose	Flat profile
Thorax	Narrow	Narrow	Narrow	Narrow	Narrow
Ilium	Normal	Hypoplastic	Normal	Normal	Normal
Femur	Short, fracture	Maximum shortening	Moderate shortening	Short, bowed	Short, bowed
Fibula	Present	Present	Present	Present	Aplastic or hypoplastic

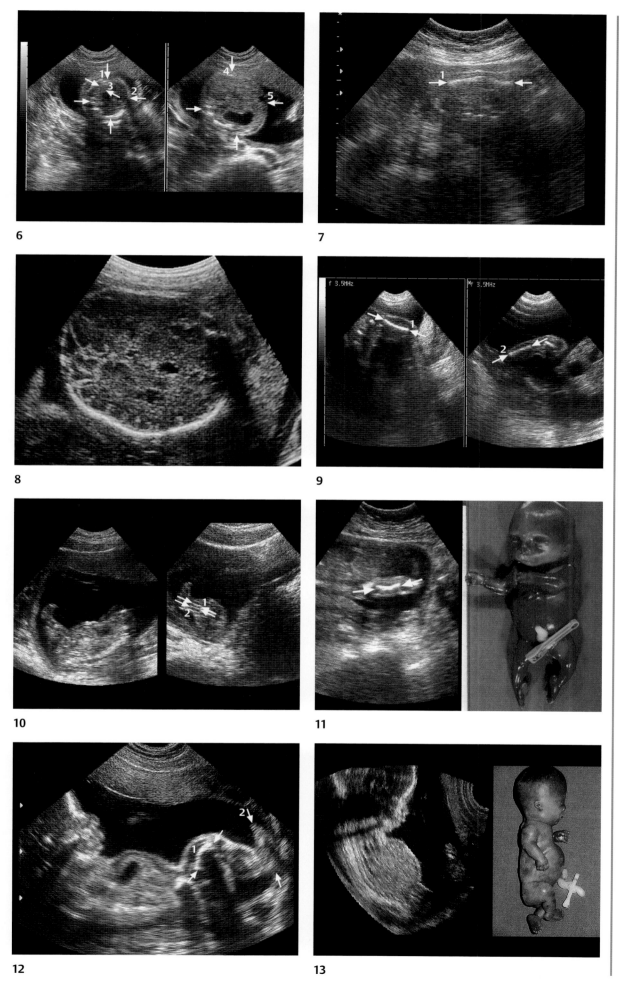

6

7

8

9

10

11

12

13

Fatal skeletal dysplasias

Fig. 30.**6** Thanatophoric dysplasia, 24 weeks. *Left:* very narrow thorax (1, 2) with a hypoplastic lung (oblique lung diameter (3) = 7 mm!). *Right:* normal-sized abdomen (4, 5).

Fig. 30.**7** Femur (arrows) in hypophosphatasia, 28 weeks. Note the ossification defect in the middle third of the bone.

Fig. 30.**8** Skull in hypophosphatasia, 34 weeks. The brain echo pattern is prominent due to poor ossification of the calvaria (sonogram courtesy of Prof. Terinde, Department of Obstetrics and Gynecology, University of Ulm).

Fig. 30.**9** Chondrodysplasia punctata, rhizomelic form, 24 weeks. There is marked shortening of the femur (1) (27 mm) and humerus (25 mm), compared with very little shortening of the distal long bones. Tibia (2).

Fig. 30.**10** Achondrogenesis at 18 weeks, 2 days. *Left:* short lower limb. *Right:* pronounced micromelia (tibia 5 mm and fibula 4 mm) (arrows).

Fig. 30.**11** Hypochondrogenesis, 22 weeks. *Left:* femur length, at 23 mm, is markedly decreased (appropriate for 17 weeks). *Right:* appearance of the fetus.

Fig. 30.**12** Thanatophoric dysplasia at 22 weeks. Note the narrow thorax and the short, bowed femur with a "telephone receiver" shape (1) (21 mm). Foot length (2) is normal (36 mm).

Fig. 30.**13** *Left:* thanatophoric dysplasia with frontal bossing and a narrow chest, 22 weeks. *Right:* appearance of the fetus.

Fig. 30.**14**   Femur length in various forms of dwarfism. The degree of bone shortening is greatest in achondrogenesis and smallest in achondroplasia.

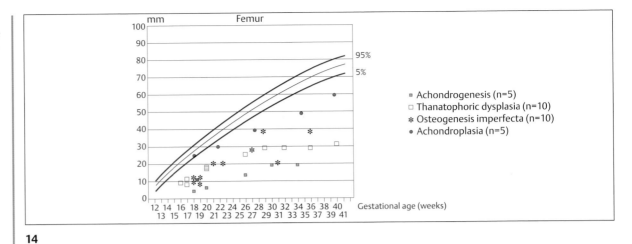

14

Fig. 30.**15**   *Left:* cloverleaf skull in thanatophoric dysplasia. *Right:* appearance of the fetus (photo courtesy of Dr. Hölzel, Bad Soden, Germany).

Fig. 30.**16**   *Left:* marked femoral shortening in short-rib syndrome, 21 weeks. *Right:* radiographic and gross appearance of the femur.

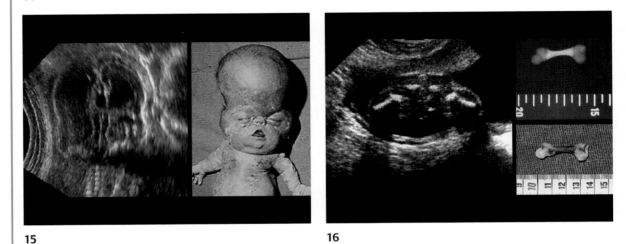

15   **16**

Fig. 30.**17**   *Left:* short upper limb in short-rib syndrome, 21 weeks. Both the humerus (21 mm) and ulna (21) show marked shortening of the ossified shaft. *Right:* appearance of the fetus.

Fig. 30.**18**   Short-rib syndrome with prominent forehead, small chest, and normal-size abdomen at 33 weeks. Comparison of sonogram, clinical appearance, and radiograph.

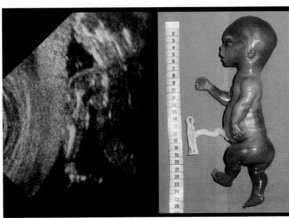
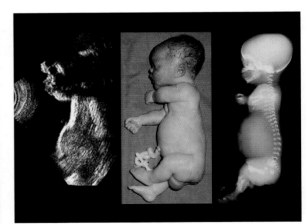

17   **18**

Fig. 30.**19**   Camptomelic dysplasia, 23 weeks. Note the bowed shafts of the long tubular bones, which are also shortened: femur (26 mm), tibia (24 mm), fibula (22 mm).

Fig. 30.**20**   Osteogenesis imperfecta II, 23 weeks. *Left:* marked angulation of the short bone due to a midshaft fracture. Center: appearance of the fetus, showing angulation of the lower limbs. *Right:* radiograph shows bilateral fractures of the femur and tibia.

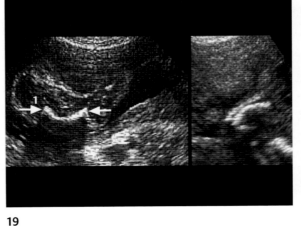
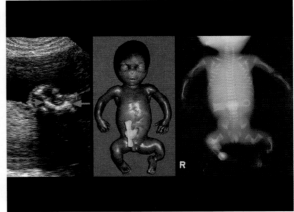

19   **20**

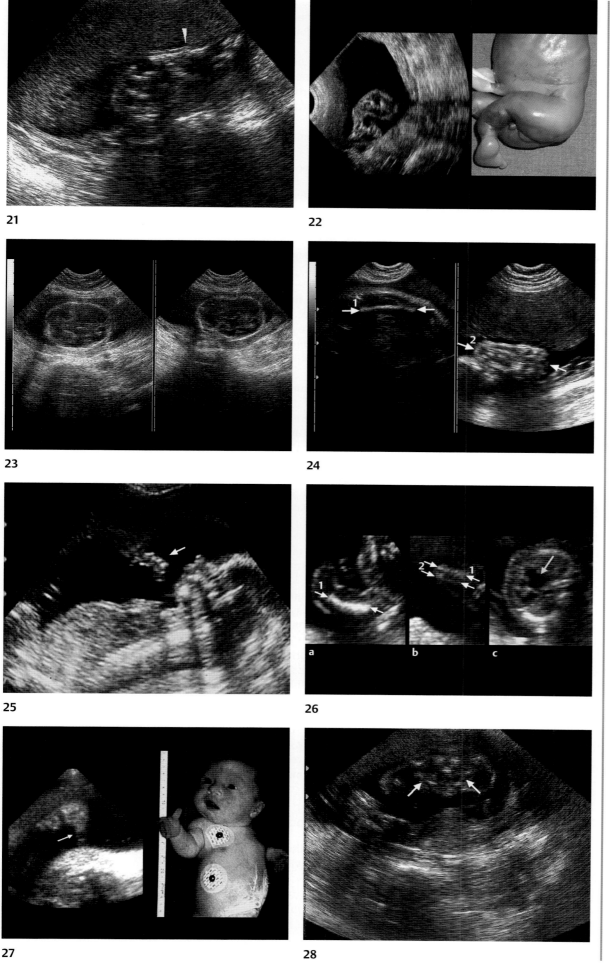

21

22

23

24

25

26

27

28

Fig. 30.**21**   Osteogenesis imperfecta II, 22 weeks. The stepoff is caused by a fracture of the femoral shaft (arrow).

Fig. 30.**22**   Osteogenesis imperfecta II at 22 weeks, 5 days. *Left:* abnormal limb shape due to multiple bone fractures. *Right:* gross appearance.

Fig. 30.**23**   Osteogenesis imperfecta II at 23 weeks, 0 days. The calvaria is thin and easily indented by external transducer pressure. *Left:* without pressure. *Right:* with pressure.

Nonfatal skeletal dysplasias

Fig. 30.**24**   Heterozygous achondroplasia, 34 weeks. *Left:* femur length, at 49 mm, is below the 5th percentile. *Right:* foot length, at 66 mm, is normal for gestational age.

Fig. 30.**25**   Ellis–van Creveld syndrome with a normal body length and very narrow thorax at 20 weeks, 5 days. Polydactyly (arrow).

Fig. 30.**26**   Ellis–van Creveld syndrome at 20 weeks, 5 days. Note the markedly reduced lengths of **(a)** the femur (22 mm), **(b)** the tibia (17 mm) and fibula (15 mm), and **(c)** an atrial septal defect.

Fig. 30.**27**   *Left:* diastrophic dysplasia with a "hitchhiker" thumb (arrow). *Right:* postnatal appearance (pictures courtesy of Prof. Gembruch, Department of Obstetrics and Gynecology, University of Lübeck, Germany).

Fig. 30.**28**   Cleidocranial dysostosis at 22 weeks, 3 days. Note the very poor ossification of the clavicles (arrows).

Chondroectodermal Dysplasia (Ellis–van Creveld Syndrome)

Definition. Disproportionate growth retardation with short distal limb segments and postaxial polydactyly.

Incidence. Rare. More than 120 cases had been described as of 1978 (20).

Etiology and pathogenesis. Autosomal-recessive inheritance with somewhat variable expressivity (131, 157). There is an array of anomalies based on the dysplasia of structures derived from the ectoderm and mesoderm (74).

Pathoanatomic findings. Disproportionate growth retardation with distal limb shortening (forearm, lower leg), a relatively narrow chest with a normal trunk length, bilateral postaxial hexadactyly of the hands and occasionally the feet, dysodontia, and hypoplastic nails (28, 155). Approximately 50% of patients have a cardiac anomaly (large atrial septal defect of ostium primum or secundum type) (157).

Ultrasound features. A prenatal ultrasound diagnosis (30, 49, 80) can be made by detecting short distal limb segments combined with polydactyly and a cardiac anomaly (Figs. 30.**25**, 30.**26**, 30.**40**).

Differential diagnosis. All thoracic dystrophy syndromes, all forms of ectodermal dysplasia syndromes.

Prognosis. In approximately one-third of cases, death occurs before 12 months of age due to congenital heart disease or pulmonary complications. Survivors display normal intelligence and attain a height of 107–160 cm (74).

Clinical management. Spontaneous delivery at term.

Chondrodysplasia punctata, Conradi–Huenermann Type

Definition. Epi-/metaphyseal bone dysplasia with stippled calcifications in the epiphyses.

Forms. The Conradi–Huenermann type of chondrodysplasia punctata is a nonfatal form, unlike the rhizomelic type.

Incidence. The overall reported incidence of chondrodysplasia punctata is 0.09 in 10,000 births (13). The Conradi–Huenermann type is more common than the fatal rhizomelic form.

Etiology and pathogenesis. The Conradi–Huenermann type has a simple dominant mode of inheritance (157).

Pathoanatomic findings. The disease is characterized by growth retardation with little shortening of the bones. There is facial dysmorphia with a low, broad nasal bridge and often a bilobed nasal tip (157). Besides slight limb shortening, there may be concomitant changes such as scoliosis and joint contractures.

Ultrasound features. In the nonfatal Conradi–Huenermann type of chondrodysplasia punctata, ultrasound has shown disorganization of the spinal column, abnormal echogenicity in the femoral epiphyses, a prominent forehead, and a depressed nasal bridge (111, 150). The occurrence of polyhydramnios and ascites has also been reported (145).

Differential diagnosis. *Chondrodysplasia punctata embryopathica* may be seen following the maternal use of dicoumarins and after various prenatal infections (74).

Prognosis. The nonrhizomelic form of chondrodysplasia punctata, unlike the rhizomelic form, is compatible with life. Possible complications include orthopedic problems, recurrent infections, and cataracts. Symptomatic orthopedic treatment is indicated.

Clinical management. Spontaneous delivery.

Diastrophic Dysplasia

Definition. Generalized skeletal dysplasia with short limbs, clubbed feet, hand deformities, joint contractures, and scoliosis (74, 131).

Etiology and pathogenesis. Autosomal-recessive mode of inheritance with the homozygous mutation of a gene located on chromosome 5q (74).

Pathoanatomic findings. Short limb bones due to a generalized chondral disturbance. The bones show metaphyseal flaring. Multiple joint contractures are present, and there is a fixed abduction contracture of the thumbs (*"hitchhiker thumbs"*). Clubbing of the feet is pronounced. Cleft palate and micrognathia are frequently noted.

Ultrasound features. Several reports have been published on the prenatal diagnosis of diastrophic dysplasia (39, 55, 65, 66, 106, 158). Most of these cases were selected for examination based on an increased risk of recurrence. Given the range of variability of this syndrome, however, it is doubtful whether prenatal diagnosis can always be accomplished even in high-risk cases. Kaitila et al. (66) and Gembruch et al. (39) reported on the prenatal detection of a fetus with short bones and abducted thumbs (Fig. 30.**27**). The detection of micrognathia and cervical kyphosis was also described (39). The head and thorax display a normal shape.

Other prenatal tests. Hastbacka et al. (52) reported on the prenatal diagnosis of diastrophic dysplasia with polymorphic DNA markers.

Differential diagnosis. The differential diagnosis includes all other disorders that are associated with joint contractures, such as arthrogryposis multiplex congenita.

Prognosis. In principle, diastrophic dysplasia is compatible with life, but it is also associated with increased perinatal mortality. Survivors experience problems related to increasing kyphoscoliosis and joint contractures.

Clinical management. In cases with pronounced micromelia that are diagnosed early, it should be considered whether it is reasonable for the patient to continue the pregnancy. After viability is reached, obstetric management should be guided by the extent of joint contractures.

Cleidocranial Dysplasia

Definition. A disease characterized by partial or complete aplasia of one or both clavicles and abnormalities of superior ossification.

Incidence. Not too rare. As of 1962, 700 cases had been described in the literature (157).

Etiology and pathogenesis. The disease is transmitted by simple dominant inheritance, with considerable variability of expression (157).

Pathoanatomic findings. A narrow upper chest cage with aplasia, hypoplasia or dysplasia of the clavicle. The superior vault is large, broad, and short.

Ultrasound features. In cases with a familial risk, targeted imaging of the clavicular region shows poor ossification or absence of the clavicles (Fig. 30.**28**). Examination of the head may reveal brachycephaly with an increased biparietal diameter.

Prognosis. Good. Short stature may become apparent after infancy. Ossification of the cranium and pelvis is considerably delayed. Dysodontia is also present.

Clinical management. Since there is no particular risk, spontaneous delivery is desired. If the woman herself is affected by the disease, she may have a narrow pelvis necessitating a cesarean delivery.

Limb Defects

Isolated Anomalies that Affect only Certain Limb Segments or Bones

Screening and targeted imaging. Abnormalities that affect only certain limb segments or individual bones and/or affect only one side can be detected sonographically only by a thorough examination of all four limbs. Experience has shown that this can be quite time-consuming. But in cases with a positive family history, targeted imaging of the proximal, middle, and distal fetal limb segments can disclose isolated anomalies. This requires favorable scanning conditions, however.

Terminology. A variety of terms are used. While one nomenclature employs more descriptive terms such as dysmelia, phocomelia, peromelia, ectromelia, etc. (Table 30.**8**, Fig. 30.**29**), the Stevenson classification (143) uses only two basic terms: amelia and meromelia (Table 30.**9**, Fig. 30.**30**). Further classification then follows the scheme outlined in Table 30.**10**.

Amelia

Definition. Amelia denotes the absence of an entire limb (arm or leg) (Fig. 30.**29**). Usually the associated shoulder girdle or, less commonly, the associated pelvic girdle is also hypoplastic. A small soft-tissue protuberance may be present at the site of the missing limb.

Incidence and Forms

Thalidomide embryopathy. Amelia is an extremely rare anomaly in the present day. Between 1958 and 1963, it occurred with some frequency in the setting of thalidomide embryopathy. Analysis of the thalidomide anomalies showed that the drug produced limb defects only when taken between the 35th and 49th days after the last menstrual period (74, 75). Exposure during the early part of the vulnerable period led to very severe arm defects such as amelia or one-finger phocomelia; later exposure led to three-finger phocomelias and femoral and tibial defects. Exposure near the end of the seventh week resulted only in minor thumb deformities (triphalangia). Exposure after 50 days postmenstruation was associated with few or no fetal abnormalities (76).

Femur–fibula–ulna syndrome. Amelia combined with a femoral and fibular defect is found in the femur–fibula–ulna syndrome (69).

Table 30.**8** Descriptive terminology of limb defects

Term	Definition
Dysmelia	Abnormal limb development
Amelia	Absence of an entire limb
Phocomelia	Proximal limb absence, with hands and feet attached directly to the shoulders or hips
Ectromelia	Hypoplasia and aplasia of single or multiple long bones with associated limb deformity (largest group of limb anomalies)
Peromelia	Congenital limb stump
Hemimelia	Absence of a longitudinal segment (e.g., radial aplasia)
Acheiria	Absence of one or both hands
Apodia	Absence of one or both feet
Acheiropodia	Absence of hands and feet

Table 30.**9** Terminology of isolated defects

Defect	Definition
Amelia	Complete absence of a limb
Meromelia	Partial absence of a limb
Segments	Major portions of the limb: proximal, middle, and distal (corre sponds in the arm to the upper arm, forearm, and hand; in the leg to the thigh, lower leg, and foot)
Intercalary defect	Absence of the proximal or middle segment
Terminal defect	Absence of all limb segments below a certain point
Transverse defect	Defect that involves the full width of the limb
Longitudinal defect	Defect that parallels the long axis of the limb
Preaxial defect	Absence of portions of the forearm, hand, leg, or foot on the radial (thumb) or tibial (big toe) side
Postaxial defect	Absence of portions of the forearm, hand, ligament, or foot on the ulnar (small finger) or fibular (small toe) side
Rudimentary	Detectable remnant of a bony structure
Ray	Longitudinal component of the middle or distal limb segments—e.g., the radius or ulna in the forearm or a finger and the corresponding metacarpal bone in the hand

Table 30.**10** Description of limb defects

Total or partial	Amelia/meromelia
Affected segment(s)	Terminal/intercalary (interposed)
Defect axis	Transverse/longitudinal
Affected limb	Upper/lower
Affected side	Right/left
Affected bones	Femur/radius/metacarpals 1–5, etc.
Location of bone defect	Proximal/middle/distal

Ultrasound features. The absence of a limb is observed in both longitudinal and transverse scans (Fig. 30.**31**).

Phocomelia

Definition. This is an anomaly in which the hands or feet are attached directly to the shoulders or hips (Fig. 30.**29**). Phocomelia occurs in the setting of certain syndromes (Table 30.**11**).

Ultrasound features. Ultrasound in all three planes shows a hand rudiment arising directly from the shoulder (Fig. 30.**32**) or a foot arising directly from the pelvic girdle.

Anomalies involving specific limb segments

Fig. 30.**29**   Descriptive terminology of isolated limb defects.

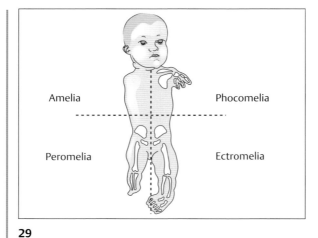

29

Fig. 30.**30**   Stevenson classification of isolated limb defects (143).

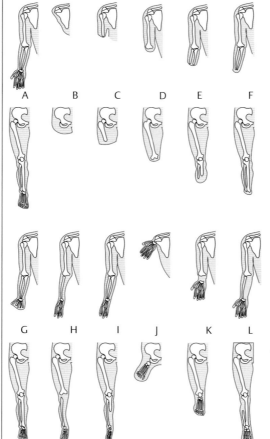

A   Normal finding

B   Amelia

C   Midhumeral and midfemoral terminal transverse meromelia

D   Radioulnar and tibiofibular transverse meromelia

E   Midradioulnar and midtibiofibular transverse meromelia

F   Carpal and tarsal transverse meromelia

G   Phalangeal transverse meromelia

H   Radial and tibial terminal longitudinal meromelia

I   Midradial and midtibial terminal longitudinal meromelia

J   Humeroradioulnar and femorotibiofibular intercalary transverse meromelia

K   Radioulnar and tibiofibular intercalary transverse meromelia

L   Ulnar and proximal fibular intercalary longitudinal meromelia

30

Fig. 30.**31**   Amelia. Complete absence of the entire right arm (arrow).

Fig. 30.**32**   Left-sided phocomelia (viewed from the dorsal aspect) at 26 weeks, etiology unknown. The rudimentary hand is attached directly to the shoulder girdle (scan courtesy of Prof. Lee, Department of Obstetrics and Gynecology, University of Vienna).

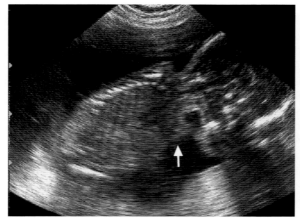

31

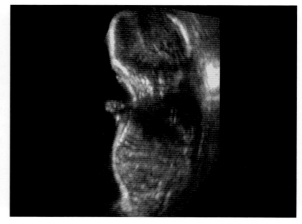

32

Table 30.11 Syndromes associated with phocomelia

> ➤ Holt–Oram syndrome
> ➤ Roberts syndrome
> ➤ Thalidomide syndrome

Table 30.12 Syndromes associated with radial aplasia

> ➤ Thrombocytopenia–radial aplasia syndrome (TAR)
> ➤ Holt–Oram syndrome
> ➤ Harris–Osborne syndrome
> ➤ Vater syndrome
> ➤ Thalidomide syndrome
> ➤ Roberts syndrome
> ➤ Edwards syndrome (trisomy 18)

In *Roberts syndrome (= Appelt–Gerken–Lenz syndrome)* (1), an autosomal-recessive disease, tetraphocomelia is accompanied by cleft lip and palate and clitoral hypertrophy.

Peromelia

Peromelia refers to the presence of a congenital limb stump (Fig. 30.**29**). It is found in the setting of *femur–fibula–ulna syndrome* (54, 69), *Hanhart syndrome* (bird face with microgenia, microglossia, and peromelia) (48), and *amniotic band syndrome,* in which strands within the amniotic fluid amputate portions of fetal limbs (Figs. 30.**33**–30.**35**).

Ectromelia

Ectromelia is a group of disorders characterized by hypoplasia and aplasia of individual long bones accompanied by limb deformity (Figs. 30.**26**, 30.**36**).

Radial Aplasia

Occurrence. Radial aplasia is often found in the setting of a complex congenital anomaly (Table 30.**12**). There is a marked axial discontinuity between the forearm and hand. In various syndromes that are associated with radial aplasia, the thumb is absent (Figs. 30.**36**, 30.**37**). By contrast, the thumb is present in thrombocytopenia–radial aplasia syndrome (29, 47, 79).

Associated anomalies. Not infrequently, radial aplasia is also associated with congenital heart disease. Tetralogy of Fallot is often found in thrombocytopenia–radial aplasia syndrome (47), atrial septal defect in Holt–Oram syndrome (10, 57), and ventricular septal defect in Harris–Osborne syndrome (50) and Edwards syndrome (113).

Sirenomelia

Inferior regression syndrome. Sirenomelia is the most severe form of inferior regression syndrome (123). It has a reported incidence of one in 60,000 births (161). The fetus is not viable.

This complex anomaly is characterized by severe regressive changes involving the lower spinal column, pelvis, and lower extremity. In pronounced cases this can lead to fusion of the legs. Other features are anal atresia and renal agenesis. A close relationship exists between inferior regression syndrome and diabetes mellitus (107).

VACTERL syndrome. Similar changes are found in VACTERL syndrome. The acronym stands for vertebral defects, anal atresia, cardiac anomalies, tracheoesophageal fistula, radial and renal anomalies, and limb anomalies (3).

Sympodia and monopodia. Sympodia refers to an incomplete fusion of the lower extremities, while monopodia denotes a complete fusion.

Symmelia. Forster (32) introduced the term symmelia (= sympodia or sympus) in 1885 and divided it into three groups based on the fusion of the lower extremities:
- Sympus apus
- Sympus monopus
- Sympus dipus

The most common form is sympus apus (apodal symmelia), in which the legs are fused together and there are no feet. One femur and one tibia are present. In sympus monopus (monopodal symmelia), the legs are partially fused. Two femora, two tibiae, and two fibulae can be observed. Only one foot is present, which may have up to ten toes. In sympus dipus (dipodal symmelia), two feet are present and form a flipper-like appendage, creating a "mermaid"- or "siren"-like appearance.

Figure 30.**38** illustrates apodal symmelia with a normal femur and a rudimentary tibia.

Prenatal diagnosis (58, 130). The prenatal diagnosis of sirenomelia is usually hampered by oligohydramnios. In a study by Sirtori et al. (130), oligohydramnios was so pronounced in five of 11 sonographically observed cases that diagnosis was extremely difficult. In a similar case, the difficulties posed by oligohydramnios prompted Fitzmorris-Glass et al. (31) to add an MRI examination. All of the cases observed by Sirtori et al. (130) had renal agenesis, ambiguous genitalia, and a single umbilical artery. Amnioinfusion is recommended in cases where ultrasound visualization is seriously hampered.

Split Hand, Split Foot

This condition is based on anomalous development of the hand or foot. The defect (aplasia or hypoplasia) affects the medial rays of the hand or foot, most commonly the third ray.

Besides an absence of fingers or toes, ultrasound demonstrates an increased distance between the rays that are present (Fig. 30.**39**).

The differential diagnosis includes the amputation of individual fingers or toes due to amniotic bands.

Polydactyly

Preaxial and postaxial polydactyly. Polydactyly is often found in the setting of various syndromes (Table 30.**13**). The condition is classified by the location of the supernumerary finger(s) or toe(s) as preaxial (= radial, affecting the thumb side or tibia/big toe side) (Fig. 30.**40a**) or postaxial (= ulnar, affecting the small finger side or fibula/small toe side) (Fig. 30.**40b, c**).

Table 30.13 Syndromes associated with polydactyly

Preaxial poly-dactyly, fingers	Postaxial poly-dactyly, fingers	Preaxial poly-dactyly, toes	Postaxial poly-dactyly, toes
➤ VATER syndrome ➤ Carpenter syndrome ➤ Patau syndrome (trisomy 13)	➤ Short rib–poly-dactyly syndrome ➤ Ellis–van Creveld syndrome ➤ Patau syndrome (trisomy 13) ➤ Meckel–Gruber syndrome ➤ Smith–Lemli–Opitz syndrome	➤ Short rib–poly	➤ Short rib–poly-dactyly syndrome ➤ Ellis–van Creveld syndrome ➤ Patau syndrome (trisomy 13) ➤ Meckel–Gruber syndrome ➤ Smith–Lemli–Opitz syndrome

Fig. 30.**33**   Right-sided peromelia at 17 weeks. The right humerus (1) is markedly shortened (18 mm) compared with the left humerus (2) (25 mm). The right forearm is absent.

Fig. 30.**34**   Left-sided peromelia due to amniotic band syndrome, 16 weeks. *Left:* ultrasound demonstrates only the upper arm. *Right:* in place of the forearm, an amniotic band (arrows) is seen between the distal stump of the upper arm and the lateral placental margin.

Fig. 30.**35**   Left-sided peromelia due to amniotic band syndrome, 23 weeks. *Left:* faint amniotic band stretching from the amputation stump below the left knee to the placenta (arrow). *Right:* postnatal appearance.

Fig. 30.**36**   Right-sided ectromelia, 22 weeks. *Left:* hand deformity accompanied by radial aplasia. *Right:* postnatal appearance.

Fig. 30.**37**   Radial aplasia in thrombocytopenia–radial aplasia syndrome at 19 weeks. The ulna (25 mm, arrows) is the only bone visible in the forearm. The thumb is present in the affected hand.

Fig. 30.**38**   Monopodal symmelia (sirenomelus) in VACTERL syndrome, 23 weeks. *Left:* normal feet and lower legs are replaced by a tapered stump. *Right:* postnatal appearance.

Fig. 30.**39**   *Left:* split hand with three fingers. *Right:* split foot with two toes (17 weeks).

Fig. 30.**40**   Polydactyly.
a   Preaxial polydactyly (hexadactyly of the left foot) in trisomy 13 (39 weeks).
b   Postaxial polydactyly (hexadactyly of the right hand) in Ellis–van Creveld syndrome (20 weeks).
c   Clinical appearance of **b**.

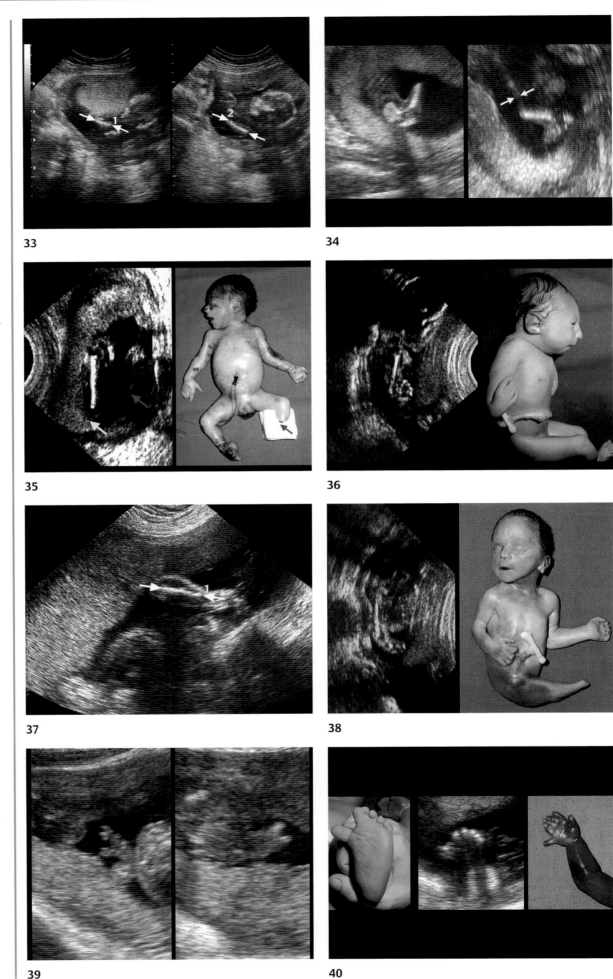

The presence of hexa- or heptadactyly in association with other anomalies can be helpful in advancing the differential diagnosis.

Syndactyly

Syndactyly is marked by the presence of a cutaneous or osseous connection between adjacent fingers or toes. Ultrasound detection is difficult but is possible when sufficient amniotic fluid is present (Fig. 30.**41**). Syndactyly can be confidently excluded only if the individual digits can be clearly identified as separate structures. Syndactyly of the fingers or toes is seen in various syndromes such as Apert syndrome (= acrocephaly–syndactyly syndrome) (8) and Mohr syndrome (= orofaciodigital syndrome) (36).

Clinodactyly

Clinodactyly refers to the radial deviation of one or more fingers (Fig. 30.**42a**). When this is detected sonographically, or when overlapping fingers are found, karyotyping should be considered since trisomy 13, 18, or 21 may be present as an underlying condition. Clinodactyly is found in Meckel–Gruber and various other syndromes.

Camptodactyly

Camptodactyly denotes a flexion contracture of one or more fingers without bony changes (Fig. 30.**42b**). This type of flexion contracture is seen in arthrogryposis multiplex congenita, trisomy 18, Meckel–Gruber syndrome, and various other syndromes.

■ *Positional Abnormalities or Restricted Motion of Fetal Limbs*

Club foot

Incidence. Club foot (pes equinovarus) is a relatively common congenital anomaly, with an incidence of one to three per 1000 live births (19). In approximately 15% of cases, there is a familial occurrence with a recessive mode of inheritance (61). Both sexes are affected with almost equal frequency (163).

Associated anomalies. Approximately 20% of these children have severe coexisting anomalies (90). The intrauterine detection of club foot should always prompt a detailed examination of the spinal column, since club foot results from spina bifida is many cases. Club foot also occurs in association with various syndromes (152) (Table 30.**14**). In trisomy 18, it is found in approximately 15% of cases (152).

Pronounced oligohydramnios and amniotic band syndrome can also cause the development of club foot (19).

Table 30.**14** Syndromes associated with pes equinovarus

> Meckel–Gruber syndrome
> Larsen syndrome
> Pena–Shokeir syndrome
> Trisomy 9p syndrome
> Partial trisomy 10q syndrome
> Edwards syndrome (trisomy 18)
> Down syndrome (trisomy 21)
> Camptomelic syndrome
> Inferior regression syndrome
> Seckel syndrome
> Robin syndrome
> Ullrich–Feichtiger syndrome

Ultrasound features. Club foot appears sonographically as a marked angular deviation of the foot in relation to the lower leg (5) (Fig. 30.**43**).

Other tests. When club foot is detected sonographically before 20 weeks, the fetus should be examined for coexisting anomalies, and karyotyping should be performed to exclude a trisomy.

Rocker-Bottom Foot

Rocker-bottom foot (62, 117) is characterized by a prominent calcaneus with a convex sole (Fig. 30.**44**). It is a feature of trisomy 18 and 18q syndrome and cerebro-oculofacioskeletal (COFS syndrome, Pena-Shokeir syndrome II) (7, 74).

Arthrogryposis Multiplex Congenita

Definition. Arthrogryposis multiplex congenita (AMC) is the term for an etiologically and clinically diverse group of disorders characterized by congenital, usually symmetrical and progressive joint contractures. Limitation of limb motion may be accompanied by clubbing of the feet.

Forms. Three groups are distinguished according to their clinical presentation (45):
● Primary involvement of the limbs (50%)
● Limb involvement combined with other congenital anomalies (cleft palate, hernia, scoliosis, etc.) (40%)
● Limb involvement combined with a CNS anomaly (microcephaly, microphthalmia) (10%)

Incidence. The incidence of AMC is between one in 5000 and one in 10,000 births (45).

Etiology and pathogenesis. Variable. All disorders that impair fetal mobility in the third month of development lead to congenital contractures (25). The etiology includes the following:
● Myopathies
● Neurogenic disorders
● Connective-tissue abnormalities
● Fetal crowding (45)

The latter problem usually results from pronounced oligohydramnios, which may be due to deficient amniotic fluid production or the prolonged leakage of amniotic fluid from the uterus.

In the group with CNS involvement, the inability to swallow leads to polyhydramnios (45). Congenital contractures usually occur sporadically, but there are documented cases with a simple dominant or autosomal-recessive mode of inheritance (45, 114). The spinal form of AMC in particular tends to have an autosomal-recessive inheritance (45).

Pathoanatomic findings. All grades of intrauterine flexion or extension contractures can occur, affecting a variable number of the joints. In one-half to two-thirds of cases, all four limbs are affected (152). Many of these children have a low birth weight. The umbilical cord tends to be wrapped around the fetus to an unusual degree, apparently due to the restriction of fetal mobility (45).

Associated anomalies. Severe accompanying anomalies may be found (microcephaly, low-set ears, hypertelorism), particularly in the group with CNS involvement.

Ultrasound features. The following ultrasound abnormalities may be seen in the spinal form of AMC: fixed limb deformities (flexion contractures at the elbow and hip, extension contracture at the knee, flex-

Fig. 30.**41** Syndactyly of the fourth and fifth rays of the left hand (arrow), 21 weeks.

Fig. 30.**42**
a Clinodactyly (radial angulation of the third and fifth fingers) with overlapping of the second and third fingers (vertical arrow). Trisomy 18, 32 weeks.
b Camptodacyly in arthrogryposis multiplex congenita, 36 weeks.

Abnormal positioning or restricted motion of the fetal limbs

Fig. 30.**43** *Left:* clubbed right foot in arthrogryposis multiplex congenita, 29 weeks. *Right:* clinical appearance.

Fig. 30.**44** Rocker-bottom foot with a convex sole and protuberant calcaneus. Trisomy 18, 22 weeks.

Fig. 30.**45** Extension contracture of the left knee joint and clubbing of the left foot in arthrogryposis multiplex congenita, 23 weeks. Polyhydramnios is also present.

Fig. 30.**46** *Left:* flexion contractures of both knees and fixed ankle dorsiflexion in arthrogryposis multiplex congenita. Polyhydramnios, 35 weeks. *Right:* postnatal appearance.

Fig. 30.**47** Flexion contracture of the right wrist in arthrogryposis multiplex congenita, Polyhydramnios, 25 weeks.

Fig. 30.**48** Pena–Shokeir syndrome at 30 weeks, 3 days.
a Markedly narrow thorax (TTD [1] = 51 mm, TSD [2] = 51 mm) with a hypoplastic lung (oblique lung diameter [3] = 11 mm).
b Club foot.

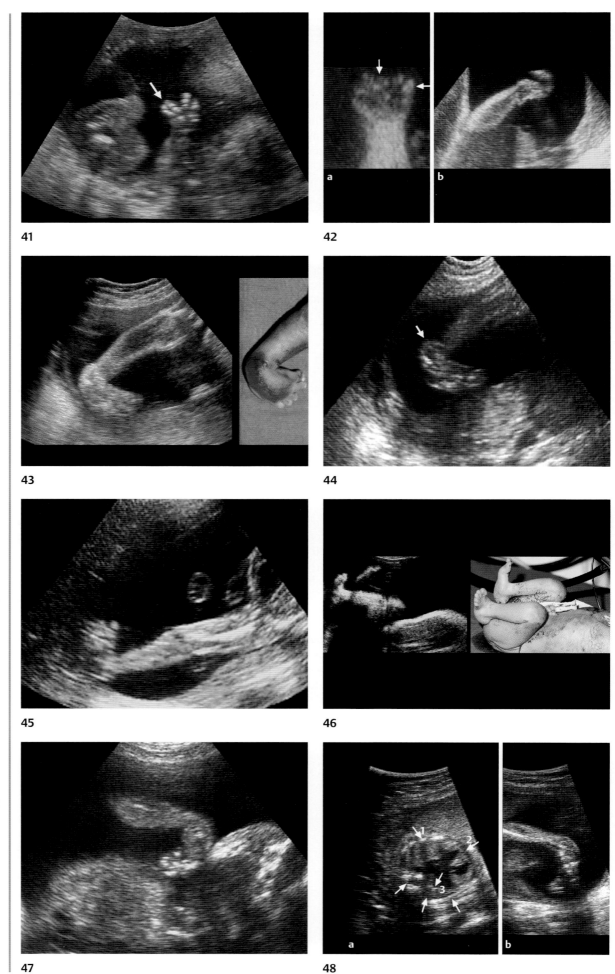

41

42

43

44

45

46

47

48

ion contractures of the fingers, clubfeet) with a definite paucity of fetal movements despite massive polyhydramnios (96) (Figs. 30.**45**–30.**47**). Growth retardation of the diaphyses of the long tubular bones is also noted.

Polyhydramnios combined with lack of fetal movement and clubfeet should always raise suspicion of AMC with CNS involvement.

Differential diagnosis. Spina bifida with limited motion of the lower extremities, diastrophic dysplasia (136).

Prognosis. The length of the pregnancy is usually normal. Five percent of all children with arthrogryposis multiplex congenita die before birth or during the first months of life (45, 110). If the cause is a CNS disorder, the mortality rate is 50% (45).

Clinical management. If a severe form of AMC is diagnosed before viability is reached, pregnancy termination may be considered. With a mature term fetus, the fixed joint positions pose a high risk of fetal trauma in a spontaneous delivery. Complications can also result from the increased coiling of the umbilical cord. Since most of these children are in a breech presentation or transverse lie, cesarean section is preferred over vaginal delivery for a viable fetus.

Pena–Shokeir Syndrome

Definition. Arthrogryposis multiplex congenita combined with pulmonary hypoplasia (10).

Incidence. More than 60 cases had been reported as of 1986 (46).

Etiology and pathogenesis. Moessinger (103) believes that the syndrome is precipitated by early akinesia, which in humans may result from a CNS defect (77). In an akinesia model (rat fetuses paralyzed with curare), Moessinger was able to produce the same abnormalities as those found in Pena–Shokeir syndrome.

Pathoanatomic findings. Features of arthrogryposis multiplex congenita with clubfeet and camptodactyly. Additional findings are pulmonary hypoplasia and facial anomalies (hypertelorism, mandibular hypoplasia, depressed nasal bridge, low-set ears).

Associated anomalies. Fetal hydrops, micropolygyria, oligogyria, cerebellar hypoplasia.

Ultrasound features. Prenatal diagnosis is possible in principle (14, 91) but depends on the extent of the changes and the gestational age. Early ultrasound diagnosis before viability is reached (up to about 24 weeks) can be accomplished only in cases with a recurrence risk that are selected for close-interval serial examinations that include biometry.

The main ultrasound findings are polyhydramnios, joint contractures, and a narrow thorax with pulmonary hypoplasia (Fig. 30.**48**). Measurements of the bony thorax and lung diameter yield valuable information on the severity of pulmonary hypoplasia (99, 101).

The signs defined by Cardwell (14) as characteristic of Pena–Shokeir syndrome are listed in Table 30.**15**.

Differential diagnosis. Potter sequence is distinguished from Pena–Shokeir syndrome by the presence of oligohydramnios.

Prognosis. Due to pulmonary hypoplasia, the prognosis is grave (110, 112). Intrauterine death may occur as early as the second trimester (16, 91). Chromosome analysis reveals a normal karyotype (16).

Clinical management. With a confident diagnosis of Pena–Shokeir syndrome, pregnancy termination may be considered at any stage because of the grave prognosis.

Table 30.**15**   Ultrasound findings in Pena–Shokeir syndrome (14)

➤ Polyhydramnios
➤ Absent or decreased fetal movements
➤ Normal fetal echocardiography
➤ Scalp edema or anasarca
➤ Pleural effusion
➤ Arthrogryposis, joint contractures
➤ Small, narrow thorax
➤ Placentomegaly
➤ Fetal hydrops, ascites
➤ Intrauterine growth retardation
➤ Unfavorable biophysical profile
➤ Micrognathia
➤ Hypertelorism
➤ Breech presentation

References

1. Appelt, H., Gerken, H., Lenz, W.: Tetraphokomelie mit Lippen-Kiefer-Gaumen-Spalte und Clitorishypertrophie – ein Syndrom. Pädiatrie u. Pädologie 2 (1966) 119–124
2. Aylsworth, A.S., Seeds, J.W., Guilford, W.B., Burns, C.B., Washburn, D.B.: Prenatal diagnosis of a severe deforming type of osteogenesis imperfecta. Amer. J. Med. Genet. 19 (1984) 707–714
3. Baumann, W., Greinacher, I., Emmrich, P., Spranger, J.: VATER- oder VACTERL-Syndrom. Klin. Pädiat. 188 (1976) 328–337
4. Benacerraf, B., Osathanondh, R., Bieber, F.R.: Achondrogenesis Type I: Ultrasound diagnosis in utero. J. Clin. Ultrasound 12 (1984) 357–359
5. Benacerraf, B.R., Frigoletto, F.D.: Prenatal ultrasound diagnosis of clubfoot. Radiology 155 (1985) 211–213
6. Berge, L.N., Marton, V., Tranebjaerg, L., Kearney, M.S., Kiserud, T., Oian, P.: Prenatal diagnosis of osteogenesis imperfecta. Acta Obstet. Gynecol. Scand. 74 (1995) 321–323
7. Bergsma, D.: Birth Defects Compendium. 2nd ed. New York: Alan R. Liss 1979
8. Blank, C.E.: Apert's syndrome (a type of acrocephalosyndactyly). Observations on a British series of 39 cases. Ann. hum. Genet. 24 (1960) 151–164
9. Brons, J.T., van der Harten, H.J., Wladimiroff, J.W. et al.: Prenatal ultrasonographic diagnosis of osteogenesis imperfecta. Amer. J. Obstet. Gynecol. 159 (1988) 176–181
10. Brons, J.T.J., Van Geijn, H.P., Wladimiroff, J.W. et al.: Prenatal ultrasound diagnosis of the Holt-Oram syndrome. Prenat. Diagn. 8 (1988) 175–181
11. Burrows, P.E., Stannard, M.W., Pearrow, J., Sutterfield, S., Baker, M.L.: Early antenatal sonographic recognition of thanatophoric dysplasia with cloverleaf skull deformity. Amer. J. Roentgenol. 143 (1984) 841–843
12. Byers, P.H., Tispouras, P., Bonadio, J.F., Starman, B.J., Schwartz, R.C.: Perinatal lethal osteogenesis imperfecta (OI type II): A biochemically heterogeneous disorder usually due to new mutations in the genes for type I collagen. Amer. J. Hum. Genet. 42 (1988) 237–248
13. Camera, G., Mastroiacovo, P.: Birth prevalence of skeletal dysplasias in the italian mulicentric monitoring system for birth defects. In: Skeletal Dysplasias. New York: Alan R. Liss 1982; S. 441–449
14. Cardwell, M.S.: Pena-Shokeir syndrome. Prenatal diagnosis by ultrasonography. J. Ultrasound Med. 6 (1987) 619–621
15. Chemke, J., Graff, G., Lancet, M.: Familial thanatophoric dwarfism. Lancet 1 (1971) 1358
16. Chen, H., Blumberg, B., Immken, L. et al.: The Pena-Shokeir syndrome: Report of five cases and further delineation of the syndrome. Amer. J. Med. Genetics 16 (1983) 213–224
17. Chervenak, F.A., Blakemore, K.J., Isaacson, G., Mayden, K., Hobbins, J.C.: Antenatal sonographic findings of thanatophoric dysplasia with cloverleaf skull. Amer. J. Obstet. Gynecol. 146 (1983) 984–985
18. Constantine, G., McCormack, J., McHugo, J., Fowlie, A.: Prenatal diagnosis of severe osteogenesis imperfecta. Prenat. Diagn. 11 (1991) 103–110
19. Cowell, H.R., Wein, B.K.: Genetic aspects of clubfoot. J. Bone Jt. Surg. 62 (1980) 1381–1384
20. Cremin, B.J., Beighton, P.: Bone dysplasias of infancy. A radiological atlas. Berlin: Springer 1978
21. Curran, J.P., Sigman, B.A., Opitz, J.M.: Lethal forms of chondrodysplastic dwarfism. Pediatrics 53 (1974) 76–85
22. De la Chapelle, A., Maroteaux, P., Havu, N., Granroth, G.: Une rare dysplasie osseuse léthale de transmission récessive autosomique. Arch. Fr. Pédiatr. 29 (1972) 759–770
23. DeLange, M., Rouse, G.A.: Prenatal diagnosis of hypophosphatasia. J. Ultrasound Med. 9 (1990) 115–117
24. De Sierra, T.M., Ashmead, G., Bilenker, R.: Prenatal diagnosis of short rib (polydactyly) syndrome with situs inversus. Amer. J. Med. Genet. 44 (1992) 555–557
25. Drachman, D.B., Sokoloff, L.: The role of movement in embryonic joint development. J. Bone Joint Surg. 57B (1975) 115
26. Elejalde, B.R., de Elejalde, M.M.: Prenatal diagnosis of perinatally lethal osteogenesis imperfecta. Amer. J. med. Genet. 14 (1983) 353–359
27. Elejalde, B.R., de Elejalde, M.M.: Thanatophoric dysplasia: fetal manifestations and prenatal diagnosis. Amer. J. Med. Genet. 22 (1985) 669–683
28. Ellis, R.W.B., van Creveld, S.: A syndrome characterized by ectodermal dysplasia, polydactyly, chondrodysplasia and congenital morbus cordis. Report of three cases. Arch. Dis. Child 15 (1940) 65–84
29. Filkins, K., Russo, J., Bilinki, I. et al.: Prenatal diagnosis of thrombocytopenia absent radius syndrome using ultrasound and fetoscopy. Prenat. Diagn. 4 (1984) 139–142
30. Filly, R.A., Golbus, M.S., Carey, J.C., Hall, J.G.: Short-limbed dwarfism: Ultrasonic diagnosis by mensuration of fetal femoral length. Radiology 138 (1981) 653–656
31. Fitzmorris-Glass, R., Mattrey, R.F., Cantrell, C.J.: Magnetic resonance imaging as an adjunct to ultrasound in oligohydramnios. Detection of sirenomelia. J. Ultrasound Med. 8 (1989) 159–162
32. Foerster, A.: Die Mißbildungen des Menschen, nebst einem Atlas. Jena, Friedrich Manke (1885)
33. Fraccaro, M.: Contributo allo studio delle melattie del mesenchima osteopoietico. I acondrogenesi. Folia Hered. Path. 1 (1952) 190–203
34. Fraser, D.: Hypophosphatasia. Amer. J. Med. 22 (1957) 730–746
35. Fryns, J.P., van den Berghe, K., van Assche, A., van den Berghe, H.: Prenatal diagnosis of campomelic dwarfism. Clin. Genet. 19 (1981) 199–201
36. Fuhrmann, W., Stahl, A.: Differentialdiagnose und Genetik von Papillon-Léage-Syndrom und Mohr-Syndrom. Humangenetik 9 (1970) 54–63
37. Gaulier, A., Chastagner, C., Lelch, H., Babin, C.: Lethal chondrodysplasia punctata, Conradi-Hünermann subtype A. One case. Path. Res. Pract. 182 (1987) 72–79
38. Gembruch, U., Hansmann, M., Födisch, H.J.: Early prenatal diagnosis of short rib-polydactyly (SRP) syndrome type I (Majewski) by ultrasound in a case at risk. Prenat. Diagn. 5 (1985) 357–362
39. Gembruch, U., Niesen, M., Kehrberg, H., Hansmann, M.: Diastrophic dysplasia: a specific prenatal diagnosis by ultrasound. Prenat. Diagn. 8 (1988) 539–545
40. Gerihauser, H., Schuster, C., Immervoll, H., Sochor, G.: Prenatal diagnosis of thanatophoric dwarfism. Ultraschall Med. 13 (1992) 41–45
41. Golbus, M., Hall, B.D., Filly, R.A., Poskanzer, L.R.: Prenatal diagnosis of achondrogenesis. J. Pediatr. 91 (1977) 464–466
42. Goncalves, L., Jeanty, Ph.: Fetal biometry of skeletal dysplasias: A multicentric study. J. Ultrasound Med. 13 (1994) 977–985
43. Graff, G., Chemke, J., Lancet, M.: Familial recurring thanatophoric dwarfism. Obstet. Gynecol. 39 (1971) 515–520
44. Graham, D., Tracey, J., Winn, K., Corson, V., Sanders, R.C.: Early second trimester sonographic diagnosis of achondrogenesis. J. clin. Ultrasound 11 (1983) 336–338
45. Hall, J.G.: Arthrogryposis. In: Spranger, J., Tolksdorf, M.: Klinische Genetik in der Pädiatrie. Stuttgart: Thieme 1980; S. 105–121
46. Hall, J.G.: Analysis of Pena-Shokeir phenotype. Amer. J. Med. Genet. 25 (1986) 99–117
47. Hall, J.G.: Thrombocytopenia and absent radius (TAR) syndrome. J. Med. Genet. 24 (1987) 79–83
48. Hanhart, E.: Über die Kombination von Peromelie mit Mikrognathie, ein neues Syndrom beim Menschen, entsprechend der Akroteriasis congenita von Wriedt und Mohr beim Rinde. Arch. Julius-Klaus-Stift, Zürich 25 (1950) 531–544
49. Hansmann, M., Gembruch, U.: Gezielte sonographische Ausschlußdiagnostik fetaler Fehlbildungen in Risikogruppen. Gynäkologe 17 (1984) 19–32
50. Harris, L.C., Osborne, W.P.: Congenital absence of hypoplasia of the radius with ventricular septal defect: Ventriculo-radial dysplasia. J. Pediat. 68 (1966) 265–272
51. Hässler, E., Schallock, G.: Chondrodystrophia calcificans. Monatschr. Kinderheilk. 82 (1940) 133–156
52. Hastbacka, J., Salonen, R., Laurila, P., de la Chapelle, A., Kaitila, I.: Prenatal diagnosis of diastrophic dysplasia with polymorphic DNA markers. J. Med. Genet. 30 (1993) 265–268
53. Heselson, N.G., Cremin, B.J., Beighton, P.: Lethal chondrodysplasia punctata. Clin. Radiol. 29 (1978) 679–684
54. Hirose, K., Koyanagi, T., Hara, K., Inoue, M., Nakano, H.: Antenatal ultrasound diagnosis of the femur-fibula-ulna-syndrome. J. Clin. Ultrasound 16 (1988) 199–203
55. Hobbins, J.C., Bracken, M.B., Mahoney, M.J.: Diagnosis of fetal skeletal dysplasias with ultrasound. Amer. J. Ostet. Gynec. 142 (1982) 306–312
56. Hoefler, S., Hoefler, G., Moser, A.B., Watkins, P.A., Chen, W.W., Moser, H.W.: Prenatal diagnosis of rhizomelic chondrodysplasia punctata. Prenat. Diagn. 8 (1988) 571–576
57. Holt, M., Oram, S.: Familial heart disease with skeletal malformations. Brit. Heart. J. 22 (1960) 236–242
58. Honda, N., Shimokawa, H., Yamaguchi, Y., Satoh, S., Nakano, H.: Antenatal diagnosis of sirenomelia (sympus apus). J. Clin. Ultrasound 16 (1988) 675–677
59. Horton, W.A., Machado, M., Chou, J.W., Campbell, D.: Achondrogenesis type II, abnormalities of extracellular matrix. Pediatr. Res. 22 (1987) 234–329
60. Houston, C.S., Opitz, J.M., Spranger, J.W. et al.: The campomelic syndrome. Amer. J. Med. Genet. 15 (1982) 3–28
61. Idelberger, K.: Der angeborene Klumpfuß. In: Schwalbe, E., Gruber, G.B.: Die Morphologie der Mißbildungen des Menschen und der Tiere, Bd. III, No. XIX. Jena: Fischer 1958; S. 939
62. Jeanty, P., Romero, R.: Obstetrical Ultrasound. New York: McGraw-Hill 1984
63. Jeune, M., Béraud, C., Carron, R.: Dystrophie thoracique asphyxiante de caractère familial. Arch. Fr. Pédiatr. 12 (1955) 886–891
64. Johnson, V.P., Petersen, L.P., Holzwarth, D.R., Messner, F.D.: Midtrimester prenatal diagnosis of short-limb dwarfism (Saldino-Noonan-syndrome). Birth Defects 18 (1982) 133–141
65. Jung, C., Sohn, C., Sergi, C.: Case report: prenatal diagnosis of diastrophic dysplasia by ultrasound at 21 weeks of gestation in a mother with massive obesity. Prenat. Diagn. 18 (1998) 378–383
66. Kaitila, I., Ammala, P., Karjalainen, O., Liukkonen, S., Rapola, J.: Early prenatal detection of diastrophic dysplasia. Prenat. Diagn. 3 (1983) 237–244
67. Kaufman, R.L., Rimoin, D.L., McAlister, W.H., Kissane, J.M.: Thanatophoric dwarfism. Amer. J. Dis. Child. 120 (1970) 53–57
68. Keats, T.E., Riddervold, H.O., Michaelis, L.L.: Thanatophoric dwarfism. Amer. J. Roentgenol. 108 (1970) 473–480
69. Kühne, D., Lenz, W., Petersen, D., Schönenberg, H.: Defekt von Femur und Fibula mit Amelie, Peromelie oder ulnaren Strahldefekten der Arme. Ein Syndrom. Humangenetik 3 (1967) 244–263
70. Kurtz, A.B., Filly, R.A., Wapner, R.J. et al.: In utero analysis of heterozygous achondroplasia: Variable time of onset as detected by femur length measurements. J. Ultrasound Med. 5 (1986) 137–140
71. Lachman, R.S.: Fetal imaging in the skeletal dysplasias: overview and experience. Pediatr. Radiol. 24 (1994) 413–417
72. Lang, N., Hansmann, M., Bellmann, M., Azubuike, J.: Thanatophorer Zwergwuchs – pränatale Diagnostik und Geburtsleitung. Gynäkologe 12 (1979) 84–87
73. Laughlin, C.L., Lee, T.G.: The prominent falx cerebri: New ultrasonic oberservation in hypophosphatasia. J. Clin. Ultrasound 10 (1982) 37–38
74. Leiber, B., Olbrich, G.: Die klinischen Syndrome. Syndrome, Sequenzen und Symptomenkomplexe. München: Urban & Fischer 1996
75. Lenz, W., Knapp, K.: Die Thalidomid-Embryopathie. Dtsch. Med. Wschr. 87 (1962) 1232–1242
76. Lenz, W.: Die sensible Phase für Mißbildungen beim Menschen. In: Tolksdorf, M., Spranger, J.: Klinische Genetik in der Pädiatrie. Stuttgart: Thieme 1979; S. 83–90
77. Lindhout, D., Hageman, G., Beemer, F.A. et al.: The Pena-Shokeir I syndrome: Report of nine Dutch cases. Amer. J. Med. Genet. 21 (1985) 655–66
78. Lipson, A., Waskey, J., Rice, J. et al.: Prenatal diagnosis of asphyxiating thoracic dysplasia. Amer. J. Med. Genet. 18 (1984) 273–277
79. Luthy, D.A., Hall, J.G., Graham, C.B.: Prenatal diagnosis of thrombocytopenia with absent radius. Clin. Genet. 15 (1979) 495–499

80. Mahoney, M.J., Hobbins, J.C.: Prenatal diagnosis of chondroectodermal dysplasia (Ellis-van Creveld syndrome) with fetoscopy and ultrasound. New Engl. J. Med. 297 (1977) 258–260

81. Mahony, B.S., Filly, R.A., Callen, P.W., Golbus, M.S.: Thanatophoric dwarfism with the cloverleaf skull: a specific antenatal sonographic diagnosis. J. Ultrasound Med. 4 (1985) 151–154

82. Majewski, F., Pfeiffer, A., Lenz, W., Müller, R., Feil, G., Seiler, R.: Polysyndaktylie, verkürzte Gliedmaßen und Genitalfehlbildungen: Kennzeichen eines selbständigen Syndroms? Z. Kinderheilk. 111 (1971) 118–138

83. Maroteaux, P., Lamy, M., Robert, J.M.: Le nanisme thanatophore. Presse méd. 75 (1967) 2519–2524

84. Maroteaux, P., Spranger, J., Opitz, J.M. et al.: Le syndrome campomélique. Presse Méd. 79 (1971) 1157–1162

85. Maroteaux, P., Fauré, C., Fessard, C., Rigault, P.: Osteogenesis imperfecta. In: Bone Diseases of Children. Philadelphia: Lippincott 1979; S. 102–109

86. Maroteaux, P., Spranger, J., Stanescu, V. et al.: Atelosteogenesis. Amer. J. Med. Genet. 13 (1982) 15–25

87. Maroteaux, P., Cohen-Solal, L.: L'Ostéogenèse imparfaite létale. Ann. Génét. 27 (1984) 11–15

88. McAlister, W.H., Crane, J.P., Bucy, R.P., Craig, R.B.: A new neonatal short limbed dwarfism. Skeletal Radiol. 13 (1985) 271–275

89. McGuire, J., Manning, F., Lange, I., Lyons, E., de Sa, D.J.: Antenatal diagnosis of skeletal dysplasia using ultrasound. 23 (1987) 367–384

90. McIntosh, R., Merritt, K.K., Richards, M.R., Samuels, M.H., Bellows, M.T.: The incidence of congenital malformations: A study of 5964 pregnancies. Pediatrics 14 (1954) 505–522

91. McMillan, R.H., Harbert, G.M., Davis, W.D., Kelly, T.E.: Prenatal diagnosis of Pena-Shokeir-syndrome, type I. Amer. J. Med. Genet. 21 (1985) 279–284

92. Meinel, K., Himmel, D.: Status of ultrasound and roentgen diagnosis in prenatal detection of osteochondrodysplasias. Zentralbl. Gynäkol. 109 (1987) 1303–1313

93. Meizner, I., Bar-Ziv, J.: Prenatal ultrasonic diagnosis of short-rib polydactyly syndrome (SRPS) type III: A case report and a proposed approach to the diagnosis of SRPS and related conditions. J. clin. Ultrasound 13 (1985) 284–287

94. Meizner, I., Bar-Ziv, J.: Prenatal ultrasonic diagnosis of short rib polydactyly syndrome, type I. A case report. J. Reprod. Med. 34 (1989) 668–672

95. Merz, E., Goldhofer, W., Ackermann, R., Brockerhoff, P., Becker, K.: Der thanatophore Zwergwuchs – pränatale Diagnostik einer letalen Osteochondrodysplasieform mittels Ultraschall. Z. Geburtsh. u. Perinat. 187 (1983) 289–292

96. Merz, E., Goldhofer, W.: Sonographisches Bild einer Arthrogryposis multiplex congenita-Form. Geburtsh. u. Frauenheilk. 45 (1985) 406–410

97. Merz, E., Goldhofer, W.: Sonographic diagnosis of lethal osteogenesis imperfecta in the second trimester: Case report and review. J. Clin. Ultrasound 14 (1986) 380–383

98. Merz, E., Kim-Kern, M.S., Pehl, S.: Ultrasonic mensuration of fetal limb bones in the second and third trimesters. J. Clin. Ultrasound 15 (1987) 175–183

99. Merz, E., Wellek, S., Bahlmann, F., Weber, G.: Sonographische Normkurven des fetalen knöchernen Thorax und der fetalen Lunge. Geburtsh. u. Frauenheilk. 55 (1995) 77–82

100. Merz, E., Wellek, S.: Das normale fetale Wachstumsprofil. Ein einheitliches Wachstumsmodell zur Berechnung von Normkurven für die gängigen Kopf- und Abdomenparameter sowie die großen Extremitätenknochen. Ultraschall in Med. 17 (1996) 153–162

101. Merz, E., Miric-Tesanic, D., Bahlmann, F., Weber, G., Hallermann, C.: Prenatal sonographic chest and lung measurements for predicting severe pulmonary hypoplasia. Prenat Diagn. 19 (1999) 614–619

102. Milsom, I., Mattsson, L.A., Dahlén-Nilsson, I.: Antenatal diagnosis of osteogenesis imperfecta by real time ultrasound: Two case reports. Brit. J. Radiol. 55 (1982) 310–312

103. Moessinger, A.C.: Fetal akinesia deformation sequence: An animal model. Pediatrics 72 (1983) 857–863

104. Mulivor, R.A., Mennuti, M., Zackai, E.H., Harris, H.: Prenatal diagnosis of hypophosphatasia: Genetic, biochemical, and clinical studies. Amer. J. Hum. Genet. 30 (1978) 271–282

105. Oberklaid, F., Danks, D.M., Mayne, V., Campbell, P.: Asphyxiating thoracic dysplasia. Arch. Dis. Child. 52 (1977) 758–765

106. O'Brien, G.C., Rodeck, C., Queenan, J.T.: Early prenatal diagnosis of diastrophic dwarfism by ultrasound. Brit. med. J. 280 (1980) 1300

107. Passarge, E., Lenz, W.: Syndrome of caudal regression in infants of diabetic mothers: Observations of further cases. Pediatrics 37 (1966) 672

108. Pazzaglia, U.E., Beluffi, G.: Radiology and histopathology of the bent limbs in campomelic dysplasia: Implications in the aetiology of the disease and review of theories. Pediatr. Radiol. 17 (1987) 50–55

109. Pena, S.D.J., Goodman, H.O.: The genetic of thanatophoric dwarfism. Pediatrics 51 (1973) 104–109

110. Pena, S.D.J., Shokeir, M.H.K.: Syndrome of camptodactyly, multiple ankylosis, facial anomalies and pulmonary hypoplasia: A lethal condition. J. Pediat. 85 (1974) 373–375

111. Pryde, P.G., Bawle, E., Brandt, F., Romero, R., Treadwell, M.C., Evans, M.I.: Prenatal diagnosis of nonrhizomelic chondrodysplasia punctata (Conradi-Hunermann syndrome). Amer. J. Med. Genet. 47 (1993) 426–431

112. Punnett, H.H., Kistenmacher, M.L., Valdes-Dapena, M., Ellison, R.T.: Syndrome of ankylosis, facial anomalies and pulmonary hypoplasia. J. Pediat. 85 (1974) 375–377

113. Rabinowitz, J.G., Moseley, J.E., Mitty, H.A. et al.: Trisomy 18, esophageal atresia, anomalies of the radius, and congenital hypoplastic thrombocytopenia. Radiology 89 (1967) 488–491

114. Radu, H., Stenzel, K., Bene, M. et al.: Das arthrogrypotische Syndrom. Deutsch. Z. Nervenheilk. 193 (1968) 118–140

115. Ramzin, M.S.: Teratogene Wirkung von Medikamenten. Gynäkologe 15 (1982) 136

116. Rathbun, J.C.: Hypophosphatasia: A new developmental anomaly. Amer. J. Dis. Child. 75 (1948) 822–826

117. Romero, R., Pilu, G., Jeanty, P., Ghidini, A., Hobbins, J.C.: Prenatal diagnosis of congenital anomalies. Norwalk: Appleton & Lange 1987

118. Saldino, R.M., Noonan, C.D.: Severe thoracic dystrophy with striking micromelia, abnormal osseous development, including the spine, and multiple visceral anomalies. Amer. J. Roentgenol. 114 (1972) 257–263

119. Sastrowijoto, S.H., Vandenberghe, K., Moerman, P., Lauweryns, J.M., Fryns, J.P.: Prenatal ultrasound diagnosis of rhizomelic chondrodysplasia punctata in a primigravida. Prenat. Diagn. 14 (1994) 770–776

120. Schaller, A.: Geburtsmedizinische Teratologie: Extremitätenfehlbildungen. München: Urban & Schwarzenberg 1975; S. 138

121. Schlensker, K.H.: Die sonographische Darstellung der fetalen Extremitäten im mittleren Trimenon. Geburtsh. u. Frauenheilk. 41 (1981) 366–373

122. Schlotter, C.M., Pfeiffer, R.A.: Pränatale Ultraschalldiagnostik bei Achondroplasie. Ultraschall 6 (1985) 229–232

123. Schönenberg, H.: Über das caudale Hypoplasiesyndrom. Mschr. Kinderheilk. 115 (1967) 18–24

124. Scott C.I. Jr.: The genetics of short stature. In: Steinberg, A.G., Bearn, A.G.: Progress in medical Genetics VIII. New York: Grune & Stratton 1972; S. 243

125. Seville, F., Carles, D., Maroteaux, P.: Letter to the editor: Thanatophoric dysplasia of identical twins. Amer. J. Med. Genet. 17 (1984) 703–706

126. Shaff, M.I., Fleischer, A.C., Battino, R., Herbert, C., Boehm, H.: Antenatal sonographic diagnosis of thanatophoric dysplasia. J. Clin. Ultrasound 8 (1980) 363–365

127. Shapiro, J.E., Phillips, J.A., Byers, P.H. et al.: Prenatal diagnosis of lethal perinatal osteogenesis imperfecta (OI Type II). Pediatrics 100 (1982) 127–133

128. Sillence, D.O., Senn, A., Danks, D.M.: Genetic heterogenecity in osteogenesis imperfecta. J. med. Genet. 16 (1979) 101–116

129. Sillence, D., Kozlowski, K., Bar-ziv, J., Fuhrmann-Rieger, A., Fuhrmann, W., Pascu, F.: Perinatally lethal short rib-polydactyly syndromes. 1. Variability in known syndromes. Pediatr. Radiol. 17 (1987) 474–480

130. Sirtori, M., Ghidini, A., Romero, R., Hobbins, J.C.: Prenatal diagnosis of sirenomelia. J. Ultrasound Med. 8 (1989) 83–88

131. Smith, D.W.: Recognizable patterns of human malformations. Genetic, embryologic and clinical aspects. Philadelphia: Saunders 1982

132. Smith, W.L., Breitweiser, T.D.: In utero diagnosis of achondrogenesis type I. Clin. Genet. 19 (1981) 51–54

133. Soothill, P.W., Vuthiwong, C., Rees, H.: Achondrogenesis type 2 diagnosed by transvaginal ultrasound at 12 weeks' gestation. Prenat. Diagn. 13 (1993) 523–528

134. Spranger, J., Langer, L.O., Maroteaux, P.: Increasing frequency of a syndrome of multiple osseous defects? Lancet 2 (1970) 716

135. Spranger, J., Opitz, J.M., Bidder, U.: Heterogeneity of chondrodysplasia punctata. Humangenetik 11 (1971) 190–212

136. Spranger, J.W., Langer, L.O., Wiedemann, H.R.: Bone Dysplasias. Stuttgart: Fischer 1974

137. Spranger, J., Grimm, B., Weller, M. et al.: Short rib-polydactyly (SRP) syndrome, types Majewski and Saldino-Noonan. Z. Kinderheilk. 116 (1974) 73–94

138. Spranger, J., Cremin, B. Beighton, P.: Osteogenesis imperfecta congenita. Features and prognosis of a heterogenous condition. Pediat. Radiol. 12 (1982) 21–27

139. Spranger, J., Maroteaux, P.: The lethal osteochondrodysplasias. In: Harris, H., Hirschhorn, K. (eds.): Advances in human genetics 19. Plenum Publishing Corporation 1990

140. Spranger, J.: Angeborene Entwicklungsstörungen des Skeletts. In: Lentze, M.J., Schaub, J., Schulte, F.J., Spranger, J. (Hrsg.): Pädiatrie. Berlin: Springer 2001; 1465–1480

141. Stamm, E.R., Pretorius, D.H., Rumack, C.M., Manco-Johnson, M.L.: Kleeblattschadel anomaly. In utero sonographic appearance. J. Ultrasound Med. 6 (1987) 319–324

142. Stephens, J.D., Filly, R.A., Callen, P.W., Golbus, M.S.: Prenatal diagnosis of osteogenesis imperfecta type II by real-time ultrasound. Hum. Genet. 64 (1983) 191–193

143. Stevenson, R.E., Meyer, L.C.: The limbs. In: Stevenson, R.E., Hall, J.G., Goodman, R.M. (eds.): Human malformations and related anomalies. Vol II. New York - Oxford: Oxford University Press 1993; pp. 699–720

144. Stoll, C., Dott, B., Roth, M.P., Alembik, Y.: Birth prevalence rates of skeletal dysplasias. Clin. Genet. 35 (1989) 88–92

145. Straub, W., Zarabi, M., Mazer, J.: Fetal ascites associated with Conradi's disease (Chondrodysplasia punctata): Report of a case. J. Clin. Ultrasound 11 (1983) 234–236

146. Stüve, A., Wiedemann, H.R.: Angeborene Verbiegungen langer Röhrenknochen. Eine Geschwisterbeobachtung. Z. Kinderheilk. 111 (1971) 184–192

147. Tenconi, R., Kozlowski, K., Largaiolli, G.: Boomerang dysplasia. Fortschr. Röntgenstr. 138 (1983) 378–380

148. Thompson, B.H., Parmley, T.H.: Obstetric features of thanatophoric dwarfism. Amer. J. Obstet. Gynec. 109 (1971) 396–400

149. Thomson, G.S., Reynolds, C.P., Cruickshank, J.: Antenatal detection of recurrence of Majewski dwarf (short rib-polydactyly syndrome type II Majewski). Clin. Radiol. 33 (1982) 509–517

150. Tuck, S.M., Slack, J., Buckland, G.: Prenatal diagnosis of Conradi's syndrome. Case report. Prenat. Diagn. 10 (1990) 195–198

151. Van Dongen, P.W., Hamel, B.C., Nijhuis, J.G., de Boer, C.N.: Prenatal follow-up of hypophosphatasia by ultrasound: case report. Eur. J. Obstet. Gynecol. Reprod. Biol. 34 (1990) 283–288

152. Warkany, J.: Congenital Malformations. Chicago: Year Book Medical Publishers 1971

153. Weiß, H., Rosseck, U., Zerres, K., Wißkirchen, I., Paulussen, F.: Pränatale Diagnose eines thanatophoren Zwergwuchses mit Kleeblattschädel – ultrasonographische Befunde, humangenetische Aspekte. Geburtsh. u. Frauenheilk. 44 (1984) 525–528

154. Wenstrom, K.D., Williamson, R.A., Hoover, W.W., Grant, S.S.: Achondrogenesis type II (Langer-Saldino) in association with jugular lymphatic obstruction sequence. Prenat. Diagn. 9 (1989) 527–532

155. Weyers, H.: Zur Kenntnis der Chondro-Ektodermaldysplasie (Ellis-van Creveld). Z. Kinderheilk. 78 (1956) 111–129
156. Whitley, C.B., Gorlin, D.J.: Achondrogenesis: New nosology with evidence of genetic heterogeneity. Radiology 148 (1983) 693–698
157. Wiedemann, H.R., Grosse, F.R., Dibbern, H.: Das charakteristische Syndrom. Blickdiagnose von Syndromen. Stuttgart: Schattauer 1982
158. Wladimiroff, J.W., Niermeijer, M.F., Laar, J., Jahoda, M., Stewart, P.A.: Prenatal diagnosis of skeletal dysplasia by real-time ultrasound. Obstet. Gynecol. 63 (1984) 360–364
159. Wladimiroff, J.W., Niermeijer, M.F., Van-der-Harten, J.J. et al.: Early prenatal diagnosis of congenital hypophosphatasia: Case report. Prenat. Diagn. 5 (1985) 47–52
160. Woo, J.S.K., Ghosh, A., Liang, S.T., Wong, V.C.W.: Ultrasound evaluation of osteogenesis imperfecta congenita in utero. J. Clin. Ultrasound 11 (1983) 42–44
161. Wright, J.C.Jr., Christopher, C.R.: Sirenomelia, Potter's syndrome and their relationship to monozygotic twinning: a case report and discussion. J. Reprod. Med. 27 (1982) 291–294
162. Wu, M.H., Kuo, P.L., Lin, S.J.: Prenatal diagnosis of recurrence of short rib-polydactyly syndrome. Amer. J. Med. Genet. 55 (1995) 279–284
163. Zimmer, J.: Das Geschlechtsverhältnis beim angeborenen Klumpfuß. Z. orthop. Chir. 70 (1940) 126–128

31 Disorders and Anomalies of the Skin

Diagnostic options. Most abnormalities of the fetal integument, unless massive, are too subtle to be detected with ordinary two-dimensional ultrasound. In cases with a suspected heritable skin disorder, fetoscopy (24, 25, 28) was long considered the only method available for detecting cutaneous abnormalities.

Today, high-resolution ultrasound transducers can detect fetal skin anomalies when used in a targeted search under favorable imaging conditions. Three-dimensional ultrasound is particularly advantageous for defining the fetal body surface in selected cases (6, 20).

Even today, however, fetoscopy or ultrasound-guided needle biopsy (7) is necessary for the definitive diagnosis of a heritable skin disorder based on the histologic analysis of skin biopsy samples.

Cutaneous Edema

▬ *Anasarca*

Definition. Massive edema of the subcutaneous cellular tissue.

Etiology and pathogenesis. Anasarca usually occurs in the setting of nonimmune fetal hydrops (10). In cases where the capillary hydrostatic and/or oncotic pressure, capillary permeability, or lymphatic drainage are impaired, a fluid shift occurs from the intravascular compartment into the interstitial extravascular compartment.

Pathoanatomic findings. The pronounced interstitial edema leads to massive swelling of the subcutaneous tissues.

Ultrasound features. Massive subcutaneous edema about the abdomen appears sonographically as a hypoechoic "life preserver" (Fig. 31.**1**). If nonimmune hydrops is present, this sign is accompanied by a marked fluid collection in body cavities (hydrothorax, pericardial effusion, ascites) (Fig. 31.**1**). Besides examining fetal anatomy, it is also necessary to evaluate fetal hemodynamics (echocardiography, arterial and venous Doppler examination) in order to make a prognosis.

Prognosis, treatment. Anasarca is usually a poor prognostic sign when observed in late pregnancy. The prognosis depends critically on the underlying disorder. With severe anemia like that occurring in parvovirus B19 infections, the treatment of choice is intrauterine transfusion via cordocentesis.

Clinical management. The detection of anasarca should always prompt a thorough diagnostic evaluation like that indicated for nonimmune hydrops (see Chapter 18).

Cutaneous Tumors

Cutaneous tumors rarely occur antenatally. Most are hemangiomas or lymphangiomas with a predominantly cystic, hypoechoic structure. They may be isolated lesions or may occur in association with syndromes, particularly the following:
- Klippel–Trenaunay–Weber syndrome (17, 32, 34)
- Sturge–Weber syndrome (17, 32, 34)
- von Hippel–Lindau syndrome (17)

▬ *Klippel–Trenaunay–Weber syndrome*

Definition. Mesodermal disease characterized by flat, segmental angiomas of the skin, usually unilateral (14).

Special form. Cases with tumor-like angiohyperplasia and angiodysplasia with arteriovenous fistulae are classified as *Parkes–Weber syndrome*.

Etiology and pathogenesis. Abnormality of embryonic venous development. Most cases occurs sporadically.

Pathoanatomic findings. Foci of varicose venectasia develop in the skin of the extremities. There may be marked swelling of the affected limb.

Ultrasound features. Several authors have described the intrauterine diagnosis of Klippel–Trenaunay–Weber syndrome (5, 12, 13, 18, 21, 26, 29, 30). A few cases have been detected before 24 weeks (13, 29). Hydrops and polyhydramnios have been described as intrauterine complications (12, 21).

In one case, the authors observed cystic expansion of the chest wall and grotesque enlargement of one arm sonographically in a 28-week fetus (2) (Fig. 31.**2**).

Even with a high-resolution color scanner (Fig. 31.**3**), ultrasound still cannot differentiate between venous and lymphatic lacunae.

Differential diagnosis. Maffucci syndrome (dyschondromatosis and multiple angiomatosis) (17).

Prognosis. The prognosis depends on the extent of the abnormalities and especially on internal organ involvement.

Clinical management. Large hemangiomas or lymphangiomas can pose an obstacle to vaginal delivery, and elective cesarean section should be considered for these cases. With smaller lesions, spontaneous delivery is possible.

Hyperechoic Focal Skin Changes

Rarely, ultrasound may reveal dense, hyperechoic, focal changes in the fetal integument (Fig. 31.**4**). The cause of these local changes is not fully understood. Possibilities include inflammatory infiltrates, focal calcifications in tuberous sclerosis, and simple physiologic changes. In two cases observed by the authors, the prenatal findings (Fig. 31.**4**) did not correlate with any postnatal abnormalities.

Bullous Skin Changes

Epidermolysis bullosa hereditaria

Definition. Epidermolysis bullosa hereditaria is a group of hereditary diseases characterized by blistering of the skin (3, 4).

Forms. The diseases are classified into three main groups (15, 23):
- Epidermolysis bullosa simplex
- Junctional epidermolyses (epidermolysis bullosa atrophicans)
- Epidermolysis bullosa dystrophica

The most severe form is Herlitz-type junctional epidermolysis bullosa (epidermolysis bullosa lethalis).

Etiology and pathogenesis. The mode of inheritance is autosomal-dominant or autosomal-recessive, depending on the form. Herlitz junctional epidermolysis bullosa has an autosomal-recessive inheritance. Parental consanguinity is often present (15).

Pathoanatomic findings. The condition is characterized by splitting and blistering of the skin. In Herlitz junctional epidermolysis bullosa, heavy blistering occurs at all skin sites exposed to mechanical stresses. The subepidermal blisters rupture to form erosive lesions (15).

Ultrasound features. With careful scrutiny of a favorably positioned fetus, it may be possible to define loosened epidermal areas with ultrasound (Fig. 31.**5**).

Invasive tests. The condition can be diagnosed by skin biopsy as early as 18 weeks (8, 27). Elevated α-fetoprotein and acetylcholinesterase levels may be found in the amniotic fluid (22). α-fetoprotein and acetylcholinesterase cannot be used for the accurate prediction of Herlitz junctional epidermolysis bullosa, however (31).

Prognosis. The life expectancy for infants with Herlitz junctional epidermolysis bullosa is less than 2 years. Affected children usually die from sepsis during the first months of life.

Clinical management. If Herlitz junctional epidermolysis bullosa is suspected, a fetal skin biopsy should be obtained. If histology confirms the disease, the parents should be referred for interdisciplinary counseling (prenatal diagnostician, dermatologist). Given the severity of the disease and the short life expectancy, the option of pregnancy termination should be discussed with the parents.

Hyperkeratotic Skin Disorders

Ichthyosis congenita

Definition. Generalized keratinizing disorder of the skin.

Forms. Ichthyosis congenita is a group of variable, genetically heterogeneous skin disorders characterized by abnormal keratinization and a historically confusing nomenclature (16). The following forms are the most common:
- A nonbullous form
- A bullous form
- A form associated with syndromes

Etiology and pathogenesis. Some cases are autosomal-recessive, others autosomal-dominant.

Pathoanatomic Findings

Collodion baby. The mild form of nonbullous ichthyosis congenita is characterized by the formation of a horny, parchment-like layer with rhagades (19). At birth, the infant is encased in a tight membrane that resembles oily parchment or collodion (16).

Harlequin fetus. The severe form of nonbullous ichthyosis congenita is a "harlequin fetus" covered with thick, armor-like plates (11, 16, 19). Other features are ectropion of the eyelids and a gaping, fish-like mouth. The bullous form is marked by hyperkeratosis and splitting in the upper epidermis.

The syndromic form is associated with various syndromes such as Sjögren–Larsson syndrome (17, 32, 34) or X-linked dominant chondrodysplasia punctata (17).

Ultrasound diagnosis. With a "harlequin fetus," the severe form of nonbullous ichthyosis congenita, ultrasound may show an abnormal facial profile with a flat nose and a fish-like mouth with prominent, gaping lips (Fig. 31.**6**). The facial abnormalities can be appreciated much more clearly with three-dimensional ultrasound than with conventional 2-D ultrasound (6).

Invasive tests. The definitive diagnosis of harlequin ichthyosis can be established antenatally by fetal skin biopsy (9, 19). The timing of the diagnosis can pose a problem, however. Because the keratinizing disorder has a relatively late onset (>24 weeks) (1), it cannot be confidently excluded before 24 weeks.

Prognosis. The prognosis depends on the extent of the abnormalities.

Collodion babies. These are high-risk neonates that require special care to prevent dehydration with hypernatremia and generalized skin infections. The mortality rate is approximately 10% (16).

Harlequin fetus. These fetuses are usually stillborn or die from respiratory failure within a few weeks after birth (16). There are isolated cases, however, in which the ichthyosis does not take a directly fatal course. Treatment with oral retinoids (etretinate) in these cases may lead to a marked decrease in keratinization with corresponding clinical improvement.

Clinical management. When ichthyosis congenita is detected in the fetus, the first step is to schedule an interdisciplinary conference (prenatal diagnostician, dermatologist) with the parents. In severe cases of ichthyosis congenita with pronounced facial abnormalities, pregnancy termination should be discussed. Genetic counseling is also indicated due to the high risk of inheritance.

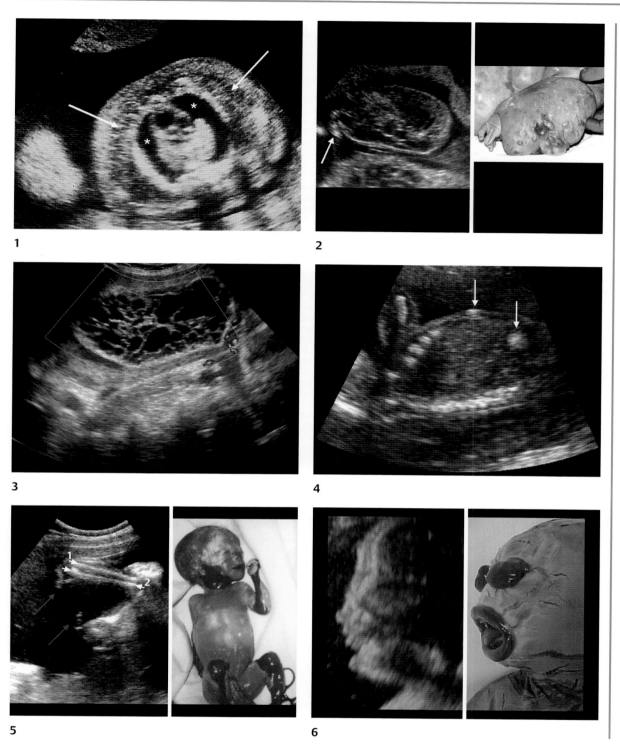

1

2

3

4

5

6

Disorders and anomalies of the skin

Fig. 31.**1** Anasarca in NIHF, 26 weeks. Note the circumferential swelling of the abdominal subcutaneous tissues, resembling a life preserver (arrows). Hydrothorax (*) is also present.

Fig. 31.**2** Klippel–Trenaunay–Weber syndrome. Left: scan at 26 weeks shows cystic expansion of the entire left arm. Arrow = hand. Right: postnatal appearance.

Fig. 31.**3** Same case as in Fig. 31.**2**. Cavernous expansion of the left arm with no detectable blood flow on color Doppler.

Fig. 31.**4** Unusual echogenic areas in the skin, 23 weeks. Inspection of the child after birth showed no corresponding abnormalities.

Fig. 31.**5** Herlitz junctional epidermolysis bullosa. Scan at 35 weeks shows loose skin tags on the fetal limbs. Right: postnatal appearance.

Fig. 31.**6** Severe nonbullous form of ichthyosis congenita ("harlequin fetus"), 30 weeks. Left: ultrasound shows a flat nasal area and a gaping, fish-like mouth with a protruding tongue. Right: clinical appearance (pictures courtesy of Dr. Bernard Benoit, Nice, France).

References

1. Arnold, M.L., Anton-Lamprecht, I.: Problems in prenatal diagnosis of the ichthyosis congenita group. Hum. Genet. 71 (1985) 301–311
2. Bahlmann, F., Merz, E., Weber, G., Kremer, W.: Pränatale Diagnose einer bullösen Lymphhämangiomatose und perinatales Management. PerinatalMedizin 8 (1996) 58–60
3. Bart, B.J.: Epidermolysis bullosa and congenital localized absence of skin. Arch. Dermatol. 101 (1970) 78–81
4. Bauer, E.A.: Epidermolysis bullosa. Birth Defects 17 (1981) 173–190
5. Becker, R., Hoffbauer, H., Entezami, M., Waldschmidt, J., Weitzel, H.K.: Thorakale Manifestation eines Klippel-Trenaunay-Syndroms. Ultraschall Med. 15 (1994) 45–48
6. Benoit, B.: Three-dimensional ultrasonography of congenital ichthyosis. Ultrasound Obstet. Gynecol. 13 (1999) 380
7. Cadrin, C., Golbus, M.S.: Fetal tissue sampling: indications, techniques, complications, and experience with sampling of fetal skin, liver, and muscle. West. J. Med. 159 (1993) 269–272
8. Eady, R.A., Tidman, M.J., Gunner, D.B. et al.: Prenatal diagnostic studies in epidermolysis bullosa. Brit. J. Dermatol. 107, Suppl. 22 (1982) 9–10
9. Elias, S., Mazur, M., Sabbagha, R., Esterly, N.B., Simpson, J.L.: Prenatal diagnosis of Harlequin ichthyosis. Clin. Genet. 17 (1980) 275–280
10. Fleischer, A.C., Killam, A.P., Boehm, F.H. et al.: Hydrops fetalis: Sonographic evaluation and clinical implications. Radiology 141 (1981) 163–168
11. Griffiths, W.A.D., Leigh, I.M., Marks, R.: Disorders of keratinisation. In: Champion, R.H., Burton, J.L., Ebling, F.J.G. (eds.): Textbook of Dermatology, Vol. 2 (5th ed.). London: Blackwell 1992
12. Hatjis, C.G., Philip, A.G., Anderson, G.G., Mann, L.I.: The in utero ultrasonographic appearance of Klippel-Trenaunay-Weber syndrome. Amer. J. Obstet. Gynecol. 139 (1981) 972–974
13. Heydanus, R., Wladimiroff, J.W., Brandenburg, H., Gaillard, J.L.J., Stewart, P.A., Niermeijer, M.F.: Prenatal diagnosis of Klippel-Trenaunay-Weber-syndrome: a case report. Ultrasound Obstet. Gynecol. 2 (1992) 360–363
14. Klippel, M., Trenaunay, P.: Du naevus variqueux osteohypertrophique. Arch. Gen. Med. Paris 3 (1900) 641–672
15. Krieg, Th., Meurer, M.: Blasenbildende Erkrankungen. In: Braun-Falco, O., Plewig, G., Wolff, H.H.: Dermatologie und Venerologie. Berlin: Springer 1996
16. Küster, W.: Keratosen. In: Braun-Falco, O., Plewig, G., Wolff, H.H.: Dermatologie und Venerologie. Berlin: Springer 1996
17. Leiber, B., Olbrich, G.: Die klinischen Syndrome. Syndrome, Sequenzen und Symptomenkomplexe. München: Urban & Fischer 1996
18. Lewis, B.D., Doubilet, P.M., Heller, V.L., Bierre, A., Bieber, F.R.: Cutaneous and visceral hemangiomata in the Klippel-Trenaunay-Weber syndrome: Antenatal sonographic detection. AJR 147 (1986) 598–600
19. Luderschmidt, C., Dorn, M., Bassermann, R., Linderkamp, O.: Kollodiumbaby und Harlekinfetus. Hautarzt 31 (1980) 154–158
20. Merz, E., Bahlmann, F., Weber, G.: Volume (3D)-scanning in the evaluation of fetal malformations – A new dimension in prenatal diagnosis. Ultrasound Obstet. Gynecol. 5 (1995) 222–227
21. Mor, Z., Schreyer, P., Wainraub, Z., Hayman, E., Caspi, E.: Nonimmune hydrops fetalis associated with angioosteohypertrophy (Klippel-Trenaunay syndrome). Amer. J. Obstet. Gynecol. 159 (1988) 1185–1186
22. Nesin, M., Seymour, C., Kim, Y.: Role of elevated alpha-fetoprotein in prenatal diagnosis of junctional epidermolysis bullosa and pyloric atresia. Amer. J. Perinatol. 11 (1994) 286–287
23. Pye, R.J.: Bullous eruptions. In: Champion, R.H., Burton, J.L., Ebling, F.J.G. (eds.): Textbook of Dermatology, Vol. 3 (5th ed.). London: Blackwell 1992
24. Rauskolb, R.: Fetoscopy: a new endoscopic approach. Endoscopy 11 (1979) 107–113
25. Rauskolb, R.: Möglichkeiten und Grenzen der Fetoskopie in der pränatalen Diagnostik. Geburtsh. u. Frauenheilk. 43 (1983) 336–338
26. Roberts, R.V., Dickinson, J.E., Hugo, P.J., Barker, A.: Prenatal sonographic appearances of Klippel-Trenaunay-Weber syndrome. Prenat. Diagn. 19 (1999) 369–371
27. Rodeck, C.H., Eady, R.A.J., Gosden, C.M.: Prenatal diagnosis of epidermolysis bullosa letalis. Lancet 1 (1980) 949–952
28. Rodeck, C.H.: Fetoscopy guided by real time ultrasound for pure fetal blood samples, fetal skin samples and examination of the fetus in utero. Brit. J. Obstet. Gynaecol. 87 (1980) 449–456
29. Seoud, M., Santos-Ramos, R., Friedman, J.M.: Early prenatal ultrasonic findings in Klippel-Trenaunay-Weber-syndrome. Prenat. Diagn. 4 (1983) 365–373
30. Shalev, E., Rotnano, S., Nseir, T., Zuckerman, H.: Klippel-Trenaunay-syndrome: ultrasonic prenatal diagnosis. J. Clin. Ultrasound 16 (1988) 268–270
31. Shulman, L.P., Elias, S., Andersen, R.N. et al.: Alpha-fetoprotein and acethylcholinesterase are not predictive of fetal junctional epidermolysis bullosa, Herlitz variant. Prenat. Diagn. 11 (1991) 813–818
32. Smith, D.W.: Recognizable patterns of human malformations. Genetic, embryologic and clinical aspects. Philadelphia: Saunders 1982
33. Warhit, J.M., Goldman, M.A., Sachs, L., Weiss, L.M., Pek, H.: Klippel-Trenaunay-Weber syndrome: Appearance in utero. J. Ultrasound Med. 2 (1983) 515–518
34. Wiedemann, H.R., Grosse, F.R., Dibbern, H.: Das charakteristische Syndrom. Stuttgart: Schattauer 1982

32 General and Specific Ultrasound Suggestive Signs of Fetal Chromosomal Abnormalities

Definitions

Suggestive signs. These are defined as sonographically detectable abnormalities of the fetus, umbilical cord, or placenta that are associated with an increased incidence of fetal chromosomal disorders. In principle, they can be detected within the framework of an extended screening examination. Suggestive signs differ from actual fetal anomalies in two major respects:
- Many suggestive signs are detectable for only a transient period (e.g., fetal nuchal translucency between 10 and 14 weeks).
- Many suggestive signs in fetuses with a normal karyotype do not affect function or viability and require no additional prenatal or postnatal follow-up (e.g., choroid plexus cysts or an echogenic intracardiac focus).

Targeted imaging. The selective search for suggestive signs, or targeted imaging, has assumed particular importance in women who are 35 or older or have a history of birth defects. The targeted imaging study expands routine ultrasound by adding a detailed search for specific stigmata of chromosomal abnormalities. This is particularly important in women at risk who refuse invasive procedures such as amniocentesis. If one or more suggestive signs are detected sonographically, the prospective parents should be informed about the possibilities of invasive prenatal karyotyping.

Risk Determination Based on Suggestive Signs

Advantage of suggestive signs. The most frequent chromosomal abnormality in newborns is trisomy 21. Up to 50% of fetuses with Down syndrome exhibit structural anomalies. But many of these anomalies, such as congenital heart defects, are difficult to detect with prenatal ultrasound and can be recognized only by an experienced examiner. On the other hand, more than 80% of all fetuses with chromosomal abnormalities have suggestive signs that can be detected at routine ultrasound screening or in a targeted imaging study.

Combinations of findings. In the past, the assessment of the risk for fetal chromosomal abnormalities was based mainly on the history (maternal age, prior pregnancies with fetal chromosomal abnormalities, family history). A more accurate and individualized risk assessment can be made by combining historical data (maternal age, prior pregnancies with fetal trisomy) with the results of biochemical maternal blood tests (triple test, 15–18 weeks) and current ultrasound findings, taking into account the current week of gestation and the presence of "suggestive signs." The exclusion of suggestive signs implies a generally lower risk of fetal chromosomal abnormalities than would be predicted by maternal age, for example.

Individual risk assessment. The individual risk of a fetal chromosomal abnormality is based on the nature and number of suggestive signs revealed by ultrasound, in addition to maternal age. For example, an isolated single umbilical cord artery is associated with a slightly increased risk, whereas bilateral renal pelvic dilatation combined with a cardiac anomaly or pericardial effusion implies a considerably higher risk. Another important factor is the week of gestation (with confirmed dates!) at the time of the examination. This is important for two reasons: (1) Early growth retardation that occurs without signs of placental insufficiency is generally an important suggestive sign of fetal chromosome anomalies. (2) Because natural selection works against fetuses with chromosome defects, the likelihood that the fetus has a chromosomal abnormality declines with increasing gestational age.

General Suggestive Ultrasound Signs of Chromosomal Abnormalities

Early Suggestive Signs: Late First or Early Second Trimester

Fetal Nuchal Translucency

Incidence. Increased fetal nuchal translucency occurs in 3% of all fetuses between 10 and 14 weeks' gestation (crown–rump length 38–80 mm).

Etiology and pathogenesis. Thickening of the subcutaneous tissue between the nuchal skin and the connective tissue enveloping the cervical spine results from a transient overperfusion of the upper body (relative aortic coarctation? early cardiac decompensation?) during the first trimester.

Ultrasound measurement. Nuchal translucency is visualized by transvaginal or transabdominal scanning in the longitudinal sagittal plane (Figs. 32.**1**, 32.**2**). The following points should be noted in the measurement of fetal nuchal translucency:
- Obtain a precise sagittal scan through the fetus (as for the measurement of crown–rump length) (Fig. 32.**2**).
- Display the fetal image on the monitor at the highest magnification.
- Do not confuse the nuchal skin with the amniotic membrane.
- Measure the nuchal translucency in its maximum thickness, and measure only the echo-free area.

Often it is helpful to measure nuchal translucency thickness two or three times in one examination before and after spontaneous fetal movements and then take the average of the measurements for risk determination. This is particularly important in women over age 35 who initially refuse an invasive test and in young women with a positive history.

Associated Disorders

Trisomies. A nuchal translucency thickness that averages 3 mm or more is associated with a fetal chromosomal abnormality (especially trisomy 21 and 18, but also trisomy 13 and Turner syndrome) in 20–30% of cases. The risk of aneuploidy correlates closely with maternal age and the maximum nuchal translucency thickness. Specifically, a thickness of 3 mm, 4 mm, 5 mm, or ≥ 6 mm is associated respectively with a 3-fold, 18-fold, 28-fold, or 36-fold increase in the basic risk (maternal age risk) for trisomies 21, 18, and 13. With a cutoff risk of one in 300 (age risk multiplied by the risk of nuchal translucency thickness), the measurement of nuchal translucency has a sensitivity of 62–84% (for comparison, risk assessment based purely on maternal age has a sensitivity of 30%).

Multiple pregnancies. Nuchal translucency measurement is particularly important in multiple pregnancies, where maternal serum screening (triple test) is of no value. Also, a discrepancy of more than 1 mm in nuchal translucency thickness between the two fetuses in a monochorionic twin pregnancy may provide the earliest predictor of a subsequent fetofetal transfusion syndrome, indicating the need for a properly timed follow-up scan (93).

Cardiac anomaly. Four percent of all fetuses with a normal karyotype who show increased nuchal translucency thickness in early pregnancy have a cardiac anomaly (indication for fetal echocardiography!). The likelihood of a cardiac anomaly in chromosomally normal fetuses increases markedly with nuchal translucency thickness between 10 and 14 weeks' gestation. For example, with a nuchal translucency thickness of 2.5–3.4 mm, 4.5–5.4 mm, and ≥ 5.5 mm, the risks increase respectively to seven in 1000, 54 in 1000, and 233 in 1000 (49, 66, 105, 108).

Cystic Hygroma

Incidence. Very rare in live births, more common (1–5%) in the early second trimester.

Ultrasound features. Ultrasound shows bilateral, often septated cysts in the region of the occiput and neck accompanied by a nuchal septum on the dorsal midline (Fig. 32.**3**).

Associated disorders. 40% to 100% of affected fetuses develop generalized hydrops, and up to 92% have a cardiac anomaly (typical: coarctation of the aorta). The aneuploidy rate in cystic hygroma is 46–90% (Turner syndrome, trisomy 21 and 18) (20, 37, 68, 120).

Fetal Hydrops

Incidence. One in 1000 births.

Ultrasound features. Ascites, pleural and/or pericardial effusion, generalized cutaneous edema.

Associated disorders. The risk of a chromosomal abnormality in nonimmune fetal hydrops is 11–78% (especially trisomy 21 and Turner syndrome) (44, 50, 62, 89, 91). The likelihood of an underlying chromosomal abnormality is highest in fetuses before 20 weeks with a coexisting cystic hygroma.

Unfused Amnion and Chorion after the First Trimester

Incidence. Approximately 2–3%. Additional fetal anomalies are detected in up to 20% of cases.

Ultrasound features. The amniotic membrane normally fuses with the chorion by the end of 12–13 weeks' gestation. If the amnion can be defined after 14 weeks as a thin, semicircular membrane around the fetus that is separated from the chorion by more than 3 mm, this is considered an indirect suggestive sign of a fetal chromosomal abnormality (Fig. 32.**4**). Often there is accompanying nuchal translucency or cystic hygroma. In approximately 40% of cases, detailed screening between 18 and 22 weeks will reveal ultrasound abnormalities (malformations or suggestive signs).

Associated disorders. Up to 6% of fetuses with no associated anomalies and 48% of fetuses with associated anomalies have a chromosomal abnormality (trisomy 21, 18 or 13, Turner syndrome).

Differential diagnosis. Subamniotic or subchorionic hemorrhage (spontaneous or after a needle procedure).

Early Growth Retardation (Second Trimester)

Importance. Nineteen percent of fetuses with severe, early growth retardation have a chromosomal abnormality, most commonly a triploidy, trisomy 18, or trisomy 13 (Fig. 32.**5**).

During the first trimester, a (small) crown–rump length can provide an additional criterion for determining a potentially increased risk only if the time of conception is known or if the patient had regular cycles before becoming pregnant.

Associated disorders. Fetuses with triploidy, trisomy 18, or trisomy 13 typically exhibit severe, early (detectable before 24 weeks), asymmetrical growth retardation. The growth retardation that is associated with other chromosomal abnormalities (trisomy 21, Turner syndrome) often is not manifested until after 24 weeks (5, 33, 41, 56, 90, 102).

The risk for a fetal chromosomal abnormality is particularly high when there are coexisting morphologic deformities, a normal or increased amniotic fluid volume, and normal Doppler flow indices in the uterine and umbilical vessels.

Differential diagnosis. Placental insufficiency is not associated with morphologic abnormalities but is associated with a decreased amniotic fluid volume and abnormal Doppler flow indices.

Suggestive Signs between 16 and 24 weeks

Choroid Plexus Cysts

Incidence. One percent of fetuses between 16 and 24 weeks' gestation.

Ultrasound features. One or more cysts are found in the region of the choroid plexus and lateral ventricles. The cysts have no functional significance and usually disappear by 26 weeks (29).

Associated disorders. On average, a chromosomal abnormality (usually trisomy 18) is found in approximately 1% of fetuses with isolated choroid plexus cysts and in 33–86% of fetuses with combined choroid plexus cysts (43, 57). This means that the risk of a chromosomal abnormality increases with the detection of associated anomalies and with maternal age. There is controversy as to whether the size and location of the cyst(s) or their bilateral occurrence affect the likelihood of an underlying chromosomal abnormality (36, 97).

Prenatal karyotyping should be offered when bilateral choroid plexus cysts are detected (Fig. 32.**6**) in an otherwise normal-appearing ultrasonogram (targeted imaging for exclusion of trisomy 18). In women under age 35 with a negative history, a triple test can be helpful in deciding for or against an invasive procedure (40). In any case, detailed ultrasound screening should be performed to rule out accompanying anomalies (67, 97).

Posterior Fossa Cyst (Cystic Expansion of the Posterior Fossa)

Incidence. Rare.

Associated disorders. Fifty percent of fetuses with a posterior fossa cyst have a chromosomal abnormality (usually trisomy 18 or 13) (11, 75, 84, 109). The risk of a chromosomal abnormality is very high in cases that are diagnosed early (before 21 weeks), in cases that show little or no ventricular dilatation, and when associated anomalies are found (Fig. 32.**7**). Accompanying intra- and extracerebral malformations are

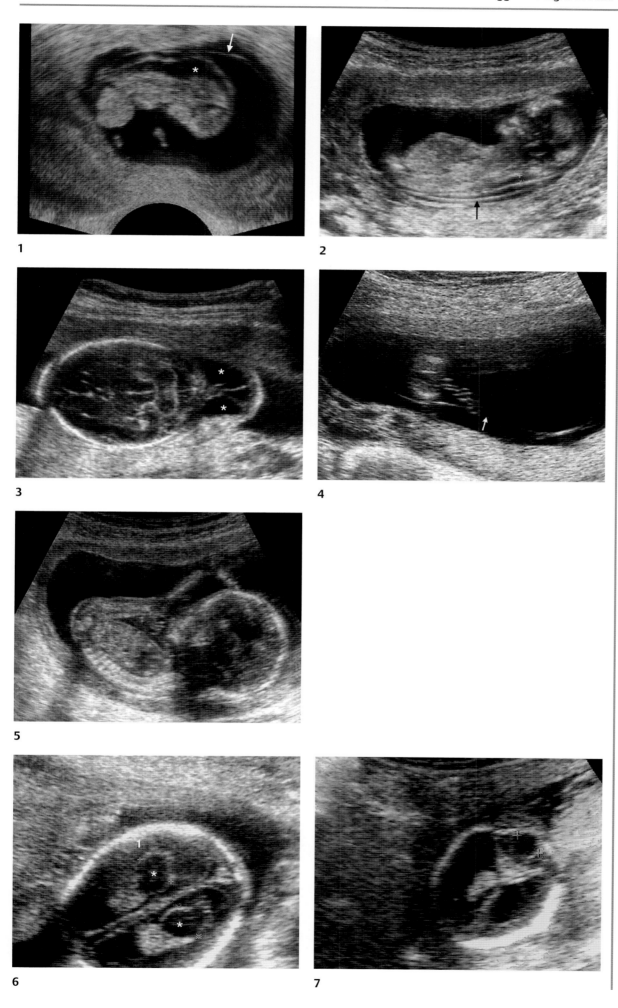

1

2

3

4

5

6

7

Early suggestive signs of chromosomal abnormalities

Fig. 32.**1** Transvaginal scan shows extensive nuchal translucency (∗) in early pregnancy. Arrow = amniotic membrane.

Fig. 32.**2** Transabdominal scan shows nuchal translucency 2.5 mm wide (++). Arrow = amniotic membrane.

Fig. 32.**3** Cystic hygroma (+) in a fetus with Turner syndrome.

Fig. 32.**4** Unfused amnion (arrow) and chorion at 14 weeks, 3 days.

Fig. 32.**5** Early disproportionate (asymmetrical) growth retardation. Note the small abdominal diameter in relation to the head diameter.

Suggestive signs between 16 and 24 weeks Superior abnormalities

Fig. 32.**6** Bilateral choroid plexus cysts (∗). Each cyst is 9 mm in diameter.

Fig. 32.**7** Posterior fossa cyst (++) 8 mm in diameter in a fetus with triploidy (69,XXX).

Fig. 32.**8**   Dandy–Walker malformation with separation of the cerebellar hemispheres (arrow) and vermian aplasia.

Cardiac abnormality

Fig. 32.**9**   Golfball phenomenon (= echogenic focus) in the left ventricle (arrow). Breech presentation, 1st breech position.

Intestinal abnormality

Fig. 32.**10**   Hyperechoic bowel (arrow).

Borderline dilatations in the second trimester

Fig. 32.**11**   Mild, bilateral ventricular dilatation at the level of the occipital horns (∗). Diameter 13 mm.

Fig. 32.**12**   Small pericardial effusion in a fetus with trisomy 21. *Left:* transverse scan shows only a thin, hypoechoic crescent around the heart (arrow). *Right:* angled oblique scan more clearly demonstrates the 3-mm pericardial effusion (arrow).

Fig. 32.**13**   Bilateral renal pelvic dilatation. The AP diameter (++) is 10 mm on each side.

Pelvic and limb abnormalities

Fig. 32.**14**   Increased pelvic bone angle (> 90°) in a fetus with trisomy 21.

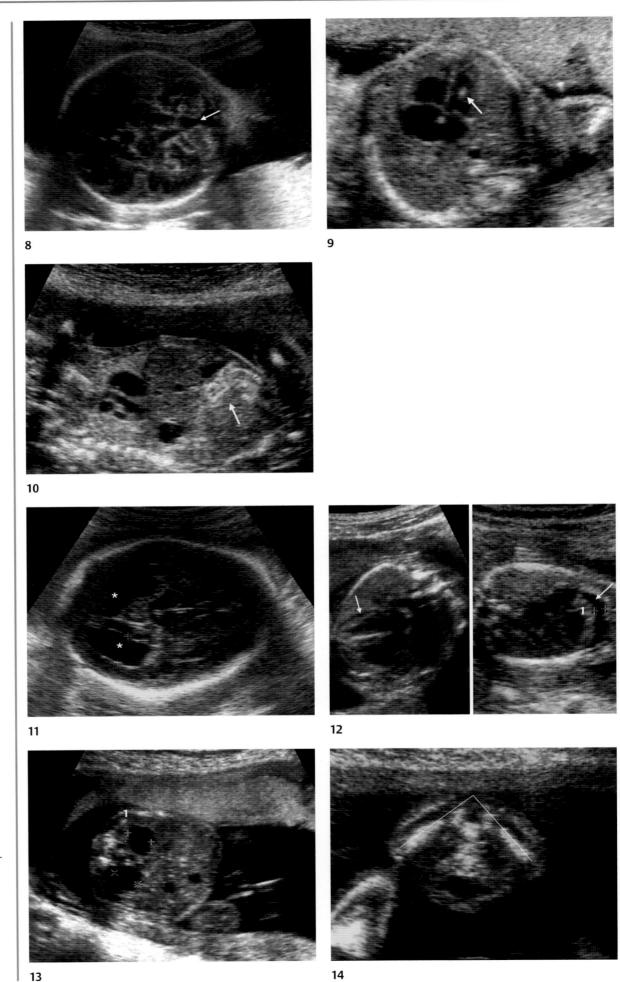

8

9

10

11

12

13

14

common and contribute greatly to the high perinatal mortality, even in fetuses with a normal karyotype.

Differential diagnosis. Differentiation is required from Dandy–Walker malformation or Dandy–Walker variant (Fig. 32.**8**), which occurs in approximately 0.03% of all fetuses. It is marked by a triad of vermian agenesis or hypoplasia, cystic dilatation of the cisterna magna, and an open communication between the cisterna magna and fourth ventricle. The prognosis is poor. Rarely, differentiation is required from cystic expansion of the posterior fossa with no cerebellar defect, or from an arachnoid cyst.

Golfball Phenomenon (Hyperechoic Intracardiac Focus)

Incidence. Two to five percent of all fetuses between 18 and 22 weeks.

Ultrasound features. Ultrasound shows a small, round, echogenic focus ("golfball," formed by thickened chordae tendineae) in the cardiac chambers (Fig. 32.**9**). It is seen much more frequently in the left ventricle than in the right. Bilateral or multiple foci are found in approximately 5% of cases.

Associated disorders. With an isolated golfball phenomenon, the risk of a fetal chromosomal abnormality (mainly trisomy 21) is approximately 1–2% when associated anomalies have been excluded. The risk of a chromosomal abnormality may be slightly higher with a right ventricular focus or bilateral foci (22). One high-risk population (amniocentesis cases over age 35) was found to have an aneuploidy rate of 6% (18). In women under age 35 with otherwise normal ultrasound findings (targeted imaging to exclude trisomy 21) and a normal serum screen (triple test), the indication for invasive testing should depend on the parents" wishes due to the relatively low risk of a chromosomal abnormality (2). The golfball phenomenon (unlike nuchal translucency or choroid plexus cysts, for example) usually remains sonographically detectable until birth. The echogenic focus is not associated with an increased risk of cardiac anomalies and has no functional significance in fetuses with a normal karyotype (30, 85).

Hyperechoic Bowel Structure

Incidence. From 0.2% to 2% of fetuses in the second trimester.

Ultrasound features and associated disorders. Bowel loops that are isoechoic or hyperechoic to the fetal iliac crests (reference echogenicity) are found mainly in association with chromosomal abnormalities and cystic fibrosis and less commonly after intra-amniotic hemorrhage or infections (CMV) (Fig. 32.**10**). In cases with fetal growth retardation and oligohydramnios, the hyperechoic bowel structure is often a reflection of severe placental insufficiency (very poor prognosis when accompanied by elevated maternal serum AFP) (1). Hence, Doppler flowmetry should be performed whenever a hyperechoic bowel structure is found.

If hyperechoic bowel is noted as an isolated ultrasound finding, the risk of a fetal chromosomal abnormality is no higher than 8% (usually trisomy 21, but other aneuploidies can occur) (4, 17, 92, 100). When hyperechoic bowel is combined with other anomalies, the risk is approximately 42%.

▀ Borderline Dilatations as Suggestive Signs in the Second Trimester

Mild Ventricular Dilatation

Ultrasound features. A value of 10 mm is considered borderline for the lateral dimension of the occipital horns of the lateral cerebral ventricles.

Associated disorders. Mild ventricular dilatation to 10–15 mm is based on an underlying fetal chromosomal abnormality (trisomy 21, 18 or 13, triploidy) in 2–3% of cases when it is an isolated finding and in up to 27% of cases when associated anomalies are present (Fig. 32.**11**). As the degree of ventricular dilatation increases, a fetal chromosomal abnormality becomes less likely, although an increasing degree of ventricular dilatation (even in the range of 10–15 mm) is associated with a rising risk of developmental delay in early childhood (12, 15, 69, 82).

Differential Diagnosis

- Hemorrhage or infection in early pregnancy (CMV: calcifications at the outer margins of the lateral ventricles)
- Aqueductal stenosis (enlargement of the lateral ventricles and third ventricle with a normal cisterna magna and normal-appearing cerebellum)
- Arnold–Chiari malformation (spinal dysraphia with cerebellar compression, predominant occipital horn dilatation)

Mild Pericardial Effusion

Ultrasound features. The physiologic cutoff is 2 mm. Unlike the pronounced pericardial effusion that occurs with generalized hydrops, cardiac anomalies or arrhythmias, autoimmune disorders, and fetal infections (e.g., parvovirus B19), it is rare to detect an isolated pericardial fluid collection larger than 2 mm with prenatal ultrasound (81, 98).

Associated disorders. A chromosomal abnormality (usually trisomy 21) is present in approximately 31% of cases (96) (Fig. 32.**12**). A mild pericardial effusion in itself has no functional significance in fetuses with a normal karyotype and is not associated with an increased risk of perinatal complications (31).

Mild Renal Pelvic Dilatation

Ultrasound features. The cutoff values for the anteroposterior renal pelvic diameter are over 4–5 mm at 20 weeks and over 10 mm at 30 weeks (Fig. 32.**13**).

Associated disorders. Isolated, unilateral renal pelvic dilatation is not associated with an increased risk of chromosomal abnormalities. When mild, isolated renal pelvic dilatation is seen bilaterally, there is an average 3% incidence of fetal chromosomal abnormalities. The basic risk for trisomy 21 associated with mild renal pelvic dilatation is increased by a factor of 3–4, depending on maternal age (7, 72, 114, 116, 117).

The risk of a fetal chromosomal abnormality is 25–32% when unilateral or bilateral renal pelvic dilatation is accompanied by other ultrasound abnormalities (cardiac anomalies are frequent).

Fig. 32.**15** *Left:* hand of a fetus with trisomy 21. The middle phalanx is absent from the fifth finger (arrow) (observation by Prof. Merz, Frankfurt). *Right:* hand of a fetus with trisomy 21. The fifth finger has a normal middle phalanx (arrow)!

Fig. 32.**16** "Sandal gap" between the first and second toes of a fetus with trisomy 21.

Umbilical Cord

Fig. 32.**17** Single umbilical artery. Transverse scan through the umbilical cord shows a large-caliber vein (LCV) adjacent to a small-caliber artery (SCA).

Fig. 32.**18** Umbilical cord cyst measuring 3.5 · 2.5 cm in a fetus with trisomy 18. *Left:* transverse scan. *Right:* longitudinal scan.

Phenotypic expression in trisomy 18

Fig. 32.**19** Strawberry-shaped skull ("strawberry sign") in the fronto-occipital plane of a fetus with trisomy 18. Vertex presentation with the spine to the right.

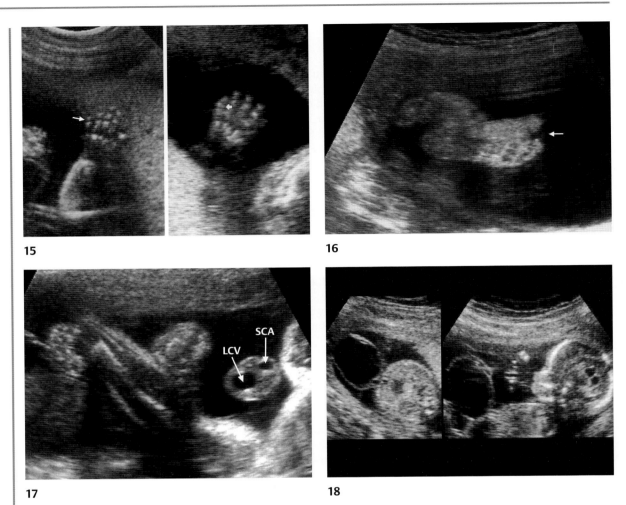

15

16

17

18

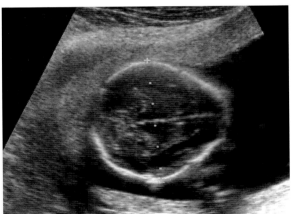

19

Suggestive Signs Involving the Pelvic Bones and Extremities

Relative Broadening of the Pelvic Bones

Ultrasound. The angle formed by the iliac crests on both sides of the lumbar spine at the level of the bladder roof (below the umbilical cord insertion) in the axial plane provides a marker for the ultrasound exclusion of chromosomal abnormalities in the early second trimester of pregnancy.

Associated disorders. In fetuses with trisomy 21, the average angle between the superior iliac crests is 79–98º (Fig. 32.**14**). The average angle in fetuses with normal karyotypes is 67–78º (14, 55, 99). The angle should be measured on the highest plane in which the iliac crests are clearly defined and show approximately equal (maximum) lengths, because even in fetuses with trisomy 21, the pelvic angles decrease inferiorly and show an increasing overlap with the angles in normal fetuses.

A cutoff value of 90º between the left and right iliac crests identifies 37–91% of fetuses with trisomy 21, with a false-positive rate of approximately 5% (normal fetuses with relatively broad pelvic bones).

Relatively Short Long Bones (Femur and Humerus)

Measurements and their significance. Fetuses with chromosomal abnormalities (especially trisomy 21) often show decreased longitudinal growth of the tubular limb bones. Differentiation from fetuses with normal karyotypes is difficult because the length measurements frequently overlap (high false-positive "detection rates"), and growth retardation due to other causes must be excluded. So instead of using normal values based on calculated gestational age, risk determinations are usually based on a biometric ratio, such as the ratio of femur length to biparietal diameter. The values listed in Table 32.**1** provide valuable additional information in targeted scans.

Deformities and Position Anomalies of the Hands and Feet

Significance. Deformities and position anomalies of the hands and feet occupy an intermediate position between the suggestive signs noted in general screening and the signs that are looked for in targeted imaging. Their detection is particularly important in young women who have a borderline triple test. While certain anomalies, such as polydactyly, can be diagnosed with high confidence toward the end of the first trimester (21), their true significance lies in their value as "associated

anomalies" that accompany other ultrasound markers or structural malformations (79).

Associated disorders. Typical sonographically detectable abnormalities are listed in Table 32.**2**.

Suggestive Signs Involving the Placenta and Umbilical Cord

Vacuolated Placenta

Significance. The "Swiss cheese" structure of the placenta that is pathognomonic for the 69,XYY form of triploidy is found in only 17% of triploid fetuses and is almost always associated with severe, early growth retardation. Triploidy in early pregnancy is typically marked by abnormally high maternal serum hCG levels (regardless of placental structure) accompanied by thick nuchal folds, significant growth retardation, and fetal structural anomalies (51, 52, 60).

Single Umbilical Artery

Incidence. One percent of all live births.

Ultrasound features. A single umbilical artery can be positively identified only in a transverse scan (Fig. 32.**17**). If doubt exists, color Doppler scanning can define the anomaly at the umbilical cord insertion above the fetal bladder.

Associated disorders. When a single umbilical artery occurs in isolation, there is only a slightly increased risk for a fetal chromosomal abnormality (approximately 1% for trisomies and structural anomalies). One-third of affected fetuses have coexisting anomalies (urogenital tract, heart, cleft anomalies). These increase the risk of a chromosomal abnormality to 12–30% (24, 83).

The risk for intrauterine growth retardation and/or prematurity is slightly increased in fetuses with a normal karyotype. The prognosis of fetuses with an isolated single umbilical artery and normal Doppler flow indices is generally rated as very favorable, however (80, 110).

Umbilical Cord Cyst

Incidence and significance in the first trimester. The incidence is 3% between 7 and 13 weeks' gestation. Approximately 25% of these fetuses display other ultrasound abnormalities, and 7% have a chromosomal abnormality (trisomy 18) (Fig. 32.**18**). The risk for structural and/or chromosomal anomalies is greatest in fetuses with a paraxial umbilical cord cyst that is located near the fetal or placental umbilical cord insertion and persists beyond 12 weeks' gestation (87).

Incidence and significance in the second trimester. Very rare. Chromosomal abnormalities are present in up to 18% of cases with an isolated umbilical cord cyst and in approximately 55% of cases (trisomy 18) where the cyst is combined with other anomalies (86, 101).

Table 32.**2** Typical hand and foot anomalies in chromosomal disorders

Trisomy 21	➢ Clinodactyly ➢ Short or absent middle phalanx of the small finger (Fig. 32.**15**) (6) ➢ "Sandal gap" between the first and second toes (Fig. 32.**16**) (118)
Trisomy 18	➢ Overlapping fingers and clubfeet
Trisomy 13 and triploidy	➢ Polydactyly

Table 32.**1** Important quantitative parameters that can signify a chromosomal abnormality

➢ Measured humeral length/normal humeral length (expected length based on biparietal diameter) < 0.90 identifies 50% of fetuses with trisomy 21 and 6.25% of fetuses with normal chromosomes (14–20 weeks) (8)

➢ Measured/normal length of humerus and femur < 0.91 identifies 44% of fetuses with trisomy 21 and 7.6% of fetuses with normal chromosomes (15–19 weeks) (10)

➢ Femur length/foot length < 0.88 identifies 35% of fetuses with trisomy 21, with a false-positive rate of 4.6% (fetuses with normal chromosomes) (39)

➢ Humerus length + femur length/foot length < 1.76 identifies 53% of fetuses with trisomy 21, with a false-positive rate of 7% (fetuses with normal karyotypes) (53)

➢ Measurement of the humerus, femur, tibia, and fibula, comparison with normal values for gestational age. When all four values are within normal limits, amniocentesis may be omitted in women under age 40 (who have no other risk factors!) (115)

Specific Ultrasound Suggestive Signs of Chromosomal Abnormalities

▬ Central Nervous System, Neural Tube

Anencephaly, Exencephaly

Incidence and significance. The incidence is one in 1000 at the end of the first trimester. Fetal aneuploidies are rare in anencephaly/exencephaly (trisomy 18). The risk is increased by maternal treatment with anticonvulsants or folic acid antagonists and in women with a folic acid deficiency or diabetes mellitus. In a few cases, amniotic bands can be detected with ultrasound. Anencephaly is invariably fatal, with a 2–3% risk of recurrence (54, 94).

Microcephaly

Incidence and associated disorders. The incidence is one in 1000 (combined) to 10,000 (isolated). The risk of an underlying chromosomal abnormality (usually trisomy 13) is 15–20%.

Differential diagnosis. Familial occurrence of a "small head" (microcephaly: head circumference or ratio of head circumference to femur or humeral length < 1st percentile in second and third trimester) (34, 41).

Holoprosencephaly

Incidence. One to two in 10,000 live births.

Associated disorders. Four percent of fetuses with isolated holoprosencephaly and 40% with combined holoprosencephaly have an underlying chromosomal abnormality (usually trisomy 13 or trisomy 18) (9, 27, 35, 59, 74). Often there are coexisting midline defects in the face or facial skeleton (proboscis, arhinia, median cleft lip and palate). With alobar holoprosencephaly, death occurs before birth or during the first 6 months of life. The recurrence risk in sporadic cases is 6%.

Agenesis of the Corpus Callosum

Incidence. Up to 1% of all live births.

Associated disorders. Isolated agenesis of the corpus callosum has a good prognosis, and the clinical picture is usually asymptomatic. In all fetuses with corpus callosum agenesis and chromosomal abnormalities (risk 10%, mainly trisomy 13 or 18) that have been described to date, associated anomalies were discovered in the heart, diaphragm, or kidneys (42, 112).

Spina bifida

Incidence. Approximately one in 1000.

Associated disorders. From 10% to 17% of fetuses with a prenatal diagnosis of spina bifida have a chromosomal abnormality (trisomy 18 or 13, triploidy, translocations). Anticonvulsants, folic acid antagonists or deficiency, and maternal diabetes mellitus increase the risk of neural tube closure defects (3, 25, 45, 119).

▬ Face

Ocular and Nasal Anomalies

Incidence. Rare.

Associated disorders. Twenty-six percent of fetuses with these anomalies have a chromosomal abnormality (trisomy 13 or 18) (73).

Facial Clefts (Cleft Lip and Palate)

Incidence. One in 1000 to five in 1000 live births.

Associated disorders. Isolated facial clefts are based on an underlying chromosomal abnormality in less than 1% of cases. When they are combined with other anomalies, the likelihood of an underlying aneuploidy (mainly trisomy 13 or 18) increases to more than 50% (73, 77, 104).

Micrognathia

Incidence. Rare.

Associated disorders. From 26% to 66% of affected fetuses have a chromosomal abnormality (typically trisomy 18, trisomy 13, or triploidy). Associated anomalies are common, and perinatal mortality is high (16, 73).

▬ Thorax

Cardiac Anomalies

Incidence. One percent of all live births.

Associated disorders. From 28% to 48% of fetuses with a cardiac anomaly diagnosed by prenatal ultrasound have a chromosomal abnormality (19, 26, 78, 107). The risk of a chromosome disorder is 16–29% with an isolated cardiac anomaly and 65–71% with combined anomalies (Table 32.**3**).

Congenital Cystic Adenomatoid Malformation (CCAM) of the Lung

Incidence. Rare.

Associated disorders. An isolated cystic adenomatoid malformation of the lung does not increase the basic risk for a chromosomal abnormality (32, 63, 65).

Table 32.**3** Cardiac anomalies and chromosomal disorders

Ventricular septal defect	10–15% Chromosomal abnormalities
Tetralogy of Fallot	When combined with other anomalies, associated with fetal trisomies (18, 13, 21) and various genetic syndromes
Coarctation of the aorta	Associated mainly with Turner syndrome
D-transposition of the great arteries	Fetal chromosomal abnormalities very rare
Hypoplastic left heart syndrome	Rarely associated with Turner syndrome, duplication on chromosome 12q, and trisomies 13, 18, and 21
Atrioventricular canal	Associated with fetal trisomy 21 in over 50% of cases

Diaphragmatic Hernia

Incidence. One in 3000 births.

Associated disorders. On average, 18% of fetuses with a diaphragmatic hernia have a chromosomal abnormality, most commonly trisomy 18. The risk of a chromosomal abnormality is 2% with an isolated diaphragmatic hernia and 34% when the hernia is combined with other anomalies. From 44% to 73% of the fetuses have accompanying anomalies, most involving the heart (13, 48, 95).

Gastrointestinal Tract and Anterior Abdominal Wall

Esophageal Atresia

Incidence. One in 2500 live births.

Associated disorders. When ultrasound shows an absence of gastric filling accompanied by polyhydramnios, a high percentage of these cases (38–75%) will have a chromosomal abnormality (mainly trisomy 18, typically without a tracheoesophageal fistula).

It is common to find an accompanying tracheoesophageal fistula that allows for slight to normal gastric filling (difficult prenatal ultrasound differential diagnosis). The risk of a chromosomal abnormality in these fetuses is only 4% (64, 106).

Duodenal Atresia and Stenosis

Incidence. One in 10,000 live births.

Ultrasound features and associated disorders. Ultrasound displays a "double bubble sign" in the fetal upper abdomen. The risk of a chromosomal abnormality (usually trisomy 21) is 30–38% in isolated cases and approximately 64% when the duodenal abnormality is combined with other anomalies (46, 71).

Omphalocele

Incidence. One in 10,000 to three in 10,000 live births.

Associated disorders. A chromosomal abnormality (mainly trisomy 18 or 13) is present in 13% of fetuses with an isolated omphalocele and in 46–50% of fetuses with a combined omphalocele.

Additional criteria. Unfavorable additional criteria for a chromosomal abnormality are advanced maternal age, the existence of other malformations (present in 40–90%), the ultrasound detection of an omphalocele before 20 weeks' gestation, an absence of liver herniation into the sac, and a small size of the umbilical hernia (diameter <3 cm in the second trimester) (28, 38, 47, 71, 103). In the first trimester, omphalocele in an aneuploid fetus is frequently associated with increased nuchal translucency thickness (111).

Differential diagnosis. Differentiation is required from a physiologic umbilical hernia in the first trimester.

Gastroschisis

Incidence. One to two in 10,000 live births.

Associated disorders. Chromosomal abnormalities are rare in fetuses with gastroschisis. Ultrasound differentiation from a ruptured om-phalocele is sometimes very difficult. Accompanying anomalies are found in 10–36% of affected fetuses (23, 47, 61, 71).

Urogenital System

Hydronephrosis

Incidence. One in 1000 to five in 1000 live births (male : female ratio = 5 : 1).

Associated disorders. Three percent of fetuses with bilateral renal pelvic dilatation or hydronephrosis (even when mild) have a chromosomal abnormality (mild dilatation: usually trisomy 21; pronounced hydronephrosis: trisomy 18, 13, and other chromosomal abnormalities). When associated anomalies are detected (cardiac), the risk of a chromosomal abnormality is 30%. This risk is higher in female fetuses with renal pelvic dilatation or hydronephrosis than in male fetuses (7, 70, 117).

Multicystic Renal Dysplasia, Renal Agenesis

Incidence. Less than one in 10,000 live births for multicystic renal dysplasia, one in 600 for unilateral renal agenesis, one in 3500 for bilateral renal agenesis.

Associated disorders. Chromosomal abnormalities (trisomy 18, 13, other anomalies) are found in 3% (isolated finding) to 30–35% (combined anomalies) of fetuses with multicystic renal dysplasia or renal agenesis.

Phenotypic Expression of Common Chromosomal Abnormalities

Trisomy 21 (Down Syndrome) (113)

Incidence. One in 710 births.

Prognosis. The mortality is 15–20% during the first year of life (cardiac anomalies, myeloproliferative diseases). The suggestive ultrasound signs of trisomy 21 are listed in Table 32.**4**.

Trisomy 18 (Edwards Syndrome) (76)

Incidence. One in 3000 births.

Prognosis. The mortality is 30% in the first month of life and 90% in the first year of life. The suggestive ultrasound signs of trisomy 18 are shown in Table 32.**5**.

Trisomy 13 (Patau Syndrome)

Incidence. One in 5000 births.

Prognosis. The mortality is 50% in the first month of life and over 80% in the first year of life. The suggestive ultrasound signs of trisomy 13 are shown in Table 32.**6**.

Triploidy

Incidence. Less than one in 2500 births.

Prognosis. 100% mortality. The suggestive ultrasound signs of triploidy are listed in Table 32.**7**.

Table 32.4 Suggestive signs of trisomy 21

General suggestive signs	➢ Nuchal translucency thickness ≥ 3 mm ➢ Unfused amnion and chorion ➢ Fetal hydrops ➢ Growth retardation ➢ Mild bilateral renal pelvic dilation ➢ Mild pericardial effusion ➢ Mild ventricular dilatation ➢ Hyperechoic bowel structure ➢ Echogenic intracardiac focus (golfball phenomenon)
Targeted search for anomalies or suggestive signs	➢ Relative shortening of femur and humerus ➢ Sandal gap between first and second toes ➢ Shortened or absent middle phalanx of fifth finger ➢ Pelvic angle > 90º ➢ Facial flattening ➢ Brachycephaly ➢ Cardiac anomalies (AV canal, VSD, ASD) ➢ Duodenal stenosis (double-bubble sign)

Table 32.5 Suggestive signs of trisomy 18

General suggestive signs	➢ Nuchal translucency thickness ≥ 3 mm ➢ Growth retardation ➢ Choroid plexus cysts ➢ Posterior fossa cyst ➢ Umbilical cord cyst ➢ Single umbilical artery ➢ Strawberry-shaped skull (Fig. 32.19)
Targeted search for anomalies or suggestive signs	➢ Hand/foot deformities (overlapping fingers) ➢ Cleft lip and palate ➢ Micrognathia ➢ Agenesis of the corpus callosum ➢ Dandy–Walker malformation ➢ Cardiac anomalies ➢ Esophageal atresia ➢ Diaphragmatic hernia ➢ Omphalocele ➢ Clubfoot

Table 32.6 Suggestive signs of trisomy 13

General suggestive signs	➢ Nuchal translucency thickness ≥ 3 mm ➢ Unfused amnion and chorion ➢ Growth retardation ➢ Posterior fossa cyst ➢ Single umbilical artery
Targeted search for anomalies or suggestive signs	➢ Hand/foot anomalies (polydactyly) ➢ Microcephaly ➢ Holoprosencephaly ➢ Facial malformations ➢ Cleft lip and palate ➢ Cardiac anomalies ➢ Renal dysplasia or agenesis ➢ Omphalocele

Table 32.7 Suggestive signs of triploidy

General suggestive signs	➢ 69, XYY: molar degeneration of placenta, abortion by 20 weeks ➢ 69, XXX: placenta usually normal at ultrasound
Targeted search for anomalies or suggestive signs	➢ Severe, early growth retardation ➢ Relative shortening of femur and humerus ➢ Hand/foot anomalies ➢ Micrognathia ➢ Cardiac anomalies

Table 32.8 Suggestive signs of Turner syndrome

General suggestive signs	➢ Lethal form: cystic hygroma, fetal hydrops ➢ Other form: growth retardation
Targeted search for anomalies or suggestive signs	➢ Relative shortening of femur and humerus ➢ Microcephaly ➢ Cardiac anomalies (coarctation of aorta)

Turner Syndrome (45,XO)

Incidence. One in 2500 live-born girls.

Prognosis. Short stature, hearing impairment (50%), cardiac anomalies (15–20% of live-born infants), infertility, rarely mental retardation. Table 32.8 lists the suggestive ultrasound signs of Turner syndrome.

References

1. Achiron, R., Seidman, D.S., Horowitz, A., Mashiach, S., Goldman, B., Lipitz, S.: Hyperechogenic fetal bowel and elevated serum alpha-fetoprotein: a poor fetal prognosis. Obstet. Gynecol. 88 (1996) 368–371
2. Achiron, R., Lipitz, S., Gabbay, U., Yagel, S.: Prenatal ultrasonographic diagnosis of fetal heart echogenic foci: no correlation with Down syndrome. Obstet. Gynecol. 89 (1997) 945–948
3. Babcook, C.J., Goldstein, R.B., Filly, R.A.: Prenatally detected fetal myelomeningocele: is karyotype analysis waranted? Radiology 194 (1995) 491–494
4. Bahado-Singh, R., Morotti, R., Cople, J.A., Mahoney, M.J.: Hyperechogenic fetal bowel: the perinatal consequences. Prenat. Diagn. 14 (1994) 981–987
5. Bahado-Singh, R.O., Lynch, L., Deren, O. et al.: First-trimester growth restriction and fetal aneuploidy: The effect of type of aneuploidy and gestational age. Amer. J. Obstet. Gynecol. 176 (1997) 976–980
6. Benacerraf, B.R., Harlow, B.L., Frigoletto, F.D.Jr.: Hypoplasia of the middle phalanx of the fifth digit. A feature of the second trimester fetus with Down's syndrome. J. Ultrasound Med. 9 (1990) 389–394
7. Benacerraf, B.R., Mandell, J., Estroff, J.A., Harlow, B.L., Frigoletto, F.D.: Fetal pyelectasis: A possible association with Down syndrome. Obstet. Gynecol. 76 (1990) 58–60
8. Benacerraf, B.R., Neuberg, D., Frigoletto, F.D.Jr.: Humeral shortening in second-trimester fetuses with Down syndrome. Obstet. Gynecol. 77 (1991) 223–227
9. Berry, S.M., Gosden, C., Snijders, R.J., Nicolaides, K.H.: Fetal holoprosencephaly: associated malformations and chromosomal defects. Fetal Diagn. Ther. 5 (1990) 92–99
10. Biagiotti, R., Periti, E., Cariati, E.: Humerus and femur length in fetuses with Down syndrome. Prenat. Diagn. 14 (1994) 429–434
11. Blazer, S., Berant, M., Sujov, P.O., Zimmer, E.Z., Bronshtein, M.: Prenatal sonographic diagnosis of vermal agenesis. Prenat. Diagn. 17 (1997) 907–911
12. Bloom, S.L., Bloom, D.D., Dellanebbia, C., Martin, L.B., Lucas, M.J., Twickler, D.M.: The developmental outcome of children with antenatal mild isolated ventriculomegaly. Obstet. Gynecol. 90 (1997) 93–97
13. Bollmann, R., Kalache, K., Mau, H., Chaoui, R., Tennstedt, C.: Associated malformations and chromosomal defects in congenital diaphragmatic hernia. Fetal Diagn. Ther. 10 (1995) 52–59
14. Bork, M.D., Egan, J.F.X., Cusick, W., Borgida, A.F., Campbell, W.A., Rodis, J.F.: Iliac wing angle as a marker for trisomy 21 in the second trimester. Obstet. Gynecol. 89 (1997) 734–737
15. Bromley, B., Frigoletto, F.D.Jr., Benacerraf, B.R.: Mild fetal lateral cerebral ventriculomegaly: clinical course and outcome. Amer. J. Obstet. Gynecol. 164 (1991) 863–867
16. Bromley, B., Benacerraf, B.R.: Fetal micrognathia: associated anomalies and outcome. J. Ultrasound Med. 13 (1994) 529–533
17. Bromley, B., Doubilet, P., Frigoletto, F.D.Jr., Krauss, C., Estroff, J.A., Benacerraf, B.R.: Is fetal hyperechogenic bowel on second-trimester sonogram an indication for amniocentesis? Obstet. Gynecol. 83 (1994) 647–651
18. Bromley, B., Lieberman, E., Laboda, L., Benacerraf, B.R.: Echogenic intracardiac focus: a sonographic sign for fetal Down syndrome. Obstet. Gynecol. 86 (1995) 998–1001
19. Bronshtein, M., Zimmer, E.Z., Gerlis, L.M., Lorber, A., Drugan, A.: Early ultrasound diagnosis of fetal congenital heart defects in high-risk and low-risk pregnancies. Obstet. Gynecol. 82 (1993) 225–229
20. Bronshtein, M., Bar-Hava, I., Blumenfeld, I., Bejar, J., Toder, V., Blumenfeld, Z.: The difference between septated and nonseptated nuchal cystic hygroma in the early second trimester. Obstet. Gynecol. 81 (1993) 683–687
21. Bronshtein, M., Stahl, S., Zimmer E.Z.: Transvaginal sonographic diagnosis of fetal finger abnormalities in early gestation. J. Ultrasound Med. 14 (1995) 591–595
22. Bronshtein, M., Jakobi, P., Ofir, C.: Multiple fetal intracardiac echogenic foci: not always a benign sonographic finding. Prenat. Diagn. 16 (1996) 131–135
23. Calzolari, E., Bianchi, F., Dolk, H., Milan, M.: Omphalocele and gastroschisis in Europe: a survey of 3 million births 1980–1990. EUROCAT Working Group. Amer. J. Med. Genet. 58 (1995) 187–194
24. Catanzarite, V.A., Hendricks, S.K., Maida, C., Westbrook, C., Cousins, L., Schrimmer, D.: Prenatal diagnosis of the two-vessel cord: implications for patient counselling and obstetric management. Ultrasound Obstet. Gynecol. 5 (1995) 98–105
25. Chan, A., Robertson, E.F., Haan, E.A., Ranieri, E., Keane, R.J.: The sensitivity of ultrasound and serum alpha-fetoprotein in population-based antenatal screening for neural tube defects. Southern Australia 1986–1991. Brit. J. Obstet. Gynaecol. 102 (1995) 370–376
26. Copel, J.A., Cullen, M., Green, J.J., Mahoney, M.J., Hobbins, J.C., Kleinman, C.S.: The frequency of aneuploidy in prenatally diagnosed congenital heart disease: an indication for fetal karyotyping. Amer. J. Obstet. Gynecol. 158 (1988) 409–413
27. Croen, L.A., Shaw, G.M., Lammer, E.J.: Holoprosencephaly: epidemiologic and clinical characteristics of a California population. Amer. J. Med. Genet. 64 (1996) 465–472
28. De Veciana, M., Major, C.A., Porto, M.: Prediction of an abnormal karyotype in fetuses with omphalocele. Prenat. Diagn. 14 (1994) 487–492
29. Digiovanni, L.M., Quilan, M.P., Verp, M.S.: Choroid plexus cysts: infant and early childhood developmental outcome. Obstet. Gynecol. 90 (1997) 191–194
30. Dildy, G.A., Judd, V.E., Clark, S.L.: Prospective evaluation of the antenatal incidence and postnatal significance of the fetal echogenic cardiac focus: a case-control study. Amer. J. Obstet. Gynecol. 175 (1996) 1008–1012

31. Di Salvo, D.N., Brown, D.L., Doubilet, P.M., Benson, C.B., Frates, M.C.: Clinical significance of isolated fetal pericardial effusion. J. Ultrasound Med. 13 (1994) 291–293
32. Dommergues, M., Louis-Sylvestre, C., Mandelbrot, L. et al.: Congenital adenomatoid malformation of the lung: when is active fetal therapy indicated? Amer. J. Obstet. Gynecol. 177 (1997) 953–958
33. Drugan, A., Johnson, M.P., Isada, N.B. et al.: The smaller than expected first-trimester fetus is at increased risk for chromosome anomalies. Amer. J. Obstet. Gynecol. 167 (1992) 1525–1528
34. Eydoux, P., Choiset, A., Le Porrier, N. et al.: Chromosomal prenatal diagnosis: study of 936 cases of intrauterine abnormalities after ultrasound assessment. Prenat. Diagn. 9 (1989) 255–269
35. Filly, R.A., Chinn, D.H., Callen, P.W.: Alobar holoprosencephaly: ultrasonographic prenatal diagnosis. Radiology 151 (1984) 455–459
36. Geary, M., Patel, S., Lamont, R.: Isolated choroid plexus cysts and association with fetal aneuploidy in an unselected population. Ultrasound Obstet. Gynecol. 10 (1997) 171–173
37. Gembruch, U., Hansmann, M., Bald, R., Zerres, K., Schwanitz, G., Födisch, H.J.: Prenatal diagnosis and management in fetuses with cystic hygromata colli. Eur. J. Obstet. Gynecol. Reprod. Biol. 29 (1988) 241–255
38. Getachew, M.M., Goldstein, R.B., Edge, V., Goldberg, J.D., Filly, R.A.: Correlation between omphalocele contents and karyotypic abnormalities: sonographic study in 37 cases. Amer. J. Roentgenol. 158 (1992) 133–136
39. Grandjean, H., Sarramon, M.F.: Femur/foot length ratio for detection of Down syndrome: results of a multicenter prospective study. Amer. J. Obstet. Gynecol. 173 (1995) 16–19
40. Gratton, R.J., Hogge, W.A., Aston, C.E.: Choroid plexus cysts and trisomy 18: risk modification based on maternal age and multiple-marker screening. Amer. J. Obstet. Gynecol. 175 (1996) 1493–1497
41. Guarglia, L., Rosati, P.: Fetal biometric ratios by transvaginal sonography as a marker for aneuploidies in early pregnancy. Prenat. Diagn. 17 (1997) 415–422
42. Gupta, J.K., Lilford, R.J.: Assessment and management of fetal agenesis of the corpus callosum. Prenat. Diagn. 15 (1995) 301–312
43. Gupta, J.K., Cave, M., Lilford, R.J. et al.: Clinical significance of fetal choroid plexus cysts. Lancet 346 (1995) 724–729
44. Hansmann, M., Gembruch, U., Bald, R.: New therapeutic aspects in nonimmune hydrops fetalis based on four hundred and two prenatally diagnosed cases. Fetal Ther. 4 (1989) 29–36
45. Harmon, J.P., Hiett, A.K., Palmer, C.G., Golichowski, A.M.: Prenatal ultrasound detection of isolated neural tube defects: is cytogenetic evaluation warranted? Obstet. Gynecol. 86 (1995) 595–599
46. Heydanus, R., Spaargaren, M.C., Wladimiroff, J.W.: Prenatal ultrasonic diagnosis of obstructive bowel disease: a retrospective analysis. Prenat. Diagn. 14 (1994) 1035–1041
47. Heydanus, R., Raats, M.A., Tibboel, D., Los, F.J., Wladimiroff, J.W.: Prenatal diagnosis of fetal abdominal wall defects: a retrospective analysis of 44 cases. Prenat. Diagn. 16 (1996) 411–417
48. Howe, D.T., Kilby, M.D., Sirry, H. et al.: Structural chromosome anomalies in congenital diaphragmatic hernia. Prenat. Diagn. 16 (1996) 1003–1009
49. Hyett, J.A., Perdu, M., Sharland, G.K., Snijders, R.S., Nicolaides, K.H.: Increased nuchal translucency at 10–14 weeks of gestation as a marker for major cardiac defects. Ultrasound Obstet. Gynecol. 10 (1997) 242–246
50. Iskaros, J., Jauniaux, E., Rodeck, C.: Outcome of nonimmune hydrops fetalis diagnosed during the first half of pregnancy. Obstet. Gynecol. 90 (1997) 321–325
51. Jauniaux, E., Brown, R., Rodeck, C., Nicolaides, K.H.: Prenatal diagnosis of triploidy during the second trimester of pregnancy. Obstet. Gynecol. 88 (1996) 983–989
52. Jauniaux, E., Brown, R., Snijders, R.J., Noble, P., Nicolaides, K.H.: Early prenatal diagnosis of triploidy. Amer. J. Obstet. Gynecol. 176 (1997) 550–554
53. Johnson, M.P., Michaelson, J.E., Barr, M.Jr. et al.: Combining humerus and femur length for improved ultrasonographic identification of pregnancies at increased risk for trisomy 21. Amer. J. Obstet. Gynecol. 172 (1995) 1229–1235
54. Johnson, S.P., Sebire, N.J., Snijders, R.J., Tunkel, S., Nicolaides, K.H.: Ultrasound screening for anencephaly at 10–14 weeks of gestation. Ultrasound Obstet. Gynecol. 9 (1997) 14–16
55. Kliewer, M.A., Hertzberg, B.S., Freed, K.S. et al.: Dysmorphologic features of the fetal pelvis in Down syndrome: prenatal sonographic depiction and diagnostic implications of the iliac angle. Radiology 201 (1996) 681–684
56. Kuhn, P., Brizot, M.L., Pandya, P.P., Snijders, R.J., Nicolaides, K.H.: Crown-rump length in chromosomally abnormal fetuses at 10 to 13 weeks' gestation. Amer. J. Obstet. Gynecol. 172 (1995) 32–35
57. Kupferminc, M.J., Tamura, R.K., Sabbagha, R.E., Parilla, B.V., Cohen, L.S., Pergament, E.: Isolated choroid plexus cyst(s): an indication for amniocentesis. Amer. J. Obstet. Gynecol. 171 (1994) 1068–1071
58. Langman, J.: Medizinische Embryologie. Die normale menschliche Entwicklung und ihre Fehlbildungen. Stuttgart: Thieme (1972)
59. Lehman, C.D., Nyberg, D.A., Winter, T.C.3rd, Kapur, R.P., Resta, R.G., Luthy, D.A.: Trisomy 13 syndrome: prenatal US findings in a review of 33 cases. Radiology 194 (1995) 217–222
60. Lockwood, C., Scioscia, A., Stiller, R., Hobbins, J.: Sonographic features of the triploid fetus. Amer. J. Obstet. Gynecol. 157 (1987) 285–287
61. Luton, D., De Lagausie, P., Guibourdenche, J. et al.: Prognostic factors of prenatally diagnosed gastroschisis. Fetal Diagn. Ther. 12 (1997) 7–14
62. McCoy, M.C., Katz, V.L., Gould, N., Kuller, J.A.: Non-immune hydrops after 20 weeks' gestation: review of 10 years' experience with suggestions for management. Obstet. Gynecol. 85 (1995) 578–582
63. McCullagh, M., MacConnachie, I., Garvie, D., Dykes, E.: Accuracy of prenatal diagnosis of congenital cystic adenomatoid malformation. Arch. Dis. Child 71 (1994) 111–113
64. McKenna, K.M., Goldstein, R.B., Stringer, M.D.: Small or absent fetal stomach. Prognostic significance. Radiology 197 (1995) 729–733
65. Miller, J.A., Corteville, J.E., Langer, J.C.: Congenital cystic adenomatoid malformation in the fetus: natural history and predictors of outcome. J. Pediatr. Surg. 31 (1996) 805–808
66. Montenegro, N., Matias, A., Areias, J.C., Castedo, S., Barros, H.: Increased fetal nuchal translucency: possible involvement of early cardiac failure. Ultrasound Obstet. Gynecol. 10 (1997) 265–268
67. Nadel, A.S., Bromley, B.S., Frigoletto, F.D.Jr., Estroff, J.A., Benacerraf, B.R.: Isolated choroid plexus cysts in the second-trimester fetus: is amniocentesis really indicated? Radiology 185 (1992) 545–548
68. Nadel, A., Bromley, B., Benacerraf, B.R.: Nuchal thickening or cystic hygromas in first- and early second-trimester fetuses: prognosis and outcome. Obstet. Gynecol. 82 (1993) 43–48
69. Nicolaides, K.H., Berry, S., Snijders, R.J., Thorpe-Beeston, J.G., Gosden, C.: Fetal lateral cerebral ventriculomegaly: associated malformations and chromosomal defects. Fetal Diagn. Ther. 5 (1990) 5–14
70. Nicolaides, K.H., Cheng, H.H., Abbas, A., Snijders, R.J., Gosden, C.: Fetal renal defects: associated malformations and chromosomal defects. Fetal Diagn. Ther. 7 (1992) 1–11
71. Nicolaides, K.H., Snijders, R.J., Cheng, H.H., Gosden, C.: Fetal gastro-intestinal and abdominal wall defects: associated malformations and chromosomal abnormalities. Fetal Diagn. Ther. 7 (1992) 102–115
72. Nicolaides, K.H., Snijders, R.J.M., Gosden, C.M., Berry, C., Campbell, S.: Ultrasonographically detectable markers of fetal chromosomal abnormalities. Lancet 340 (1992) 704–707
73. Nicolaides, K.H., Salvesen, D.R., Snijders, R.J.M., Gosden, C.M.: Fetal facial defects: associated malformations and chromosomal abnormalities. Fetal Diagn. Ther. 8 (1993) 1–9
74. Nyberg, D.A., Mack, L.A., Bronstein, A., Hirsch, J., Pagon, R.A.: Holoprosencephaly: prenatal sonographic diagnosis. Amer. J. Roentgenol. 149 (1987) 1051–1058
75. Nyberg, D.A., Mahony, B.S., Hegge, F.N., Hickok, D., Luthy, D.A., Kapur, R.: Enlarged cisterna magna and the Dandy-Walker malformation: factors associated with chromosomal abnormalities. Obstet. Gynecol. 77 (1991) 436–442
76. Nyberg, D.A., Kramer, D., Resta, R.G. et al.: Prenatal sonographic findings of trisomy 18: review of 47 cases. J. Ultrasound Med. 12 (1993) 103–113
77. Nyberg, D.A., Sickler, G.K., Hegge, F.N., Kramer, D.J., Kropp, R.J.: Fetal cleft lip with and without cleft palate: US classification and correlation with outcome. Radiology 195 (1995) 677–684
78. Paladini, D., Calabro, R., Palmieri, S., D'Andrea, T.: Prenatal Diagnosis of Congenital Heart Disease and Fetal Karyotyping. Obstet. Gynecol. 81 (1993) 679–682
79. Paluda, S.M., Comstock, C.H., Kirk, J.S., Lee, W., Smith, R.S.: The significance of ultrasonographically diagnosed fetal wrist position anomalies. Amer. J. Obstet. Gynecol. 174 (1996) 1834–1837
80. Parilla, B.V., Tamura, R.K., MacGregor, S.N., Geibel, L.J., Sabbagha, R.E.: The clinical significance of a single umbilical artery as an isolated finding on prenatal ultrasound. Obstet. Gynecol. 85 (1995) 570–572
81. Parilla, B.V., Tamura, R.K., Ginsberg, N.A.: Association of parvovirus infection with isolated fetal effusions. Amer. J. Perinatol. 14 (1997) 357–358
82. Patel, M.D., Filly, A.L., Hersh, D.R., Goldstein, R.B.: Isolated mild fetal cerebral ventriculomegaly: clinical course and outcome. Radiology 192 (1994) 759–764
83. Persutte, W.H., Hobbins, J.: Single umbilical artery: a clinical enigma in modern prenatal diagnosis. Ultrasound Obstet. Gynecol. 6 (1995) 216–219
84. Persutte, W.H., Coury, A., Hobbins, J.C.: Correlation of fetal frontal lobe and transcerebellar diameter measurements: the utility of a new prenatal sonographic technique. Ultrasound Obstet. Gynecol. 10 (1997) 94–97
85. Petrikovski, B.M., Challenger, M., Wyse, L.J.: Natural history of echogenic foci within ventricles of the fetal heart. Ultrasound Obstet. Gynecol. 5 (1995) 92–94
86. Ramirez, P., Haberman, S., Baxi, L.: Significance of prenatal diagnosis of umbilical cord cyst in a fetus with trisomy 18. Amer. J. Obstet. Gynecol. 173 (1995) 955–957
87. Ross, J.A., Jurkovich, D., Zosmer, N., Jauniaux, E., Hacket, E., Nicolaides, K.H.: Umbilical cord cysts in early pregnancy. Obstet. Gynecol. 89 (1997) 442–445
88. Sanders, R.C.: Structural Fetal Abnormalities. The Total Picture. St. Louis: Mosby-Year Book 1996
89. Santolaya, J., Alley, D., Jaffe, R., Warsof, S.L.: Antenatal classification of hydrops fetalis. Obstet. Gynecol. 79 (1992) 256–259
90. Schemmer, G., Wapner, R.J., Johnson, A., Schemmer, M., Norton, H.J., Anderson, W.E.: First-trimester growth patterns of aneuploid fetuses. Prenat. Diagn. 17 (1997) 155–159
91. Schwanitz, G., Zerres, K., Gembruch, U., Bald, R., Hansmann, M.: Rate of chromosomal aberrations in prenatally detected hydrops fetalis and hygroma colli. Hum. Genet. 84 (1989) 81–82
92. Scioscia, A.L., Pretorius, D.H., Budorick, N.E., Cahill, T.C., Axelrod, F.T., Leopold, G.R.: Second-trimester echogenic bowel and chromosomal abnormalities. Amer. J. Obstet. Gynecol. 167 (1992) 889–894
93. Sebire, N.J., D'Ercole, C., Hughes, K., Carvalho, M., Nicolaides, K.H.: Increased nuchal translucency thickness at 10–14 weeks of gestation as a predictor of severe twin-to-twin transfusion syndrome. Ultrasound Obstet. Gynecol. 10 (1997) 86–89
94. Sepulveda, W., Sebire, N.J., Fung, T.Y., Pipi, E., Nicolaides, K.H.: Crown-chin length in normal and anencephalic fetuses at 10 to 14 weeks' gestation. Amer. J. Obstet. Gynecol. 176 (1997) 852–855
95. Sharland, G.K., Lockhart, S.M., Heward, A.J., Allan, L.D.: Prognosis in fetal diaphragmatic hernia. Amer. J. Obstet. Gynecol. 166 (1992) 9–13
96. Sharland, G., Lockhart, S.: Isolated pericardial effusion: an indication for fetal karyotyping? Ultrasound Obstet. Gynecol. 6 (1995) 29–32
97. Sharony, R.: Fetal choroid plexus cysts – is a genetic evaluation indicated? Prenat. Diagn. 17 (1997) 519–524
98. Shenker, L., Reed, K.L., Anderson, C.F., Kern, W.: Fetal pericardial effusion. Amer. J. Obstet. Gynecol. 160 (1989) 1505–1507
99. Shipp, T.D., Bromley, B., Lieberman, E., Benacerraf, B.R.: The iliac angle as a sonographic marker for Down syndrome in second-trimester fetuses. Obstet. Gynecol. 89 (1997) 446–450
100. Slotnick, R.N., Abuhamad, A.Z.: Prognostic implications of fetal echogenic bowel. Lancet 347 (1996) 85–87

101. Smith, G.N., Walker, M., Johnston, S., Ash, K.: The sonographic finding of persistent umbilical cord cystic masses is associated with lethal aneuploidy and/or congenital anomalies. Prenat. Diagn. 16 (1996) 1141–1147

102. Snijders, R.J., Sherrod, C., Gosden, C.M., Nicolaides, K.H.: Fetal growth retardation: associated malformations and chromosomal abnormalities. Amer. J. Obstet. Gynecol. 168 (1993) 547–555

103. Snijders, R.J., Sebire, N.J., Souka, A., Santiago, C., Nicolaides, K.H.: Fetal exomphalos and chromosomal defects: relationship to maternal age and gestation. Ultrasound Obstet. Gynecol. 6 (1995) 250–255

104. Snijders, R.J., Sebire, N.J., Psara, N., Souka, A., Nicolaides, K.H.: Prevalence of fetal facial cleft at different ages of pregnancy. Ultrasound Obstet. Gynecol. 6 (1995) 327–329

105. Snijders, R.J.M., Nicolaides, K.H.: Ultrasound markers for fetal chromosomal defects. New York: Parthenon Publishing Group 1996

106. Stringer, M.D., McKenna, K.M., Goldstein, R.B., Filly, R.A., Adzick, N.S., Harrison, M.R.: Prenatal diagnosis of esophageal atresia. J. Pediatr. Surg. 30 (1995) 1258–1263

107. Stümpflen, I., Stümpflen, A., Wimmer, M., Bernaschek, G.: Effect of detailed fetal echocardiography as part of routine prenatal ultrasonographic screening on detection of congenital heart disease. Lancet 348 (1996) 854–857

108. Taipale, P., Hiilesmaa, V., Salonen, R., Ylostalo, P.: Increased nuchal translucency as a marker for fetal chromosomal defects. New Engl. J. Med. 337 (1997) 1689–1690

109. Ulm, B., Ulm, M.R., Deutinger, J., Bernaschek, G.: Dandy-Walker malformation diagnosed before 21 weeks of gestation: associated malformations and chromosomal abnormalities. Ultrasound Obstet. Gynecol. 10 (1997) 167–170

110. Ulm, B., Ulm, M.R., Deutinger, J., Bernaschek, G.: Umbilical artery Doppler velocimetry in fetuses with a single umbilical artery. Obstet. Gynecol. 90 (1997) 205–259

111. Van Zalen-Sprock, R.M., Vugt, J.M., van Geijn, H.P.: First-trimester sonography of physiological midgut herniation and early diagnosis of omphalocele. Prenat. Diagn. 17 (1997) 511–518

112. Vergani, P., Ghiaini, A., Strobelt, N. et al.: Prognostic indicators in the prenatal diagnosis of agenesis of corpus callosum. Amer. J. Obstet. Gynecol. 170 (1994) 753–758

113. Vintzileos, A.M., Egan, J.F.: Adjusting the risk for trisomy 21 on the basis of second-trimester ultrasonography. Amer. J. Obstet. Gynecol. 172 (1995) 837–844

114. Vintzileos, A.M., Campbell, W.A., Rodis, J.F., Guzman, E.R., Smulian, J.C., Knuppel, R.A.: The use of second-trimester genetic sonogram in guiding clinical management of patients at increased risk for fetal trisomy 21. Obstet. Gynecol. 87 (1996) 948–952

115. Vintzileos, A.M., Egan, J.F., Smulian, J.C., Campbell, W.A., Guzman, E.R., Rodis, J.F.: Adjusting the risk for trisomy 21 by a simple ultrasound method using fetal long-bone biometry. Obstet. Gynecol. 87 (1996) 953–958

116. Vintzileos, A.M., Campbell, W.A., Guzman, E.R., Smulian, J.C., McLean, D.A., Ananth, C.V.: Second-trimester ultrasound markers for detection of trisomy 21: which markers are the best? Obstet. Gynecol. 89 (1997) 941–944

117. Wickstrom, E.A., Thangavelu, M., Parilla, B.V., Tamura, R.K., Sabbagha, R.E.: A prospective study of the association between isolated fetal pyelectasis and chromosomal abnormality. Obstet. Gynecol. 88 (1996) 379–382

118. Wilkins, I.: Separation of the great toe in fetuses with Down syndrome. J. Ultrasound Med. 13 (1994) 229–231

119. Williamson, P., Alberman, E., Rodeck, C., Fiddler, M., Church, S., Harris, R.: Antecedent circumstances surrounding neural tube defect births in 1990–1991. The Steering Committee of the National Confidential Enquiry into Counselling for Genetic Disorders. Brit. J. Obstet. Gynaecol. 104 (1997) 51–56

120. Zimmer, E.Z., Drugan, A., Ofir, C., Blazer, S., Bronshtein, M.: Ultrasound imaging of fetal neck anomalies: implications for the risk of aneuploidy and structural anomalies. Prenat. Diagn. 17 (1997) 1055–1058

33 Ultrasound Features of Infectious Diseases in Pregnancy

Possible sequelae of intrauterine infections. Whether intrauterine exposure to viruses or microorganisms will lead to embryopathy or fetopathy depends not only on the infecting organism and the pathogenesis of the infection but also to a large degree on the gestational age at the time of the infection (70). Additional factors are the maternal and fetal immune status and the concentration and virulence of the pathogens. A maternal infectious disease during pregnancy does not necessarily lead to an embryonic or fetal infection. If an intrauterine infection does occur, it may take an asymptomatic course. But some organisms can produce a disseminated, sepsis-like condition that can lead to ultrasound abnormalities such as intrauterine growth retardation, microcephaly, ventriculomegaly, fetal hydrops, and hyperechoic foci in the cerebrum, liver, or bowel. Infection of the embryo can also induce organ malformations.

Awareness of typical stigmata. The attending gynecologist should be familiar with the sonomorphologic stigmata that are typical of the most common prenatal infections. This is important in two respects:
1. The detection or exclusion of sonomorphologic abnormalities in cases of known maternal infection can provide an additional criterion that is useful in counseling pregnant women on possible fetal consequences, and it may modify further diagnostic and therapeutic procedures.

For example, if a maternal varicella infection is contracted during the first half of pregnancy, the risk of intrauterine infection is approximately 10%. But the risk that the fetus will develop a prognostically unfavorable varicella syndrome, which includes unilateral limb hypoplasias, scarification of the skin, and ocular and CNS abnormalities, is only about 2% (8). At the same time, the ultrasound detection of joint contractures or limb hypoplasias is virtually pathognomonic for a congenital varicella syndrome.

Another example relates to the ultrasound surveillance of pregnancies with a confirmed parvovirus B19 infection. Finding nonimmune fetal hydrops in these cases is the key criterion for proceeding with a life-saving intrauterine fetal transfusion.

2. If ultrasound screening reveals nonimmune fetal hydrops or other stigmata that may be associated with a fetal infection, the differential diagnosis should go beyond chromosomal abnormalities, cardiac anomalies, malformation syndromes, and various metabolic disorders to include the group of congenital infections known under the acronym TORCH (Table 33.1). Armed with a precise infection history and maternal serologic findings, the physician can then consult with the patient to decide whether further invasive tests (amniocentesis, cordocentesis) should be performed.

Principal signs. Table 33.2 lists the principal sonomorphologic signs of congenital infections that are accessible to prenatal diagnosis. It is generally true that even a meticulous ultrasound examination cannot confirm or exclude a prenatal infection with complete confidence (48). Nevertheless, the detection or exclusion of ultrasound abnormalities that are typical of prenatal infections can provide an important criterion for counseling the patient and planning further management. A knowledge of these typical signs also contributes to the efficient use of serologic studies.

Table 33.1 List of TORCH infections that can cause fetal disease through transplacental (*) and/or perinatal transmission (adapted from 7). Bold type indicates the prenatal infections for which ultrasound abnormalities have been described

T	**Toxoplasmosis*** *(Toxoplasma gondii)*

O	Other infectious microorganisms:
	 Parvovirus B19*
	 Varicella*/herpes zoster (varicella-zoster virus)
	 Coxsackie infection* (coxsackie ECHO viruses)
	 Lymphocytic choriomeningitis* (LCM virus)
	 Syphilis* *(Treponema pallidum)*
	 Measles* (measles virus)
	 Mumps* (mumps virus)
	 Hepatitis* (hepatitis viruses B, C, D, E, G)
	 HIV* (human immunodeficiency virus)
	 Malaria* (plasmodia)
	 Influenza* (influenza A virus)
	 Mononucleosis* (Epstein–Barr virus)
	 Borreliosis* *(Borrelia burgdorferi)*
	 Listeriosis* *(Listeria monocytogenes)*
	 Gonorrhea (gonococci)
	 Urogenital colonization with chlamydia *(Chlamydia trachomatis)*
	     Papillomaviruses (HPV), mycoplasma (Mycoplasma hominis,
	     Ureaplasma urealyticum), and streptococci (group B)

R	**Rubella*** (rubella virus)
C	**Cytomegalovirus***
H	Herpes simplex (herpes simplex virus)

Table 33.2 Principal ultrasound signs of the most common infections that can be diagnosed prenatally

Infection	Main ultrasound signs
Toxoplasmosis	Hydrocephalus Intracranial calcifications Fetal hydrops
Parvovirus B19 infection	Fetal hydrops
Varicella	Limb hypoplasia Joint contractures Cutaneous edema
Coxsackie infection	Cardiomegaly Pericardial effusion Fetal hydrops
Lymphocytic choriomeningitis	Hydrocephalus Growth retardation
Syphilis	Fetal hydrops Hepatomegaly
Rubella	Growth retardation Microcephaly Cardiac anomalies
Cytomegalovirus	Fetal hydrops Growth retardation Microcephaly Hydrocephalus Intracranial calcifications

The Most Common Infectious Diseases

▬ *Toxoplasmosis*

Causative Organism

Route of infection. Toxoplasmosis is caused by the coccidian protozoon *Toxoplasma gondii.* The definitive host is the cat, in which the obligate intracellular parasite reproduces. Humans, numerous mammals, and birds serve as intermediate hosts. Humans acquire the infection from the oocysts contained in cat feces, which may be ingested in contaminated fruits, vegetables, etc. The disease may also be transmitted by ingesting bradyzoites in meats or sausages that have not been adequately heated.

Initial infection. In a new infection, the presence of tachyzoites in the blood induces antibody formation and immobilization of the pathogens, which persist for the life span of the host, mainly in muscle tissue and in the brain. The toxoplasmosis infection confers lifelong immunity, and reinfection generally does not occur in immunocompetent individuals. The seroprevalence in women of childbearing age is between 30% and 40% (7). Toxoplasmosis poses a threat to the unborn only when contracted as an initial infection during pregnancy, for it is only during the parasitemic phase that the organisms can cross the placental barrier.

Clinical Aspects and Treatment

Transmission rate. Approximately two to four in 1000 live-born infants have a congenital toxoplasmosis infection. The transmission rate depends on the gestational age and the time of the initial infection. It is 15% in the first trimester, approximately 30% in the second trimester, and 60–70% in the third trimester. Initial infections in the first trimester are transmitted to the fetus less often than infections acquired later, but they tend to take a less favorable course than later infections.

Complete picture. The relatively rare complete picture of congenital toxoplasmosis includes a florid meningoencephalitis with intracerebral calcifications, hydrocephalus, and chorioretinitis. Infected fetuses may also develop sepsis-like symptoms such as jaundice, hepatosplenomegaly, thrombocytopenia, and pulmonary involvement.

Late manifestations. Some 90% of infants with a prenatal infection are asymptomatic at birth. No reliable data are available on the incidence of late manifestations such as chorioretinitis, intellectual deficits, and cerebral seizures (9).

Treatment. With an acute toxoplasmosis infection, intrauterine transplacental therapy (administration of spiramycin, 2–3 g/day, or pyrimethamine and sulfonamide) can probably reduce the risk of congenital toxoplasmosis by one-half. All infants with serologically confirmed congenital toxoplasmosis, whether clinically overt or subclinical, should be treated with cycles of pyrimethamine, sulfadiazine, corticosteroids, and folic acid during the first year of life (7).

Main Ultrasound Signs

Ventriculomegaly. The main ultrasound sign of a prenatal toxoplasmosis infection is ventriculomegaly. By comparison, intracranial calcifications are not commonly seen. This is also true of fetal hydrops. Among our own patients, we found sonomorphologic abnormalities in only four of 73 cases that were referred to us for ultrasound evaluation over a 5-year period for an acute toxoplasmosis infection contracted during pregnancy. We observed hydrocephalus in two cases, intracerebral calcifications and hepatomegaly in one case, and subtle signs of fetal hydrops in one case.

Diagnosis

Based on the nonspecific signs that are associated with a new infection, serologic tests are the primary tool for the diagnosis of acute toxoplasmosis (21).

Screening. In Germany, unlike France and Austria, toxoplasmosis screening has not become a routine part of prenatal care. An early toxoplasmosis test at the pregnancy planning stage would be ideal for screening purposes. A positive Sabin–Feldman test or positive indirect immunofluorescence test would signify immunity. Seronegatives, meanwhile, would be urged to take certain precautions after conceiving (avoid contact with cats, wash fruits and vegetables thoroughly, avoid raw meats) and should receive additional serologic tests in the second and third trimesters to exclude a primary infection during pregnancy (14). Arguments against general screening are the existence of many diverse tests with different units of measurement and the fact that IgM titers can persist for up to 14 months.

Testing and detection in suspected cases. All pregnant women who present with lymph node swelling or flu-like symptoms should be given an immediate serologic test for toxoplasmosis (15). In the diagnosis of toxoplasmosis, the referring physician must rely on the interpretation of the laboratory technologist (9). When it is found that a woman has contracted toxoplasmosis during pregnancy, fetal infection can be diagnosed by determining IgM in the fetal blood or detecting tachyzoites in the amniotic fluid by PCR; the latter method is preferred (13). Pregnant women with a primary toxoplasmosis infection should always be treated and the fetuses monitored by close-interval serial scans. Normal ultrasound anatomy does not exclude congenital toxoplasmosis or late sequelae, however.

Management of Primary Toxoplasmosis Infection with Ultrasound Abnormalities

If toxoplasmosis-associated abnormalities are found at prenatal ultrasound, the likelihood of congenital toxoplasmosis is increased. In cases with hydrocephalus and hydrops, the option of pregnancy termination should be discussed due to the very poor prognosis. If the pregnancy is continued, transplacental therapy with pyrimethamine and sulfonamides is indicated.

▬ *Parvovirus B19 Infection (Erythema Infectiosum)*

Causative Organism

Parvovirus B19 infection is caused by the human parvovirus (B19), first identified as the cause of erythema infectiosum in 1983 (1). Parvoviruses are a group of extremely small, nonenveloped, icosahedral viruses that contain a single DNA strand as genetic material and show a pronounced tropism for erythropoid precursor cells (7).

Clinical Aspects

Anemia and fetal hydrops. Parvovirus B19 can be transmitted to the fetus across the placenta throughout pregnancy. Parvoviruses were first identified as a possible cause of nonimmune fetal hydrops in 1984 (5).

The viruses compromise the function of the hematopoietic organs through the infection and lysis of erythropoid precursor cells. Because normal hematopoiesis quickly resumes in healthy children and adults following the initial synthesis of specific IgM and IgG, and normal erythrocytes have a life span of 120 days, the hematologic effects of the disease are detectable but clinically unimportant (28). Hemoglobin levels may fall dramatically, however, in patients with various underlying hematologic disorders and in fetuses. Infected fetuses may become hydropic due to severe anemia and, if untreated, are at high risk for intrauterine death.

Incidence. Tercanli et al. (46) reported an approximately 10% risk that a parvovirus B19 infection would lead to severe fetal anemia with hydrops based on published data available at the time. Enders (10) found a 17.5% rate of fetal hydrops in 874 pregnant women with a primary parvovirus B19 infection. Recent prospective data have shown that the risk of hydrops is probably lower than previously thought: Miller et al. (32) found only 7 cases of hydrops in 367 cases of confirmed maternal infection. The risk was highest (3.8%) for maternal infections contracted between 13 and 16 weeks' gestation. No cases of fetal hydrops were found in this series when infection was contracted after 20 weeks. Intrauterine death occurred in just 10% of fetuses infected during the first half of pregnancy. Among our own cases, 58 women with a primary parvovirus infection were referred for further testing during the past 5 years, and 16 of these cases were found to have fetal hydrops. Intrauterine fetal death occurred in four cases.

Risk of fetal anomalies. No fetal anomalies were documented in our own case material. Parvovirus B19 infection does not appear to be associated with a clinically significant risk of malformations. There are isolated case reports on meconium peritonitis and intestinal anomalies following fetal parvovirus infection, which may have been secondary to vasculitis (40). There is speculation as to whether the B19 virus can directly infect cells of mesoendodermal origin that express the receptor P antigen (10). This could account for the organ malformations that have been described in association with parvovirus infections (34, 37, 47, 49). However, prospective and retrospective data in large clinical populations have shown no significant risk of anomalies secondary to fetal parvovirus infections (20, 32).

Main Ultrasound Signs

The ultrasound hallmark of prenatal parvovirus B19 infection is generalized fetal hydrops, which may assume extreme proportions when hemoglobin values are low.

Diagnosis

It is estimated that parvovirus B19 infections are responsible for approximately 10–15% of nonimmune fetal hydrops cases (33). This means that parvovirus B19 infection is an extremely important differential diagnosis in all fetuses that exhibit nonimmune hydrops.

History and serology. An accurate history can corroborate the suspicion of infection. Often, patients must be carefully questioned before they will recall a characteristic, fleeting maculopapular rash on the trunk and limbs. Fifty percent of infected adults also complain of joint pain in the hands and feet. But because the disease runs a subclinical course in about one-third of adults, finding nonimmune fetal hydrops should trigger a parvovirus B19 IgG and IgM antibody determination in the maternal blood even in patients who give no history of infection. After 17 weeks' gestation, cordocentesis should additionally be performed for a hemoglobin determination. In 80% of cases the virus can be directly detected in the fetal blood by PCR. By comparison, an IgM assay in the fetal blood is of minor importance because only 20% of infected

fetuses show an elevated IgM (10). If the history is suspicious for a maternal infection but fetal hydrops is not found, serologic testing of the maternal blood is sufficient. The same applies to contact cases that present no symptoms.

Ultrasound follow-ups. If maternal serologic testing detects a primary parvovirus B19 infection, fetal anomalies and subtle signs of hydrops should be excluded by a qualified sonographer, and weekly follow-up scans should be scheduled. The sonomorphologic examination can be supplemented by Doppler scanning to determine the peak systolic flow velocities in the middle cerebral artery (31). Increased flow velocities in the fetal cerebral blood vessels, like the presence of hydrops, are considered to be a sign of fetal anemia.

Management of Primary Parvovirus B19 Infection with Ultrasound Abnormalities

Umbilical cord transfusion. The treatment of choice for fetal hydrops caused by parvovirus B19 infection is the umbilical cord transfusion of packed red blood cells. Spontaneous remissions can occur with conservative treatment (12, 26, 38), but intrauterine therapy leads to significantly higher rates of fetal survival (11). The lowest hemoglobin value that we found in our own cases was 1.7 g%. Twelve of 13 fetuses that were transfused for parvovirus infection survived. One hydropic fetus died during an umbilical cord transfusion performed in the 19th week of gestation. Two fetuses with extremely low hemoglobin values (2.2 and 2.0 g%) died in the interval between diagnostic cordocentesis and the transfusion scheduled for the next day. In another case, intrauterine fetal death occurred at only 14 weeks.

Number of transfusions. In contrast to the regimen for erythroblastosis, one or two transfusions are usually sufficient, since the erythrocytes formed by the fetus itself after recovery of the hematopoietic organs are not lysed and the hemoglobin values gradually rise again on their own. In a few cases, however, four or five transfusions may be necessary. The precise reason for this is still unknown. All surviving fetuses have developed normally thus far, including those with extremely low hemoglobin values.

Timing the transfusion. It is our practice to draw maternal and fetal blood simultaneously in all cases of nonimmune fetal hydrops detected after 16 weeks' gestation. If low hemoglobin values are found and a parvovirus infection is a diagnostic possibility, we do not await the results of serologic tests but proceed with an umbilical cord transfusion as soon as possible—on the same day if hemoglobin values are extremely low. We accept the fact that, in a few cases, the serologic findings will show that the umbilical cord transfusion was not indicated. There were two anemic, hydropic fetuses in our series that had a primary cytomegalovirus infection. Both fetuses died later in the pregnancy after undergoing a single intrauterine transfusion.

Prognosis. It is our view that the high mortality risk of severe, untreated fetal anemia and the good prognosis of parvovirus B19 infection treated by intrauterine therapy justify the use of this procedure. Parents and referring physicians should be informed about the excellent success rates of intrauterine transfusions and the good long-term prognosis of parvovirus B19 infection, even with pronounced fetal hydrops and severe fetal anemia, and should be encouraged to apply this type of therapy.

■ *Varicella (Chickenpox)*

Causative Organism

The varicella-zoster virus belongs to the group of herpes viruses. The highly contagious pathogen is transmitted by droplet infection and confers a stable, life-long immunity, virtually eliminating the risk of second infections. The virus does persist in sensory ganglia, however, and it can be reactivated as herpes zoster in immunocompromised patients.

Clinical Aspects

Given the high endemicity of varicella in the general population, it is unlikely that an infection will be contracted during pregnancy. Some 93–94% of all women of childbearing age have already had chickenpox during childhood and are immune (7).

Congenital varicella syndrome. When a varicella infection occurs in the first half of pregnancy, there is risk of congenital varicella syndrome marked by cutaneous scarring and ulcerations, limb hypoplasias, muscular atrophy, chorioretinitis, and cerebral seizures. Though it has a high mortality, this syndrome is rare. Enders et al. (9) showed in a prospective multicenter study that when a primary varicella infection is contracted during the first half of pregnancy, a congenital varicella syndrome develops in only about 2% of cases. Infection near term is problematic, as it carries a risk of severe neonatal varicella.

Herpes zoster. By contrast, herpes zoster does not have a viremic phase. As a result, herpes zoster during pregnancy is not associated with embryopathy or perinatal infection (16).

Main Ultrasound Signs

Limb hypoplasias. The main ultrasound findings are limb hypoplasias and joint contractures. In one of our patients who contracted varicella about one week after conception, we noted hypoplasia of the fetal left hand in the 18th week of gestation (Fig. 33.**1**). When serologic tests confirmed a recent varicella infection, the patient opted for pregnancy termination based on the high risk of a congenital varicella syndrome indicated by the ultrasound findings. Viral hybridization in various fetal tissues yielded positive results.

Tercanli et al. (46) described one case of varicella syndrome in which ultrasound revealed massive cutaneous edema. In another case report, a congenital varicella syndrome was manifested by early growth retardation, limb hypoplasias, and multiple intra-abdominal and thoracic calcifications (22).

Diagnosis

Serologic tests. Chickenpox is easily diagnosed by its clinical presentation. Serologic confirmation is based on IgG and IgM antibody detection and high complement fixation titers (46). If a pregnant woman has had contact with infected individuals during the first half of pregnancy or near term, her immune status can be quantitatively determined by the detection of IgG antibodies. A very rapid determination can be made with the varicella agglutination test. Seronegative women exposed to varicella up to 22 weeks or near term should receive passive immunization.

Ultrasound examination. When varicella is contracted during the first half of pregnancy, invasive testing is not recommended due to the low rate of varicella embryopathy (46). The effects of this embryopathy are very severe, however (16), and so a qualified ultrasound examination should be performed at about 20 weeks to check for typical stigmata.

Management of Primary Varicella Infection with Ultrasound Abnormalities

If sonomorphologic stigmata such as limb hypoplasias, joint contractures, or cutaneous edema are noted in the first half of pregnancy with a serologically confirmed varicella infection, pregnancy termination is indicated. There is no need for further invasive studies.

■ *Coxsackie Infection*

Causative Organism

Coxsackie and enteric cytopathic human orphan (ECHO) viruses belong to the group of enteroviruses. These viruses occur in a variety of types and produce only nonspecific cold-like symptoms that may include myalgia.

Clinical Aspects

Two case control studies published by the same group of authors indicate that coxsackievirus infection acquired during pregnancy is associated with increased rates of miscarriages and stillbirths (2, 17). Infections contracted in the third trimester can be transmitted across the placenta and may produce sepsis-like manifestations in the fetus (42). Individual case reports and data from animal studies indicate that coxsackieviruses can cause fetal myocarditis (25, 39). Coxsackievirus infections in pregnancy have also been related to the occurrence of juvenile diabetes (6, 27). Perinatally acquired coxsackie and ECHO virus infections can cause severe meningoencephalitis and myocarditis with a high mortality, especially in premature infants.

Main Ultrasound Signs

The cardinal ultrasound signs of an intrauterine coxsackie infection are cardiomegaly, pericardial effusion, and decreased myocardial contractility. Coxsackie infection should also be included in the differential diagnosis of nonimmune fetal hydrops (35).

Diagnosis

Viral isolation is the principal method used in the laboratory diagnosis of enteroviral infections (7). Due to a lack of epidemiologic data, we do not know the frequency of infections during pregnancy. No prospective data are available on pregnancy outcomes in coxsackievirus infections. Coxsackieviruses should be sought in all unexplained cases of nonimmune fetal hydrops, especially if there are concomitant signs of fetal myocarditis.

Management of Coxsackie Infection with Ultrasound Abnormalities

If a coxsackie infection is found during the investigation of fetal hydrops or fetal pericardial effusion, the prognosis is uncertain. We recommend a conservative approach with serial scans obtained at frequent intervals. The surveillance should be intensified in the third trimester, and the timing of the delivery should be planned according to the fetal status evaluated in consultation with a neonatologist and pediatric cardiologist.

Lymphocytic Choriomeningitis

Causative Organism

The lymphocytic choriomeningitis (LCM) virus belongs to the group of arenaviruses. The natural host is the domestic mouse. Another source of infection is the Syrian hamster, which can transmit the virus through bites or in its urine (7).

Clinical Aspects

Transplacental transmission of the LCM virus to the fetus can occur at any stage of pregnancy (3). The symptoms in most cases are nonspecific, and therefore a clinical diagnosis usually cannot be made. Infections in the first trimester lead to an increased spontaneous abortion rate. LCM infections in the second and third trimesters can cause fetal hydrocephalus and chorioretinitis (29).

Main Ultrasound Signs

The ultrasound hallmark of a prenatal LCM infection is hydrocephalus after toxoplasmosis and cytomegalovirus have been excluded as the cause.

Diagnosis

The diagnosis is established by viral isolation and antibody detection in the maternal blood (7).

Management of LCM Infection with Ultrasound Abnormalities

If the extended serologic investigation of prenatal hydrocephalus indicates an LCM infection, the prognosis is uncertain. As with cytomegalovirus infection, prenatal therapy is not possible. Because no prospective data are available on the anticipated rate of fetal harm and the extent of potential disabilities, a conservative approach is recommended. Pregnancy termination is reasonable only in fetuses who exhibit very pronounced hydrocephalus of early onset.

Syphilis

Causative Organism

Syphilis is caused by the spirochetal bacterium *Treponema pallidum*, which is transmitted almost exclusively by sexual contact.

Clinical Aspects and Treatment

Congenital syphilis. Congenital syphilis, which still had a shockingly high incidence in the last century, has become rare today owing to effective prevention programs and modern diagnostic and therapeutic options. In 1966, for example, only three cases of congenital syphilis were documented in Germany (36). The majority of infected infants appear healthy at birth and present initial symptoms at 2–12 weeks, consisting of a maculopapular rash, persistent rhinitis, and hepatosplenomegaly. Typical late manifestations of congenital syphilis are interstitial keratitis, sensorineural hearing loss, dental changes, and foci of inflammatory periosteal thickening on the tibiae. In untreated cases, cardiovascular or neurologic symptoms may appear following a latent period of several years.

Maternal syphilis infection. With a maternal syphilis infection, *Treponema pallidum* may be transmitted to the fetus via the placenta at any time during the pregnancy, but usually not before 18 weeks. As the bacterial burden increases, the risk of fetal infection rises. The transmission risk is highest when the pregnant woman is in the secondary stage marked by systemic symptoms and mucocutaneous lesions. Pregnant women with syphilis have increased rates of spontaneous abortion, stillbirth, and premature delivery.

Treatment. The treatment of choice for maternal syphilis infection is 2.4 million units/day of penicillin G for 14 days, administered by intramuscular injection. For safety, the same regimen can be applied 1–2 months before the due date.

Main Ultrasound Signs

Generally a syphilis infection is diagnosed not from sonomorphologic signs but from the clinical examination and serologic findings. But since hydrops has been described in infected fetuses (7), congenital syphilis should be included in the differential diagnosis of nonimmune fetal hydrops.

Diagnosis

Screening. The customary screening test is the *Treponema pallidum* hemagglutination (TPHA) test, which can detect IgG and IgM antibodies by only the second week after infection. This test is positive in all stages of the disease. IgG antibodies can also be detected for life following successful therapy or spontaneous recovery, but they do not protect against recurrent infection. The TPHA test is performed routinely in early pregnancy. If it is negative, there is no need for further studies unless there is clinical evidence suspicious for an early infection.

High-risk groups. A second TPHA test in the third trimester is recommended for high-risk populations (36). If the test is positive, a fluorescence treponemal antibody absorption (FTA-ABS) test or TP-ELISA test should be done for confirmation. The cardiolipin test (Venereal Disease Research Laboratory test) and quantitative IgM antibody assay can determine the need for treatment and can also assess therapeutic response.

Management of Syphilis Infection with Ultrasound Abnormalities

Every newly acquired or inadequately treated old syphilis infection that is diagnosed during pregnancy should be treated at once with penicillin, regardless of whether the fetus appears sonographically normal or fetal hydrops is observed. Given the rarity of syphilis-induced hydrops, the full spectrum of diagnostic possibilities should be considered when a syphilis infection is detected.

Rubella

Causative Organism

Rubella is caused by the rubella virus, which is a small RNA togavirus. It is transmitted by direct contact with infected droplets.

Clinical Aspects

Gregg syndrome. The triad of cataract, cardiac anomalies, and deafness first described in 1941 by the ophthalmologist Sir Norman Gregg (18), often referred to as "Gregg's syndrome," is a classic example of embryopathy caused by maternal infection. The classic triad may be accompanied by mental and psychomotor retardation, occasional signs of generalized infection (hepatosplenomegaly, thrombocytopenic purpura, rash), and growth retardation.

Incidence. With more effective inoculation strategies and improved laboratory methods, the incidence of rubella embryopathy has declined in most industrialized countries from approximately one in 1000 live births to a rate between one in 6000 and over one in 12,000 (46). A rubella infection in early pregnancy entails a high risk of embryopathy. When the infection is contracted during the first 6 weeks of gestation, approximately two-thirds of fetuses will develop a rubella syndrome. Infections acquired in later weeks are associated with lower risks: approximately 25% between 7 and 9 weeks, 20% between 10 and 12 weeks, and 10% between 13 and 17 weeks. Periconceptional infections and infections after 18 weeks' gestation do not pose a risk to the conceptus.

Main Ultrasound Signs

Cardiac anomalies, microcephaly, and IUGR. The anomaly typically found in rubella embryopathy is a ventricular septal defect or tetralogy of Fallot. Additional stigmata seen at ultrasound are growth retardation and microcephaly. It should be emphasized that ultrasound is less important than serology in rubella infections, especially when the infection is diagnosed during the first 12 weeks of pregnancy. But if a cardiac anomaly, microcephaly, or early growth retardation is noted at the second ultrasound screening, the rubella findings obtained in previous routine antenatal tests should be checked and updated if necessary to exclude an occult rubella infection.

Diagnosis

Serologic tests in pregnant women. Women who exhibit possible rubella symptoms (swollen lymph nodes, especially in the neck; a patchy, nonconfluent rash that starts behind the ear and spreads quickly to the face, back, and extensor surfaces of the extremities) should undergo serologic testing with antibody determination. Rubella-specific IgG and IgM antibodies can be detected just 3–6 days after the rash appears (46). But because IgM antibodies can persist for a long time, the presence of elevated IgM antibodies without clinical symptoms requires additional tests to distinguish a new, clinically asymptomatic infection from an older infection with persistent antibodies. Today most serologic problems can be solved by means of short-interval follow-ups and test combinations for IgG avidity, IgA antibody detection, and immunoblot testing performed in a specialized laboratory (10).

Invasive tests. In pregnant women with a primary rubella infection, the detection of IgM antibodies in the fetal blood provides an index for diagnosing fetal rubella infection. But since IgM antibody production may still be too low before 21 weeks' gestation, cordocentesis should be performed no earlier than 22 weeks to avoid false-negative results (10). Another current option is viral detection in chorionic villi or amniotic fluid. But considering the extremely high risk of embryopathy when rubella infection is detected serologically during the first 10 weeks of pregnancy, it is also reasonable to terminate the pregnancy in these circumstances and avoid further invasive testing. An alternative is to begin the testing with amniocentesis or chorion villus sampling. But a negative finding should be confirmed by cordocentesis at 22 weeks (46). The diagnostic accuracy of prenatal testing is as high as 94%. The parents should be informed that even when the amniotic fluid, chorionic villi, and cord blood are negative, rubella embryopathy still cannot be ruled out with absolute certainty. A normal ultrasound examination cannot exclude fetal rubella infection.

Management of Primary Rubella Infection with Ultrasound Abnormalities

If ultrasound abnormalities such as cardiac defects, microcephaly, or early growth retardation are found in association with a rubella infection contracted in early pregnancy, the amniotic fluid, chorionic villi, or fetal blood should be tested for rubella virus to obtain further confirmation. Cordocentesis to determine IgM titers should be done no earlier than 22 weeks. Given the potential for false-negative serologic and virologic findings in the fetal blood, however, pregnancy termination should be considered in cases where a rubella infection has been contracted in early pregnancy and ultrasound abnormalities are found. This option should be discussed with the parents even in cases with negative viral detection or negative fetal IgM values.

Cytomegalovirus Infection

Causative Organism

Belonging to the group of herpes viruses (41), cytomegalovirus is composed of double-stranded DNA. As with all herpes viruses, the primary infection is followed by lifelong persistence of the genome with a potential for reactivation.

Clinical Aspects

Incidence. Cytomegalovirus is the most frequent viral cause of congenital infections leading to pediatric diseases and late sequelae. The incidence of congenitally infected newborns in Germany is approximately 0.3–1%. An initial infection acquired in the first or second trimester carries the greatest risk of fetal harm. Although new infections contracted during pregnancy have an intrauterine infection rate of 40%, only one-third of infected infants display symptoms at birth or develop late sequelae.

Abnormal findings. Infected infants may exhibit low birth weight, petechiae, jaundice, as well as microcephaly and seizures. Typical laboratory findings are thrombocytopenia and elevated liver values. Chorioretinitis and intracranial calcifications also aid in making a diagnosis. Children who already manifest clinical signs of cytomegalovirus infection as newborns exhibit a high mortality (30%). Approximately 70% of the survivors have psychomotor or mental retardation.

Reactivated infections. In contrast to primary CMV infections, reactivated infections in the presence of maternal IgG antibodies apparently pose little fetal risk. It is difficult in laboratory tests to distinguish between primary and reactivated infections, however, because long-persisting IgM antibodies and reinfections with new IgM formation are common in cytomegalovirus infections. As a result, the virologic differentiation between a usually asymptomatic primary CMV infection and a reactivated infection is not currently possible unless seroconversion can be demonstrated (19). Based on the diagnostic inadequacies with a high rate of false-positive findings, general screening is not currently recommended as a routine part of prenatal care in Germany.

Main Ultrasound Signs

Cytomegalovirus infections may present sonographically with nonimmune fetal hydrops, hydrocephalus, intracranial calcifications, microcephaly, and intrauterine growth retardation. Sonomorphologic abnormalities are not always found in prenatal CMV infections, however, and often do not appear until the late second or third trimester. Hence, a normal ultrasound examination does not exclude a congenital CMV infection. Our own experience is based mainly on 22 women with a suspected new or reactivated CMV infection who were referred to us during the past 5 years for further testing. We observed microcephaly in two fetuses, and the other fetuses were sonographically normal. In four other cases that were referred for hydrocephalus (two cases) and early growth retardation (two cases), serologic tests confirmed a primary CMV infection.

Diagnosis

Serologic tests in pregnant women. If a CMV infection is suspected clinically—either from maternal symptoms such as fever and swollen lymph nodes (which not specific and may be absent even in primary infections) or from abnormal ultrasound findings—cytomegalovirus should be considered in the differential diagnosis and the maternal blood tested for antibodies. If there is serologic suspicion of a primary CMV infection, the direct detection of viruses in the urine, saliva, pharyngeal mucus, or cervical secretions can support the diagnosis although viral detection in maternal secretions is of limited use in distinguishing between acute primary and reactivated infections (45).

Invasive tests. If the overall findings cannot rule out a primary CMV infection, viral detection in the amniotic fluid or chorionic villi prior to 20 weeks is the method of choice (30). An IgM determination and viral detection in fetal blood at 22 weeks can further support the diagnosis of an intrauterine CMV infection, especially in cases where pregnancy termination is considered.

Management of Primary CMV Infection with Ultrasound Abnormalities

An abnormal ultrasound examination with positive viral detection in the amniotic fluid or fetal blood or elevated IgM titers in the fetal blood imply a poor prognosis. Intrauterine fetal death is particularly common when fetal hydrops is present. To prevent additional hypoxic injury at the time of delivery, obstetric management is the same as for a healthy fetus despite the poor prognosis. If the diagnosis is made before viability is reached, pregnancy termination may be considered.

Differential Diagnosis of the Most Common Ultrasound Features of Infectious Diseases

None of the sonomorphologic stigmata that may be seen in fetal infections are specific for a particular disease, but they are important in terms of differential diagnosis. This section deals with the differential diagnosis of the principal infection-association ultrasound signs that are listed in Table 33.**2**. A differential diagnostic protocol is suggested for each of these signs.

▬ *Nonimmune Fetal Hydrops (NIHF)*

Definition and pathogenesis. The term "fetal hydrops" refers to an abnormal collection of fetal body fluid in the interstitium, in the subcutaneous tissue, and/or in serous cavities such as pleural cavity, pericardium, or peritoneal cavity (4). Fetal anemia, hypoproteinemia, malformations, chromosomal abnormalities, and infections can lead to increased hydrostatic pressure (heart failure, decreased venous return) or decreased colloidal osmotic pressure (capillary damage or protein loss), resulting in fetal hydrops.

Immune hydrops. Rh incompatibility has become a less important cause of fetal hydrops owing to improved prophylactic measures, but erythroblastosis ("immune" hydrops) should still be considered first whenever fetal hydrops is diagnosed.

Ultrasound examination. If a negative antibody screening test of the maternal blood excludes immune hydrops, a difficult situation arises since any of a number of diseases with varying prognoses could be responsible for "nonimmune" fetal hydrops (23, 24). The differential diagnosis that Shah and Hadlock (43) compiled for nonimmune hydrops covers almost 100 diseases. As always, the process of differential diagnosis begins with a detailed ultrasound examination. In many cases this examination can significantly narrow the etiologic possibilities.

Chromosomal abnormality. A cystic hygroma combined with ascites and pleural effusion (Fig. 33.**2**) should raise suspicion of a chromosomal abnormality. Costly serologic tests to check for infection may be postponed until the result of karyotyping is available. Further tests are necessary only if the suspicion of a chromosomal abnormality is not confirmed.

Parvovirus B19 infection. When generalized nonimmune fetal hydrops with pronounced ascites is detected at about 20 weeks (Fig. 33.**3**), a parvovirus B19 infection is the first cause that should be considered. A corroborative history (contact with infected persons, transient skin eruption) increases the likelihood of a parvovirus infection. The priority tests in this situation are cordocentesis to determine the fetal hemoglobin content, parvovirus isolation, and IgG and IgM antibody assays in the maternal and fetal blood. If significant fetal anemia is present, a prompt umbilical cord transfusion is life-saving for the fetus.

Cardiac anomalies. If cardiac anomalies are responsible for fetal hydrops, generally the prognosis is poor. An example is the Ebstein anomaly (Fig. 33.**4**), which is not associated with an abnormal karyotype or with fetal infections. Further invasive tests are necessary, therefore.

Syndromes and rare metabolic disorders. The differential diagnosis of nonimmune fetal hydrops concludes with syndromes and rare metabolic defects, which often cannot be diagnosed until after birth (Fig. 33.**5**).

Diagnostic algorithm. The flowchart in Fig. 33.**6** shows the sequence in which the major diagnostic steps are applied in the investigation of fetal hydrops. Serologic tests have an important role in the diagnosis of infections but should be applied selectively and are not necessary in all cases.

▬ *Hydrocephalus*

Enlargement of the fetal CSF spaces is associated with chromosomal abnormalities in approximately 10% of cases (44). The most important infectious diseases in the differential diagnosis are toxoplasmosis and cytomegalovirus infection. When ventriculomegaly is detected (Fig. 33.**7**), we recommend karyotyping along with the determination of maternal toxoplasmosis and cytomegalovirus antibodies. Cordocentesis is the method of choice after 22 weeks' gestation, because by that time IgM determination in the fetal blood can be performed as well as karyotyping. If the findings are negative, lymphocytic choriomeningitis should also be excluded.

▬ *Growth Retardation*

If growth retardation is already noted at the second ultrasound screening, it is essential to rule out cytomegalovirus, rubella and varicella infections, as well as chromosome anomalies. Also, a full TORCH serology should be obtained in all cases of intrauterine fetal death.

Microcephaly

Microcephaly is the term used when fetal head circumference is well below the fifth percentile. These cases require a detailed examination of the fetal brain to exclude anomalies such as holoprosencephaly (Fig. 33.**8**). It should also be determined whether a primary rubella or CMV infection exists. Enlargement of the lateral ventricles is particularly apt to occur in CMV infections.

Cardiac Anomalies

Chromosomal abnormalities. Only a small percentage of cardiac anomalies are due to infectious diseases. The recommended diagnostic measures depend on what kind of cardiac anomaly is present. Karyotyping is generally recommended, especially in fetuses with an AV canal or double-outlet right ventricle, since chromosomal abnormalities are commonly found in association with these defects. Karyotyping is not necessary when an Ebstein anomaly is found.

Infections. Rubella embryopathy can lead to cardiac anomalies, most notably ventricular septal defects and the tetralogy of Fallot. If rubella immunity was not present during the first trimester, rubella serology of the maternal blood should be repeated. If an isolated pericardial effusion is found (Fig. 33.**9**), a coxsackie infection should be excluded, especially when signs of myocarditis are present.

Intra-abdominal Calcifications, Hepatomegaly

Intraperitoneal calcifications (Fig. 33.**10**) have been observed in association with meconium peritonitis. The cause may be meconium ileus secondary to cystic fibrosis or mechanical problems (volvulus, bowel atresias) (35). The differential diagnosis for hepatomegaly includes erythroblastosis, storage diseases, and various syndromes (Beckwith–Wiedemann syndrome, Zellweger syndrome). The differential diagnosis for intraperitoneal calcifications and hepatomegaly includes the following infectious diseases: toxoplasmosis, parvovirus B19 infection, varicella, syphilis, rubella, and CMV infection.

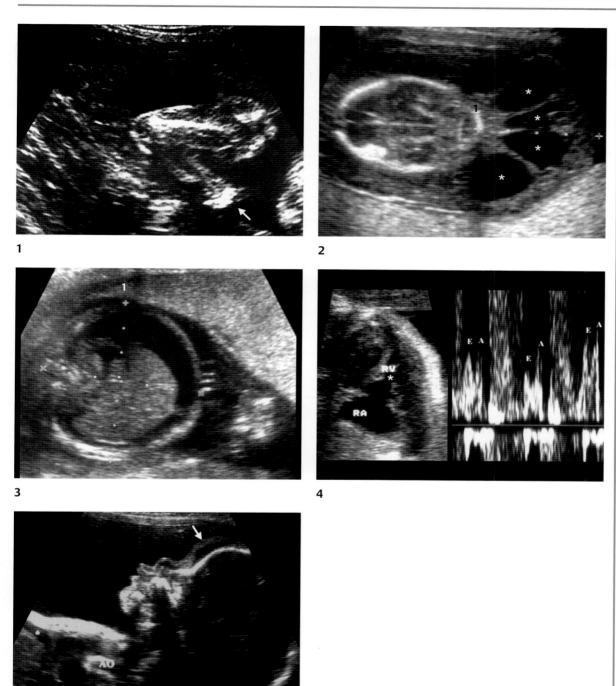

1

2

3

4

5

Differential diagnosis of infection-associated findings

Fig. 33.1 View of the left upper extremity at 18 weeks. The elbow joint is fixed in a flexed position, and the hand is hypoplastic (arrow). The patient was exposed to varicella during early pregnancy. The ultrasound finding is consistent with a congenital varicella syndrome.

Fig. 33.2 Large, septated cystic hygroma (∗). Transverse scan, 17 weeks.

Fig. 33.3 Pronounced ascites in parvovirus B19 infection. Transverse scan at the level of the liver, 21 weeks.

Fig. 33.4 Ebstein anomaly. *Left:* the tricuspid valve plane (∗) is displaced far into the right ventricle. *Right:* pronounced holosystolic AV valvular insufficiency.

Fig. 33.5 Fetal hydrops diagnosed in the third trimester. There is moderate ascites (∗) and pronounced frontal edema of the head (arrow). The walls of the ascending aorta (AO) are hypoechoic. A sialine storage disease was diagnosed after birth.

Fig. 33.**6** Algorithm for the diagnostic evaluation of fetal hydrops.

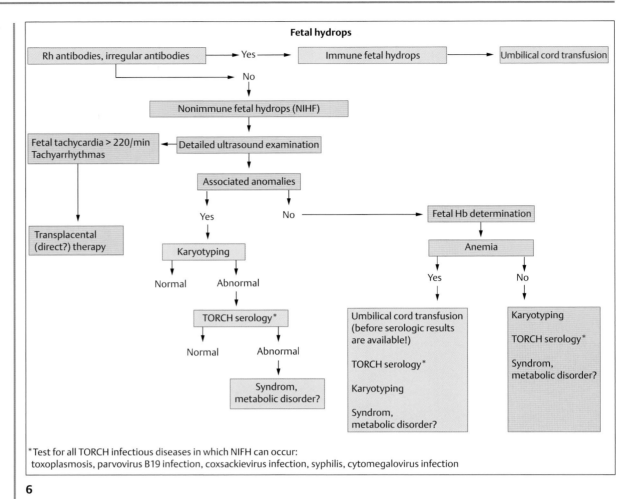

Fetal hydrops

Rh antibodies, irregular antibodies → Yes → Immune fetal hydrops → Umbilical cord transfusion

No

Nonimmune fetal hydrops (NIHF)

Fetal tachycardia > 220/min
Tachyarrhythmas ← Detailed ultrasound examination

Associated anomalies

Yes   No → Fetal Hb determination

Transplacental
(direct?) therapy   Anemia

Karyotyping   Yes   No

Normal   Abnormal

Umbilical cord transfusion   Karyotyping
(before serologic results
TORCH serology*   are available!)   TORCH serology*

Normal   Abnormal   TORCH serology*   Syndrom,
metabolic disorder?

Karyotyping

Syndrom,
metabolic disorder?   Syndrom,
metabolic disorder?

*Test for all TORCH infectious diseases in which NIFH can occur:
toxoplasmosis, parvovirus B19 infection, coxsackievirus infection, syphilis, cytomegalovirus infection

6

Fig. 33.**7** Bilateral ventriculomegaly (∗) in toxoplasmosis infection.

Fig. 33.**8** *Left:* microcephaly diagnosed at 25 weeks. Note the abnormal configuration of the cerebrum. Semilobar holoprosencephaly was present. *Right:* normally developed abdomen.

Fig. 33.**9** Subtle pericardial effusion (++) (3 mm), cardiomegaly.

Fig. 33.**10** Transverse scan at the level of the fetal liver demonstrates multiple foci of calcification (arrow).

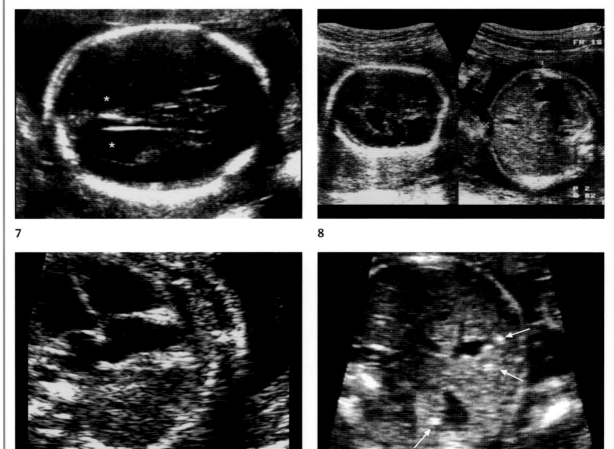

7   **8**

9   **10**

References

1. Anderson, M.J., Jones, S.E., Fisher-Hoch, S.P. et al.: Human parvovirus, the cause of erythema infectiosum (fifth disease)? Lancet I (1983) 1378
2. Axelsson, C., Bondestam, K., Frisk, G., Bergstrom, S., Diderholm, H.: Coxsackie B virus infections in women with miscarriage. J. Med. Virol. 39 (1993) 282–285
3. Barton, L.L., Peters, C.J., Ksiazek, T.G.: Lymphocytic choriomeningitis virus: an unrecognized teratogenic pathogen. Emerg. Infect. Dis. 1 (1995) 152–153
4. Becker, R., Fuhrmann, W., Holzgreve, W., Sperling, K.: Pränatale Diagnostik und Therapie. Stuttgart: Wiss. Verl.-Ges. 1995
5. Brown, T., Anand, A., Ritchie, L.D., Clewley, J.P., Reid, T.M.S.: Intrauterine parvovirus infection associated with hydrops fetalis. Lancet 2 (1984) 1033–1034
6. Dahlquist, G., Frisk, G., Ivarsson, S.A., Svanberg, L., Forsgren, M., Diderholm, H.: Indications that maternal coxsackie B virus infection during pregnancy is a risk factor of childhood-onset IDDM. Diabetologia 38 (1995) 1371–1373
7. Enders, G.: Infektionen und Impfungen in der Schwangerschaft. 2. Auflage. München: Urban & Schwarzenberg 1991
8. Enders, G., Miller, E., Cradock-Watson, J., Bolley, I., Ridehalgh, M.: Consequences of varicella and herpes zoster in pregnancy: prospective study of 1739 cases. Lancet 343 (1994) 1547–1550
9. Enders, G.: Infektionen von Mutter, Fetus und Neugeborenen. In: Wulf, K.H., Schmidt-Matthiesen, H. (Hrsg.): Klinik der Frauenheilkunde und Geburtshilfe. Bd. 5, 3. Auflage. München: Urban & Schwarzenberg 1994
10. Enders, G.: Röteln und Ringelröteln. In: Friese, K., Kachel, W. (Hrsg.): Infektionskrankheiten der Schwangeren und des Neugeborenen. Berlin: Springer 1998; S. 67–89
11. Fairley, C.K., Smoliniec, J.S., Caul, O.F., Miller, E.: An observational study of the effect of intrauterine transfusion on the outcome of fetal hydrops from parvovirus B19. Lancet 346 (1995) 1335–1337
12. Faure, J.-M., Giacalone, P. L., Deschamps, F., Boulot, P.: Nonimmune hydrops fetalis caused by intrauterine human parvovirus B19 infection: A case of spontaneous reversal in utero. Fetal Diagn. Ther. 12 (1997) 66–67
13. Fricker-Hidalgo, H., Pelloux, H., Muet, F. et al.: Prenatal diagnosis of congenital toxoplasmosis: Comparative value of fetal blood and amniotic fluid using serological techniques and cultures. Prenat. Diagn. 17 (1997) 831–835
14. Friese, K., Beichert, M., Hof, H.: Untersuchungen zur Häufigkeit konnataler Infektionen. Geburtsh. Frauenheilk. 51 (1991) 890–896
15. Friese, K., Hlobil, H.: Pränatale Toxoplasmose – brauchen wir ein Screening in der Schwangerschaft? Frauenarzt 39 (1998) 271–278
16. Friese, K., Kachel, W. (Hrsg.): Infektionskrankheiten der Schwangeren und des Neugeborenen. Berlin: Springer 1998
17. Frisk, S., Diderholm, H.: Increased frequency of coxsackie B virus in women with spontaneous abortion. J. Infect. 24 (1992) 141–145
18. Gregg, N.M.: Congenital cataract following German measles in mothers. Trans. ophthal. Soc. Aust. 3 (1941) 35
19. Hagay, Z.J., Biran, G., Ornoy, A., Reece, E.A.: Congenital cytomegalovirus infection: A long-standing problem still seeking a solution. Amer. J. Obstet. Gynecol. 174 (1996) 241–245
20. Harger, J.H., Adler, S.P., Koch, W.C., Harger, G.F.: Prospective evaluation of 618 pregnant women exposed to parvovirus B19: risks and symptoms. Obstet. Gynecol. 91 (1998) 413–420
21. Hezard, N., Marx-Chemla, C., Foudrinier, F. et al.: Prenatal diagnosis of congenital toxoplasmosis in 261 pregnancies. Prenat. Diagn. 17 (1997) 1047–1054
22. Hofmeyr, G.J., Moolla, S., Lawrie, T.: Prenatal sonographic diagnosis of congenital varicella infection – a case report. Prenat. Diagn. 16 (1996) 1148–1151
23. Holzgreve, W., Curry, C.J.R., Golbus, M.S., Callen, P.W., Filly, R.A., Smith, J.C.: Investigation of nonimmune hydrops fetalis. Amer. J. Obstet. Gynecol. 150 (1984) 805–812
24. Holzgreve, W., Holzgreve, B., Curry, J.R.: Non-immune hydrops fetalis: Diagnosis and management. Semin. Perinatol. 9 (1985) 52–62
25. Hu, W.L., Lu, J.H., Meng, C.C., Hwang, B.: Neonatal myocardial infarction: a case report. Chung Hua I Hsueh Tsa Chih Taipei 61 (1998) 110–115
26. Humphrey, W., Magoon, M., O'Shaughnessy, R.: Severe nonimmune hydrops secondary to parvovirus B19 infection: Spontaneous reversal in utero and survival of a term infant. Obstet. Gynecol. 78 (1991) 900–902
27. Hyoty, H., Hiltunen, M., Knip, M. et al.: A prospective study of the role of coxsackie B and other enterovirus infections in the pathogenesis of IDDM. Childhood Diabetes in Finland (DiMe) Study Group. Diabetes 44 (1995) 652–657
28. Jäger, G.R., Schwarz, T.F.: Hämatologische Bedeutung der Parvovirus B19-Infektion. Die gelben Hefte 34 (1994) 81–84
29. Larson, P.D., Chartrand, S.A., Tomashek, K.M., Hauser, L.G., Ksiazek, T.G.: Hydrozephalus complicating lymphocytic choriomeningitis virus infection. Pediatr. Infect. Dis. J. 12 (1993) 528–531
30. Lipitz, S., Yagel, S., Shalev, E., Arichon, R., Mashicach, S., Schiff, E.: Prenatal diagnosis of fetal primary cytomegalovirus infection. Obstet. Gynecol. 89 (1997) 763–767
31. Mari, G., Adrignolo, A., Abuhamad, A.Z.: Diagnosis of fetal anemia with Doppler ultrasound in the pregnancy complicated by maternal blood group immunization. Ultrasound Obstet. Gynecol. 5 (1995) 400–405
32. Miller, E., Fairley, C.K., Cohen, B.J., Seng, C.: Immediate and long term outcome of human parvovirus B19 infection in pregnancy. Brit. J. Obstet. Gynaecol. 105 (1998) 174–178
33. Modrow, S., Hernauer, A., Gigler, A.: Die Parvovirus B19-Infektion. Die gelben Hefte 38 (1998) 26–36
34. Morey, A.L., Keeling, J.W., Porter, H.J., Fleming, K.A.: Clinical and histopathological features of parvovirus B19 infection in the human fetus. Brit. J. Obstet. Gynecol. 99 (1992) 566–574
35. Nyberg, D.A., Mahony, B.S., Pretorius, D.H.: Diagnostic ultrasound of fetal anomalies. St. Louis: Mosby Year Book 1990
36. Pieringer-Müller, E., Hof, H.: Syphilis. In: Friese, K., Kachel, W. (Hrsg.): Infektionskrankheiten der Schwangeren und des Neugeborenen. Berlin: Springer 1998; S. 235–256
37. Porter, H.J., Quantril, A.M., Fleming, K.A.: B19 parvovirus infection in myocardial cells. Lancet I (1988) 535–536
38. Pryde, P.G., Nugent, C.E., Pridjian, G., Barr, M.Jr., Faix, R.G.: Spontaneous resolution of nonimmune hydrops fetalis secondary to human parvovirus B19 infection. Obstet. Gynecol. 79 (1992) 859–861
39. Rozee, K.R., Klassen, G.A., Ahmad-Raza, A., Lee, S.H.: A mouse model of coxsackievirus myocarditis. Can. J. Cardiol. 8 (1992) 145–148
40. Schild, R.L., Plath, H., Thomas, P., Schulte-Wissermann, H., Eis-Hübinger, A.M., Hansmann, M.: Fetal parvovirus B19 infection and meconium peritonitis. Fetal Diagn. Ther. 13 (1998) 15–18
41. Scott, L.L.: Perinatal herpesvirus infections. Herpes simplex, varicella, and cytomegalovirus. Infect. Dis. Clin. North. Amer. 11 (1997) 27–53
42. Shah, S.S., Gallagher, P.G.: Neonatal sepsis due to echovirus 18 infection. J. Perinat. Med. 25 (1997) 381–384
43. Shah, Y.P., Hadlock, F.P.: Hydrops and ascites. In: Nyberg, D.A., Mahony, B.S., Pretorius, D.H.: Diagnostic ultrasound of fetal anomalies. St. Louis: Mosby Year Book 1990; S. 563–591
44. Snijders, R.J.M., Nicolaides, K.H.: Ultrasound markers for fetal chromosomal defects. New York: The Parthenon Publishing Group 1996
45. Stagno, S.: Cytomegalovirus. In: Remington, J.S., Klein, J.O. (eds.): Infectious diseases of the Fetus and Newborn Infant. Philadelphia: Saunders 1992
46. Tercanli, S., Enders, G., Holzgreve, W.: Aktuelles Management bei mütterlichen Infektionen mit Röteln, Toxoplasmose, Zytomegalie, Varizellen und Parvovirus B19 in der Schwangerschaft. Gynäkologe 29 (1996) 144–163
47. Tiessen, R.G., van Elsacker-Niele, A.M., Vermeij-Keers, C., Oepkes, D., van Roosmalen, J., Gorsira, M.C.: A fetus with a parvovirus B19 infection and congenital anomalies. Prenat. Diagn. 14 (1994) 173–176
48. Weigel, M.: Sonographische und invasive Diagnostik bei Infektionserkrankungen in der Schwangerschaft. In: Friese, K., Kachel, W. (Hrsg.): Infektionskrankheiten der Schwangeren und des Neugeborenen. Berlin: Springer 1998; S. 47–66
49. Weiland, H.T., Vermey-Keers, C., Salimans, M.M.M., Fleuren, G.F., Verwey, R.A., Anderson, M.J.: Parvovirus B19 associated with fetal abnormality (Letter). Lancet I (1987) 682–683

Ultrasound of the Placenta, Umbilical Cord, and Amniotic Fluid

34 Placenta

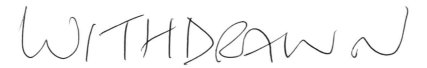

Normal Placenta

The placenta, as an extracorporeal fetal organ, is subject to both fetal and maternal regulation. Its structure and function can be understood only in terms of its ongoing development and transformation as gestation proceeds.

"The placenta is an organ like any other, yet it is also more and something different" (6) because it is formed by two organisms, functions without nerves, must link two different circulations and pressure systems, and has its own unique morphologic and immunologic responses (Fig. 34.1).

▬ *Morphology*

Fetal part and maternal part. Morphologically, the placenta consists of a fetal part, which develops from the chorion, and a maternal part, which is derived from the endometrium. The fetal part is composed of the chorionic plate and the chorionic villi. The villi arise from the chorionic plate and project into the intervillous spaces, which are filled with maternal blood. The maternal part of the placenta is formed by the decidua basalis, whose compact boundary layer is called the decidual plate (46) (Fig. 34.1).

Cotyledons. The mature placenta in humans has a rounded to discoid shape. The villi extend into the decidua basalis, leaving intervening decidual segments that form the placental septa. Ultimately these septa subdivide the fetal placenta into 10–38 irregular lobes or lobules, called the cotyledons, each of which contains two or more villous stems and their branches (46).

Chorion frondosum. The fetal placenta (chorion frondosum) is anchored to the maternal placenta (decidua basalis) by a cytotrophoblastic shell and the anchoring villi (Fig. 34.1), which extend from the chorionic plate through the intervillous spaces and are firmly attached to the decidua basalis via the cytotrophoblastic shell (46).

▬ *Placental Circulation*

The placenta has a large internal surface area available for the exchange of substances between the fetal and maternal blood.

Fetal circulation. Deoxygenated blood from the fetus flows through the umbilical arteries to the placenta. At the site where the umbilical cord inserts on the placenta, the umbilical arteries divide into numerous, radially arranged vessels that arborize in the chorionic plate and enter the villous stems. Within the villi they form an extensive capillary network through which the fetal blood comes into intimate contact with the maternal blood. Mixing of fetal and maternal blood normally does not occur. The oxygen-enriched fetal blood then enters the thin-walled veins of the villi, which pass with the arteries to the chorionic plate where they converge to form the umbilical vein. Finally the umbilical vein carries the oxygenated blood back to the fetus through the umbilical cord (46).

Maternal placental circulation. The blood in the intervillous spaces is derived from the maternal vascular system (open circulation). It enters the intervillous spaces from the basal side through approximately 80–100 spiral arteries in the uterine mucosa. As the spiral arteries pulsate, they inject their contents into the placenta in jet-like spurts. The blood of the spiral arteries, which is under considerably higher pressure than the blood of the intervillous spaces, flows rapidly to the chorionic plate, which caps the intervillous spaces like a roof or "lid." The pressure drops quickly at this point, and the blood flows slowly past the surfaces of the villi, allowing for a more intensive interchange of gas and substances. Finally the maternal blood drains through the veins of the decidua basalis (the "floor" of the intervillous spaces) to the collecting veins of the endometrium, where it reenters the maternal circulation (46). A sufficient volume of maternal blood must bathe the chorionic villi in order for the conceptus to thrive (46).

Ultrasound. Not only can modern ultrasound evaluate the anatomy and development of the placenta, but Doppler and power Doppler imaging can provide insights into the physiology and pathophysiology of this organ. As a result, placental ultrasound has become an integral part of the obstetric ultrasound examination. Aside from the evaluation of normal placental development, targeted imaging of the placenta may be done to investigate certain maternal symptoms or fetal abnormalities, or it may be indicated before or after an invasive procedure (Table 34.1).

Table 34.1 Indications for targeted ultrasound imaging of the placenta

➢ Uterine hemorrhage
➢ Unexplained lower abdominal pain
➢ Premature contractions, labor
➢ Diabetes mellitus
➢ GEPH disorder
➢ Multiple pregnancy
➢ Suspected growth retardation
➢ Abnormal fetal position
➢ Suspected NIHF or Rh incompatibility
➢ Suspected placental abnormality (shape, location)
➢ Polyhydramnios
➢ Before and after an invasive procedure (especially transplacental puncture)

The present section deals with the ultrasound evaluation of the normal and abnormal placenta. The evaluation of blood flow in the placental and umbilical vessels with ultrasound is discussed in the chapter on Doppler ultrasound.

▬ *Ultrasound anatomy*

Development. The placenta begins to develop from the chorion frondosum and decidua basalis in the eighth week of intrauterine life (55). Sonographically, the chorion frondosum can be distinguished by its thickness from the thinner, opposing chorion laeve as early as 8–9 weeks (Fig. 34.2). Starting at about 10 weeks, the placenta is clearly distinguishable from its surroundings as a disk-shaped organ (Fig. 34.3). The chorionic plate forms the interface of the placenta with the amniotic cavity, while the basal plate marks its boundary with the uterine wall. Both plates come together in the marginal zone. Between them is the placental substance, which is composed of villous structures (58%) and intervillous spaces (42%). The placenta at term has a weight of approximately 500 g, a basal area of approximately 200 cm², and a thickness of approximately 1–2.5 cm (7, 66).

Ultrasound visualization. Between 8 and 20 weeks' gestation, the placenta appears sonographically as a homogeneous, moderately echogenic, granular organ that contrasts with the hypoechoic myometrium. After 20 weeks, the placenta contains increased numbers of venous lakes, which appear as hypoechoic areas, and increasing calcium deposits.

Placental location. The placenta may be located chiefly on the anterior uterine wall (Fig. 34.**4**), posterior uterine wall (Fig. 34.**5**), uterine side wall (Fig. 34.**6**), or on the uterine fundus (Fig. 34.**7**).

Complete visualization. In the third trimester, the placenta can no longer be completely visualized with conventional ultrasound technology because of its size. This can be done only by SieScape imaging, in which compound and real-time ultrasound are combined (Fig. 34.**8**).

Problems. Occasionally it can be difficult to visualize a posterior placenta because of the interposed fetus. If a placenta at this location cannot be seen in longitudinal section, it can be at least partially visualized with a transverse scan.

With a low-lying placenta, a slightly distended maternal bladder is necessary to make an accurate evaluation of the lower placental margin and avoid misinterpretation.

▬ *Placental Biometry*

Placental thickness. In a normal pregnancy the placental thickness increases steadily between 15 and 37 weeks. Thereafter, the placental thickness decreases slightly until the 40th week (56) (Fig. 34.**9**). Hoddick et al. (28) found a maximum placental thickness of 3 cm up to 20 weeks and a maximum of 4–5 cm thereafter.

Rule of thumb. The maximum placental thickness is measured from the chorionic plate to the interface of the basal plate and myometrium (Fig. 34.**10**). As a general rule of thumb, the placental thickness in millimeters approximately equals the gestational age in weeks. Normally the placenta covers one-fourth of the myometrial surface at 20 weeks and approximately one-eighth at term (41).

Placental diameter. The mean placental diameter is 70 mm between 13 and 16 weeks and reaches 220 mm by the end of pregnancy (36).

▬ *Placental Structure and Placental Maturation*

Grading by placental maturity. Winsberg (69) was the first author, in 1973, to observe differences in placental structures with ultrasound. In 1979, Grannum et al. (20) proposed a ultrasound classification based on four grades (0–III) of placental maturity. The criteria for evaluating placental maturity are the chorionic plate, placental substance, and basal plate (Figs. 34.**11**–34.**15**):

- **Grade 0** (Fig. 34.**12**). This placenta exhibits a smooth chorionic plate and a homogeneous, granular internal structure. The basal plate shows no echogenic areas.
- **Grade I** (Fig. 34.**13**). This grade shows the first ultrasound signs of placental maturation. The chorionic plate appears as a smooth, slightly wavy line. Scattered echogenic areas approximately 1–4 mm long are seen within the placental substance, their long axes directed parallel to the basal plate. The basal plate itself contains no echogenic areas.

- **Grade II** (Fig. 34.**14**). The changes in this grade affect all three zones. The chorionic plate shows marked indentations. The placental substance is subdivided by comma-like densities that connect with the notches in the chorionic plate but do not extend to the basal plate. The echogenic areas in the placental substance appear larger and more numerous than in grade I. There are also short, linear, basal echogenic densities directed along the axis of the basal plate.
- **Grade III** (Fig. 34.**15**). The chorionic plate is interrupted by indentations that now extend to the basal plate and compartmentalize the placenta into different segments, corresponding to the cotyledons. Each of the cotyledons has a hypoechoic center. Additional irregular densities with acoustic shadowing are visible near the chorionic plate. Near the basal plate, the echogenic areas become larger and confluent. Overall, the grade III placenta displays a garland-like appearance.

Since changes of variable degree may be found, Grannum et al. (20) recommend grading the placenta according to the most mature area that is seen.

Grading by gestational age. Petrucha and Platt (50) used gestational age as a basis for placental grading (Fig. 34.**16**). Grade 0 is almost always found in the first and second trimesters, and grade I may occasionally be seen. Grade I and II become increasingly common after 26 weeks' gestation. Grade III normally appears only after 35 weeks. At the same time, complete placental maturation to grade III is seen in only 15% of cases. The remaining cases reach only grade I or II by term.

Placental and lung maturity. Grannum et al. (20, 21) found that in 86 cases as the grade of placental maturity increased, the lecithin/sphingomyelin (L/S) ratio rose to 2.0 or more, leading them to conclude that placental maturation correlated with fetal lung maturity. Other investigators using a similar study design were unable to confirm these findings (25, 38, 52).

Placental maturity and growth retardation. There appears to be a significant link between premature placental maturation (grade II before 32 weeks or grade III before 35 weeks) and fetal growth retardation (31). Kazzi et al. (37) found that small fetuses (< 2700 g) with a grade III placenta had a four times higher risk of intrauterine growth retardation than fetuses without a grade III placenta.

Placental calcification. Hills et al. (27) discovered a correlation between placental calcification, hypertension, and intrauterine growth retardation in a study of 128 high-risk pregnancies. In another study, Brown et al. (10) found a strong correlation between early placental calcification and cigarette smoking.

Failure of maturation. The failure of placental maturation, defined as the presence of a grade 0 placenta after 32 weeks' gestation, is suspicious for gestational diabetes (21).

Subchorionic cystic spaces. Subchorionic cystic spaces are found in approximately 10–15% of pregnancies (Figs. 34.**17**–34.**19**). The majority are blood-filled spaces (35, 47). An echo-free space at the margin of the placenta is a blood-filled marginal sinus (Fig. 34.**20a**). It requires differentiation from a subchorionic hematoma at the placental margin. Centrally located, subchorionic blood sinuses may become relatively large and extend to the base of the placenta (Fig. 34.**20b**). Large subchorionic spaces are not associated with other placental or fetal abnormalities (35).

Placentones and spiral arteries. Especially after 28 weeks, round echo-free areas appear in the placental substance. Each of these areas represents the center of a placentone (= smallest flow unit). It is the site

Ultrasound anatomy of the normal placenta

Fig. 34.**1** Schematic diagram of a mature placenta. Jets of maternal blood spurt into the intervillous spaces and bathe the chorionic villi, where substances are exchanged with the fetal blood. The inflowing arterial blood pushes the venous blood into the endometrial veins, which are dispersed over the entire surface of the decidua basalis. Note that the umbilical arteries carry deoxygenated blood (blue) to the placenta while the umbilical vein returns oxygenated blood (red) to the fetus. The individual cotyledons are separated from one another by the decidual septa of the maternal placenta. Each cotyledon consists of two or more villous stems and their branches. For simplicity, only one villous stem is shown in each cotyledon in the diagram, but the origins of the other villous stems are shown in the chorionic plate (from [46]).

Fig. 34.**2** Posterior placenta (arrows) at 8 weeks, 5 days. Transvaginal longitudinal scan.

Fig. 34.**3** Left sidewall placenta with cord insertion at 12 weeks. Transvaginal transverse scan through the uterus.

Fig. 34.**4** Anterior placenta at 20 weeks, 2 days. Longitudinal scan.

Fig. 34.**5** Posterior placenta at 27 weeks, longitudinal scan. Color Doppler shows the umbilical cord vessels on the fetal surface of the placenta.

Fig. 34.**6** Right sidewall placenta. Transverse scan at 21 weeks.

Fig. 34.**7** Fundal placenta. Longitudinal scan at 22 weeks.

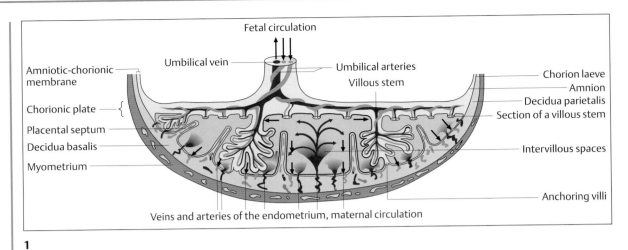

Fetal circulation

Umbilical vein — Umbilical arteries
Amniotic-chorionic membrane — Villous stem
Chorionic plate — Chorion laeve
Placental septum — Amnion
Decidua basalis — Decidua parietalis
Myometrium — Section of a villous stem
— Intervillous spaces
— Anchoring villi
Veins and arteries of the endometrium, maternal circulation

1

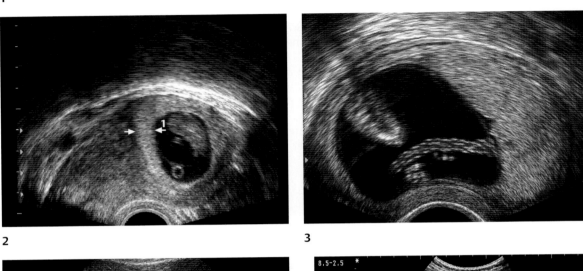

2   **3**

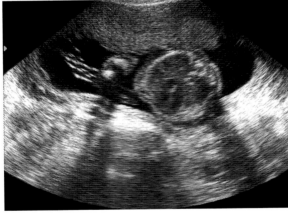 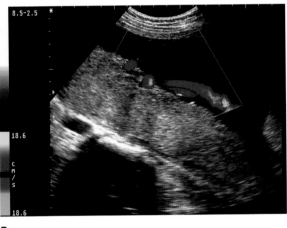

4   **5**

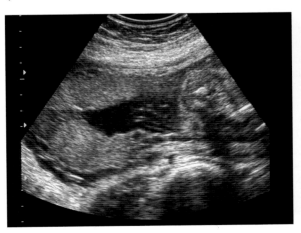 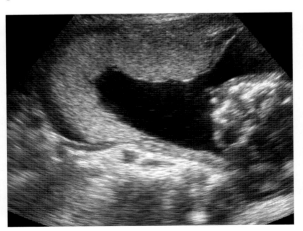

6   **7**

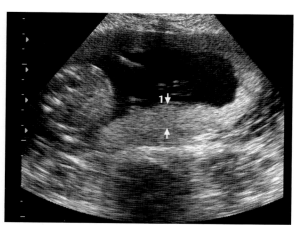

8

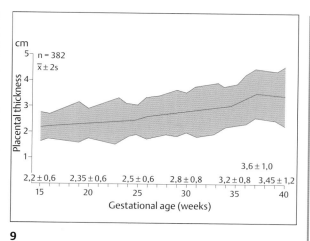

9

Fig. 34.**8** SieScape image (Siemens) at 32 weeks defines the full length of the placenta along the anterior uterine wall.

Fig. 34.**9** Placental thickness versus gestational age (after 57).

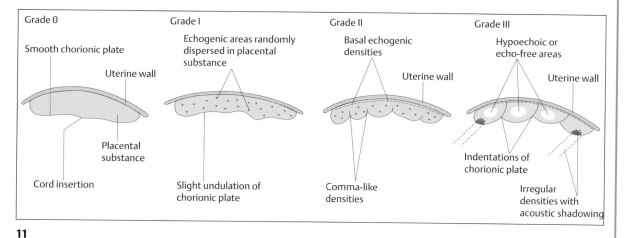

Graph axis labels:
cm
Placental thickness
n = 382
x̄ ± 2s
3,6 ± 1,0
2,2 ± 0,6   2,35 ± 0,6   2,5 ± 0,6   2,8 ± 0,8   3,2 ± 0,8   3,45 ± 1,2
15   20   25   30   35   40
Gestational age (weeks)

10

Fig. 34.**10** Ultrasound measurement of placental thickness (arrows) in a posterior and left sidewall placenta at 20 weeks, 0 days.

Placental grades

Fig. 34.**11** Placental maturation during pregnancy. Ultrasound appearance of grades 0—III (after 20).

Grade 0
Smooth chorionic plate
Uterine wall
Placental substance
Cord insertion

Grade I
Echogenic areas randomly dispersed in placental substance
Slight undulation of chorionic plate

Grade II
Basal echogenic densities
Uterine wall
Comma-like densities

Grade III
Hypoechoic or echo-free areas
Uterine wall
Indentations of chorionic plate
Irregular densities with acoustic shadowing

11

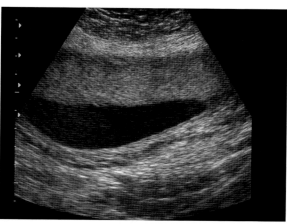

12

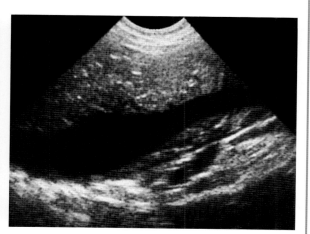

13

Fig. 34.**12** Grade 0 placenta at 16 weeks. Posterior placenta, longitudinal scan.

Fig. 34.**13** Grade I placenta at 33 weeks. Anterior placenta, transverse scan.

Fig. 34.**14**   Grade II placenta at 36 weeks. Posterior placenta, transverse scan.

Fig. 34.**15**   Grade III anterior placenta at 39 weeks shows typical echogenic, garland-like areas of calcification. *Left:* lateral view. *Right:* overall view in tangential scan.

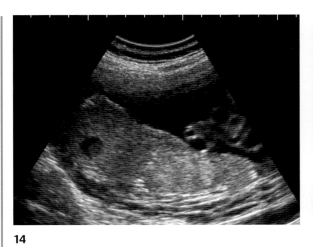

14

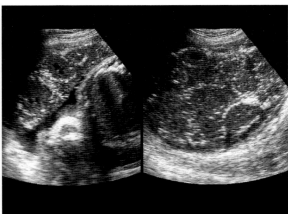

15

Fig. 34.**16**   Frequency distribution of the four placental grades with progressive gestational age, after Grannum (50).

16

Placental perfusion

Fig. 34.**17**   Posterior placenta with a cyst-like, subchorionic blood-filled space ("placental cyst"), 19 weeks.

Fig. 34.**18**   Anterior placenta with hypoechoic, subchorionic blood lakes. Longitudinal scan at 33 weeks. Not an abnormal finding!

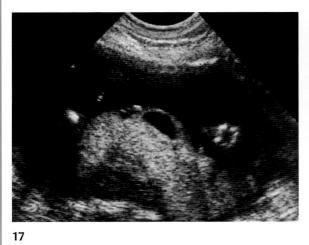

17

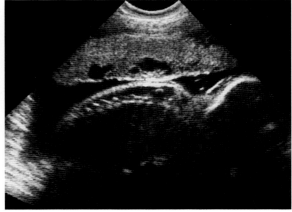

18

Fig. 34.**19**   Anterior placenta at 34 weeks contains multiple, hypoechoic blood lakes located at slightly deeper levels.

Fig. 34.**20**   Blood-filled marginal sinus and subchorionic blood sinus.
a Hypoechoic marginal sinus at the lower placental margin. Longitudinal scan at 22 weeks.
b Large, centrally located subchorionic sinus extending to the base of the placenta. The fine internal echoes within the sinus are caused by the slow blood flow. Longitudinal scan at 20 weeks.

19

20

where a spiral artery ejects its blood, which then flows toward the periphery (4, 64) (Fig. 34.**21**).

Color Doppler or power Doppler imaging can be used to define and quantitatively evaluate the perfusion of the placenta (Figs. 34.**22**, 34.**23**). These techniques can also demonstrate the inflow of blood from the spiral artery (Fig. 34.**24**).

Uterine wall vascularity. A copious blood supply to the uterine wall behind the placenta, which is particularly common in the third trimester, can lead to a misdiagnosis of retroplacental hematoma (Figs. 34.**25**, 34.**26**). In equivocal cases, color Doppler can be used to visualize flow in the uterine wall vessels, excluding a retroplacental hematoma (Fig. 34.**27**).

Placental Abnormalities

Abnormalities of Placental Shape

No increase in fetal risk. Generally the placenta has a rounded to slightly oval shape. A reniform, heart-shaped, or biscuit-shaped placenta is not harmful to the fetus, nor is a bilobed or multilobed placenta.

Increased fetal risk. Morphologic abnormalities of the placenta that are associated with increased fetal risk are a bipartite or tripartite placenta and a succenturiate (accessory) placenta lobe (Fig. 34.**28**), whose ultrasound appearance was described by Jeanty et al. (34) (Fig. 34.**29**, 34.**30**).

If a succenturiate lobe is present, color Doppler scanning can define the vessel that connects the accessory lobe to the main placenta (Fig. 34.**31**).

Fetal risk is also increased by a circumvallate placenta (8), whose fetal surface is smaller than the maternal surface (Fig. 34.**28**), and by a placenta membranacea, which is abnormally thin and may not provide an adequate fetal supply.

All of these abnormalities are detectable with ultrasound. These diagnoses are clinically important due to an increased risk of maternal hemorrhage and fetal mortality (32).

Abnormalities of Placental Location

Vaginal bleeding in the second or third trimester is always suspicious for an abnormal placental location with premature abruption or marginal sinus hemorrhage. The main positional abnormalities are as follows:
- **Low-lying placenta.** A low-lying placenta is one whose lower margin is located between 0.5 and 5 cm from the internal cervical os (29).
- **Marginal placenta previa.** This describes a placenta whose lower margin extends to the internal os.
- **Partial placenta previa.** The edge of the placenta partially covers the internal os.
- **Complete placenta previa.** The placenta completely covers the internal os (Fig. 34.**32**).

Incidence. The incidence of placenta previa varies with gestational age. Ultrasound in the second trimester can demonstrate placenta previa in more than 5% of all pregnancies, but the incidence of placenta previa at term is only 0.5% (68). This is attributable to placental growth processes and the changes that occur in the lower uterine segment as gestation proceeds. The phenomenon of superior placental migration appears to result from the longitudinal and transverse growth of the lower uterine segment, which alters the relationship of the placenta to the internal cervical os (21).

When a marginal or partial placenta previa is detected in early pregnancy, follow-up scans should be scheduled. A definitive placenta previa should not be diagnosed until the third trimester.

The incidence of placenta previa is one in 20 in multiparous women and one in 1500 in primiparae (22). The incidence is higher in older mothers, in multiple pregnancies, after miscarriages, and after cesarean section. The recurrence risk of placenta previa is 4–8%, and the incidence in patients with prior cesarean section is over 10% (13).

Ultrasound verification. For the ultrasound verification of a low-lying placenta (Fig. 34.**33**), the distance is measured from the lower placental margin to the internal cervical os. Often it is difficult sonographically to distinguish a marginal placenta previa (Fig. 34.**34**) from a partial previa (Fig. 34.**35**). A complete previa is usually easy to identify, however (Fig. 34.**36**).

Problems of placental localization. Especially with a posterior placenta, localization can be hampered by the interposed position of the fetus. The diagnosis of placenta previa requires a moderately distended maternal bladder. The internal os is difficult to define clearly on an empty bladder, and a low-lying placenta may be mistaken for placenta previa. An overdistended bladder or focal uterine contractions can also mimic placenta previa by displacing the lower uterine segment (62). Finally, an organized hematoma at the lower pole of a low-sited placenta can create the erroneous appearance of placenta previa. If findings are equivocal, a transvaginal scan should be performed. Several studies have documented the value of transvaginal ultrasound in the diagnosis of placenta previa (42, 59, 60).

Uterine anomalies. An abnormal placental location is also occasionally seen in patients with uterine anomalies. With a uterus subseptus, for example, the placenta may be partially implanted in the area of the septum as well as on the uterine wall (Fig. 34.**37**).

Abnormal Placental Biometry

Thick placenta. An abnormally thick placenta is found in cases where the basal plate has a very small area of myometrial attachment. Placentomegaly can occur in association with numerous disorders including maternal diabetes mellitus, maternal anemia, hydrops, placental hemorrhage, intrauterine infection, congenital neoplasms, Beckwith–Wiedemann syndrome, sacrococcygeal teratoma, hydatidiform mole, and chromosomal abnormalities (Figs. 34.**38**–34.**40**).

Placental hydrops. The thickest placentas are found in cases of Rh incompatibility and nonimmune fetal hydrops. The increased fluid retention associated with these conditions leads to a spongy, expanded placental structure (57). A placental thickness greater than 5 cm is termed placental hydrops (Fig. 34.**39**).

Large, vacuolated placenta. When combined with oligohydramnios, this type of placenta is suspicious for triploidy (14) (Fig. 34.**40**).

Small or thin placenta. A small placenta is found in cases of intrauterine growth retardation, intrauterine infection, and chromosomal abnormalities (Fig. 34.**41**). Very thin placentas may be found when the basal plate has a large area of myometrial attachment or in association with massive polyhydramnios (Fig. 34.**42**).

Other parameters. In addition to placental thickness, sectional imaging of the placenta provides length and width measurements that can be used to calculate placental volume (19, 33, 70), area of attachment (40), and placental surface area (30).

Fig. 34.**21**   Fallout areas within the placenta at 35 weeks. Each represents the center of the placentone into which the corresponding spiral artery ejects its blood.

Fig. 34.**22**   Color Doppler demonstrates normal placental perfusion in the third trimester.

Fig. 34.**23**   Power Doppler image demonstrates normal placental perfusion (green box) at 36 weeks, 4 days.

Fig. 34.**24**   Color Doppler shows blood flow from a spiral artery into the center of a placentone, 37 weeks.

Fig. 34.**25**   A copious blood supply to the uterine wall behind the placenta (arrow) mimics placental abruption. Longitudinal scan at 24 weeks.

Fig. 34.**26**   A hypoechoic marginal sinus at the lower edge of the placenta (arrow), combined with a richly vascularized uterine wall behind the placenta, mimics placental abruption at 34 weeks.

Fig. 34.**27**   Color Doppler demonstrates a copious blood supply in the uterine wall behind an anterior placenta. Longitudinal scan.

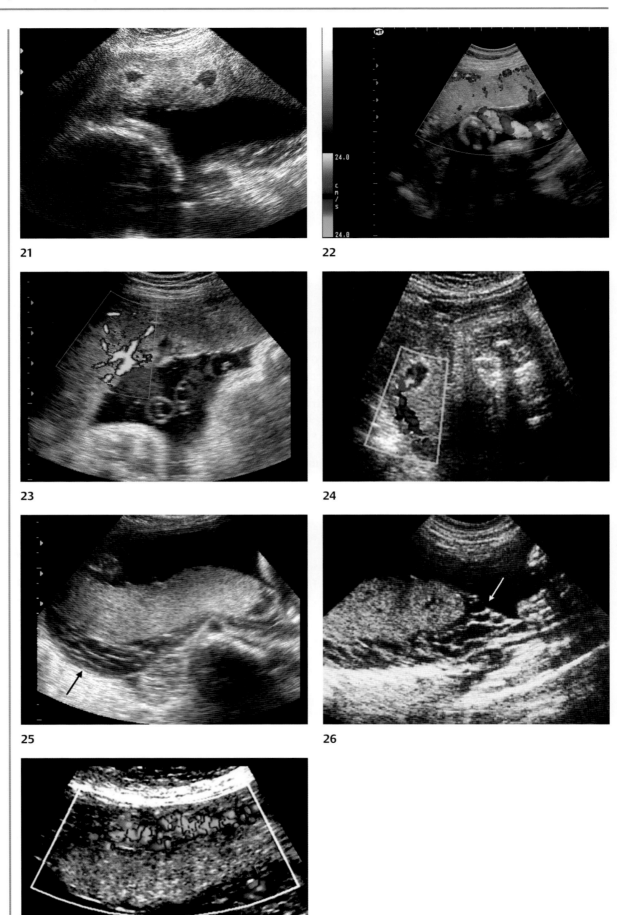

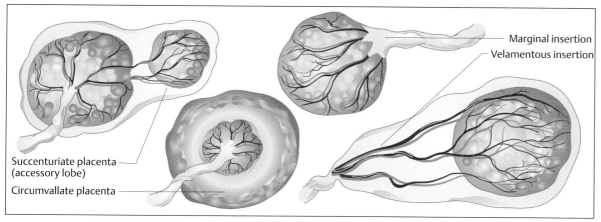

Marginal insertion
Velamentous insertion

Succenturiate placenta
(accessory lobe)
Circumvallate placenta

28

Abnormalities of placental shape and location

Fig. 34.**28** Diagrams of abnormal placental variants and cord insertions: succenturiate placenta, circumvallate placenta, marginal insertion, and velamentous insertion.

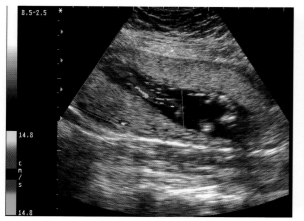

29

30

Fig. 34.**29** Bipartite placenta on the anterior and posterior uterine walls, longitudinal scan. The cord insertion is located between the two halves of the placenta.

Fig. 34.**30** Succenturiate placenta.
1 = Main placenta on the anterior uterine wall.
2 = Succenturiate lobe on the posterior wall, transverse scan.

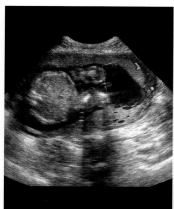
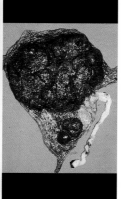

31

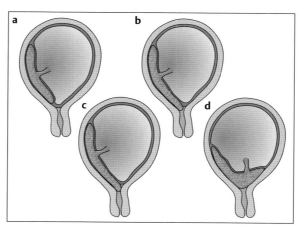

32

Fig. 34.**31** Same case as in Fig. 34.**30**. *Left:* color Doppler demonstrates the vessels connecting the two placentas, transverse scan. *Right:* postpartum appearance of the main placenta and succenturiate lobe.

Fig. 34.**32** Diagrams of abnormal placental locations.
a Low-lying placenta.
b Marginal placenta previa.
c Partial placenta previa.
d Complete placenta previa.

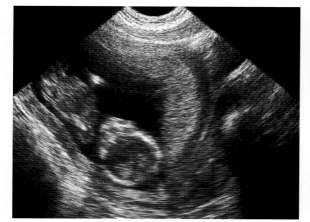

33

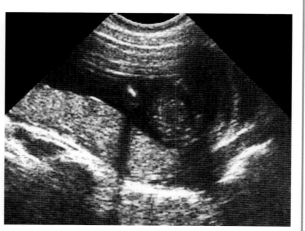

34

Fig. 34.**33** Low-lying anterior placenta, longitudinal scan at 18 weeks. The lower edge of the placenta is located 2.0 cm from the internal cervical os.

Fig. 34.**34** Marginal placenta previa on the posterior uterine wall. Longitudinal scan at 17 weeks.

Fig. 34.**35**   Partial placenta previa on the anterior uterine wall. Longitudinal scan at 14 weeks.

Fig. 34.**36**   Complete placenta previa. Longitudinal scan at 17 weeks, acquired with a wide-angle transducer.

Fig. 34.**37**   Abnormal placental location in uterus septus. Most of the placenta is situated on the posterior wall in the left half of the uterus, but its medial portion (∗) extends onto the septum (arrow). Transverse scan through the uterus at 21 weeks.

Abnormal placental biometry and implantation depth

Fig. 34.**38**   Thick, globular-shaped placenta measuring 7.4 cm in diabetes mellitus. Posterior placenta, 36 weeks.

Fig. 34.**39**   Hydropic posterior placenta (placental thickness 6.4 cm) in nonimmune fetal hydrops, 32 weeks.

Fig. 34.**40**   *Left:* abnormally large placenta (5 cm in diameter) with conspicuous vacuoles (Swiss cheese pattern) in a partial molar pregnancy, 19 weeks. Karyotype: XXX triploidy. *Right:* clinical appearance of the placenta and associated fetus.

Fig. 34.**41**   *Left:* abnormally thin anterior placenta (placental thickness 1.7 cm) at 33 weeks, with marked fetal growth retardation by 4 weeks. *Right:* appearance of the placenta. Placental weight 170 g, placental size 10 × 8 cm.

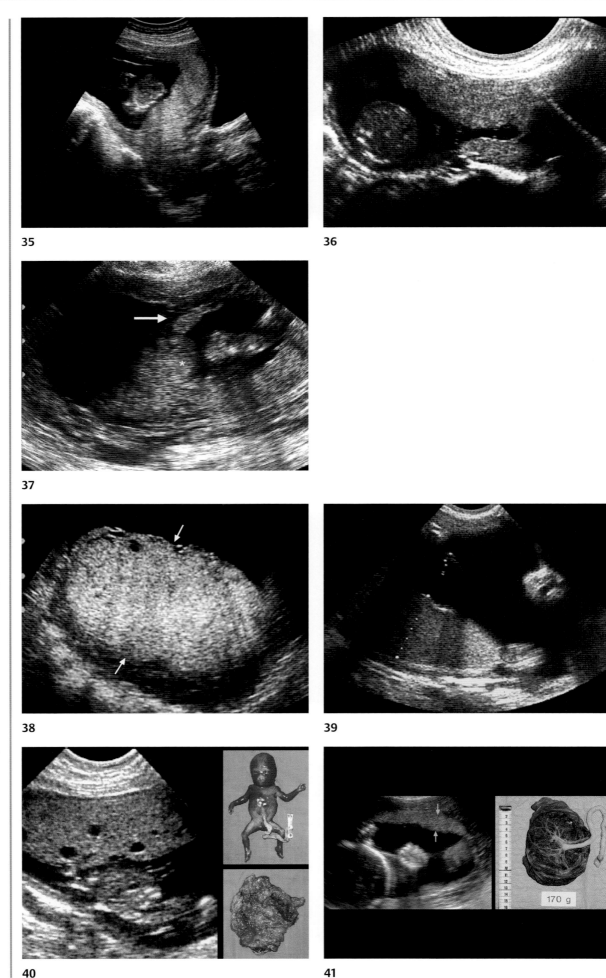

35

36

37

38

39

40

41

Placental area. Hoogland et al. (30) showed that placental area measurements can be useful in predicting fetal growth retardation. The weight and size of the organ provide an index for recognizing placental growth disturbances. For equal weights, the basal area of the placenta has pathogenetic significance. A placenta with a larger area contains more spiral artery terminations and is believed to be more favorable for fetal nutrition than a placental with a small area (6).

Placental perfusion. Color Doppler is useful for the qualitative evaluation of placental blood flow. It is common to find a marked reduction of perfusion in cases of fetal growth retardation (Fig. 34.**43**).

▬ *Placenta Accreta, Placenta Increta, Placenta Percreta*

Definition. These are conditions in which the chorion frondosum is implanted too deeply, with a partial or complete absence of the decidua basalis.

Forms. Three main forms are distinguished (Fig. 34.**44**):
- **Placenta accreta.** The basal villi are directly adherent to the myometrium without an interposed decidual layer. This condition may involve all or part of the placenta.
- **Placenta increta.** Villi and trophoblastic islands are located within the myometrium.
- **Placenta percreta.** The villi penetrate the myometrium all the way to the serosa.

Incidence. Reported incidence data range from one in 500 to one in 70,000 pregnancies (9).

Predisposing factors and pathogenesis. Predisposing factors are high parity, prior inflammations, scarring of the uterine corpus, prior cesarean section, and placenta previa.

The pathogenesis is based on the absence or poor development of the decidua, with an excessive depth of placental implantation. The clinical importance of this abnormal placentation is reflected in the fact that placenta accreta was present in 50% of all patients who required a postpartum hysterectomy (54).

Ultrasound criteria. *Placenta accreta* is marked sonographically by an absence of the hypoechoic, subplacental venous complex that normally occurs between the placenta and myometrium (16, 49) (Fig. 34.**45**). With *placenta increta*, placental tissue can be seen infiltrating the myometrium (Fig. 34.**46**). The detection of placental vessels in the bladder wall signifies *placenta percreta*. Color Doppler can help confirm this diagnosis by demonstrating placental vessels in the bladder wall.

Finberg and Williams (17) describe several ultrasound criteria for diagnosing placenta accreta, increta, or percreta: absence of the hypoechoic myometrium between the placenta and echogenic uterine-bladder serosa, thinning or irregularity of the echogenic uterine-bladder serosa, and the extension of tissue of placental echogenicity into the myometrium or behind the uterine serosa. Applying these criteria, they were able to make a true-positive diagnosis in 14 of 18 cases and a true-negative diagnosis in 15 of 16 cases.

▬ *Placental Hematomas*

In patients with uterine bleeding, ultrasound permits the rapid detection of a fresh placental hemorrhage or organized hematoma. Fresh blood appears sonographically as an echo-free area. As the collection becomes organized it shows increasing echogenicity, until finally the hematoma may exhibit a placenta-like structure.

Forms. Hematomas can be classified into several forms based on their location.

Retroplacental hematoma. A fresh retroplacental hematoma appears as an echo-free area between the placenta and uterine wall, causing the placenta to bulge toward the uterine cavity (Figs. 34.**47**–34.**49**). The presence of this hematoma leads to separation of the placental villi from the maternal blood vessels. If more than 30–40% of the maternal placental surface is affected by the hematoma, it is likely that significant fetal hypoxia will occur (18). Retroplacental hematomas usually result from the rupture of spiral arteries leading to a "high-pressure hemorrhage," while most peripheral hematomas are due to bleeding from peripheral veins, resulting in a low-pressure hemorrhage (23, 24, 48). Thus, placental abruption and retroplacental hematoma are closely related to hypertension and vascular disease, whereas placental abruption due to a peripheral hematoma is most commonly due to heavy maternal smoking during pregnancy. This leads to a decrease in uterine blood flow, especially at the less well-perfused placental margins, with subsequent necrosis and hemorrhage (48).

Retroplacental hematoma mainly requires differentiation from a well-vascularized uterine wall (Figs. 34.**25**, 34.**26**) and from intramural myoma (Fig. 34.**50**).

Intraplacental hematoma (intervillous thrombosis). Intervillous thrombi can be detected in 36% of placentas at term. They result from intraplacental hemorrhage due to the rupture of villous capillaries, causing extravasation from both the fetal and maternal systems (18). Sonographically, the thrombi usually appear as rounded intraplacental hypoechoic areas that may contain fine internal echoes (Fig. 34.**51**). Differentiation from placental infarction can be difficult. Intervillous thrombosis is distinguished from "placental lakes" by the inability to detect blood flow.

Marginal sinus hematoma. A marginal sinus hematoma is a subchorionic hematoma. It appears sonographically as a hypoechoic, crescent-shaped separation of the membranes from the uterine wall directly adjacent to the placenta (Figs. 34.**47**, 34.**52**–34.**54**). Differentiation is required from a large placental marginal sinus. Serial scans will usually document a reduction in the bulge.

Subamniotic hematoma. This collection on the placental surface is from fetal vessels that have spontaneously ruptured or have been punctured by an invasive procedure (Fig. 34.**47**). Ultrasound shows a hemorrhagic area on the placental surface that bulges into the amniotic cavity (Fig. 34.**55**).

Older hematomas. Older hematomas can acquire an echogenic, placenta-like structure due to the organization process. Fibrin strands are sometimes visible within the hematoma (Fig. 34.**56**).

▬ *Placental Abruption*

The premature separation of a normally positioned placenta from the myometrium is a major cause of maternal and perinatal morbidity and mortality. The incidence of placental abruption in the third trimester is 0.5–1.3%. It may be caused by pathologic processes involving the placental attachment site or the uterine vessels (22, 23). The reported perinatal mortality rate is 17–50% (3, 43). Mortality rates higher than 70% have been observed in some series (51).

Risk factors. The risk of placental abruption is increased by a prior history of abnormal pregnancy, multiparity, low birth weight, and especially by cigarette smoking and drug use.

Other risk factors are rapid uterine decompression after premature

Fig. 34.**42** Abnormally thin anterior placenta (placental thickness 1.6 cm) with pronounced polyhydramnios in a monoamniotic twin pregnancy, 32 weeks.

Fig. 34.**43** Placental perfusion.
a Normal placental perfusion (power Doppler image), 20 weeks.
b Deficient placental perfusion in GEPH disorder (power Doppler image), 28 weeks.

42

43

Fig. 34.**44** Schematic representation of placenta accreta, placenta increta, and placenta percreta.

Fig. 34.**45** Placenta accreta. A clear line of demarcation cannot be discerned between the placenta and uterine wall.

44

45

Fig. 34.**46** Left-sided placenta increta. The echogenic placenta has infiltrated the hypoechoic myometrium (arrows).

Placental hematomas

Fig. 34.**47** Possible sites of occurrence of placental hematomas.

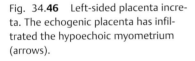

46

47

Fig. 34.**48** Retroplacental hematoma (4.5 x 3 cm) bordering a posterior placenta. Transverse scan at 26 weeks.

Fig. 34.**49** Gross specimen corresponding to Fig. 34.**48**.

48

49

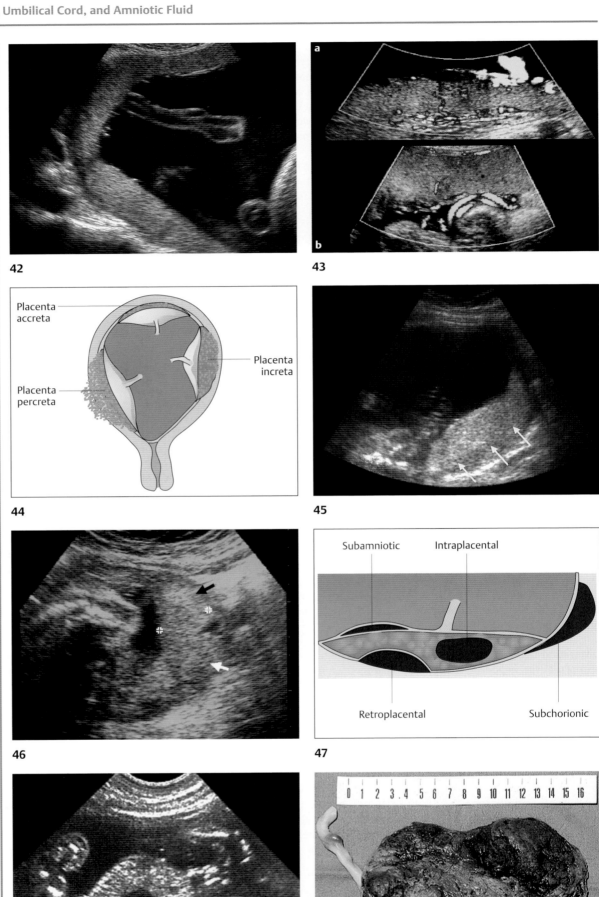

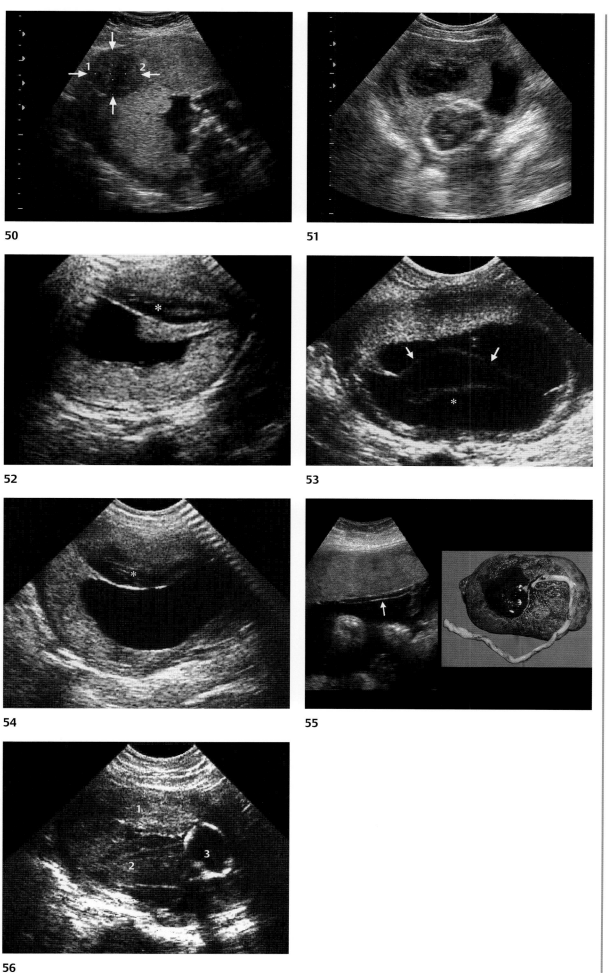

50

51

52

53

54

55

56

Fig. 34.**50** Hypoechoic intramural fundic myoma (3.5 × 3.1 cm) located behind the placenta mimics a retroplacental hematoma at 15 weeks, 3 days.

Fig. 34.**51** Hypoechoic intraplacental hematoma (4.3 × 3 cm) at 17 weeks. Fetal growth is at the lower limit of normal for gestational age.

Fig. 34.**52** Subchorionic hematoma on the anterior uterine wall (∗) with partial placental separation.

Fig. 34.**53** Large marginal sinus hematoma (∗) with separation of the membranes from the posterior uterine wall (arrows). Transverse scan at 18 weeks.

Fig. 34.**54** Marginal sinus hematoma (∗) with separation of the membranes from the anterior uterine wall. Transverse scan at 17 weeks. The streak-like echoes signify initial organization of the hematoma.

Fig. 34.**55** Separation of the amniotic membrane by a subamniotic 4-cm hematoma located at the lower margin of a low-lying posterior placenta. Longitudinal scan at 18 weeks.

Fig. 34.**56** Old placental hematoma at the lower placental margin with intrauterine fetal death. Echogenic fibrin strands are already visible within the organized hematoma. Transverse scan at 20 weeks.
1 = Placenta
2 = Organized hematoma
3 = Fetal head

Placental abruption and placental infarction

Fig. 34.**57** Almost complete placental abruption with intrauterine fetal death. Longitudinal scan at 34 weeks. 1 = Uterine wall, 2 = fresh hematoma, 3 = detached placenta. Emergency ultrasound was performed in the delivery room.

Fig. 34.**58** Placental abruption with a large retroplacental hematoma. Specimen corresponding to Fig. 34.**57**.

Fig. 34.**59** Above: GEPH placenta with a large, fresh, hypoechoic, hemorrhagic infarct and a small, older, echogenic infarct (arrow) at 31 weeks. Below: corresponding specimen.

Fig. 34.**60** GEPH placenta on the right sidewall with a conspicuous infarction (arrows) at 35 weeks. There is marked concomitant fetal growth retardation.

Tumors of the placenta

Fig. 34.**61** Chorioangioma with a hypoechoic cavernous structure.

Fig. 34.**62** Chorioangioma. Color Doppler demonstrates well-vascularized areas of the tumor.

Fig. 34.**63** Circumscribed bulge with scattered lacunae in an otherwise normal placenta, mimicking a placental tumor.

Unfused amnion, amniotic bands

Fig. 34.**64** Failure of the amniotic epithelium (arrows) to fuse with the chorion, 13 weeks. Karyotype: trisomy 21.

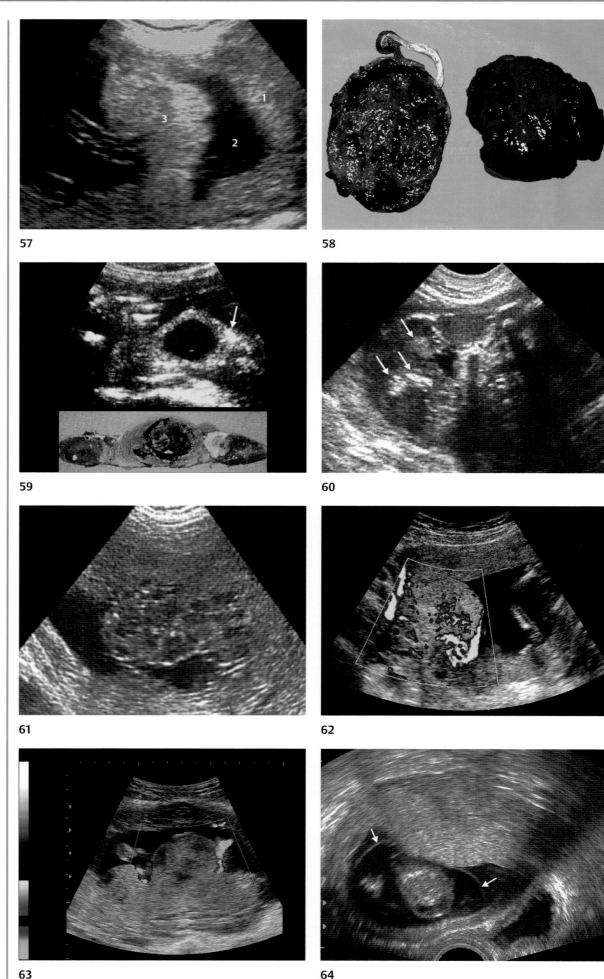

57

58

59

60

61

62

63

64

rupture of the membranes (especially with concomitant polyhydramnios), rapid delivery of the first child in a multiple pregnancy, premature labor, and premature deliveries.

Diagnosis. The diagnosis of placental abruption is made from clinical manifestations (bleeding, premature labor, pain, faintness), which can vary greatly in degree, and by direct ultrasound visualization of the detached placenta.

A complete or almost complete abruption is characterized by a large hematoma, which appears as a broad, hypoechoic crescent separating most or all of the placenta from the uterine wall (Figs. 34.**57**, 34.**58**).

Placental Infarction

Infarcts occur in up to 25% of all placentas at term. Most infarcts are small and have no clinical consequences (18). Extensive placental infarction in the first and second trimesters usually results from a maternal vascular disease. In a few cases, large myomas can lead to adjacent placental infarction. Sonographically, the placenta contains areas of variable size, sometimes confluent, that are initially hypoechoic and become more echogenic with passage of time (Figs. 34.**59**, 34.**60**).

Tumors of the Placenta

The following types are distinguished:
- Trophoblastic diseases
- Chorioangiomas
- Teratomas
- Metastatic lesions

Chorioangioma

This is a vascular tumor arising from the amniotic surface of the placenta. It is not observed until the third trimester (67). The incidence is approximately one in 250 pregnancies. About four-fifth of chorioangiomas are incidental microscopic findings. Tumors that produce clinical manifestations or ultrasound changes are very rare, with an incidence of one in 3500 to one in 20,000 births. Grossly, the lesions are solitary or multiple, sharply marginated, occasionally pedunculated tumors weighing up to 500 g. Both hyper- and hypovascular areas can occur in the same tumor, along with cellular and fibrous areas.

Complications. Potential complications of chorioangioma are polyhydramnios, premature labor, fetal hydrops, and intrauterine growth retardation. Several causes besides tumor size have been suggested for polyhydramnios and hydrops associated with placental chorioangioma: umbilical cord obstruction, protein loss, and especially intratumoral arteriovenous shunting, which directs blood past the placenta and leads to fetal volume overload and congestive failure.

Ultrasound diagnosis. Asokan et al. (1) published the first report on the ultrasound diagnosis of chorioangioma in 1978. The tumor appears sonographically as a circumscribed, solid (hyperechoic or hypoechoic) mass that often arises from the fetal side of the placenta and is usually located near the umbilical cord insertion (Fig. 34.**61**). Richly vascularized areas of the tumor can be defined with color Doppler ultrasound (Fig. 34.**62**). Polyhydramnios occurs in approximately one-third of cases (63). Fetal hydrops is a poor prognostic sign, usually occurring in association with large tumors that involve the placenta or umbilical cord. Quintero et al. (53) reported on initial therapeutic experience with intrauterine endoscopic tumor devascularization using a laser technique.

Differential diagnosis. Circumscribed bulges in an otherwise normal placenta (Fig. 34.**63**) and intraplacental hemorrhages are sometimes difficult to distinguish from a chorioangioma. Doppler scanning can advance the differential diagnosis by defining arterial blood flow in the chorioangioma.

Teratomas

Placental teratomas are usually solid, nonhomogeneous masses that are detectable in the chorionic plate or umbilical cord.

Metastatic Lesions

Placental metastases from malignant primary tumors have been described for both maternal and fetal malignancies.
- Maternal primary
  - Tumor cells can embolize to the intervillous spaces from various carcinomas (ovarian, mammary, gastric, pulmonary), lymphatic leukemia, Ewing sarcoma, and angioplastic sarcoma of the vagina. Metastases from malignant melanoma can infiltrate the villous stroma and may even invade the fetus through transplacental spread.
- Fetal primary:
  - Neuroblastoma, hepatoblastoma, congenital leukosis (66).

Unfused Amnion

Under normal circumstances the amniotic membrane fuses with the chorion between 12 and 13 weeks' gestation and can no longer be distinguished from it. If this fails to occur, the unfused amnion may be identified as a thin, semicircular membrane surrounding the fetus (Fig. 34.**64**). When noted after 14 weeks' gestation, this is considered an indirect sign of a fetal chromosomal abnormality (see Chapter 32).

Amniotic Bands

Occasionally an echogenic strand can be seen within the amniotic fluid, stretching between the placenta and uterine wall. These strands are usually produced by a partial separation of the amnion and chorion (12) (Figs. 34.**65**, 34.**66**), but some result from partial uterine septation or a synechia (44). In contrast to amniotic band syndrome, these strands are not attached to the fetus and do not constrain fetal movements.

Amniotic Band Syndrome

Definition. The amniotic band syndrome or ADAM syndrome (*amniotic deformity, adhesions, mutilations*) is a type of disruption in which fibrous amniotic strands form between the amnion and fetus in early pregnancy, causing a significant disturbance of fetal development marked by ectodermal, craniofacial, or visceral defects.

Findings. Depending on the location of the amniotic bands, constrictions around the fetal extremities may be the only abnormalities that occur in mild cases. Severe cases may involve the amputation of fingers, toes or an entire limb (Figs. 30.**33**–30.**35**), or the bands may strangulate whole portions of the brain (2, 11). A band wrapped around the umbilical cord may cause intrauterine fetal death (15, 39).

Pathogenesis. Torpin (61) attributes the syndrome to an early rupture of the amnion followed by amniochorionic separation, allowing the fetus to come into contact with the chorion. Both the exposed chorion and the outer surface of the amnion have the ability to produce meso-dermal strands, and these can extend toward the fetus after the chorion has absorbed the amniotic fluid. The chorion thickens as gestation proceeds and is then able to retain the fluid that is newly formed.

Incidence. Incidence data on amniotic band syndrome range from one in 1200 (58) to one in 10,000 (2) live births.

Ultrasound detection. Severe cases can be detected sonographically as early as 24 weeks' gestation (44, 45). Typically, oligohydramnios is found in association with fine echogenic strands that stretch between the placenta or uterine wall *and* the fetus and restrict fetal movements. The fetal abnormalities caused by amniotic bands, unlike genetic fetal anomalies, tend to be asymmetrical (61).

A unilateral encephalocele or a large defect in the anterior abdominal wall with the evisceration of liver and bowel (see Chapter 26), possibly combined with thoracoschisis, should raise suspicion of amniotic band syndrome, even if the amniotic bands cannot be directly visualized with ultrasound due to pronounced oligohydramnios (44).

Prognosis. The prognosis depends on the severity of the entrapments that have occurred. If large defects are detected sonographically before 24 weeks, termination should be considered due to the dismal prognosis. Occurrence of the syndrome does not appear to increase the risk of recurrence (26).

References

1. Asokan, S., Chadalavada, K., Gardi, R., Sastry, V.: Prenatal diagnosis of placental tumor by ultrasound. J. Clin. Ultrasound 6 (1978) 180–181
2. Baker, C.J., Rudolph, A.J.: Congenital ring constrictions and intrauterine amputations. Amer. J. Dis. Child. 121 (1971) 393–400
3. Balde, M., Grischke, E.M., Stolz, W., Kaufmann, M., Bastert, G.: Die vorzeitige Plazentalösung. Geburtsh. u. Frauenheilk. 50 (1990) 199–202
4. Beck, T.: Der venöse Blutfluß der intervillösen Mikrozirkulation in der menschlichen Plazenta. Z. Geburtsh. Perinat. 186 (1982) 114–118
5. Becker, V.: Pathologie der Plazenta. Spezielle pathologische und diagnostische Probleme. In.: Födisch, H.J. (Hrsg.): Neue Erkenntnisse über die Orthologie und Pathologie der Plazenta. Stuttgart: Enke 1977; S. 26–44
6. Becker, V.: Plazenta. In: Doerr, W., Seifert, S.: Pathologie der weiblichen Genitalorgane I. Pathologie der Plazenta und des Abortes. Berlin: Springer 1989; S. 1–140
7. Benirschke, K., Kaufmann, P.: Pathology of the human placenta. 2nd ed. Berlin: Springer 1990
8. Bey, M., Dott, A., Miller, J.M.Jr.: The sonographic diagnosis of circumvallate placenta. Obstet. Gynecol. 78 (1991) 515–517
9. Breen, J.L., Neubecker, R., Gregori, C.A., Franklin, J.E.Jr.: Placenta accreta, increta and percreta. A survey of 40 cases. Obstet. Gynecol. 49 (1977) 43–47
10. Brown, H.L., Miller, J.M.J, Khawli, O., Gabert, H.A.: Premature placental calcification in maternal cigarette smokers. Obstet. Gynecol. 71 (1988) 914–917
11. Burck, U., Held, K.R.: Amnionbändersyndrom – Zwei Fallbeschreibungen. In: Tolksdorf, M., Spranger, J.: Klinische Genetik in der Pädiatrie. Stuttgart: Thieme 1979; S. 133
12. Burrows, P.E., Lyons, E.A., Phillips, H.J., Oates, I.: Intrauterine membranes: Sonographic findings and clinical significance. J. Clin. Ultrasound 10 (1982) 1–8
13. Clark, S.L., Koonings, P.P., Phelan, J.P.: Placenta praevia/accreta and prior cesarean section. Obstet. Gynecol. 66 (1985) 89–92
14. Claussen, U., Hansmann, M.: Die „Pipettenmethode" zur schnellen Karyotypisierung bei sonographischen Verdachtskriterien für eine Chomosomenanomalie. Gynäkologie 17 (1984) 33–40
15. Cody, M.L., Uetzmann, I.F.: Amniotic bands as a cause of intrauterine fetal death. Amer. J. Obstet. Gynec. 74 (1957) 1102–1105
16. De Mendoncu, L.K.: Sonographic diagnosis of placenta accreta: Presentation of six cases. J. Ultrasound Med. 7 (1988) 211–215
17. Finberg, H.J., Williams, J.W.: Placenta accreta: Prospective sonographic diagnosis in patients with placenta previa and prior cesarean section. J. Ultrasound Med. 11 (1992) 333–343
18. Fox, H.: Pathology of the placenta. London: Saunders 1978; S. 95–148
19. Geirssson, R.T., Ogston, S.A., Patel, N.B., Christie, A.D.: Growth of the total intrauterine, intraamniotic and placental volume in normal singleton pregnancy measured by ultrasound. Brit. J. Obstet Gynaecol. 92 (1985) 46–53
20. Grannum, P.A., Berkowitz, R.L., Hobbins, J.C.: The ultrasonic changes in the maturing placenta and their relation to fetal pulmonic maturity. Amer. J. Obstet. Gynecol. 133 (1979) 915–922
21. Grannum, P.A., Hobbins, J.C.: The placenta. Radiol. Clin. North Amer. 20 (1982) 353–365
22. Green, J.R.: Placenta praevia and abruptio placentae. In: Creasy, R.K., Resnik, R. (eds.): Maternal-Fetal Medicine: Principles and Practice. Philadelphia: Saunders 1992; p. 592
23. Green-Thompson, R.W.: Antepartum haemorrhage. Clin. Obstet. Gynecol. 9 (1982) 479–515

Fig. 34.**65**   Transverse amniotic band 5 mm thick at the lower placental margin. Transverse scan at 17 weeks.

Fig. 34.**66**   Amniotic band between the lower edge of the anterior placenta and the posterior uterine wall. Longitudinal scan at 16 weeks. Below the amniotic band is the fetus, whose movements are not constrained.

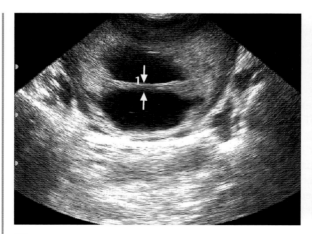

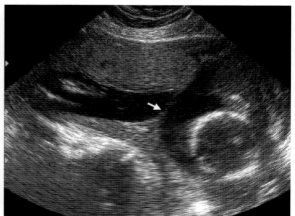

65   **66**

24. Grünwald, P., Levin, H., Yousem, H.: Abruption and premature separation of the placenta. Amer. J. Obstet. Gynecol. 102 (1968) 604–610
25. Harman, C.R., Manning, F.A., Stearns, E., Morrison, I.: The correlation of ultrasonic placental grading and fetal pulmonary maturation in 563 pregnancies. Amer. J. Obstet. Gynecol. 143 (1982) 941–943
26. Higginbottom, M.C., Jones, K.L., Hall, B.D., Smith, D.W.: The amniotic band disruption complex: timing of amniotic rupture and variable spectra of consequent defects. J. Pediat. 95 (1979) 544–549
27. Hills, D., Irwin, G.A.L., Tuck, S.: Distribution of placental grade in high-risk gravidity. AJR 143 (1984) 1011–1013
28. Hoddick, W.K., Mahony, B.S., Callen, P.W.: Placental thickness. J. Ultrasound Med. 4 (1985) 479–482
29. Holländer, H.J.: Die Ultraschalldiagnostik während der Schwangerschaft. In: Döderlein, G., Wulf, H.H.: Klinik der Frauenheilkunde und Geburtshilfe, Bd. VI. München: Urban & Schwarzenberg 1975
30. Hoogland, H.J., de Haan, J., Martin, C.B.Jr.: Placental size during early pregnancy and fetal outcome: a preliminary report of a sequential ultrasonographic study. Amer. J. Obstet. Gynecol. 138 (1980) 441–443
31. Hopper, K.D., Komppa, G.H., Williams, B.P.: A reevaluation of placental grading and its clinical significance. J. Ultrasound Med. 3 (1984) 261–266
32. Hurley, V.A., Beischer, N.A.: Placenta membranacea: Case reports. Brit. J. Obstet. Gynaecol. 94 (1987) 798–802
33. Jauniaux, E., Ramsay, B., Campbell, S.: Ultrasonographic investigation of placental morphologic characteristics and size during the second trimester of pregnancy. Amer J. Obstet. Gynecol. 170 (1994) 130–137
34. Jeanty, P., Kirkpatrick, C., Verhoogen, C., Struyven, J.: The succenturiata placenta. J. Ultrasound 2 (1983) 9–12
35. Katz, V.L., Blanchard, G.F., Watson, W.J., Miller, R.C., Chescheir, N.C., Thorp, J.M.: The clinical implications of subchorionic placental lucencies. Amer. J. Obstet. Gynecol. 164 (1991) 99–100
36. Kaufmann, P.: Placentation und Placenta. In: Hinrichsen, K.V. (Hrsg.): Human-Embryologie. Berlin: Springer 1993; S. 159–204
37. Kazzi, G.M., Gross, T.L., Sold, R.J.: Detection of intrauterine growth retardation: A new use for sonographic placental grading. Amer. J. Obstet. Gynecol. 145 (1983) 733–737
38. Kazzi, G.M., Gross, T.L., Rosen, M.G., Jaatoul-Kazzi, N.Y.: The relationship of placental grade, fetal lung maturity and neonatal outcome in normal and complicated pregnancies. Amer. J. Obstet. Gynecol. 148 (1984) 54–58
39. Kotz, H.L., Vidone, R.A.: Intrauterine death due to amniotic bands. Obstet. Gynecol. 13 (1959) 717–722
40. Kozlowski, P., Terinde, R., Schmitt, H.: Bestimmung des Plazentawachstums aus Ultraschallschnittbildern. Ultraschall 1 (1980) 116–132
41. Laing, F.C.: Ultrasound evaluation of obstetric problems relating to the lower uterine segment and cervix. In: Sanders, R.C., James, A.E.Jr. (eds): The principles and practice of ultrasonography in obstetrics and gynecology. 3rd ed. Norwalk, CT 1985; pp. 355–367
42. Leerentfeld, R.A., Gilberts, E.C., Arnold, M.J., Wladimiroff, J.W.: Accuracy and safety of transvaginal sonographic placental localisation. Obstet. Gynecol. 76 (1990) 759–762
43. Lowe, T.W., Cunningham, F.G.: Placental abruption. Clin. Obstet. Gynecol. 33 (1990) 406–413
44. Mahony, B.S., Filly, R.A., Callen, P.W., Golbus, M.S.: The amniotic band syndrome: Antenatals sonographic diagnosis and potential pitfalls. Amer. J. Obstet. Gynecol. 152 (1985) 63–68
45. Merz, E., Gerlach, R., Hoffmann, G., Goldhofer, W.: Das Amnionbändersyndrom im Ultraschall. Geburtsh. u. Frauenheilk. 44 (1984) 576–578

46. Moore, K.L.: Embryologie. Stuttgart: Schattauer 1985
47. Morin, F., Winsberg, F.: Real-time identification of blood flow in the placental and umbilical cord. J. Clin. Ultrasound 10 (1982) 21–24
48. Naeye, R.L.: Abruptio placentae and placenta praevia: frequency, perinatal mortality and cigarette smoking. Obstet. Gynecol. 55 (1980) 701–704
49. Pasto, M.E., Kurtz, A.B., Rijkin, M.D.: Ultrasonographic findings of placenta increta. J. Ultrasound Med. 2 (1983) 155–159
50. Petrucha, R.A., Platt, L.D.: Relationship of placental grade to gestational age. Amer. J. Obstet. Gynecol. 144 (1982) 733
51. Psychrembel, W., Dudenhausen, J.W.: Praktische Geburtshilfe. Berlin: de Gruyter 1989; S. 588
52. Quinlan, R.W., Cruz, A.C.: Ultrasonic placental grading and fetal pulmonary maturity. Amer. J. Obstet. Gynecol. 142 (1982) 110–111
53. Quintero, R.A., Reich, H., Romero, R., Johnson, M.P., Goncales, L., Evans, M.L.: In utero endoscopic devascularisation of a large choriangioma. Ultrasound Obstet. Gynecol. 8 (1996) 48–52
54. Ramin, S.M., Gilstrap, L.C.: Placental abnormalities: previa, abruption and accreta. In: Plauch, W.C., Morrison, J.C., O'Sullivan, M. (eds): Surgical obstetrics. Philadelphia: Saunders 1992; S. 203
55. Reynols, S.R.M.: On growth and form in the hemochorial placenta: An essay on the physical forces that shape the chorionic throphoblast. Amer. J. Obstet. Gynecol. 114 (1972) 115–132
56. Schlensker, K.H.: Plazentographie mittels Ultraschall-Schnittbildverfahren. Geburtsh. u. Frauenheilk. 31 (1971) 879–897
57. Schlensker, K.H.: Ultraschallplazentographie. Gynäkologie 9 (1976) 156–165
58. Seeds, J.W., Cefalo, R.C., Herbert, W.N.P.: Amniotic band syndrome. Amer. J. Obstet. Gynec. 144 (1982) 243–248
59. Sherman, S.J., Carlson, D.E., Platt, L.J., Medearis, A.L.: Transvaginal ultrasound: does it help in the diagnosis of placenta praevia? Ultrasound Obstet. Gynecol. 2 (1992) 256–260
60. Smith, S., Lauria, M.R., Comstock, L.H. et al.: Transvaginal ultrasonography for all placentas that appear to be low-lying or over the internal cervical os. Ultrasound Obstet. Gynecol. 9 (1997) 22–24
61. Torpin, R.: Amniochorionic mesoblastic fibrous strings and amniotic bands. Amer. J. Obstet. Gynec. 91 (1965) 65–75
62. Townsend, R.T., Laing, F.C., Nyberg, D.A.: Technical factors responsible for „placental migration": sonographic assessment. Radiology 160 (1986) 105–108
63. van Wering, J.H., van der Slikke, J.W.: Prenatal diagnosis of choriangioma associated with polyhydramnions using ultrasound. Eur. J. Obstet. Gynecol. Reprod. Biol. 19 (1985) 255–259
64. Vermeulen, R.C.W., Lambalk, N.B., Exalto, N., Arts, N.F.: An anatomic basic for ultrasound images of the human placenta. Amer. J. Obstet. Gynecol. 153 (1985) 806–810
65. Vogel, M.: Atlas der morphologischen Plazentadiagnostik. 2. Auflage. Berlin: Springer 1996
66. Vogel, M.: Pathologie der Schwangerschaft, der Plazenta und des Neugeborenen. In: Remmele, W. (Hrsg.): Pathologie, Bd. 4. Berlin: Springer 1997; S. 369–461
67. Wallenburg, H.C.S.: Choriangioma of the placenta. Obstet. Gynecol. Surv. 26 (1971) 411–428
68. Wexler, M.D., Gottesfeld, K.R.: Second trimester placenta praevia: An apparently normal placentation. Obstet. Gynecol. 50 (1977) 706–709
69. Winsberg, F.: Echographic changes with placental aging. J. Clin. Ultrasound 1 (1973) 52
70. Wolf, H., Oosting, H., Treffers, P.E.: Placental volume measurement by ultrasonography: Evaluation of the method. Amer. J. Obstet. Gynecol. 156 (1987) 1191–1194

35 Umbilical Cord

Normal Umbilical Cord

Anatomy and Physiology

Length. The umbilical cord at the end of pregnancy is approximately 50–70 cm long and 1–1.5 cm thick. Longitudinal growth of the cord is probably stimulated by stretching of the cord during fetal movements. Accordingly, a short umbilical cord is often associated with a lack of fetal movement during the first half of pregnancy (6). A long umbilical cord (> 90 cm) is found in 0.2–1% of pregnancies (21). This increases the risk of cord coiling and prolapse and of true knotting of the cord. A short umbilical cord (< 40 cm) is described in 0.3–0.9% of placentas (34). A short cord is associated with an increased risk of breech presentation, placental abruption during fetal descent, and vasospasms in the cord caused by extensive traction during delivery.

Vessels. The umbilical cord contains two arteries, which carry deoxygenated blood from the fetus to the placenta, and one vein, which returns oxygenated blood from the placenta to the fetus. Even in the first trimester, both longitudinal and transverse ultrasound scans can demonstrate the three umbilical vessels with their hypoechoic lumina, with color Doppler providing the most detailed views (Fig. 35.1). As the pregnancy proceeds, the vein is clearly distinguishable from the two arteries by its larger caliber (Fig. 35.2).

Umbilical Cord Biometry

Cord diameter. Measurement of the cord diameter is an outer-to-outer measurement that can be performed in both longitudinal and transverse scans (Fig. 35.4). Weissman et al. (33) recommend using the highest possible magnification for measuring the umbilical cord and the umbilical vessels. If the cord does not have an approximately round cross section, its diameter is obtained by averaging the largest and smallest cross sections. The cord diameter increases steadily during pregnancy and plateaus at about 36 weeks. This results from a reduction in the Wharton jelly volume due to a decreased water content (31).

Umbilical vessel diameters. Unlike the cord itself, the diameters of the umbilical vessels are taken as inner-to-inner measurements. The diameter of the umbilical vein (Fig. 35.5) is consistently greater than that of the two arteries (Fig. 35.6).

If a discrepancy is noted between the arterial calibers, the artery with the smaller diameter is considered to be the normal vessel while the larger artery represents abnormal dilatation (33). An arterial diameter greater than 4 mm between 20 and 36 weeks is considered strong evidence of a single umbilical artery (22). Dilatation of the single umbilical artery, with a corresponding decrease in flow resistance, is viewed as a compensatory mechanism to maintain adequate fetoplacental blood flow (27).

Raio et al. (26) suggest that discordant umbilical arterial diameters are a mild form of the single umbilical artery syndrome.

Abnormalities of the Umbilical Cord

Single Umbilical Artery

Incidence. The most frequent abnormality of the umbilical cord is a single umbilical artery, which has an incidence of 0.5–2.5% of all pregnancies (23) (Figs. 35.7, 35.8).

Etiology and pathogenesis. Three pathogenetic theories have been advanced:

- Primary agenesis of one umbilical artery
- Secondary atrophy or atresia of an originally normal umbilical artery
- Persistence of an original allantoic artery

Risk factors. The risk of a single umbilical artery is increased in maternal diabetes, epilepsy, hypertension, and in oligo- and polyhydramnios. Twin pregnancies show a significantly higher risk for a single umbilical artery than singleton pregnancies (13).

Ultrasound evaluation. Ultrasound evaluation of the umbilical arteries should be part of every examination for fetal anomalies. It is easiest to evaluate the umbilical vessels in a cross-sectional scan of the cord, which displays the three vessels in a "Mickey Mouse" pattern. Color Doppler may be helpful if the examination is difficult (15). Jeanty (16) deals with difficult situations by defining the umbilical arteries in the fetal pelvis to exclude a single umbilical artery (Fig. 35.9).

Associated anomalies. In 1955, Benirschke and Brown (1) were the first to report that 27 of 55 patients (49%) with a single umbilical artery exhibited congenital anomalies. Since then, numerous studies have documented an association between a single umbilical artery and congenital anomalies, perinatal mortality, premature delivery, intrauterine growth retardation, and chromosomal abnormalities (18, 30).

The overall reported incidence of associated anomalies is between 20% and 50%. One-fifth of these cases have multiple anomalies. The organ systems most commonly affected are the musculoskeletal system (23%), genitourinary tract (20%), cardiovascular system (19%), gastrointestinal tract (10%), and central nervous system. No consistent pattern of anomalies is seen, and any organ may be affected.

Chromosomal abnormalities. Fetuses with a single umbilical artery show an increased incidence of chromosomal disorders (3, 20). The most common is trisomy 18, but other chromosomal abnormalities such as trisomy 13, Turner syndrome, and triploidies are also associated with a single umbilical artery. The risk of a chromosome disorder depends on the presence of associated anomalies, so when concomitant malformations are detected along with a single umbilical artery, karyotyping should be performed.

Growth retardation. Intrauterine growth retardation and low birth weight are present in 28% of fetuses with a single umbilical artery. Fifteen to 20% of these cases have no accompanying anomalies (18).

Perinatal mortality. Fetuses with a single umbilical artery have a reported perinatal mortality rate of 8–60%, with an average of 20% (13, 18). It is unclear at present whether the increased mortality rate applies only to cases that have associated anomalies.

Management. Based on the figures presented above, the detection of a single umbilical artery has the following implications for further obstetric management:

- Detailed ultrasound examination of the fetus
- Fetal echocardiography
- Karyotyping
- Regular monitoring of fetal growth and condition
- Thorough examination of the neonate

Persistent Right Umbilical Vein

In very rare cases, a cross-sectional view of the umbilical cord may reveal an extra vessel (Fig. 35.**10**) (14). This is a persistent right umbilical vein, which normally is obliterated in the sixth week of embryonic life (8). The detection of an extra umbilical vessel, like the absence of a vessel, should trigger a detailed examination for fetal anomalies.

Knotting of the Umbilical Cord

True knotting. True knotting of the umbilical cord is seen in approximately 0.04–1% of all births (2). Predisposing factors are a long cord, polyhydramnios, a small fetus, and monoamniotic twins (32). Generally there is an increased risk of fetal hypoxia due to traction on the initially loose knot. Perinatal mortality is increased, with a rate of approximately 10% (4).

False knotting. The ultrasound diagnosis of true knotting of the cord is difficult (Fig. 35.**11**) because of its resemblance to the much more frequent condition of false knotting. A false knot results from the varicose dilatation of vascular loops or a circumscribed excess of Wharton jelly with pseudocystic degeneration.

Coiling of the Umbilical Cord

Coiling of the umbilical cord has an overall incidence of 20–33% (Fig. 35.**12**). In most cases it does not have a clinical or morphologic correlate. In other cases the coiling can restrict the fetal blood supply, producing characteristic changes in the cardiotocogram (25). In a study of 137 cases by Ertan, color Doppler ultrasound could detect coiling of the cord with a sensitivity of 97%, a positive predictive value of 89%, and a negative predictive value of 96% (9). The authors conclude that when coiling of the umbilical cord is detected sonographically, intrapartal monitoring should be intensified.

Umbilical Cord Cysts

For reasons unknown, the fluid content of the umbilical cord is highly variable. It is common to detect fluid-filled pseudocysts that do not have an epithelial lining. It is rare to find true umbilical cord cysts as remnants of the allantoic duct, the omphaloenteric duct, or superficial epithelial inclusion cysts (Fig. 35.**13**). The ultrasound appearance of these cysts has been documented in case reports (10, 24). Fink and Filly described several cases in which an umbilical cord cyst was associated with an omphalocele (10). Hence, when an umbilical cord cyst is detected sonographically, other cord abnormalities such as vascular anomalies, hemangioma, or omphalocele should be excluded.

Umbilical Cord Hematoma, Umbilical Cord Venous Thrombosis

Umbilical cord hematomas are usually secondary to an invasive procedure such as amniocentesis or cordocentesis (Fig. 35.**14**). Spontaneous hematomas caused by bleeding from umbilical vessels, hemangiomas, or persistent omphalomesenteric vessels are rare findings with an incidence between one in 5000 and one in 12,700 deliveries (11).

The high fetal mortality of up to 50% usually results from a fatal blood loss or compression of the umbilical vessels by the hematoma (29).

Thrombosis of the umbilical vein is most commonly a result of cordocentesis or intrauterine transfusion.

Tumors of the Umbilical Cord

Hemangiomas. Tumors of the umbilical cord are rare. They include hemangiomas, for which sporadic cases have been reported (28). These tumors appear sonographically as solid, echogenic, sometimes cystic masses of the umbilical cord that are frequently combined with an umbilical cord cyst. Like chorioangiomas of the placenta, hemangiomas of the umbilical cord can cause the shunting of blood with fetal hydrops.

Teratomas. Teratomas of the umbilical cord incorporating elements of all three germ layers are rare.

Variations of the Umbilical Cord Insertion

The normal umbilical cord insertion may be central (Fig. 35.**15**) or lateral (Fig. 35.**16**) in its location. Several abnormal types of cord insertion (17) are described below.

Marginal cord insertion. A marginal cord insertion has important fetal implications (Fig. 35.**17**) because kinking of the vessels at the placental margin can compromise the fetoplacental circulation. From 2% to 10% of all pregnancies exhibit a marginal cord insertion.

Velamentous insertion. The velamentous insertion, present in up to 1% of all pregnancies, poses a considerably greater risk to the fetus (11) (Fig. 35.**18**). Risk factors for this condition are multiparity, uterine anomalies, and pregnancies with an IUD in place. Since the cord vessels lie separately in a membrane, rupture of the membranes prematurely or at delivery can cause vascular tearing with risk of fetal death due to blood loss.

Vasa previa. This is a rare but very dangerous condition in which the cord vessels are located in the fetal membrane over the internal cervical os. The incidence is 0.1% of all pregnancies and is usually associated with a velamentous insertion. A succenturiate placental lobe is present in 3–6% of cases (7). The fetal mortality in cases of vasa previa rupture is between 33% and 100%. The clinical hallmarks are intrapartum hemorrhage and fetal distress after amniotomy. The early prenatal diagnosis of vasa previa is desirable to avoid hazardous situations. The first report on the diagnosis of vasa previa with Doppler ultrasound was published in 1987 (12). Today, transvaginal color Doppler scanning can detect vasa previa with a high degree of confidence so that a cesarean delivery can be planned (5, 19).

References

1. Benirschke, K., Brown, W.H.: A vascular anomaly of the umbilical cord. Obstet. Gynecol. 6 (1955) 399–404
2. Benirschke, K., Kaufmann, P.: Pathology of the human placenta. 2nd ed. Berlin: Springer 1990
3. Byrne, J.W.A.: Malformations and chromosome anomalies in spontaneously aborted fetuses with single umbilical artery. Amer. J. Obstet. Gynecol. 1 (1985) 340–342
4. Chasnoff, J., Fletcher, M.A.: True knot of the umbilical cord. Amer. J. Obstet. Gynecol. 117 (1997) 425–427
5. Clerici, G., Burnelli, L., Lauro, V., Pilu, G.L., Di Renzo, G.L.: Prenatal diagnosis of vasa previa presenting as amniotic band. „A not so innocent amniotic band". Ultrasound Obstet. Gynecol. 7 (1996) 61–63
6. De Sa, D.J.: Pathology of neonatal intensive care. London: Chapman and Hall 1995
7. Dougall, A., Baird, L.H.: Vasa previa – report of three cases and review of the literature. J. Obstet. Gynecol. 94 (1987) 712–715
8. England, M.A.: Farbatlas der Embryologie. Stuttgart: Schattauer 1985
9. Ertan, K., Schmidt, W.: Umbilical cord enlargement and color-coded Doppler ultrasound. Geburtsh. Frauenheilk. 54 (1994) 196–203
10. Fink, J.J., Filly, R.A.: Omphalocele associated with umbilical cord allantoic cyst; sonographic evaluation in utero. Radiology 194 (1983) 473–476
11. Fox, H.: Pathology of the placenta. Philadelphia: Saunders 1978
12. Gianopoulos, J.G., Carver, T., Tomych, P.G., Karlmann, R., Gadwood, U.: Diagnosis of vasa previa with ultrasonography. Obstet. Gynecol. 69 (1987) 488–491
13. Heifitz, G.A.: Single umbilical artery: a statistical analysis of 237 autopsy cases and review of the literature. Perspect. Pediatr. Pathol. 8 (1984) 345–378
14. Hill, L.M., Kislak, S., Runco, C.: An ultrasonic view of the umbilical cord. Obstet. Gynecol. Surv. 42 (1987) 82–88
15. Jauniaux, E., Campbell, S., Vyas, S.: The use of color Doppler imaging for prenatal diagnosis of umbilical cord abnormalities: report of three cases. Amer. J. Obstet. Gynecol. 161 (1989) 1195–1197
16. Jeanty, P.: Fetal and funicular vascular anomalies: identification with prenatal ultrasound. Radiology 173 (1989) 367–370
17. Kloos, K., Vogel, M.: Pathologie der Plazentarperiode. Stuttgart: Thieme 1974
18. Leuny, A.K.C., Robson, W.L.M.: Single umbilical artery. Amer. J. Dis. child. 143 (1989) 108–111
19. Meyer, W.J., Blumenthal, L., Cadhin, A., Gauthin, D.W., Rotmensch, S.: Vasa previa: prenatal diagnosis with transvaginal color Doppler flow imaging. Amer. J. Obstet. Gynecol. 169 (1993) 1627–1629
20. Nyberg, D.A., Mahony, B.S., Luthy, D., Kapur, R.: Single umbilical artery. Prenatal detection of concurrent anomalies. J. Ultrasound Med. 10 (1991) 247–253
21. Perrin, E.V.D.M.: Pathology of the placenta. New York: Churchill, Livingston 1984
22. Persutte, W.H., Lenke, R.R.: Transverse umbilical arterial diameter: Technique for the prenatal diagnosis of single umbilical artery. Ultrasound Med. 13 (1994) 763–766
23. Persutte, W.H., Hobbins, J.: Single umbilical artery: a clinical enigma in modern prenatal diagnosis. Ultrasound Obstet. Gynecol. 6 (1995) 216–219
24. Petrikowsky, B.M., Nochimson, D.J., Campbell, W.A.: Fetal jejunal atresia with persistent omphalomesenteric duct. Amer. J. Obstet. Gynecol. 158 (1988) 173–175
25. Polin, R.A., Fox, W.W.: Fetal and neonatal physiology. Vol. 1 and 2. Philadelphia: Saunders 1992
26. Raio, L., Saile, G., Brühwiler, H.: Diskordante Nabelschnurarterien: Pränatale Diagnostik und Bedeutung. Ultraschall in Med. 18 (1997) 229–232
27. Raio, L., Müller, M., Schumacher, A., Ghezzi, F., Di Naro, E., Brühwiler, H.: Gefäßdurchmesser und Resistance-Indices bei unauffälligen Feten mit singulärer Nabelschnurarterie. Ultraschall in Med. 19 (1998) 187–191
28. Resta, R.G., Luthy, D.A., Mahony, B.S.: Umbilical cord haemangioma associated with extremely high alpha-fetoprotein levels. Obstet. Gynecol. 72 (1988) 488–491
29. Ruvinsky, E.D., Wiley, T.L., Morrison, J.C.: In utero diagnosis of umbilical cord haematoma. Amer. J. Obstet. Gynecol. 140 (1981) 833–834
30. Shalev, E.: Placenta and umbilic cord. In: Chervenak, F.A., Isaacson, G.C., Campbell, S. (eds.): Ultrasound in Obstetrics and Gynecology, Lippincott, Philadelphia 1993; pp. 1089–1091
31. Sloper, K.S., Brown, R.S., Baum, J.D.: The water content of the human umbilical cord. Early Hum. Dev. 3 (1979) 205–210
32. Spellacy, W.N., Graven, H., Fisch, R.V.: The umbilical cord complications of true knots, nucheal coils and cord around the body. Amer. J. Obstet. Gynecol. 94 (1996) 425–427
33. Weissman, A., Jakobi, P., Bronsthein, M., Goldstein, I.: Sonographic measurement of the umbilical cord and vessels during normal pregnancies. J. Ultrasound Med. 13 (1994) 11–14
34. Wigglesworth, J.S., Singer, D.B. (eds.): Textbook of fetal and perinatal pathology. Vol. 1 and 2. Oxford: Blackwell 1991

Normal umbilical cord

Fig. 35.**1** Sidewall placenta with umbilical cord insertion. Color Doppler demonstrates flow in the cord vessels. Uterine transverse scan at 10 weeks.

Fig. 35.**2** Cross-sectional view of the umbilical cord at 27 weeks demonstrates the large-caliber vein and the two smaller-caliber arteries.

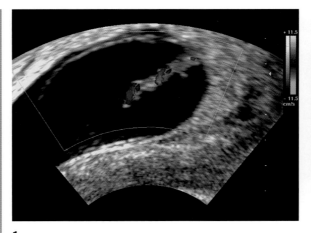

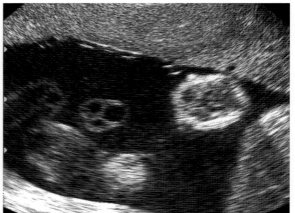

1

2

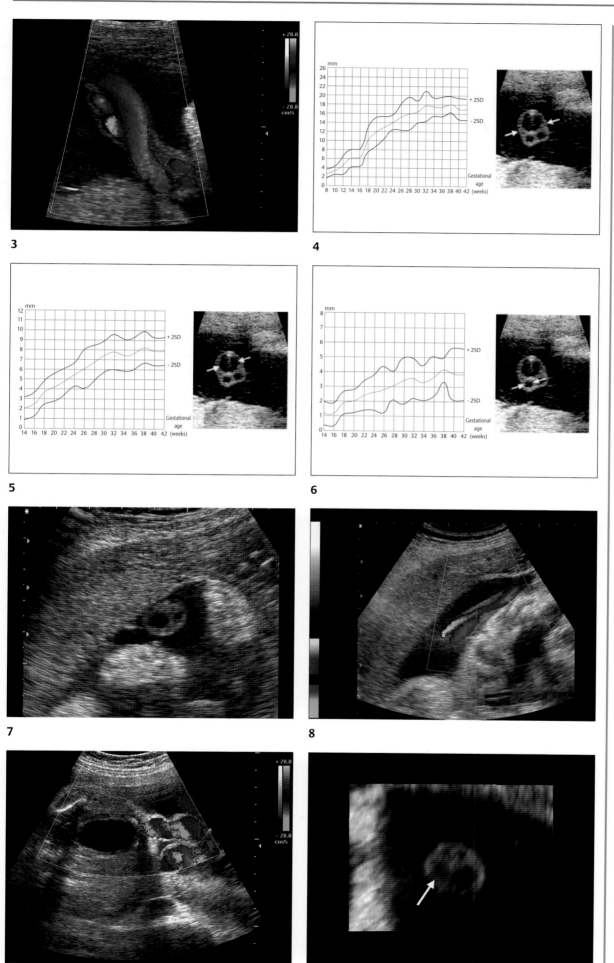

3

4

Fig. 35.**3**   Color Doppler image of the umbilical cord. Longitudinal scan at 35 weeks. The umbilical vein is shown in blue, the two umbilical arteries in red.

Umbilical cord biometry

Fig. 35.**4**   *Left:* normal growth curves for umbilical cord diameter after Weissman et al. (33). *Right:* outer-to-outer ultrasound measurement of the cord diameter.

5

6

Fig. 35.**5**   *Left:* umbilical vein biometry. Normal growth curves after Weissman et al. (33). *Right:* inner-to-inner ultrasound measurement of the venous diameter.

Fig. 35.**6**   *Left:* umbilical artery biometry. Normal growth curves after Weissman et al. (33). *Right:* inner-to-inner ultrasound measurement of the arterial diameter.

7

8

Abnormalities of the umbilical cord

Fig. 35.**7**   Atypical cord with a single umbilical artery. Trisomy 21, transverse scan, 29 weeks.

Fig. 35.**8**   Single umbilical artery in a longitudinal scan of the cord, 29 weeks. Color Doppler image of the umbilical vessels. The artery is shown in red, the vein in blue.

9

10

Fig. 35.**9**   When both umbilical arteries are present, color Doppler demonstrates an artery on each side of the fetal bladder. With a single umbilical artery, a vessel is seen on only one side of the bladder.

Fig. 35.**10**   Atypical umbilical cord with a persistent right umbilical vein (arrow). Instead of one vein, two veins are seen alongside the two umbilical arteries. Fetal hydrocephalus was also present. Transverse scan at 28 weeks.

Fig. 35.**11**   True knotting of the umbilical cord (arrow).

Fig. 35.**12**   Coiling of the umbilical cord around the fetal neck. The umbilical vessels can be rapidly visualized with color Doppler.

Fig. 35.**13**   Umbilical cord cyst (∗) measuring 6.5 × 5.4 × 5.2 cm, 35 weeks.

Fig. 35.**14**   Small umbilical cord hematoma (arrow) following cordocentesis (puncture of a free loop of umbilical cord).

Fig. 35.**15**   Central cord insertion in a posterior placenta. The vessels at the insertion site are visualized with color Doppler.

Fig. 35.**16**   Lateral cord insertion in a placenta implanted on the posterior and right uterine walls. Transverse scan.

Fig. 35.**17**   Marginal cord insertion in a posterior placenta. Transverse scan.

Fig. 35.**18**   Velamentous insertion (arrow) in an anterior placenta.

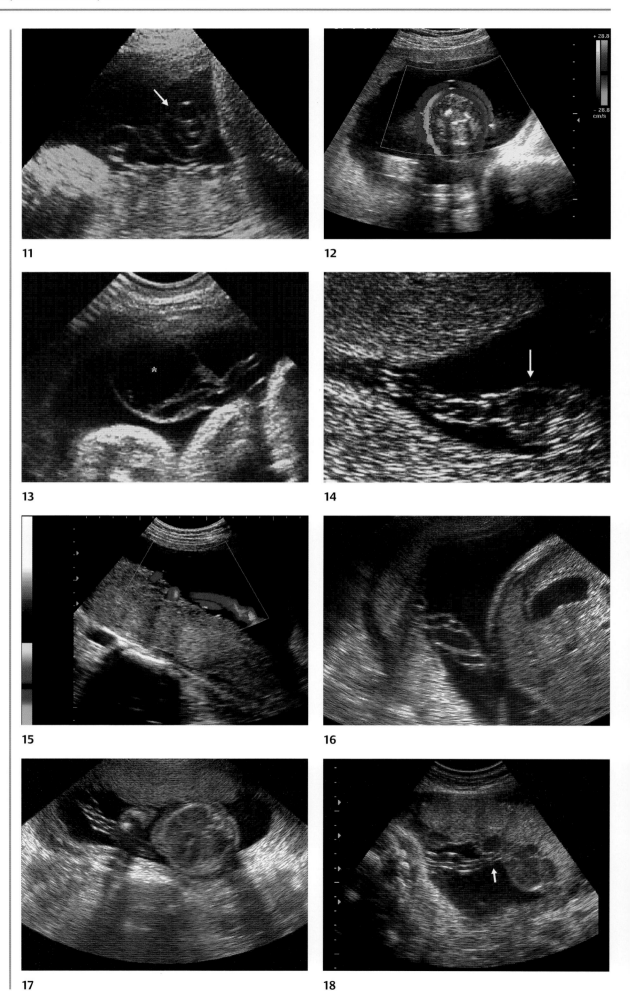

36 Amniotic Fluid

Physiology and Pathophysiology

The maintenance of a normal amniotic fluid volume is essential for normal fetal development. An excess or deficiency of amniotic fluid is associated with an increased incidence of fetal and neonatal morbidity and mortality (4).

Functions. The amniotic fluid enables the fetus to move freely, cushions against fetal injuries, ensures the maintenance of a constant temperature, contributes to the enlargement and expansion of the uterine cavity, critically influences the symmetrical development of the conceptus (especially the musculoskeletal system), and promotes cervical dilatation during birth.

Production and absorption. Under normal circumstances, the amniotic fluid is in a state of dynamic equilibrium between production and absorption. Available exchange surfaces are the amniotic epithelium, umbilical cord, fetal skin, gastrointestinal tract, respiratory tract, and urogenital tract (41).

▬ Production of Amniotic Fluid

Many theories have been advanced on the production of amniotic fluid. So far, however, no satisfactory explanation has been found to account for its production in all stages of pregnancy.

Amniotic fluid production is attributed initially to the amniotic epithelium and later to the fetal kidneys (1, 41). The fetal membranes and umbilical cord are the most important structures for the continuous exchange of water and electrolytes, while the swallowing of amniotic fluid by the fetus and fetal urine output into the amniotic fluid are intermittent processes (41).

Fetal urine production. Even before Hippocrates, it was believed that fetal urine production contributed to the formation of the amniotic fluid. This has been confirmed by more recent studies. Hypotonic urine can be detected in the fetal bladder as early as 12 weeks' gestation (20). The 24-hour fetal urinary output has been calculated at 7–17 mL based on ultrasound studies at 18 weeks (2). The daily urine output increases to 600–800 mL by the end of pregnancy.

▬ Regulation of Amniotic Fluid Volume

Fetal swallowing. An important factor in amniotic fluid regulation is fetal swallowing, which can be demonstrated as early as 12 weeks' gestation (2). The swallowed fluid volume increases during pregnancy to 200–450 mL/day (30). Approximately half of the daily fetal urine output is eliminated by fetal swallowing.

Aspiration and exchange through the skin. The amniotic fluid volume is also regulated by the fetal aspiration of amniotic fluid. The capillary bed in the fetal skin is also utilized as an exchange surface until the skin keratinizes. When keratinization is complete (at about 24 weeks), the skin is no longer permeable to water and electrolytes (41). Transfer through the umbilical vessels is also believed to play a role in amniotic fluid production (10).

Maternal plasma volume. Goodlin et al. (14) showed that the amniotic fluid volume depends on the extent of maternal plasma expansion between 29 and 36 weeks' gestation and that an acute increase in the maternal plasma volume can improve existing oligohydramnios.

Normal values. The total amniotic fluid volume is replaced approximately once every 24 hours. The amniotic fluid volume is approximately 60 mL at 12 weeks (41) and rises steadily to approximately 1000 mL by 34 weeks. It then decreases to an average of 840 mL by term (31) (Fig. 36.**1**). If the pregnancy is carried past the due date, the amniotic fluid volume continues to decline and averages only 540 mL at 42 weeks (31).

The amniotic fluid volume is not only related to gestational age but also correlates with fetal and placental weight (31).

Vernix caseosa. Bright, punctate echoes can be seen within the amniotic fluid in the second and third trimesters (Fig. 36.**2**). These floating echoes represent desquamated epithelial cells and small flakes of vernix caseosa.

Ultrasound Assessment of Amniotic Fluid Volume

Importance. An abnormal increase or decrease in the amniotic fluid volume correlates with fetal anomalies and maternal diseases and is therefore considered an important ultrasound suggestive sign of a fetal abnormality or maternal disorder (42).

Hence, ultrasound assessment of the amniotic fluid should be part of every obstetric ultrasound examination. The goal is to classify the amniotic fluid volume as normal, polyhydramnios, oligohydramnios, or severe oligohydramnios.

▬ Methods of Quantification

Various methods are available for quantitating the amniotic fluid volume with ultrasound. They include purely subjective assessments, the semiquantitative determination of the largest amniotic fluid pocket, the four-quadrant amniotic fluid index, planimetric measurement of the intrauterine volume, and mathematical models for calculating the amniotic fluid volume.

However, none of these methods, which are described below, can provide a "gold standard" for quantitating the fluid volume. Ultimately, a subjective assessment by an experienced examiner using real-time ultrasound will direct the diagnostic decision.

Subjective Assessment of Amniotic Fluid Volume

Examining the entire uterus, the sonographer evaluates the amniotic fluid volume based on his or her own subjective experience (13). The fluid volume is classified as normal (Figs. 36.**3**–36.**5**), copious (Figs. 36.**6**, 36.**7**), polyhydramnios (Figs. 36.**11**–36.**13**), scant (Figs. 36.**14**, 36.**15**), oligohydramnios (Fig. 36.**16**), or severe oligohydramnios (Figs. 36.**17**, 36.**18**).

According to Holländer (17), polyhydramnios should be diagnosed in the last 2 months of pregnancy if a second fetus would fit comfortably within the amniotic cavity.

Semiquantitative Determination of the Largest Amniotic Fluid Pocket

In this method the amniotic fluid volume is assessed by measuring the largest dimension of an echo-free fluid pocket between the fetus and uterine wall. The result is categorized as shown in Table 36.**1**.

Four-Quadrant Amniotic Fluid Index

Amniotic fluid index. Phelan et al. (28) expanded the semiquantitative four-quadrant technique and made it more precise by introducing the amniotic fluid index (AFI) for use in the third trimester. In this method the maternal abdomen is divided into four quadrants (Fig. 36.**8**). The quadrants are centered on the maternal umbilicus, and the linea alba forms the vertical axis. The vertical diameters of the largest fluid pocket in each of the four quadrants are determined in millimeters (Fig. 36.**9**) and are then added together to obtain the AFI (Table 36.**2**). Moore and Cayle (24) determined the AFI values as percentiles for 16–42 weeks of gestation (Fig. 36.**10**).

Planimetric Measurement of Intrauterine Volume

In this method, numerous scan planes are directed through the uterus at designated intervals. The intrauterine area of each plane is determined sonographically and multiplied by the thickness of the interval. The values are then added together to obtain the fetal intrauterine volume (8, 19).

Other Mathematical Calculations of Amniotic Fluid Volume

Various mathematical formulas have been devised for use with ultrasound data. The formulas are based on the largest amniotic fluid pocket or the intrauterine volume minus the fetal and placental volumes (12, 34).

■ *Abnormal Amniotic Fluid Volume*

Polyhydramnios (Hydramnios)

Chronic and acute hydramnios. Hydramnios refers to an amniotic fluid volume in excess of 2000 mL (Figs. 36.**11**–36.**13**). An amniotic fluid volume that increases markedly over a period of weeks (chronic hydramnios) is distinguished from a rapid volume increase in a matter of days (acute hydramnios).

Incidence. Polyhydramnios is found in 1.1–2.8% of all pregnancies, and 8–18% of cases are associated with a fetal anomaly (16, 35, 43). The rate of chromosomal abnormalities ranges from 9.6% to 22% (6, 11, 27).

Causes. Polyhydramnios can have numerous causes (Table 36.**3**). The main fetal abnormalities that lead to polyhydramnios are neural tube defects (anencephaly, iniencephaly, spina bifida), digestive tract anomalies (esophageal, duodenal or jejunal atresia), cardiac anomalies, and immune or nonimmune fetal hydrops. In particular, any defect that interferes with fetal swallowing (e.g., arthrogryposis multiplex congenita) or hampers fluid reabsorption in the small bowel can cause polyhydramnios (4, 5, 41, 36).

Other potential causes of polyhydramnios are placental chorioangioma, sacrococcygeal teratoma, and a fetofetal transfusion syndrome in twin pregnancies.

Polyhydramnios of maternal origin is found in diabetes mellitus and Rh incompatibility.

On the whole, polyhydramnios has a fetal cause in 20% of cases and a maternal cause in another 20%. The remaining 60% of cases are classified as *idiopathic polyhydramnios* (15, 16, 37).

Treatment. Definite clinical symptoms such as abdominal pain or dyspnea are indications for the treatment of polyhydramnios. Serial amniotic fluid decompressions removing 2–4 liters of amniotic fluid are the treatment of choice in many cases. Larger fluid volumes should not be removed in one sitting, as excessive decompression can lead to placental abruption.

Indomethacin, a prostaglandin synthetase inhibitor, is available for the medical treatment of polyhydramnios. It acts by decreasing the fetal urine output (22, 23). Except in fetofetal transfusion syndrome, indomethacin therapy yields good results in idiopathic polyhydramnios, providing a significant reduction in amniotic fluid volume (18). There is a risk, however, that indomethacin therapy will cause premature constriction of the fetal ductus arteriosus as well as mild endocardial ischemia and papillary muscle dysfunction (22).

Oligohydramnios

Incidence. Oligohydramnios is found in 1.7–7% of all pregnancies (16, 29) (Fig. 36.**16**). Generally speaking, oligohydramnios is considered to be an unfavorable prognostic sign (38).

Causes. A decreased amniotic fluid volume can have numerous causes (Table 36.**4**) such as fetal anomalies, intrauterine growth retardation, postmaturity, and premature rupture of the membranes. Rare causes may include placental dysfunction and medical therapy with prostaglandin synthetase inhibitors (e.g., indomethacin).

When fetal anomalies are responsible for oligohydramnios, the most frequent cause is a urogenital anomaly (4, 5), particularly bilateral renal agenesis, multicystic renal dysplasia, infantile polycystic kidneys, and obstructions of the ureters and urethra. Especially for fetuses with urethral stenosis, it is true that the smaller the amniotic fluid volume,

Table 36.1   Semiquantitative determination of the largest amniotic fluid pocket

> 2 cm, < 8 cm	Normal amniotic fluid volume
> 8 cm ● 8–12 cm ● 12–16 cm ● > 16 cm	Polyhydramnios ● Mild polyhydramnios ● Moderate polyhydramnios ● Severe polyhydramnios
≥ 1 cm, ≤ 2 cm	Borderline low amniotic fluid volume
< 1 cm	Oligohydramnios

Table 36.2   Amniotic fluid assessment using the four-quadrant amniotic fluid index

50–200 mm	Normal
> 200 mm	Polyhydramnios
< 50 mm	Oligohydramnios

Table 36.3   Possible causes of polyhydramnios

Fetal causes	➢ Neural tube defects ➢ Obstruction of the upper and middle digestive tract ➢ Cardiac anomalies ➢ Immune fetal hydrops ➢ Nonimmune fetal hydrops ➢ Arthrogryposis multiplex congenita
Maternal causes	➢ Diabetes mellitus ➢ Rh incompatibility
Other causes	➢ Chorioangioma ➢ Fetofetal transfusion syndrome

the poorer the prognosis (21). The complete absence of amniotic fluid, termed anhydramnios, is usually associated with an original Potter syndrome unless rupture of the membranes has occurred (Figs. 36.**17**, 36.**18**).

Growth-retarded fetuses. Oligohydramnios is commonly associated with fetal growth retardation, especially when the latter is due to placental insufficiency. The decreased amniotic fluid volume is attributed to diminished fetal urine output (7). Placental insufficiency leads to fetal hypoxia with a redirecting of blood flow away from the kidneys toward the brain, resulting in decreased urine production.

Eutrophic fetuses. With a eutrophic fetus, the amniotic fluid volume declines physiologically toward the end of the pregnancy (28, 31). This

Table 36.**4**   Possible causes of oligohydramnios

Fetal causes	➢ Urogenital anomalies
Maternal causes	➢ (Undetected) rupture of the membranes ➢ GEPH disorder ➢ Postmaturity
Placental causes	➢ Placental insufficiency ➢ Amniotic band syndrome

decline is also thought to be accompanied by decreased urine production (40), but this is controversial (32). Zimmermann et al. (44) conclude that the decreased amniotic fluid volume at term does not have a renovascular cause but is based on intra- and extrarenal causes.

Premature rupture of the membranes. When oligohydramnios is due to premature rupture of the membranes, the clinically detected membrane defect cannot always be documented objectively.

Search for fetal anomalies. Whenever oligohydramnios is detected, a targeted search for fetal anomalies should be carried out due to the association between oligohydramnios and fetal abnormalities. Unfortunately, the decreased amniotic fluid volume often makes it difficult to conduct an accurate examination. Hence, the scans should be performed by an experienced examiner and should be supplemented by invasive measures such as amnioinfusion.

Complications. Potential complications of oligohydramnios are pulmonary hypoplasia, skeletal and facial deformities, intrauterine growth retardation, and a significantly higher incidence of fetal morbidity and mortality (4, 5, 39). Correcting oligohydramnios by amnioinfusion not only improves imaging conditions (9) but can also improve the condition of the fetus in some cases (25).

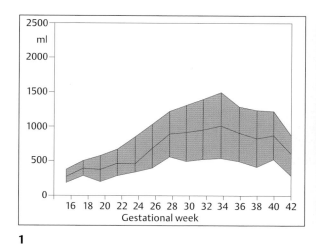

1

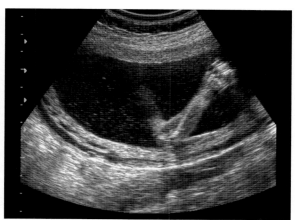

2

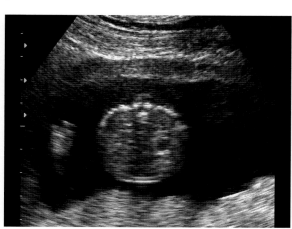

3

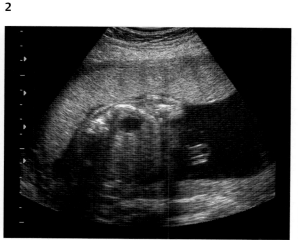

4

Assessment of amniotic fluid volume

Fig. 36.**1**   Amniotic fluid volume versus gestational age, mean ± 1 SD (modified from 31).

Fig. 36.**2**   Vernix flakes appear as punctate echoes in the amniotic fluid, 21 weeks.

Fig. 36.**3**   Normal amniotic fluid volume in the second trimester. Transverse scan at 17 weeks.

Fig. 36.**4**   Normal amniotic fluid volume in the second trimester. Transverse scan at 22 weeks.

Fig. 36.**5**   Normal amniotic fluid volume in the third trimester. Transverse scan at 32 weeks.

Fig. 36.**6**   Copious amniotic fluid. Longitudinal scan at 22 weeks.

Fig. 36.**7**   Copious amniotic fluid. Transverse scan at 24 weeks.

Fig. 36.**8**   Diagram of the four-quadrant technique for determining the amniotic fluid index.

Fig. 36.**9**   Ultrasound measurement of the four-quadrant amniotic fluid index. The vertical fluid pockets are measured in all four quadrants (in millimeters) and added together.

Fig. 36.**10**   Amniotic fluid index versus gestational age. The data are shown as percentiles (5th to 95th percentiles) from 16 to 42 weeks (after 24).

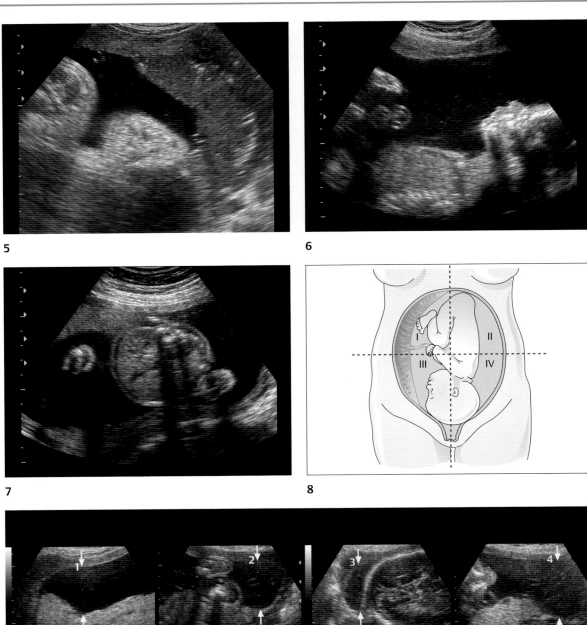

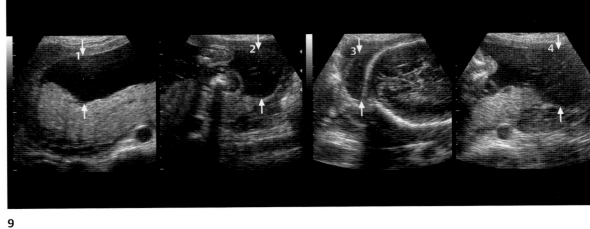

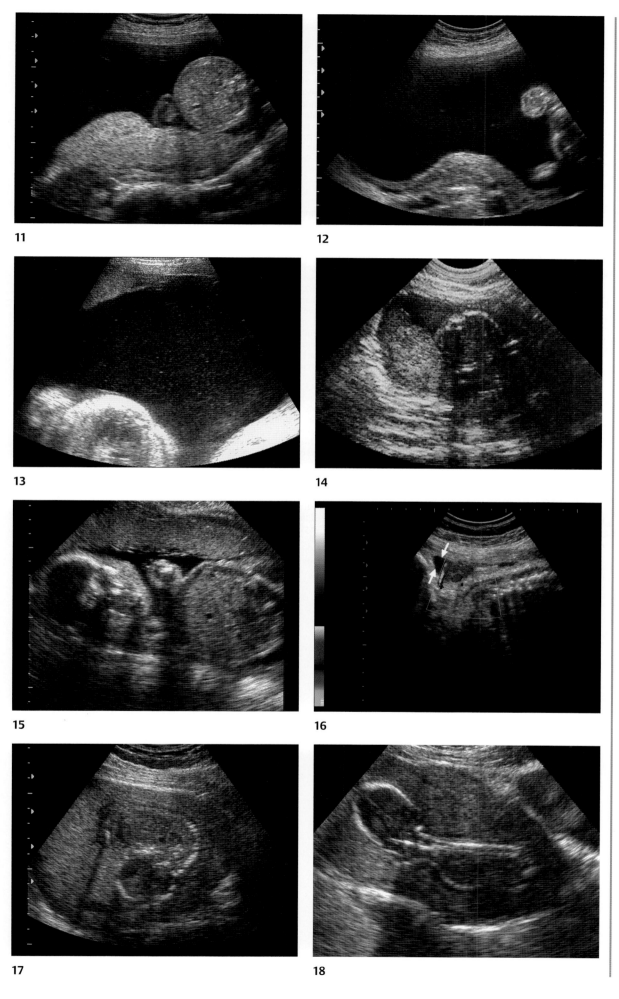

11

12

13

14

15

16

17

18

Abnormal amniotic fluid volume

Fig. 36.**11** Polyhydramnios with a left diaphragmatic hernia. Transverse scan at 21 weeks. The stomach is not visualized.

Fig. 36.**12** Marked polyhydramnios. Transverse scan at 22 weeks.

Fig. 36.**13** Massive polyhydramnios in diabetes mellitus. Transverse scan at 37 weeks.

Fig. 36.**14** Scant amniotic fluid in early placental insufficiency. Transverse scan at 22 weeks.

Fig. 36.**15** Scant amniotic fluid. Longitudinal scan at 26 weeks. The largest fluid pocket measures 1.8 cm.

Fig. 36.**16** Oligohydramnios in placental insufficiency. Longitudinal scan at 34 weeks. The amniotic fluid pocket measures 9 mm (arrows). Color Doppler shows that the umbilical cord occupies most of the fluid pocket.

Fig. 36.**17** Severe oligohydramnios in original Potter syndrome. Longitudinal scan at 16 weeks.

Fig. 36.**18** Severe oligohydramnios due to premature rupture of the membranes. Longitudinal scan at 23 weeks.

References

1. Abramovich, D.R.: Fetal factors influencing the volume and composition of liquor amnii. J. Obstet. Brit. Cwlth. 77 (1970) 865–877
2. Abramovich, D.R., Garden, A., Jandial, L., Page, K.R.: Fetal swallowing and voiding, the relation to hydramnios. Obstet. Gynecol. 54 (1979) 15–20
3. Arduini, D., Rizzo, G.: Fetal renal artery velocity waveforms and amniotic fluid volume in growth-retarded and postterm fetuses. Obstet. Gynecol. 77 (1991) 370–373
4. Chamberlain, P.F., Manning, F.A., Morrison, I., Harman, C.R., Lange, I.R.: Ultrasound evaluation of amniotic fluid volume. I. The relationship of marginal and decreased amniotic fluid volumes and perinatal outcome. Amer. J. Obstet. Gynecol. 150 (1984) 245–249
5. Chamberlain, P.F., Manning, F.A., Morrison, I., Harman, C.R., Lange, I.R.: Ultrasound evaluation of amniotic fluid volume. II. The relationship of increased amniotic fluid volume to perinatal outcome. Amer. J. Obstet. Gynecol. 150 (1984) 250–254
6. Damatu, N., Filly, R.A., Goldstein, R.B., Callen, P.W., Goldberg, J., Golbus, M.: Frequency of fetal anomalies in sonographically detected polyhydramnios. J. Ultrasound Med. 12 (1993) 11–15
7. Deutinger, J., Bartl, W., Pfersmann, C., Neumark, J., Bernaschek, G.: Fetal kidney volume and urine production in cases of fetal growth retardation. J. Perinat. Med. 15 (1987) 307–315
8. Geirsson, R.T., Patel, N.B., Christie, A.D.: In-vivo accuracy of ultrasound measurements of intrauterine volume in pregnancy. Brit. J. Obstet. Gynaecol. 91 (1984) 37–40
9. Gembruch, U., Hannsmann, M.: Artificial instillation of amniotic fluid as a new technique for the diagnostic evaluation of cases of oligohydramnios. Prenat. Diagn. 8 (1988) 33–45
10. Genbrane-Youmes, J., Hoang, N.M., Orcel, L.: Ultrastructure of human umbilical vessels: a possible role in amniotic fluid formation. Placenta 7 (1986) 173–185
11. Glantz, J., Abramowicz, J.S., Sherer, D.M.: Significance of idiopathic midtrimester polyhydramnios. Amer. J. Perinat. 11 (1994) 305–308
12. Gohari, P., Berkowitz, R.L., Hobbins, J.C.: Prediction of intrauterine growth retardation by determination of total intrauterine volume. Amer. J. Obstet. Gynecol. 127 (1977) 255–260
13. Goldstein, R.B., Filly, R.A.: Sonographic estimation of amniotic fluid volume: subjective assessment versus pocket measurements. J. Ultrasound Med. 7 (1988) 363–369
14. Goodlin, R.C., Anderson, J.C., Gallagher, T.F.: Relationship between amniotic fluid volume and maternal volume expansion. Amer. J. Obstet. Gynecol. 146 (1983) 505–511
15. Hill, L.M., Breckle, R., Thomas, M.L., Fries, J.K.: Polyhydramnios: Ultrasonically detected prevalence and neonatal outcome. Obstet. Gynecol. 69 (1987) 21–25
16. Hobbins, J.C., Grannum, A.T., Berkowitz, R.L., Silvermann, R., Mahony, M.J.: Ultrasound in the diagnosis of congenital anomalies. Amer. J. Obstet. Gynecol. 134 (1979) 331–345
17. Holländer, H.J.: Die Ultraschalldiagnostik in der Schwangerschaft. München: Urban & Schwarzenberg 1984
18. Kirshon, B., Mari, G., Moise, K.J.: Indomethacin therapy in the treatment of symptomatic polyhydramnios. Obstet. Gynecol. 75 (1990) 202–205
19. Kurtz, A.B., Kurtz, R.J., Rifkin, M.D. et al.: Total uterine volume: A new graph and its clinical applications. J. Ultrasound Med. 3 (1984) 299–308
20. Lind, T.: The biochemistry of amniotic fluid. In: Sandler, M. (ed.): Amniotic fluid and its clinical significance. New York: Dekker 1981
21. Mahony, B.S., Callen, P.W., Filly, R.A.: Fetal urethral obstruction: US evaluation. Radiology 157 (1985) 221–224
22. Moise, K.J., Huhta, J.C., Sharif, D.S.: Indomethacin in the treatment of premature labour: Effects on the fetal ductus arteriosus. New Engl. J. Med. 319 (1988) 327–331
23. Moise, K.J.: Indomethacin therapy in the treatment of symptomatic polyhydramnios. Clin. Obstet. Gynecol. 34 (1991) 310–318
24. Moore, T.R., Cayle, J.E.: The amniotic fluid index in normal human pregnancy. Amer. J. Obstet. Gynecol. 162 (1990) 1168–1173
25. Nageolte, M., Bertucci, M.P., Towes, D.L.K., Lagrow, D.L., Modanlow, H.: Prophylactic amnion infusion in pregnancies complicated by oligohydramnios: a prospective study. Obstet. Gynecol. 77 (1991) 677–680
26. Nwosu, E.C., Welch, C.R., Manasse, P.R., Walkinshaw, S.A.: Longitudinal assessment of amniotic fluid index. Brit. J. Obstet. Gynaecol. 100 (1993) 816–819
27. Okamura, K.J., Morutsuki, J., Kosnye, S., Tanigawara, S., Yajiman, A.: Diagnostic use of cordocentesis in twin pregnancy. Fetal Diagn. Ther. 9 (1994) 385–390
28. Phelan, J.P., Smith, C.V., Broussard, P., Small, M.: Amniotic fluid volume assessment with the four quadrant technique at 36–42 weeks gestation. J. Reprod. Med. 32 (1987) 540
29. Philipson, E.H., Sokol, R.J., Williams, T.: Oligohydramnios: Clinical association and predicitve value for intrauterine growth retardation. Amer. J. Obstet. Gynecol. 146 (1983) 271–278
30. Pritchard, J.A.: Fetal swallowing and amniotic fluid volume. Obstet. Gynecol. 28 (1969) 606–610
31. Queenan, J.T., Thompson, W., Whitfield, C.R., Shah, S.J.: Amniotic fluid volumes in normal pregnancies. Amer. J. Obstet. Gynecol. 114 (1972) 34–38
32. Rabinowitz, R., Peters, M.T., Vyas, S., Campbell, S., Nicolaides, K.H.: Measurement of fetal urine production in normal pregnancy by real-time ultrasonography. Amer. J. Obstet. Gynecol. 161 (1985) 1264–1266
33. Rutherford, S.E., Phelan, J.P., Smith, C., Jacobs, N.: The four-quadrant assessment of amniotic fluid volume: An adjunct to antepartum fetal heart rate testing. Obstet. Gynecol. 70 (1987) 353–356
34. Schiff, E., Ben-Baruch, G., Kushnir, U., Mashiach, S.: Standardized measurement of amniotic fluid volume by correlation of sonography with dye dilution technique. Obstet. Gynecol. 76 (1990) 44–46
35. Schmidt, W., Hendrik, J.H., Heberlin, D., Kubli, E.: Mißbildungsdiagnostik mittels Ultraschall. In: Rettenmeyer, G., Loch, E.G., Hansmann, M.: Ultraschalldiagnostik in der Medizin. Stuttgart: Thieme 1981; S. 212
36. Seeds, A.E.: Current concepts of amniotic fluid dynamics. Amer. J. Obstet. Gynecol. 138 (1980) 575–586
37. Sivit, C.J., Hill, M.C., Larsen, J.W., Lande, I.M.: Second trimester polyhydramnios: Evaluation with US. Radiology 165 (1987) 467–469
38. Sviges, J.M.: Early midtrimester oligohydramnios: a sign of poor fetal diagnosis. Aust. N.-Z. J. Obstet. Gynecol. 27 (1987) 90–92
39. Thibeault, D.W., Beatty, E.C., Hall, R.T.: Neonatal pulmonary hypoplasia with premature rupture of fetal membranes and oligohydramnios. J. Pediatr. 107 (1985) 273–277
40. Trimmer, K.J., Leveno, K.J., Peters, M.T., Kelly, M.A.: Observations on the cause of oligohydramnios in prolonged pregnancy. Amer. J. Obstet. Gynecol. 163 (1990) 1900–1903
41. Wallenburg, H.C.S.: The amniotic fluid. I. Water and electrolyte homeostasis. J. Perinat. Med. 5 (1977) 193–205
42. Wallenburg, H.C.S., Wladimiroff, J.W.: The amniotic fluid. II. Polyhydramnios and oligohydramnios. J. Perinat. Med. 6 (1977) 233–243
43. Zamah, N.M., Gillieson, M.S., Walters, J.H., Hall, P.E.: Sonographic detection of polyhydramnios. A five year experience. Amer. J. Obstet. Gynecol. 143 (1982) 523–527
44. Zimmermann, R., Eichhorn, K.-H., Huch, A., Huch, R.: Zusammenhang zwischen verminderter Fruchtwassermenge und Dopplerspektren fetaler Gefäße am Termin. Geburtsh. u. Frauenheilk. 53 (1993) 479–482

Ultrasound in Multiple Pregnancy

37 Multiple Pregnancies

Special Features of Multiple Pregnancies

▰ *High-Risk Pregnancy*

Multiple pregnancies are characterized by a significantly higher fetal morbidity and mortality than singleton pregnancies. This places them in the category of high-risk pregnancies.

Chorionicity and amnionicity. The 4 to 10 times higher morbidity and mortality rates of twin pregnancies relate critically to the chorionicity and amnionicity of the pregnancy (dichorionic diamniotic, monochorionic diamniotic, monochorionic monoamniotic) (7, 8, 10). The higher risk of monochorionic twins is due mainly to the presence of vascular anastomoses between the shared portions of the placenta. A hydrodynamic imbalance may develop between the two fetal circulations, causing a twin-to-twin transfusion syndrome. By contrast, this type of vascular anastomosis is almost never seen in dichorionic pregnancies.

Perinatal mortality, prematurity. The early ultrasound diagnosis of multiple gestation has done much in recent years to reduce perinatal mortality and preterm deliveries. Owing to the more selective and intensive surveillance of multiple pregnancies, the perinatal mortality has been reduced from approximately 12–14% (57, 92) to 0.6–3.9% (40, 43), and the incidence of preterm delivery has been lowered from 33% to 10% (43).

▰ *Frequency of Multiple Pregnancy*

Hellin (49) established a rule in 1895 for estimating the frequency of multiple pregnancies: one birth in every 85 is twins, one in every 85^2 is triplets, one in every 85^3 is quadruplets, and so on (Table 37.1).

Vanishing twin. Today we know that the frequency of primary multiple pregnancies is considerably higher than predicted by the Hellin rule. This is because in the era before ultrasonography, a large percentage of early twin pregnancies were undiagnosed, and one of the twins died or was reabsorbed during the first trimester ("vanishing twin") without ever being detected (61). As early as 1932, Von Verschuer (109) reported that 32 of 100 primary twin gestations reduced spontaneously to a singleton pregnancy.

With the advent of ultrasonography and especially of transvaginal scanning, it became possible for the first time to make an early, detailed evaluation of twin pregnancies. Ultrasound studies by various groups of authors (39, 60, 63) indicate that 20–50 of every 100 primary twin pregnancies (with two detectable embryos) convert to a singleton pregnancy during the first trimester.

Assisted reproductive technologies. The Hellin rule (49) pertains only to multiple pregnancies that occur spontaneously. With the increasing use of assisted reproductive technologies in recent years—ovarian hyperstimulation, in-vitro fertilization (IVF), gamete intrafallopian transfer (GIFT), intracytoplasmic sperm injection (ICSI)—there has been a rising incidence of twin pregnancies and higher-order multiple gestation (12). In the 1996 national IVF registry of Germany (31), there was a 24.5% reported incidence of twins after IVF and a 7.5% incidence of triplets.

Maternal age. Current modes of reproductive behavior also affect the incidence of twin pregnancies. As more women choose to have their first pregnancy after 30 years of age, there is a natural age-associated rise in the incidence of twins (55, 98).

Genetic predisposition. Besides maternal age, the prevalence of twins is also influenced by other factors such as parity and race (7). Higher rates of twin births in certain populations and in various families suggest that there is a genetic predisposition for twinning.

Current rate of twin births. Studies in the United States indicate that the rate of twin births doubled between 1973 and 1990 (66), reaching a frequency of one in 43 births (2.3%) in 1990. If vanishing twins are also factored in, the current incidence of primary twin pregnancies is approximately 5%. Three-fourths of all twins are dizygotic, and the remaining one-fourth are monozygotic (Fig. 37.1).

Table 37.1 Frequency of spontaneous multiple pregnancies in Europe, calculated from the Hellin rule (49)

Twins	1 : 85	1 : 85 births
Triplets	1 : 85^2	1 : 7 225 births
Quadruplets	1 : 85^3	1 : 614,125 births
Quintuplets	1 : 85^4	1 : 52,200,625 births

▰ *Chorionicity and Amnionicity*

Chorionicity in Dizygotic Twins

Dichorionic diamniotic pregnancy. Dizygotic twins arise from two different oocytes that were each fertilized by a different sperm. They are not genetically identical, therefore, and they may be of the same or different gender, making them equivalent to singleton siblings. Since each embryo has its own placenta, amnion, and chorion, the pregnancy is always dichorionic and diamniotic.

Fused placentas. The placentas of dizygotic twins may be separate or they may be fused if the implantation sites are close together. Even fused placentas can be differentiated histologically, however. On the gross inspection of fused dizygotic twin placentas, chorionic tissue is always visible between the two amniotic membranes–i.e., the fusion is confined to the villous layer (Fig. 37.2, Table 37.2). Careful inspection of the delivered placenta reveals four layers: two amnions and two chorions. Vascular anastomoses almost never occur in dichorionic placentas (10), but exceptions have been reported (87).

Chorionicity in Monozygotic Twins

Monozygotic twinning is a more complex process than dizygotic twinning. Monozygotic twins result from the division of a single oocyte fertilized by one sperm. Hence the twins are genetically identical and are always of the same sex. The chorionicity and placentation depend on the time at which the fertilized oocyte divides. Under normal circum-

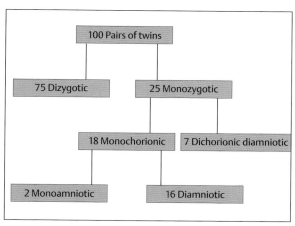

1

Chorionicity and amnionicity

Fig. 37.**1** Frequency distribution of dizygotic and monozygotic twins.

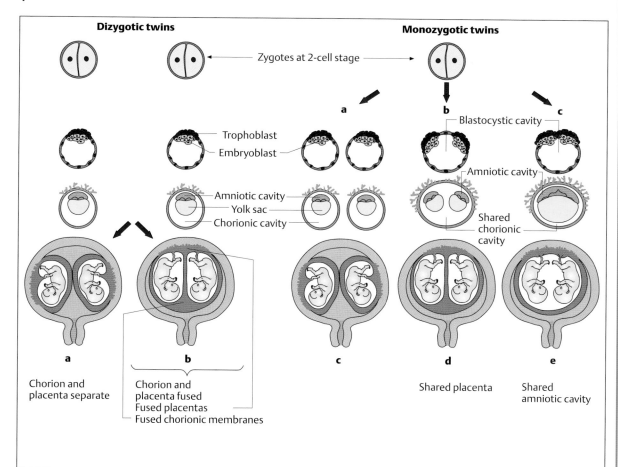

2

Fig. 37.**2** *Left:* development of dizygotic twins. *Right:* development of monozygotic twins (after 89).
a Dichorionic diamniotic twins with separate placentas.
b Dichorionic diamniotic twins with a fused placenta.
c Dichorionic diamniotic twins.
d Monochorionic diamniotic twins.
e Monochorionic monoamniotic twins.

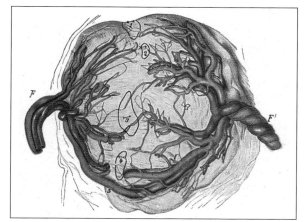

3 a

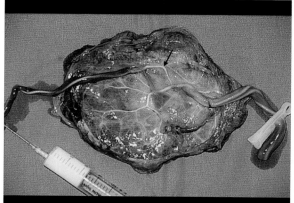

3 b

Fig. 37.**3** Vascular anastomoses.
a Monozygotic twin placenta, after Schatz (91). As the arrows indicate, arterial blood at sites 1 and 4 flows from fetus F′ through villous capillaries to the veins of fetus F. Arterial blood at sites 2 and 3 flows from fetus F to the veins of fetus F′. At point 5 there is a large superficial anastomosis between the veins of both twins (usually there is only one arterial anastomosis between the twins) (after 79).
b Monochorionic diamniotic placenta. Milk was injected into an umbilical artery to define the arterioarterial shunt (arrow).

stances, this division occurs between the 2nd and 12th day of development.

Dichorionic diamniotic twins. If the zygote divides at the two-cell stage, segmentation is already complete. Two embryos develop, each having its own placenta and enclosed in its own amniotic and chorionic sac (dichorionic diamniotic). This placentation is the same as that in a dizygotic multiple pregnancy. After birth, the membranes are found to consist of four layers: two amnions and two chorions (Fig. 37.**2**, Table 37.**2**).

Monochorionic diamniotic twins. In the great majority of cases, the division occurs in the early blastocyst stage between the fourth and seventh days of development. In this case only the embryoblast splits into two separate groups of cells within the blastocyst; the trophoblast is already formed. This results in a common placenta with a shared chorion but two separate amniotic sacs (monochorionic diamniotic). When inspected after birth, the membranes consist of only two layers (two amnions) (Fig. 37.**2**, Table 37.**2**).

Monochorionic monoamniotic twins. Less commonly, the blastocyst divides at the stage of the two-layer embryonic disk shortly before the appearance of the primitive streak, starting on about the eighth day of development. This results in twins with a shared placenta and a common chorionic and amniotic sacrococcygeal (monochorionic monoamniotic pregnancy) (Fig. 37.**2**, Table 37.**2**).

Conjoined twins. Incomplete division of the blastocyst or the secondary fusion of two originally separate zygotes along the long axis of the embryonic disk after the 12th day of development can lead to conjoined twins, known also as Siamese twins (99). This term is derived from the brothers Chang and Eng Bunker from Siam (1811–1874), who were joined at the sternum by a band of hepatic tissue.

Fetofetal vascular anastomoses. One characteristic of the monochorionic placenta is that it contains fetofetal vascular anastomoses in approximately 90% of cases (10). They may occur in the chorionic plate as arterioarterial, venovenous, or arteriovenous anastomoses or in the form of a deep intercotyledon arteriovenous shunt (Fig. 37.**3a**). The connections that are most commonly and easily detected in the delivered placenta are arterioarterial shunts. They are easily detected by stroking the blood from one vascular segment into the other with the fingers or by the injection of milk (10) (Fig. 37.**3b**).

The deep arteriovenous shunt is the most difficult to detect but has the greatest clinical significance. The artery that supplies a cotyledon originates from one twin, and the vein that drains the cotyledon leads to the second twin.

Twin–twin transfusion syndrome. This syndrome develops from the vascular anastomoses that exist in a monochorionic placenta (10).

Although both twins share the monochorionic placenta, both fetuses

generally receive an adequate, balanced blood supply. But there are isolated cases in which a twin–twin transfusion syndrome develops. The unequal blood supply leads to increasingly discordant twin growth and, without treatment, frequently ends in the intrauterine death of both fetuses (26, 108).

Chorionicity in Triplet and Higher-Order Multiple Pregnancies

Monochorionic and dichorionic placentation may coexist in higher-order pregnancies due to simultaneous monozygosity and dizygosity of the different fetuses (10).

Ultrasound of Multiple Pregnancy in the First Trimester

Normal Multiple Pregnancy

Number, Viability, and Growth of Multiple Fetuses

Diagnosis. Multiple gestation can be diagnosed with transvaginal ultrasound as early as the fifth week of development by detecting two or more gestational sacs (Fig. 37.**4**). An exception is the rare monochorionic monoamniotic multiple pregnancy, in which only one gestational sac is seen. But the definitive diagnosis of an intact multiple pregnancy requires more than the detection of multiple sacs. It is also necessary to detect a viable embryo in each sac. This can be done as early as the sixth or seventh week by documenting embryonic heart activity (Fig. 37.**5**).

Before the parents are notified of an intact multiple pregnancy, the examiner should confirm viability and also make certain that the growth of the individual embryos is equal and appropriate for dates during early pregnancy. The growth of multiple embryos during the first trimester is the same as that of singletons, and so standard growth curves for CRL, BPD, and AC can be used to monitor growth in a multiple pregnancy.

Search for more embryos. There is very little chance that an experienced examiner using modern ultrasound equipment will overlook a twin pregnancy. But whenever a twin gestation or any other multiple pregnancy is found (Figs. 37.**6**, 37.**7**), the examiner should always look for additional embryos.

Higher-order multiple pregnancies (quintuplets, sextuplets) are considerably more difficult to diagnose, as it is virtually impossible to define all the gestational sacs in one plane. It is much easier to evaluate these cases by multiplanar three-dimensional transvaginal scanning (73). After storing the entire uterine corpus and all the intrauterine sacs as volume data, the examiner can make a detailed survey of the uterus by scrolling through the volume in all three planes. This technique is also used to resolve equivocal cases.

False-positive diagnosis of twin pregnancy. With an intrauterine hematoma that has roughly the same size and echogenicity of a chorionic sac, the less experienced examiner may mistake the hematoma for a second gestational sac (Fig. 37.**8**).

Uterine anomalies can also cause confusion. For example, a pseudogestational sac in the second horn of a bicornuate uterus can mimic a twin gestation (Fig. 37.**9**). The septum in a subseptate uterus (Fig. 37.**10**) or a solitary amniotic band (Fig. 37.**11**) can also mimic twin sacs.

Polyhydramnios can lead to a false-positive diagnosis of twin pregnancy even in the second trimester. The examiner may see an active

Table 37.**2** Placentation and chorionicity and their prevalence in monozygotic and dizygotic twins (adapted from 79 and 18)

Type of twins	Sex	Placentation	Chorionicity	Frequency
Dizygotic (75%)	Same or different	2 placentas or 1 fused placenta	Dichorionic diamniotic	
Monozygotic (25%)	Same	2 placentas or 1 fused placenta	Dichorionic diamniotic	30%
	Same	1 placenta	Monochorionic diamniotic	62%
	Same	1 placenta	Monochorionic monoamniotic	8%

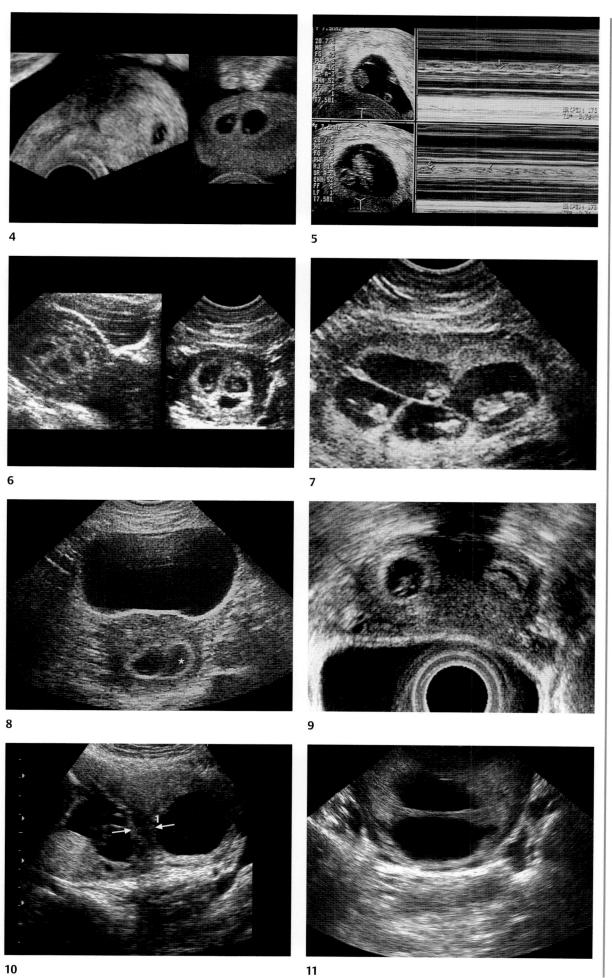

4

5

6

7

8

9

10

11

Normal multiple pregnancy in the first trimester

Fig. 37.4 Dichorionic diamniotic twin pregnancy at 5 weeks, 5 days gestation. *Left:* longitudinal scan shows the yolk sac in one of the two gestational sacs. There is free fluid in the cul-de-sac. *Right:* transverse uterine scan of the same pregnancy shows the two adjacent gestational sacs.

Fig. 37.5 M-mode tracings of twin heart activity at 7 weeks, 0 days. The heart rates are 176 bpm for twin I and 173 bpm for twin II.

Fig. 37.6 Triplets at 7 weeks' gestation. *Left:* longitudinal scan of the uterus. *Right:* transverse scan of the uterus showing all three gestational sacs.

Fig. 37.7 Quadruplets following hormonal stimulation therapy. Transverse scan of the uterus at 11 weeks, 1 day.

Fig. 37.8 Hematoma (∗) next to the gestational sac mimics a twin pregnancy. Transverse scan of the uterus at 6 weeks.

Fig. 37.9 Singleton pregnancy in the right cornu of a bicornuate uterus The thickened endometrium and central fluid collection in the left cornu mimics a twin gestation. Transverse scan of the uterus at 7 weeks, 2 days.

Fig. 37.10 A 13-mm wide septum in a subseptate uterus (arrows) mimics a twin pregnancy. Transverse scan through the upper uterine corpus at 24 weeks, 3 days.

Fig. 37.11 A 5-mm thick amniotic band at the inferior end of the placenta mimics a twin pregnancy.

Fig. 37.**12** Chorionicity.
a, b Chorionicity of dichorionic diamniotic twins.
a Separate placentas.
b Fused placentas.
c, d Chorionicity of monochorionic twins.
c Monochorionic diamniotic twins.
d Monochorionic monoamniotic twins.

Fig. 37.**13** Dichorionic diamniotic twins. Transverse scan of the uterus at 5 weeks.

Fig. 37.**14** Dichorionic diamniotic twins. Longitudinal scan of the uterus at 9 weeks.

Fig. 37.**15** Dichorionic diamniotic twins with a fused placenta and positive lambda sign (large arrow). Each gestational sac has a separate amniotic membrane (small arrows). Transverse scan of the uterus at 16 weeks.

Fig. 37.**16** Positive lambda sign (arrow) in a dichorionic diamniotic twin pregnancy.

Fig. 37.**17** Half twin peak (arrow) in a dichorionic diamniotic twin pregnancy with separate placentas (1 = anterior placenta, 2 = posterior placenta). Transverse scan of the uterus at 15 weeks.

Fig. 37.**18** T sign (arrow) in a monochorionic diamniotic twin pregnancy.

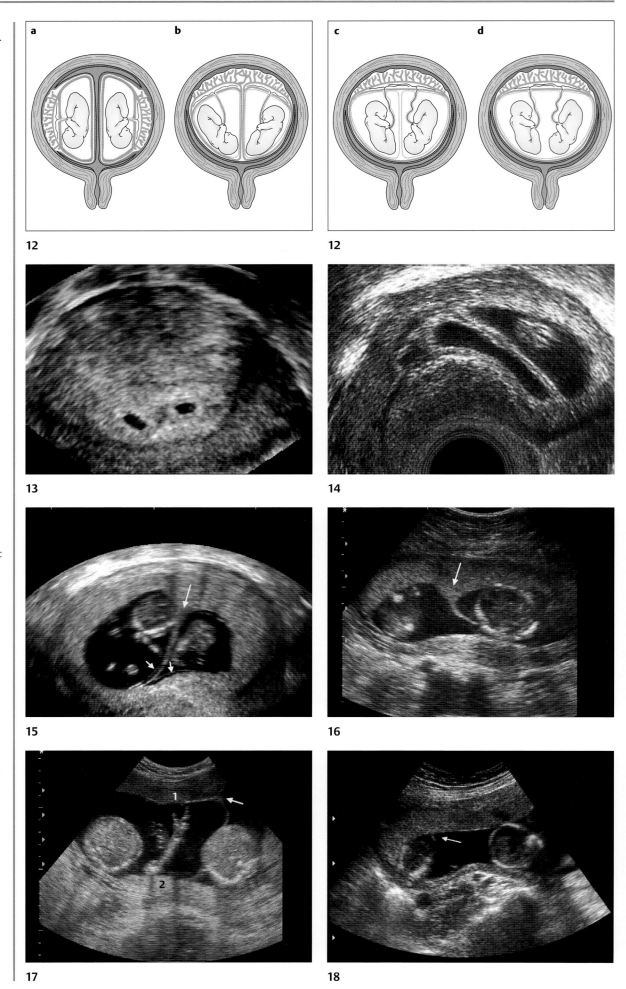

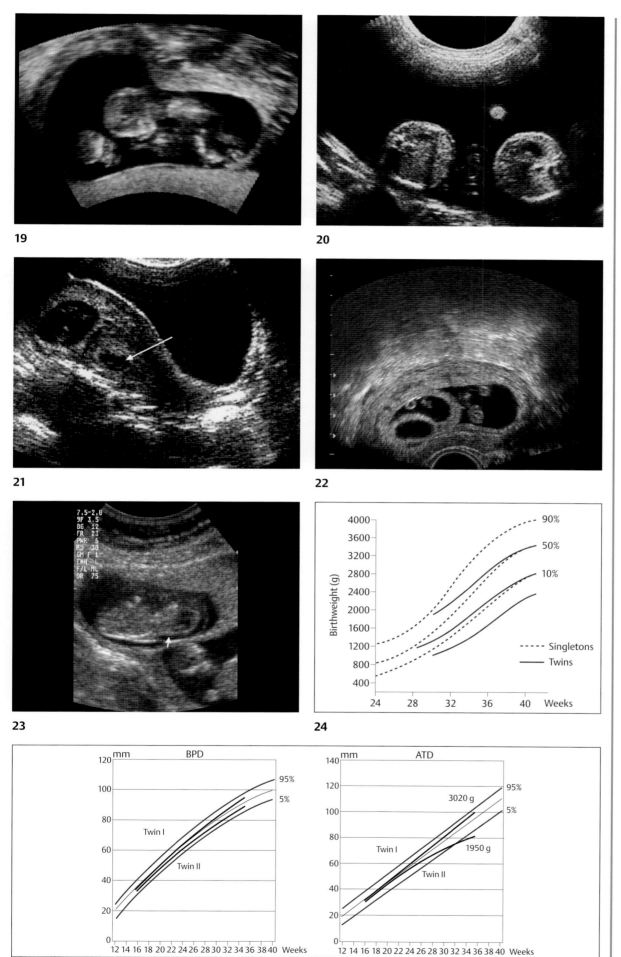

19

20

21

22

23

24

25

Fig. 37.19 Monochorionic monoamniotic twins at 12 weeks. The twins are in overlying positions in one cavity. They are not separated by an amniotic membrane.

Fig. 37.20 Monochorionic monoamniotic twins with polyhydramnios at 23 weeks. Ultrasound does not show a dividing amniotic membrane.

Abnormal multiple pregnancy in the first trimester

Fig. 37.21 Longitudinal scan of the uterus demonstrates a normal gestational sac in the upper part of the uterine corpus and an abnormal sac in the lower corpus (arrow). The lower sac is considerably smaller, and the embryo is also markedly smaller than the one in the upper sac.

Fig. 37.22 Partially abnormal triplet gestation in a transverse scan of the uterus at 8 weeks. The apparent size of the embryonic structures varies with the level of the transverse scan plane and the intrauterine location of the gestational sacs.

Fig. 37.23 Nuchal translucency thickness of 7 mm in one twin at 12 weeks, 5 days.

Normal development in the second and third trimesters

Fig. 37.24 Intrauterine growth of singletons and twins (after 3).

Growth discordance

Fig. 37.25 Graphic representation of discordant growth in twins. *Left:* biparietal diameter (BPD). *Right:* abdominal transverse diameter (ATD).

singleton fetus on one side of the uterus, then move the transducer and observe the same fetus on the opposite side.

Differentiating Monochorionic and Dichorionic Placentas with Ultrasound

Risk profiles. When the number, viability, and growth of multiple fetuses have been evaluated in the first part of the ultrasound examination, the next step is to determine chorionicity and amnionicity (Fig. 37.**12a–d**). While the prospective parents are concerned mainly with whether the infants are monozygotic or dizygotic, the examiner is more interested in their chorionicity, since monochorionic twins are at considerably higher risk than dichorionic twins (Table 37.**3**). Monochorionic monoamniotic twins have the highest risk, while dichorionic twins have the same risk as singletons.

A reliable ultrasound assessment of chorionicity can be made only in early pregnancy.

Ultrasound detection of two separate placentas. This finding confirms a dichorionic pregnancy, as does the detection of different-sex fetuses. But gender cannot be reliably determined in the first trimester with ultrasound, and the only remaining option is to evaluate the placentation and the membrane that separates the gestational sacs (Table 37.**2**, Fig. 37.**12 a–d**).

Ultrasound detection of a single placenta. With this finding, the gestation may be either monochorionic (Fig. 37.**12c, d**) or dichorionic (Fig. 37.**12b**). The latter results from the fusion of two placentas at adjacent implantation sites. Same-sex twins with a shared placenta may be either monozygotic or dizygotic.

Study results. Since the early 1980s, various groups of authors have used antenatal ultrasound in an effort to predict the chorionicity and amnionicity of twin pregnancies (53, 58, 68). A review of these studies may be found in Tutschek et al. (103).

Mahony et al. (68) conducted comparative ultrasound and pathoanatomic studies of 66 twin pregnancies. They found that when a single placenta was detected sonographically, subsequent pathologic analysis revealed a monochorionic placenta in 49% of the cases, while the rest were dichorionic. When ultrasound revealed a dividing membrane between the twins, a diamniotic pregnancy was subsequently confirmed in all cases. Conversely, when a dividing membrane was not visualized, a monoamniotic pregnancy was actually present in only one of 11 cases (9%). This means that in the remaining 10 cases (91%), a dividing membrane was present but was not defined with ultrasound.

Another approach to differentiating monochorionic and dichorionic placentation is based on the fact that the membrane separating monochorionic diamniotic twins consists of only two layers, while that separating dichorionic diamniotic twins consists of four layers and is therefore thicker. This has led various authors (51, 58, 102) to perform ultrasound measurements of the intertwin membrane thickness. When

Kurtz et al. (58) measured membrane thickness in 85 dichorionic diamniotic twin pregnancies, they found that a thick membrane was present in 78 (92%). In 16 monochorionic diamniotic pregnancies, a thin membrane was identified in 14 (88%). These authors used a cutoff of 2 mm or more for dichorionic placentas and < 1 mm for monochorionic placentas. On the whole, this method shows high intra- and inter-observer variability and is also affected by gestational age.

Other groups of authors (24, 105) have tried to count the number of membrane layers, but this has proved to be a time-consuming procedure (Fig. 37.**15**).

Lambda sign. Today the most widely used method of identifying a dichorionic placenta is based on the detection of two separate gestational sacs (Figs. 37.**13**, 37.**14**) or, if the sacs are fused, on the detection of the lambda sign described in 1981 (11), which was later called the "twin peak" sign (33). This sign consists of a moderately echogenic triangle that is located at the fusion site of the two placentas and whose apex projects into the gap between the two amniotic cavities (Figs. 37.**15**, 37.**16**). The term "lambda sign" is based on the resemblance of the intertwin membrane-placental junction to the Greek letter ?. Sepulveda et al. (95) found it to be a very reliable sign for diagnosing dichorionic gestation. In another study, the same authors (96) found that the optimum gestational age for demonstrating the lambda sign was between 10 and 14 weeks.

Half twin peak. Wood et al. (113) found that separate placentas were also associated with a triangular but more sharply tapered junctional area, which they called the "half twin peak" (Fig. 37.**17**).

T sign. Twin pregnancies without a lambda sign (absent twin peak) (113) are classified as monochorionic and are therefore monozygotic. With monochorionic diamniotic twins, the base of the dividing membrane is thin and T-shaped, giving rise to the descriptive term "T sign" for this type of pregnancy (Fig. 37.**18**).

If only one placenta is found bordering a single cavity, with no evidence of a dividing membrane or a T sign at mid-placenta, it may be concluded that the pregnancy is monochorionic and monoamniotic (Figs. 37.**19**, 37.**20**).

The ultrasound criteria that are used in the prenatal differentiation of monochorionic and dichorionic placentas are summarized in Table 37.**4**.

Differentiating Monozygotic and Dizygotic Twins with Ultrasound

The parents in twin pregnancies usually want to know whether their babies are monozygotic or dizygotic. Although the ultrasound detection of various parameters can give information on the monozygosity of twins, a definite prenatal diagnosis can be made only in a certain percentage of cases.

Definite dizygosity. Twins are definitely dizygotic if they are of different sexes. In such cases it does not matter whether ultrasound shows two separate placentas or a shared placenta (secondary fusion of two adjacent placental sites).

In women who undergo assisted reproduction by IVF, ICSI or some other technique, multiple offspring generally are heterozygous due to the implantation of multiple fertilized oocytes. But this fact alone does not guarantee dizygotic twins. The blastocyst may divide secondarily after it has implanted, resulting in monozygotic twins.

Monozygotic twins. A confident antenatal ultrasound diagnosis of monozygotic twins can be made only (1) if there is a single gestational sac with only one placenta and (2) either the two umbilical cords are intertwined or the twins are conjoined.

Table 37.3   Potential complications of monochorionic twinning

Complications of monochorionic diamniotic twinning
➤ Vanishing twin
➤ Twin–twin transfusion syndrome
➤ Parasitic twin (acardius acranius)
➤ Fetal death syndrome in the surviving twin

Complications of monochorionic monoamniotic twinning
➤ Twin–twin transfusion syndrome
➤ Conjoined twins
➤ Tangled umbilical cords

Table 37.**4** Suggestive ultrasound signs of dichorionic and monochorionic pregnancy from 10 to 14 weeks' gestation

Dichorionic diamniotic pregnancy	Visualization of two placentas and a dividing membrane ("half twin peak" sign) or Visualization of one placenta and a dividing membrane, plus a lambda sign
Monochorionic diamniotic pregnancy	Visualization of one placenta and a dividing membrane, plus a T sign
Monochorionic monoamniotic pregnancy	Visualization of one placenta; dividing membrane and T sign are not visualized

Equivocal diagnosis. The diagnosis is equivocal in the case of same-sex twins with a morphologically dichorionic-diamniotic placenta. Approximately four-fifths of these cases are dizygotic and one-fifth are monozygotic (19). The zygosity can be determined only by using nonmorphologic methods such as chromosome analysis (70) or blood group determination (16) or ultimately by testing the twins for similarities when they reach childhood.

▪ Abnormal Multiple Pregnancy in the First Trimester

Hematoma. Two adjacent, hypoechoic areas within the uterus do not always signify twins. They may represent a singleton pregnancy with an adjacent intrauterine hematoma (Fig. 37.**8**).

Unequal sac sizes. If a disparity of gestational sac sizes is noted during the first trimester (Fig. 37.**21**), the smaller sac is almost certainly an abnormal gestation that will either be expelled or reabsorbed. On the other hand, this finding may simply result from an oblique scan through the second sac, which is then found to be of normal size when imaged in the correct plane. An early growth discordance between the embryos also signifies an abnormality that may result in the death of the smaller embryo (Fig. 37.**22**).

Blighted twin. The term "blighted twin" is used when the second gestational sac is empty (26). It is analogous to the "blighted ovum" that can occur in a singleton pregnancy.

▪ Early Detection of Fetal Anomalies

Gross anomalies. In multiple pregnancies as in singleton pregnancies, it is possible to detect gross fetal anomalies or their suggestive signs during the first trimester by transvaginal ultrasound. The anomalies that can be detected at this early stage include conjoined twins (67, 90) as well as anencephaly or omphalocele in one of the twins.

Chromosomal abnormalities. A chromosomal abnormality in a twin may be manifested by a marked growth discrepancy between the two twins or by the presence of abnormal nuchal translucency (Fig. 37.**23**) (76, 80). Nuchal translucency is not only a suggestive sign of a possible chromosomal abnormality, but it may also signify a cardiac anomaly or an early or impending twin–twin transfusion syndrome (94).

Ultrasound of Multiple Pregnancy in the Second and Third Trimesters

▪ Normal Development

Growth curves. The longitudinal growth of twins and multiples during the first two trimesters shows no significant difference relative to the growth of singleton fetuses (35, 85) (Fig. 37.**24**). For this reason, the same standard growth curves can be used as for singletons (72).

Flattening of the growth curve. During the third trimester, however, twins and multiples show a somewhat slower growth pattern characterized mainly by a smaller biparietal diameter and less trunk growth (42, 45, 75, 88, 97). As a result of this, the growth curve is flatter than in singletons (Fig. 37.**25**). The difficulty is that this somewhat physiologic flattening of growth in twins and multiples during the third trimester can be difficult to distinguish from early intrauterine growth retardation.

Triplet growth curves. Mordel et al. (75) addressed this problem by plotting normal growth curves for biparietal diameter, abdominal circumference, and femur length in 108 triplet pregnancies. They showed that the growth curve of a triplet in the third trimester follows that of a singleton with a time lag of approximately 1–3 weeks. Growth curves that are below these reference values are easily and quickly recognized, prompting close-interval serial scans or an early interventional procedure. Fountain et al. (35) and Weissman et al. (111) advocate the use of special triplet growth curves based on their retrospective studies, which involved relatively small case numbers.

Polyhydramnios. Polyhydramnios is a fairly common finding in the second or third trimester of a twin pregnancy, especially with monozygotic twins (110) (Fig. 37.**20**).

Assessment of Chorionicity and Amnionicity in the Second and Third Trimesters

Lambda sign. Chorionicity and amnionicity are more difficult to assess in the second and third trimesters than in the first trimester because the lambda sign becomes more difficult to detect as the pregnancy proceeds and the dichorionic placentas fuse together. In 7% of cases, the lambda sign disappears completely by 20 weeks' gestation (96).

Sex determination. One advantage of a later assessment is that gender can be determined sonographically with higher confidence. The fact that the fetuses are of the same or different sex can be included in the overall evaluation. If ultrasound findings from the first trimester are not available, the features currently detectable can be used in an attempt to distinguish between a monochorionic and dichorionic pregnancy.

Suggestive signs. The suggestive signs at ultrasound that are helpful in determining the chorionicity, amnionicity, and zygosity of twin pregnancies are summarized in Table 37.**5**.

Fetal positions. It is good practice in every twin or multiple pregnancy to rescan the uterus and evaluate the fetal positions prior to delivery. Similarly, the position of the second twin should be checked after the delivery of the first twin.

Abnormal Multiple Pregnancy in the Second and Third Trimesters

Growth Discordance

If growth discordance is noted in multiple fetuses, consideration must be given to what still constitutes a normal variant and what constitutes early pathology (Fig. 37.**26**). Generally the smaller twin is at higher risk (26, 44, 61, 108).

Intrauterine fetal death. Leveno et al. (62) found that a discordance of 7 mm or more in BPD was associated with the subsequent intrauterine death of the smaller twin in 20% of cases. With a smaller growth discordance, this rate was between 2% and 5%.

Head shape. Discordant head growth does not necessarily reflect an underlying disorder. For example, a dolichocephalic head shape in a twin or multiple like that seen in breech presentations may be responsible for the biparietal discordance. If head circumference is used instead of BPD, it is easier to recognize true discordant growth.

Causes. True growth retardation affecting only one twin may be caused by circumscribed placental insufficiency, a twin–twin transfusion syndrome, or a fetal anomaly (Figs. 37.**26**, 37.**27**). In pregnancies with two separate placentas, it is possible that local changes such as infarctions or placental abruption or a primarily small placenta may cause a deficient supply to one fetus while the second fetus continues to receive a normal supply from the second placenta. But if only one placenta is visualized at ultrasound, the growth retardation of one twin may be a result of twin-to-twin transfusion.

Blood flow conditions. The blood flow conditions in such cases can be investigated by a comparative Doppler examination of the major vessels in both twins.

Twin–Twin Transfusion Syndrome

Occurrence. A twin–twin transfusion syndrome occurs almost exclusively in monochorionic (monozygotic) twin pregnancies. Most cases are diamniotic, and occurrence in monoamniotic twins is rare. Isolated cases of twin–twin transfusion syndrome with a dichorionic placenta have been reported (56, 59).

Acute and chronic form. An acute form of twin–twin transfusion syndrome is distinguished from a chronic form. While the acute form usually occurs in connection with delivery, the chronic form develops in utero, most commonly during the second trimester.

Superficial and deep vascular anastomoses. Twin–twin transfusion syndrome is made possible by the presence of placental vascular anastomoses between the two fetal circulations (7, 87). These connections occur almost exclusively in monochorionic placentas and are rare in dichorionic placentas (87). As early as 1882, Schatz (91) described anastomoses of varying calibers which he called the "third circulation." The vascular anastomoses may be superficial, deep, or both (Fig. 37.**3**). Most superficial connections are either arterioarterial anastomoses (28%) or a combination of arterioarterial and arteriovenous anastomoses (28%) (6). Other forms such as venovenous anastomoses (87) and other combinations are much less common (14). The deep anastomoses are arteriovenous shunts in a shared cotyledon, consisting of an artery arising from one twin and a vein draining to the other twin.

Table 37.**5**   Suggestive ultrasound signs for determining the chorionicity, amnionicity, and zygosity of twins (adapted from Mahony et al. [68])

No. of placentas	Membrane visible	Other features	Dichorionic	Monochorionic	Diamniotic	Monoamniotic	Dizygotic	Monozygotic	Remarks
2	Yes	Sex different	x		x		x		
2	Yes	Sex same	x		x		x	x	
2	No	Sex different	x		x		x		Membrane present but not visible
2	No	Sex same	x		x		x	x	Membrane present but not visible
2	Yes/No	One fetus is hydropic, the other normal	x		x		x	x	No twin–twin transfusion syndrome, different cause of NIHF
1	Yes	Sex different	x		x		x		
1	Yes	Sex same, positive lambda sign	x		x		x		
1	Yes	Sex same, T sign		x	x			x	
1	Yes	One fetus is hydropic, the other small		x	x			x	Twin–twin transfusion syndrome
1	No	Sex different	x		x		x		Membrane may be present but not visible
1	No	Sex same	x	x	x	x	x	x	Membrane may be present but not visible
1	No	One fetus can move freely, the other is immobile	x	x	x		x	x	Oligohydramnios in one sac, stuck twin in twin–twin transfusion syndrome
1	No	Both umbilical cords intertwined		x		x		x	
1	No	Conjoined twins		x		x		x	

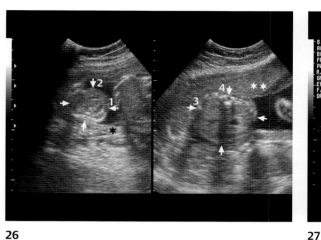

26

27

Twin–twin transfusion syndrome

Fig. 37.**26** Growth discordance in dichorionic diamniotic twins. Twin II (left image) shows deficient development with abnormal placental maturation (∗), while twin I (right image) shows normal development with normal placental maturation (∗∗).

Fig. 37.**27** Twin–twin transfusion syndrome with a marked growth discordance at 24 weeks. Left image: donor with oligohydramnios. Right image: recipient with polyhydramnios.

Fig. 37.**28** Pathophysiology of the twin–twin transfusion syndrome. Because of a common cotyledon with an arterial supply from the donor and venous drainage to the recipient ("third circulation"), there is a transient or sustained shunting of blood to the recipient. This leads to an increased circulating blood volume in the recipient twin with cardiac overload and polyuria (hydramnios). The donor twin has decreased circulatory volume and urine output (oligohydramnios) and is frequently underdeveloped (modified from 81).

Fig. 37.**29** Development of a twin–twin transfusion syndrome.

Fig. 37.**30** Development of polyhydramnios in the recipient.

Shunt

Common cotyledon ("third circulation")

Recipient:
Volume +
Diuresis +
Hydramnios
AV valvular incompetence
Fetal hydrops
AGA

Donor:
Volume –
Diuresis –
Oligohydramnios
Stuck twin
SGA

28

Donor twin	Recipient twin
Hypovolemia	Hypervolemia
Hypotension, decreased venous return	Hypertension, increased venous return
Growth retardation, anemia	Myocardial hypertrophy, plethora
Heart failure	Heart failure
Hydrops	Hydrops
Intrauterine death	Intrauterine death

29

Hypervolemia

↓

Atrial dilatation, increased arterial pressure

↓

Release of ANF (atrial natriuretic factor) (77, 112)

↙ ↘

Blockage of aldosterone   Inhibition of renal renin synthesis, Inhibition of angiotensin

↓   ↓

Natriuresis   Increased glomerular filtration

↘ ↙

Increased diuresis

↓

Polyhydramnios

30

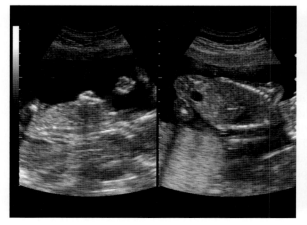

31

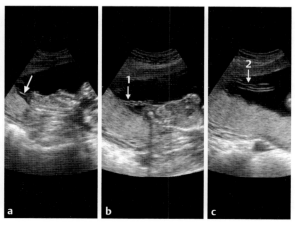

32

Fig. 37.**31** Typical features of twin–twin transfusion syndrome. *Left:* "stuck twin" tightly enclosed in an amniotic sac. The bladder is not visualized. The hypoechoic area represents amniotic fluid surrounding the second twin. *Right:* recipient with a full bladder and polyhydramnios.

Fig. 37.**32** Twin–twin transfusion syndrome at 17 weeks, 5 days.
a View of the amniotic membrane tightly enclosing the stuck twin (arrow).
b Markedly thin umbilical cord diameter of the donor (arrow).
c Thick, engorged umbilical cord of the recipient (arrow).

Balanced or unbalanced circulation. Although vascular anastomoses exist in most monochorionic placentas, a twin-to-twin transfusion syndrome develops only in 15–20% of monochorionic twins (26, 108). This means that a balanced circulation exists in most monochorionic placentas. A transfusion syndrome occurs only when the blood flow between the two circulations becomes unbalanced. As blood is shunted between the two placental circulations, the donor always gives up more blood than is transfused back by the recipient.

Recipient. As a result of this transfusion, the recipient twin becomes hypervolemic. This volume overload leads in turn to hypertension, cardiac hypertrophy, fetal pleural effusions, and eventual hydrops culminating in the death of the fetus (44, 91, 108). Plethora and hypertension additionally cause polyuria, which Schatz (91) identifies as the main cause of polyhydramnios (Figs. 37.**28**–37.**30**).

Donor. The donor twin, meanwhile, becomes hypovolemic, hypotensive, and restricted in its growth. Its anemic condition can lead to heart failure, generalized edema, and cavitary effusions. Eventually the progressive anemia leads to intrauterine fetal death (Fig. 37.29). With a monochorionic diamniotic placenta, the anemic half of the placenta is generally associated with oligohydramnios while the hyperemic half is associated with polyhydramnios. This is referable to decreased urine output by the donor and increased urine output by the recipient (Figs. 37.**28**–37.**30**).

Unanswered questions. While some of the pathophysiologic mechanisms of twin–twin transfusion syndrome are understood, there are several points that remain unclear. We do not know the precipitating factor that triggers an imbalance between the two circulations. The timing of the syndrome onset is also uncertain, therefore. It is reasonable to assume that the imbalance between the two circulations is due to an increased number of vascular anastomoses. However, when Bajoria et al. (2) studied the angioarchitecture in monochorionic twin placentas, they found that the placentas from pregnancies with twin–twin transfusion syndrome had significantly fewer anastomoses than those without the syndrome, and that the connections in twin–twin transfusion syndrome were more likely to be deep, solitary arteriovenous anastomoses.

Diagnosis of Chronic Twin–Twin Transfusion Syndrome

The diagnosis of chronic twin–twin transfusion syndrome is made sonographically based on a combination of various parameters, all of which need not be present. This depends on the gestational age and on the severity of the transfusion syndrome.

Monochorionicity. Because the twin–twin transfusion syndrome occurs chiefly in monochorionic pregnancies, the first step is to identify monochorionicity. With a monochorionic diamniotic placenta, this is done by detecting a thin dividing membrane over the chorionic plate (T sign). Additionally, it should be confirmed that the fetuses are of the same sex.

Growth discordance. For growth discordance to be diagnosed, more than a 20% weight discrepancy must be present between the two twins (17). But since weight estimation in twins can be problematic and has a large range of error, especially when the two compartments have different amniotic fluid volumes, a more reliable method is to use the difference between the two abdominal circumferences. A difference of 20 mm is the recommended cutoff point (13, 52).

Urine output. The increased urine output by the hypervolemic recipient leads to polyhydramnios (typically between 20 and 30 weeks' gestation), usually accompanied by a well-distended fetal bladder (Fig. 37.**31**). The donor, on the other hand, shows a decreased urine output—usually reflected in a small or nonvisualized bladder (Fig. 37.**31**)—accompanied by oligohydramnios.

Stuck twin. When massive polyhydramnios develops, the donor becomes a "stuck twin" (18, 36) that is affixed to the uterine wall by a tight membrane that resembles clear plastic wrap. The recipient, meanwhile, can move freely in the surrounding polyhydramnios. Because the dividing membrane tightly encloses the stuck twin, usually the outline of the sac is not visible (Fig. 37.**32 a**). The examiner may fail to notice the lack of movement by the stuck fetus and diagnose a normal monochorionic monoamniotic twin pregnancy. A monochorionic placenta in a twin–twin transfusion syndrome is not the only condition in which a stuck twin can occur. It may also be found in association with a dichorionic placenta in original Potter syndrome or in cases of pronounced placental insufficiency.

Umbilical cords. When the umbilical cords are examined in twin–twin transfusion syndrome, the recipient may be found to have a considerably thicker cord than the donor (Fig. 37.**32 b, c**). Also, the donor may have a velamentous cord insertion. This is a more common finding in twin–twin transfusion syndrome than in normal monochorionic diamniotic twins (36). Presumably the membranous insertion in the donor is compressed, causing a restriction of blood flow leading in turn to decreased renal perfusion and a diminished urine output (36).

Heart failure and hydrops. In advanced cases the circulatory overload in the recipient leads to myocardial hypertrophy, characterized by a rising preload and AV valvular incompetence (38). Eventually the cardiac failure results in hydrops. In the hypovolemic donor, the decreased venous return also leads to heart failure (46).

Doppler. Doppler and color Doppler ultrasound can detect disparities of vascular resistance in the umbilical cord arteries and can help to detect AV valvular incompetence. Comparative studies of both umbilical arteries in pregnancies with twin–twin transfusion syndrome showed that the difference in the ratio of peak systolic velocity (S) to end diastolic velocity (D) (the S/D ratio) between the two twins was greater than 0.4 in all of the cases examined (82). Finally, it may be possible to define the vascular anastomoses in the chorionic plate directly by color Doppler imaging (Fig. 37.**33**).

Hemoglobin concentration. The hemoglobin difference of > 5 g% stated in several publications (101) should no longer be used as a definitive criterion. Antenatal and intrapartum measurements have revealed both large and small hemoglobin differences in chronic twin–twin transfusion syndrome (34). Moreover, Danskin and Neilson (25) found that hemoglobin differences > 5 g% could be detected with similar frequency in both monochorionic and dichorionic twins.

The ultrasound parameters that are relevant in the diagnosis of twin–twin transfusion syndrome are reviewed in Table 37.**6**.

Treatment of Twin–Twin Transfusion Syndrome

Serial amniotic drainage or laser therapy. When a twin–twin transfusion syndrome is suspected on the basis of ultrasound findings, early treatment is indicated due to the high mortality (> 70%) that occurs with a wait-and-see approach (28, 41, 69). If increasing growth retardation is noted in one twin with the development of polyhydramnios around the recipient, intrauterine therapy may consist of serial amniocentesis (28, 48, 69) with maternal digitalization or the fetoscopic laser coagulation of superficial placental vascular connections (48, 108) (see Chapter 46), depending on gestational age and the severity of the growth discordance.

Table 37.6 Ultrasound signs of twin–twin transfusion syndrome

> ➢ Detection of monochorionic placenta with different echogenicities
> ➢ Detection of concordant external genitalia
> ➢ Growth discordance between the twins
>   • Discrepancy in abdominal circumference > 20 mm or
>   • Weight discrepancy > 20% relative to the larger twin
> ➢ Unequal amniotic fluid volumes
>   • Donor: oligohydramnios (stuck twin)
>   • Recipient: polyhydramnios
> ➢ Unequal bladder filling
>   • Donor: little or no visible bladder filling
>   • Recipient: well-distended bladder
> ➢ Unequal umbilical cord thickness
>   • Donor: thin umbilical cord, sometimes with a velamentous insertion
>   • Recipient: thick umbilical cord
> ➢ Hydrops of one fetus
> ➢ Marked discrepancy in Doppler findings (umbilical artery) between the two umbilical cords
>   • S/D ratio discrepancy > 0.4
> ➢ Color Doppler: development of tricuspid insufficiency in the recipient
> ➢ Vascular anastomoses in the chorionic plate may be directly visualized with color Doppler

If signs of twin–twin transfusion syndrome are noted early, during the period from 18 to 22 weeks' gestation, laser therapy is the current preference for achieving the best prognosis. Regardless of whether laser therapy or serial amniocentesis is performed, further surveillance of the fetuses should include Doppler examinations.

Intrauterine Death of One Twin

Incidence and causes. The incidence of the intrauterine death of one twin after 20 weeks' gestation was reported at 0.5–6.8% in a 1985 review (29).

The intrauterine death of one twin is three times more common with a monochorionic placenta than with a dichorionic placenta (5). Whereas coiling of the umbilical cord has been identified as the main cause of death in monochorionic monoamniotic twins (23, 54), twin–twin transfusion syndrome is the principal cause in monochorionic diamniotic twins.

Fetus papyraceus. The death of one twin in the first or second trimester does not always lead directly to a premature delivery. Litschgi and Stucki (64) observed the premature intrauterine death of one twin with continuation of the pregnancy in 6.8% of their twin gestations. The interval between the death of the twin and delivery ranged from 12 hours to 20 weeks. If the dead twin remains in utero for a prolonged period, the fetus becomes mummified while its amniotic fluid is reabsorbed. Pressure from the live twin flattens the dead fetus against the uterine wall (61) (Fig. 37.**34**). Finally the dead twin is delivered with the afterbirth in the form of a fetus papyraceus or fetus compressus (79) (Fig. 37.**34**).

Complications of Intrauterine Fetal Death

Neurologic injury. When one twin dies in a pregnancy with monochorionic placentation, there is a danger that so much blood will enter the vascular system of the dead twin from the living twin that the latter becomes severely anemic, causing foci of cerebral necrosis and brain damage or provoking the death of the second fetus (10). The risk of neurologic injury in the surviving fetus of a monochorionic twin pregnancy has not been accurately determined. In a review by Beinder (4), it is estimated at 18%.

Disseminated intravascular coagulation. Another risk to the surviving twin, according to Benirschke (5), is that the vascular anastomoses may transmit thromboplastic material from the dead twin to the live twin, inciting a disseminated intravascular coagulation that can cause multiple organ damage. It appears, however, that hypotension and anemia are more important than coagulopathy in producing the CNS lesions that are observed (78).

Risks of premature delivery and cesarean section. If the intrauterine death of one twin occurs late in the pregnancy, during the second or third trimester, Prömpeler et al. (84) found that the risk of premature delivery or cesarean section for the surviving fetus was substantially increased (50% and 59%, respectively). Twenty-two percent of the surviving twins developed growth retardation, and the perinatal mortality was 13%.

Maternal coagulopathy. A maternal clotting disorder in the form of hypofibrinogenemia is rare (106). According to Pritchard and Ratnoff (83), it does not occur before the fifth week after an intrauterine fetal death. These authors recommend induction of labor if the maternal fibrinogen level falls below 150 mg/dL.

Management of Intrauterine Fetal Death

Surveillance. If the intrauterine death of a twin occurs before the second twin has reached viability (< 24 weeks' gestation), the surviving twin should be checked sonographically at intervals of 1 week. If there is dichorionic placentation and the fetus continues to grow normally, the surveillance may be continued as in a singleton pregnancy. With monochorionic placentation, however, the surviving fetus should be closely watched for abnormalities such as possible CNS disorders or abnormal Doppler findings.

Timing and mode of delivery. After the surviving twin has reached viability, further management depends on the gestational age and the degree of demonstrable fetal compromise. Since early delivery in a monochorionic pregnancy does not necessarily protect the survivor from serious morbidity (20), significant prematurity should be considered acceptable only if definite fetal compromise (FHR monitoring, Doppler) can be documented. To exclude encephalomalacia, every surviving twin should undergo a detailed neonatologic examination after delivery.

Coagulation tests. Maternal coagulation tests should be performed at 1- to 2-week intervals. If a test is abnormal and the pregnancy is still significantly premature, an attempt can be made to prolong the pregnancy by hospitalizing the patient and administering heparin.

▀ Detection of Fetal Anomalies

The incidence of congenital anomalies in twins, at 6–10% (65), is generally higher than in singletons. Depending on chorionicity, the anomalies may be like those found in singletons or may be specific for monochorionic twins.

Anomalies in Dizygotic Twins

Basically, all anomalies that occur in singletons can also occur in dizygotic twins. Besides structural anomalies such as neural tube defects (anencephaly, spina bifida) (37), cardiac anomalies, hydrocephalus, omphalocele, and urogenital anomalies (Figs. 37.**35**–37.**37**), chromosomal abnormalities are also found.

Chromosomal abnormalities. According to Rodis et al. (88), the risk of having a child with Down syndrome is increased in twin pregnancies.

Fig. 37.**33**   *Left:* color Doppler image of a superficial vascular shunt between the two placentas. Pulsed Doppler trace indicates pulsatile blood flow. *Right:* postmortem appearance of the twins with a severe, early twin–twin transfusion syndrome.

Intrauterine fetal death

Fig. 37.**34**   *Left:* fetus papyraceus following intrauterine fetal death (arrow). The adjacent image shows the normal-size head of the normally developed twin for comparison. *Right:* postpartum appearance of the fetus papyraceus.

Anomalies in multiple fetuses

Fig. 37.**35**   Dichorionic diamniotic twin pregnancy with an anencephalic second twin (17 weeks, 6 days). Left image: normally developed head of the first twin. Right image: absent superior vault of the anencephalic twin.

Fig. 37.**36**   Dichorionic diamniotic twin pregnancy with the development of hydrocephalus in the second twin (28 weeks, 6 days). *Left:* first twin. *Right:* second twin.

Fig. 37.**37**   Dichorionic diamniotic twin pregnancy with an omphalocele in the second twin (arrow) (19 weeks, 2 days).

Fig. 37.**38**   Pathogenesis of the parasitic twin (TRAP sequence) (modified from 81).
a   Phase I: the arterial pressure in the twin on the left exceeds that in the twin on the right, causing a reversal of blood flow in the right twin with a deficient supply to the upper body.
b   Phase II: the reversal of blood flow in the right twin leads to atrophy of the heart and upper-body organs. This causes an increased cardiac load in the second twin, which now must provide for its own circulation plus that of the parasitic fetus.

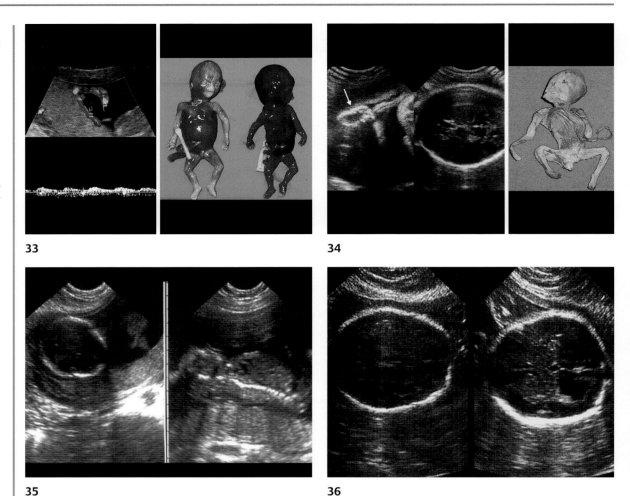

33   **34**

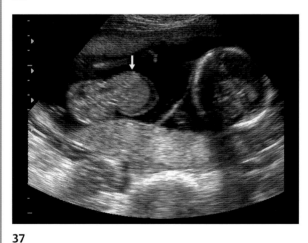

35   **36**

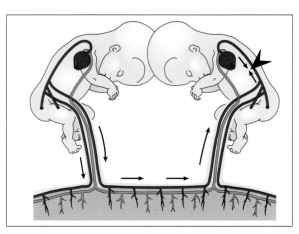

37

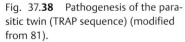
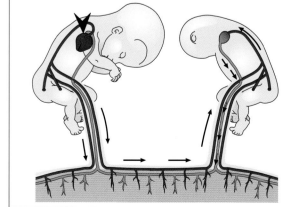

38 a   **38 b**

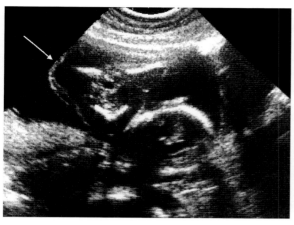

39

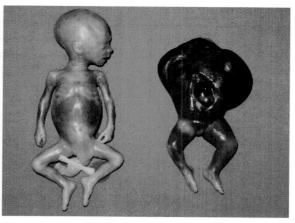

40

Fig. 37.**39** Acardiac acephalic twin. Scan demonstrates both the amorphous twin (arrow) and the normally developed twin (24 weeks).

Fig. 37.**40** Postpartum appearance of the fetuses in Fig. 37.**39**.

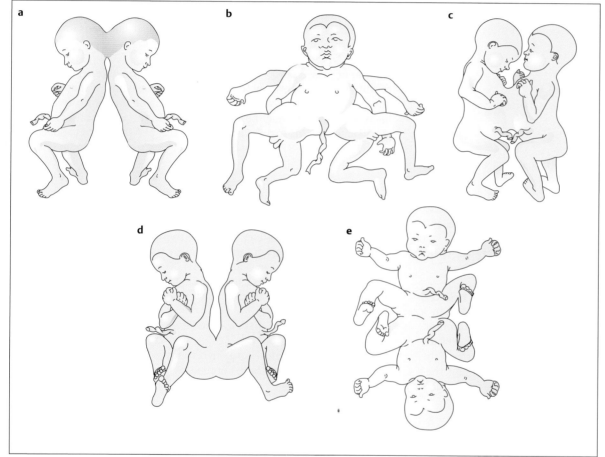

41

Fig. 37.**41** Various forms of conjoined twinning. **a—d** Vertical plane of symmetry. **e** Horizontal plane of symmetry.
a Craniopagus occipitalis.
b Cephalothoracopagus monosymmetros.
c Thoracopagus.
d Pygopagus.
e Ischiopagus.

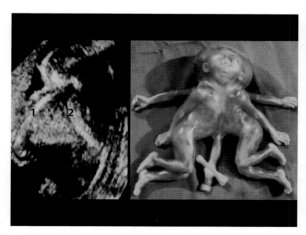

42

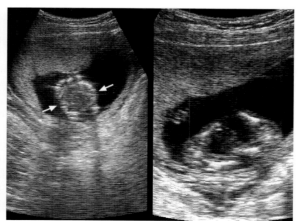

43

Fig. 37.**42** Cephalothoracopagus with fusion of the head and face. *Left:* ultrasound view of the two spinal columns. *Right:* postpartum appearance (observation by Dr. Hölzel, Bad Soden Hospital, Bad Soden, Germany).

Fig. 37.**43** Thoracopagus at 17 weeks. Left image shows the two adjacent spinal columns (arrows) with a common thorax. Right image shows the pelvic regions of the both fetuses, which are not fused.

Their calculations show that the risk in a 33-year-old woman with a twin pregnancy is comparable to that in a 35-year-old woman with a singleton pregnancy. Unilateral growth retardation in one twin is always suspicious for a chromosome disorder and should prompt a detailed ultrasound evaluation and chromosome analysis.

Management of a detected anomaly. The detection of an anomaly in one twin with a normal-appearing co-twin poses a difficult situation for the parents and the diagnostician. When a structural anomaly is found, it is advisable to obtain a chromosome analysis for both fetuses before any further decision is made. If a chromosome disorder is excluded and the structural defect is surgically correctible, the pregnancy should be closely monitored but can be continued without difficulty. If the anomaly in one twin is incompatible with life, the risk of continuing the pregnancy should be weighed against the risk of fetocide (27).

Anomalies in Monozygotic Twins

In the classification of Schwalbe (93), monozygotic twinning anomalies are divided into two main groups:
1. Asymmetrical free twins (acardiac twin)
2. Conjoined twins, subdivided into:
   a) symmetrical conjoined twins (diplopagus)
   b) asymmetrical conjoined twins (heteropagus, parasitic twin).

1. Asymmetrical Free Twins

Acardia (TRAP sequence, parasitic chorioangiopagus). Acardia refers to a group of anomalies in which the vascular systems of the free twins are interconnected and the circulation of the acardiac fetus is driven by the heart of the second twin. Acardius ("heartless fetus") is an anatomically misleading term in that many acardiac fetuses have at least a rudimentary heart, though it is never fully functional (93).
Forms. Schwalbe (93) identified four subtypes of acardiac twins (Table 37.**7**).

Pathogenesis. Some authors in the late nineteenth century believed that acardia developed from initially normal twin embryos due to a secondary redistribution of blood flow through vascular anastomoses, causing blood flow to be reversed in the acardiac twin (93). Authors had known about reversed blood flow in acardiac fetuses since the works of Hempel (50) in 1850 and Claudius (22) in 1859. Claudius theorized that the reversal of blood flow was the key factor in understanding the pathogenesis of acardia.

TRAP sequence. Today this anomaly is considered to be the most severe form of an early twin-to-twin transfusion at the embryonic stage, in which a rise of pressure in one circulation, acting through large vascular connections, causes a reversal of blood flow in the other circulation (Fig. 37.**38**) (81). This creates a circulatory pattern in which the normal twin supplies the acardiac twin with blood through one arterioarterial and one venovenous anastomosis. Pulsatile blood flow from the normal twin enters the umbilical artery of the acardius (generally there is only one artery), travels into the iliac arteries and descending aorta, and then returns via the umbilical vein (TRAP sequence = *twin reversed arterial perfusion*) (104). The copious blood supply to the lower

body half and the scant supply to the upper body half leads to secondary atrophy of the heart and upper-body organs. Development of the upper body and head is severely compromised. The extent of the developmental abnormality is highly variable and leads to bizarre anomalies of the parasitic twin, which may be only a shapeless mass of tissue in extreme cases (93).

Cardiac decompensation. Due to the excessive demands on its circulation, the healthy "pump twin" undergoes early cardiac decompensation followed by intrauterine death (mortality approximately 50%) (74, 104). The risk of decompensation appears to correlate with the size of the parasitic twin (74).

Ultrasound diagnosis. Ultrasound diagnosis is based on the detection of a deformed second twin with an absent or rudimentary heart (Figs. 37.**39**, 37.**40**), the detection of reversed arterial perfusion (directed toward the parasite), and signs of cardiac overload in the pump twin (cardiomegaly, secondary AV valvular incompetence, hydramnios). As the pump twin undergoes cardiac decompensation, it becomes hydropic.

Treatment. The choice of treatment depends on the severity of the condition. Treatment may be conservative, consisting of maternal digitalis therapy with close-interval serial scans of the pump twin, or an invasive procedure may be done to occlude the umbilical cord of the acardiac fetus. This may be done by the use of *N*-butyl-2-cyanoacrylate glue (Histoacryl) (81), endoscopic ligation (71), or endoscopic laser coagulation (47, 107).

2. Conjoined Twins

a. Symmetrical conjoined twins ("Siamese twins"). Symmetrical conjoined twins are complete, same-sex twins that are joined at certain body sites. They are often called "Siamese twins" after the twins Chang and Eng Bunker, born in Siam in 1811. These brothers were joined at the sternum (xiphopagus), lived until 1874, were married to two sisters, and fathered nine children each (93).

Forms. Schwalbe (93) distinguished two forms of symmetrical conjoined twins:
- Complete symmetrical conjoined twins
- Incomplete symmetrical conjoined twins.

In the complete form, both twins are equally well developed and are conjoined at certain body regions. In the incomplete form, the superior or inferior part of the body is duplicated in varying degrees (Table 37.**8**, Fig. 37.**41**).

Incidence. Conjoined twins occur in approximately one of every 50,000 births (9, 99, 100). The most common type is thoracopagus (93).

Ultrasound diagnosis (1, 21, 30). The ultrasound diagnosis of conjoined twins is based on an observed lack of separation in the ultrasound anatomy, synchrony of fetal movements, and detection of possible single, shared organs such as a common heart or liver (Figs. 37.**42**–37.**48**).

Prognosis and management. With the early ultrasound detection of conjoined twins, further management depends on the prognosis, which in turn depends on the type of connection between the twins. The extent of the fusion is highly variable, ranging from a simple skin connection to the sharing of a common organ such as the liver or heart (99, 100).

Early prenatal diagnosis. This is of key importance in planning interdisciplinary prenatal and postnatal management. Conjoining by a sim-

Table 37.**7**   Schwalbe classification of acardiac twins (93)

Hemiacardius anceps	Fetus with recognizable body forms and parts
Holoacardius amorphus	Fetus with unrecognizable body forms and organs
Holoacardius acephalus	Fetus lacking the superior half (or more) of the body
Holoacardius acormus	Fetus lacking the inferior half (or more) of the body

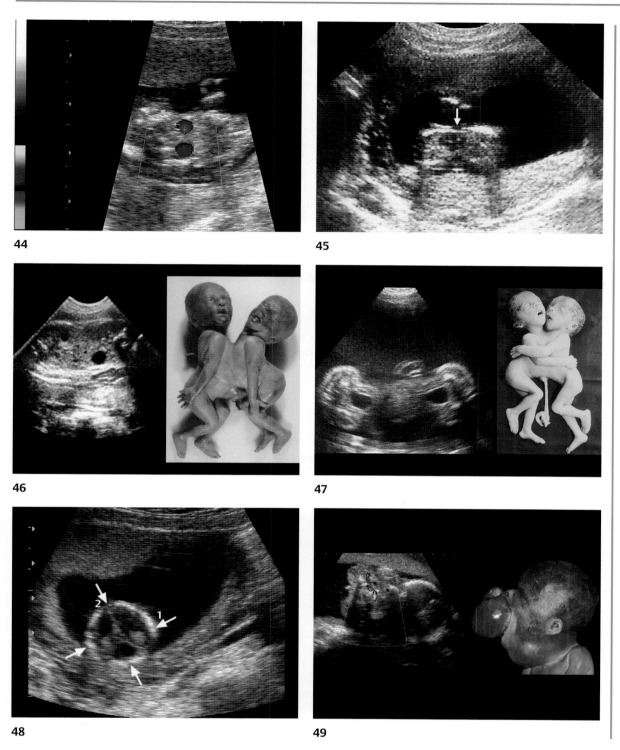

44

45

46

47

48

49

Fig. 37.**44** Thoracopagus with two separate, beating hearts (color Doppler view), 16 weeks.

Fig. 37.**45** Thoracopagus with a common heart (arrow), 14 weeks.

Fig. 37.**46** Thoracopagus at 27 weeks. *Left:* transverse scan at the level of the thoracoabdominal junction. *Right:* postpartum appearance.

Fig. 37.**47** Thoracopagus at 28 weeks. *Left:* ultrasound view of the fused thorax and upper abdomen with the origin of a shared umbilical cord. A full urinary bladder is visible on each side. *Right:* appearance after cesarean section.

Fig. 37.**48** Common head (syncephalus) in cephalothoracopagus monosymmetros at 15 weeks. 1 = BPD, 2 = OFD

Fig. 37.**49** Epignathus. *Left:* color Doppler shows a vessel supplying the tumor mass protruding from the fetal mouth. Longitudinal scan at 22 weeks. *Right:* pathoanatomic correlate.

Table 37.8 Schwalbe classification of complete symmetrical conjoined twins (93)

I. Vertical plane of symmetry (forms with single or double symmetry)	
A. *Ventral union*	
➢ Supraumbilical	
• Complete supraumbilical union • Partial supraumbilical union	Cephalothoracopagus (janus) Prosopothoracopagus Thoracopagus Sternopagus Xiphopagus (or frontal craniopagus)
➢ Infraumbilical	Ilioxiphopagus
➢ Supra- and infraumbilical	Iliothoracopagus Cephalothoracoiliopagus
B. *Dorsal union*	Pygopagus Occipital craniopagus
II. Horizontal plane of symmetry (forms with single or double symmetry)	
A. *Superior union*	Parietal craniopagus (from which occipital and frontal craniopagus are derived)
B. *Inferior union*	Ischiopagus
III. Median planes of individual parts (parallel to plane of symmetry, may coincide with it or diverge from it: duplicitas parallela)	
➢ Superior divergence of median planes	Catadidymus (duplicitas anterior)
➢ Corresponding inferior divergence ➢ Divergence in mid-body region ➢ Combined forms	Anadidymus (duplicitas posterior) Duplicitas media

Table 37.9 Schwalbe classification of parasitic twins (93)

I. Parasite attached to the head of the autosite	➢ Epignathus ➢ Parasitic craniopagus ➢ Parasitic janus ➢ Parasitic dicephalus
II. Parasite attached to the front of the trunk (or neck) of the autosite	➢ Parasitic thoracopagus ➢ Epigastrius ➢ Parasitic dipygus
III. Parasite attached to the back of the autosite	➢ Notomelus
IV. Parasite attached to the inferior end of the autosite	➢ Parasitic pygopagus ➢ Sacral parasites

Table 37.10 Important parameters in the ultrasound evaluation of multiple pregnancy

First trimester	➢ Detection of all embryos ➢ Determination of gestational age ➢ Size comparison of embryos (CRL) ➢ Early detection of anomalies ➢ Detection of a vanishing twin ➢ Determination of chorionicity and amnionicity
Second trimester	➢ Biometry ➢ Detection of anomalies ➢ Invasive testing as indicated ➢ Amniotic fluid volumes ➢ Detection of twin–twin transfusion syndrome ➢ Doppler examinations (from about 20 weeks) in monochorionic twins or if growth discordance is noted
Third trimester	➢ Biometry ➢ Amniotic fluid volumes ➢ Fetal lie ➢ Placental location
At delivery	➢ Fetal lie ➢ Lie of the second twin after delivery of the first twin

ple skin connection implies a favorable prognosis, but the prognosis is poor if multiple organs are shared. For example, while xiphopagus is operable in principle, surgical separation is not feasible for a cephalothoracopagus with a single heart and liver. Edmonds and Layde (27) reported a survival rate of 4.3% in a total of 81 conjoined twins.

Decision on pregnancy termination. The question of whether to continue the pregnancy following the ultrasound diagnosis depends on the extent of the anomaly. If there is a chance of later surgical separation, the parents should be told that an accurate disease evaluation and risk assessment cannot be made until after the delivery. But if there is no reasonable prospect for surgical separation of the conjoined twins, termination should be considered.

If conjoined twins are not detected until the third trimester, a planned abdominal delivery will at least prevent maternal complications such as dystocia and uterine rupture.

b. Asymmetrical conjoined twins (autosite and parasite). In this condition one twin (the parasite) is smaller and less complete than the other, fully developed twin (autosite). The reduction anomaly may be such that the parasitic twin lacks entire body parts, but in some cases it may show relatively complete development. All gradations may occur between these extremes (93). The parasitic twin may be attached to a certain body region of the autosite, appearing for example as a pharyngeal polyp (Fig. 37.**49**) or a sacral parasite.

Forms. The Schwalbe classification (93) is shown in Table 37.**9**.

Prognosis and management. The prognosis depends on the location and extent of the parasite. With an extensive anomaly that is detected early, the option of pregnancy termination should be discussed with the parents.

Summary of the Management of Multiple Pregnancies

For practical purposes, it is helpful to note the points that should be covered in the ultrasound examination at different stages in the pregnancy (Table 37.**10**).

First trimester. The priorities in the first trimester are to detect the multiple pregnancy and count the embryos, compare the growth of the embryos by measuring the crown–rump lengths, and confirm the gestational age. Chorionicity should be determined between 10 and 14 weeks' gestation so that a risk assessment can be made.

Dichorionic diamniotic twins. In a dichorionic diamniotic pregnancy where the twins show comparable growth, further surveillance is like that for a singleton pregnancy up to about 20 weeks' gestation. After 20 weeks, follow-up scans should be obtained at 3-week intervals. If growth discordance is noted during the first trimester or early second trimester, amniocentesis or chorionic villus sampling is recommended to exclude a chromosomal abnormality in the smaller twin. If discordant growth is noted later in the pregnancy, close-interval biometric scans should be obtained. Further surveillance should also include Doppler examinations. With an increasing growth disparity between the twins, early delivery in the third trimester may be considered depending on the gestational age and the amount of the disparity.

Monochorionic diamniotic twins. If monochorionic diamniotic placentation is detected with ultrasound, a careful biometric analysis (head, trunk, long bones) should be accompanied by an assessment of amniotic fluid volumes and bladder filling in the same-sex fetuses to permit the early detection of a twin–twin transfusion syndrome. Starting at 20 weeks, biometric scans should be obtained at 2-week intervals in this type of pregnancy. Doppler flowmetry of the major vessels and echocardiography are also helpful in assessing risk.

Higher-order multiples. In higher-order multiple pregnancies, basically the same recommendations apply as for monochorionic twins, bearing in mind that monozygosity and dizygosity may coexist in higher-order multiples. Close-interval ultrasound and Doppler surveillance should be initiated at 20 weeks.

Delivery. An ultrasound scanner should be available in every twin delivery, not only to check the lie of the fetuses but also to verify the position of the second twin after the first twin has been delivered.

References

1. Apuzzio, J.J., Ganesh, V., Landau, I., Pelosi, M.: Prenatal diagnosis of conjoined twins. Amer. J. Obstet. Gynecol. 148 (1984) 343–344
2. Bajora, R., Wigglesworth, J., Fisk, N.M.: Angioarchitecture of monochorionic placentas in relation to the twin–twin transfusion syndrome. Amer. J. Obstet. Gyneocl. 172 (1995) 856–863
3. Bazso, J., Dolhany, B., Pohanka, Ö.: Gewichtszunahme bei Zwillingskindern in den 28. bis 42. Schwangerschaftswochen. Zbl. Gynäk. 92 (1970) 628–633
4. Beinder, E.: Besondere fetale Risikosituationen bei Mehrlingen im 2. und 3. Trimenon. Gynäkologe 31 (1998) 245–253
5. Benirschke, K.: Twin placenta in perinatal mortality. N. Y. State J. Med. 61 (1961) 1499–1508
6. Benirschke, K., Driscoll, S.G.: The pathology of the human placenta. Berlin: Springer 1967
7. Benirschke, K., Kaufmann, P.: Multiple pregnancies. In: Pathology of the human placenta. 2nd ed. Berlin: Springer 1990; S. 636–753
8. Benirschke, K: The plazenta in twin gestation. Clin. Obstet. Gynecol. 33 (1990) 18–31
9. Benirschke, K.: Sonographic diagnosis of conjoined twinning. Ultrasound Obstet. Gynecol. 11 (1998) 241
10. Benirschke, K.: Klassifikation und Plazentationsverhältnisse bei der Mehrlingsgravidität. Gynäkologe 31 (1998) 198–202
11. Bessis, R., Papiernik, E.: Echographic imagery of amniotic membranes in twin pregnancies. In: Gedda, L., Parisi, P. (eds.): Twin Research 3: Twin Biology and Multiple Pregnancy. New York: Alan R. Liss 1981; S. 183–187
12. Bielfeld, P., Krüssel, J.: Einfluß der assistierten Reproduktion auf die Inzidenz von Mehrlingsschwangerschaften. Gynäkologe 31 (1998) 203–208
13. Blickstein, I., Freidman, A., Caspi, B., Lancet, M.: Ultrasonic prediction of growth discordancy by intertwin difference in abdominal circumference. Int. J. Gynecol. Obstet. 29 (1989) 121–124
14. Blickstein, I.: The twin–twin transfusion syndrome. Obstet. Gynecol. 76 (1990) 714–722
15. Bollmann, R., Jahnke, F.: Erfahrungen mit der nicht-selektiven Embryoreduktion und dem selektiven Fetozid. Gynäkologe 31 (1998) 254–260
16. Bolte, A., Breuker, K.H.: Diagnose der Zwillingsschwangerschaft und Geburtsverlauf. Arch. Gynäk. 228 (1979) 172–174
17. Brennan, J.N., Diwan, R.V., Rosen, M.G., Bellon, E.M.: Fetofetal transfusion syndrome: prenatal ultrasonographic diagnosis. Radiology 143 (1982) 535–536
18. Cameron, A.H.: The Birmingham twin survey. Proc. Roy. Soc. Med. 61 (1968) 229–234
19. Campbell, S., Grundy, M., Singer, J.D.: Early antenatal diagnosis of spina bifida in a twin fetus by ultrasonic examination and alpha-fetoprotein estimation. Brit. med. J. (1976) II 676
20. Carlson, N.J., Towers, C.V.: Multiple gestation complicated by the death of one fetus. Obstet. Gynecol. 73 (1989) 685–689
21. Chen, H.Y., Hsieh, F.J., Huang, L.H.: Prenatal diagnosis of conjoined twins by real time sonography: a case report. J. clin. Ultrasound 11 (1983) 94–96
22. Claudius: Die Entwicklung der herzlosen Mißgeburten (1859). Zitiert nach: Schwalbe, E.: Die Morphologie der Mißbildungen des Menschen und der Tiere. II. Teil: Die Doppelbildungen. Jena: Fischer 1907
23. Colburn, D.W., Pasquale, S.A.: Monoamniotic twin pregnancy. J. reprod. Med. 27 (1982) 165–168
24. D'Alton, M.E., Dudley, D.K.: The ultrasonographic prediciton of chorionicity in twin gestation. Amer. J. Obstet. Gynecol. 160 (1989) 557–561
25. Danskin, F.H., Neilson, J.P.: Twin-to-twin transfusion syndrome: What are appropriate diagnostic criteria? Amer. J. Obstet. Gynecol. 161 (1989) 365–369
26. Denbow, M.L., Cox, P., Taylor, M., Hammal, D.M., Fisk, N.M.: Placental angioarchitecture in monochorionic twin pregnancies: relationship to fetal growth, fetofetal transfusion syndrome and pregnancy outcome. Amer. J. Obstet. Gynecol. 182 (2000) 417–426
27. Edmonds, L.D., Layde, P.M.: Conjoined twins in the United States 1970–1977. Teratology 25 (1982) 301–308
28. Elliott, J.R., Urig, M.A., Clewell, W.H.: Aggressive therapeutic amniocentesis for treatment of twin–twin transfusion syndrome. Obstet. Gynecol. 77 (1991) 537–540
29. Enbom, J.A.: Twin pregnancy with intrauterine death of one twin. Amer. J. Obstet. Gynecol. 152 (1985) 424–429
30. Fagan, C.J.: Antepartum diagnosis of conjoined twins by ultrasonography. Amer. J. Roentgenol. 129 (1977) 921–922
31. Felderbaum, R., Dahnke, W.: D.I.R. – Deutsches IVF-Register: Ergebnisse der Datenerhebung für das Jahr 1996. Fertilität 13 (1997) 99
32. Finberg, H.J., Birnholz, J.C.: Ultrasound observations with first trimester bleeding: the blighted twin. Radiology 132 (1979) 137–142
33. Finberg, H.J.: The „twin peak sign": reliable evidence of dichorionic twinning. J. Ultrasound Med. 11 (1992) 571–577
34. Fisk, N.M., Borrell, A., Hubinont, C., Tannirandorn, Y., Nicolini, U., Rodeck, C.H.: Fetofetal transfusion syndrome: do the neonatal criteria apply in utero? Arch. Dis. Childh. 65 (1990) 657–661
35. Fountain, S.A., Morrison, J.J., Smith, S.K., Winston, R.M.: Ultrasonographic growth measurements in triplet pregnancies. J. Perinat. Med. 23 (1995) 257–263
36. Fries, M.H., Goldstein, R.B., Kilpatrick, S.J., Golbus, M.S., Callen, P.W., Filly, R.A.: The role of velamentous cord insertion in the etiology of twin–twin transfusion syndrome. Obstet. Gynecol. 81 (1993) 569–574
37. Garrett, W.J., Fisher, C.C., Kossoff, G.: Anencephaly in one of twins diagnosed by ultrasonic echography. Med. J. Aust. 11 (1975) 587–589
38. Gembruch, U., Bald, R., Fahnenstich, H., Hansmann, M.: Chronic twin–twin transfusion syndrome: a Doppler-sonographic and Doppler-echocardiographic longitudinal study. J. Matern. Fetal Invest. 3 (1993) 201
39. Gindoff, P.R., Yen, M.N., Jewelewicz, R.: The vanishing sac syndrome. Ultrasound evidence of pregnancy failure in multiple gestations, induced and spontaneous. J. Reprod. Med. 31 (1986) 322–325
40. Goeschen, K.: Sonographische Befunde bei Mehrlingen und ihre Konsequenzen. Geburtsh. u. Frauenheilk. 40 (1980) 836–838
41. Gonsoulin, W., Moise, K.J.Jr., Kirshon, B., Cotton, D.B., Wheeler, J.M., Carpenter, R.J.: Outcome of twin–twin transfusion diagnosed before 28 weeks of gestation. Obstet. Gynecol. 75 (1990) 214–216
42. Göttlicher, S., Madjaric, J., Krone, H.A.: Der biparietale Durchmesser des fetalen Kopfes bei Zwillingen und Einlingen im Verlauf der Schwangerschaft. Eine vergleichende Studie. Geburtsh. u. Frauenheilk. 37 (1977) 762–767
43. Grennert, I., Persson, P.H., Gennser, G.: Benefits of ultrasonic screening of a pregnant population. Acta obstet. gynec. scand. 78, Suppl. (1978) 5–14
44. Harrison, S.D., Cyr, D.R., Patten, R.M., Mack, L.A.: Twin growth problems: causes and sonograhic analysis. Semin. Ultrasound CT MR 14 (1993) 56–67
45. Hata, T. Deter, R.L., Hill, R.M.: Individual growth curve standards in triplets: prediction of third trimester growth and birth characteristics. Obstet. Gynecol. 78 (1991) 379–384
46. Hecher, K., Ville, Y., Snijders, R., Nicolaides, K.: Doppler studies of the fetal circulation in twin–twin transfusion syndrome. Ultrasound Obstet. Gynecol. 5 (1995) 318–324
47. Hecher, K., Reinold, U., Gbur, K., Hackelöer, B.J.: Unterbrechung des umbilikalen Blutflusses bei einem akardischen Zwilling durch endoskopische Laserkoagulation. Ultrasound Obstet. Gynecol. 5 (1996) 97–100
48. Hecher, K., Plath, H., Bregenzer, T., Hansmann, M., Hackelöer, B.J.: Endoscopic laser surgery versus serial amniocentesis in the treatment of severe twin–twin transfusion syndrome. Amer. J. Obstet. Gynecol. 180 (1999) 717–724
49. Hellin, D.: Die Ursache der Multiparität der unipaaren Tiere überhaupt und der Zwillingsschwangerschaft beim Menschen insbesondere. München (1895)
50. Hempel: De monstris acephalis. Diss. Hafniae (1850). Zitiert nach: Schwalbe, E.: Die Morphologie der Mißbildungen des Menschen und der Tiere. II. Teil: Die Doppelbildungen. Jena: Fischer 1907
51. Hertzberg, B.S., Kurtz, A.B., Choi, H.Y. et al.: Significance of membrane thickness in the sonographic evaluation of twin gestations. Amer. J. Roentgenol. 148 (1987) 151–153
52. Hill, L.M., Guzick, D., Chenevey, P., Boyles, D., Nedzesky, P.: The sonographic assessment of twin growth discordancy. Obstet. Gynecol. 84 (1994) 501–504
53. Hill, L.M., Chenevey, P., Hecker, J., Martin, J.G.: Sonographic determination of first trimester twin chorionicity and amnionicity. J. Clin. Ultrasound 24 (1996) 305–308
54. Holländer, H.J.: Monoamniotische Zwillinge. Z. Geburtsh. 171 (1969) 292–300
55. Jewell, S.E., Yip, R.: Increasing trends in plural births in the United States. Obstet. Gynecol. 85 (1995) 229–232
56. King, A.D., Soothill, P.W., Montemagno, R., Young, M.P., Sams, V., Rodeck, C.H.: Twin-to-twin blood transfusion in a dichorionic pregnancy without the oligohydramnios-polyhydramnios sequence. Brit. J. Obstet. Gynaec. 102 (1995) 334–335
57. Kucera, H., Reinhold, E., Schönswetter P.: Zur Bedeutung der Ultraschalldiagnostik für das perinatale Schicksal von Mehrlingsschwangerschaften. In: Hinselmann, M., Anliker, M., Merudt, R.: Ultraschalldiagnostik in der Medizin. Stuttgart: Thieme 1980; S. 157
58. Kurtz, A.B., Wapner, R.J., Mata, J., Johnson, A., Morgan, P.: Twin pregnancies: accuracy of first-trimester abdominal US in predicting chorionicity and amnionicity. Radiology 185 (1992) 759–762
59. Lage, J.M., Vanmarter, L.J., Mikhail, E.: Vascular anastomoses in fused, dichorionic twin placentas resulting in twin transfusion syndrome. Placenta 10 (1989) 55–59
60. Landy, H.J., Weiner, S., Corson, S.L., Batzer, F.R., Bolognese, R.J.: The „vanishing twin": ultrasonographic assessment of fetal disappearance in the first trimester. Amer. J. Obstet. Gynecol. 155 (1986) 14–19
61. Landy, H.J., Keith, L.G.: The vanishing twin: a review. Hum. Reprod. Update 4 (1998) 177–183
62. Leveno, K.J., Santos-Ramos, R., Duenhoelter, J.H., Reisch, J.S., Whalley, P.J.: Sonar cephalometry in twin pregnancy: Discordancy of the biparietal diameter after 28 weeks gestation. Amer. J. Obstet. Gynecol. 138 (1980) 615–619
63. Levi, S.: Ultrasonic assessment of the high rate of human multiple pregnancy in the first trimester. J. clin. Ultrasound 4 (1976) 3–5
64. Litschgi, M., Stucki, D.: Verlauf von Zwillingsschwangerschaften nach intrauterinem Fruchttod eines Föten. Z. Geburtsh. Perinat. 184 (1980) 277–230
65. Little, J., Bryan, E.: Congenital anomalies on twins. Semin. Perinat. 10 (1986) 50–64
66. Luke, B.: The changing pattern of multiple births in the United States: maternal and infant characteristics, 1973 and 1990. Obstet. Gynecol. 84 (1994) 101–106
67. Maggio, M., Callan, N.A., Hamod, K.A., Sanders, R.C.: The first-trimester ultrasonographic diagnosis of concoined twins. Amer. J. Obstet. Gyneocl. 152 (1985) 833–835
68. Mahony, B.S., Filly, R.A., Callen, P.W.: Amnionicity and chorionicity in twin pregnancies: prediction using ultrasound. Radiology 155 (1985) 205–209
69. Mahony, B.S., Petty, C.N., Nyberg, D.A., Luthy, D.A., Hickok, D.E., Hirsch, J.H.: The „stuck twin" phenomen: ultrasonographic findings, pregnancy outcome and management with serial amniocentesis. Amer. J. Obstet. Gynecol. 163 (1990) 1513–1522
70. McCracken, A.A., Daly, P.A. Zolnik, M.R., Clark, A.M.: Twins and Q-banded chromosome polymorphisms. Hum. Genet. 45 (1978) 253–258
71. McCurdy, C.M., Childers, J.M., Seeds, J.W.: Ligation of the umbilical cord of an acardiac-acephalus twin with an endoscopic intrauterine technique. Obstet. Gynecol. 82 (1993) 708–711
72. Merz, E., Wellek, S.: Normal fetal growth profile – a uniform model for calculating normal curves for current head and abdomen parameters and long limb bones. Ultraschall Med. 17 (1996) 153–162
73. Merz, E., Bahlmann, F., Welter, C., Miric-Tesanic, D.: Transvaginale 3D-Sonographie in der Frühgravidität. Gynäkologe 32 (1999) 213–219
74. Moore, T.R., Gale, S. Benirschke, K.: Perinatal outcome of forty-nine pregnancies complicated by acardiac twinning. Amer. J. Obstet. Gynecol. 163 (1990) 907–912

75. Mordel, N., Laufer, N., Zajicek, G. et al.: Sonographic growth curves of triplet conceptions. Amer. J. Perinatol. 10 (1993) 239–242
76. Nicolaides, K.H., Azar, G., Gosden, C.M.: Fetal nuchal edema: associated malformations and chromosomal defects. Fetal Diagn. Ther. 7 (1992) 123–131
77. Nimrod, C., Keane, P., Harder, J. et al.: Atrial natriuretic peptide production in association with nonimmune fetal hydrops. Amer. J. Obstet. Gynecol. 159 (1988) 625–628
78. Okamura, K., Murotsuki, J., Tanigawara, S., Uehara, S., Yajima, A.: Funipuncture for evaluation of hematologic and coagulation indices in the surviving twin following cotwin's death. Obstet. Gynecol. 83 (1994) 975–978
79. Ottow, B.: Die Mehrlingsschwangerschaft und die Mehrlingsgeburt. In Stoeckel, W.: Lehrbuch der Geburtshilfe. 9. Aufl. Jena: Fischer 1945; S. 250
80. Pandya, P.P., Hilbert, F., Snijders, R.J.M., Nicolaides, K.H.: Nuchal translucency and crown-rump length in twin pregnancies with chromosomally abnormal fetuses. J. Ultrasound Med. 14. (1995) 565–568
81. Plath, H., Hansmann, M.: Diagnostik und Therapie zwillingsspezifischer Anomalien. Gynäkologe 31 (1998) 229–244
82. Pretorius, D.H., Manchester, D., Barkin, S., Parker, S., Nelson, T.R.: Doppler ultrasound of twin transfusion syndrome. J. Ultrasound Med. 7 (1988) 117–124
83. Pritchard, J.A., Ratnoff, O.P.: Studies of fibrinogen and other hemostatic factors in women with intrauterine death and delayed delivery. Surg. Gynec. Obstet. 101 (1955) 467–477
84. Prömpeler, H.J., Madjar, H., Klos, W. et al.: Twin pregnancies with single fetal death. Acta Obstet. Gynecol. Scand. 73 (1994) 205–208
85. Reece, E.A., Yarkoni, S., Abdalla, M. et al.: A prospective longitudinal study of growth in twin gestation compared with growth in singleton pregnancies. I. The fetal head. J. Ultrasound Med. 10 (1991) 439–443
86. Reisner, D.P., Mahony, B.S., Petty, C.N. et al.: Stuck twin syndrome: Outcome in thirty-seven consecutive cases. Amer. J. Obstet. Gynecol. 169 (1993) 991–995
87. Robertson, E., Neer, K.: Placental injection studies in twin gestation. Amer. J. Obstet. Gynecol. 147 (1983) 170–173
88. Rodis, J.F., Vintzileos, A.M., Campbell, W.A., Pinette, M.G., Nochimson, D.J.: Intrauterine fetal growth in concordant twin gestation. Amer. J. Obstet. Gynecol. 162 (1990) 1025–1029
89. Sadler, T.W.: Medizinische Embryologie. 9. Aufl. Stuttgart: Thieme 1998
90. Scharl, A., Schlensker, K.H., Wohlers, W., Heymans, L.: Frühe Ultraschalldiagnose des Thorakopagus. Z. Gburtsh. Perinat. 192 (1988) 38–41
91. Schatz, F.: Eine besondere Art von einseitiger Polyhydramnie mit andersseitiger Oligohydramnie bei eineiigen Zwillingen. Arch. Gynäkol. 19 (1882) 329–326
92. Scholtes, G.: Überwachung und Betreuung der Mehrlingsschwangerschaften. Geburtsh. Frauenheilk. 37 (1977) 747–755
93. Schwalbe, E.: Die Morphologie der Mißbildungen des Menschen und der Tiere. II. Teil: Die Doppelbildungen. Jena: Fischer 1907
94. Sebire, N.J., D'Ercole, C., Hughes, K., Carvalho, M., Nicolaides, K.H.: Increased nuchal translucency at 10–14 weeks of gestation as a predictor of severe twin-to-twin transfusion syndrome. Ultrsound Obstet. Gynecol. 10 (1997) 86–89
95. Sepulveda, W., Sebire, N.J., Hughes, K., Odibo, A., Nicolaides, K.H.: The lambda sign at 10–14 weeks of gestation as a predictor of chorionicity in twin pregnancies. Ultrasound Obstet. Gynecol. 7 (1996) 421–423
96. Sepulveda, W., Sebire, N.J., Hughes, K., Kalogeropoulos, A., Nicolaides, K.H.: Evolution of the lambda or twin-chorionic peak sign in dichorionic twin pregnancies. Obstet. Gynecol. 89 (1997) 439–441
97. Socol, M.L., Tamura, R.K., Sabbagha, R.E., Chen, T., Vaisrub, N.: Diminished biparietal diameter and abdominal circumference growth in twins. Obstet. Gynecol. 64 (1984) 235–238
98. Spellacy, W.N., Handler, A., Ferre, C.D.: A case-control study of 1253 twin pregnancies from a 1982–1987 perinatal data base. Obstet. Gynecol. 75 (1990) 168–171
99. Spencer, R.: Theoretical and analytical embryology of conjoined twins. Part I. Clin. Anat. 13 (2000) 36–53
100. Spencer, R.: Theoretical and analytical embryology of conjoined twins. Part II. Clin. Anat. 13 (2000) 97–120
101. Tan, K.L., Tan, R., Tan, S.H., Tan, A.M.: The twin transfusion syndrome. Clin. Pediatr. 18 (1979) 111–114
102. Townsend, R.R., Simpson, G.F., Filly, R.A.: Membrane thickness in ultrasound prediction of chorionicity of twin gestations. J. Ultrasound Med. 7 (1988) 327–332
103. Tutschek, B., Reihs, T., Crombach, G.: Diagnostik und Prognose von Mehrlingsgraviditäten im I. Trimenon. Gynäkologe 31 (1998) 209–217
104. Van Allen, M.I., Smith, D.W., Shepard, T.H.: Twin reversed arterial perfusion (TRAP) sequence: A study of 14 twin pregnancies with acardius. Sem. Perinat. 7 (1983) 285–293
105. Vayssiere, C.F., Heim, N., Camus, E.P., Hillion, Y.E., Nisand, I.F.: Determination of chorionicity in twin gestations by high-frequency abdominal ultrasonography. Counting the layers of the dividing membrane. Amer. J. Obstet. Gynecol. 175 (1996) 1529–1533
106. Vial, Y., Hohlfeld, P.: Intrauterine death in twin pregnancies. Schweiz. Rundsch. Med. Prax. 88 (1999) 1435–1438
107. Ville, Y., Hyett, J., Vandenbusche, F.P.A., Nicolaides, K.H.: Endoscopic laser coagulation of umbilical cord vessels in twin reversed arterial perfusion sequence. Ultrasound Obstet. Gynecol. 4 (1994) 396–398
108. Ville, Y.: Twin transfusion syndrome. J. Gynecol. Obstet. Biol. Reprod. (Paris) 27 (1998) 255–257
109. Von Verschuer, O.: Biologische Grundlagen der menschlichen Mehrlingsforschung. Z. Abstammungs- und Vererbungslehre 61 (1932) 147
110. Wallenburg, H.C., Wladimiroff, J.W: The amniotic fluid. II. Polyhydramnios and oligohydramnios. J. Perinat. Med. 6 (1977) 233–243
111. Weissman, A., Jacobi, P., Yofe, N., Zimmer, E.Z., Paldi, E., Brandes, J.M.: Sonographic growth measurements in triplet pregnancies. Obstet. Gynecol. 75 (1990) 324–348
112. Wieacker, P., Wilhelm, C., Prömpeler, H., Petersen, K.G., Schillinger, H., Breckwoldt, M.: Pathophysiology of polyhydramnios in twin transfusion syndrome. Fetal Diag. Ther. 7 (1992) 87–92
113. Wood, S.L., Onge, R.St., Connors, G., Elliot, P.D.: Evaluation of the twin peak or lambda sign in determining chorionicity in multiple pregnancy. Obstet. Gynecol. 88 (1996) 6–9

38   Diagnosis of Maternal Disorders by Abdominal Ultrasound

The uterine corpus and adnexa can no longer be evaluated by transvaginal scanning in late pregnancy, as they are located too far from the transducer. They are accessible to transabdominal ultrasound, which is not restricted in its cephalad range and permits convenient evaluation of the uterus, abdominal cavity, and retroperitoneum.

Cervical Incompetence

Incompetent closure of the uterine cervix is one of the most common precipitating factors of habitual late abortion.

Causes. Cervical incompetence may be caused by a constitutional connective-tissue weakness of the cervix, which becomes incompetent when strained to a certain degree, or the incompetence may result from a cervical lesion that was sustained in a previous delivery. Cervical incompetence is most common between the third and fifth months of pregnancy.

Transvaginal and abdominal ultrasound. Ultrasound examination of the cervix has become the standard method for diagnosing cervical incompetence. Transvaginal scanning is used in most cases (7, 8, 10, 11, 12, 23) (see Chapter 7), as the uterine closure apparatus can be defined more clearly and evaluated more accurately than with transabdominal scanning.

Nevertheless, routine abdominal ultrasound in the second and third trimesters still affords a rewarding view of the cervix (Fig. 38.**1**). If cervical incompetence is present, it can usually be diagnosed without difficulty by transabdominal scanning. If findings are equivocal, however, a transvaginal examination should always be added.

In cases with premature rupture of the membranes and incipient cervical incompetence, transvaginal scanning can be withheld to avoid an ascending infection, and cervical surveillance can be continued with abdominal ultrasound. The dimensions that are used (cervical length, funnel width, funnel length; Fig. 38.**2**) are measured in the same way as in transvaginal ultrasound.

Bladder distension. To better evaluate the internal os, care should be taken that the maternal bladder is only slightly distended. An overdistended bladder can alter the shape of the uterine cervix and compress the cervical canal, in some cases making it impossible to detect cervical incompetence (16). The degree of bladder distension should be approximately the same in each subsequent examination.

Cervical length. The ultrasound monitoring of cervical length can not only aid in the early detection of cervical incompetence but can also help to avoid cerclage in cases where reduced cervical length has been detected clinically but follow-up scans do not show further shortening.

Conversely, in cases where cerclage has already been applied to the cervix, the cervical length can be checked sonographically to assess the efficacy of the procedure (6).

Uterine Leiomyomas during Pregnancy

Growth. In patients with known uterine leiomyomas, regular ultrasound examinations during pregnancy furnish information not only on the number, location, structure, shape, and size of the leiomyomas (Figs. 38.**3**–38.**8**) but also on their growth. In a prospective longitudinal study, Aharoni et al. (1) noted growth in 22% of 32 leiomyomas observed during pregnancy, while the rest showed no change in size.

Submucous leiomyomas. Large submucous leiomyomas are associated with a high incidence of obstetric complications. A submucous leiomyoma located directly below the placenta (Fig. 38.**6**) increases the risk of subsequent placental insufficiency, abruptio placentae (57%), and difficult placental separation following the delivery (9, 18).

Occasionally, a local uterine contraction wave can mimic a submucous leiomyoma (Fig. 38.**9**). The absence of the feature on subsequent scans distinguishes it from a true leiomyoma.

Subserous leiomyomas. Subserous leiomyomas in the uterine corpus can cause significant discomfort as a result of tumor growth and capsular tension, but they rarely cause obstetric interference even when of substantial size. On the other hand, a large subserous leiomyoma located in the cervical region is almost certain to cause obstetric complications. When the location and size of the leiomyoma are checked by serial ultrasound scans, it can be determined at an early stage whether cesarean section will be required.

Follow-up. Follow-up scans of a uterine leiomyoma may demonstrate marked structural changes in the tumor over time, depending on its blood supply. A disruption in the blood supply leads to degenerative changes ranging to necrosis (Fig. 38.**8**).

Pain during Pregnancy

Abdominal ultrasound has proven to be an important tool for investigating abdominal pain during pregnancy. For example, abdominal ultrasound can confirm (Fig. 38.**10**) or exclude (Fig. 38.**11**) the torsion of an ovarian mass as the cause of unilateral midabdominal pain.

When a cystic mass is detected in the lower abdomen, transvaginal scanning should additionally be performed as it usually provides better discrimination of the mass (Figs. 38.**12**, 38.**13**).

Upper abdominal pain. Ultrasound in these cases provides a quick and easy means of checking for liver problems such as cholecystolithiasis (20) (Fig. 38.**14**) or hepatic hemorrhage in the setting of a HELLP syndrome (15, 19) (Figs. 38.**15**, 38.**16**).

Flank pain. Urinary stasis with renal pelvic dilatation can often be demonstrated as a cause of flank pain (5, 14, 24) (Fig. 38.**17**). It is important, however, to distinguish a physiologic pregnancy-specific dilatation of the pyelocaliceal system from a pathologic distension. In ultrasound examinations of normal pregnant women, Schmoller (20) found that more than 80% showed dilatation of the pyelocaliceal system during the third trimester. The dilatation was unilateral in more 60% of the cases and predominantly affected the right side.

When pyelocaliceal dilatation exceeds 2 cm in the largest sagittal diameter, serial scans should be obtained at intervals of 1–2 weeks. This permits the early detection of any further increase, allowing for prompt treatment by stent insertion or percutaneous nephrostomy to prevent pressure atrophy of the renal parenchyma.

Lower abdominal pain. Lower abdominal pain may be caused by appendicitis (4, 17), diverticulitis, an incarcerated hernia, adhesive bowel obstruction, nephrolithiasis (13), or in rare cases by a pelvic kidney (Fig. 38.**18**). An inexperienced sonographer may mistake the latter structure for a "mass." The prompt detection of a pelvic kidney is important due to the risk of tearing or avulsion of a dystopic sacral kidney, especially in a surgically assisted vaginal delivery (2).

Ultrasound Diagnosis of Symphyseal Distension during Pregnancy

Definition. A predominantly estrogen-induced loosening of the pelvic joints normally occurs during pregnancy (21). Unphysiologic loosening of the pubic symphysis during pregnancy and especially during delivery leads to "symphyseal distension," which is associated with suprasymphyseal pain and a waddling gait.

Diagnosis. Symphyseal distension is usually demonstrated by an AP pelvic radiograph during the puerperium, but abdominal ultrasound can easily detect it prior to delivery and without radiation exposure. There may be a marked widening of the symphyseal gap (> 10 mm) as well as a visible stepoff in the pelvic girdle (> 5 mm) (3) (Figs. 38.**19**, 38.**20**).

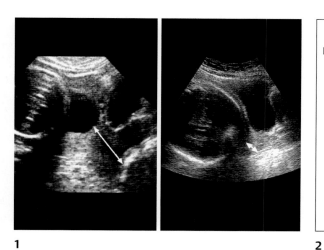

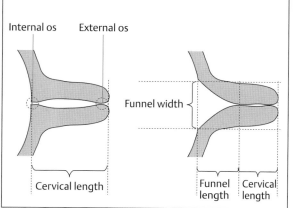

1

2

Cervical incompetence

Fig. 38.**1** *Left:* normal cervical length (4.2 cm) at 27 weeks. *Right:* cervical incompetence, with a cervical length of 1.8 cm (33 weeks, 3 days).

Fig. 38.**2** Diagram showing the various linear measurements of the cervix (cervical length, funnel width, funnel length).

Uterine leiomyomas

Fig. 38.**3**   Subserous leiomyoma in the anterior uterine wall (34 x 20 mm) at 21 weeks, 4 days.

Fig. 38.**4**   Large subserous leiomyoma in the anterior uterine wall (82 x 42 mm) at 28 weeks.

Fig. 38.**5**   Two adjacent, hypoechoic, anterior intramural leiomyomas (26 x 20 mm and 35 x 29 mm) at 24 weeks.

Fig. 38.**6**   Retroplacental intramural leiomyoma at 17 weeks.

Fig. 38.**7**   Intramural leiomyoma of the right posterior uterine wall (36 x 35 mm) shows a mixed hypoechoic-hyperechoic pattern due to regressive changes. Transverse scan of the uterus at 20 weeks.
S = spinal canal.

Fig. 38.**8**   Subserous leiomyoma in the posterior uterine wall (50 x 46 mm) with hypoechoic necrotic foci and hyperechoic calcific foci at 21 weeks, 4 days.

Fig. 38.**9**   Contraction wave (∗) in the posterior uterine wall at 16 weeks, simulating a uterine leiomyoma.

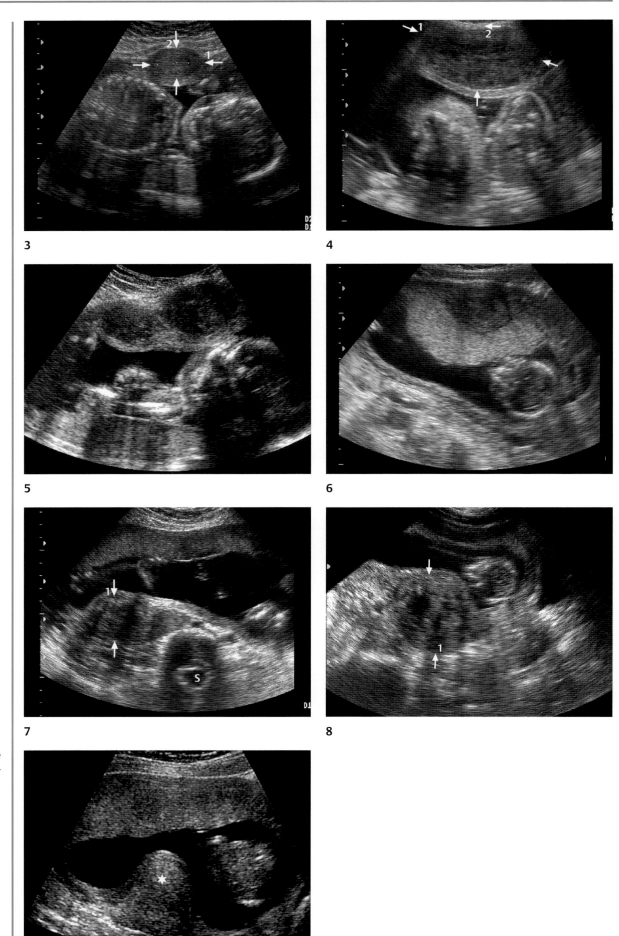

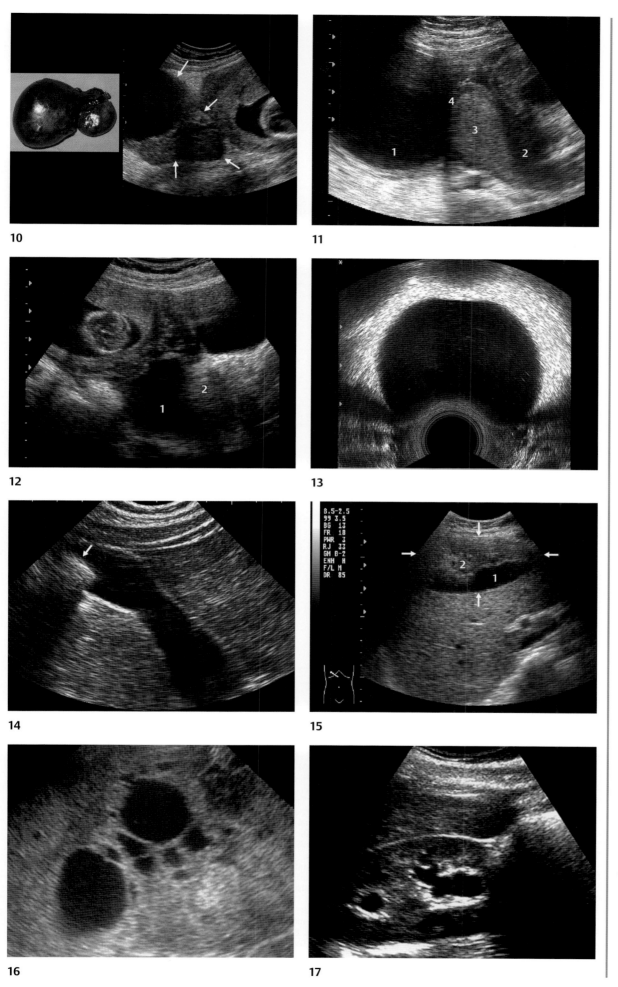

10

11

12

13

14

15

16

17

Pain

Fig. 38.**10** Torsion of a left-sided adnexal mass (arrows). Oblique sagittal scan through the left midabdomen at 18 weeks.

Fig. 38.**11** Subseptate uterus mimics a right-sided ovarian mass. Transverse scan at 31 weeks. 1 = Right half of uterus, 2 = left half of uterus, 3 = placenta (partially abuts the septum!), 4 = central septum.

Fig. 38.**12** Mixed cystic (1) and solid (2) dermoid in the cul-de-sac. Longitudinal scan at 13 weeks.

Fig. 38.**13** Transvaginal scan at 17 weeks demonstrates a cul-de-sac abscess with fine internal echoes following perityphlitic abscess formation.

Fig. 38.**14** Solitary gallstone (arrow) (7 mm diameter) in a pregnant woman with upper abdominal pain. Transverse scan at 6 weeks.

Fig. 38.**15** HELLP syndrome with a large, subcapsular hepatic hematoma on the right side (160 mL) (arrows). The collection is partly liquid (1) and partly organized (2). Oblique scan through the upper abdomen.

Fig. 38.**16** HELLP syndrome with sites of severe intrahepatic hemorrhage, appearing as hypoechoic round zones with fine internal echoes, at 26 weeks.

Fig. 38.**17** Borderline-pathologic urinary stasis on the right side. Longitudinal scan of the kidneys at 30 weeks. The renal calices are distended to 18 mm in their AP diameter.

Fig. 38.**18**   Unilateral pelvic kidney on the right side (arrows). Longitudinal scan through the right lower abdomen at 12 weeks.

Symphyseal distension

Fig. 38.**19**   Measurement of symphyseal width.

a Measurement of the hypoechoic symphyseal gap in a transverse scan.

b Symphyseal laxity is evidenced by 16 mm of symphyseal dehiscence with a 6-mm stepoff, 26 weeks.

Fig. 38.**20**   Normal values of symphyseal width during pregnancy (n = 211) (after 3).

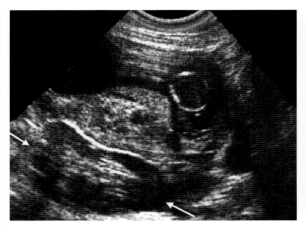

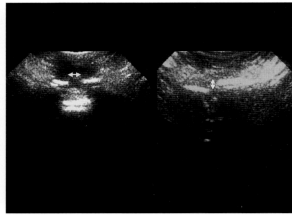

18   **19**

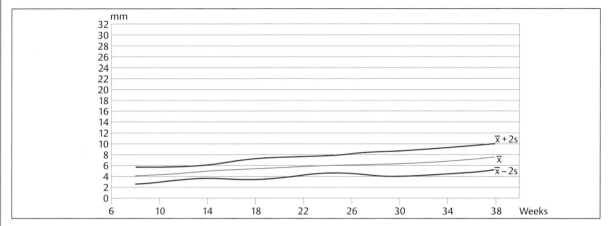

20

References

1. Aharoni, A., Reiter, A., Golan, D., Paltiely, Y., Sharf, M.: Patterns of growth of uterine leiomyomas during pregnancy. Brit. J. Obstet. Gynaecol. 5 (1988) 510–513
2. Altwein, J.E.: Urologie. Stuttgart: Enke 1979; S. 410
3. Bahlmann, F., Merz, E., Macchiella, D., Weber, G.: Sonographische Darstellung des Symphysenspaltes zur Beurteilung eines Symphysenschadens in der Schwangerschaft und post partum. Z. Geburtsh. Perinat. 197 (1993) 27–30
4. Bau, A., Atri, M.: Acute female pelvic pain: ultrasound evaluation. Semin. Ultrasound CT MR. 21 (2000) 78–93
5. Bernaschek, G., Kratochwil, A.: Graviditätsbedingte Erweiterungen am Nierenhohlraumsystem. Sonographische Diagnose und Verlaufskontrollen. Geburtsh. u. Frauenheilk. 41 (1981) 208–212
6. Bernstine, R.L., Lee, S.H., Crawford, W.L., Shimek, M.P.: Sonographic evaluation of the incompetent cervix. J. Clin. Ultrasound 9 (1981) 417–420
7. Cook, C.M., Ellwood, D.A.: A longitudinal study of the cervix in pregnancy using transvaginal ultrasound. Brit. J. Obstet. Gynaecol. 103 (1996) 16–18
8. Eppel, W., Schurz, B., Frigo, P., Reinold, E.: Vaginosonographische Beobachtung des zervikalen Verschlußapparates unter besonderer Berücksichtigung der Parität. Geburtsh. u. Frauenheilk. 52 (1992) 148–151
9. Exacoustos, C., Rosati, P.: Ultrasound diagnosis of uterine myomas and complications in pregnancy. Obstet. Gynecol. 82 (1993) 97–101
10. Hösli, I., Tercanli, S., Holzgreve, W.: Ultraschalldiagnostik der Zervix zur Früherkennung der drohenden Fehlgeburt. Gynäkologe 33 (2000) 361–369
11. Iams, J.D., Paraskos, J., Landon, M.B., Teteris, J.N., Johnson, F.F.: Cervical sonography in preterm labor. Obstet. Gynecol. 84 (1994) 40–46
12. Iams, J.D., Goldenberg, R.L., Meis, P.J. et al.: The length of the cervix and the risk of spontaneous premature delivery. New Engl. J. Med. 334 (1996) 567–572
13. Marlow, R.A.: Nephrolithiasis in pregnancy. Amer. Fam. Physician 40 (1989) 185–190
14. Muller-Suur, R., Tyden, O.: Evaluation of hydronephrosis in pregnancy using ultrasound and renography. Scand. J. Urol. Nephrol. 19 (1985) 267–273
15. Ochs, A.: Akute Hepatopathien in der Schwangerschaft: Diagnostik und Therapie. Schweiz. Rundsch. Med. Prax. 18 (1992) 980–982
16. Pfersmann, C., Deutinger, J., Bernaschek, G.: Die Zervixlänge gegen Ende der Schwangerschaft – eine sonographische Studie. Geburtsh. u. Frauenheilk. 46 (1986) 213–214
17. Retzke, U., Graf, H., Schmidt, M.: Appendizitis in der Schwangerschaft. Zentralbl. Chir. 123, S4 (1998) 61–65
18. Rice, J.P., Kay, H.H., Mahony, B.S.: The clinical significance of uterine leiomyoma in pregnancy. Amer. J. Obstet. Gynecol. 160 (1989) 1212–1216
19. Rinehart, B.K., Terrone, D.A., Magann, E.F., Martin, R.W., May, W.L., Martin, J.N.Jr.: Preeclampsia-associated hepatic hemorrhage and rupture: mode of management related to maternal and perinatal outcome. Obstet. Gynecol. Surv. 54 (1999) 196–202
20. Schmoller, H.: Die Ultraschalluntersuchung der Nieren in der Schwangerschaft. Röntgenpraxis 35 (1982) 69–73
21. Schmorell, E.: Die orthopädischen Besonderheiten der Frau durch ihre Fortpflanzungsaufgaben. In: Hohmann, G., Hackenbroch, M., Lindemann, K.: Handbuch der Orthopädie. Band II. Stuttgart: Thieme 1958; S. 1120–1136
22. Scott, L.D.: Gallstone disease and pancreatitis in pregnancy. Gastroenterol. Clin. North. Amer. 21 (1992) 803–815
23. Smith, C.V., Anderson, J.C., Matamoros, A., Rayburn, W.F.: Transvaginal sonography of cervical width and length during pregnancy. J. Ultrasound Med. 11 (1992) 465–467
24. Spernol, R., Riss, P., Bernaschek, G.: Echographische Untersuchung des Nierenbeckens bei klinischer Diagnose Pyelitis gravidarum. Geburtsh. u. Frauenheilk. 42 (1982) 717–719

39 Abdominal Ultrasound in the Puerperium

Ultrasound can be a valuable tool during the puerperium, especially in monitoring the progression of uterine involution and investigating the cause of uterine bleeding or unexplained fever. Abdominal ultrasound of the puerpera usually does not require a full bladder, because the enlarged uterus directly abuts the anterior abdominal wall and can be scanned without difficulty.

Uterine Involution

As ultrasound studies by Klug (5) and Meyenburg and Schulze-Hagen (8) have shown, postpartum involution of the uterus is a continuous process that occurs at different rates in different individuals (Fig. 39.**1**).
Length and angulation. Uterine involution can be evaluated more precisely with ultrasound than by manual examination, since the length of the uterus can be accurately measured (Fig. 39.**2**–39.**4**). Moreover, the degree of uterine angulation cannot be assessed by external palpation.

Factors that affect uterine involution. Klug (5) and Meyenburg and Schulze-Hagen (8) found no difference in the rate of uterine involution following spontaneous and cesarean deliveries. The apparent subinvolution that follows cesarean section is caused by swelling in the area of the isthmic suture (Figs. 39.**5**, 39.**6**), which delays straightening of the uterus during the first few days.

The rate of uterine involution is greatest during the first week after delivery and becomes slower thereafter. By 28 days after delivery, uterine size has reached the upper limit for the nongravid uterus (1). With an increase in maternal parity, Wachsberg et al. (9) found significantly larger uterine dimensions during the first four postpartum weeks. Birth weight and nursing had no effect on uterine involution. In a study by Galli et al. (4), however, early nursing led to an acceleration of uterine involution during the first four days after delivery.

Complications in the Puerperium

Retained Products and Lochial Retention

The most frequent complications in the puerperium include disturbances of uterine involution, heavy bleeding, and fever. They may be caused by retained products of conception or lochial retention.

Retained membranes or placenta. Remnants of the fetal membranes or placenta that are retained in utero can be detected sonographically by their echo structure, allowing for their removal by curettage (which may be done under ultrasound guidance). Retained membranes appear as a markedly hyperechoic, sheet-like area while placental remnants appear as dense, irregular echoes. If the findings are equivocal by abdominal ultrasound, transvaginal scanning should be performed (Fig. 39.**7**). Generally speaking, retained placental remnants in the uterus cannot be compared to the typical structural appearance of the placenta during pregnancy. The same is true of placental remnants following a spontaneous or induced abortion (2) (Fig. 39.**8**).

Lochial retention. The retention of lochia in the puerperium is manifested by a pronounced separation of the structures of the uterine cavity. The intrauterine fluid collection leads to an essentially uniform enlargement of the uterine cavity, which contains hypoechoic material that may show honeycomb-like septation (Figs. 39.**9**, 39.**10**). This represents an accumulation of fresh blood, lochia, and clotted blood. A large blood collection with hematoma formation can cause significant expansion of the uterine cavity, in which case transvaginal scanning is usually better for distinguishing the material from retained placenta (Fig. 39.**11**).

Treatment. The persistence of these findings is important in febrile puerperae and may necessitate cervical dilatation and the administration of oxytocic agents. If the uterine cavity appears smooth at ultrasound, curettage may be omitted in favor of conservative treatment with oxytocic drugs (6). Malvern and Campbell (7) concluded in 1973 that curettage could be avoided in 74% of women with postpartum bleeding by the use of ultrasound.

Bladder Dysfunction

Residual urine determination. Ultrasound permits the uncomplicated determination of residual urine volumes in women who have bladder dysfunction during the puerperium.

Follow-Up of Cesarean Section

In patients who report increasing pain after a cesarean section, ultrasound can be used to exclude or detect a hematoma in the wound area or suture dehiscence. Transvaginal scanning should be performed if the findings are equivocal (Fig. 39.**12**). Today many centers dispense with manual intrauterine probing in women who want to deliver spontaneously after a prior cesarean section, instead using ultrasound to evaluate the uterine suture line. If uterine rupture is suspected, ultrasound findings can be combined with clinical parameters to provide a prompt indication for operative treatment.

Trauma to the Pelvic Floor

3-D ultrasound. With recent developments such as 3-D ultrasound, it is now possible to conduct a detailed ultrasound survey of the pelvic floor and detect any obstetric trauma to the pelvic floor that has resulted from a spontaneous or surgically assisted vaginal delivery (10).

Uterine involution

Fig. 39.**1**   Uterine involution in the puerperium (adapted from [5]).

Fig. 39.**2**   Uterus 1 day postpartum. Uterine length is 21.3 cm (scan taken with a wide-angle transducer).

Fig. 39.**3**   Same uterus as in Fig. 39.**2**, 6 days postpartum. Uterine length is 14.3 cm. Echogenic membrane remnants (arrow) are visible in the isthmic region of the uterus.

Fig. 39.**4**   Same uterus as in Figs. 39.**2** and 39.**3**, 4 weeks postpartum. Uterine length is 8.1 cm. Following spontaneous expulsion of the membranes shown in Fig. 39.**3**, ultrasound demonstrates a normal-appearing uterine cavity.

Fig. 39.**5**   Uterine involution 5 days after cesarean section. Edema has developed around the isthmic suture (arrow).

Fig. 39.**6**   Same uterus as in Fig. 39.**5**, 13 days postpartum. There has been marked regression of wound edema (arrow).

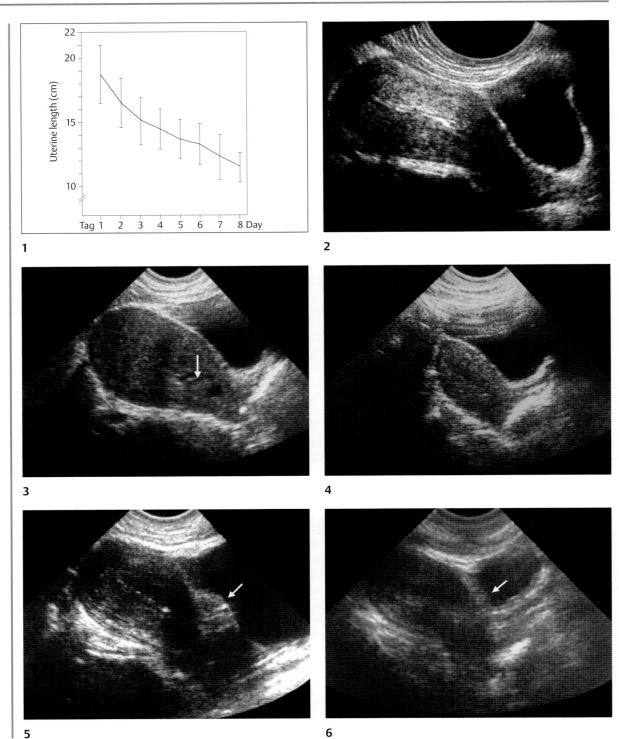

1

2

3

4

5

6

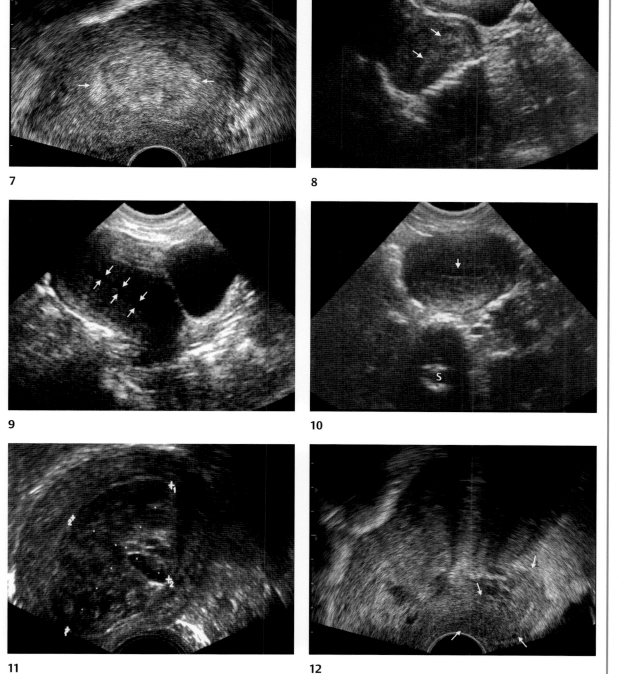

7

8

9

10

11

12

Retained placenta and lochia

Fig. 39.**7** Placental remnants postpartum (arrows), longitudinal transvaginal scan of the uterus.

Fig. 39.**8** Placental remnants (arrows) following pregnancy termination. Retroflexed uterus, longitudinal scan.

Fig. 39.**9** Intrauterine fluid collection (arrows). Longitudinal scan 11 days postpartum.

Fig. 39.**10** Transverse scan of the uterus in Fig. 39.**9**. The spinal canal (S) is visible behind the uterus, which shows a fluid collection within the uterine cavity (arrow).

Fig. 39.**11** Large postpartum clot in the uterine cavity, measuring 71 × 44 × 52 mm. Transvaginal scan.

Follow-up of cesarean section

Fig. 39.**12** Following cesarean section, marked hematoma formation (arrows) is evident about the surgical wound. Transvaginal scan.

References

1. Buisson, P., Tomikowski, J., Santarelli, J., Kapitaniak, B.: Clinical and ultrasonographic study of uterine involution in postpartum physiology. Rev. Fr. Gynecol. Obstet. 88 (1993) 12–18
2. Dalicho, F.H.: Mütterliche Organveränderungen, Pelvimetrie, Ultraschall post partum. In: Meinel, K., Issel, E.P., Watzek, H. (Hrsg.): Geburtshilfliche und gynäkologische Ultraschalldiagnostik. Stuttgart: Thieme 1991; S. 121–123
3. Demečko, D., Slezák, P., Hubková, B., Vaničková, Z., Táborský, D.: Anwendungsmöglichkeiten der Ultrasonographie im Puerperium. Zentralbl. Gynäkol. 111 (1989) 211–216
4. Galli, D., Groce, P., Chiapparini, I., Dede, A.: Ultrasonic evaluation of the uterus during puerperium. Minerva ginecol. 45 (1 V) (1993) 473–478
5. Klug, P.W.: Die Bedeutung der Sonographie im frühen Puerperium. Geburtsh. u. Frauenheilk. 44 (1984) 425–427
6. Lee, C.Y., Madrazo, B., Drukker, B.H.: Ultrasonic evaluation of the postpartum uterus in the management of postpartum bleeding. Obstet. Gynecol. 58 (1981) 227–232
7. Malvern, J., Campbell, S.: Ultrasonic scanning of the puerperal uterus following secondary post partum hemorrhage. J. Obstet. Gynaecol. Brit. Cwlth. 80 (1973) 320–324
8. Meyenburg, M., Schulze-Hagen, K.: Involution des Uterus nach Kaiserschnitt und Spontangeburt. In: Otto, R.C., Jann, F.X.: Ultraschalldiagnostik 82. Stuttgart: Thieme 1983; S. 185–186
9. Wachsberg, R.H., Kurtz, A.B., Levine, L.D., Solomon, P., Wapner, R.J.: Real-time ultrasonographic analysis of the normal postpartum uterus: technique, variability and measurements. Ultrasound Med. 13 (1994) 215–222
10. Wisser, J., Schulz, G., Kurmanavicius, J., Huch, R., Huch, A.: Use of 3 D ultrasound as a new approach to assess obstetrical trauma to the pelvic floor. Ultraschall Med. 20 (1999) 15–18

Doppler Ultrasound

40 Basic Principles of Doppler Ultrasound

Historical Development

The methodologic principles of present-day Doppler ultrasound are based on the discoveries of the Austrian mathematician and physicist Christian Johann Doppler (1803–1853). In 1842, Doppler (3) published his treatise "On the Colored Light of Binary Stars," in which he described the phenomenon in which the frequency of light waves changes according to whether the light source is moving toward or away from the observer. Another century passed until Satomura (29), in 1959, first utilized this "Doppler effect" to record blood flow velocities in human peripheral arteries. Doppler investigation of the fetoplacental vascular system was first described by Fitzgerald (5) in 1977. In subsequent years Doppler ultrasound was widely used in the surveillance of high-risk pregnancies, and today it permits the evaluation and analysis of the smallest vessels in the fetomaternal circulation. Doppler ultrasound provides a noninvasive method for evaluating the fetal cardiovascular system and, when used discriminatingly, can provide a significant reduction in perinatal morbidity and mortality. This development was recognized in 1995 when Doppler was added to the standard antenatal care program in Germany. Table 40.1 lists the risks that constitute indications for fetal Doppler ultrasound in this program.

Basic Concepts

Doppler effect, Doppler shift. Spectral Doppler technology can be used for the continuous analysis of blood flow velocities (cm/s). A frequency shift occurs when the sound waves emitted from an ultrasound transmitter at a specific frequency encounter moving corpuscular elements in the blood, are reflected from them, and are detected by an ultrasound receiver (the "Doppler effect") (6, 24, 34) (Fig. 40.1). The velocity of the moving elements is displayed on the ultrasound monitor in the form of a gray-scale amplitude trace, generated by a Fourier transform process. The Doppler frequency spectrum is displayed in a coordinate system in which velocity is plotted over an adjustable time scale. The recorded frequency shift is called the Doppler frequency spectrum or Doppler shift. This Doppler effect is described mathematically by the Doppler equation, which defines the dependence of the frequency shift (f_d) on the transmitted frequency (f_0), blood flow velocity (V), sound propagation velocity (c), and insonation angle (cos α).

Doppler formula:

$$V = \frac{f_d \cdot c}{2f_0 \cdot \cos \alpha}$$

Table 40.1 Indications for fetal Doppler ultrasound

- Suspected intrauterine growth retardation
- Pregnancy-induced hypertension, eclampsia/preeclampsia
- Prior history of fetal growth retardation or intrauterine fetal death
- Prior history of eclampsia/preeclampsia
- Abnormal fetal heart rate
- Strong suspicion of fetal disease or anomaly
- Growth discordance in multiple pregnancy
- Investigation of a suspected cardiac anomaly or disease

Table 40.2 Doppler indices

Index	Formula	Author
Pulsatility index	$= \frac{S - D}{V_{mean}}$	Pourcelot 1976 (19)
Resistance index	$= \frac{S - D}{S}$	Gosling 1974 (7)
S/D ratio	$= \frac{S}{D}$	Stuart 1980 (28)

S = maximum systolic flow velocity;
D = maximum diastolic flow velocity;
V_{mean} = mean flow velocity

f_d = Doppler frequency
f_0 = Ultrasound transmission frequency
V = Blood flow velocity
c = Sound velocity in tissue (approximately 1540 m/s)
cos α = Insonation angle

Antegrade and retrograde flow. Blood flow is defined as antegrade when it is directed toward the ultrasound transducer and retrograde when it is directed away from the transducer. When the recorded Doppler frequency spectrum appears above the zero baseline on the ultrasound monitor, then by definition it represents antegrade flow (toward the transducer). Frequencies displayed below the baseline indicate retrograde flow. The magnitude of the frequency shift is proportional to the observed velocity.

Resistance indices. Specific resistance indices are used in obstetric practice for the qualitative interpretation of Doppler spectra (22, 23). These indices describe the pulsatility of the blood flow, and so they reflect the flow resistance within the sampled vessel. They are calculated from the maximum flow velocities during systole (S) and diastole (D) and also from the mean flow velocity (V_{mean}) (Fig. 40.2). Because these indices are ratios, they are not angle-dependent and allow estimation of the peripheral vascular resistance. The diastolic flow velocities are proportional to the magnitude of the peripheral vascular resistance. High diastolic flow velocities signify a low peripheral resistance while low diastolic velocities reflect a high peripheral resistance or vasoconstriction. The most commonly used resistance indices in obstetrics are the pulsatility index (PI) of Gosling, the resistance index (RI) of Pourcelot, and the S/D ratio (7, 19, 28) (Table 40.2).

Pulsatility index. To calculate the pulsatility index (PI), it is necessary to know the mean intensity-weighted flow velocity (V_{mean}). This quantity depends on the width and amplitude values of the velocity distribution within the Doppler sample volume. The pulsatility index is calculated by subtracting the diastolic frequency shift (D) from the maximum systolic frequency shift (S) divided by the mean velocity (V_{mean}).

Resistance index and S/D ratio. The resistance index (RI) is also a ratio and describes by how much the end-diastolic peak velocity declines in relation to the systolic peak. The higher the vascular resistance, the greater the value of RI. The S/D ratio is the ratio of peak systolic velocity to peak diastolic velocity. It has the same diagnostic value as the resistance index.

Advantages and disadvantages of the indices. Small changes in resistance are reflected earlier in the RI, because the mathematically more complex V_{mean} used to determine PI shows a greater range of normal variation. To make an accurate determination of V_{mean}, therefore, it is necessary to record an optimum frequency spectrum in which the Doppler envelope curve is sharply outlined. This requirement leads to somewhat higher intra- and interobserver variability compared with the resistance index. But in cases that have severely abnormal Doppler signals with absent end-diastolic flow, a further reduction in flow (absent end-diastolic flow versus absent early diastolic flow, reverse flow) can no longer be detected by calculating the RI (in both cases RI = 1), and the PI is more useful for this purpose. In clinical practice and especially in Doppler follow-up examinations, the same index should be consistently used.

Doppler Techniques

Continuous-Wave Doppler

In continuous-wave (CW) Doppler, the transducer contains two crystals or piezoelectric elements (29, 34), one of which constantly emits signals at a certain frequency while the other continuously receives the returning echoes. All movements along the Doppler beam are registered and displayed as a frequency spectrum.

Advantages and disadvantages. The main advantage of this method, besides its low cost and ease of handling, is its ability to detect relatively high flow velocities, since aliasing problems do not occur. The disadvantage is that CW Doppler does not discriminate among signals from different depths, and so it cannot localize the signals to specific vessels.

Use in obstetrics. For these reasons, CW Doppler has limited applications in obstetric examinations and is used only in some departments to record uterine and umbilical flow patterns. Additionally, CW Doppler can be used in fetal echocardiography to detect high flow velocities like those associated with severe valvular stenosis. The Doppler indices (PI, RI, S/D) are the same whether they are determined by CW Doppler or pulsed Doppler (8, 16).

Pulsed Doppler

In pulsed Doppler systems, the same crystal alternately transmits sound pulses and receives the returning echoes (29, 34) (Fig. 40.**1**). A specific volume of interest, called the sample volume or Doppler gate, can be defined, making it possible to record flow information from a targeted vascular segment. The pulse repetition frequency (PRF) setting determines the range of velocities that can be recorded. Pulsed Doppler affords a significantly better signal-to-noise ratio than CW Doppler.

Duplex and triplex mode. Today, blood flow velocities are usually investigated by the combined use of pulsed spectral Doppler and real-time imaging (duplex mode) or by combining real-time imaging with spectral and color Doppler (triplex mode) (12, 27). Before performing clinical Doppler flow measurements, however, it is necessary to know the basic principles of Doppler ultrasound so that optimum Doppler frequency spectra can be recorded from the various fetomaternal vessels (4). The accurate recording of Doppler waveforms is essential for clinical interpretation (14, 15).

Color Doppler Ultrasound

Color duplex ultrasound provides a simultaneous display of soft-tissue structures and moving blood. Flow information is acquired by activating multiple successive sample volumes along adjacent scan lines, in a process known as multigate Doppler (18). The number of color samples along the individual color scan lines affects the "quality" of the color image while the number of color lines within the color box affects the "density" of the image. From 5 to 15 individual analyses (or more with newer systems) are performed for each color line, depending on the size of the color box.

Color encoding. In color Doppler, colors are assigned to the moving red cells according to the mean value of the frequency shift. Instead of being plotted as a frequency spectrum, the received Doppler signals are color encoded and displayed in the gray-scale image as an intensity-weighted mean blood flow velocity with the aid of an autocorrelation algorithm (9, 10). This color encoding often makes it easier for the examiner to locate the vessels of interest, while also providing information on the direction and variance of the flow. Color Doppler thus provides insights into the physiology and pathophysiology of blood flow. The instruments in current use employ color scales in which velocities in the positive range are displayed as red to yellow-orange, for example, while flows in the negative velocity range are displayed as dark blue to light blue or turquoise (Fig. 40.**3**). By definition, flow directed toward the transducer is encoded in red while flow away from the transducer is encoded in blue (Fig. 40.**4**). The magnitude of the frequency shift (velocities) is proportional to the brightness of the hues. When turbulence is present, the laminar blood flow is replaced by a large number of different measured velocities (= high variance). In most current instruments, turbulent flow is indicated by the presence of green pixels, although other colors may be assigned (Fig. 40.**5**). For example, turbulence may produce a mosaic pattern in which turquoise pixels (blue + green) represent negative Doppler shifts while yellow pixels (red + green) represent positive Doppler shifts (Fig. 40.**6**).

Equipment settings. As in pulsed Doppler, an optimum insonation angle is necessary to obtain a good color signal. Ideally, the angle setting of the color box should be less than 45° relative to the long axis of the vessel. The color frequency range is adjusted with the PRF control so that the highest expected velocity components in the targeted vessel will be just below the threshold for color aliasing. Velocity information (in cm/s or kHz) is presented on the color information scale in most color Doppler instruments. This scale provides only a crude virtual impression of the velocity range, however, and is not comparable to the velocities measured by pulsed Doppler. The gain setting for the B-mode image has no effect on the color-encoded display, but it should not be set too high as this will give poorer delineation of the vessels.

Equipment-Related Factors that Affect the Doppler Spectrum

Pulse Repetition Frequency and Aliasing

Pulse repetition frequency. The pulse repetition frequency (PRF) is the number of pulses that are transmitted per second. It is indirectly proportional to the depth setting of the sample volume. If the region of interest is deeply situated (e.g., due to polyhydramnios), more time must be allowed for a returning signal, and so a lower PRF is required. The PRF setting should conform to the flow velocities that are expected to occur in the vessels of interest. Higher velocities require a higher PRF, and lower velocities require a lower PRF. The velocity range and the height of the baseline should be adjusted so that the Doppler spectra

Doppler techniques

Fig. 40.1   Principle of pulsed Doppler ultrasound. SV = sample volume.

Fig. 40.2   Example of a normal Doppler frequency spectrum recorded from the umbilical artery. S = systole, D = diastole, V~mean~ = intensity-weighted mean flow velocity.

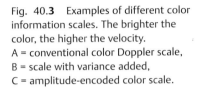

1

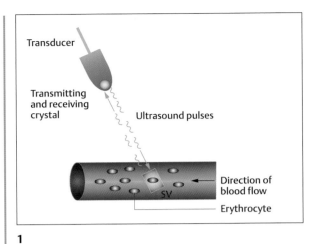

2

Fig. 40.3   Examples of different color information scales. The brighter the color, the higher the velocity.
A = conventional color Doppler scale,
B = scale with variance added,
C = amplitude-encoded color scale.

Fig. 40.4   Color Doppler image of a normal umbilical cord with three vessels. Flow directed toward the transducer is encoded in red, flow away from the transducer in blue.

3

4

Fig. 40.5   Color scale with a symmetrically positioned baseline and variance encoding.

Fig. 40.6   Four-chamber view with color-encoded display of turbulent flow (= color aliasing) in a fetus with holosystolic tricuspid insufficiency due to an Ebstein anomaly.

+ 57.7 cm/s → Nyquist limit

Red
Blood flow toward the transducer
(= positive Doppler shift)

Blue
Blood flow away from the transducer
(= negative Doppler shift)

Green
Reflects the degree of turbulence

→ Nyquist limit
– 57.7 cm/s

5

6

Equipment-related effects

Fig. 40.7   Example of aliasing in spectral Doppler. A = baseline set too high, B = pulse repetition frequency set too low.

Fig. 40.8   Aliasing in color Doppler, illustrated for a single umbilical artery.
A = optimum PRF setting at 2500 Hz. This setting results in good color filling of the umbilical vessels. B = PRF setting is too low (1000 Hz), causing a color reversal. C = PRF setting is too high (5000 Hz), causing incomplete color filling of the vessels.

7

8

are displayed without aliasing. The same applies to the settings used in color Doppler ultrasound.

Aliasing. Aliasing occurs when the pulse repetition frequency is less than twice the Doppler frequency shift. In this case the Doppler shift is displayed above the Nyquist limit (= one half the PRF) by a whole multiple of the pulse repetition frequency. This physical limit is also termed the Nyquist limit:

$$Fd_{max} = \frac{PRF}{2}$$

When this limit is exceeded, aliasing occurs—i.e., the peaks in the Doppler spectrum are truncated and "wrapped around," appearing below the baseline. Aliasing can be prevented by lowering the baseline, increasing the pulse repetition frequency, or using a lower-frequency transducer (2.5 or 3.5 MHz instead of 5 MHz) (Fig. 40.**7**). Another option is to reposition the transducer relative to the area of interest in an effort to increase the PRF. Aliasing in color Doppler is characterized by a color reversal from bright colors at one end of the scale to bright colors at the opposite end of the scale (Fig. 40.**8**).

Variance encoding. The laminar flow that normally prevails in vessels can become turbulent as a result of stenosis, valvular incompetence, etc. This type of flow is characterized by the formation of vortices in which the blood particles no longer move parallel to the vessel wall but at right angles to it. When variance encoding is switched on, non-laminar turbulent flow is marked by the presence of green pixels, making the turbulence easier to detect (Fig. 40.**6**). The degree of turbulence is directly proportional to the radius of the vessel lumen or stenosis, proportional to the mean flow velocity, and inversely proportional to the blood viscosity. Turbulence also greatly alters the shape of the flow profile. Turbulence appears as a mosaic in the color Doppler image. This is seen with high-velocity flow across stenotic valves, for example, or it may occur physiologically at sites such as the ductus venosus. The green component is proportional to the square of the standard deviation of the measured frequency shift (= variance). The degree of turbulence is influenced in a complex way by the degree of the stenosis, the geometry of the stenosis, the surface characteristics of the vessel wall, the prestenotic flow velocity, the viscosity of the blood, and the pulsatility of the flow. Besides vascular stenoses, color changes may also be caused by a faulty instrument setting, such as improper selection of the pulse repetition frequency (Fig. 40.**8**).

Gain

Doppler gain. The Doppler gain should be adjusted to provide a clear, well-defined frequency spectrum that is free of background noise (Fig. 40.**9**). If the signals are weak, however, it may be necessary to use a high gain setting and increase the power output to amplify the Doppler signal. Before color flow is switch on, care should be taken to obtain a good B-mode image with the lowest possible B-mode gain. The imaged vessels should be free of internal echoes, as this can make it difficult to localize the flow information.

Color gain. The color gain should be adjusted so that the surrounding structures are free of color signals, color completely fills the vessel lumen without bleeding across the vessel wall, and an acute insonation angle (< 60°) is used. Incomplete color filling of the vessel can have several causes:
- Priority set too low
- Color wall filter set too high
- Color velocity range (PRF) set too high
- Angle between the vessel and color box too large
- Color gain set too low (Fig. 40.**10**)

Flow Profile, Sample Volume, Pulsatility

Plug flow and profile flow. Under physiologic conditions, almost all portions of the fetal vessels are perfused by laminar flow. The flow profile during the acceleration phase in very pulsatile vessels tends to be flat (= plug flow) and then becomes paraboloid during the slower velocity phase (= profile flow). Plug flow typically occurs in large vessels with high velocities and high pulsatility, while profile flow is more apt to occur in small vessels with low-velocity flow. Both of these flow patterns can be detected in the fetal aorta, which exhibits plug flow during systole and profile flow in diastole (Fig. 40.**11**). In plug flow, the mean flow velocity is approximately equal to the maximum flow velocity. In profile flow, on the other hand, the mean velocity is only about half of the maximum velocity. This pattern is characteristic of the umbilical artery and middle cerebral artery, for example (Fig. 40.**11**).

Positioning the sample volume. The sample volume is the area from which Doppler signals are recorded. The size and position of the sample volume are adjustable and should conform to the specific examination conditions. The sample volume should cover approximately two-thirds of the vessel lumen (Fig. 40.**12a**), although this is of minor importance in obstetric studies due to the small vascular calibers. The vessel wall itself should be outside the sample volume. If the sample volume does not adequately cover the vessel lumen, it will sample an incomplete frequency spectrum with a distorted flow profile (Fig. 40.**12b**). This leads to a faulty calculation of V_{mean}, which in turn distorts the calculated pulsatility index.

Vessels with high pulsatility. If the sample volume does not fit the lumen of a vessel with high pulsatility (e.g., the fetal aorta, plug flow) but is too small or too large, the central flow velocities will not be detected. As a result, the maximum flow velocities in the display will be too low, and consequently the resistance indices (PI, RI) will be too high.

Vessels with low pulsatility. In these vessels, which carry profile flow, improper placement of the sample volume will again cause the central flow velocities to be missed. But because the flow profile is paraboloid, this will not affect the ratio of the systolic and diastolic flow velocities.

Intracardiac waveforms. A small sample volume (1–2 mm) is needed to record intracardiac Doppler waveforms, especially in the area of the atrioventricular and semilunar valves (Fig. 40.**17**). In the interest of recording an optimum frequency spectrum, no effort is made to display slow flows since only rapid flows carry the necessary information. By contrast, a larger sample volume is necessary for simultaneous sampling of the inferior vena cava and abdominal aorta in the diagnosis of fetal arrhythmias.

Insonation Angle, Angle Setting

Acute angle. The failure to obtain an optimum angle setting is one of the most common errors in recording both spectral and color Doppler signals. As a consequence of the cosine function, the smaller the angle of incidence of the sound beam (= insonation angle), the higher the frequency shift for a given flow velocity (Fig. 40.**13**). To obtain useful spectra, then, the vessel of interest should first be located in an optimum B-mode image, and then the Doppler frequency spectrum should be recorded at a low acute angle. The best Doppler signals are acquired when the insonation angle is less than 60°, and preferably less than 45°. When the beam–vessel angle is 90°, no signals are received (cos 90° = 0 in the Doppler equation). The insonation angle can be checked or defined in the frozen image with the angle-correct bar. However, angle correction after the image is acquired has no effect on the

Fig. 40.**9** Adjusting the signal-to-noise ratio. Ideally, no background noise should be displayed.

Fig. 40.**10** Adjusting the color gain.
A = optimum color gain setting.
B = too much color gain, leading to vessel-wall unsharpness and color bleed from the vessel lumen.
C = mosaic pattern caused by too much color gain.

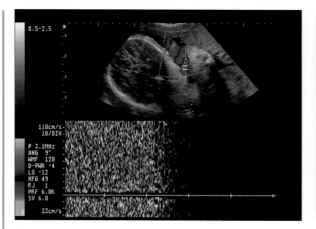

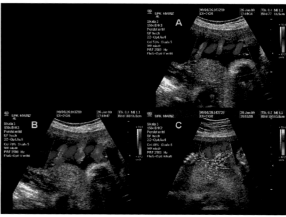

9

10

Fig. 40.**11** The paraboloid flow profile in the umbilical artery (profile flow) contrasts with the flat profile in the thoracic descending aorta (plug flow).

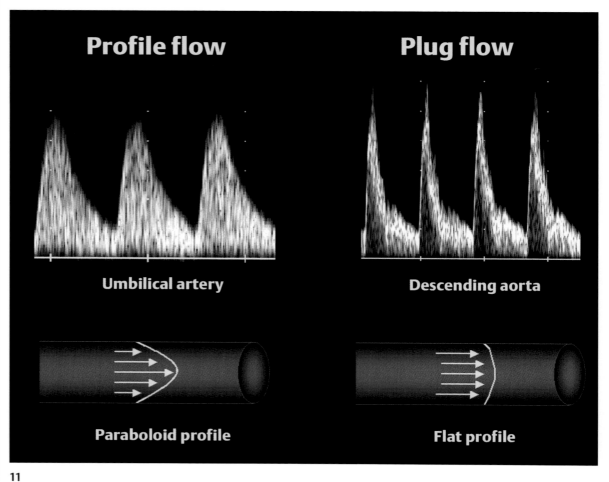

11

Fig. 40.**12**
a Correct positioning of the sample volume.
b The sample volume on the left samples a complete flow profile across the vessel lumen, while the volume on the right provides an incomplete sample.

Fig. 40.**13** Effect of insonation angle on the magnitude of the frequency shift.

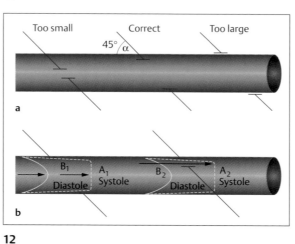

12

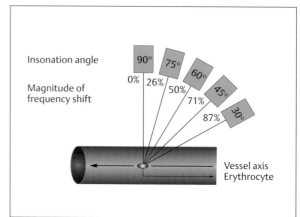

13

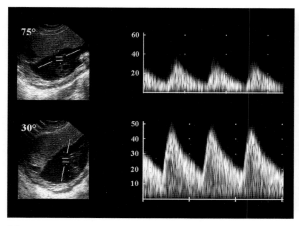

14

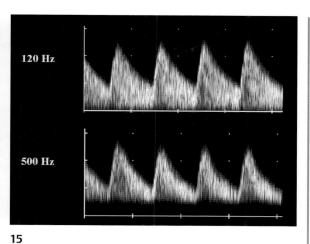

15

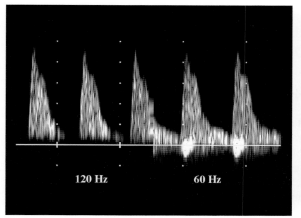

16

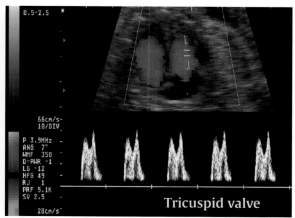

17

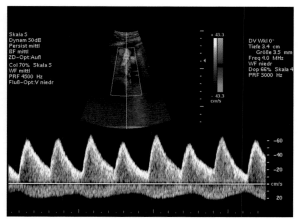

18

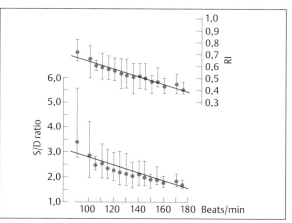

19

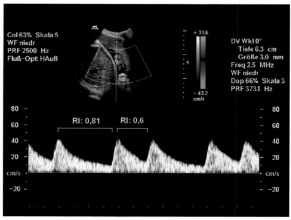

20

Fig. 40.**14**   Effect of insonation angle on the Doppler frequency spectrum, illustrated for the umbilical artery. Top: 75°. Bottom: 30°.

Fig. 40.**15**   Effect of wall filter setting on the Doppler frequency spectrum. Top: 120 Hz. Bottom: 500 Hz.

Fig. 40.**16**   If the end-diastolic velocities are poorly displayed, the wall filter should be reduced to permit optimum waveform analysis.

Fig. 40.**17**   In recording tricuspid valve velocities and other fetal echocardiographic studies, a high wall filter setting should be used for suppression of low-frequency echoes.

Fetal factors affecting the Doppler spectrum

Fig. 40.**18**   Doppler spectrum in the presence of fetal breathing movements, illustrated for the umbilical artery and vein.

Fig. 40.**19**   Effect of fetal heart rate on the resistance indices RI and S/D (after 17).

Fig. 40.**20**   Sporadic supraventricular extrasystoles. The prolonged cardiac cycle results in decreased end-diastolic flow velocities and higher resistance indices.

Doppler spectrum and only changes the flow velocity scale on the monitor. It is important, therefore, to have an optimum insonation angle during the examination.

Angle too large. In theory, the insonation angle does not affect the qualitative analysis of the frequency spectrum. But angles greater than 60° will not detect higher flow velocities as precisely as smaller angles, resulting in a flatter Doppler trace with lower mean flow velocities (Fig. 40.**14**). As a result, the pulsatility index is the only resistance index that is affected by larger angles.

Wall Filter (High-Pass Filter)

Choosing the right setting. The wall filter serves to eliminate unwanted low-frequency components of the Doppler spectrum that are generated by pulsatile movements of the vessel wall. Low-frequency echoes are suppressed on both sides of the baseline. The threshold of the wall filter is adjustable and should conform to the examination conditions. The filter setting, which ranges from 30 to 2000 Hz depending on the type of system used, should not be higher than the frequency of the pulsating vessel. A wall filter setting of 100 Hz or less is usually recommended for obstetric Doppler examinations (22). If the filter is set too high, it can cause an apparent absence of end-diastolic velocities (Fig. 40.**15**). For this reason, the wall filter should be decreased by one setting if end-diastolic flow velocities are not detected (Fig. 40.**16**). By contrast, high wall filter settings (200–350 Hz) are recommended for fetal echocardiography to eliminate interference from moving valves (Fig. 40.**17**).

Color filter. The same principle underlies the color filter, which is used to adjust color sensitivity. There should be good color filling of the vessel with no spurious color outside the vessel wall. Generally this adjustment is made with the color gain control. The color filter should be set to approximately 200–300 Hz. The optimum color filter setting is based on the expected blood flow velocities in the vessels of interest and is tailored to the individual case. For example, a high color filter is used in examining the fetal heart while a low color filter is used to define placental or pulmonary vessels. Color sensitivity is also influenced by the pulse repetition frequency, the color gain, and by the quality, density and priority settings.

Displaying the Frequency Spectrum

Initial instrument settings. Before a Doppler examination is performed, the signal-to-noise ratio should be correctly adjusted on the monitor (Fig. 40.**9**). First the gain control is turned up until conspicuous background noise, composed of white pixels, appears on the screen. Then the gain is gradually lowered until only the true Doppler frequency spectrum is seen, with no trace of background noise. Lowering the Doppler gain any further would lead to poor registration of the frequency spectrum. An optimum display of the frequency spectrum is essential for calculating the resistance indices (14). For this reason, the wall filter should be set to 100 Hz or less. Otherwise the calculated mean intensity-weighted flow velocity (V_{mean}) would be too high, resulting in a faulty calculation of the pulsatility index, especially when abnormal flow patterns are present. The baseline should be displayed in the lower third of the screen to provide a visually appealing image (Figs. 40.**17**, 40.**18**).

Examination procedure. When the vessel of interest has been identified on the screen, the B-mode image should be frozen for Doppler interrogation, as this will ensure a better quality of the recorded Doppler signal compared with the duplex mode. Whenever possible, a precise longitudinal scan of the vessel should be displayed in the B-mode image. This is not always possible, however, especially with the umbilical

artery. With vessels that are difficult to image (e.g., the uterine arteries), color Doppler should also be activated to make the vessels easier to locate. When the vessel of interest has been identified, the sample volume is positioned at the site of interest within the color flow signal, the angle-correct bar is aligned with the vessel axis, and pulsed Doppler is switched on. The angle-correct bar provides information only on the current insonation angle and does not affect the flow profile. Frequency spectra that are moving toward the transducer are displayed above the baseline, and spectra that are moving away from the transducer and displayed below the baseline. The Doppler trace is analyzed in the frozen image over at least 3–5 uniform cycles with a built-in software program that allows both automated and manual waveform analysis (25). Kurmanavicius (11) even recommends waveform analysis over 5–7 cardiac cycles. It is good practice to document the frequency spectrum of each vessel of interest with the associated velocity ranges and to use resistance indices for waveform analysis.

Effects of Examination Technique on the Doppler Spectrum

Maternal Factors

Medications and diseases. When interpreting Doppler frequency spectra, it is important to take into account pharmacologic effects (e.g., fenoterol, beta blockers, antihypertensive drugs, "recreational" drugs), maternal diseases (e.g., pregnancy-induced hypertension, preeclampsia, diabetes mellitus, connective-tissue diseases, cardiovascular diseases), and emotional states. To obtain valid Doppler findings, the examination should be performed with the patient at rest in a semilateral position. For this reason, it is best to start with a sonomorphologic evaluation and fetal biometry and then proceed with Doppler scanning.

Obesity. Severe maternal obesity often makes it difficult to define the fetus with ultrasound and record Doppler waveforms. The umbilicus provides a relatively good acoustic window in these cases. Imaging conditions can also be improved by elevating the obese abdominal wall and placing the transducer on the side of the lower abdomen above the inguinal ligament.

Respiratory movements. Maternal respiratory excursions can also be a serious hindrance in recording Doppler spectra. It is often helpful in this situation to have the patient hold her breath for a brief period.

Fetal Factors

Fetal movements. Fetal breathing movements and body movements are the most frequent obstacle to recording a useful frequency spectrum (31). Fetal breathing movements cause a decrease in systolic and diastolic flow velocities during inspiration and an increase in flow velocities during expiration (26) (Fig. 40.**18**). Significant variations and irregularities can be seen in Doppler frequency spectra due to fetal breathing activity. Like fetal body movements, breathing movements can make it difficult or even impossible to record useful Doppler spectra. For this reason, accurate Doppler flowmetry and waveform analysis should be attempted only under conditions of fetal rest.

Fetal heart rate. A fetal heart rate between 120 and 160 bpm has no apparent effect on the Doppler spectrum, so it does not alter the individual resistance indices (30). It is still true, however, that the resistance indices are indirectly proportional to the fetal heart rate (17) (Fig. 40.**19**). For example, when the heart rate increases due to paroxysmal supraventricular tachycardia or some other cause, the diastolic phase of the cycle is shortened, causing less of a decrease in end-diastolic flow velocities. As a result, higher values are calculated for the resistance indices. On the other hand, fetal bradycardia affects the Doppler spectral analysis by prolonging the diastolic phase, leading to an increase in resistance indices. Fetal supraventricular extrasystoles also affect the frequency spectrum and the qualitative analysis of the envelope curve (Fig. 40.**20**).

Checklist. The checklist in Table 40.**3** is helpful for troubleshooting problems that may arise in Doppler examinations.

Newer Methods of Color Imaging

Power Doppler

Amplitude analysis. In power Doppler imaging (power color Doppler, color perfusion imaging), the flow information within a selected area is color encoded based on the energy content of the Doppler signal that is returned by reflection and scattering. Unlike conventional color Doppler, in which a Fourier transform is used to analyze the frequency spectrum, power Doppler is based on the amplitude or intensity of the echoes received (13). Signals of lower intensity are encoded in a darker color, while signals of higher intensity are encoded in a brighter color. Unlike conventional color Doppler, flow information is displayed in only one color, and so power Doppler does not provide directional information (Fig. 40.**21**).

Advantages. Aliasing does not occur, and the insonation angle has very little effect on vascular imaging. Thus, power Doppler is very sensitive to blood flow in small vessels and to low-velocity flows. Initial studies of the placenta have shown that power Doppler can provide an excellent view of the placental angioarchitecture in normal pregnancies and in pregnancies with placental insufficiency (20). The color sensitivity and signal-to-noise ratio can be further enhanced by deleting the grayscale image from the color box and replacing it with a dark background (Fig. 40.**22**). This provides a starker image in which it is easier for the human eye to perceive the vessels.

Disadvantages. Vascular stenoses and turbulent flows cannot be visualized. Another drawback is that power Doppler does not provide velocity or directional discrimination. Also, it is highly susceptible to motion artifacts. This can be a particular problem when imaging around the heart. But the most serious problem with power Doppler at present lies in the quantification of the color-encoded information.

Outlook. Power Doppler imaging, including three-dimensional color power imaging, is definitely opening up new approaches in the investigation of vascular anatomy and pathology (1) (Fig. 40.**23**). Moreover, it appears that vascular imaging can be improved by the administration of ultrasound contrast agents. To date, however, only a few scientific studies have appeared on the use of these agents in the fetomaternal vascular system (2).

Tissue Doppler Echocardiography, Tissue Doppler

Myocardial motion imaging. Tissue Doppler echocardiography (TDE) is a modification of conventional color Doppler in which signals from cardiac wall movements of sufficiently high amplitude but slower than 10 cm/s are color encoded to create a two-dimensional image. The pulse repetition frequency and color gain are considerably lower than in conventional color Doppler: the PRF is set at approximately 200 Hz and the color gain at 14–24 dB (32). The best results are provided by an apical scan of the heart in the four-chamber view. Myocardial movements directed toward the transducer are encoded in red, movements away from the transducer in blue (Fig. 40.**24**). Although the frame rate seems very low, at 8 images/second, it is fully adequate for the color imaging of myocardial motion.

Advantages. The main advantage of TDE is its ability to evaluate the function of the myocardium and atrioventricular valves. Initial experience with TDE shows that it can furnish new information on myocardial function in conditions such as hypoplastic left heart syndrome, cardiomyopathies, and cardiac tumors (32).

Table 40.**3**   Troubleshooting checklist for Doppler examinations

Poor delineation of the Doppler frequency spectrum
➢ Check for adequate coupling gel
➢ Check the scan plane
➢ Check the insonation angle
➢ Check for excessive transducer pressure
➢ Increase the Doppler gain
➢ Increase the power output
➢ Switch on the duplex mode

Irregular display of the Doppler frequency spectrum
➢ Patient at rest?
➢ Patient agitated?
➢ Fetal breathing movements?
➢ Fetal body movements?
➢ Fetal arrhythmia?

Peaks in the frequency spectrum are displayed below the baseline
➢ Change the scan plane
➢ Lower the baseline
➢ Increase the PRF
➢ Use a lower-frequency transducer (if the PRF cannot be increased)

Amplitudes too low
➢ Increase the insonation angle
➢ Decrease the PRF

Little or no capacity for automated waveform analysis
➢ Check for adequate coupling gel
➢ Unsharp Doppler spectrum due to poor recording?
➢ Check the scan plane
➢ Doppler gain set too high?
➢ Too much background noise?

Incomplete color filling of the vessels
➢ Check for adequate coupling gel
➢ Check the insonation angle
➢ Increase color priority
➢ Increase color persistence
➢ Increase color gain
➢ Decrease color velocity range (PRF)
➢ Reduce color wall filter

Spurious color outside the vessel
➢ Decrease color gain
➢ Increase PRF
➢ Optimize the insonation angle
➢ Decrease color persistence

Color mosaic within the vessel
➢ Increase PRF
➢ Rule out vascular anomaly

Newer color Doppler techniques

Fig. 40.**21** Color information scale for amplitude-encoded blood flow analysis (power Doppler).

Fig. 40.**22** Power Doppler image of placental blood flow.

Fig. 40.**23** Three-dimensional color power image of a vein of Galen aneurysm (1).

Fig. 40.**24** Tissue Doppler images of the fetal heart. Apical four-chamber view in systole (left) and diastole (right).

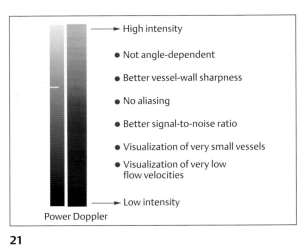

→ High intensity

- Not angle-dependent
- Better vessel-wall sharpness
- No aliasing
- Better signal-to-noise ratio
- Visualization of very small vessels
- Visualization of very low flow velocities

→ Low intensity

Power Doppler

21

22

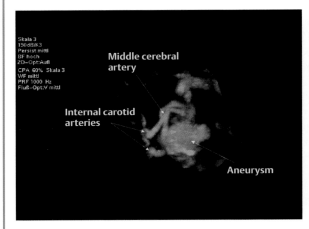

23

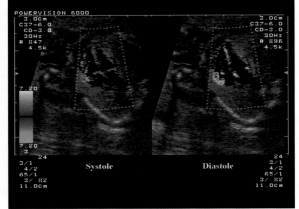

24

References

1. Bahlmann, F.: Three-dimensional color power imaging of an aneurysm of the vein of Galen. Ultrasound Obstet. Gynecol. 15 (2000) 341
2. Denbow, M.L., Blomley, M.J.K., Cosgove, D.O., Fisk, N.M.: Ultrasound microbubble contrast angiography in monochorionic twin fetuses. Lancet 346 (1997) 773
3. Doppler, C.: Über das farbige Licht der Doppelsterne und einiger anderer Gestirne des Himmels. Abhandl. Königl. Böhm. Gesellsch. 2 (1842) 465–482
4. European Association of Perinatal Medicine Study Group „Doppler Technology in Perinatal Medicine": B. Doppler technology. J. Perinat. Med. 22 (1994) 458–462
5. Fitzgerald, D.E., Drumm, J. E.: Non-invasive measurement of the fetal circulation using ultrasound: a new method. Brit. Med. J. 2 (1977) 1450–1451
6. Fobbe, F., Klews, P.M., Kubale, R., Landwehr, P.: Geräteeinstellung und Untersuchungstechnik. In: Wolf, K.J., Fobbe, F. (Hrsg.): Farbkodierte Duplexsonographie. Grundlagen und klinische Anwendung. Stuttgart: Thieme 1993; S. 37–44
7. Gosling, R.G., King, D.H.: Ultrasound angiology. In: Marcus, W., Adamson, L. (eds.): Arteries and veins. Edingburgh: Churchill Livingstone 1975; pp. 61–69
8. Gudmundson, S., Fairlie, F., Lingman, G., Marsal, K.: Recording of blood flow velocity waveforms in the uteroplacental circulation: Reproducibility study and comparison of pulsed and continuos wave Doppler ultrasonography. J. Clin. Ultrasound 18 (1990) 97–101
9. Klews, P.M.: Einführung in die farbkodierte Duplexsonographie (FKDS). In: Wolf, K.J., Fobbe, F. (Hrsg.): Farbkodierte Duplexsonographie. Grundlagen und klinische Anwendung. Stuttgart: Thieme 1993; S. 1–13
10. Klews, P.M.: Physik und Technik der farbkodierten Duplexsonographie (FKDS). In: Wolf, K.J., Fobbe, F. (Hrsg.): Farbkodierte Duplexsonographie. Grundlagen und klinische Anwendung. Stuttgart: Thieme 1993; S. 248–295
11. Kurmanavicius, J., Baumann, H., Huch, R., Huch, A.: Determination of the minimum number of cardiac cycles necessary to ensure representative blood flow velocity measurements. J. Perinat. Med. 17 (1989) 33–39
12. Landwehr, P.: Hämodynamische Grundlagen. In: Wolf, K.J., Fobbe, F. (Hrsg.): Farbkodierte Duplexsonographie. Grundlagen und klinische Anwendung. Stuttgart: Thieme 1993; S. 19–36
13. Macsweeney, J.E., Cosgove, D.O., Arenson, J.: Colour Doppler energy (power) mode ultrasound. Clin. Radiol. 51 (1996) 387–390
14. Maulik, D., Yarlagadda, A.P., Youngblood, J.P., Willoughby, L.: Components of variability of umbilical arterial Doppler velocimetry – a prospective analysis. Amer. J. Obstet. Gynecol. 160 (1989) 1406–1412
15. Maulik, D.: Hemodynamic interpretation of the arterial Doppler waveform. Ultrasound Obstet. Gynecol. 3 (1993) 219–227
16. Mehalek, K.E., Berkowitz G.S., Chitkara, U., Rosenberg, J., Berkowitz, R.L.: Comparison of continuous-wave and pulsed Doppler S/D ratios of umbilical and uterine arteries. Obstet. Gynecol. 72 (1988) 603–606
17. Mires, G., Dempster, J., Patel, N.B., Crowford, J.W.: The effect of fetal heart rate on umbilical artery flow velocity waveforms. Brit. J. Obstet. Gynecol. 94 (1987) 665–669
18. Mitchell, D.G.: Color Doppler Imaging: Principles, limitations and artifacts. Radiology 177 (1990) 1–10
19. Pourcelot, L.: Applications cliniques de l'examen Doppler transcutane. In: Peronneau, P.: Velocimetrie Ultrasonor Doppler Inserm (1974) 212–218
20. Pretorius, D.H., Nelson, T.R., Baergen, R.N., Pai, E., Cantrell, C.: Imaging of placental vascular using three-dimensional ultrasound and color power Doppler: a preliminary study. Ultrasound Obstet. Gynecol. 12 (1998) 45–49
21. Satomura, S.: Study of the flow patterns in peripheral arteries by ultrasound. J. Acoust. Soc. Jpn. 15
22. Schmidt, W., Rühle, W., Braun, W., Auer, L.: Verläßlichkeit der Duplexsonographie zur nichtquantitativen Messung des Durchflusses im Vergleich zur induktiven Flußmessung einer in vitro-Studie. Z. Geburtsh. Perinat. 192 (1988) 19–23
23. Schneider, K.T.M.: Standards in der Perinatalmedizin. Dopplersonographie in der Schwangerschaft. Geburtsh. u. Frauenheilk. 56 (1996) M69–M73
24. Scoutt, L.M., Zawin, M.L., Taylor, K.J.: Doppler US. Part II. Clinical Applications. Radiology 174 (1990) 309–319
25. Spencer, J.A., Price, J.: Intraobserver variation in Doppler ultrasound indices of placental perfusion derived from different number of waveforms. J. Ultrasound Med. 8 (1989) 197–199
26. Spencer, J.A., Price, J., Lee, A.: Influence of fetal breathing and movements on variability of umbilical Doppler indices using different numbers of waveforms. J. Ultrasound Med. 10 (1991) 37–41
27. Strauss, A.L.: Farbduplexsonographie der Arterien und Venen. Leitfaden und Atlas. Berlin: Springer 1994
28. Stuart, B., Drumm, J., Fitzgerald, D.E., Duigan, N.M.: Fetal blood velocity waveforms in normal pregnancy. Brit. J. Obstet. Gynecol. 88 (1981) 865–869
29. Taylor, K.J., Holland, S.: Doppler US: Part I. Basic principles, instrumentation and pitfalls. Radiology 174 (1990) 297–307
30. Thompson, R.S., Trudinger, B.J., Cook, C.M.: A comparison of Doppler ultrasound waveform indices in the umbilical artery. I. Indices derived from the maximum velocity waveform. Ultrasound Med. Biol. 12 (1986) 835–840
31. Trudinger, B.J.: The umbilical circulation. Semin. Perinatol. 4 (1987) 311–321
32. Twinning, P.: Myocardial motion imaging: A new application of power color flow and frequency-based color flow Doppler in fetal echocardiography. Ultrasound Obstet. Gynecol. 13 (1999) 255–259
33. Vetter, K.: Dopplersonographie in der Schwangerschaft. Edition Medizin VHC 1991
34. Wells, P.N.T.: Review article: Doppler ultrasound in medical diagnosis. Brit. J. Radiol. 62 (1989) 399–420

41 Hemodynamic Evaluation of Early Pregnancy

WITHDRAWN

Transvaginal color Doppler examination. It has not been too many years since ultrasound in early pregnancy was used only to confirm the integrity of the pregnancy by detecting positive heart activity. With the introduction of transvaginal scanning, the transducer was moved closer to the embryo, permitting the use of higher frequencies for higher image resolution. With transvaginal Doppler scanning, it became possible to examine the uterine and embryonic circulations from the start of oocyte implantation.

Transvaginal Doppler scanning can provide color images of the uteroplacental and embryonic vessels in addition to spectral waveforms.

Color Doppler is helpful in early pregnancy owing to its ability to demonstrate arterial blood flow as well as intracardiac and venous flows. While this technique has not become a routine part of early pregnancy evaluations, it has yielded important information on the development of the uteroplacental circulation.

In this chapter we shall present study results on the physiology of the uteroplacental and embryonic circulations, the development of the intervillous circulation and yolk sac blood supply, and abnormalities of early pregnancy.

Normal Early Pregnancy

▬ *Development of the Intervillous Circulation*

Classic Theory

Implantation. There is only a brief period following ovulation in which the endometrium is highly receptive to implantation. Only during these few days can a blastocyst enter the uterine cavity, establish contact with the endothelial layers, and implant (65). The ideal implantation time is between the fifth and seventh days after ovulation. Implantation of the blastocyst occurs on about the 21st day of the cycle and is completed by day 26, when the endometrium has closed over the blastocyst. At the time of its initial attachment, the inner cell mass of the blastocyst is directed toward the endometrium (65). The trophoblast synthesizes proteolytic enzymes that induce erosion and penetration of the uterine mucosa. During implantation, the trophoblast causes erosion of the adjacent maternal capillaries, causing maternal blood to come into direct contact with the conceptus. This communicating lacunar network becomes the intervillous space of the placenta (Fig. 41.**1**).

Changes in the spiral arteries. During the fourth week, the migrating trophoblast penetrates the uterine wall and invades larger venous sinusoids and superficial arterioles. The extravillous cytotrophoblastic cells expand from the tips of the anchored villi into the lumina of the spiral arteries. They transform the thick-walled, muscular arteries into lax, sac-like uteroplacental vessels that are passively distended and adapted to the increasing maternal blood flow that is necessary for fetal oxygen delivery and embryonic growth (13).

Trophoblastic cells can be found in the spiral arteries around the sixth week after conception. The disruption of the muscle cells and the elastic fibers of the spiral arteries by the trophoblasts has two effects:
1. The increasing blood flow leads to a progressive expansion of the spiral arteries that extends to the uteroplacental arteries, adapting the vessels to the increasing blood flow.
2. The uteroplacental arteries at this stage are not affected by the autonomic nervous system (33).

Opening of the spiral arteries. During the second month of gestation, the intervillous space enlarges due to extensive sprouting of the villi. At this stage many terminal portions of the spiral arteries near the intervillous space contain cytotrophoblastic plugs. Meanwhile, many large central connections are found between the decidual veins. After 40 days (crown–rump length 15 mm) the spiral arteries open into the intervillous space, and cytotrophoblastic cells appear within the lumina. Maternal blood reaches the intervillous space through gaps between the cells of the endovascular trophoblasts. The continued presence of cytotrophoblastic plugs in the lumina of the spiral arteries suggests that the blood pressure in the arteries is not very high, for otherwise the plugs would be dislodged. Maximum trophoblast activity is found at the center of the placental bed and spreads centrifugally from there toward the periphery.

During the third month of gestation, cytotrophoblastic plugs fill the lumina at the terminal ends of most of the spiral arteries. None of the spiral arteries open directly into the intervillous space. Later in this developmental stage, the plugs are more loosely arranged and are less able to restrict the entry of maternal blood into the intervillous space.

Definitive placenta. By the end of 4 months' gestation, the chorion frondosum has been transformed into the definitive placenta. The chorionic villi of the decidua capsularis degenerate, and the adjacent intervillous space disappears. The thin, avascular chorion laeve is formed (33). Trophoblast regression occurs at sites where the rows of cytotrophoblastic cells degenerate.

Trophoblastic infiltration of the myometrium occurs between 8 and 18 weeks' gestation (13). The endovascular cytotrophoblast partially replaces the endometrium and invades the muscle cells of the myometrial vessels. The result is a progression expansion of the radial arteries within the myometrium.

Low-pressure system. The uteroplacental circulation is a low-pressure system in which the vascular calibers increase as they near the intervillous space. A substantial pressure drop occurs from the proximal, nondilated portions of the uteroplacental arterioles to the distal, dilated portions. This keeps the full arterial blood pressure from being transmitted to the intervillous space.

Varying Study Results

No intervillous blood flow before 12 weeks' gestation. The classic theory on the development of the uteroplacental circulation (15, 67) was altered by the results of Hustin and Shaaps (18, 19). Their in vivo studies of the placenta using transvaginal ultrasound, intervillous hysteroscopy, and phase contrast examinations of chorionic villi showed that there was no true continuous blood flow in the intervillous space during the first 3 months of pregnancy. When these authors examined tomograms of perfused hysterectomy specimens with an in situ pregnancy obtained at 7, 8, and 9 weeks' gestation, they found no contrast material in the intervillous space. But when this examination was done at 13 weeks' gestation, the placenta quickly filled with contrast material. Histologic examination of these hysterectomy specimens revealed occlusion of the uteroplacental arteries by trophoblastic cells up until 12 weeks' gestation. The reconstruction of serial spiral artery sections also showed that blood circulation did not occur in the intervillous space prior to 12 weeks. On the other hand, the uteroplacental arteries at 13 weeks were free of trophoblastic plugs, and contrast material was found in the intervillous space, where it bathed the chorionic villi. These results indicate that the early placenta is bathed chiefly by fluid derived from the maternal plasma and uterine glandular secretions. The authors believe that blood flow in the intervillous space is either absent or incomplete prior to 12 weeks' gestation. According to this theory, the transformation of the spiral arteries continues during the first trimester through a progressive widening of the arteries. By the end of 12 weeks, all of the trophoblastic plugs are loosened and dislodged, allowing the free influx of maternal blood into the intervillous space so that a fully developed placental circulation can be established.

Placental Po₂ levels. This theory is supported by a more recent study (70) in which a polarographic oxygen electrode was introduced under ultrasound guidance. It was found that the placental Po_2 levels between 8 and 10 weeks' gestation were significantly lower than the Po_2 levels in the endometrium. By 12–13 weeks, however, these levels were identical, indicating a significant rise of intraplacental Po_2 between 8–10 and 12–13 weeks' gestation. This rise in the placental Po_2 correlates with the development of continuous maternal blood flow in the intervillous space at the end of the first trimester.

Color Doppler Studies

Transvaginal color Doppler imaging has made it possible to perform hemodynamic studies in all portions of the embryonic, fetal, and uteroplacental circulation (36, 38, 39, 40, 43, 44, 46, 47) (Fig. 41.**2**). The interest shown by various groups of authors in the maturing embryo has greatly improved our knowledge and understanding of the embryonic circulation. Nevertheless, our current knowledge on the anatomy and physiology of the uteroplacental circulation is based largely on the classic studies of earlier authors, and therefore is it important to review the various Doppler theories on the development of the intervillous circulation.

Intervillous blood flow during the first trimester. In 1991 and 1992, Jauniaux et al. (26, 29) and Jaffe and Warsof (22) were still unable to detect intraplacental blood flow before 12 weeks' gestation by transvaginal color Doppler scanning. They were first able to detect this flow at about 14 weeks. This coincided with the appearance of pandiastolic flow in the umbilical artery and an abrupt rise of peak systolic flow in the umbilical artery. Consistent with the theories of Hustin and Shaaps (18, 19), they concluded that the simultaneous appearance of intraplacental flow and pandiastolic umbilical artery flow could be attributed to an abrupt rise of blood flow velocity in the umbilical artery due to the sudden dislodgement and clearance of the trophoblastic plugs from the spiral arteries.

At this time Kurjak et al. (41) were still unable to show an abrupt change in the uteroplacental circulation between 12 and 14 weeks' gestation. But with the advent of more sensitive color Doppler instruments, several authors reported the positive detection of intervillous blood flow during the first trimester.

In 1995, Kurjak et al. (50) published the first report on a combined Doppler and histomorphologic study of the intervillous circulation. Using transvaginal color Doppler, they identified two types of continuous intervillous blood flow in all of the patients examined: pulsatile artery-like flow (Fig. 41.**3**) and continuous vein-like flow (Fig. 41.**4**). Parallel histologic studies showed that the lumina of the spiral arteries were never completely occluded by trophoblastic plugs (Fig. 41.**5**). These data indicate that the development of the intervillous circulation is

more of a continuous process than a sudden event at the end of the first trimester.

Since then, many other groups of authors have reported similar results. Valentin et al. (78) conducted a study on uteroplacental and luteal blood flow with subsequent histomorphologic analysis. Color Doppler examinations in normal pregnancies detected an intervillous circulation at 6 weeks' gestation. The two same types of Doppler signals (pulsatile and continuous) were detected and measured in more than 90% of the 64 pregnancies examined between 5 and 11 weeks. The authors found that the high blood flow velocities measured in the subchorionic arteries were inconsistent with complete arterial occlusion by trophoblastic plugs. The histomorphologic studies showed that the trophoblastic plugs were incomplete, leaving room for the passage of red blood cells. This led the authors to conclude that an intervillous circulation is already present in the first trimester.

Merce et al. (58) reported similar results in 108 normal single pregnancies between 4 and 15 gestational weeks. They were able to detect intervillous blood flow as early as 5 weeks, 6 days. They recorded a slightly undulating, vein-like signal that tended to show increasing flow velocities over the course of the first trimester. The authors also recorded flow signals in retrochorionic segments of the uteroplacental vessels. They concluded that their results were consistent with the classic embryologic concept of an intervillous circulation developing between the fourth and seventh weeks of gestation. According to Merce et al. (58), the uteroplacental circulation undergoes pronounced changes starting at 4 weeks. An intervillous circulation and a primitive umbilical cord circulation could be demonstrated as early as 5 weeks.

Comparison with monkeys. Experimental studies in animal models, especially monkeys from the *Macaca* genus, have played a key role in research on the development of the placenta and the uteroplacental circulation. The classic study by Elisabeth Ramsey (67, 68) on the circulation in the intervillous space of the primate placenta laid the groundwork for all current research in this area. Nimrod et al. (60, 61) recently reported on color Doppler investigations of the early uteroplacental circulation in the cynomolgus monkey *(Macaca fascicularis)*. These authors were able to detect an intervillous circulation as early as 18 days postconception. Despite known differences between humans and monkeys in the depth of trophoblast invasion of the spiral arteries, these discoveries can be considered important evidence for the early development of an intervillous circulation in all primate placentas, though one must be careful in drawing analogies.

Comparison of normal and abnormal early pregnancies. In further studies, Kurjak et al. (51, 53) examined a group of 60 normal pregnancies from 6 to 12 weeks' gestation and also a group of 34 abnormal early pregnancies (22 missed abortions and 12 blighted ova) between 7 and 12 weeks' gestation. In all of the pregnancies, the same Doppler signals were detected in the intervillous space—i.e., pulsatile artery-like signals with characteristic spiking and continuous vein-like signals. No differences in Doppler parameters were found between the missed abortion group and the group with normal early pregnancies (Fig. 41.**6**).

A lower impedance (RI and PI) was found in the blighted ovum group (Fig. 41.**7**). These results differ significantly from those published by Jauniaux et al. (31), who found increased intervillous blood flow in 70% of abnormal pregnancies before 12 weeks. Histomorphologic analysis in these cases showed that the trophoblastic layer was thinner and interrupted and that the intervillous space contained massive amounts of maternal blood. The authors assume that trophoblastic plugs in the spiral arteries prevent the maternal blood from entering the intervillous space in order to protect the vulnerable chorionic villi from the high-pressure arterial blood. Accordingly, the premature entry of maternal blood into the intervillous space can rupture the embryo-maternal interface, causing separation of the early placenta and

Development of the intervillous space

Fig. 41.1 Transvaginal scan of an early gestational sac. Note the eccentric location of the sac near the uterine fundus, the oval shape of the sac, and its double wall structure. Color Doppler defines the vascular network around the gestational sac.

Fig. 41.2 Transvaginal color Doppler image of an early gestational sac. Blood flow signals are clearly recorded in the uterine, radial and spiral arteries.

Fig. 41.3 A pulsatile, artery-like blood flow pattern (right) sampled isolated from the intervillous space (left) is characterized by a low vascular resistance (RI = 0.43).

Fig. 41.4 Another spectrum sampled from the intervillous space (left) exhibit a continuous, vein-like flow pattern (right).

Fig. 41.5 The progressive disruption of the spiral artery wall by trophoblast invasion leads to vascular expansion with a decrease in resistance (left). The pulsed Doppler flow signal shows high end-diastolic flow velocities and a characteristic "spike-like" waveform resulting from a low impedance to blood flow (right).

Fig. 41.6 Transvaginal color Doppler scan of a missed abortion at 7 weeks' gestation (left). Pulsatile, artery-like flow signals are recorded from the intervillous space (right).

Fig. 41.7 Transvaginal color Doppler scan of a blighted ovum (left). The blood flow signals from the intervillous space (right) show a low-resistance pattern (RI = 0.39).

Yolk sac and vitelline duct

Fig. 41.8 Transvaginal scan of a gestational sac at 8 weeks (left). Vascular signals are sampled from the umbilical cord and live embryo (right). The low flow velocity and the absence of end-diastolic blood flow are typical findings in the yolk sac and vitelline duct vessels.

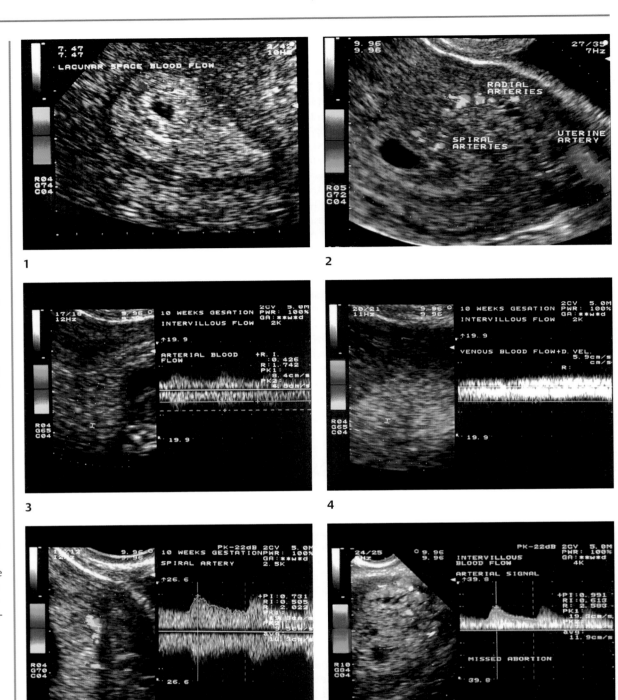

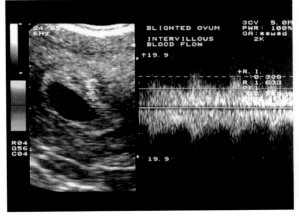

eventual abortion. Conversely, this concept does not preclude the detection of continuous intervillous blood flow during the first trimester.

Conclusions. It appears that the early placenta contains areas in which trophoblastic plugs in the spiral arteries are loose enough to permit the intervillous circulation of blood. Apparently only a few of these flow areas exist initially to provide sufficient oxygen and nutrients for the continued development of the pregnancy. At this time the intervillous space is not as isolated as in the mature placenta. There are still areas with limited blood flow allowing nutrients and oxygen to diffuse through the intercellular fluid. The number of areas with developing intervillous blood flow increase steadily with embryonic and placental growth to maintain a state of metabolic equilibrium. This process ends with the fully developed intervillous space of the mature placenta. Thus, the theory of a continuously developing intervillous space is consistent with the fact that lower oxygen levels are found in placental tissue than in the endometrium between 8 and 10 weeks' gestation (70). Also, this theory does not weaken the hypothesis that the free entry of maternal blood into the intervillous space at this stage of pregnancy can mechanically rupture the embryo-maternal interface, leading to spontaneous abortion (31).

The use of transvaginal pulsed and color Doppler ultrasound is yielding new insights into the functional development of the intervillous space, advancing research not only on the intervillous blood supply but also on the mechanisms of blood circulation in the interior of the space.

▣ *Blood Flow in the Yolk Sac and Vitelline Duct*

A variety of ultrasound parameters such as the size of the gestational sac, the embryonic growth pattern, and the size of an accompanying intrauterine hematoma have been used in an effort to predict pregnancy outcome (30). The yolk sac is the earliest embryonic structure that can be detected within the gestational sac at the start of the fifth postmenstrual week. According to Levi et al. (54), the yolk sac should be detectable sonographically at a mean gestational sac size of 8 mm. If the contours of the yolk sac are closely scrutinized, an embryo with heart activity can be identified next to the yolk sac as early as the sixth week.

Vascular development in the yolk sac. The diameter of the yolk sac increases steadily from 3.4 to 5.4 mm between the 6th and 12th weeks of gestation. An abnormal size and morphology of the yolk sac may be suggestive of subsequent early pregnancy failure. The yolk sac is connected to the embryo by the yolk stalk (vitelline duct), which transmits the blood vessels (26). The vascular system begins to develop in the walls of the yolk sac approximately 2 weeks after ovulation. The vessels develop in the mesonephros surrounding the vitelline duct and communicate with the primitive cardiovascular system of the embryo through paired vitelline veins and arteries. The wall of the yolk stalk appears to have the same embryonic origin as the wall of the yolk sac, and so blood vessels are found in the stalk. The mesenchyma that is normally seen in the wall of the yolk sac at all stages is not observed between the mesothelium and the vitelline duct. This suggests that blood corpuscles and vessels develop earlier than the mesenchyma. As a result, hematopoiesis can precede the formation of the mesenchyma in the yolk sac wall. With further growth of the amnion and elongation of the vitelline duct, the yolk sac moves away from the embryo. The embryonic coelom is obliterated in stages, while the amnion encases the connecting stalk and forms the epithelium of the later umbilical cord (27).

Detectability with color Doppler. Because the yolk sac is the earliest vascular and hematopoietic organ in the embryo, our group of authors

(43, 44, 45) has investigated the vascular development of the yolk sac and of the vitelline duct using transvaginal color Doppler (42). The study group consisted of 105 pregnant women between 5 and 10 weeks' gestation. The first color and pulsed Doppler signals from the yolk sac were found between 5 and 6 weeks. The highest detection rate, at 85.71%, was achieved between weeks 7 and 8. A characteristic flow pattern was recorded in all of the yolk sacs examined, consisting of a low flow velocity (5.8 ± 1.7 cm/s) with absent end-diastolic flow (Fig. 41.**8**). The PI had a mean value of 4.24 ± 0.94. As the function of the yolk sac declined, its ultrasound detection rate also decreased, falling to 78.26% by 9 weeks and 61.11% by 10 weeks. Color and pulsed Doppler signals could be recorded from the vitelline duct in 85.71% of the patients during the seventh week of pregnancy. The vitelline vessels showed similar peak systolic flow velocities and pulsatility indices as those of the yolk sac. The best detection rate of these vessels (89.3%) was achieved during the eighth week of gestation.

Elongation of the vitelline duct, causing a progressive separation of the yolk sac from the embryo, was accompanied by a decrease in the detectability of the vitelline duct (73.9% in week 9 and 55.6% in week 10). Abnormal patterns of yolk sac development and vascular development in the vitelline duct were observed in pregnancies that later miscarried (Fig. 41.**9**).

▣ *Changes in Uterine Blood Flow after Placentation*

Anatomy. The maternal part of the placental circulation consists of the two uterine arteries and their branches, which spread over the uterus until they reach the decidua of the placenta (21). Arising from the internal iliac artery, the uterine artery runs along the lateral pelvic wall to the uterus at the level of the cervix. From the cervix, it ascends in a tortuous course along the uterine side wall and anastomoses with the tubal branch of the ovarian artery. The main uterine artery then branches into the arcuate arteries, from which the smaller radial arteries pass toward the uterine cavity where they become the basal arteries. The spiral arteries arise in continuity with the basal arteries to supply the endometrium. These vessels can be visualized at the myometrial-endometrial boundary. The uterine circulation is rich in anastomoses (66). Branches of the uterine arteries anastomose with branches of the ovarian and vaginal arteries to form a vascular arcade that supplies all of the internal genital organs. Vascular connections are also found between the main and side branches of the uterine artery.

Intrauterine placental development requires adaptive changes in the uterine vasculature. The fact that the uterine vascular network elongates and dilates during pregnancy has long been known by anatomists (66). With transvaginal pulsed and color Doppler, it is possible to identify these uterine vascular changes.

Uterine artery. Numerous Doppler studies (22, 26, 38, 39, 41, 43, 44, 46) have documented a gradual decline in the resistance index of the uterine artery during the first trimester of pregnancy. This decline continues during the second and third trimesters and can be demonstrated in all portions of the uteroplacental circulation.

Spiral arteries. During early pregnancy the spiral arteries are progressively transformed into nonmuscular, dilated, tortuous channels (28, 64). Turbulent blood flow of low impedance is typical of the transformed spiral arteries and can often be detected at the placental implantation site (37). With the invasion of larger maternal blood vessels that carry flow at higher pressure, higher flow velocities develop and a larger diastolic component appears in the Doppler signal. Jaffe and Warsof (22) investigated these vascular changes with Doppler ultrasound starting at 5 weeks' gestation.

Waveform changes. The uteroplacental circulation has been thoroughly investigated at all stages of gestation. As the pregnancy progresses, the impedance of the blood flow declines steadily from the uterine artery to the spiral arteries (Fig. 41.**10**). This is accompanied by an increase in blood flow with a shift in the peak systolic values. The peak systolic flow velocity shows a declining trend from the uterine artery across the arcuate arteries to the radial arteries.

Pulsed Doppler waveforms recorded from the uterine artery display a typical pattern: a high peak systolic velocity with a characteristic notch in the systolic downstroke and low end-diastolic flow. Waveforms from the spiral arteries show higher peak flow velocities and a lower vascular impedance than in the rest of the uteroplacental circulation. These changes may result from the dilatation of the spiral arteries induced by trophoblast invasion, a hormonally mediated vasodilatation, and a decrease in the viscosity of the maternal blood. As the wall structure of the spiral arteries is transformed during pregnancy, the vessels acquire hemodynamic properties that are very different from those found in other arteries of the uteroplacental circulation. It is known that the normal early development of the embryo depends on uterine perfusion, implantation mechanism, and chromosome structure.

Possible applications. Doppler techniques provide a noninvasive means of detecting abnormal implantation and a deficient uterine blood supply. As a result, Doppler ultrasound could be an important method for the investigation of hemodynamic disturbances.

Three morphologic studies (20, 34, 69) have shown an association between abnormal transformation of the spiral arteries and the occurrence of spontaneous abortion. There is also evidence that decreased trophoblast invasion of the decidua and spiral arteries may be linked to a chromosomal abnormality. For this reason, examinations of blood flow in the intervillous space and at the level of the placental bed may provide additional parameters that can be used in the prediction of pregnancy outcomes.

▬ *Early Embryonic Circulation*

Documentation of heart rate. Approximately 21 days after ovulation, at the end of 5 weeks' gestation, the primitive heart begins to beat. Embryonic heart activity has been detected in utero as early as 36 days' menstrual age (57). The heart rate rises from an initial 80–90 bpm to 150–170 bpm at the end of 9 weeks. Parasympathetic nerve development most likely accounts for the occurrence of beat-to-beat variations (Fig. 41.**11**). The heart rate falls again after 9 weeks, reaching an average rate of 158 bpm by the end of 14 weeks. Some studies suggest that the assessment of embryonic heart rate variability is useful in the prediction of pregnancy outcome (7, 57, 59). A heart rate below 85 bpm detected between 5 and 7 weeks or a declining heart rate in two successive ultrasound examinations are suspicious signs for impending pregnancy failure.

Transvaginal fetal echocardiography. Transvaginal fetal echocardiography has proved to be an effective method for defining normal early fetal cardiac anatomy. It is also useful for diagnosing severe cardiac anomalies during the last first trimester and early second trimester.

Intracardiac waveforms. When diastolic flow velocities are measured at the level of the atrioventricular plane and in the outflow tract, characteristic intracardiac flow patterns are recorded (80). The E wave (early diastolic filling) and A wave (atrial contraction) can be measured over both the mitral and tricuspid valves. The E/A ratio expresses the relationship between the passive and active phases of ventricular filling. The ratio increases during pregnancy from 0.5 in the first trimester to 0.9 at term. Presumably this reflects the increasing ventricular compliance that develops with advancing gestation.

Examination of embryonic vessels. Embryonic vessels that are used in the assessment of embryonic status include the aorta, the umbilical arteries, the carotid arteries, and the middle cerebral artery.

Aorta and umbilical arteries. Pulsations of the embryonic aorta and umbilical artery can be detected as early as the sixth week of gestation (Fig. 41.**12**). By the end of 10 weeks, there is still no detectable end-diastolic flow in the umbilical arteries (Fig. 41.**13**) or fetal aorta (Fig. 41.**14**). Diastolic flow velocities do appear between the 11th and 14th weeks, but they are irregular and incomplete. Pandiastolic frequencies are consistently present after this period, however (4, 44, 45). Chorionic and intraplacental arterioles, which are branches of the umbilical artery, can also be detected in many pregnancies. The impedance of the blood flow falls steadily from the umbilical artery to its branches (16, 26).

Intracranial vessels. The intracranial circulation can be defined as early as the seventh week of gestation. At this time subtle pulsations of the internal carotid artery can be detected at the skull base. During weeks 9 and 10, color signals representing blood flow can be recorded in the anterolateral quadrants of the skull base. Starting in week 9, arterial pulsations can be detected lateral to the mesencephalon and cerebral flexure on transverse scans. Often it is not possible to distinguish clearly between the internal carotid artery and middle cerebral artery. A characteristic flow pattern showing a systolic component with absent end-diastolic flow can be seen from the 7th to 10th week of gestation (Fig. 41.**15**). This reflects a high vascular resistance in the embryo, umbilical cord, and placenta compared with late pregnancy. End-diastolic blood flow is present only irregularly between the 11th and 12th weeks. From the 12th week on, end-diastolic flow is consistently observed in the middle cerebral artery. A significant decrease in the pulsatility index (PI) has been noted in intracranial vessels with advancing gestational age. This decrease is seen two weeks earlier than in other areas of the fetal circulation (40, 79, 81). End-diastolic flow velocities are also present in the cerebral vessels earlier than in the fetal aorta or the umbilical artery (Fig. 41.**16**). This signifies a low vascular resistance in the fetal brain that is independent of vascular resistance changes occurring in the fetal trunk or in the uteroplacental circulation. This seemingly independent, autoregulatory mechanism helps to ensure an adequate blood supply to the growing fetal brain. After 12 weeks' gestation, end-diastolic flow patterns also appear in the umbilical artery and the descending aorta, signifying a decrease in fetal vascular resistance. It was only recently that we were able to detect continuous diastolic flow in the middle cerebral artery between 9 and 10 weeks' gestation using newer Doppler equipment.

Choroid plexus. Blood flow in the choroid plexus can also be investigated with transvaginal color Doppler ultrasound (49). Blood vessels can be clearly visualized in the choroid plexus as early as the ninth week, appearing as color signals at the inner margin of the lateral ventricle. Aside from venous color signals, the blood flow with an absent diastolic component is easily identified. Low RI values can be measured in these vessels after 11 weeks. The vascular network of the choroid plexus is most easily demonstrated at 13 weeks. It becomes more difficult to define as morphologic development continues. Like the other cerebral vessels, the arteries of the choroid plexus show a steady decline of vascular resistance with an increase in blood flow as pregnancy progresses.

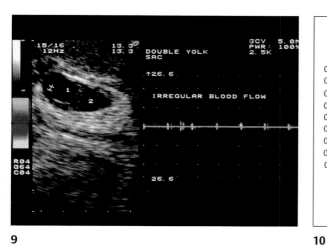

9

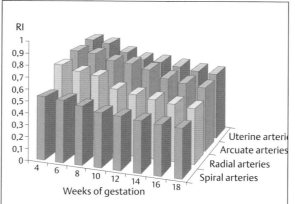

10

Fig. 41.**9**   Irregular blood flow pattern in the yolk sac of an early missed abortion.

Maternal and embryonic vessels

Fig. 41.**10**   Mean resistance indices (RI) in the uteroplacental vessels in normal pregnancies.

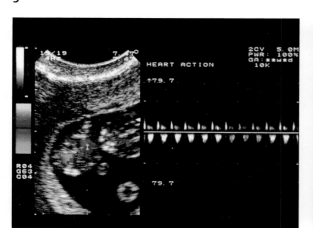

11

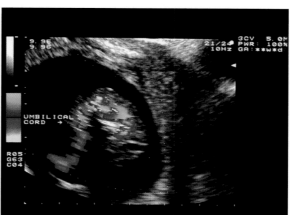

12

Fig. 41.**11**   Trunk of an embryo at 9 weeks' gestation (left). Pulsed Doppler flowmetry demonstrates irregular embryonic heart activity (right).

Fig. 41.**12**   Common view of the whole umbilical cord and the embryonic aorta at 10 weeks' gestation.

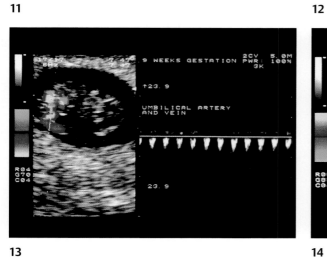

13

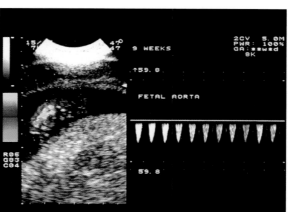

14

Fig. 41.**13**   Pulsed Doppler flow signals from the umbilical artery show an absence of end-diastolic blood flow. Venous flow is constantly present above the baseline.

Fig. 41.**14**   Pulsed Doppler flow signals from the fetal aorta at 9 weeks show an absence of end-diastolic blood flow.

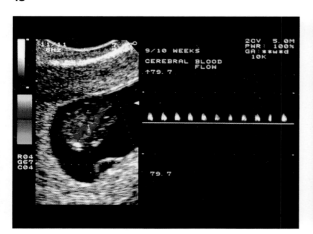

15

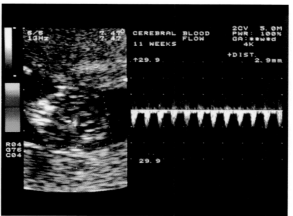

16

Fig. 41.**15**   Cerebral artery at 9–10 weeks (left). Pulsed Doppler examination shows an absence of end-diastolic blood flow (right).

Fig. 41.**16**   Cerebral blood flow at 11 weeks (left). The pulsed Doppler flow signals (right) show continuous diastolic blood flow and a significantly lower impedance compared with the flow in other fetal vessels.

Early Pregnancy Loss

Most cases of early pregnancy loss present clinically with uterine bleeding. Approximately 25% of pregnant women experience uterine bleeding during the first trimester, and more than 50% of these pregnancies miscarry (5). Uterine bleeding, however, is only the clinical manifestation of diverse pathologic events such as subchorionic hematoma, incomplete or complete abortion, blighted ovum, missed abortion, or a disturbance of trophoblastic development.

▬ Subchorionic Hematoma

Volume and location. A transparent crescent- or wedge-shaped structure between the uterine wall and chorion usually signifies a subchorionic hematoma. Anatomically, it represents a separation of the chorionic plate from the underlying decidua caused by a collection of blood between the chorion and decidua. In the past, a number of studies were published on subchorionic hematomas, often reporting contradictory results (35). Most authors investigated the volume of the hematoma. The results published by various groups of investigators are summarized in Table 41.**1** (1, 6, 8, 9, 14, 25, 32, 56, 62, 63, 71, 73, 74, 82). In some studies it was found that the location of the hematoma had prognostic implications with regard to pregnancy outcome. Most hematomas that were associated with spontaneous abortion were located in the uterine corpus or fundus rather than near the cervix.

Hemodynamic effects. It was also found that hematomas alter the blood flow in the spiral arteries due to mechanical compression. This was interpreted as a secondary effect with no impact on pregnancy outcome (52). The results of serial transvaginal color and pulsed Doppler examinations could assume prognostic importance because they provide a direct look at the pathophysiology of bleeding during pregnancy. Vascular resistance is increased and blood flow decreased by the presence of a hematoma (Fig. 41.**17**). As the pregnancy progresses and the hematoma is reabsorbed, the impedance of the blood flow returns to normal. An improvement of blood flow in such cases is predictive of a normal pregnancy outcome. These studies are helpful in the clinical management and follow-up of patients with vaginal bleeding in early pregnancy.

▬ Incomplete and Complete Abortion

Increased perfusion and low blood flow signals are typical of retained gestational products. They are easily detected following an incomplete abortion, while intracavitary vascular imaging no longer shows an increase after a complete abortion has occurred.

▬ Blighted Ovum and Missed Abortion

Blighted ovum. A few color Doppler studies have dealt with blighted ovum. The results are inconsistent, however, and vary from author to author (23, 24, 36). It has been shown that some blighted ova have a copious blood supply, in which case the intensity of the color pattern correlates with the activity of the trophoblast. For this reason, the persistence of increased color signals may suggest that the blighted ovum will under molar change (36).

Missed abortion. In patients with a questionable missed abortion, transvaginal color Doppler is helpful for detecting heart activity in the embryo (Fig. 41.**18**). In one study where this technique was used, significantly higher mean uterine PI values were found in missed abortion

cases than in normal pregnancies (31). Intervillous flow was detected before 12 weeks in 69.6% of the missed abortions but in none of the normal pregnancies. However, more recent Doppler studies using more sensitive instruments have also detected continuous intervillous blood flow during the first trimester of normal pregnancies (51, 78). This technique can demonstrate two different blood flow patterns within the intervillous space: a pulsatile artery-like flow pattern and a continuous vein-like pattern.

Regarding the RI and PI of the intervillous arterial blood flow, no differences in these indices have been found between missed abortions and normal pregnancies (53) (Fig. 41.**6**). Low intervillous blood flow like that found in anembryonic pregnancies may reflect changes in the placental stroma, where some villi are prone to edema formation (Fig. 41.**7**). The loss of the embryonic component of the placental circulation has little impact on trophoblastic function, because the trophoblast continues to be supplied with maternal intervillous blood (75). As a result, trophoblastic fluid in the villous stroma is no longer drained by the embryonic circulation. The progressive accumulation of fluid can lead to a significant reduction of intervillous blood flow. Low blood flow in the spiral arteries means that a massive, continuous in-

Table 41.**1** Clinical outcome of pregnancies complicated by subchorionic hematoma

Author, year	n	Pregnancy outcome	Remarks
Abu-Yousef et al. 1987 (1)	21	7 SpAb 3 Pd 5 severe hemorrhage, therapeutic abortion	A large SCH is associated with an increased risk of unfavorable pregnancy outcome
Baxi and Pearlstone 1991 (6)	5	1 Pd at 24 weeks	Selected patient group with autoantibodies
Bloch et al. 1989 (8)	31	2 SpAb 2 Pd 26 Dt	No correlation between size of SCH and pregnancy outcome
Borium et al. 1989 (9)	86	19 SpAb	SCH volume was < 30 mL in 85% of the patients
Goldstein et al. 1983 (14)	10	2 SpAb	No correlation between size of SCH and pregnancy outcome
Jakab et al. 1994 (25)	35	8 SpAb	No correlation between size of SCH and pregnancy outcome
Jouppila 1985 (32)	33	6 SpAb 3 Pd	Size of SCH unrelated to pregnancy outcome
Mantoni and Pedersen 1981 (56)	12	2 SpAb 1 Pd	Larger SCHs associated with an increased risk of adverse pregnancy outcome
Nyberg et al. 1987 (62)	46	3 Intrauterine fetal deaths 6 Pregnancy terminations 12 Pd	No correlation between size of SCH and pregnancy outcome
Pedersen and Mantoni 1990 (63)	23	1 SpAb 2 Pd	Large SCH (> 50 mL) is not associated with an increased risk of adverse pregnancy outcome
Saurbrei and Pham 1986 (71)	30	3 SpAb 4 Stillbirths 7 Pd	Large SCH (> 60 mL) is associated with an increased risk of adverse pregnancy outcome
Spirit et al. 1979 (73)	4	2 Pd 2 Dt	
Stabile et al. 1989 (74)	20	0 SpAb	Volume of SCH < 16 mL in all study patients
Ylostalo et al. 1984 (82)	16	5 Placental abruptions	Mean pregnancy duration shortened in patients with a hematoma

SCH = subchorionic hematoma, SpAb = spontaneous abortion, Pd = premature delivery, Dt = delivery at term

flux of maternal blood in the absence of effective drainage will rupture the embryomaternal interface, ultimately leading to abortion (53).

All of these results indicate that the development of the intervillous circulation is more of a continuous process than a sudden event at the end of the first trimester. Studies of the yolk sac and vitelline vessels in patients with spontaneous abortion have also yielded some interesting initial results. A vein-like flow signal, irregular velocity waveforms, or increased diastolic flow are possible signs indicating deficient embryonic development or the resorption of embryonic remnants (Fig. 41.**9**).

▬ *Trophoblastic Diseases*

Trophoblastic diseases encompass a variety of clinical and histomorphologic entities ranging from a simple molar pregnancy or invasive mole to chorionic carcinoma.

Diagnosis. Ultrasound has proven to be a useful modality in the diagnosis of hydatidiform mole. It can also be helpful in the follow-up of patients who have undergone uterine evacuation. Some studies have shown, however, that the persistence of a trophoblastic disease cannot be predicted with ultrasound. Trophoblastic diseases are characterized by vascular abnormalities that may include neoangiogenesis or increased vascular resistance. Arteriographic studies have demonstrated an abnormal uterine circulation in patients with an invasive mole or chorionic carcinoma. It was concluded, however, that this circulatory change does not affect clinical management (10). Doppler ultrasound, especially transvaginal color Doppler, has been recognized as a useful tool in the evaluation of trophoblastic diseases (2, 3, 11, 12, 17, 48, 55, 72, 76, 77, 83).

Myometrial infiltration. A trophoblastic disease is often associated with increased blood flow to the placenta. For this reason, color Doppler can be useful in patients with an invasive mole or chorionic carcinoma, particularly in terms of evaluating myometrial infiltration (Fig. 41.**19**). The detection of increased blood flow in the myometrium can aid in the diagnosis of early invasion, even before it becomes visible in the B-mode image. With invasive moles and chorionic carcinoma, myometrial trophoblast invasion can be recognized as intense color-encoded areas within the myometrium (35) (Fig. 41.**20**). These areas represent dilated spiral arteries as well as newly formed tumor-feeding vessels (Fig. 41.**21**). Being a malignant tumor, chorionic carcinoma contributes to the neovascularization by producing its own blood vessels. All of these vessels are characterized by a high flow velocity and low-resistance flow pattern.

Resistance values. The resistance values in the uteroplacental vessels are significantly lower in patients with a trophoblastic disease than in patients with a normal pregnancy (48, 55, 76). The highest resistance values are found in patients with a complete mole, while the lowest values are observed in chorionic carcinoma (12). Table 41.**2** shows the resistance values of uteroplacental vessels in patients with different types of trophoblastic disease.

Monitoring of chemotherapy. Transvaginal color Doppler is also useful for monitoring patients who are on chemotherapy for a trophoblastic disease (3, 11, 17, 72, 77, 83). A disappearance of color signals from neovascularized areas was documented in patients who received chemotherapy for trophoblastic disease. A negative correlation was found between β-hCG titers and the vascular indices.

▬ *Conclusion*

On the whole, blood flow studies in early pregnancy have expanded our knowledge and understanding of the hemodynamic changes that occur during placentation. In early pregnancies with a subchorionic hematoma, detailed Doppler examinations can furnish additional information that may influence maternal management. It has also been shown that the Doppler technique can be used effectively in the early diagnosis of trophoblastic diseases, in defining the extent of these diseases (comparable to angiography), and in predicting and monitoring their response to chemotherapy. Doppler cannot, however, replace β-hCG measurements as a routine first-line study in the follow-up of these patients. On the other hand, Doppler is excellent for distinguishing among the different types of trophoblastic disease. For this reason, a color Doppler examination should be added to the work-up of all cases where there is suspicion of trophoblastic disease.

Despite the results published to date, further prospective, controlled clinical studies are needed to define more clearly the prognostic value of Doppler criteria in early pregnancy.

Table 41.**2** Resistance index (RI) and pulsatility index (PI) measured in the uterine, arcuate, radial and spiral arteries in patients with trophoblastic diseases

Group of patients	n	Uterine artery RI	PI	Arcuate artery RI	PI	Radial artery RI	PI	Spiral artery RI	PI	Peritumoral blood flow RI	PI
Hydatidiform mole	20	0.75* (0.03)	1.71* (0.41)	0.62* (0.08)	1.15* (0.35)	0.47* (0.07)	0.81* (0.23)	0.39* (0.05)	0.54* (0.18)	– –	– –
Partial mole	2	0.73 0.75	1.64 1.69	0.60 0.61	1.19 1.28	0.48 0.49	0.88 0.69	0.35 0.38	0.53 0.60	– –	– –
Invasive mole	2	0.70 0.71	1.24 1.26	– –	– –	– –	– –	– –	– –	0.33 0.30	0.48 0.53
Chorionic carcinoma	6	0.64* (0.05)	1.23* (0.21)	– –	– –	– –	– –	– –	– –	0.29 (0.05)	0.43 (0.27)
Control group	23	0.82* (0.04)	2.18* (0.55)	0.68* (0.05)	1.46* (0.52)	0.52* (0.06)	0.92* (0.38)	0.48* (0.04)	0.58* (0.29)	– –	– –

( ) = 2 SD * = Statistically significant (p < 0.01)

Retrochorionic hematoma and missed abortion

Fig. 41.**17** Transvaginal scan of an early pregnancy at 10 weeks, complicated by a retrochorionic hematoma (left). Doppler scan shows the alteration of spiral arterial blood flow on the side of the hematoma (RI = 1.0) (right).

Fig. 41.**18** Transvaginal scan of a missed abortion. Dilated spiral arteries are seen very close to the cavity of the gestational sac. Fetal blood circulation is absent!

Trophoblastic diseases

Fig. 41.**19** Transvaginal color Doppler image of an invasive mole. Conspicuous flow signals are evident within the myometrium.

Fig. 41.**20** Color Doppler demonstrates increased blood flow within the myometrium, consistent with an invasive mole.

Fig. 41.**21** Transvaginal ultrasound of an invasive mole. The cyst-like area (3 cm in diameter) does not appear to be vascularized. By contrast, the heavily perfused area within the myometrium (left side of image) signifies invasion. Low vascular resistance (RI = 0.40) is detected within the richly vascularized area (right side of image).

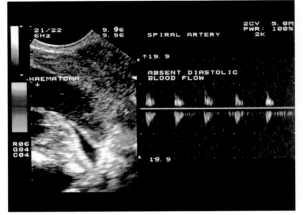

17

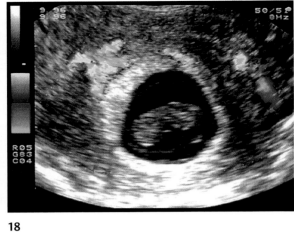

18

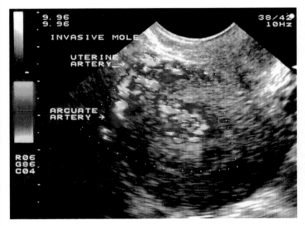

19

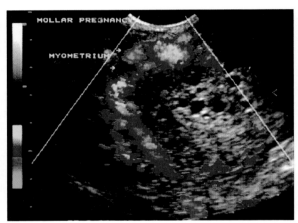

20

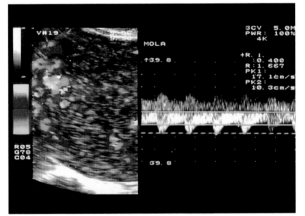

21

References

1. Abu-Yousef, M.M., Bleicher, J.J., Williamson, R.A.: Subchorionic hemorrhage: sonographic diagnosis and clinical significance. Amer. J. Roentgenol. 149 (1987) 737–740
2. Achiron, R., Goldenberg, M., Lipitz, S., Mashiach, S.: Transvaginal duplex Doppler ultrasonography in bleeding patients suspected of having residual trophoblastic tissue. Obstet. Gynecol. 81 (1993) 507–511
3. Aoki, S., Hata, T., Hata, K. et al.: Doppler color flow mapping of an invasive mole. Gynecol. Obstet. Invest. 27 (1989) 52–54
4. Arduini, D., Rizzo, G.: Umbilical artery velocity waveforms in early pregnancy: a transvaginal color Doppler study. J. Clin. Ultrasound 19 (1991) 335–339
5. Barnea, E.: Epidemiology and etiology of early pregnancy disorders. In: Barnea, E., Hustin, J., Jauniaux, E. (eds.): The First Twelve Weeks of Gestation. Berlin: Springer 1992; S. 263–279
6. Baxi, L., Pearlstone, M.: Subchorionic hematomas and the presence of autoantibodies. Amer. J. Obstet. Gynecol. 165 (1991) 1423–1426
7. Birnholz, J.C.: First trimester fetal arrhythmias. Fetal. Diagn. Ther. 8, Suppl.2 (1990) 6
8. Bloch, C., Altchek, A., Levy-Ravetch, M.: Sonography in early pregnancy: the significance of subchorionic hemorrhage. M. Sinai. J. Med. 56 (1989) 290–293
9. Borlum, K.G., Thomsen, A., Clausen, I., Eriksen, G.: Long-term prognosis of pregnancies in women with intrauterine hematomas. Obstet. Gynecol. 74 (1989) 231–234
10. Brewis, R.A.L., Bagshave, K.D.: Pelvic arteriography in invasive trophoblastic neoplasia. Brit. J. Radiol. 41 (1968) 481–495
11. Carter, J., Fowler, J., Carlson, J. et al.: Transvaginal color flow Doppler sonography in the assessment of gestational trophoblastic disease. J. Ultrasound Med. 12 (1993) 595–599
12. Flam, F., Lindholm, H., Bui, T.H., Lundstrom-Lindstedt, V.: Color Doppler studies in trophoblastic tumors: a preliminary report. Ultrasound Obstet. Gynecol. 1 (1991) 349–352
13. Fox, H.: Current topic: trophoblastic pathology. Placenta 12 (1991) 479–486
14. Goldstein, S.R., Subramanyam, B.M., Raghavendra, B.N., Horii, S.C., Hilton, S.: Subchorionic bleeding in threatened abortion: sonographic findings and clinical significance. Amer. J. Radiol. 141 (1983) 975–978
15. Hamilton, W.J., Boyd, J.D., Mossman, M.W.: Human embryology. Cambridge: Heffer 1972
16. Hsieh, F.J., Kuo, P.L., Ko, T.M., Chang, F.M., Chen, H.Y.: Doppler velocimetry of intraplacental fetal arteries. Obstet. Gynecol. 77 (1991) 478–482
17. Hsieh, F.J., Wu, C.C., Chen, C.A., Hsieh, C.Y., Chen, H.Y.: Correlation of uterine hemodynamics with chemotherapy response in gestational trophoblastic tumors. Obstet. Gynecol. 83 (1994) 1021–1025
18. Hustin, J., Shaaps, J.P.: Echographic and anatomic studies of the maternotrophoblastic border during the first trimester of pregnancy. Amer. J. Obstet. Gynecol. 157 (1987) 162–168
19. Hustin, J., Shaaps, J.P., Lambotte, R.: Anatomical studies of the uteroplacental vascularization in the first trimester of pregnancy. Troph. Res. 3 (1988) 49–60
20. Hustin, J., Jauniaux, E., Shaaps, J.P.: Histological study of the materno-embryonic interference in spontaneous abortion. Placenta 11 (1990) 477–486
21. Itskovitz, J., Lindenbaum, E.S., Brandes, J.M.: Arterial anastomosis in the pregnant human uterus. Obstet. Gynecol. 1 (1980) 3–19
22. Jaffe, R., Warsof, S.L.: Transvaginal color Doppler imaging in the assessment of uteroplacental blood flow in the normal first-trimester pregnancy. Amer. J. Obstet. Gynecol. 164 (1991) 781–785
23. Jaffe, R., Warsof, S.L.: Color Doppler imaging in the assessment of uteroplacental blood flow in abnormal first trimester intrauterine pregnancies: an attempt to define etiologic mechanism. J. Ultrasound Med. 11 (1992) 41–44
24. Jaffe, R.: Investigation of abnormal first-trimester gestations by color Doppler imaging. J. Clin. Ultrasound 21 (1993) 521–526
25. Jakab, A.Jr., Juhasz, B., Toth, Z.: Outcome of the first trimester subchorial hematomas. Presented at the Tenth International Congress, The Fetus as a Patient. Brijuni, Croatia 1994; abstract 54
26. Jauniaux, E., Jurkovic, D., Campbell, S.: In vivo investigations of anatomy and physiology of early human placental circulations. Ultrasound Obstet. Gynecol. 1 (1991) 435–445
27. Jauniaux, E., Jurkovic, D., Henriet, Y.: Development of the secondary yolk sac: correlation of sonographic and anatomic features. Hum. Reprod. 6 (1991) 1160–1165
28. Jauniaux, E., Jurkovic, D., Kurjak, A., Hustin, J.: Assessment of placental development and function. In: Kurjak, A. (ed.): Transvaginal color Doppler. New Jersey: Parthenon 1991
29. Jauniaux, E., Jurkovic, D., Campbell, S., Hustin, J.: Doppler ultrasonographic features of the developing placental circulation: correlation with anatomic findings. Amer. J. Obstet. Gynecol. 166 (1992) 585–587
30. Jauniaux, E., Jurkovic, D., Campbell, S.: Pathophysiology and diagnosis of early pregnancy complications. In: Barnea, E.R., Check, J.H., Grudzinskas, J.G., Maruo, T. (eds.): Implantation and Early Pregnancy in Humans. London: Parthenon 1992; pp. 465–485
31. Jauniaux, E., Zaidi, J., Jurkovic, D., Campbell, S., Hustin, J.: Comparison of color Doppler features and pathohistological finding in complicated early pregnancy. Hum. Reprod. 9 (1994) 2432–2437
32. Jouppila, P.: Clinical consequences after ultrasound diagnosis of intrauterine hematoma in threatened abortion. J. Clin. Ultrasound 13 (1985) 107–110
33. Khong, T.Y., Liddel, H.S., Robertson, W.B.: Infective haemochorial placentation as a cause of miscarriage: a preliminary study. Brit. J. Obstet. Gynecol. 94 (1987) 649–655
34. Khong, T.Y., Pearce, J.M.: Development and investigation of the placenta and its blood supply. In: Lavery, J.P. (ed.): The Human Placenta. Clinical Perspectives. Rockville: Aspen 1987; pp. 25–45
35. Kupesic, S., Kurjak, A., Chervenak, F.: Doppler studies of subchorionic hematomas in early pregnancy. In: Chervenak, F., Kurjak, A. (eds.): Current Perspectives on the Fetus as a Patient. New York: Parthenon 1996; pp. 33–39

36. Kurjak, A., Zalud, I., Salihagic, A., Crvenkovic, G., Matijevic, R.: Transvaginal color Doppler in the assessment of abnormal early pregnancy. J. Perinat. Med. 19 (1991) 155–165
37. Kurjak, A., Kupesic-Urek, S., Predanic, M., Zudenigo, D., Matijevic, R., Salihagic, A.: Transvaginal color Doppler in the study of early pregnancies associated with fibroids. J. Matern. Fetal. Invest. 2 (1992) 81–87
38. Kurjak, A., Predanic, M., Kupesic, S., Zudenigo, D., Matijevic, R., Salihagic, A.: Transvaginal color Doppler in the study of early normal pregnancies and pregnancies associated with uterine fibroids. J. Matern. Fetal Invest. 3 (1992) 81–85
39. Kurjak, A., Kupesic, S., Predanic, M., Salihagic, A.: Transvaginal color Doppler assessment of the uteroplacental circulation in normal and abnormal early pregnancy. Early Hum. Dev. 29 (1992) 385–389
40. Kurjak, A., Predanic, M., Kupesic, S., Funduk-Kurjak, B., Demarin, V., Salihagic, A.: Transvaginal color Doppler study of middle cerebral artery blood flow in early normal and abnormal pregnancy. Ultrasound Obstet. Gynecol. 2 (1992) 424–428
41. Kurjak, A., Predanic, M., Kupesic-Urek, S.: Transvaginal color Doppler in the assessment of placental blood flow. Eur. J. Obstet. Gynecol. Reprod. Biol. 49 (1993) 29–32
42. Kurjak, A., Crvenkovic, G., Salihagic, A., Zalud, I., Miljan, M.: The assessment of normal early pregnancy by transvaginal color Doppler ultrasonography. J. Clin. Ultrasound 21 (1993) 3–8
43. Kurjak, A., Zudenigo, D., Funduk-Kurjak, B., Shalan, H., Predanic, M., Sosic, A.: Transvaginal color Doppler in the assessment of the uteroplacental circulation in normal early pregnancy. J. Perinat. Med. 21 (1993) 25–34
44. Kurjak, A., Zudenigo, D., Predanic, M., Kupesic, S.: Recent advances in the Doppler study of early fetomaternal circulation. J. Perinat. Med. 22 (1994) 419–439
45. Kurjak, A., Chervenak, F., Zudenigo, D., Kupesic, S.: Early fetal hemodynamics assessed by transvaginal color Doppler. In: Kurjak, A., Chervenak, F. (eds.): The Fetus as a Patient. London: Parthenon 1994; pp. 435–457
46. Kurjak, A., Zudenigo, D., Predanic, M., Kupesic, S., Funduk-Kurjak, B.: Transvaginal color Doppler study of fetomaternal circulation in threatened abortion. Fetal. Diagn. Ther. 9 (1994) 341–347
47. Kurjak, A., Kupesic, S., Kostovic, Lj.: Vascularization of yolk sac and vitelline duct in normal pregnancies studied by transvaginal color Doppler. J. Perinat. Med. 22 (1994) 433–440
48. Kurjak, A., Zalud, I., Predanic, M., Kupesic, S.: Transvaginal color and pulsed Doppler study of uterine blood flow in the first and early second trimester of pregnancy: normal versus abnormal. J. Ultrasound Med. 13 (1994) 43–47
49. Kurjak, A., Schulman, H., Predanic, M., Kupesic, S., Zalud, I.: Fetal chorioid plexus vascularization assessed by color and pulsed Doppler. J. Ultrasound Med. 13 (1994) 841–844
50. Kurjak, A., Laurini, R., Kupesic, S., Kos, M., Latin, V., Bulic, K.: A combined Doppler and morphopathological study of intervillous circulation. In The Fifth World Congress of Ultrasound in Obstetrics and Gynecology. Ultrasound Obstet. Gynecol. 6 (Suppl. 2) (1995) 116
51. Kurjak, A., Kupesic, S., Kos, M., Latin, V., Zudenigo, D.: Early hemodynamics studied by transvaginal color Doppler. Prenat. Neonat. Med. 1 (1996) 38–49
52. Kurjak, A., Schulman, H., Zudenigo, D., Kupesic, S., Kos, M., Goldenberg, M.: Subchorionic hematomas in early pregnancy: clinical outcome and blood flow patterns. J. Matern. Fetal. Med. 5 (1996) 41–44
53. Kurjak, A., Kupesic, S.: Doppler assessment of the intervillous blood flow in normal and abnormal early pregnancy. Obstet. Gynecol. 89 (1997) 252–256
54. Levi, C.S., Lyons, E.A., Lindsay, D.J.: Early diagnosis of nonviable pregnancy with endovaginal ultrasound. Radiology 167 (1988) 383–387
55. Long, M.G., Boultbee, J.E., Begent, R.H., Hanson, M.E., Bagshave, K.D.: Preliminary Doppler study on the uterine artery and myometrium in trophoblastic tumors requiring chemotherapy. Brit. J. Obstet. Gynaecol. 97 (1990) 686–689
56. Mantoni, M., Pedersen, J.F.: Intrauterine hematoma: an ultrasound study of threatened abortion. Brit. J. Obstet. Gynaecol. 88 (1981) 47–50
57. May, D.A., Sturtevant, N.V.: Embryonic heart rate as a predictor of pregnancy outcome: A prospective analysis. J. Ultrasound Med. 10 (1991) 591–593
58. Merce, L.T., Barco, M.J., Bau, S.: Color Doppler sonographic assessment of placental circulation in the first trimester of normal pregnancy. J. Ultrasound Med. 15 (1996) 135–142
59. Merchiers, E.H., Dhont, M., De Sutter, P.A., Beghin, C.J., Vandekerckhove, D.A.: Predictive value of early embryonic cardiac activity for pregnancy outcome. Amer. J. Obstet. Gynecol. 165 (1991) 11–14
60. Nimrod, C., Simpson, N., De Vermette, R., Fournier, J.: Placental and early fetal haemodynamics: the suitability of the monkey model. The Fetus as a Patient, XII International Congress, Grado, Italy, May 1996; 68
61. Nimrod, C., Simpson, N., Hafner, T. et al.: Assessment of early placental development in the cynomolgus monkey (Macaca fascicularis) using color and pulsed wave Doppler sonography. J. Med. Primatol. 25 (1996) 106–111
62. Nyberg, D.A., Laurence, A.M., Benedetti, T.J., Cyr, D.R., Schulman, W.P.: Placental abruption and placental hemorrhage: correlation of sonographic findings with fetal outcome. Radiology 164 (1987) 457–460
63. Pedersen, J.F., Mantoni, N.: Large intrauterine hematoma in threatened miscarriage. Frequency and clinical consequences. Brit. J. Obstet. Gynaecol. 97 (1990) 75–78
64. Pijnenborg, R., Dixon, G., Robertson, W.B., Brosens, I.: Trophoblastic invasion of human decidua from 8 to 18 weeks of pregnancy. Placenta 1 (1980) 3–19
65. Pijnenborg, R., Bland, J.M., Robertson, W.B., Dixon, G., Brosens, I.: The pattern of interstitial invasion of the myometrium in early human pregnancy. Placenta 2 (1981) 303–316
66. Pijnenborg, R., Bland, J.M., Robertson, W.B., Brosens, I.: Utero-placental arterial changes related to interstitial trophoblast migration in early human pregnancy. Placenta 4 (1983) 397–414
67. Ramsey, E.M.: Circulation in the intervillous space of the primate placenta. Amer. J. Obstet. Gynecol. 84 (1962) 1649–1663

68. Ramsey, E.M., Chez, R.A., Doppman, J.L.: Radioangiographic measurement of the internal diameters of the uteroplacental arteries in Rhesus monkeys and man. Carnegie Inst. Contrib. Embryol. 38 (1979) 59–70
69. Rockelein, G., Ulmer, R., Schwille, R.: Surface and branching of placental villi in early abortion: relationship to karyotype. Wirchows Arch. A. Pathol. Anatom. 417 (1990) 151–158
70. Rodesh, F., Simon, P., Donner, C., Jauniaux, E.: Oxygen measurements in endometrial and trophoblastic tissues during early pregnancy. Obstet. Gynecol. 80 (1992) 283–285
71. Saurbrei, E.E., Pham, D.H.: Placental abruption and subchorionic hemorrhage in the first half of pregnancy: US appearance and clinical outcome. Radiology 160 (1986) 109–111
72. Shimamoto, S., Sakuma, S., Ishigaki, T., Makino, N.: Intratumoral blood flow: evaluating with color Doppler echography. Radiology 165 (1987) 445–448
73. Spirit, B.A., Kagan, E.H., Rozanski, R.M.: Abruptio placentae: sonographic and pathologic correlation. Amer. J. Roentgenol. 133 (1979) 877–880
74. Stabile, I., Campbell, S., Grudzinskas, J.G.: Threatened miscarriage and intrauterine hematomas. Sonographic and biochemical studies. J. Ultrasound Med. 8 (1989) 289–292
75. Szhulman, A.E.: The natural history of early human spontaneous abortion. In: Barnea, E.R., Check, J.H., Grudzinkas, J.G., Marvo, T. (eds.): Implantation and Early Pregnancy in Humans. London: Parthenon 1993; pp. 309–321
76. Taylor, K.J.W., Schwartz, P.E., Kohorn, E.I.: Gestational trophoblastic neoplasia: diagnosis with color Doppler ultrasound. Radiology 165 (1987) 445–448
77. Tepper, R., Shulman, A., Altaras, M., Goldberger, S., Maymon, R., Holzinger, M.: The role of color Doppler flow in the management of nonmetastatic gestational trophoblastic disease. Gynecol. Obstet. Invest. 38(1) (1994) 14–17
78. Valentin, L., Sladkevicius, P., Laurini, R., Sodeberg, H., Marsal, K.: Uteroplacental and luteal circulation in normal first trimester pregnancies: Doppler ultrasonographic and morphologic study. Amer. J. Obstet. Gynecol. 174 (1996) 768–775
79. Van Zalen-Sprock, M.M., Van Vugt, J.M.G., Colenbrander, G.J., Geijn, H.P.: First-trimester uteroplacental and fetal blood flow velocity waveforms in normally developing fetuses: a longitudinal study. Ultrasound Obstet. Gynecol. 4 (1994) 284–288
80. Wladimiroff, J.W., Huisman, T.W.A., Stewart, P.A.: Cardiac Doppler flow velocities in the late first trimester fetus: a transvaginal Doppler study. J. Amer. Coll. Cardiol. 17 (1991) 1357–1359
81. Wladimiroff, J.W., Huisman, T.W.A., Stewart, P.A.: Intracerebral, aortic and umbilical artery flow velocity waveforms in the late-first-trimester fetus. Amer. J. Obstet. Gynecol. 166 (1992) 46–49
82. Ylostalo, P., Ammala, P., Seppala, M.: Intrauterine hematoma and placental protein 5 in patients with uterine bleeding during pregnancy. Brit. J. Obstet. Gynaecol. 91 (1984) 353–356
83. Zanetta, G., Lissoni, A., Colombo, M., Marzola, M., Cappelini, A., Mangioni, C.: Detection of abnormal intrauterine vascularization by color Doppler imaging: a possible additional aid for the follow up of patients with gestational trophoblastic tumors. Ultrasound Obstet. Gynecol. 7 (1996) 32–37

42 Uteroplacental Circulation

Doppler ultrasound has become a very promising tool for investigating the conditions of intrauterine fetal life. As a simple, noninvasive method of determining blood flow velocities, Doppler has been used in obstetric diagnosis for more than 20 years. Campbell et al. (27) were the first to report on Doppler studies of the uteroplacental vasculature in 1983. Even then, the study results indicated that abnormal uterine Doppler spectra were associated with an increased rate of preeclampsia, low birth weight, and premature delivery. The noninvasive Doppler evaluation of uteroplacental blood flow is becoming a subject of growing scientific and clinical interest among obstetricians.

Development of the Uteroplacental Vascular System

Anatomy. The uteroplacental vascular system is supplied by the two uterine arteries and ovarian arteries, which communicate with one another through vascular arcades. These arteries give rise to the arcuate vessels, which form a circumferential vascular plexus in the myometrium. These vessels in turn give rise to approximately 100 radial arteries, which subsequently divide into the basal arteries, which remain in the myometrium, and the spiral arteries, which are distributed to the endometrium and decidua (Fig. 42.5). The spiral arteries are responsible for supplying the individual placental functional units. The placenta is subdivided functionally into fetomaternal flow units called placentones. Described morphologically as cotyledons, approximately 40–60 of these units occur in the human placenta (107).

Transformation processes in placentation. Normal placentation is associated with critical morphologic and hemodynamic changes by which the maternal spiral arteries are transformed into uteroplacental vessels (see also Chapter 41). The invasion of trophoblastic cells causes an increasing dilatation of the spiral arteries in two stages. Trophoblast invasion in the first trimester initially involves the decidual segments of the spiral arteries, and then in the second trimester it spreads to the myometrial segments with vascular diameters of approximately 500 µm. As a result of this endovascular invasion process, the endometrium of the spiral arteries becomes lined by trophoblastic cells while the musculoelastic media is broken down and replaced by fibrinoid. This physiologic transformation process leads to vasodilatation in the terminal portions of the spiral arteries and intervillous inflow tract (22, 96, 103). The diameters of the spiral arteries undergo a 4- to 6-fold increase. The result of this transformation is a marked slowing of blood flow, which causes the maternal arterial blood pressure to fall to the level of the intervillous blood pressure. The pressure in the intervillous space is approximately 10 mmHg. The net result of the morphologic changes in the uteroplacental vessels is an approximately 10-fold increase in uteroplacental blood flow (43). As term approaches, the uterus is perfused at a rate of approximately 500–800 mL/min.

Exchange processes. Maternal arterial blood reaches the center of the fetoplacental unit through approximately 100 spiral arteries. This inflow, first described by Borell (11), can be accurately visualized with modern color Doppler systems (Fig. 42.2) (58, 74). The maternal blood flows radially from the center of the placentone into a peripheral zone of low villous density in the intervillous space, where it bathes the surface of the villous trees (Fig. 42.3). The fetomaternal exchange of gas and other substances in this area is promoted by the development of a great many mature intermediate and tertiary villi, by the local decrease in blood flow velocity, and by the presence of short diffusion paths in the small intervillous spaces. Venous blood finally exits the placenta via the subchorionic space and intercotyledon drainage pathway, entering the venous ostia of the basal plate (5) (Figs. 42.3, 42.4). Maternal intervillous blood circulation in the hemochorionic placenta is modulated by the luminal width of the uteroplacental vascular system (uterine arteries, arcuate arteries, basal arteries, radial arteries, spiral arteries).

Doppler Ultrasound of the Uteroplacental Vessels

Examination of the uterine arteries. Doppler ultrasound of the uterine arteries has become an established method in recent years for evaluating the total resistance of uteroplacental blood flow. With color Doppler, it is also possible to record blood flow velocities from circumscribed areas such as the spiral artery and arcuate artery (91) (Figs. 42.5, 42.6). This type of study show a significant decline in systolic and diastolic flow velocities, with a decrease in pulsatility, from the uterine artery to the spiral arteries. Since each uterine artery divides into 12–15 arcade arteries, it is apparent that Doppler measurements of the arcuate arteries reflect the hemodynamic function of only a circumscribed, terminal supply area. Hence they are of little diagnostic value, especially when one considers their lack of reproducibility. By contrast, flowmetry in both uterine arteries reflects the overall status of uterine perfusion. Bilateral Doppler scanning is recommended for the general assessment of uterine perfusion.

Transducer handling and instrument settings. In principle, either CW Doppler or pulsed gray-scale Doppler can be used to evaluate the uteroplacental vessels (27, 41, 49, 59, 85, 108). Color Doppler, however, is the simplest and most effective technique of uterine artery examination (14, 15). Color Doppler significantly shortens the examination time while yielding more reproducible results. Signal patterns are recorded from the main trunk of the uterine artery on each side. The artery is located by sweeping the transducer from medially to laterally into the lower outer quadrant of the uterus. The uterine artery will appear as a red-encoded vessel coursing toward the uterine fundus (Fig. 42.7). The uterine artery and external iliac artery may appear to cross paths, but this phenomenon is seen only during pregnancy and results from increased uterine growth causing a lateral shift of both uterine arteries. To record uterine blood flow velocities, the sample volume is placed on the uterine artery approximately 1–2 cm medial to the crossing site, and pulsed Doppler is activated (7, 14, 53). Good-quality uterine artery spectra can be acquired at an insonation angle of 15–50° and should present a sharp, clear envelope curve (Fig. 42.8). The optimum PRF setting for most examinations is between 4 and 6 kHz, using a wall filter setting of 60–120 Hz.

Sample volume. A clearly defined sample volume location is essential for the reproducible acquisition of high-quality Doppler spectra. This is particularly important when we consider that the resistance indices of

Normal uterine Doppler findings

Fig. 42.**1** Uteroplacental vascular system with physiologic dilatation of the spiral arteries (after 67).

Fig. 42.**2** Color-encoded images of uteroplacental blood flow within a placentone at 31 weeks' gestation. *Left:* power Doppler image. *Right:* conventional color Doppler image. The spiral artery with Borell inflow (blue) into the placentone is clearly defined.

Fig. 42.**3** Intervillous hemodynamics within a placentone (after 5). Blood flow from the spiral artery (red) bathes the surface of the villous tree. Fetomaternal exchange of gases and nutrients occurs between the mature intermediate villi and tertiary villi. Blood depleted of oxygen and nutrients leaves the placenta through the subchorionic space and intercotyledon drainage tract, passing to the venous ostia of the basal plate (blue).

Fig. 42.**4** Color Doppler image of intracotyledon blood flow. Blue = Borell inflow. Red = venous outflow.

Fig. 42.**5** Appearance of Doppler frequency spectra recorded at different sites in the uteroplacental vascular system.

Fig. 42.**6** Normal Doppler signal pattern recorded from the spiral artery at 28 weeks. Note the low systolic and diastolic flow velocities.

Fig. 42.**7** Color Doppler image of the left uterine artery in the lateral uterine wall. Cephalad blood flow is encoded in red.

Fig. 42.**8** Normal Doppler frequency spectrum of the uterine artery, recorded by color Doppler at 32 weeks.

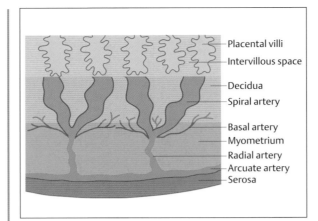

Placental villi
Intervillous space
Decidua
Spiral artery
Basal artery
Myometrium
Radial artery
Arcuate artery
Serosa

1

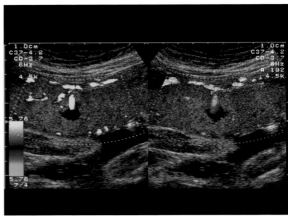

2

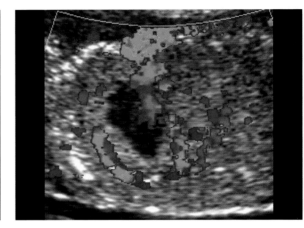

3

4

Arcuate artery

Uterine artery

External iliac artery

5

6

7

8

the uterine vessels are higher than the indices of the arcuate arteries and subplacental arteries (7). Faulty positioning of the sample volume in the uterine vessels, like superimposed waveforms from the external and internal iliac arteries, can lead to errors of interpretation. The external iliac artery is characterized by high pulsatility and a bidirectional frequency spectrum with early diastolic flow reversal (Fig. 42.**9**). The external iliac vein is distinguished from the artery by its greater diameter, an absence of pulsatile flow, and a monophasic Doppler spectrum.

Physiologic notch. At the start of pregnancy, the uterine signal pattern shows high pulsatility with high systolic and low diastolic flow velocities in addition to an early diastolic (postsystolic) notch (Fig. 42.**10**). This notch represents a pulse wave reflection due to increased peripheral vascular resistance and is the spectral counterpart of incomplete trophoblast invasion. Under physiologic conditions, the end-diastolic velocities increase with continued gestation while vascular resistance decreases as placentation progresses (Fig. 42.**10**). The Doppler changes described above are most pronounced at the start of the second trimester (35, 45). After 24–26 weeks' gestation, no additional Doppler changes are generally found in the uterine signal pattern (3, 40, 113) (Figs. 42.**11**, 42.**12**). Similar findings are seen in the spiral arteries (91).

Resistance index and pulsatility index. The resistance index (RI) and pulsatility index (PI) are the most widely used criteria for determining the impedance to flow in the downstream vessels and for the qualitative analysis of uterine waveforms. The intraobserver variability in color Doppler imaging of the uterine artery ranges from 4% to 7%, with an interobserver variability of 6.6% (16, 92).

Persistent notch. Another useful analytical criterion is a persistent early diastolic notch in the spectral waveform (29, 88) (Fig. 42.**15**). Table 42.**1** reviews the frequency of unilateral and bilateral notches and of abnormally high resistance indices. An early diastolic notch may still be a normal finding at 24–26 weeks' gestation (see above) (40, 113). But persistence of the notch thereafter suggests deficient trophoblast invasion with insufficient dilatation of the spiral arteries and an impending deficiency of uterine blood flow (78) (Fig. 42.**16**).

Placental pathology and location. Bilateral abnormal Doppler velocity spectra in the uterine arteries have a high association with abnormal histopathologic placental findings in the form of accelerated villous maturation and patchy reticular infarcts (57). At the same time, the flow velocities found in the uterine arteries can vary markedly with the location of the placenta. Thus, with a lateral placenta location, significantly lower resistance indices are found on the placental side than on the contralateral side (68) (Figs. 42.**13**, 42.**14**). Also, it is common to detect a notch on the contralateral side, although this does not appear to have clinical significance when flow in the ipsilateral uterine artery is normal (8, 69, 92). Studies have shown, however, that an increased resistance index or early diastolic notch on the placental side is associated with an increased rate of pregnancy complications, especially with regard to hypertensive disorders (47, 69, 80).

Transvaginal ultrasound. Transvaginal ultrasound can be used in the Doppler examination as an alternative to transabdominal scanning (34, 56). After insertion of the vaginal transducer, the paracervical region is imaged in a coronal plane, taking care to apply as little transducer pressure as possible. The uterine artery can generally be identified as a hypoechoic structure 2–4 mm in diameter with longitudinal pulsations.

Reproducibility. To obtain valid and reproducible measurements, it is advantageous to image the uterine artery with color Doppler. Different study results in abnormal uterine Doppler spectra are based partly on varying definitions of the patient population and partly on differences in how the frequency spectra are analyzed.

Table 42.**1** Frequency of abnormal uteroplacental Doppler waveforms

Author	Weeks gestation	n	Doppler	RI↑ (%)	Unilateral notch (%)	Bilateral notches (%)	Notch + RI↑ (%)
Steel 1990 (112) (unselected)	24	1014	CW	12 (RI > 0.58)	–	–	–
Kurmanavichius 1990 (76) (unselected)	18–21 / 31–33	129 / 157	CW / –	– / 8.3	10.9 / 1.9	3.1 / –	– / –
Bower 1993 (16) (unselected)	18–22 / 24	2058	CW / Color	– / –	– / –	– / –	16 / 5.1
Valensise 1993 (123) (unselected)	22	272	Color	9.5 (RI > 0.58)	–	–	–
North 1994 (92) (unselected)	19–24	458	Color	17 (RI > 90th percentile)	–	–	–
Konchak 1995 (72) (AFP↑)	17–22	103	Color	10.6 (RI = 0.7)	–	–	6.8
Mires 1995 (88) (unselected)	18 / 24	1412	Color	– / –	1.9 / –	4.2 / 2.1	– / –
Murakoshi 1996 (91)	18–26 / > 26	160	Color	– / –	40.7 / 6.9	– / –	– / –
Harrington 1996 (55) (unselected)	19–21 / 24	1326	Color	– / –	– / 4.7	– / 3.6	– / –
Harrington 1997 (56) (unselected)	12–16	652	TVS	–	22.8	32.7	–
Zimmermann 1997 (128) - High-risk	21–24	175	PW	–	–	17.6	–
- Low-risk		172		–	–	8	–
Mires 1998 (89) (unselected)	18–20 / 22–24	6579	Color	– / –	2.9 / 0.3	1.6 / 0.5	– / –
Kurdi 1998 (75) (unselected)	19–21	946	Color	–	–	12.4	–

Clinical Significance of Uterine Doppler Ultrasound

The measurement of uterine flow velocities with Doppler ultrasound is an important step in the evaluation of the maternofetal unit (16, 27, 54, 109, 112, 119). But while it cannot be used as a primary study for detecting fetal compromise, abnormal uterine blood flow velocities do correlate well with existing or impending fetal growth retardation, preeclampsia, and increased rates of prematurity, placental abruption, cesarean section, and low birth weight (8, 27, 55, 56, 59, 63, 92, 118).

Resistance indices and bilateral notches. The presence of bilateral notches appears to be a particularly good predictor for these complications (Fig. 42.**15**), as are increased uterine resistance indices. The recommended cutoff levels for increased vascular resistance in the uterine artery are RI values above the 90th percentile (92) or above the 95th percentile (8, 16, 53) of the individual uterine reference curves. RI values above 0.58–0.68 have also been classified as pathologic (8, 50, 110, 112, 128). An early diastolic notch is usually associated with increased RI values but may also be seen when the resistance indices are normal (Fig. 42.**17**–42.**19**). The combination of RI values above the 90th percentile and the presence of bilateral diastolic notches appears to be the best parameter for predicting serious pregnancy complications (29).

Current studies do not document a relationship between nicotine abuse and abnormal uterine Doppler waveforms (62).

Fig. 42.**9** Normal biphasic Doppler signal pattern of the right external iliac artery.

Fig. 42.**10** Doppler spectra recorded from the uterine artery at different gestational ages. The progressive increase in diastolic flow velocity is a result of normal trophoblast invasion.

Fig. 42.**11** Doppler reference range for the pulsatility index (PI) of the uterine artery for a central placental location. The 90% confidence interval is shown. The upper curve represents the approximate 95th percentile, the middle curve the 50th percentile, and the lower curve the approximate 5th percentile (3).

Fig. 42.**12** Doppler reference range for the resistance index (RI) of the uterine artery for a central placental location. The 90% confidence interval is shown. The upper curve represents the approximate 95th percentile, the middle curve the 50th percentile, and the lower curve the approximate 5th percentile (3).

Fig. 42.**13** Doppler reference range for the resistance index (RI) of the uterine artery on the placental side of a unilateral placental location. The 95% confidence interval is shown. The upper curve represents the 95th percentile, the middle curve the 50th percentile, and the lower curve the 5th percentile (76).

Fig. 42.**14** Doppler reference range for the resistance index (RI) of the uterine artery on the nonplacental side of a unilateral placental location. The 95% confidence interval is shown. The upper curve represents the 95th percentile, the middle curve the 50th percentile, and the lower curve the 5th percentile (76).

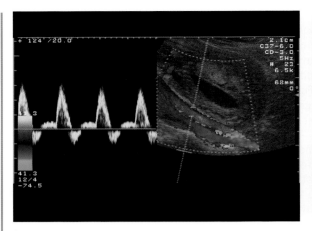

9

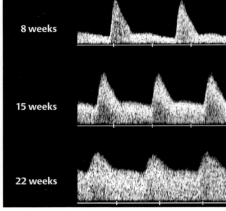

10

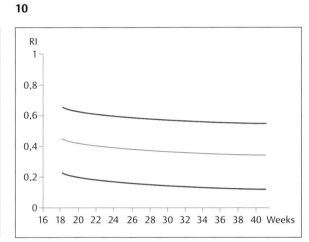

11

12

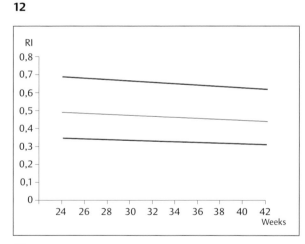

13

14

Intrauterine Growth Retardation

Etiology and pathogenesis. Intrauterine growth retardation (IUGR) occurs in a setting of chronic placental insufficiency and results mainly from a reduction of maternal blood flow in the fetomaternal unit (83). Analogous to the etiology of preeclampsia, the main pathogenic cause of this perfusion deficit is impaired trophoblast invasion with an absence of spiral artery dilatation (24, 25, 87) (Fig. 42.**16**). When Brosens et al. (24) performed placental bed biopsies from normotensive pregnancies with SGA fetuses, they observed a partial or complete impairment of trophoblast invasion in more than 50% of the cases. The severity of the intrauterine growth retardation is proportional to the severity of the placental abnormality (46). The spiral arteries located in the decidua often exhibit typical histopathologic features: endothelial disruption, intimal thickening, and atheromatous-like lesions ranging to complete vascular obliteration. The results are multiple placental infarctions accompanied by a reduction of placental parenchyma and villous surface area (18). Histomorphologic studies have shown that the diameters of the spiral arteries measured in intrauterine growth retardation are only about 40% of the diameters found in healthy pregnancies (67). Spiral arteries may also be completely obliterated by fibrin in pregnancies that are complicated by fetal growth retardation (111). Intrauterine growth retardation, then, can be considered a secondary result of uteroplacental insufficiency.

Role of Doppler ultrasound. These histologic vascular changes correlate with Doppler findings in the uterine and umbilical arteries (42, 57, 93). It should be considered, however, that the etiology of intrauterine growth retardation is very diverse. This accounts for the varying reports on the sensitivity and positive predictive value of uterine artery Doppler examinations (Table 42.**2**). Although Doppler scanning of the uterine arteries does not presently meet the criteria of a screening examination, the detection of abnormal uterine artery waveforms is associated with a 3- to 9-fold increase in risk for intrauterine growth retardation due to chronic placental insufficiency (8, 15, 35, 53, 56, 61, 91, 92). Thus, when abnormal uterine artery waveforms are detected, serial biometry scans should be performed at frequent intervals. Conversely, Doppler evaluation of the umbilical artery and fetal vascular system is indicated when signs of intrauterine growth flattening are observed.

Preeclampsia

Preeclampsia, defined as an initial occurrence of hypertension and proteinuria during the second half of pregnancy, is associated with significant perinatal morbidity and mortality. The main problems on the fetal side are intrauterine growth retardation and premature delivery. Moreover, pregnancy-induced hypertensive diseases continue to be a major cause of maternal mortality in the United States, Scandinavia, England, and many other countries—despite appropriate antihypertensive treatment and active obstetric therapy (100, 102).

Etiology and pathogenesis. While the clinical manifestations of pregnancy-induced hypertension and preeclampsia arise chiefly during the middle of the second half of pregnancy, the underlying pathophysiologic changes occur much earlier. In the current hypothesis on the pathogenesis of pregnancy-induced hypertension and preeclampsia, it is believed that endothelial dysfunction causes an imbalance to develop between the vasoactive eicosanoids prostacyclin (prostaglandin I_2, PGI_2) and thromboxane A_2 (TXA_2) (33, 44, 127). Thromboxane A_2, which is synthesized by the platelets, caused increased platelet aggregation (= platelet hyperactivity), increased vasoconstriction, and a stimulation of phospholipase A_2 activity. This leads to rise of peripheral vascular resistance and a pronounced reduction of uterine blood flow. Prostacyclin (PGI_2), which is synthesized in the vascular endothelium, is an antagonist of TXA_2. PGI_2 mainly causes increased vasodilatation, decreased platelet aggregation, and decreased platelet adhesion to the vascular endothelium. Additionally, it often interferes with trophoblast invasion, causing histomorphologic features similar to those seen in intrauterine growth retardation.

A lateral placental location correlates with an increased rate of preeclampsia (48, 69).

Role of Doppler ultrasound. Doppler examination of the uterine arteries appears to be useful in predicting the risk for preeclampsia and its severity, even before clinical manifestations appear. The Doppler crite-

Table 42.**2** Value of uterine Doppler ultrasound in predicting intrauterine growth retardation (< 10th percentile)

Author	Weeks gestation	Doppler	Criterion	n	Sensitivity (%)	Specificity (%)	PPV (%)	NPV (%)	RR
Steel 1990 (112) (unselected)	16–22	CW	RI	1014	33	91	27	–	–
Bewley 1991 (8) (unselected)	16–22	CW	AVRI > 95th percentile	913	15	96	35	88	3.0
Valensise 1993 (123) (unselected)	22	Color	RI	272	66	96	53	97	–
North 1994 (92) (unselected)	19–24	Color	A/C ratio > 90th percentile, RI > 90th percentile	458	47 50	89 90	23 27	96 91	– –
Todros 1995 (117) (unselected)	19–24	CW	S/D ratio	916	12	92	8	96	–
Konchak 1995 (72) (AFP ↑)	17–22	Color	Notch (uni. + bil.), RI ≥ 0,7	103	28.6 35.7	94.4 93.3	44.4 45.5	89.4 90.2	– –
Harrington 1996 (55) (unselected)	24	Color	Uni. notch Bil. notch Notch + RI > 95th percentile	1326	13.7 21.8 32	95.9 97.8 93.6	29 50 91.8	90.1 90.8 91.8	3.0 5.5 6.7
Irion 1998 (62) (unselected)	26	Color	A/C ratio ≥ 2.5 RI ≥ 0.58	1194	29 29	86 89	21 25	– –	– –
Mires 1998 (89) (unselected)	18–20 22–24	Color	Bil. notch Uni. notch Bil. notch Uni. notch	6579	7.4 13.7 4.0 8.5	98.7 96.1 99.6 98.4	15.2 10.1 26.7 14.5	97.1 97.2 97.0 97.1	5.2 3.6 9.0 5.1
Kurdi 1998 (75) (unselected)	19–21	Color	Bil. notch	946	36.8	89.2	17.9	95.7	–
Benedetto 1998 (6)	24	Color	RI > 0.58	180	70	53	16	93	–

PPV = positive predictive value
NPV = negative predictive value
RR = relative risk

uni. = unilateral
bil. = bilateral

ria that are thought to imply an increased risk for preeclampsia are increased resistance indices and the presence of an early diastolic notch (27, 40, 60). Bower et al. (16) found that the risk of preeclampsia was increased 68-fold in a low-risk population at 24 weeks when a persistent early diastolic notch was found in both uterine artery waveforms or if the resistance indices were above the 95th percentile. Other authors were unable to confirm this level of preeclampsia risk, however (62) (Table 42.**3**).

Histopathologic findings in placentas and placental bed biopsies from preeclamptics show a good correlation with Doppler findings in the uterine artery (57, 81, 93, 125). There is no correlation, however, between abnormal uterine artery waveforms and maternal blood pressure.

On the whole, Doppler scanning of the uterine arteries can help to confirm suspicion of preeclampsia or provide a better clinical assessment of the severity of overt preeclampsia.

Aspirin Therapy

The rationale for the prophylactic use of low-dose aspirin therapy (50–150 mg/day acetylsalicylic acid) is based on the fact that aspirin selectively inhibits the synthesis of thromboxane A2 by inhibiting platelet cyclooxygenase, thereby shifting the relationship between TXA_2 and PGI_2 in favor of PGI_2 (30, 127).

Study results. Based on this pathophysiologic working hypothesis, various investigators between the mid-1980s and early 1990s were able to show that low-dose aspirin therapy was effective in the treatment of pregnancy-induced hypertension and especially of preeclampsia (4, 106, 120, 121, 126). Moreover, a meta-analysis by Dekker and Sibai (33)

showed that low-dose aspirin therapy in a high-risk population could reduce the incidence of pregnancy-induced hypertension by 40%, preeclampsia by 85%, and intrauterine growth retardation by 50%. Thomas et al. (116) had similar results in their meta-analysis, finding a 44% reduction in the risk for intrauterine growth retardation.

On the other hand, several multicenter studies and the Collaborative Low-dose Aspirin Study in Pregnancy (CLASP) in particular (31) found that prophylactic aspirin use was of little benefit in preventing preeclampsia or improving perinatal outcome in low-risk and high-risk populations (28, 31).

These controversial findings are based largely on the fact that, for the present, there are no sensitive test procedures for predicting or assessing the risk of preeclampsia, and that different studies have used different inclusion and exclusion criteria for defining preeclampsia and intrauterine growth retardation. Thus it is very difficult to divide patients into high- and low-risk categories, making it difficult to compare different studies.

Doppler studies. Doppler ultrasound studies of the uterine arteries have shown that prophylactic aspirin use in patients with a bilateral early diastolic notch or resistance indices above the 95th percentile at 20 weeks of pregnancy is associated with a significant reduction in the severity of preeclampsia and with significantly higher birth weights and less prematurity (17, 86).

At the same time, a randomized controlled study found that low-dose aspirin prophylaxis in patients with abnormal uterine waveforms was of no apparent benefit in reducing pregnancy complications (90) (Table 42.**4**).

Although there continues to be disagreement on the efficacy of aspirin prophylaxis in a high-risk population, Uzan et al. (122) recom-

Table 42.3   Value of uterine Doppler ultrasound in predicting preeclampsia

Author	Weeks gestation	Doppler	Criterion	n	Sensitivity (%)	Specificity (%)	PPV (%)	NPV (%)	RR
Steel 1990 (112) (unselected)	16–22	CW	RI > 0.58	1014	63	89	10	–	–
Bewley 1991 (8) (unselected)	16–22	CW	RI > 95th percentile	917	24	95	20	96	5.3
Bower 1993 (16) (unselected)	18–22	CW	Bil. notch	2058	82	86.7	12	99.5	–
			RI > 95th percentile		37	95	–	–	
	24	Color	Bil. notch	273	78	96	28	99.5	68
			RI > 95th percentile		45	96	–	–	
Valensise 1993 (123) (unselected)	22	Color	RI > 0.58	272	88	93	30	99	–
North 1994 (92) (unselected)	19–24	Color	A/C ratio > 90th percentile,	458	53	88	14	98	–
			RI > 90th percentile		27	89	8	97	–
Konchak 1995 (72) (AFP ↑)	17–22	Color	Notch (uni. + bil.),	103	83.3	95.6	55.6	98.9	–
			RI ≥ 0.7		83.3	93.8	45.5	98.9	–
Todros 1995 (117) (unselected)	19–24	CW	S/D ratio	916	40	92	3	99.5	–
	26–31	CW			60	92	5	99.7	–
Mires 1995 (88) (unselected)	18	Color	Bil. notch	1412	73.7	67.8	37.3	–	14
Chan 1995 (29)	20	CW	Notch + RA > 90th percentile	334	21.7	96.9	35.7	93.9	5.9
Harrington 1996 (55) (unselected)	24	Color	Notch uni.	1326	22.7	95.5	16.1	97	5.6
			Bil. notch		54.5	97.9	50	98.3	40.8
			Notch + RI > 95th percentile		77.3	93.9	30.9	99.1	34.7
Harrington 1997 (56) (unselected)	12–16	TVU	Bil. notch	652	93	69	–	–	–
Kurdi 1998 (75) (unselected)	19–21	Color	Bil. notch + RI > 0.55	946	61.9	88.7	11.1	99.0	–
Irion 1998 (62) (unselected)	18	Color	A/C ratio ≥ 2.5	1000	50	57	5	–	–
	26		A/C ratio ≥ 2.5	1194	34	85	8	–	–
			RI ≥ 0.58		26	88	7	–	–
Benedetto 1998 (6)	24	Color	RI ≥ 0.58	180	73	55	27	90	–
Mires 1998 (89) (unselected)	18–20	Color	Bil. notch	6579	13.9	98.5	9.3	99.0	9.7
			Uni. notch		30.6	95.7	7.3	99.2	9.2
	22–24		Bil. notch		5.6	99.6	12.5	98.9	12.0
			Uni. notch		16.7	98.2	9.5	99.1	10.1

PPV = positive predictive value   uni. = unilateral
NPV = negative predictive value   bil. = bilateral
RR = relative risk

mend that prophylactic aspirin therapy (60–150 mg/day) be considered early in women who have a history of pregnancy complications and who also have an early diastolic notch and/or elevated resistance indices in both uterine arteries. The results of large multicenter studies indicate that low-dose aspirin will not produce adverse side effects with an increase in fetal or maternal risk (31, 38).

Elevated Maternal Serum AFP Levels and Uterine Artery Waveforms

Abnormal uterine artery waveforms (increased resistance indices, early diastolic notch) are found in 11–19% of women with elevated alpha-fetoprotein levels (2, 72, 104). It appears that elevated maternal serum alpha-fetoprotein levels (MSAFP) in association with a sonographically normal-appearing fetus, when combined with abnormal uterine Doppler spectra, are associated with increased perinatal mortality and increased rates of premature delivery and low birth weight (2, 21). An 11% incidence of placental abruption has also been reported in these cases (104). When elevated MSAFP levels are detected and the Doppler spectrum shows an early diastolic notch, these findings are diagnostic of preeclampsia with a sensitivity of 83% and a positive predictive value of 56% (72). It is assumed that a prostacyclin-thromboxane imbalance in favor of thromboxane leads to increased platelet aggregation, which in turn leads to increased vascular thrombosis and placental infarctions (82). Histologic studies of placentas have shown a relationship between elevated MSAFP levels and placental vascular pathology (19, 105).

At present we do not know for certain whether prophylactic low-dose aspirin therapy should be instituted in patients who have elevated MSAFP levels accompanied by abnormal uterine artery waveform patterns. On the one hand, improvements in perinatal outcomes have been achieved with this therapy, but it was found that significantly more babies died from placental abruption in the aspirin-treated patients than in a placebo group (52).

Raised human chorionic gonadotropin levels combined with elevated resistance indices (RI) also appear to be associated with an adverse pregnancy outcome (9, 10).

Effect of Uterine Contractions on Uterine Artery Waveform

Radioangiographic studies in humans have demonstrated that uterine contractions cause a rise of intrauterine pressure and a reduction of uteroplacental blood flow (12).

Intrauterine pressure > 30 mmHg. If uterine contractions raise the intrauterine pressure above 30 mmHg, there is an arrest of intervillous blood flow due to vascular obliteration in the villous capillary system and in the spiral and radial arteries. This decrease in blood flow appears to occur even during mild uterine contractions such as focal Braxton Hicks contractions (13, 94). Kofinas et al. (71) found in color Doppler studies that the resistance indices of the arcuate and uterine arteries did not change at the level of the subplacental myometrium during these contractions. They found a significant increase in resis-

tance indices only in response to contractions occurring in the nonplacental myometrium. These findings show that a "functional asymmetry" of the myometrium exists during Braxton Hicks contractions (71).

Oxytocin stress test. A relationship has also been found between oxytocin-induced uterine contractions and the level of the end-diastolic uterine artery flow velocity (94). Olofson et al. (93) showed that an abnormal oxytocin stress test was associated with significantly higher pulsatility indices in the uterine artery than a normal oxytocin stress test (PI 3.9 ± 0.28 versus 2.62 ± 0.24). The increased Doppler indices also correlate with the occurrence of decelerations in FHR monitoring. The end-diastolic uterine artery blood flow velocities are inversely proportional to the intensity of the uterine contraction (20, 41) (Fig. 42.**20**).

Intrauterine pressure > 60 mmHg. The end-diastolic velocities in the uterine arteries are reduced when the intrauterine pressure exceeds 35 mmHg, and they are completely absent when the pressure exceeds 60 mmHg (41). Especially during labor, the uterine contractions that occur intermittently and with growing intensity cause a reduction in uterine blood flow. This decrease has been documented with Doppler ultrasound in both uterine arteries and in the arcuate arteries based on a rise in the resistance and pulsatility indices (41, 64, 71). In the interval between contractions, there is a recovery or normalization of uteroplacental blood flow with a corresponding increase in end-diastolic velocities. No differences are found in the Doppler spectra of the uterine arteries during early and late dilatation (39). It has been shown, however, that when abnormal Doppler waveforms (increased RI, early diastolic notch) were recorded prior to labor, there is an increased incidence of decelerations, lower Apgar scores, and a higher rate of secondary cesarean sections (112, 114, 118).

Effect of Medications on Uterine Artery Waveform

Doppler provides a noninvasive method for the evaluation of uteroplacental hemodynamics. One area of interest is the effect of vasoactive medications on uterine blood flow. In comparing published results, however, it should be considered that differences in dosages and clinical populations can lead to controversial findings on the effects of certain agents (65).

Beta mimetics. Preterm labor is most commonly treated with intravenous beta mimetic drugs. Several groups of authors have documented a decrease in uterine artery resistance indices and an improvement of uterine blood flow with Doppler ultrasound (20, 36). The decrease in resistance indices is caused partly by a simultaneous rise in maternal heart rate (the shortened diastole causes an increase in end-diastolic velocities, with a fall in resistance indices) and partly by the decrease in uterine tone, making the uterus less contractile. Activation of the β_2 receptors in the uterus may also play a role, lowering the resistance in the uteroplacental vascular system by relaxing the vascular smooth muscle (20). All of these factors lead to an increase in uteroplacental blood flow.

Table 42.**4** Frequency of preeclampsia and intrauterine growth retardation in patients taking aspirin or a placebo

Author	Weeks gestation	Doppler	Cutoff	n	Preeclampsia Aspirin	Placebo	p	IUGR Aspirin	Placebo	p
McParland 1990 (86)	18–20 24	CW	RI > 0.58	100	2%	19%	0.02	14%	14%	n.s.
Bower 1996 (17)	18–22 24	CW Color	RI > 95% Notch	60	13%	38%	0.03	26%	41%	0.2
Morris 1996 (90)	18	Color	S/D > 90% Notch	102	8%	14%	n.s.	27%	22%	n.s.

Indomethacin and magnesium. Magnesium or indomethacin can be used as an alternative to beta mimetics to inhibit labor. While indomethacin does not affect uteroplacental hemodynamics, intravenous magnesium sulfate therapy tends to lower the resistance indices in the uterine vessels (65, 85).

α-Methyldopa and dihydralazine. Hypertensive pregnancy disorders are associated with an increase in peripheral vascular resistance. Antihypertensive therapy in pregnancy relies mainly on the drugs α-methyldopa and dihydralazine. While α-methyldopa does not affect uteroplacental blood flow in healthy, normotensive pregnant women, its use in patients with preeclampsia or chronic hypertension causes a significant fall of uteroplacental resistance indices (101). Results on the effect of dihydralazine on uteroplacental blood flow have been contradictory. While one study found no changes in uterine resistance indices (37), another study reported increased resistance indices.

Calcium antagonists. Calcium antagonists such as nifedipine are another option in the treatment of pregnancy-induced hypertension (97, 98). Pirhonen et al. (97, 98) observed a fall of resistance indices in the uterine arteries after the oral administration of nifedipine, while the resistance indices in the arcuate arteries remained unchanged.

NO donors. Lately there have been isolated reports on the intravenous or transdermal administration of NO donors in the treatment of preeclampsia (26, 51, 77, 79, 99, 115). In normal pregnancies, nitric oxide (NO) formed in the endothelium relaxes the vascular smooth muscle and inhibits platelet aggregation. In preeclampsia, on the other hand, there is greater endothelial dysfunction leading to an increase in vasoconstriction and platelet aggregation. Although only a few studies have been done to date on NO effects in very small numbers of patients, most of the studies showed an improvement of uteroplacental blood flow after the administration of NO donors, with a fall of resistance indices in the uterine arteries.

◾ Doppler Screening of Uterine Vessels

Requirements. Despite many attempts to establish a reliable method for the prediction of preeclampsia and intrauterine growth retardation, so far researchers have been unable to devise a suitable screening test for this purpose (32). A test procedure for the prediction of pregnancy complications must meet several criteria: it must be cost-effective, reproducible, easy to use, noninvasive, and it must provide high sensitivity combined with a high positive predictive value.

Doppler ultrasound of the uterine arteries. For the present, Doppler scanning of the uterine arteries appears to be the best available method for the prediction of preeclampsia and intrauterine growth retardation (9, 16, 62). The goal of Doppler screening of the uterine arteries is early risk identification (8, 92). Studies of this kind have already been done in the first trimester, but the results to date have not contributed to the early detection of these disorders (45). A number of Doppler studies of the uterine artery between 16 and 24 weeks' gestation suggest that the persistence of elevated uterine resistance indices and especially the persistence of a bilateral early diastolic notch are important clinical criteria for the prediction of preeclampsia and intrauterine growth restriction (15, 55, 95, 128). The data indicate that a unilateral notch implies a relatively low risk of pregnancy complications whereas a bilateral notch, especially when combined with high RI values above the 95th percentile, is associated with a significantly higher rate of pregnancy complications (29, 55). North et al. (92) and Irion et al. (62) attempted to characterize the notch more precisely by calculating the ratio of peak systolic to peak early-diastolic velocities, called the A/C ratio. Their results, however, did not improve the prediction of preeclampsia or intrauterine growth retardation.

Sensitivity and predictive value. On the whole, published reports on the sensitivity and positive predictive value of uterine Doppler ultrasound are very sobering and somewhat controversial (Tables 42.**2** and 42.**3**). The discrepancies in published results have several causes: the use of different Doppler equipment, differences in the timing of the examinations, differences in the sizes and definitions of the patient groups, varying definitions of abnormal Doppler waveforms, poor definition of the Doppler reference planes used in the studies, and varying definitions of the outcome criteria.

◾ Conclusion

In summary, it may be said that a bilateral notch and/or increased resistance indices in the uterine vessels are associated with a markedly increased risk of pregnancy complications, especially preeclampsia, intrauterine growth retardation, and placental abruption.

General Doppler screening of the uterine vessels between 18 and 22 weeks' gestation cannot be recommended at present due to inadequate sensitivity and a low positive predictive value. On the other hand, Doppler scans of the uteroplacental vessels in pregnant women with a positive history are useful for predicting the development of a hypertensive pregnancy disorder and intrauterine growth retardation at an early stage.

Practical approach. Figure 42.**21** presents a flowchart for evaluating the uterine vessels in high-risk patients.
- The detection or persistence of abnormal uterine artery waveforms is associated with a 58% incidence (seven-fold greater risk) of preeclampsia and/or IUGR later in the pregnancy (128). These findings warrant close surveillance of the subsequent pregnancy, relying mainly on serial ultrasound scans to evaluate growth.
- Doppler monitoring of the fetoplacental and fetal vascular system is not strictly necessary in these cases, but if fetal growth flattens it should be done for further assessment of fetal well-being.
- Fetal Doppler ultrasound is also indicated in very anxious and distressed patients. Doppler scanning of the maternofetal unit in these cases can help to allay the patient's concerns.
- Prophylactic low-dose aspirin therapy (50–150 mg/day) may be considered in patients with abnormal uterine artery waveforms (17, 86). The value of aspirin therapy in pregnancy has not been definitively established, however.

For the future, it is reasonable to expect that the combination of biophysical test procedures and biochemical markers with uteroplacental Doppler ultrasound will further improve our ability to predict preeclampsia and intrauterine growth retardation (6, 124).

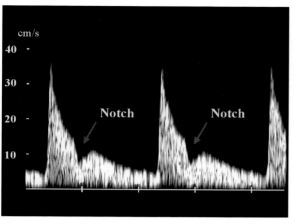

15

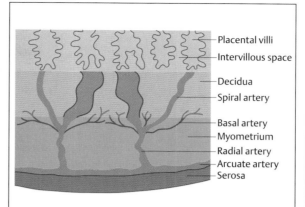

Placental villi
Intervillous space
Decidua
Spiral artery
Basal artery
Myometrium
Radial artery
Arcuate artery
Serosa

16

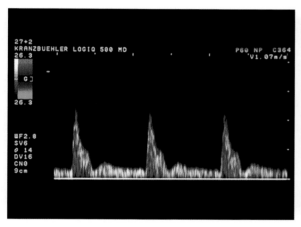

17

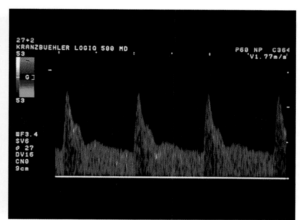

18

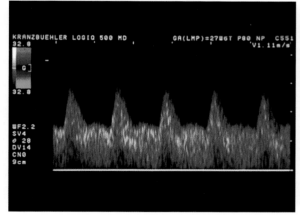

19

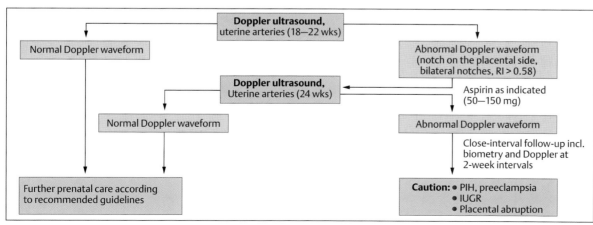

Uterine contraction

20

Doppler ultrasound,
uterine arteries (18—22 wks)

Normal Doppler waveform

Abnormal Doppler waveform
(notch on the placental side,
bilateral notches, RI > 0.58)

Doppler ultrasound,
Uterine arteries (24 wks)

Aspirin as indicated
(50—150 mg)

Normal Doppler waveform

Abnormal Doppler waveform

Close-interval follow-up incl.
biometry and Doppler at
2-week intervals

Further prenatal care according
to recommended guidelines

Caution: • PIH, preeclampsia
• IUGR
• Placental abruption

21

Abnormal findings

Fig. 42.**15**   Abnormal uterine artery waveform. Note the v-shaped early diastolic notch and the low end-diastolic flow velocities. This spectral pattern has a high association with an increased risk for preeclampsia and with increased rates of intrauterine growth retardation, prematurity, cesarean section, and placental abruption.

Fig. 42.**16**   Abnormal uteroplacental vascular system, with lack of dilatation of the spiral arteries (after 67).

Fig. 42.**17**   Very abnormal color Doppler frequency spectrum from the left uterine artery in a patient with severe preeclampsia (27 weeks, 2 days).

Fig. 42.**18**   Spectrum from the right uterine artery in the same patient as in Fig. 42.**17**. This spectrum, also abnormal, contains a typical V-shaped early diastolic notch. The diastolic flow velocities are higher than in Fig. 42.**17**. The bilateral notches imply a high risk for serious pregnancy complications.

Fig. 42.**19**   This uterine artery waveform contains a notch but shows normal diastolic flow velocities (20 weeks, 2 days). When found unilaterally, this spectral pattern is considered normal.

Fig. 42.**20**   Uterine artery waveforms recorded during uterine contractions. As the intensity of the contraction builds, the pulsatility of the flow increases with a resulting decline of end-diastolic flow velocities.

Fig. 42.**21**   Flowchart for Doppler evaluation of the uterine artery in high-risk patients.

References

1. Arduini, D., Rizzo G., Romanini, C., Mancuso, S.: Uteroplacental blood flow velocity waveforms as predictors of pregnancy-induced hypertension. Eur. J. Obstet. Gynecol. Reprod. Biol. 26 (1987) 335–341
2. Aristidou, A., van den Hof, M.C., Campbell, S., Nicolaides, K.: Uterine artery Doppler in the investigation of pregancies with raised maternal serum alpha-fetoprotein. Brit. J. Obstet. Gynaecol. 97 (1990) 431–435
3. Bahlmann, F., Neubert, S., Steiner, E., Trautmann, K., Wellek, S.: Das uteroplazentare Dopplerflußprofil in einem Normalkollektiv – Berechnung von Referenzbereichen für Widerstandsindizes der A. uterina. (In Vorbereitung)
4. Beaufils, M., Uzan, S., Donsimoni, R., Colau, J.C.: Prevention of preeclampsia by early anti-platelet therapy. Lancet 1 (1985) 840–842
5. Beck, T.: Der materne Blutfluß durch die menschliche Plazenta. Z. Geburtsh. u. Perinat. 186 (1982) 65–71
6. Benedetto, C., Valensie, H., Marozio, L., Giarola, M., Massobrio, M., Romanini, C.: A two-stage screening test for pregnancy-induced hypertension and preeclampsia. Obstet. Gynecol. 92 (1998) 1005–1011
7. Bewley, S., Campbell, S., Cooper, D.: Uteroplacental Doppler flow velocity waveforms in the second trimester. A complex circulation. Brit. J. Obstet. Gynaecol. 96 (1989) 1040–1046
8. Bewley, S., Cooper, D., Campbell, S.: Doppler investigation of uteroplacental blood flow resistance in the second trimester: a screening study for pre-eclampsia and intrauterine growth retardation. Brit. J. Obstet. Gynaecol. 98 (1991) 871–879
9. Bewley, S., Chard, T., Grudzinskas, G., Cooper, D., Campbell, S.: Early prediction of uteroplacental complications of pregnancy using Doppler ultrasound, placental function tests and combination testing. Ultrasound Obstet. Gynecol. 2 (1992) 333–337
10. Bewley, S., Chard, T., Grudzinskas, G., Campbell, S.: The relationship of uterine and umbilical Doppler resistance to fetal and placental protein synthesis in the second trimester. Placenta 14 (1993) 663–670
11. Borell, U., Fernström, I., Westman, A.: Eine arteriographische Studie des Plazentarkreislaufes. Geburtsh. u. Frauenheilk. 18 (1958) 1–9
12. Borell, U., Fernstrom, I., Ohlson, L., Wiquist, N.: Influence of uterine contractions on the uteroplacental blood flow at term. Amer. J. Obstet. Gynecol. 93 (1965) 44–57
13. Bower, S., Campbell, S., Vyas, S., McGirr, C.: Braxton-Hicks contractions can alter uteroplacental perfusion. Ultrasound Obstet. Gynecol. 1 (1991) 46–49
14. Bower, S., Vyas, S., Campbell, S., Nicolaides, K.H.: Color Doppler imaging of the uterine artery in pregnancy: normal ranges of impedance to blood flow, mean velocity and volume of flow. Ultrasound Obstet. Gynecol. 2 (1992) 261–265
15. Bower, S., Schuchter, K., Campbell S.: Doppler ultrasound screening as part of routine antenatal scanning: prediction of pre-eclampsia and intrauterine growth retardation. Brit. J. Obstet. Gynaecol. 100 (1993) 989–994
16. Bower, S., Bewley, S., Campbell, S.: Improved prediction of preeclampsia by two-stage screening of uterine arteries using the early diastolic notch and color Doppler imaging. Obstet. Gynecol. 82 (1993) 78–83
17. Bower, S.J., Harrington, K.F., Schuchter, K., McGirr, C., Campbell, S.: Prediction of pre-eclampsia by abnormal uterine Doppler ultrasound and modification by aspirin. Brit. J. Obstet. Gynaecol. 103 (1996) 625–629
18. Boyd, P.A., Scott, A.: Quantitative structural studies on human placentas associated with preeclampsia, essential hypertension and intrauterine growth retardation. Brit. J. Obstet. Gynaecol. 92 (1985) 714–721
19. Boyd, P.A.: Why might maternal serum AFP be high in pregnancies in which the fetus is normally formed? Brit. J. Obstet. Gynaecol. 99 (1992) 93–95
20. Brar, H.S., Medearis, A.L., DeVore, G.R., Platt, L.D.: Maternal and fetal blood flow velocity waveforms in patients with preterm labor: Effects of tocolytics. Obstet. Gynecol. 72 (1988) 209–214
21. Bromley, B., Frigoletto, F.D., Harlow, B.L., Pauker, S., Benacerraf, B.R.: The role of Doppler velocimetry in the structurally normal second-trimester fetus with elevated levels of maternal serum α-fetoprotein. Ultrasound Obstet. Gynecol. 4 (1994) 377–380
22. Brosens, I., Robertson, W.B., Dixon, H.G.: The physiological response of the vessels of the placental bed to normal pregnancy. J. Pathol. Bacteriol. 93 (1967) 569–579
23. Brosens, I., Robertson, W.B., Dixon, H.G.: The role of spiral arteries in the pathogenesis of pre-eclampsia. Obstet. Gynecol. Annu. 1 (1972) 177–180
24. Brosens, I., Dixon, H.G., Robertson, W.B.: Fetal growth retardation and the arteries of the placental bed. Brit. J. Obstet. Gynaecol. 84 (1977) 656–663
25. Brosens I.: The utero-placental vessels at term – the distribution and extent of physiological changes. Trophoblast Res. 3 (1988) 61–68
26. Cacciatore, B., Halmesmäki, E., Kaala, R., Teramo, K., Ylikorkala: Effects of transdermal nitroglycerin on impedance to flow in the uterine, umbilical, and fetal middle cerebral arteries in pregnancies complicated by preeclampsia and intrauterine growth retardation. Amer. J. Obstet. Gynecol. 179 (1998) 140–145
27. Campbell, S., Diaz-Recasens, J., Griffin, D.R. et al.: New Doppler technique for assessing uteroplacental blood flow. Lancet 1 (1983) 675–677
28. Caritis, S., Sibai, B., Hauth, J. et al. and the National Institute of Child Health and Human Development Network of Maternal-Fetal Medicine Units: Low-dose Aspirin to prevent preeclampsia in women at high risk. New Engl. J. Med. 338 (1998) 701–705
29. Chan, F.Y., Pun, T.C., Lam, C., Khoo, J., Lee, C.P., Lam, Y.H.: Pregnancy screening by uterine artery Doppler velocimetry – which criterion performs best? Obstet. Gynecol. 85 (1995) 596–602
30. Clarke, R.J., May, G., Price, P., Fitzgerald, G.A.: Suppression of thromboxane A2 but not of systemic prostacyclin by controlled-release aspirin. New Engl. J. Med. 325 (1991) 1137–1141
31. CLASP trial: Collaborative low dose aspirin study in pregnancy. MRC collaborative group on low dose aspirin in pregnancy. Lancet 343 (1993) 619–629
32. Conde-Agudelo, A., Lede, R., Belizan, J.: Evaluation of methods used in the prediction of hypertensive disorders of pregnancy. Obstet. Gynecol. Surv. 49 (1994) 210–222
33. Dekker, G.A., Sibai, B.M.: Early detection of pre-eclampsia. Amer. J. Obstet. Gynecol. 165 (1991) 160–172
34. Deutinger, J., Rudelstorfer, R., Bernaschek, G.: Vaginosonographic velocimetry of both main uterine arteries by visual vessel recognition and pulsed Doppler method during pregnancy. Amer. J. Obstet. Gynecol. 159 (1988) 1072–1076
35. Deutinger, J., Rudelstorfer, R., Bernaschek, G.: Vergleich von Doppler-Strömungsmessungen in Arteria arcuata und in Arteria uterina bei fetaler Wachstumsretardation. Geburtsh. u. Frauenheilk. 48 (1988) 863–868
36. Deutinger, J., Rudelsdorfer, R., Pattermann, A., Bernaschek, G.: Vaginosonographic velocimetry in uterine arteries before and after administration of beta-mimetics. Brit. J. Obstet. Gynaecol. 99 (1992) 417–421
37. Duggan, P.M., McCovan, L.M.E., Stewart, A.W.: Antihypertensive velocity waveforms in pregnant women with severe hypertension. Aust. NZ. J. Obstet. Gynaecol. 32 (1992) 335–338
38. ECPPA: randomised trial of low dose aspirin for the prevention of maternal and fetal complications in high risk pregnant women. Brit. J. Obstet. Gynaecol. 103 (1996) 39–47
39. Fendel, H., Fettweis, P., Billet, P. et al.: Doppleruntersuchungen des arteriellen utero-feto-plazentaren Blutflusses vor und während der Geburt. Z. Geburtsh. u. Perinat. 191 (1987) 121–129
40. Fleischer, A., Schulman, H., Faramakides, G. et al.: Uterine artery Doppler velocimetry in pregnant women with hypertension. Amer. J. Obstet. Gynecol. 154 (1986) 806–813
41. Fleischer, A., Anyaegbunam, A., Schulman, H., Farmakides, G., Randolph G.: Uterine and umbilical artery velocimetry during normal labor. Amer. J. Obstet. Gynecol. 157 (1987) 40–43
42. Fok, R.Y., Pavlova, Z., Benirschke, K.: The correlation of arterial lesions with umbilical artery Doppler velocimetry in the placentas of small-for-dates pregnancies. Obstet. Gynecol. 75 (1990) 578–583
43. Freese, U.: The uteroplacental vascular relationship in the human. Amer. J. Obstet. Gynecol. 101 (1968) 8–16
44. Friedman, S.A.: Preeclampsia: a review of the role of prostaglandins. Obstet. Gynecol. 71 (1988) 122–137
45. Funk, A., Rath, W.: Dopplersonographie der uterinen Gefäße in der Frühschwangerschaft. Geburtsh. u. Frauenheilk. 57 (1997) 479–485
46. Gerretsen, G., Huisjes, H.J., Elema, J.G.: Morphological changes of the spiral arteries in the placental bed in relation to pre-eclampsia and fetal growth retardation. Brit. J. Obstet. Gynaecol. 88 (1981) 876–881
47. Gonser, M., Pfeiffer, K.H., Dietl, J., Hofstaetter C., Gross, M.: Effect of placental location on uteroplacental Doppler measurements and perinatal risk estimation. J. Matern. Fetal. Invest. 3 (1993) 9–13
48. Gonser, M., Tillack, N., Pfeiffer, K.H., Mielke, G.: Plazentalokalisation und Inzidenz der Präeklampsie. Ultraschall Med. 17 (1996) 236–238
49. Grab, D., Hütter, W., Keim, T., Stahl, C., Terinde, R.: Der Einfluß der Plazentalokalisation auf die uteroplazentare Durchblutung. Ultraschall Klin. Prax. 6 (1991) 105–108
50. Grunewald, C., Carlström, K., Lunell, N.O., Nisell, H., Nylund, L.: Dihydralazin in preeclampsia: acute effects on atrial natriuretic peptide concentration and fetomaternal hemodynamics. J. Matern. Fetal Invest. 3 (1993) 21–24
51. Grunewald, C., Kublickas, M., Carlström, K., Lunell, N.O., Nisell, H.: Effects of nitroglycerin on the uterine and umbilical circulation in severe preeclampsia. Obstet. Gynecol. 86 (1995) 600–604
52. Hamid, R., Robson, M., Pearce, J.M.: Low dose aspirin in women with raised maternal serum alpha-fetoprotein and abnormal Doppler waveform patterns from the uteroplacental circulation. Brit. J. Obstet. Gynaecol. 101 (1994) 481–484
53. Harrington, K., Campbell, S., Bewley, S., Bower, S.: Doppler velocimetry studies of the uterine artery in the early prediction of pre-eclampsia and intrauterine growth retardation. Eur. J. Obstet. Gynecol. Reprod. Biol. 42 (1991) 14–20
54. Harrington, K., Carpenter, R.G., Nguyen, M., Campbell, S.: Changes observed in Doppler studies of the fetal circulation in pregnancies complicated by pre-eclampsia or the delivery of a small-for-gestational-age baby. I. Cross-sectional analysis. Ultrasound Obstet. Gynecol. 6 (1995) 19–28
55. Harrington, K., Cooper, D., Lees, C., Hecher, K., Campbell, S.: Doppler ultrasound of the uterine arteries: the importance of bilateral notching in the prediction of pre-eclampsia, placental abruption or delivery of a small-for gestational-age baby. Ultrasound Obstet. Gynecol. 7 (1996) 182–188
56. Harrington, K., Carpenter, R.G., Goldfrad, C., Campbell, S.: Transvaginal Doppler ultrasound of the early prediction of pre-eclampsia and intrauterine growth retardation. Brit. J. Obstet. Gynaecol. 104 (1997) 674–681
57. Hitschold, T., Ulrich, S., Kalder, M., Müntefering, H., Berle, P.: Blutströmungsprofile der Arteria uterina. Korrelation zur Plazentamorphologie und zu klinisch-geburtshilflichen Daten im Rahmen der Präeklampsie. Z. Geburtsh. u. Neonat. 199 (1995) 8–12
58. Hsieh, F.J., Kuo, P.L., Ko, T.M., Chang, F.M., Chen, H.Y.: Doppler velocimetry of intraplacental fetal arteries. Obstet. Gynecol. 77 (1991) 478–482
59. Hütter, W., Grab, D., Sterzik, K., Terinde, R., Wolf, A.: Methodenkritische Anwendung des continuous-wave Dopplers in der Geburtsmedizin. Perinatal Medizin 3 (1991) 103–108
60. Hütter, W., Grab, D., Sterzik, K., Terinde, R., Wolf, A.: Uteroplacental diastolic notching in 510 uneventful pregnancies. J. Perinat. Med. 20 (1992) 387–395
61. Hütter, W., Grab, D., Schneider, D., Terinde, R., Wolf, A.: Continuous-wave Doppler investigation of uteroplacental vessels in high-risk pregnancies as predictor of fetal growth retardation and pregnancy-induced hypertension. Gynecol. Obstet. Invest. 38 (1994) 90–95
62. Irion, O., Masse, J., Forest, L.C., Moutquin, J.M.: Prediction of pre-eclampsia, low birth-weight for gestation and prematurity by artery blood flow velocity waveforms analysis in low risk nulliparous women. Brit. J. Obstet. Gynaecol. 105 (1998) 422–429

63. Jacobson, S.L., Imhof, R., Manning, N. et al.: The value of Doppler assessment of the uteroplacental circulation in predicting preeclampsia or intrauterine growth retardation. Amer. J. Obstet. Gynecol. 162 (1990) 110–114
64. Janbu, T., Nesheim, B.: Uterine artery blood velocities during contractions in pregnancy and labour related to intrauterine pressure. Brit. J. Obstet. Gynaecol. 94 (1987) 1150–1155
65. Jouppila, P.: New information obtained by Doppler and color Doppler methods on the effects of vasoactive agents in obstetrics. Ultrasound Obstet. Gynecol. 5 (1995) 289–293
66. Keeley, M.M., Wade, R.V., Laurent, S.L., Hamann, V.: Alterations in maternal-fetal Doppler flow velocity waveforms in preterm labor patients undergoing magnesium sulfate tocolysis. Obstet. Gynecol. 81 (1993) 191–194
67. Khong, T.Y., DeWolf, F., Robertson, W.B., Brosens, I.: Inadequate maternal vascular response to placentation in pregnancies complicated by pre-eclampsia and by small-for-gestational age infants. Brit. J. Obstet. Gynaecol. 93 (1986) 1049–1059
68. Kofinas, A.D., Penry, M., Greiss, F.C., Meis, P.J., Nelson, L.H.: The effect of placental location on uterine artery flow velocity waveforms. Amer. J. Obstet. Gynecol. 159 (1988) 1504–1508
69. Kofinas, A.D., Penry, M., Swain, M., Hatjis, C.G.: Effect of placental laterality on uterine artery resistance and development of preeclampsia and intrauterine growth retardation. Amer. J. Obstet. Gynecol. 161 (1989) 1536–1539
70. Kofinas, A.D., Espeland, M.A., Penry, M., Swain, M., Hatjis, C.G.: Uteroplacental Doppler flow velocity waveform indices in normal pregnancy: A statistical exercise and the development of appropriate reference values. Amer. J. Perinatol. 9 (1992) 94–101
71. Kofinas, A.D., Simon, N.V., Clay, D., King, K.: Functional asymmetry of the human myometrium documented by color and pulsed-wave Doppler ultrasonographic evaluation of uterine arcuate arteries during Braxton Hicks contractions. Amer. J. Obstet. Gynecol. 168 (1993) 184–188
72. Konchak, P.S., Bernstein, I.M., Capeless, M.D.: Uterine artery Doppler velocimetry in the detection of adverse obstetric outcomes in women with unexplained elevated maternal serum α-fetoprotein levels. Amer. J. Obstet. Gynecol. 173 (1995) 1115–1119
73. Kurjak, A., Dudenhausen, J.W., Kos, M. et al.: Doppler information pertaining to the intrapartum period. J. Perinat. Med. 24 (1996) 271–276
74. Kurjak, A., Dudenhausen, J.W., Hafner, T., Kupesic, S., Latin, V., Kos, M.: Intervillous circulation in all three trimesters of normal pregnancy assessed by color Doppler. J. Perinat. Med. 25 (1997) 373–380
75. Kurdi, W., Campbell, S., Aquilina, J., England, P., Harrington, K.: The role of color Doppler imaging of the uterine arteries at 20 weeks gestation in stratifying antenatal care. Ultrasound Obstet. Gynecol. 12 (1998) 339–345
76. Kurmanavichius, J., Baumann, H., Huch, R., Huch, A.: Uteroplacental blood flow velocity waveforms as a predictor of adverse fetal outcome and pregnancy-induced hypertension. J. Perinat. Med. 18 (1990) 255–260
77. Lees, C.C., Langford, E., Brown, A.S. et al.: The effect of S-Nitrosogluthatione on platelet activation, hypertension and uterine and fetal Doppler in severe preeclampsia. Obstet. Gynecol. 88 (1996) 14–19
78. Lees, C.C., Brown, A.S., Harrington, K.F., Beacon, H.J., Martin, J.F., Campbell, S.: A cross-sectional study of platelet volume in healthy normotensive women with bilateral uterine artery notches. Ultrasound Obstet. Gynecol. 10 (1997) 277–281
79. Lees, C., Valensise, H., Black, R. et al.: The efficacy and fetal-maternal cardiovascular effects of transdermal glyceryl trinitrate in the prophylaxis of pre-eclampsia and its complications: a randomized double-blind placebo-controlled trial. Ultrasound Obstet. Gynecol. 12 (1998) 334–338
80. Liberati, M., Rotmensch, S., Zannolli, P. et al.: Uterine artery Doppler velocimetry in pregnant women with lateral placentas. J. Perinat. Med. 25 (1997) 133–138
81. Lin, S., Shimuzu, I., Suehara, N., Nakayama, M., Aono, T.: Uterine artery Doppler velocimetry in relation to trophoblast migration in the myometrium of the placental bed. Obstet. Gynecol. 85 (1995) 760–765
82. Louden, K.A.: The use of low dose aspirin in pregnancy. Clin. Pharmacokinet. 23 (1992) 90–92
83. Lunell, N.O., Nylund, I.: Uteroplacental blood flow. Clin. Obstet. Gynecol. 35 (1992) 108–118
84. Mari, G., Kirshon, B., Wasserturm, N., Moise, K.J., Deter, R.L.: Uterine blood flow velocity waveforms in pregnant women during Indomethacin therapy. Obstet. Gynecol. 76 (1990) 33–36
85. McCowan, L.M., Ritchie, K., Mo, L.Y., Bascom, P.A., Sherret, H.: Uterine artery flow velocity waveforms in normal and growth-retarded pregnancies. Amer. J. Obstet. Gynecol. 158 (1988) 499–504
86. McParland, P., Pearce, J.M., Chamberlain, G.V.P.: Doppler ultrasound and aspirin in recognition and prevention of pregnancy-induced hypertension. Lancet 335 (1990) 1552–1555
87. Meekins, J.W., Pijnenborg, R., Hanssens, M., McFayden, I.R., Van Asshe, A.: A study of placental bed spiral arteries and trophoblastic invasion in normal and severe pre-eclamptic pregnancies. Brit. J. Obstet. Gynaecol. 101 (1994) 669–674
88. Mires, G.J., Christie, A.D., Leslie, J., Lowe, E., Patel, N.B., Howie, P.W.: Are "notched" uterine arterial waveforms of prognostic value for hypertensive and growth disorders of pregnancy. Fetal Diagn. Ther. 10 (1995) 111–118
89. Mires, G.J., Williams, F.L., Leslie, J., Howie, P.W.: Assessment of uterine arterial notching as a screening test for adverse pregnancy outcome. Amer. J. Obstet. Gynecol. 179 (1998) 1317–1323
90. Morris, J.M., Fay, R.A., Ellwood, D.A., Cook, C.M., Devonald, K.J.: A randomized controlled trial of aspirin in patients with abnormal uterine artery blood flow. Obstet. Gynecol. 87 (1996) 74–78
91. Murakoshi, T., Sekizuka, N., Takakuwa, K., Yoshizawa, H., Tanaka, K.: Uterine and spiral artery flow velocity waveforms in pregnancy-induced hypertension and/or intrauterine growth retardation. Ultrasound Obstet. Gynecol. 7 (1996) 122–128
92. North, R.A., Ferrier, C., Long, D., Townend, K., Kincaid-Smith, P.: Uterine Artery Doppler Flow velocity waveforms in the second trimester for the prediction of preeclampsia and fetal growth retardation. Obstet. Gynecol. 83 (1994) 378–386
93. Olofson, P., Laurini, R.N., Marsal, K.: A high uterine artery pulsatility index reflects a defective development of placental spiral arteries in pregnancies complicated by hypertension and fetal growth retardation. Eur. J. Obstet. Gynecol. 49 (1993) 161–168
94. Oosterhof, H., Dijkstra, K., Aarnoudse, J.G.: Uteroplacental Doppler velocimetry during Braxton Hicks' contraction. Gynecol. Obstet. Invest. 34 (1992) 155–158
95. Park, Y.W., Cho, J.S., Kim, H.S., Song, C.H.: The clinical implications of early diastolic notch in third trimester Doppler waveform analysis of the uterine artery. J. Ultrasound. Med. 15 (1996) 47–51
96. Pijnenborg, R., Dixon, G., Robertson, W.B., Brosens, I.: Trophoblastic invasion of human decidua from 8 to 18 weeks of pregnancy. Placenta 1 (1980) 3–19
97. Pirhonen, J.P., Erkkola, R.U., Ekblad, U.U., Nyman, L.: Single dose of nifedipine in normotensive pregnancy: Nifedipine concentrations, hemodynamic responses, and uterine and fetal flow velocity waveforms. Obstet. Gynecol. 76 (1990) 807–811
98. Pirhonen, J.P., Erkkola, R.U., Ekblad, U.U.: Uterine and fetal flow velocity waveforms in hypertensive pregnancy: The effect of a single dose of nifedipine. Obstet. Gynecol. 76 (1990) 37–41
99. Ramsey, B., De Belder, A., Campbell, S., Moncada, S., Martins, J.F.: A nitric oxide donor improves uterine artery diastolic blood flow in normal early pregnancy and in women at high risk of preeclampsia. Eur. J. Clin. Invest. 24 (1994) 76–78
100. Report on Confidential Enquiries into Maternal Deaths in the United Kingdom 1991–1994. London: HMSO, 1996
101. Rey, E.: Effects of methyldopa on umbilical and placental artery blood flow velocity waveforms. Obstet. Gynecol. 80 (1992) 783–787
102. Roberts, J.M.: Pre-eclampsia: more than pregnancy-induced hypertension. Lancet 341 (1993) 1447–1450
103. Robertson, W.B., Path, F.R.C., Khong, T.Y. et al.: The placental bed biopsy: Review from three European centers. Amer. J. Obstet. Gynecol. 155 (1986) 401–412
104. Robson, M., Hamid, R., McParland, P., Pearce, J.M.: Doppler ultrasound of the uteroplacental circulation in the prediction of pregnancy outcome in women with raised maternal serum alpha-fetoprotein. Brit. J. Obstet. Gynaecol. 101 (1994) 477–480
105. Salafia, C.M., Silberman, L., Herrera, N., Mahoney, J.: Placental pathology at term associated with elevated midtrimester maternal serum α-fetoprotein concentration. Amer. J. Obstet. Gynecol. 158 (1988) 1064–1066
106. Schiff, E., Peleg, E., Goldenberg, M. et al.: The use of aspirin to prevent pregnancy-induced hypertension and lower the ratio of thromboxane A2 to prostacyclin in relatively high risk pregnancies. New Engl. J. Med. 321 (1989) 351–356
107. Schuhmann, R.A.: Placenton: Begriff, Entstehung, funktionelle Anatomie. In: Becker, V., Schiebler, T., Kubli, F. (Hrsg.): Die Plazenta des Menschen. Stuttgart: Thieme 1981
108. Schulman, H., Fleischer, A., Farmakides, G., Bracero, L., Rochelson, B., Grunfeld, L.: Development of uterine artery compliance in pregnancy as detected by Doppler ultrasound. Amer. J. Obstet. Gynecol. 155 (1986) 1031–1036
109. Schulman, H., Ducey, J., Farmakides, G., Guzman, E., Winter, D., Penny, B.: Uterine artery Doppler velocimetry: The significance of divergent systolic/diastolic ratios. Amer. J. Obstet. Gynecol. 157 (1987) 1539–1542
110. Schulman, H., Winter, D., Farmakides, G. et al.: Pregnancy surveillance with doppler velocimetry of uterine and umbilical arteries. Amer. J. Obstet. Gynecol. 160 (1989) 192–196
111. Sheppard, B., Bonnar, J.: An ultrastructural study of utero-placental spiral arteries in hypertensive and normotensive pregnancy and fetal growth retardation. Brit. J. Obstet. Gynaecol. 88 (1981) 695–705
112. Steel, S.A., Pearce, J.M., McParland, P., Chamberlain, G.V.P.: Early doppler ultrasound screening in prediction of hypertensive disorders of pregnancy. Lancet 335 (1990) 1548–1551
113. Thaler, I., Manor, D., Itskovitz, J. et al.: Changes in uterine blood flow during human pregnancy. Amer. J. Obstet. Gynecol. 162 (1990) 121–125
114. Thaler, I., Weiner, Z., Itskovitz, J.: Systolic or diastolic notch in uterine artery blood flow velocity waveforms in hypertensive pregnant patients: Relationship to outcome. Obstet. Gynecol. 80 (1992) 277–282
115. Thaler, I., Amit, A., Jakobi, P., Itskovitz-Eldor, J.: The effect of isosorbide dinitrate on uterine artery and umbilical artery flow velocity waveforms at mid-pregnancy. Obstet. Gynecol. 88 (1996) 838–843
116. Thomas, F., Petrulis, A.S.: A meta-analysis of low dose aspirin for the prevention of pregnancy induced hypertensive desease. JAMA 266 (1991) 261–265
117. Todros, T., Ferrazzi, E., Arduini, D. et al.: Performance of Doppler ultrasonography as a screening test in low risk pregnancies results of a multicentre study. J. Ultrasound Med. 14 (1995) 343–348
118. Trudinger, B.J., Giles, W.B., Cook, C.M.: Uteroplacental blood flow velocity-time waveforms in normal and complicated pregnancy. Brit. J. Obstet. Gynaecol. 92 (1985) 39–45
119. Trudinger, B.J., Giles, W.B., Cook, C.M.: Flow velocity waveforms in the maternal uteroplacental and fetal umbilical placental circulations. Amer. J. Obstet. Gynecol. 152 (1985) 155–163
120. Trudinger, B.J., Cook, C.M., Thompson, R.S., Giles, W.B., Connelly, A.: Low dose aspirin therapy improves weight in umbilical placental insufficiency. Amer. J. Obstet. Gynecol. 161 (1988) 681–685
121. Uzan, S., Beaufils, M., Breart, G., Bazin, B., Capitant, C., Paris, J.: Prevention of fetal growth retardation with low-dose aspirin: findings of the EPREDA trial. Lancet 337 (1991) 1427–1431
122. Uzan, M., Haddad, B., Breart, G., Uzan, S.: Uteroplacental Doppler and aspirin therapy in the prediction and prevention of pregnancy complications. Ultrasound Obstet. Gynecol. 4 (1994) 342–349
123. Valensise, H., Bezzeccheri, V., Rizzo, G., Tranquilli, A.L., Garzetti, G.G., Romanini, C.: Doppler velocimetry of the uterine artery as a screening test for gestational hypertension. Ultrasound Obstet. Gynecol. 3 (1993) 18–22

124. Valensise, H.: Uterine artery Doppler velocimetry as a screening test: where we are and where we go? Ultrasound Obstet. Gynecol. 12 (1998) 81–83

125. Voigt, H.J., Becker, V.: Uteroplacental insufficiency comparison of uteroplacental blood flow velocity and histomorphology of placental bed. J. Matern. Invest. 2 (1992) 251–255

126. Wallenburg, H.C.S., Dekker, G.A., Markovitz, J.W., Rotmans, P.: Low-dose aspirin prevents pregnancy-induced hypertension and preeclampsia in angiotensin-sensitive primigravidae. Lancet 1 (1986) 1–3

127. Walsh, S.W.: Physiology of low-dose aspirin therapy for the prevention of preeclampsia. Sem. Perinat. 14 (1990) 152–170

128. Zimmermann, P., Eiriö, V., Koskinen, J., Kujansuu, E., Ranta, E.: Doppler assessment of the uterine and uteroplacental circulation in the second trimester in pregnancies at high risk for pre-eclampsia and/or intrauterine growth retardation: comparison and correlation between different Doppler parameters. Ultrasound Obstet. Gynecol. 9 (1997) 330–338

43 Fetal Circulation

Surveillance of high-risk pregnancies. Doppler ultrasound of the fetal vascular system is an important adjunct for the evaluation of high-risk pregnancies in obstetrics and prenatal medicine. Various studies have shown that fetal Doppler ultrasound, especially of the uterine artery, plays an important role in the management of high-risk pregnancies (51). Other studies have shown that umbilical Doppler ultrasound in a normal population of pregnant women has no effect on the pregnancy outcome and consequently is not recommended for routine prenatal care (61, 62). The selective use of fetal Doppler leads to a significant reduction in prenatal mortality and morbidity (50, 127) (Fig. 43.**1**). For example, Korsdorp et al. (90) found in a multicenter study that when Doppler velocimetry was included in the surveillance of high-risk pregnancies, there was a significant reduction in antepartum testing, labor induction, cesarean sections for fetal distress, and neurologic injuries.

To interpret Doppler findings correctly and integrate them into obstetric management, it is essential to know the physiologic and pathophysiologic aspects of fetal hemodynamics and the proper clinical use of the Doppler technique.

Aspects of Fetal Physiology

The exchange of gas and nutrients in the placenta occurs partly through passive diffusion and partly through active transport processes. The oxygen- and nutrient-enriched blood enters the fetal circulation from the placenta via the umbilical vein. The fetal circulation, unlike the postnatal circulation, is characterized by the presence of three major shunts through the ductus venosus, foramen ovale, and ductus arteriosus, and by a parallel functional arrangement of the pulmonary and systemic cardiac circulations (Fig. 43.**2**).

Right heart dominance. The hemodynamics of the fetal circulation results in a dominance of the right heart. In experiments in fetal sheep, the right ventricular stroke volume accounted for approximately two-thirds of the combined ventricular output while the left ventricular stroke volume supplied about one-third (157, 172). Right heart dominance has also been found in human fetuses, but the right ventricular stroke volume exceeds the left ventricular stroke volume by only 28% (91).

Specific shunts and streamlining effect. The ductus venosus represents the first of three specific shunts in the fetal circulation. It performs an important regulatory function in the distribution of oxygen-enriched blood. Experiments in fetal sheep have shown that approximately 55% of the oxygenated umbilical vein blood flows through the ductus venosus while approximately 45% flows into the left and right halves of the liver (52). The funnel-shaped narrowing of the ductus venosus causes a marked acceleration of blood flow, which causes a streamlining of blood flow in the dorsal, medial part of the inferior vena cava. About 27% of the stream that enters the right atrium passes directly through the foramen ovale into the left atrium. Additional deoxygenated blood from the pulmonary veins flows into the left atrium, accounting for 8% of the total output. The left ventricle, then, receives 35% of the total output. Approximately 8% of the left ventricular output in the fetus is distributed to the coronary arteries, 63% enters the cerebral circulation,

and the remaining 29% is pumped through the aortic arch into the descending aorta. This ensures an optimum oxygen supply to the brain and myocardium. The much slower blood flow velocities in the distal inferior vena cava create a stream in the ventral, lateral part of the inferior vena cava that is directed into the right atrium (157, 172) (Fig. 43.**3**). The crista dividens, located at the lower part of the foramen ovale, helps to separate the two streams. Deoxygenated blood from the superior vena cava, inferior vena cava, and coronary sinus enters the right atrium and passes into the right ventricle through the tricuspid valve. The right ventricle supplies approximately 65% of the combined ventricular output in fetal sheep (172).

Due to the high vascular resistance in the pulmonary vascular system, only about 13% of the right ventricular output enters the pulmonary arteries while 87% enters the descending aorta through the ductus arteriosus. In fetal sheep, approximately 60% of the deoxygenated right ventricular output and 19% of the oxygenated left ventricular output are returned to the placenta for a renewed exchange of gas and nutrients.

Doppler Ultrasound of the Arterial System

▬ *Umbilical Artery*

Normal findings. The two umbilical arteries are used in evaluating fetoplacental hemodynamics (Fig. 43.**4**). Doppler sampling of the uterine artery waveform is the simplest vascular examination for the assessment of fetal condition. The frequency spectrum of the umbilical artery displays a sawtooth pattern and is characterized by a relatively low pulsatility compared with the fetal aorta (Fig. 43.**5**). During the course of a normal pregnancy, the end-diastolic flow velocity in the umbilical artery increases in relation to the systolic velocity (Fig. 43.**6**). This physiologic increase in diastolic blood flow reflects a reduction of peripheral vascular resistance due to increasing villous differentiation in the placenta. It is also caused by an increase in vascular calibers, increased cardiac output and compliance, and by the progressive rise of fetal blood pressure that occurs during pregnancy. As a result of these mechanisms, the resistance indices PI and RI decline with advancing gestational age (Fig. 43.**7**). Resistance indices within the 90% confidence interval and values below the 5% confidence limit are interpreted as normal findings.

Sources of error. Resistance indices above the 95th percentile are abnormal and suggestive of fetal distress. It is important, however, to rule out common sources of error such as a too-low insonation angle, fetal breathing movements and body movements, wall filter setting > 120 Hz, poorly defined Doppler waveform, or a heart rate outside normal limits (Fig. 43.**8**). It is also important to obtain a standard recording of umbilical blood flow velocities, particularly since the resistance indices in the umbilical artery normally decrease from the fetus to the placenta (119). For simplicity, the Doppler spectrum is sampled from a free loop of umbilical cord. In cases where standard reference curves are used for the umbilical artery, care should be taken that the method of measurement is applied accurately so that valid data are obtained. Because the umbilical cord is often twisted, an optimum umbilical artery

Fig. 43.**1**   Effect of Doppler ultrasound of the umbilical artery on perinatal mortality in a high-risk population. Cumulative meta-analysis (from 50).

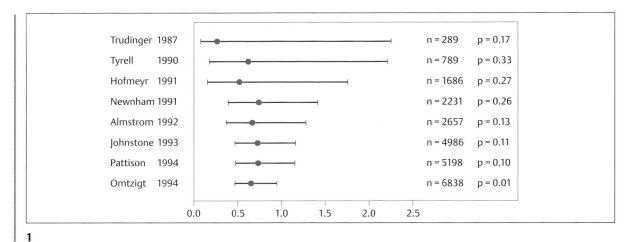

1

Fig. 43.**2**   Parallel arrangement of the fetal circulation (after 172).

Fig. 43.**3**   Percentage distribution of output from the fetal cardiac chambers, great vessels, and central shunts in the sheep (after 172).

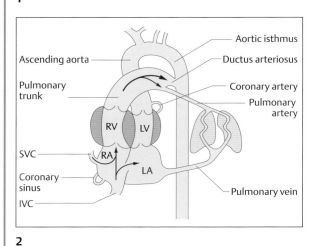

2

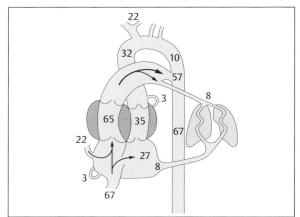

3

Umbilical artery

Fig. 43.**4**   Color Doppler image of a normal free loop of umbilical cord, demonstrating the two arteries (blue) and one vein (red) at 28 weeks.

Fig. 43.**5**   Normal color Doppler frequency spectrum sampled from the umbilical artery (shown here in red) at 27 weeks.

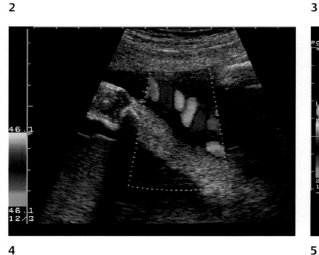

4

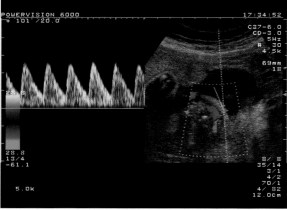

5

Fig. 43.**6**   Umbilical artery waveform patterns as a function of gestational age. Note the steady, physiologic increase in peak systolic flow velocities and especially in diastolic velocities with advancing gestational age. The absence of diastolic flow at 10 weeks' gestation is a normal finding.

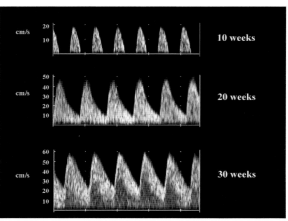

6

waveform cannot always be acquired. An alternative in these cases is to sample the descending aorta. Fetal breathing movements can produce variable wave-like distortions in spectra recorded from the umbilical artery and vein and in extreme cases can cause a phasic absence of end-diastolic flow. These distortions are caused by changes in the intra-abdominal pressure.

Abnormal waveforms. Histopathologic studies of the placenta have shown that a greater than 60% obliteration of the placental vascular bed leads to increased impedance in the umbilical cord arteries with a consequent decrease in end-diastolic flow or even reverse flow (57, 107).

An abnormal umbilical waveform is characterized by a decrease, absence, or reversal of end-diastolic flow (Figs. 43.**9**, 43.**11**, 43.**12**). These changes basically reflect a progressive deterioration of fetal well-being in the setting of intrauterine growth retardation, which is usually a result of chronic placental insufficiency. The functional disturbance in the fetomaternal unit is a continuous process characterized by a progressive loss of compensatory reserve capacity. The timing of cardiovascular decompensation in the fetus varies considerably from case to case and depends on the severity of the placental pathology, the compensatory capacity of the individual fetus, the gestational age, and the underlying maternal disease.

Absent end-diastolic flow and reverse flow. When absent or reverse end-diastolic flow is noted in the Doppler spectra, it should be confirmed that the spectra have been optimally recorded under resting conditions. This includes the use of a low wall filter setting (< 100 Hz, Fig. 43.**10**) and an acute insonation angle less than 60° and preferably less than 30°. Also, it is good practice to repeat the Doppler measurement once or twice to confirm an abnormal flow pattern. Absent end-diastolic flow has an estimated incidence of 5–8%, reverse end-diastolic flow approximately 0.5%. Absence of end-diastolic flow can often be detected prior to 32 weeks (190). Perinatal mortality is markedly increased in these cases and ranges from 30% to 50%, especially when reverse flow is present (90). When reverse flow is detected in the umbilical artery, it is predictive of fetal death within a few days in more than 50% of cases. There are isolated reports of cases being followed for several weeks (25, 90, 190).

Cordocentesis. Abnormal waveforms have been objectively documented by cordocentesis and correlated with the results of fetal blood gas analysis and fetal biochemistry (3, 30, 150, 151). It has been shown that severely abnormal waveforms are associated with a high rate of decreased pH and pO_2 levels and elevated pCO_2, lactate and erythropoietin levels in the fetus. Conversely, normal waveforms appear to correlate with a good fetal outcome (35).

Conclusion. Abnormal umbilical artery waveforms provide early evidence of fetal compromise and correlate with an increased rate of obstetric and neonatal problems and with impaired neuromotor development (13, 28). Abnormal umbilical artery waveforms have a strong association with pregnancy-induced hypertension and preeclampsia (51, 73, 176). A planned cesarean delivery should be considered whenever absent end-diastolic flow is detected in the umbilical artery after 32 weeks' gestation, and a primary cesarean section is definitely indicated in cases where reverse flow is found.

Doppler Umbilical Artery Velocimetry Compared with Fetal Heart Rate Monitoring

Useful adjunct. Electronic fetal heart rate (FHR) monitoring, while controversial in a scientific sense, continues to be the mainstay for antepartum fetal surveillance in obstetric departments. Doppler velocimetry of the umbilical artery is an effective adjunct to FHR

Table 43.1   Comparison of fetal surveillance by Doppler and CTG (4)

	Doppler group (n = 214)	CTG group (n = 212)	p-value
Number of antenatal examinations (mean)	4.1	8.2	< 0.001
Hospital stay in days (mean)	9.0	9.6	0.48
Hospitalizations for surveillance (%)	69 (31.3%)	97 (45.8%)	< 0.01
Induction of labor (n)	22 (10.3%)	46 (21.7)	< 0.01
Emergency cesarean sections for impending fetal asphyxia (%)	11 (5.1%)	30 (14.2%)	< 0.01

monitoring in cases where fetal compromise is recognized (175). In a randomized prospective study by Swedish authors comparing electronic FHR monitoring with Doppler umbilical artery velocimetry in small-for-gestational-age fetuses, the group that received Doppler velocimetry was found to have fewer antepartum tests, shorter antenatal hospital stays, fewer inductions, fewer emergency cesarean sections, and fewer transfers to neonatal ICU with no increase in perinatal mortality and morbidity (4) (Table 43.**1**). Moreover, both open and blind prospective studies have shown that fetal compromise and impending intrauterine asphyxia can be detected significantly earlier by Doppler umbilical artery velocimetry than by FHR monitoring (11, 110) (Fig. 43.**11**). On the other hand, abnormal FHR patterns can be found in approximately 6% of IUGR fetuses that have normal-appearing umbilical artery Doppler waveforms (27). Consequently, fetal Doppler velocimetry should not be used as a solitary method for fetal surveillance, but it does provide a useful adjunct to FHR monitoring in the assessment of fetal well-being.

Earlier onset of changes. The time interval between the appearance of abnormal umbilical artery waveforms and the initial occurrence of FHR decelerations varies considerably in different fetuses. It has been shown by multivariant analysis that gestational age, the presence of pregnancy-induced hypertension or preeclampsia, and the detection of umbilical vein pulsations are the major factors that determine the interval to the onset of late decelerations (14). FHR pattern changes in cases with abnormal umbilical artery waveforms are found to consist initially of a decrease in oscillation frequency and amplitude, followed by decelerations (Fig. 43.**12**). Decreased variability and the absence of accelerations may also be noted as unfavorable FHR criteria. Oligohydramnios also appears to adversely affect the FHR pattern (26).

Conclusion. A major drawback of antepartum FHR monitoring is the high rate of false-positive findings. In addition, FHR monitoring is less reproducible than Doppler velocimetry and shows higher interobserver variability (161). For these reasons, it is reasonable to expect that as Doppler ultrasound becomes more widely utilized in ambulatory and inpatient prenatal care, there will be further improvements in the quality of antepartum fetal surveillance.

Umbilical Cord Complications

Umbilical cord compression. A postsystolic notch can sometimes be recognized in the umbilical artery waveform (1, 99, 154) (Fig. 43.**13**). This appears to be a sign of cord compression, which may be caused by knotting or coiling of the cord. The pathophysiologic mechanism is not yet fully understood, but it is assumed that narrowing of the arterial lumen leads to prestenotic turbulence that facilitates reverse flow, resulting in a postsystolic notch. The clinical significance of this abnormality is also unclear, but it appears to be useful for the prediction of umbilical cord complications, especially in the management of monoamniotic twin pregnancies (1, 99).

Coiling of the umbilical cord. One or more coils in the umbilical cord are observed around the time of delivery in approximately 20–30% of all pregnancies. This condition is known to correlate with obstetric complications, abnormal FHR patterns, protracted labor, increased rates of acidosis, and abnormalities of neurologic development (103). Coiling of the umbilical cord can be diagnosed in more than 90% of cases with color Doppler ultrasound (134). It is most clearly appreciated in a transverse scan of the bladder neck region. The umbilical vessels appear as colored, ring-like structures on both sides of the neck (see Chapter 35). Abnormal umbilical artery waveforms are not commonly detected antenatally, occurring chiefly in the intrapartum period or when multiple coils are present. Coiling of the cord is most likely to be missed or misinterpreted when oligohydramnios or anhydramnios is present or when the fetal head is deeply engaged. Color-flow imaging of the umbilical vessels to exclude coiling of the cord is mainly indicated in the intrapartum period when type I decelerations and variable decelerations have been noted. Color Doppler in this setting can help to evaluate the obstetric situation and assist in the planning of further management.

Single Umbilical Artery

Incidence and associated complications. Single umbilical artery has a reported incidence of 0.5% to 2.5% in the literature (133). Absence of the left umbilical artery (73%) is more common than absence of the right artery (27%) (2). Due to the markedly increased rate of congenital anomalies, chromosomal abnormalities, intrauterine growth retardation, prematurity, and increased perinatal mortality, the affected fetuses are considered high-risk and should undergo a detailed ultrasound evaluation. If ultrasound reveals morphologic abnormalities, invasive cytogenetic testing should be performed (2, 133). If the fetus shows no morphologic abnormalities, the obstetric risk and perinatal outcome do not appear to be increased (132).

Evaluation of the pelvic vessels. If it is difficult to visualize the umbilical vessels with B-mode ultrasound, color Doppler can be added (Fig. 43.**14**) (162, 178). Color imaging of the fetal pelvic vessels can also be a useful adjunct (Fig. 43.**15**) (162, 163). In Doppler studies of the common iliac arteries and femoral arteries, significantly higher pulsatility indices have been found on the side of the absent umbilical artery—i.e., the side that does not contribute to the fetoplacental circulation (162, 163). It has also been shown that the pulsatility index of the common iliac artery on the side where the umbilical artery is present declines significantly during the course of pregnancy, while on the side where the artery is absent it remains high and shows a markedly higher vascular resistance, especially in the third trimester (165). Besides having a larger caliber, the common iliac artery that contributes to the fetoplacental circulation has been found to exhibit degenerative histopathologic changes in the form of calcifications and atherosclerotic lesions (122, 125). These findings have prompted speculation on a possible association with later cardiovascular changes (e.g., early atherosclerotic lesions, arterial hypertension, iliac vein thrombosis) in childhood and adulthood (165). Developmental disturbances of the lower extremities based on abnormal intrauterine hemodynamics have not been observed, however.

Compensatory arterial dilatation. Based on studies published to date, Doppler flow measurements in the single umbilical artery, both in fetuses with normal somatic development and in SGA fetuses, have shown no significant differences relative to fetuses with two umbilical arteries (162, 178). However, PI values below the 50th percentile have been demonstrated in 84% of fetuses with a single umbilical artery (44). This tendency toward somewhat lower fetoplacental vascular resistance is best explained by the slightly larger caliber of the single umbilical artery (approximately 1 mm) due to compensatory dilatation

(44). While normal Doppler indices in the single umbilical artery imply a normal obstetric course and a good fetal and neonatal outcome, abnormal umbilical Doppler indices correlate with a less favorable prognosis in the fetal and neonatal period (178). Abnormal Doppler indices are found chiefly in fetuses with growth retardation, an anomaly, or a chromosomal abnormality (178).

▬ *Descending Aorta*

Quantitative analysis of blood flow. The first quantitative studies of blood flow in the fetal aorta were performed in the mid-1980s by Eik-Nes et al. (53, 54) and Griffin et al. (65). These studies indicate that volume flow in the aorta correlates with the diameter of the vessel. Values for the third trimester range from 191 to 246 mL/min/kg (106) (Table 43.**2**). Both the aortic volume flow and the mean flow velocity increase slightly toward the end of pregnancy (Table 43.**2**), while the mean diameter of the fetal aorta increases markedly from 4.9 mm to 7.6 mm between 28 and 40 weeks' gestation (55). However, the blood flow in the fetal aorta can be difficult to assess quantitatively due to imprecise intrauterine weight estimation, the effect of the insonation angle on flow velocities, and especially the imprecise determination of the aortic diameter (55). Errors of up to 35% have been found in the determination of fetal aortic volume flow. It appears that an optimum frequency spectrum can be recorded in only 82% of cases (55). Based on the large scatter of the measurements and the poor reproducibility of the test results, most investigators have abandoned this quantitative analysis in favor of a semiquantitative waveform analysis based on the resistance indices RI and PI (54).

Accurate B-mode visualization. A spectrum can be recorded from the fetal aorta using either gray-scale or color Doppler. First, however, the aorta must be accurately defined in the B-mode image (Figs. 43.**16**–43.**20**). After piercing the diaphragm, the aorta runs immediately anterior or to the left of the spinal column. It is most easily located when the fetus is in a dorsoposterior lie. Starting from a transverse scan through the fetal abdomen, the transducer is rotated to the sagittal plane to give a longitudinal view of the aorta. A frequency spectrum is recorded from the fetal descending aorta by placing the Doppler gate at the level of the diaphragm (54, 105, 118, 173) using an insonation angle < 60° and preferably < 30° (Figs. 43.**19**, 43.**20**). It is important to use a standard plane of measurement, as the aortic vascular resistance and flow velocity decrease with greater distance from the heart (Fig. 43.**21**) (20). This is caused by the vessels arising below the diaphragm (celiac trunk, superior and inferior mesenteric arteries, renal artery) and by the morphologic change in the aortic wall. The wall filter should be set to 120 Hz or less, depending the instrument. When the fetal aorta has been located and defined, the scanning angle is adjusted relative to the course of the vessel (Figs. 43.**19**, 43.**20**). In this way the size of the insonation angle can be accurately controlled. With a dorsoanterior fetus, it can be difficult or impossible to visualize the aorta because of acoustic shadowing from the fetal spine. The be-

Table 43.**2** Fetal aortic blood flow in the third trimester

Author	Year	Number of cases (n)	Weeks' gestation	Blood flow mL/kg/min
Eik-Nes	1980	26	32–41	191 ± 12.2
Wladimiroff	1981	4	34–40	168
Eldrige	1981	22		166 ± 6
Marsal	1981	64	27–40	240
Griffin	1983	45	24–42	246 ± 3.5
Van Lierde	1984	20	37–40	216 ± 24
Erskine	1985	15	28–40	206
Lingman	1986	21	28	241
Lingman	1986	21	40	213

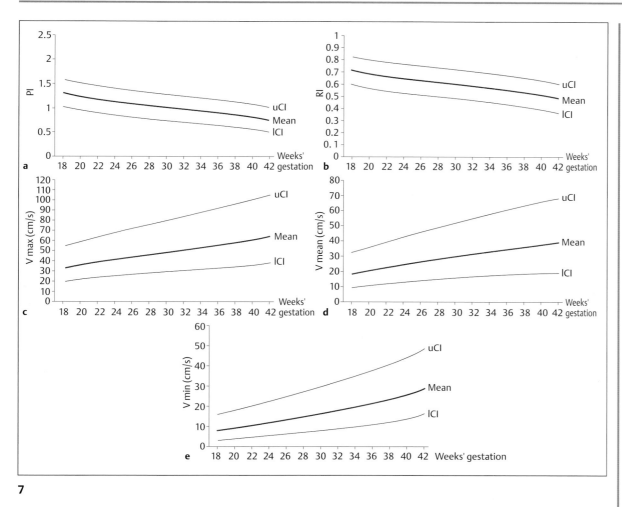

7

Fig. 43.**7** Reference ranges for resistance indices and blood flow velocities in the umbilical artery. uCI = upper confidence interval, lCI = lower confidence interval (90% of normal values are within the confidence intervals) (after 22).
a Reference range for the pulsatility index (PI).
b Reference range for the resistance index (RI).
c Reference range for the peak systolic blood flow velocity (cm/s).
d Reference range for the mean intensity-weighted blood flow velocity (cm/s).
e Reference range for end-diastolic blood flow velocity (cm/s).

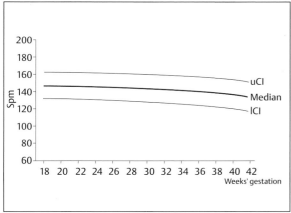

8

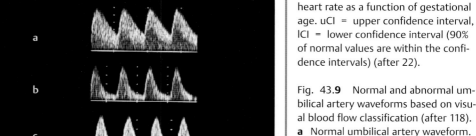

9

Fig. 43.**8** Reference range for fetal heart rate as a function of gestational age. uCI = upper confidence interval, lCI = lower confidence interval (90% of normal values are within the confidence intervals) (after 22).

Fig. 43.**9** Normal and abnormal umbilical artery waveforms based on visual blood flow classification (after 118).
a Normal umbilical artery waveform.
b Decreased end-diastolic velocity.
c Absent end-diastolic velocity.
d Reverse end-diastolic flow (reverse flow).

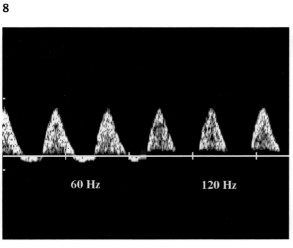

10

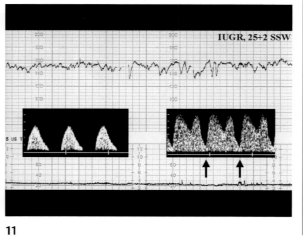

11

Fig. 43.**10** Effect of wall filter setting on end-diastolic flow velocity in a case with absent diastolic flow. With the higher wall filter setting, the end-diastolic velocities are filtered out, creating the appearance of absent flow instead of reverse flow.

Fig. 43.**11** FHR recording compared with Doppler frequency spectra from a severely growth-retarded fetus at 25 weeks, 2 days. The umbilical artery (left) shows absent end-diastolic flow. The flow velocities in the ductus venosus (right) are decreased but still positive during atrial contraction (A wave, arrows). The FHR recording shows a normal pattern of oscillations and accelerations.

Fig. 43.**12** FHR recording compared with arterial and venous Doppler spectra from a growth-retarded fetus at 28 weeks, 2 days. The spectra indicate reverse flow in the umbilical artery and descending aorta with a brain-sparing effect in the middle cerebral artery. The venous system also shows a very abnormal Doppler frequency pattern. The ductus venosus shows high pulsatility with a retrograde component during atrial contraction. The other spectra show double pulsations in the umbilical vein and an increased retrograde component in the inferior vena cava during atrial contraction. The FHR recording is abnormal, showing decreased variability and slight deceleration.

Fig. 43.**13** Simultaneous Doppler spectra recorded from the umbilical artery and vein. Note the postsystolic notch in the umbilical artery, which may signify a knotted or coiled umbilical cord.

Fig. 43.**14** Color Doppler view of the umbilical cord, showing one artery (red) and one vein (blue) at 29 weeks. This finding indicates a single umbilical artery.

Fig. 43.**15** Same fetus as in Fig. 43.**14**. Color Doppler view of the right umbilical artery adjacent to the fetal bladder. The left umbilical artery on the other side of the bladder neck is absent.

Aorta

Fig. 43.**16** Color Doppler view of blood flowing from the left ventricle into the ascending aorta.

Fig. 43.**17** Color Doppler view of the fetal aortic arch with the origins of the brachiocephalic trunk (1), left common carotid artery (2), and left subclavian artery (3). The fetus is in a dorsoposterior lie.

Fig. 43.**18** Color Doppler view of the descending aorta with the origin of the celiac trunk (1) and superior mesenteric artery (2).

Fig. 43.**19** Normal Doppler spectrum of the fetal aorta at 26 weeks, 4 days, with an excellent insonation angle (35°).

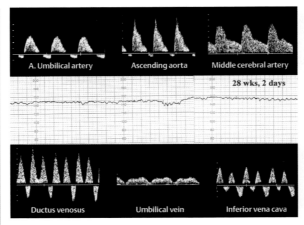

12

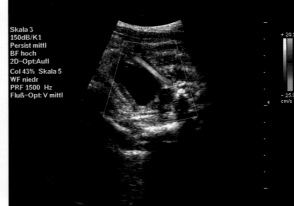

13

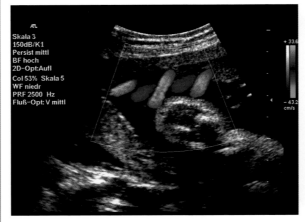

14

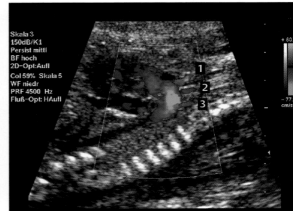

15

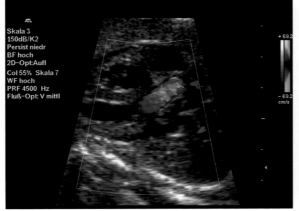

16

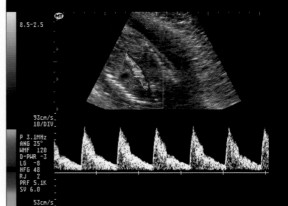

17

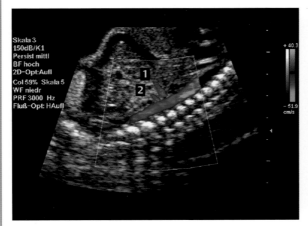

18

19

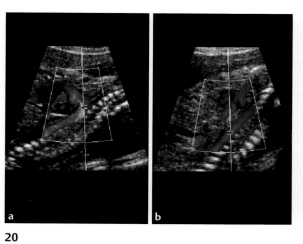

20

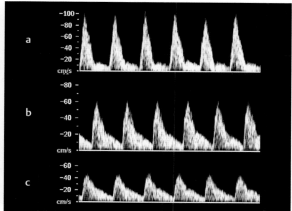

21

Fig. 43.**20** Placement of the sample volume for recording an aortic Doppler spectrum.
a In the aortic arch.
b In the descending aorta at the level of the diaphragm (= reference plane).

Fig. 43.**21** Doppler spectra recorded from various sites in the fetal aorta.
a = Level of the aortic arch, **b** = level of the diaphragm, **c** = below the renal vessels. The pulsatility of the aortic blood flow decreases with increasing distance from the heart.

Fig. 43.**22** Reference ranges for resistance indices and blood flow velocities in the descending aorta.
uCI = upper confidence interval, lCI = lower confidence interval (90% of normal values are within the confidence intervals) (after 20).
a Pulsatility index (PI).
b Resistance index (RI).
c Peak systolic blood flow velocity (cm/s).
d Mean intensity-weighted blood flow velocity (cm/s).
e End-diastolic blood flow velocity (cm/s).

22

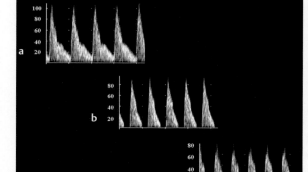

23

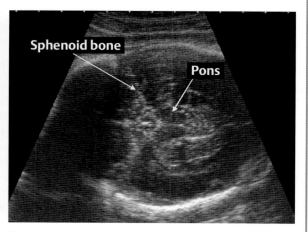

24

Fig. 43.**23** Normal and abnormal Doppler spectra recorded from the fetal aorta at the level of the diaphragm.
a Normal Doppler spectrum.
b Zero diastolic flow.
c Reverse flow.

Cerebral vessels

Fig. 43.**24** Normal B-mode ultrasound image of the circle of Willis. The real-time image clearly demonstrates the rhomboid-shaped vascular structures anterior to the pons.

ginner in particular can find it difficult to define the fetal aorta accurately and record an optimum Doppler velocity spectrum. For these reasons, the fetal aorta should not be considered a "learner's vessel."

Typical waveform. The waveform of the fetal aorta is characterized by a steep systolic up slope with a postsystolic notch and by relatively low antegrade end-diastolic flow velocities (Figs. 43.**19**, 43.**21**). The systolic upstroke phase (acceleration time) reflects the contractility of the heart, and the subsequent diastolic phase reflects the peripheral vascular resistance. Viewed over the cardiac cycle, the aortic waveform changes from profile flow in systole to paraboloid flow in diastole. The postsystolic notch is caused by aortic valve closure during early ventricular diastole and marks a slight decrease in blood flow velocity. It is most conspicuous at the thoracic level (Fig. 43.**21**). The frequency spectrum is influenced by the stroke volume and contractility of the fetal heart and by the compliance of the vessel, the viscosity of the blood, and the impedance of the downstream arterial system.

Resistance indices and flow velocities. The resistance indices (RI, PI) are used to evaluate vascular resistance and fetal condition. The resistance indices show no significant changes during the second half of pregnancy (Fig. 43.**22**) (20, 174). The determination of absolute flow velocities (Fig. 43.**22**) can be helpful in the assessment of fetal anemia and to evaluate hemodynamics following intrauterine blood transfusions. In particular, a fetal Hb level below 5 g% is associated with an increase in blood flow velocities. The accurate assessment of fetal anemia requires the use of a standard measurement plane and a constant, defined insonation angle. Intrauterine growth retardation, meanwhile, is associated with decreased mean flow velocities and severely abnormal Doppler flow patterns. Much as in the umbilical artery, a decrease in end-diastolic flow velocities is considered a sign of fetal compromise (Fig. 43.**23**).

Blood flow classes. Joupilla et al. first reported on absent or reversed end-diastolic flow velocities in 1984 and 1986 (86, 87). Based on these observations, Jaurin et al. (102) and Marsal et al. (118) proposed in 1987 a semiquantitative visual classification of the aortic Doppler spectrum into various blood flow classes. These classes, numbered 0 through IV, are characterized as follows:

- Blood flow class 0:   Normal frequency spectrum of the fetal aorta with normal resistance indices
- Blood flow class I: End-diastolic flow velocities decreased, resistance indices increased above normal
- Blood flow class II: Slight loss of end-diastolic flow
- Blood flow class III: Complete loss of end-diastolic flow
- Blood flow class IV: Reverse end-diastolic flow

Blood flow classes III and IV in particular appear to correlate with abnormal FHR patterns and a decrease in the mean aortic flow velocity (Fig. 43.**12**). In one study, FHR abnormalities were recorded after an average of 3 days, with a range between 0 and 43 days (102). Abnormal aortic flow patterns appear to precede abnormal FHR recordings by a period of days to weeks (86). It has also been shown that declining mean flow velocities in the aorta correlate with the severity of hypoxemia, hypercapnia, and lactic acidosis (168).

Cerebral Vessels

Cerebral blood flow. Cerebral blood flow in the fetus is modulated by a variety of factors. Besides autoregulatory mechanisms, the interaction among pO_2, pCO_2, pH, and blood pressure plays a key role in the hemodynamics of the cerebral blood supply (45). Experimental studies in fetal lambs have shown that cerebral blood flow near term is approximately 125 mL/100 g/min and that approximately 22% of the total car-

diac stroke volume is delivered to the brain. Oxygen saturation, as measured by the fetal hemoglobin, is estimated at approximately 60%.

Pulsed Doppler studies. Besides improved B-mode resolution, the evolution of Doppler techniques from CW scanning to pulsed and color Doppler has enabled the simultaneous visualization of the fetal cerebrovascular system and the associated blood flow velocities. The first pulsed Doppler examinations of the fetal internal carotid artery were performed by Wladimiroff et al. in 1986 (193). Working with a small population, these authors found different Doppler frequency spectra in normal and growth-retarded fetuses. They also found a correlation between increased end-diastolic flow velocities in the internal carotid artery and adverse perinatal outcomes (193). This prompted further Doppler studies of various cerebral vessels such as the common carotid artery, anterior cerebral artery, posterior cerebral artery, and especially the middle cerebral artery (6, 29, 111, 129, 196). A common feature of all the cerebral vessels is that the end-diastolic velocities increase toward the end of pregnancy while the resistance indices (RI, PI) decline.

Middle Cerebral Artery

Vessel of first choice. In recent years the middle cerebral artery has become the vessel of first choice for evaluating fetal intracranial blood flow owing to the good reproducibility of the findings (111, 129). This vessel is advantageous for Doppler scanning because with a transverse fetal head position, the course of the vessel and the direction of its blood flow are parallel to the ultrasound beam. This permits the use of a very small insonation angle, which is particularly useful for the assessment of absolute flow velocities. In contrast to other cerebral vessels, the Doppler spectrum of the middle cerebral artery shows much less variation in response to fetal activity states (129). But for the precise evaluation of the middle cerebral artery waveforms and to avoid false-positive findings, it is important to be familiar with cerebrovascular anatomy, especially around the circle of Willis. Variations of vascular anatomy are a relatively common finding in this region (5).

Visualization of the artery. The middle cerebral artery is most easily visualized in a transverse plane. First the fetal head is imaged in the standard biometry plane, and then the plane is shifted downward toward the skull base. This brings into view the circle of Willis, which appears as a diamond-shaped vascular structure located anterior and inferior to the pons (Figs. 43.**24**–43.**26**). The middle cerebral artery branches laterally from the circle of Willis on each side. Each artery runs anterolaterally toward the orbit at the level of the sphenoid bone (111). The cerebral vessels can also be defined in a sagittal plane using color Doppler. The pericallosal arteries can also be imaged in this plane (Fig. 43.**27**). Visualization or nonvisualization of the pericallosal artery is helpful in recognizing agenesis of the corpus callosum.

Recording the frequency spectrum. The best site for recording a Doppler spectrum is the midpoint of the middle cerebral artery, approximately 1 cm from the circle of Willis or at the origin of the internal carotid artery (15, 111) (Fig. 43.**28**). Although good and reproducible Doppler spectra can be recorded from the individual cerebral vessels with conventional pulsed gray-scale Doppler, the cerebrovascular system of the fetus can be defined much more quickly and accurately with color Doppler (187). In this way cerebral Doppler frequency spectra can be recorded quickly, accurately, and in conformance with safety requirements (see Chapter 48). Cerebral blood flow velocities are usually recorded with a curved-array transducer operating at a frequency of 2.5–5 MHz. The width of the sample volume is set between 2 and 4 mm. The wall filter should be set to 120 Hz or less. The insonation angle is generally = 20° for the optimum visualization of middle cerebral artery anatomy. This will permit the optimum recording of flow velocities in more than 95% of cases.

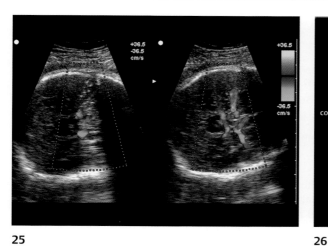

25

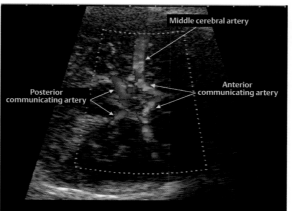

26

Fig. 43.**25**   Color Doppler images of the internal carotid arteries (left) and the circle of Willis (right), which is located at a slightly higher level.

Fig. 43.**26**   Color Doppler image of the circle of Willis (right).

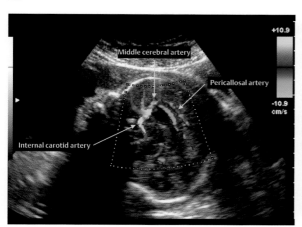

27

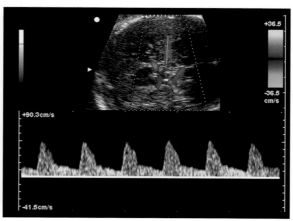

28

Fig. 43.**27**   Color Doppler image of the internal carotid artery, middle cerebral artery, and pericallosal artery in a parasagittal scan.

Fig. 43.**28**   Normal spectrum recorded from the middle cerebral artery with color Doppler in a 29-week fetus.

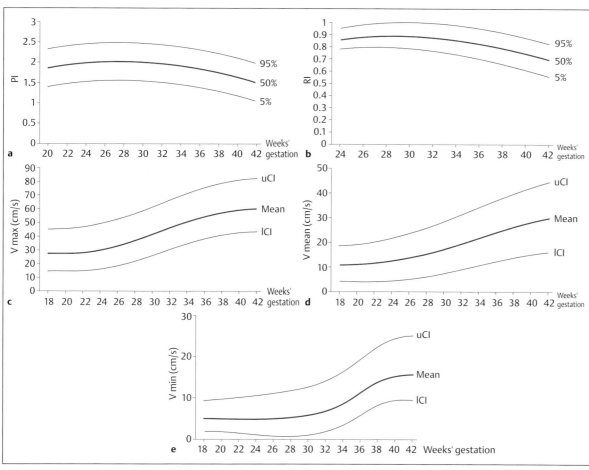

29

Fig. 43.**29**   Reference ranges for resistance indices and blood flow velocities in the middle cerebral artery.
% = percentiles. uCI = upper confidence interval, lCI = lower confidence interval (90% of normal values are within the confidence intervals).
a   Pulsatility index (PI) (after 9).
b   Resistance index (RI) (after 100).
c   Peak systolic blood flow velocity (cm/s) (after 21).
d   Mean intensity-weighted blood flow velocity (cm/s) (after 21).
e   End-diastolic blood flow velocity (cm/s) (after 21).

Normal and abnormal waveforms. The normal Doppler frequency spectrum is characterized by a sharp systolic upstroke followed by a steep postsystolic downstroke and a low diastolic flow component (Fig. 43.**28**). The middle cerebral artery shows the highest resistance indices of all the cerebral vessels (111, 180). The reference curve for the resistance and pulsatility index of the middle cerebral artery shows a typical parabolic shape with a maximum between 25 and 30 weeks' gestation (Fig. 43.**29**) (21). A physiologic decline in the resistance indices occurs during the closing weeks of pregnancy.

Abnormal waveforms are characterized by high flow velocities in diastole. This phenomenon is called the brain-sparing effect (Fig. 43.**30**).

Increased resistance indices. If the fetal head is in a very low position, middle cerebral artery Doppler spectra can be recorded by transvaginal scanning (104). This is an important option, since abdominal pressure on the fetal head can decrease the cerebral end-diastolic flow velocities, resulting in higher calculated resistance indices (188). Increased cerebral resistance indices have also been found in association with pronounced oligohydramnios and in some fetuses with severe hydrocephalus (185). However, increased cerebrovascular resistance indices in hydrocephalus do not correlate with a poorer perinatal outcome or with the need for ventriculoperitoneal shunt insertion (67).

Absolute blood flow velocities. Owing to the favorable insonation angle between the Doppler beam and the middle cerebral artery, absolute blood flow velocities can be determined for the assessment of fetal anemia. An inverse correlation exists between the peak systolic and mean blood flow velocities and the fetal hemoglobin and hematocrit levels (117, 189). Besides an accurate recording of the Doppler spectrum, the detection of abnormal absolute flow velocities requires a knowledge of the reference ranges for the individual absolute cerebral blood flow velocities (Fig. 43.**29**).

Internal Carotid Artery

The internal carotid artery is visualized just below the circle of Willis (Figs. 43.**25**, 43.**27**) (193). It is located by starting at the circle of Willis and moving the probe slightly downward toward the skull base. The internal carotid artery appears as a small, pulsating hypoechoic area on each side of the optic chiasm. But because the cerebral vessels are so close together, the accurate differentiation and recording of flow velocities is very difficult and requires the use of color Doppler. The magnitude of the resistance indices in the individual cerebral vessels can vary considerably, resulting in misinterpretations (111).

Common Carotid Artery

The common carotid artery is visualized in a longitudinal plane in the lateral part of the neck (Fig. 43.**31**). A very high degree of probe angulation is usually needed to acquire optimum Doppler spectra with an insonation angle of 30°–60°. Because this artery is relatively difficult to visualize, it is less clinically important than other cerebral vessels. On the other hand, its close proximity to the jugular vein allows for simultaneous Doppler velocimetry of the jugular vein and common carotid artery. This can be useful in the diagnosis and accurate classification of fetal arrhythmias.

Cerebroplacental Ratio (C/U Ratio)

The ratio of the Doppler pulsatility indices of the middle cerebral artery and umbilical artery, called the cerebroplacental ratio, can be used to describe the redistribution of fetal blood volume in the setting of chronic fetal hypoxemia (15, 17, 38, 65). When a cutoff value of = 1 or a value below the 5th percentile is used, the cerebroplacental ratio ap-

Table 43.3 Normal and abnormal cerebroumbilical ratios related to perinatal outcome (15)

	C/U-Ratio > 1	C/U-Ratio ≤ 1	P-value
Cases of intrauterine growth retardation (n/N) (%)	3/39 (7.6%)	10/22 (45.4%)	0.0009
Birthweight < 25th percentile	17/39 (43.5%)	17/22 (77.2%)	0.008
Stay in neonatal ICU (days)	14,5 ± 19.3	26,0 ± 22.3	0.03
Cesarean sections (n)	20/39 (51.2%)	19/22 (86.3%)	0.01

pears to be a better predictor of intrauterine growth retardation and increased neonatal morbidity than evaluation of the umbilical artery or middle cerebral artery alone (15, 17) (Table 43.**3**). Apparently this applies only to fetuses with a gestational age less than 34 weeks, however. If the cerebroplacental ratio is below the 5th percentile in these cases, it has a reported sensitivity of 73.1%, a specificity of 89.4%, and respective positive and negative predictive values of 76% and 77% in the prediction of intrauterine growth retardation and increased neonatal morbidity (17).

Brain-Sparing Effect

Compensatory mechanism. Studies in experimental animals have shown that fetal hypoxemia evokes a dilatation of the cerebral vessels that increases the blood flow to the brain (41, 167). Cohn et al. (41) measured a 2- to 3-fold increase in cerebral blood flow in hypoxic fetal lambs. Similar observations have been made in Doppler studies of various cerebral vessels in human fetuses (3, 187, 194, 150). Particularly in fetuses with asymmetrical growth retardation due to chronic placental insufficiency, Doppler has revealed increased diastolic flow velocities and decreased resistance indices in the internal carotid artery, anterior cerebral artery, posterior cerebral artery, superior cerebellar artery, and especially in the middle cerebral artery (Figs. 43.**12**, 43.**30**) (177, 189). This phenomenon, called the brain-sparing effect, involves a hypoxemia-induced redistribution of the fetal blood volume in favor of the brain. It is a protective compensatory mechanism aimed at maintaining an adequate cerebral blood supply. The lowered pO2 values in the fetal umbilical vein detected by cordocentesis correlate with increased end-diastolic flow velocities and decreased resistance indices (32, 187).

Loss of cerebral autoregulation. A loss of the brain-sparing effect, or a normalization of the resistance indices in the cerebral vessels, following hypoxemia-induced vasodilatation appears to be associated with a very high risk of intrauterine fetal death and may immediately precede it (114, 155). In extreme cases, the Doppler frequency spectrum in the cerebral vessels may even show a retrograde flow component during diastole (Fig. 43.**32**) (166). These fetuses are very likely to have severe intrauterine asphyxia. From a pathophysiologic standpoint, it has been suggested that brain edema due to severe, increasing hypoxemia leads to a rise of intracranial pressure with a consequent rise in the resistance indices (187). An imbalance between thromboxane and prostacyclin in favor of thromboxane has also been postulated. In one study, rat brains with severe hypoxemic-ischemic injury were found to have elevated thromboxane levels, which may have caused the cerebral vasoconstriction (63). It is also believed that severe hypoxemia and acidemia induce a state of general circulatory collapse leading to a loss of cerebral autoregulation (144). The decompensation of cerebral hemodynamics results from increasing acidemia. This acidemia is accompanied by an alteration of brain metabolism, which in turn can lead to severe brain damage and intrauterine fetal death.

Predictive value for pregnancy outcome. Lowered resistance indices in the middle cerebral artery appear to be associated with a poorer perinatal outcome (179, 191). This is a highly controversial issue, however

(158). Mari et al. (116) found in 43 preterm infants between 25 and 33 weeks' gestation that the detection of a brain-sparing effect was not associated with an increased risk of intraventricular hemorrhage, but that preterm labor was a risk factor in the occurrence of cerebral hemorrhage. The quality of neonatal primary care also appears to affect the risk of cerebral hemorrhage. In particular, strong blood pressure fluctuations should be avoided during primary care whenever possible. When an isolated brain-sparing effect is detected in the middle cerebral artery, accompanied by normal Doppler indices in the umbilical artery or descending aorta, current evidence does not indicate that there is an increased risk of cerebral hemorrhage or adverse perinatal outcome (158, 171). Consequently, finding lowered resistance indices in the middle cerebral artery is not an indication for early delivery. Adding Doppler examination of the middle cerebral artery in high-risk pregnancies does not furnish additional information compared with umbilical velocimetry alone and does not improve the sensitivity for predicting an SGA infant or adverse pregnancy outcome (171). But if abnormal umbilical artery waveforms are found, Doppler examination of the middle cerebral artery should be added so that the degree of the brain-sparing effect can be better appreciated (15, 65, 129, 171).

Cerebral Arteriovenous Malformations

Vein of Galen malformation. Congenital arteriovenous malformations most commonly occur in the territory of the middle cerebral artery. Only a few reports have been published on the antenatal diagnosis of vein of Galen malformations, consisting mostly of case studies. In a review of 18 fetuses diagnosed prenatally with a vein of Galen malformation, one-third of the fetuses exhibited cardiomegaly and signs of destruction of the brain parenchyma (164).

Doppler findings. Arteriovenous shunts can be identified with color Doppler by their greatly increased flow velocities and their typical mosaic color pattern (Figs. 43.**33**, 43.**34**). If the shunt volume is high enough, an increase in systolic and especially end-diastolic flow can be detected. The resistance and pulsatility indices in the vessels feeding the angioma are decreased. The signal from the aneurysm presents acoustically as a systolic-diastolic machine sound. The increasing cardiac volume load imposed by the cerebral arteriovenous shunts presents a serious problem with increasing gestational age. Intrauterine heart failure can develop, and further cardiac decompensation can lead to generalized fetal hydrops and intrauterine death. These cases may respond positively to transplacental therapy by maternal digitalization.

▬ *Pulmonary Vessels*

Volume flow in the pulmonary vascular system. Animal studies have shown that only about 9% of the fetal cardiac output flows through the pulmonary arteries to the lung (78). Approximately twice that amount has been detected in human fetuses by Doppler flowmetry (136, 137). The generally low perfusion of the fetal pulmonary vascular system is caused by a high arterial pressure and high vascular resistance in the pulmonary arteries. This promotes a greater amount of right ventricular flow through the pulmonary trunk to the ductus arteriosus. Velocimetry of the pulmonary vessels can be performed with pulsed gray-scale Doppler in principle, but color Doppler is best for detailed imaging of the pulmonary vessels and identifying them as venous or arterial (39, 40) (Fig. 45.**35**). Color Doppler also permits the selective sampling of flow spectra out to the peripheral pulmonary vessels.

Pulmonary artery. The pulmonary artery waveform is characterized by a steep early systolic upstroke to the peak velocity (V_{max}). The systolic downstroke exhibits a biphasic notch that may even show negative deflections at the end of systole (Fig. 43.**36**). The flow velocities in the

diastolic phase show low values that are consistent with the high pulmonary resistance. Accordingly, relatively high resistance indices are found, and these remain constant throughout the pregnancy (Fig. 43.**37**) (101). The peripheral pulmonary vessels show markedly lower flow velocities than the central vessels.

Doppler scanning of the pulmonary arteries could be clinically important in predicting the development of intrauterine pulmonary hypoplasia. But this presupposes the occurrence of pathomorphologic changes in the pulmonary vascular system, like those found in association with congenital diaphragmatic hernia, Potter sequence, hydrothorax, or anhydramnios (Fig. 43.**38**).

Pulmonary veins. Doppler studies of the pulmonary veins furnish information on left ventricular pressure. Similar to the ductus venosus, the pulmonary veins have a unidirectional frequency spectrum that is characterized by a triphasic cycle (Fig. 43.**39**). But the pulmonary veins show considerably lower flow velocities in their Doppler spectra than the ductus venosus. Increased preload indices or a reverse flow component in the pulmonary vein during atrial contraction are found in conditions such as severe aortic stenosis or hypoplastic left heart (Fig. 43.**40**). Studies currently underway may provide the data needed to support the clinical value of this examination (152).

▬ *Ductus arteriosus*

Cardiac hemodynamics. Doppler examination of the ductus arteriosus permits a quantitative assessment of blood flow velocities and yields important insights into the physiology and pathophysiology of cardiac hemodynamics. This information is useful in the diagnosis of severe ductus-associated heart defects, such as severe pulmonary valvular stenosis or atresia, and in monitoring the response to indomethacin therapy (120, 121). Doppler measurements in the ductus arteriosus can be performed as early as 10 weeks' gestation by transvaginal scanning, but they require a very specific indication at this early stage of pregnancy (33).

Recording the frequency spectrum. The Doppler frequency spectrum is best recorded in a sagittal scan of the right ventricular outflow tract ("short basal axis" view). The sample volume is positioned in the distal part of the ductus arteriosus, in line with the pulmonary trunk, and the frequency spectrum is recorded with the aid of color Doppler using an insonation angle < 10° (34) (Fig. 43.**41**). While the systolic, mean and diastolic blood flow velocities are dependent on gestational age, the pulsatility and resistance indices show no changes (121). Another view of the ductus arteriosus can be obtained in an oblique transverse scan superior to the four-chamber view (48). This plane is mainly useful for evaluating the blood flow direction with color Doppler, e.g., detecting retrograde perfusion caused by a severe obstruction of the right ventricular outflow tract.

Interpreting the frequency spectrum. The indices used in interpreting the frequency spectrum are the pulsatility index and the peak systolic and diastolic flow velocities. The systolic blood flow velocities in the ductus arteriosus are the highest anywhere in the fetal circulation. Doppler measurements show acceptable inter- and intraobserver reproducibility, regardless of gestational age (34, 64). The peak systolic velocities in the ductus arteriosus appear to have the greatest clinical significance (34, 64).

Constriction in response to indomethacin. Doppler examinations of the ductus arteriosus are particularly indicated in cases where indomethacin is being used for the treatment of preterm labor or polyhydramnios. Constriction of the ductus arteriosus in response to indomethacin therapy occurs in approximately 50% of cases, depending

Fig. 43.**30** Abnormal frequency spectrum recorded from the middle cerebral artery with color Doppler in a fetus with severe intrauterine growth retardation at 27 weeks. This waveform pattern, called the brain-sparing effect, is characterized by increased end-diastolic flow velocities.

Fig. 43.**31** Color Doppler image of the common carotid artery (reverse end-diastolic flow) and jugular vein (blue), longitudinal scan.

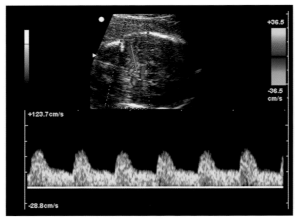

30

31

Fig. 43.**32** The retrograde end-diastolic flow component in the middle cerebral artery is caused by severe fetal acidemia in an acute HELLP syndrome (29 weeks).

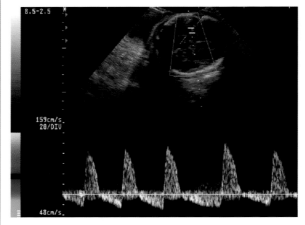

32

Fig. 43.**33** Vein of Galen aneurysm. The mosaic color pattern is caused by turbulent blood flow associated with the aneurysm.

Fig. 43.**34** Abnormal Doppler spectra recorded from the umbilical vein (lower left) and ductus venosus (lower right) of a fetus with a vein of Galen aneurysm. A large shunt volume results from the cerebral arteriovenous anastomoses (28 weeks, 4 days).

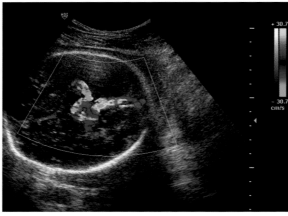

33

34

Pulmonary vessels

Fig. 43.**35** Color Doppler images of the pulmonary artery (left) and pulmonary vein (right).

Fig. 43.**36** Normal frequency spectrum recorded from the pulmonary artery with color Doppler.

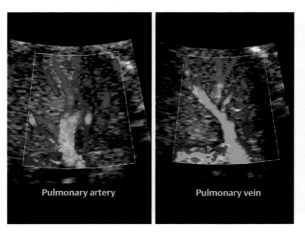

35

36

on gestational age (124, 183). Because the risk of ductus arteriosus constriction increases with advancing gestational age, indomethacin should not be administered after 32 weeks' gestation (124, 183). Also, weekly fetal echocardiography with ductus arteriosus velocimetry is warranted for the duration of the therapy (93, 123, 183). Doppler signs of indomethacin-induced constriction of the ductus arteriosus consist mainly of increased systolic flow velocities, which are seen an average of 5 days after the start of treatment (183). Peak systolic and diastolic flow velocities greater than 140 cm/s and 35 cm/s, respectively, and a pulsatility index < 1.9 appear to signify incipient ductal constriction (123, 141, 183). With its better reproducibility, however, the peak systolic velocity appears to be the most useful parameter for detecting ductal obliteration (34, 64, 183). If Doppler shows evidence of premature ductal constriction, the indomethacin therapy should be discontinued. It appears that indomethacin-induced constriction of the ductus arteriosus is fully reversible after the drug is withdrawn (123, 183). Indeed, recent evidence indicates that the ductal constriction is only a transient response (141). Rarely, intrauterine closure of the ductus arteriosus can occur spontaneously, with a high mortality rate. There are also rare reports of ductal constriction occurring in response to prenatal betamethasone therapy to induce fetal lung maturation (16).

Renal Artery

Regulation of renal blood flow. Experimental studies in fetal sheep have shown that only 2–4% of the fetal cardiac output reaches the kidney during the last trimester (159). Renal blood flow at this stage is equal to 1.5–2.0 mL/min/g kidney weight. This low rate of renal blood flow compared with neonates is associated with a high vascular resistance and low glomerular filtration rate (153). Fetal diuresis is regulated by the interaction between hemodynamic and endocrine factors (41, 159, 195). Besides renal blood flow, it appears that the hormonal parameters prostaglandin E$_2$ (PGE$_2$), arginine vasopressin (AVP), cortisol, and atrial natriuretic factor (ANF) play a particularly important role in this process (195). The fetus responds to hypoxemia and concomitant acidemia with an increase in these hormonal parameters, while hemodynamic modulation is produced by a rise of renovascular resistance causing a decrease in renal blood flow (41, 153).

Recording the frequency spectrum. Both pulsed Doppler and color Doppler have been used in examinations of the fetal renal vessels (115). The fetal renal vessels are most easily visualized by locating the kidney in the coronal plane. Color Doppler can then be used to define the renal artery and vein from the renal hilum to the abdominal aorta (Fig. 43.**42**). The sample volume is positioned in the hilar area for renal blood flow interrogation. The insonation angle is generally less than 30° in this view. As with all other vessels, the wall-filter setting should be less than 125 Hz.

Interpreting the frequency spectrum. Waveform analysis is based on the use of the pulsatility index or resistance index (Fig. 43.**43**). Doppler frequency spectra can be successfully recorded from the renal artery in 90% of cases (186). Since renovascular blood flow increases during pregnancy, vascular resistance is decreased (9, 115, 186). Using a wall filter setting of 120 Hz, Vyas et al. (186) were able to detect end-diastolic flow in the renal artery in only 46% of cases. This showed a marked dependence on gestational age, however. End-diastolic flow could be detected in just 11% of cases between 18 and 25 weeks' gestation, in 19% between 26 and 34 weeks, and in 86% between 35 and 43 weeks (186). But when the wall filter was set to 50 Hz, end-diastolic flow was consistently detected (181). An intraobserver variability of 6.7% has been reported for the renal artery pulsatility index (115).

Changes in vascular resistance. Increased renal vascular resistance has been described in association with intrauterine growth retardation and oligohydramnios (12, 115, 181, 186). Studies in fetal lambs (153) have shown that vasopressin is elevated in the setting of fetal hypoxia. Raised vasopressin levels lead to an increase in vascular resistance, causing a reduction in renal blood flow. They also alter the tubular reabsorption capacity of the kidney, explaining the development of oligohydramnios and other effects. On the other hand, postdate pregnancy and polyhydramnios have not found to be associated with changes in fetal renovascular resistance (12, 115, 182). Moreover, no Doppler changes have been found in response to indomethacin therapy for polyhydramnios (112), although animal studies have shown a decrease in urine production and amniotic fluid volume in response to prostaglandin synthesis inhibitors (94). No relationship was found between a decreased amniotic fluid volume at term and renal Doppler values (198).

Renal agenesis. Imaging of the renal vessels is particularly important for the exclusion of unilateral or bilateral renal agenesis. While renal agenesis is detected in only 69–73% of cases using conventional real-time ultrasound, a 100% detection rate is reported for nonvisualization of the renal vessels with color Doppler ultrasound (49) (see Chapter 27). In this examination it is helpful to know the normal length of the aortic segment located between the aortic bifurcation and the renal vessels. The length of this aortic segment correlates with femur length (49). The diagnosis of renal agenesis with color Doppler ultrasound has been reported as early as 14 weeks' gestation (108).

Cystic renal diseases. Whereas Doppler examinations of the renal vessels in fetuses with hydronephrosis have shown no effect on renovascular resistance, increased renovascular resistance indices have been found in fetuses with multicystic kidneys (Potter IIA) and decreased renal artery resistance indices in fetuses with polycystic dysplastic kidneys (e.g., Meckel–Gruber syndrome) (68, 88, 71). At present, however, these findings appear to have little clinical relevance in terms of making a prognostic assessment of these renal disorders.

Peripheral Vessels

With the new color Doppler instruments, it is possible to define even the smallest fetal blood vessels. While it appears at present that the Doppler scanning of peripheral arterial vessels has no special clinical importance, it will be mentioned briefly in order to complete our discussion of arterial Doppler and acknowledge its relevance to potential scientific studies in the future (Figs. 43.**44**–43.**46**).

Hypoxemia-induced redistribution. Experimental animal studies have shown that the peripheral arterial blood volume decreases during fetal hypoxia (41, 60), with hypoxia-induced peripheral vasoconstriction occurring in fetal sheep only during the third trimester (84). It is unclear at present whether Doppler measurements of peripheral vessels are feasible for detecting hypoxia-induced hemodynamic redistribution in human fetuses. Clinical studies are currently underway to resolve this issue.

Femoral artery and anterior tibial artery. The vascular resistance in both the femoral artery (113) and the anterior tibial artery (192) shows a linear increase during normal pregnancies. Because of the increasing vascular tonus in the peripheral vessels, the pulsatility index of the anterior tibial artery increases slightly from an average of 3.29 to 4.09 during the second half of pregnancy (Fig. 43.**46**) (192). A comparison of the sides shows no difference between the right and left anterior tibial arteries. On the other hand, significant differences have been found between the pulsatility indices of the right and left femoral arteries in fetuses with a single umbilical artery (163).

Fig. 43.**37**   Reference range for the pulsatility index (PI) of the pulmonary artery (after 101).
Upper limit = 95th percentile.
Lower limit = 5th percentile.

Fig. 43.**38**   This fetus has a postero-lateral congenital diaphragmatic hernia on the left side. In the Doppler frequency spectrum of the pulmonary artery, no blood flow velocities are recorded at end diastole. This signifies a high vascular resistance in the pulmonary artery secondary to chronic pulmonary hypoplasia. The risk of postnatal pulmonary hypertension is extremely high.

Fig. 43.**39**   Normal frequency spectrum recorded from the pulmonary vein with color Doppler.

Fig. 43.**40**   Doppler frequency spectrum from the pulmonary vein of a fetus with hypoplastic left heart syndrome and aortic atresia. The reverse flow component during atrial contraction reflects an elevated left atrial pressure.

Ductus arteriosus

Fig. 43.**41**   Longitudinal color Doppler scan of the ductus arteriosus shows a normal-appearing Doppler spectrum.

Renal artery

Fig. 43.**42**   Color Doppler scan of the abdominal aorta with the origins of the renal arteries and renal vein. The renal artery Doppler spectrum appears normal. Despite a low wall filter setting, the end-diastolic velocities are not displayed.

Fig. 43.**43**   Reference ranges for the resistance indices of the renal artery.
a Pulsatility index (PI) (after 9).
b Resistance index (RI) (after 109).
Upper limit = 95th percentile.
Lower limit = 5th percentile.

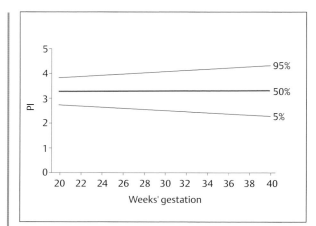

37

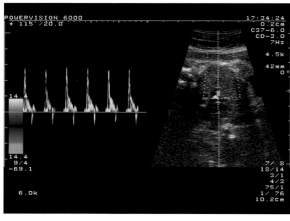

38

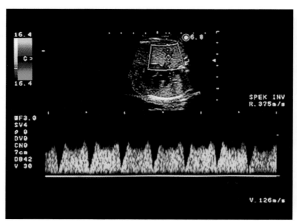

39

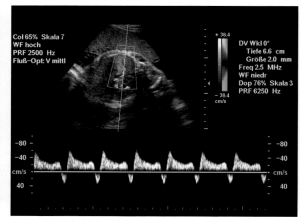

40

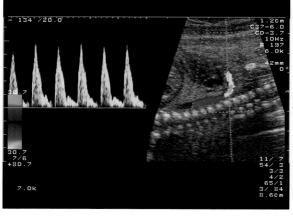

41

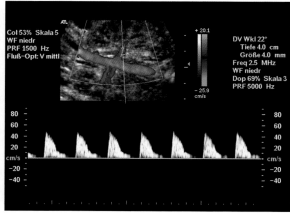

42

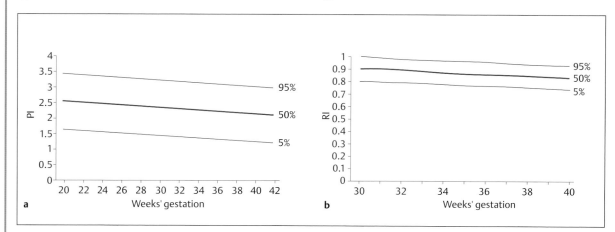

43

▦ *Doppler Ultrasound of the Venous System*

Doppler ultrasound has become increasingly important in recent years for investigating physiologic and pathophysiologic changes in the fetal cardiovascular system, especially with regard to the cardiac and venous systems. Although volume flow in the umbilical vein was already being investigated with Doppler in the early 1980s, this method did not become widely utilized due to its relatively low accuracy and reproducibility. A detailed evaluation of the fetal venous system had to await further technical refinements in ultrasound instrumentation and especially the introduction of color Doppler scanning. Besides studies of the umbilical vein, inferior vena cava, and hepatic veins, Doppler examination of the ductus venosus has become a subject of current scientific interest.

▦ *Umbilical Vein*

Quantitative blood flow analysis. Doppler examinations of the umbilical vein to assess fetal blood volume were first performed by Eik-Nes et al. (53, 54) and Gill et al. (58, 59) in the early 1980s. These authors calculated a relatively constant mean volume flow of 110–125 mL/kg/min for the third trimester, which declines to 90 mL/kg/min as term approaches (53, 55, 59). The quantitative analysis of umbilical blood flow, like the calculation of fetal aortic volume flow, is problematic because, as in the aorta, slight fluctuations in vessel diameter lead to a large variation of blood flow values (54). This quantitative method of determining blood volume did not become widely established due to its poor reproducibility (55).

Recording the frequency spectrum. The Doppler spectrum is recorded from either the intra-amniotic or intrahepatic segment of the umbilical vein. The intrahepatic segment is preferred owing to better reproducibility. The fetal abdomen is imaged in a transverse plane, and the sample volume is placed in the midportion of the intrahepatic umbilical vein using an insonation angle less than 30°.

Umbilical vein pulsations. The umbilical vein waveform generally shows a monophasic pattern with a mean flow velocity of 10–15 cm/s (Fig. 43.**47**). Under physiologic conditions, umbilical vein pulsations occur until the end of the first trimester and during fetal breathing movements (83, 146). After 13 weeks' gestation, pulsations are no longer detected under normal conditions. The presence of umbilical vein pulsations in the second or third trimester may signify a cardiac anomaly, arrhythmia, or congestive heart disease. Also, these pulsations are commonly associated with absent end-diastolic flow in the umbilical artery as a result of chronic placental insufficiency (69, 126) (Figs. 43.**12**, 43.**61**, 43.**62**). The umbilical vein pulsations in these cases coincide with atrial systole and are an expression of myocardial insufficiency. Pulsations in the umbilical vein may occur as single or double pulsations or may produce a triphasic Doppler spectrum (Fig. 43.**47**). A markedly increased mortality rate of 50–60% is reported in cases where these flow patterns are detected (69, 83, 126).

▦ *Ductus venosus*

Recording the frequency spectrum. Both two-dimensional real-time ultrasound and color Doppler can be used to image the ductus venosus and obtain a spectral sample (Figs. 43.**48**–43.**50**). Of all the precardial veins, the ductus venosus yields the best and most reliable information on fetal myocardial hemodynamics and cardiac function while providing reproducible spectra (18, 19, 47, 72, 149). Doppler signals are acquired most easily and quickly when the fetus is in a dorsoposterior lie. The intrahepatic segment of the umbilical vein should be imaged first to gain rapid venous orientation. The vein is optimally visualized either in the midsagittal plane or in an oblique transverse scan through the fetal abdomen (95). The intrahepatic segment of the umbilical vein points to the site where the vein enters the ductus venosus (Fig. 43.**48**). The diameter of the ductus venosus rarely exceeds 2 mm and shows a slight funnel-shaped expansion, with a total length of up to 20 mm (96). To record flow signals, the sample volume is positioned directly at the junction of the umbilical vein with the ductus venosus (Fig. 43.**54**). The width of the sample volume (approximately 2.5–6 mm) should just span the vessel; otherwise it would detect unwanted signals from the closely adjacent hepatic veins and umbilical vein. The use of color Doppler makes it considerably easier to locate the ductus venosus and accurately position the sample volume. The color-flow image will clearly reveal the difference in flow velocity between the umbilical vein and ductus venosus (Fig. 43.**50**). The 3–4 times higher blood flow velocity in the ductus venosus leads to a color reversal with aliasing (Fig. 43.**54**). The spectrum is always sampled at the origin of the ductus venosus, which is the site where the color reversal occurs (Fig. 43.**54**). Due to the funnel-like shape of the ductus venosus, the flow velocities are higher at the ductal inlet than at the outlet (Fig. 43.**51**). An insonation angle less than 30° (or 50°) is recommended to obtain an optimum waveform (19, 72). The wall filter should be set as low as possible—between 125 Hz and 50 Hz depending on the instrument. An experienced examiner can record distinct Doppler signals from the ductus venosus in more than 90% of cases (19, 72).

Interpreting the frequency spectrum. The normal waveform of the ductus venosus shows continuous, triphasic forward flow throughout the cardiac cycle (Figs. 43.**50**–43.**52**, 43.**54**). Very little or no pulsatility occurs in some cases as a normal variant, due for example to subtle fetal breathing movements (Fig. 43.**53**) (96). This problem can be eliminated by waiting a few minutes and then continuing the examination. The peak flow velocities in the ductus venosus are the highest anywhere in the fetal venous system and appear to be responsible for the "streamlining" effect. Analogous to the arterial system, the blood flow velocities in the ductus venosus are dependent on gestational age, fetal breathing and body movements, and fetal heart rate (82). On average, the mean blood flow velocity (V_{mean}) increases from 19 to 34 cm/s between 14 and 41 weeks' gestation (19) (Fig. 43.**52**). The blood flow velocity in the ductus venosus may be double or triple the normal value during inspiration, depending on the amplitude of the fetal breathing movements.

The peak flow velocities during ventricular systole (= S), early ventricular diastole (= D), and late ventricular diastole (= atrial contraction [a]) are determined for waveform analysis (Fig. 43.**54**). Hemodynamically, these phases reflect the rapidly time-varying pressure gradient between the umbilical vein and the right atrium (Fig. 43.**55**). The highest pressure gradient that develops between the ductus venosus and right atrium occurs during ventricular systole. It is caused by the descent of the AV valve plane, resulting in antegrade flow with filling of the atria. This is followed by early diastole, marked by opening of the AV valves and passive filling of the ventricles. This corresponds to the E phase of the biphasic atrioventricular waveform. During atrial contraction, which coincides with the A phase of the atrioventricular waveform, the foramen ovale closes and the rest of the atrial blood volume is actively pumped into the right ventricle. These processes can

Table 43.4   Venous Doppler indices for the qualitative evaluation of cardiac preload and central venous pressures

Author	Year	Index
Reed et al. (138)	1990	a/S
Rizzo et al. (149)	1994	S/a
Huisman et al. (80)	1991	S/D
DeVore et al. (47)	1993	(S-a)/S
Hecher et al. (72)	1994	(S-a)/D
Hecher et al. (72)	1994	(S-a)/Tamx
Bahlmann et al. (19)	2000	(S-a)/V$_{mean}$

Peripheral arterial vessels

Fig. 43.**44** Color Doppler image of the femoral artery, with associated Doppler frequency spectrum. Note the high pulsatility of the femoral artery waveform and the very low velocities displayed below the baseline.

Fig. 43.**45** Color Doppler image of the tibial and fibular arteries.

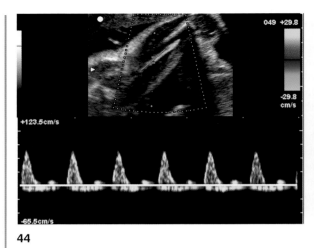

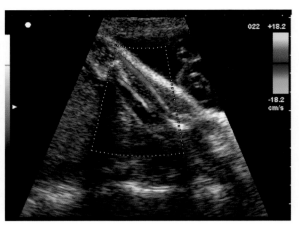

44

45

Fig. 43.**46** Reference ranges for the pulsatility index (PI) of the tibial artery (after 192).
Upper limit = 95th percentile.
Lower limit = 5th percentile.

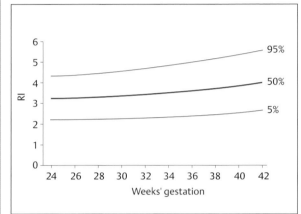

46

Venous system

Fig. 43.**47** Doppler frequency spectra of the umbilical vein in various fetal states.

Fig. 43.**48** Longitudinal scan of the umbilical vein and ductus venosus within the liver.

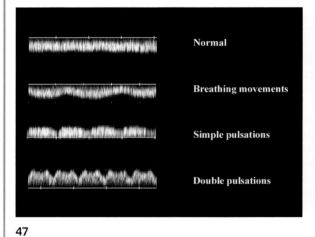

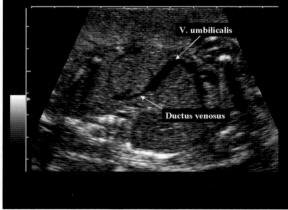

47

48

Fig. 43.**49** B-mode image (left) and power Doppler image (right) of the umbilical vein, ductus venosus, and hepatic veins.

Fig. 43.**50** Simultaneous display of the different flow velocities in the umbilical vein and ductus venosus.

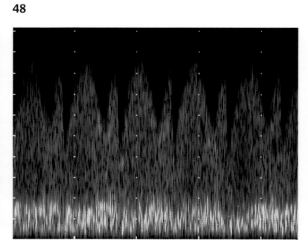

49

50

supply information on the end-diastolic right ventricular pressure and central venous pressure. The Doppler indices listed in Table 43.**4**, which are independent of insonation angle, are useful for the qualitative description of pulsatility.

Evaluating the cardiac preload. These Doppler indices can be used to evaluate the cardiac preload. The corresponding reference ranges are shown in Figs. 43.**56** and 43.**57**. With advancing gestational age, placental maturation processes cause a reduction in placental resistance, with a corresponding fall in the end-diastolic ventricular pressure. This pressure decrease, caused mainly by a rise of flow velocities during atrial contraction, is reflected in decreased venous pulsatility and smaller preload indices. An increase in preload indices is the result of increased end-diastolic ventricular pressure in the heart. In the healthy fetus, the umbilical venous pressure during atrial contraction is greater than the central venous pressure.

When there is severe centralization of the fetal circulation, due for example to chronic placental insufficiency or hypovolemia, the hypoxemia leads to myocardial insufficiency, which causes a rise of central venous pressure in the fetal right heart. This lowers the peak flow velocities in the ductus venosus during atrial contraction, possibly to the point of flow reversal (Figs. 43.**11**, 43.**12**, 43.**58**, 43.**61**, 43.**62**, 43.**64**–43.**66**).

Inferior Vena Cava

Recording the frequency spectrum. There is disagreement as to the best sampling site for Doppler examination of the inferior vena cava (81, 72, 138, 147). It appears that scanning the vessel just below the right atrium (Fig. 43.**59**) can distort the recorded waveform due to the varying flow directions at the level of the subdiaphragmatic veins (80). Rizzo et al. (147) compared different sampling sites for recording velocity waveforms from the inferior vena cava. They found that recording the Doppler spectrum between the renal vessels and the subdiaphragmatic hepatic veins or below the ductus venosus provided the best reproducibility, the most favorable beam–vessel angle, and the least variation (Fig. 43.**60**) (147). At this site the inferior vena cava is scanned in a longitudinal parasagittal plane at a low insonation angle (< 30°). An alternative is to place the sample volume just below the termination of the inferior vena cava at the right atrium (138), but this leads to greater variability in the flow patterns (80).

Interpreting the frequency spectrum. As in the ductus venosus, the waveform of the inferior vena cava reflects the systolic and diastolic phases of the cardiac cycle and therefore reflects the intracardiac pressures (140, 142). Unlike the ductus venosus, the inferior vena cava waveform exhibits a bidirectional, triphasic flow pattern with a retrograde component during atrial contraction. Additionally, the flow velocities in the inferior vena cava are one-half to one-third the velocities in the ductus venosus (Fig. 43.**60**). As in the ductus venosus, qualitative analysis of the inferior vena cava spectrum is based on the indices listed in Table 43.**4**. With advancing gestational age, the retrograde component during atrial contraction shows a relative decline (148). This is associated with a decrease in pulsatility and other Doppler indices and is attributable to the decline in fetoplacental resistance and an increasing differentiation of diastolic ventricular function. An increase of pulsatility and retrograde flow is often seen in hypoxic fetuses with marked blood flow centralization and also in fetuses with congestive heart disease or cardiac arrhythmias (73, 75, 151) (Figs. 43.**61**, 43.**62**).

Evaluation of fetal arrhythmias. Simultaneous Doppler tracings of the inferior vena cava and descending aorta can be obtained to evaluate fetal arrhythmias (37, 89, 138) (Fig. 43.**63**). For this purpose the sample volume is enlarged so that flow velocities are recorded simultaneously from both vessels (Fig. 43.**63**).

Indications for Doppler Ultrasound

IUGR in a Setting of Chronic Placental Insufficiency

B-mode imaging. The diagnosis of intrauterine growth retardation is based primarily on sonographically determined biometric parameters. The fetal abdominal circumference appears to be the best parameter for detecting intrauterine growth restriction (36, 169). Besides biometry, attention should be given to placental morphology and amniotic fluid volume, and the fetal organs should be closely scrutinized to exclude anomalies. Also, it should be considered that intrauterine growth retardation is caused by an underlying chromosomal abnormality in approximately 10–20% of cases. Doppler scanning of the uteroplacental and fetoplacental vessels can provide further differentiation and, more importantly, aids in the assessment of fetal well-being.

Doppler findings. Elevated resistance indices and absent or reverse end-diastolic flow velocities in the umbilical artery signify a markedly increased risk of intrauterine growth retardation, fetal hypoxemia, and acidemia ranging to severe asphyxia. They also correlate closely with a high perinatal mortality and morbidity and with later neuromotor deficits (51). The main difficulty in assessing fetal compromise is that growth-retarded fetuses vary considerably in their ability to adapt to chronic hypoxemia, which is critically influenced by coexisting maternal diseases such as preeclampsia and type I diabetes mellitus.

Adaptive processes. Hypoxemia and acidemia induce a centralization of the fetal circulation with a rise of peripheral vascular resistance and a rerouting of blood flow to the brain, myocardium, and adrenals (41). In a setting of chronic placental insufficiency, a growth-retarded fetus can apparently compensate for its chronic hypoxemic state through specific adaptive processes that include an increase in maximum myocardial blood flow, new blood vessel formation in the myocardium, and changes in energy metabolism. The hemodynamic changes include an increase in erythropoiesis, increased anaerobic glycolysis, and appropriate adaptive processes aimed at preventing serious fetal injury. When the fetus reaches the limit of its ability to compensate, acidemia increases leading to irreversible damage that is reflected in high prenatal mortality and morbidity.

Centralization of the fetal circulation and myocardial insufficiency. As resistance increases in the placental vascular bed, the fetal circulation becomes more centralized to conserve the oxygen supply to vital organs. Doppler shows a corresponding increase of resistance indices in the umbilical artery and fetal aorta and a lowering of the cerebral resistance indices. The increasing resistance in the fetal aorta (afterload ↑) leads to a rise of end-diastolic pressure in the right ventricle. Over time this leads to greater pulsatility in the venous vessels and the occurrence of umbilical vein pulsations (139, 140, 142). The increase in pulsatility and preload indices in the venous vessels, as well as the appearance of pulsations in the umbilical vein, are the expression of a hypoxia-induced myocardial insufficiency. These signs are especially pronounced in fetuses with progressive acidemia (75, 98, 150, 151).

Correlation with FHR changes. Abnormally high preload indices in the ductus venosus and inferior vena cava and pulsations in the umbilical vein correlate with abnormal FHR changes and may precede them in some cases (Figs. 43.**11**, 43.**12**, 43.**61**, 43.**62**) (42, 73). The FHR changes consist mainly of decreased variability and silent oscillations. Increased decelerations are most likely to occur as a result of elevated preload indices in the ductus venosus and a reverse flow component during atrial contraction.

Fig. 43.**51** Effect of the sampling site on flow velocities in the ductus venosus. Due to the funnel-shaped expansion of the ductus, blood flow velocities are considerably lower at its outlet.

Fig. 43.**52** Normal ductus venosus spectra as a function of gestational age. With advancing gestational age, the absolute flow velocity increases while pulsatility declines.

Fig. 43.**53** Color Doppler image of the sinus venosus with the origin of the ductus venosus in a dorsoanterior fetus. The Doppler spectrum shows low pulsatility and is considered a normal variant.

Fig. 43.**54** *Right:* Color Doppler image of the of the umbilical vein and ductus venosus (arrow). The different blood flow velocities are clearly recognized. The 3–4 times higher velocities in the ductus venosus cause aliasing to occur in the initial part of the vessel. That is the site where the flow velocities are sampled. The Doppler spectrum (left) is characterized by a unidirectional, triphasic pattern.
VS = ventricular systole, EVD = early ventricular diastole, ac = atrial contraction.

Fig. 43.**55** Schematic representation of the fetal cardiac cycle.

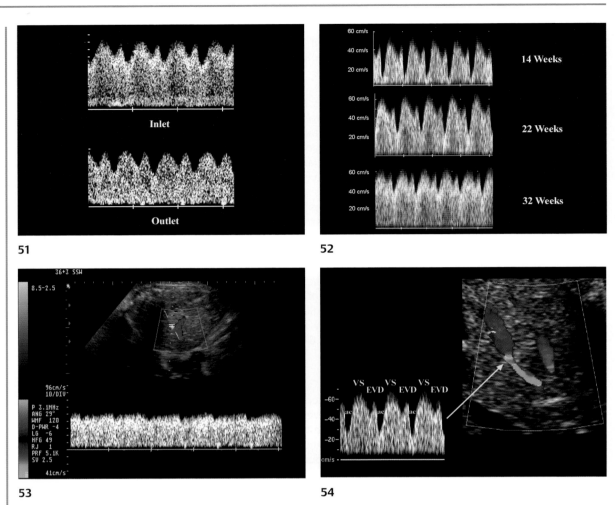

51

52

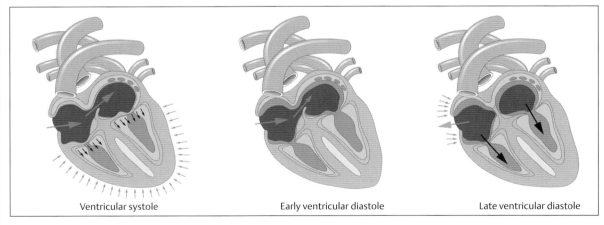

53

54

55

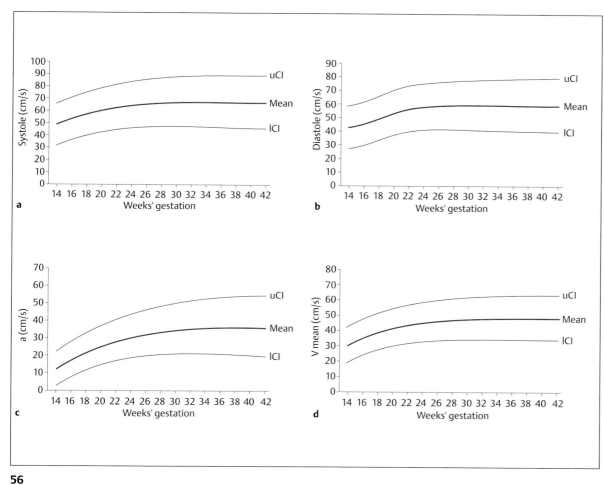

Fig. 43.**56** Reference ranges for the various flow velocities in the ductus venosus at different points in the cardiac cycle. The normal limits cover 90% of the normal population (after 19).
uCI = upper confidence interval,
lCI = lower confidence interval
(90% of normal values are within the confidence intervals).

a Peak flow velocities during ventricular systole (= S).
b Peak flow velocities during early ventricular diastole (= D).
c Peak flow velocities during atrial contraction (= a).
d Mean intensity-weighted flow velocity (V_{mean}).

56

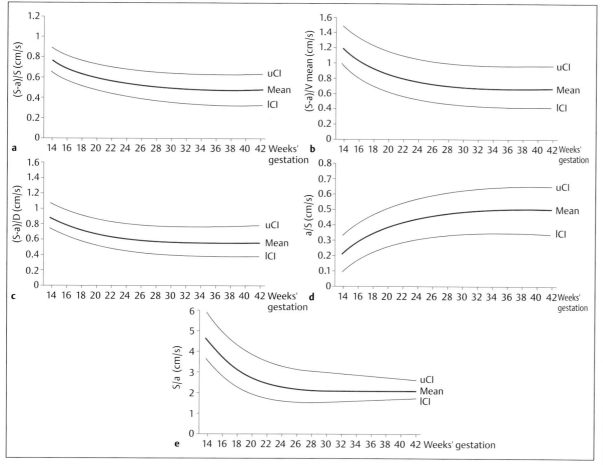

Fig. 43.**57** Reference ranges for the various preload indices of the ductus venosus. The normal limits cover 90% of the normal population (after 19).
uCI = upper confidence interval,
lCI = lower confidence interval.

a Preload index (S-a)/S.
b Preload index (S-a)/V_{mean}.
c Preload index (S-a)/D.
d Preload index a/S.
e Preload index S/a.

57

Fig. 43.**58** Doppler frequency spectra of the ductus venosus show increasing pathology (a–d) as a result of myocardial insufficiency.

Fig. 43.**59** Inflow tract of the superior vena cava and inferior vena cava into the right atrium.

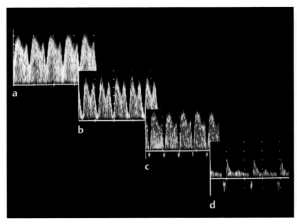

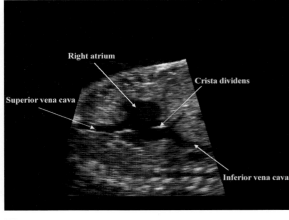

58

59

Fig. 43.**60** Normal Doppler frequency spectrum recorded from the inferior vena cava. S = Ventricular systole, D = early ventricular diastole, a = atrial contraction.

Fig. 43.**61** Very abnormal Doppler spectra recorded from the inferior vena cava, ductus venosus, and umbilical vein of a fetus with severe intrauterine growth retardation (28 weeks, 5 days). The spectra are temporally aligned for comparison. The hypoxemic myocardial insufficiency causes an increase in right atrial pressure during atrial contraction (= a). This is reflected in an increased retrograde component in the inferior vena cava, a reverse flow component in the ductus venosus, and a twin-peak pulsation pattern with a deep second notch in the umbilical vein.

Fig. 43.**62** Correlation of individual venous Doppler spectra with the FHR recording. (Same fetus as in Fig. 43.**61**).

Fig. 43.**63** Normal Doppler frequency spectra recorded simultaneously from the fetal aorta and inferior vena cava.

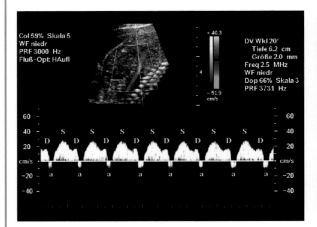

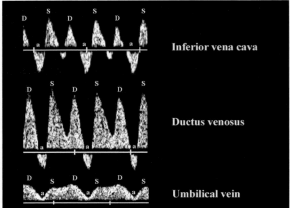

60

61

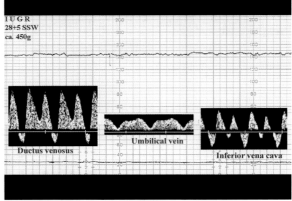

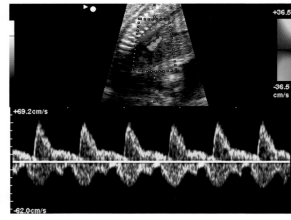

62

63

Venous Doppler. Venous Doppler scanning is mainly indicated in cases that have shown absent or reverse end-diastolic flow in the umbilical artery (70). The goal of venous Doppler in these cases is to provide additional, noninvasive information on the functional capacity of the fetal heart to help determine the optimum timing of the delivery. This is particularly important before 30 weeks' gestation in severely growth-retarded fetuses in a setting of chronic placental insufficiency. The essential goal in these cases is to prolong the pregnancy by at least 1–2 days to allow for therapy to accelerate fetal lung maturation. Clinical studies are currently underway to assess the practical implications of venous Doppler for clinical management.

Multiple Pregnancies

In cases where fetal anomalies or chromosomal abnormalities can be excluded, growth discordance in multiple fetuses is most commonly associated with intrauterine growth retardation due to chronic placental insufficiency or a fetofetal transfusion syndrome.

Fetofetal transfusion syndrome. In fetofetal transfusion syndrome, generally there are arteriovenous anastomoses that allow chronic shunting of blood from one twin (the donor) to the other twin (the recipient). This leads to progressive hypervolemia in the recipient with a variable degree of hypovolemia in the donor. The result is an increase of diuresis in the recipient and impaired diuresis in the donor, with the concomitant development of poly- and oligohydramnios, known also as a "stuck twin" (see Chapter 37).

If the recipient becomes unable to compensate for the increased blood volume, it develops congestive heart failure. The resulting rise of central venous pressure in the heart leads to cardiomegaly, which is reflected in increased preload indices in the venous vessels and, in severe cases, umbilical vein pulsations. Once congestive heart failure has developed, tricuspid valve incompetence can be detected in the recipient in 49% of cases, and elevated preload indices are found in 37% (197) (Fig. 43.**64**). Tricuspid valve incompetence need not always be accompanied by increased pulsatility in the venous vessels. This is explained by the time difference in the flows: whereas the reflux (regurgitation) in tricuspid valve incompetence occurs mainly during ventricular systole, the reverse flow (= a) in venous vessels occurs during late ventricular diastole or atrial contraction.

Implications of Doppler findings. In cases where the fetoscopic laser coagulation of placental arteriovenous anastomoses is proposed, elevated preload indices in the recipient prior to the treatment appear to be associated with a markedly reduced survival rate. On the other hand, elevated venous preload indices in the donor are found in only 9% of cases and apparently do not affect the survival rate. Elevated preload indices may reflect hypovolemia as well as increased placental resistance. The incidence of fetal hydrops, usually in the recipient, is approximately 7%, depending on cardiac adaptation capacity. Interestingly, these cases frequently show normal resistance indices in the arterial vessels (76). Abnormal umbilical artery waveforms with absent or reversed end-diastolic flow are found in 5% of recipient twins and 19% of donor twins.

Fetal Hydrops

Venous Doppler. It is common to find abnormal Doppler flow patterns in the venous vessels of fetuses with hydrops based on an underlying cardiovascular disease (56, 97). A decrease in right ventricular stroke volume may be found in nonimmune fetal hydrops, manifested by elevated preload indices in the venous vessels and the presence of umbilical vein pulsations (Figs. 43.**65**, 43.**68**) (69).

Causes. Abnormal Doppler venous spectra in fetuses with a sacrococcygeal teratoma or vein of Galen aneurysm, for example, may be caused by the development of arteriovenous anastomoses with high shunt volumes (Fig. 43.**34**). A progressive rise of pulsatility in the venous vessels can also develop in the setting of endocardial fibroelastosis and can lead to fetal hydrops as cardiac compliance continues to deteriorate (Fig. 43.**66**). In some congenital heart diseases, particularly those associated with anomalies of the ventricular inflow or outflow tract, abnormal venous flow patterns may be detected despite normal waveforms in the arterial system (Fig. 43.**65**) (97).

Cardiac arrhythmias. Fetal arrhythmias, especially supraventricular tachyarrhythmias, atrial fibrillation, atrial flutter, and severe bradyarrhythmias, may also be associated with fetal heart failure and the development of fetal hydrops in cases where the arrhythmias are of long duration (Fig. 43.**67**) (13, 89). Tachycardia leads to hypoxia-induced cardiomyopathy with the development of AV valvular incompetence, which in turn leads to generalized hydrops and possible intrauterine fetal death. Above a critical heart rate of 210 bpm, both the ductus venosus and the inferior vena cava display monophasic flow patterns with forward flow during systole and reverse flow during diastole (Fig. 43.**68**) (56). With successful cardioversion, the venous blood flow spectra quickly return to normal and the hydrops clears. In rare cases, fetal hydrops may correlate with agenesis of the ductus venosus (56, 97).

Isolated supraventricular extrasystoles, on the other hand, are considered harmless in the great majority of cases. The postextrasystolic phase is marked by a brief interval of raised right atrial pressure based on the increased blood volume (Fig. 43.**69**). In the cardiac cycle that follows, this volume is pumped into the circulation by an increased stroke volume, and the right atrial pressure returns to normal. The increased stroke volume that follows the postextrasystolic pause is manifested in the umbilical vein, for example, by higher systolic flow velocities (Fig. 43.**67**). The underlying effect is based on the Frank Starling law, which states that the force of cardiac contraction depends indirectly on the end-diastolic volume.

Rh Incompatibility

Hyperdynamic circulation. Severe, acute fetal anemia induces vasoconstriction in the splanchnic and renal vascular beds, thereby increasing the oxygen supply to the brain, heart, and adrenals. On the other hand, fetuses with severe chronic anemia, due for example to blood group incompatibility or an acute parvovirus B19 infection, can mount specific humoral, rheologic, and cardiovascular adaptive responses that are able to maintain an adequate oxygen supply for a certain period of time. Although there is no overall change of vascular resistance in the fetoplacental circulation, the anemic fetus responds with a progressive increase in cardiac output and blood flow velocity (74, 92, 131). Flow properties in the fetal blood vessels are also affected by the low viscosity of the blood. The term "hyperdynamic circulation" has been applied to this anemia-induced cardiovascular adaptation.

Resistance indices and flow velocities. Severe fetal anemic states are typically manifested by sinusoidal oscillation patterns in the FHR trace (Fig. 43.**70**). Increased flow velocities are found predominantly in the middle cerebral artery, descending aorta, and ductus venosus (Fig. 43.**70**) (74, 117). As in the arterial system, there is no increase of pulsatility in the venous vessels (74, 131). Consequently, the resistance indices in the arterial vessels and the preload indices in the venous vessels cannot be used to predict the degree of anemia. These findings are supported by experimental studies in fetal lambs with induced chronic anemia. It has been shown, for example, that progressive anemia accompanied by fetal hydrops is not associated with a rise of right ventricular pressure but does lead to an increase in right ventricular

Doppler ultrasound of cardiac complications

Fig. 43.64 Doppler frequency spectra from the umbilical artery and ductus venosus in fetofetal transfusion syndrome.

Fig. 43.65 Arterial and venous Doppler spectra in a fetus with severe hypoplastic left heart.

Fig. 43.66 Arterial and venous Doppler spectra in a fetus with pronounced endocardial fibroelastosis and a hypoplastic right heart.

Fig. 43.67 Doppler spectra recorded from the umbilical artery in various forms of fetal arrhythmia. In supraventricular tachycardia (here 222 bpm), the end-diastolic flow velocities are markedly increased due to the shortened cardiac cycle. Umbilical vein pulsations can often be demonstrated but are not present in all cases. With a complete AV block (here 66 bpm), on the other hand, the end-diastolic flow velocity is decreased due to the prolonged diastolic phase of the cycle. The increased cardiac blood volume is reflected in synchronous pulsations of the umbilical vein during the early systolic phase of the cycle. With supraventricular extrasystoles, there is a noncompensatory postextrasystolic pause in which the end-diastolic flow velocities decline. The peak systolic blood flow velocities that follow are elevated due to the increased stroke volume, which may be interpreted as a consequence of the Frank Starling law.

Fig. 43.68 Doppler spectra recorded from the umbilical vein, ductus venosus, and inferior vena cava of a fetus with supraventricular tachycardia (222 bpm). Note the monophasic pulsations in the umbilical vein and the monophasic waveform of the ductus venosus and inferior vena cava.

Fig. 43.69 Doppler frequency spectrum from the ductus venosus in a fetus with supraventricular extrasystoles. The intracardiac blood volume is increased immediately after the extrasystole and returns to normal in two cardiac cycles.

Fig. 43.70 Cardiogram, aortic Doppler spectrum, and ductus venosus Doppler spectrum in a fetus with severe anemia.

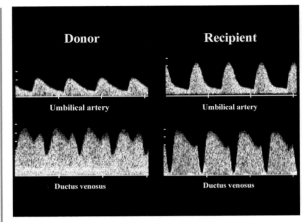

64

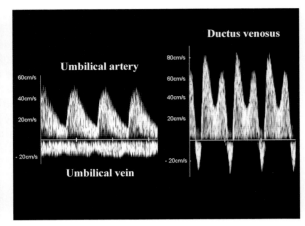

65

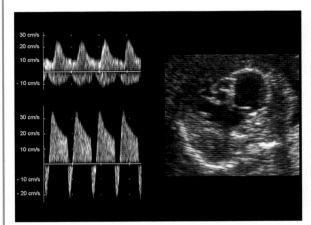

66

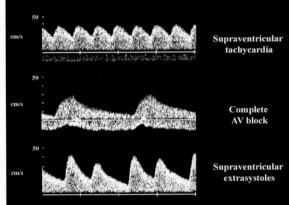

67

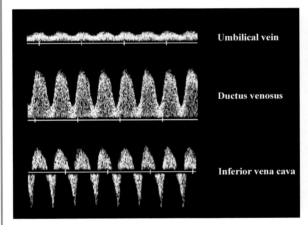

68

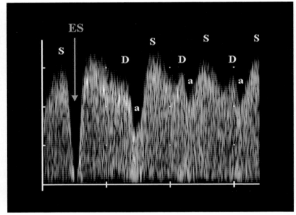

69

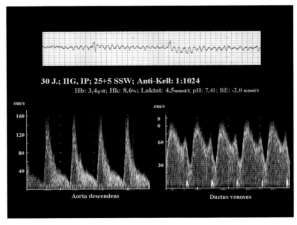

70

stroke volume and myocardial blood flow (43). Fetal hydrops, then, does not appear to be the primary cause of congestive heart failure but more likely results from changes in the colloidal osmotic pressure and/or hypoxemia-induced endothelial lesions in the fetal vessels. The hematocrit must fall below 10% before cardiovascular compensatory mechanisms are exhausted, at which point the declining cardiac stroke volume and rising ventricular pressures result in congestive failure (43).

Transfusion monitoring. Doppler examinations of the ductus venosus in the setting of an intrauterine intravascular blood transfusion can furnish information on hemodynamic changes during or immediately following the transfusion (130).

Oxygen Therapy

Improvement of fetal oxygenation. The transmaternal administration of oxygen for a specified period (maternal hyperoxygenation) is one option for the treatment of SGA and/or IUGR fetuses. Cordocentesis has confirmed that transmaternal oxygen administration leads to improved fetal oxygenation (128). The therapy consists of 6–8 L of 50–70% oxygen administered by mask inhalation (24, 46, 128).

Effect on fetal hemodynamics. Besides improving fetal oxygenation, maternal oxygen therapy also appears to affect fetal hemodynamics (7, 170). Transient improvement of abnormal fetal blood flow patterns has been observed with the therapy (7). The fetal hemodynamic response apparently depends on gestational age, however. For example, no change in cerebral blood flow was found in fetuses before 30 weeks' gestation (31, 143), whereas fetuses after 30 weeks showed a definite response to oxygen administration (8). Meanwhile, it has been shown that IUGR fetuses that do not respond to oxygen therapy have a markedly higher risk for acute fetal distress with a poorer prognosis (8, 31).

Clinical efficacy. The clinical efficacy of this therapy is debated. While some authors reported a 30–50% reduction in mortality (24, 128), other authors found no effect on mortality rate, instead reporting an increase in morbidity (143). Experiments in animals have even shown that changing the status of fetal oxygenation tends to cause a deterioration of fetal condition. Because of small case numbers and different study designs, the studies published to date do not permit a conclusive assessment of the benefits of this therapy.

Prolonged Pregnancy

Incidence and risks. The incidence of prolonged pregnancy is approximately 5% in cases where gestational age is assigned by ultrasound examination in early pregnancy.

Perinatal mortality increases markedly as the pregnancy is prolonged. For example, the incidence of intrauterine fetal death rises sixfold from 0.35 per 1000 at 37 weeks' gestation to 2.12 per 1000 at 43 weeks (79). To interpret Doppler indices based on the calculated due date, it is important to know the exact gestational age and also the Doppler reference curves for the final weeks of pregnancy. Although prolonged pregnancy is associated with an increased risk of relative uteroplacental insufficiency, this condition cannot be detected with Doppler ultrasound (85).

Changes after term. No significant changes in resistance indices occur in the uteroplacental vascular system after term in postdate pregnancies (85, 145). A slight decrease in mean blood flow velocity has been measured in the fetal aorta, but the resistance indices are unchanged (145, 184). On the other hand, a decline in resistance indices has been found in the fetoplacental vascular compartment (i.e., the umbilical artery), which is attributed to the progressive differentiation of the placenta (77, 160). A decline in resistance indices has also been found in the cerebrovascular system in pregnancies carried past the due date (10). The end-diastolic velocity in the middle cerebral artery at term equals approximately one-half the systolic velocity (85). This physiologic fall of resistance in the cerebral vessels should not be confused with the brain-sparing effect in severely growth-retarded fetuses, however, and therefore it is not considered a criterion for fetal compromise.

The amniotic fluid volume normally decreases toward the end of the pregnancy. However, there is no relationship between an increased amniotic fluid volume and the Doppler spectra recorded from the fetal vessels at term (198).

Conclusion. In summary, it may be said that abnormal Doppler spectra are very rarely recorded toward the end of pregnancy or in prolonged pregnancies. Also, Doppler findings are not useful in predicting fetal compromise in pregnancies that are carried past term (85). Although severely abnormal Doppler waveforms with absent end-diastolic flow in the umbilical artery have been reported after 42 weeks' gestation in isolated cases, evidence to date indicates that fetal Doppler ultrasound does not aid in clinical decision-making in true postdate pregnancies and does not supply additional information on increased perinatal risk (23, 85, 145, 184). In the great majority of cases, then, the use of Doppler ultrasound will be based on psychological indications as a means of reassuring the parents and often the attending physician.

References

1. Abuhamad, A.Z., Mari, G., Copel, J.A., Cantwell, J.C., Evans, A.T.: Umbilical artery flow velocity waveforms in monoamniotic twins with cord entanglement. Obstet. Gynecol. 86 (1995) 674–677
2. Abuhamad, A.Z., Shaffer, W., Mari, G., Copel, J.A., Hobbins, J.C., Evans, A.T.: Single umbilical artery: Does it matter which artery is missing? Amer. J. Obstet. Gynecol. 173 (1995) 728–732
3. Akalin-Sel, T., Nicolaides, K.H., Peacock, J., Campbell, S.: Doppler dynamics and their complex interrelation with fetal oxygen pressure, carbon dioxide pressure, and pH in growth-retarded fetuses. Obstet. Gynecol. 84 (1994) 439–444
4. Almström, H., Axelsson, O., Cnattingius, S. et al.: Comparison of umbilical-artery velocimetry and cardiotocography for surveillance of small-for gestational-age fetuses. Lancet 340 (1992) 936–940
5. Alpers, B.J., Berry, R.G., Paddison, R.M.: Anatomical studies of the Circle of Willis in normal brain. Arch. Neurol. Psych. 81 (1959) 409–418
6. Arabin, B., Bergmann, P.L., Saling, E.: Simultaneous assessment of blood flow velocity waveforms in uteroplacental vessels, the umbilical artery, the fetal aorta, and the fetal common carotid artery. Fetal Ther. 2 (1987) 17–26
7. Arduini, D., Rizzo, G., Mancuso, S., Romanini, C.: Short-term effects of maternal oxygen administration on blood flow velocity waveforms in healthy and growth-retarded fetuses. Amer. J. Obstet. Gynecol. 159 (1988) 1077–1080
8. Arduini, D., Rizzo, G., Romanini, C., Mancuso, S.: Fetal haemodynamic response to acute maternal hypertension as predictor of fetal distress in intrauterine growth retardation. Brit. Med. J. 298 (1989) 1561–1562
9. Arduini, D., Rizzo, G.: Normal values of pulsatility index from fetal vessels: a cross sectional study on 1556 healthy fetuses. J. Perinat. Med. 18 (1990) 165–172
10. Arduini, D., Rizzo, G., Romanini, C., Mancuso, S.: Doppler assessment of fetal blood flow velocity waveforms during acute maternal oxygen administration as predictor of fetal outcome in post-term pregnancy. Amer. J. Perinat. 7 (1990) 258–262
11. Arduini, D., Rizzo, G., Soliani, A., Romanini, C.: Doppler velocimetry versus nonstress test in the antepartum monitoring of low-risk pregnancies. J. Ultrasound Med. 10 (1991) 331–335
12. Arduini, D., Rizzo, G.: Fetal renal artery velocity waveforms and amniotic fluid volume in growth-retarded and post-term fetuses. Obstet. Gynecol. 77 (1991) 370–373
13. Arduini, D., Rizzo, G.: Prediction of fetal outcome in small for gestational age fetuses. Comparison of Doppler measurements obtained from different fetal vessels. J. Perinat. Med. 20 (1992) 29–38
14. Arduini, D., Rizzo, G., Romanini, C.: The development of abnormal heart rate patterns after absent end-diastolic velocity in umbilical artery: Analysis of risk factors. Amer. J. Obstet. Gynecol. 168 (1993) 43–50
15. Arias, F.: Accuracy of the middle-cerebral-to-umbilical artery resistance index ratio in prediction of neonatal outcome in patients at high rsik for fetal and neonatal complications. Amer. J. Obstet. Gynecol. 171 (1994) 1541–1545
16. Azancot-Benisty, A., Benifla, J.L., Matias, A., De Crepy, A., Madelenat, P.: Constriction of the fetal ductus arteriosus during prenatal betamethasone therapy. Obstet. Gynecol. 85 (1995) 847–876
17. Bahado-Singh, R.O., Kovanci, E., Jeffres, A. et al.: The Doppler cerebroplacental ratio and perinatal outcome in intrauterine growth restriction. Amer. J. Obstet. Gynecol. 180 (1999) 750–756

18. Bahlmann, F., Merz, E.: Insights into normal and abnormal fetal ductus venosus blood velocities. Ultrasound Obstet. Gynecol. 6 (Suppl. 2) (1995) 72
19. Bahlmann, F., Wellek, S., Reinhardt, I., Merz, E., Steiner, E., Welter, E.: Reference values of ductus venosus flow velocity waveforms and various calculated waveform indices. Prenat. Diagn. 20 (2000) 623–634
20. Bahlmann, F., Wellek, S., Reinhard, I., Krummenauer, F., Merz, E., Welter, C.: Reference values of fetal aortic flow velocity waveforms and associated intra-observer reliability in normal pregnancies. Ultrasound Obstet. Gynecol. 17 (2001) 42–49
21. Bahlmann, F., Reinhardt, I., Krummenauer, F., Neubert, S., Macchiella, D., Wellek, S.: Blood flow velocity waveforms of the fetal middle cerebral artery in a normal population: reference values from 18 weeks to 42 weeks of gestation. Perinat. Med. (2001) in press
22. Bahlmann, F., Reinhardt, I., Krummenauer, F., Neubert, S., Macchiella, D., Wellek, S.: Blood flow velocity waveforms of the umbilical artery in a normal population: reference values from 18 weeks to 42 weeks of gestation. In Vorbereitung
23. Battaglia, C., Larocca, E., Lanzani, A., Coukos, G., Genazzani, A.R.: Doppler velocimetry in prolonged pregnancy. Obstet. Gynecol. 77 (1991) 213–216
24. Battaglia, C., Artini, P.G., D'Ambrogio, G., Galli, P.A., Segre, A., Genazzani, A.R.: Maternal hyperoxygenation in the treatment of intrauterine growth retardation. Amer. J. Obstet. Gynecol. 167 (1992) 430–435
25. Battaglia, C., Artini, P.G., Galli, P.A., D'ambrogio, G., Droghini, F., Genazzani, A.R.: Absent or reversed end-diastolic flow in umbilical artery and severe intrauterine growth retardation. Acta. Obstet. Gynecol. Scand. 72 (1993) 167–171
26. Behrens, O., Wedeking-Schöhl, H., Goeschen, K.: Prognostischer Wert der Kardiotokographie bei Schwangerschaften mit pathologischem Dopplerbefund. Geburtsh. u. Frauenheilk. 56 (1996) 272–277
27. Bekedam, D.J., Visser, G.H.A., van der Zee, A.G.J., Snijders, R.J.M., Poelmann-Weesjes, G.: Abnormal velocity waveforms of the umbilical artery in growth retarded fetuses: relationship to antepartum late heart rate deceleration and outcome. Early Hum. Dev. 24 (1990) 79–89
28. Berkowitz, G.S., Mehalek, K.E., Chitkara, U., Rosenberg, J., Cogswell, C., Berkowitz, R.L.: Doppler velocimetry in the prediction of adverse outcome in pregnancies at risk for intrauterine growth retardation. Obstet. Gynecol. 71 (1988) 742–746
29. Bilardo, C.M., Campbell, S., Nicolaides, K.H.: Mean blood velocities and flow impedance in the fetal descending thoracic aorta and common carotid artery in normal pregnancy. Early Hum. Dev. 18 (1988) 213–221
30. Bilardo, C.M., Nicolaides, K.H., Campbell, S.: Doppler measurements of fetal and uteroplacental circulations: Relationship with umbilical venous blood gases measured at cordocentesis. Amer. J. Obstet. Gynecol. 162 (1990) 115–120
31. Bilardo, C.M., Snijders, R.M., Campbell, S., Nicolaides, K.H.: Doppler study of the fetal circulation during long-term maternal hyperoxygenation for severe early onset intrauterine growth retardation. Ultrasound Obstet. Gynecol. 1 (1991) 250–257
32. Bonnin, P., Guyot, B., Bailliart, O., Benard, C., Blot, P., Martineaud, J.P.: Relationship between umbilical and fetal cerebral blood flow velocity waveforms and umbilical venous blood gases. Ultrasound Obstet. Gynecol. 2 (1992) 18–22
33. Brezinka, C., Huisman, T.W.A., Stijnen, T., Wladimiroff, J.W.: Normal Doppler flow velocity waveforms in the fetal ductus arteriosus in the first half of pregnancy. Ultrasound Obstet. Gynecol. 2 (1992) 397–401
34. Brezinka, C., Stijnen, T., Wladimiroff, J. W.: Doppler flow velocity waveforms in the fetal ductus arteriosus during first half of pregnancy: a reproducibility study. Ultrasound Obstet. Gynecol. 4 (1994) 121–123
35. Burke, G., Stuart, B., Crowley, P., Scanuill, S.N., Drumin, J.: Is intrauterine growth retardation with normal umbilical artery blood flow a benign condition? Brit. Med. J. 300 (1990) 1044–1045
36. Chambers, S.E., Hoskins, P.R., Haddad, N.G., Johnstone, F.D., McDicken, W.N., Muir, B.B.: A comparison of fetal abdominal circumference measurements and Doppler ultrasound in the prediction of small-for-dates babies and fetal compromise. Brit. J. Obstet. Gynecol. 96 (1989) 803–808
37. Chan, F.Y., Woo, S.K., Ghosh, A., Tang, M., Lam, C.: Prenatal diagnosis of congenital fetal arrhythmias by simultaneous pulsed Doppler Velocimetry of the fetal abdominal aorta and inferior vena cava. Obstet. Gynecol. 76 (1990) 200–204
38. Chan, F.Y., Pun, T.C., Lam, P., Lam, C., Lee, C.P., Lam, Y.H.: Fetal cerebral Doppler studies as a predictor of perinatal outcome and subsequent neurologic handicap. Obstet. Gynecol. 87 (1996) 981–988
39. Chaoui, R., Taddei, F., Bast, C. et al.: Sonographische Untersuchung des fetalen Lungenkreislaufs. Der Gynäkologe 30 (1997) 230–239
40. Chaoui, R., Taddei, F., Rizzo, G., Bast, C., Lenz, F., Bollmann, R.: Doppler echocardiography of the main stems of the pulmonary arteries in the normal human fetus. Ultrasound Obstet. Gynecol. 11 (1998) 173–179
41. Cohn, E.H., Sacks, E.J., Heymann, M.A., Rudolph, A.M.: Cardiovascular responses to hypoxemia and acidemia in fetal lambs. Amer. J. Obstet. Gynecol. 120 (1974) 817–824
42. Damron, D.P., Chaffin, D.G., Anderson, C.F., Reed, K.L.: Changes in umbilical arterial and venous blood flow velocity waveforms during late decelerations of the fetal heart rate. Obstet. Gynecol. 84 (1994) 1038–1040
43. Davies, L.E., Hohimer, A.R., Giraud, G.D., Reller, M.D., Morton, M.J.: Right ventricular function in chronically anemic fetal lambs. Amer. J. Obstet. Gynecol. 174 (1996) 1289–1294
44. De Catte, L., Burrini, D., Mares, C., Waterschoot, T.: Single umbilical artery: analysis of Doppler flow indices and arterial diameters in normal and growth-retarded fetuses. Ultrasound Obstet. Gynecol. 8 (1996) 27–30
45. Degani, S., Lewinsky, R.M., Shapiro, I.: Doppler studies of fetal cerebral blood flow. Ultrasound Obstet. Gynecol. 4 (1994) 158–165
46. De Rochambeau, B., Poix, D., Mellier, D.: Maternal hyperoxygenation: a fetal blood flow velocity prognosis test in small-for gestational-age fetuses? Ultrasound Obstet. Gynecol. 2 (1992) 279–282
47. DeVore, G.R., Horenstein, J.: Ductus venosus index: a method for evaluating right ventricular preload in the second-trimester fetus. Ultrasound Obstet. Gynecol. 3 (1993) 338–342
48. DeVore, G.R.: Color Doppler examination of the outflow tracts of the fetal heart: a technique for identification of cardiovascular malformations. Ultrasound Obstet. Gynecol. 4 (1994) 463–471
49. DeVore, G.R.: The value of color Doppler sonography in the diagnosis of renal agenesis. J. Ultrasound Med. 14 (1995) 443–449
50. Divon, M.Y.: Randomized controlled trials of umbilical artery Doppler velocimetry: how many are too many? Ultrasound Obstet. Gynecol. 6 (1995) 377–379
51. Divon, M.V.: Umbilical artery Doppler velocimetry: Clinical utility in high-risk pregnancies. Amer. J. Obstet. Gynecol. 174 (1996) 10–14
52. Edelstone, D.I., Rudolph, A.M.: Preferential streaming of ductus venosus blood to the brain and heart in fetal lambs. Amer. J. Physiol. 237 (1979) H724–H729
53. Eik-Nes, S.H., Brubakk, A., Ulstein, M.: Measurement of human fetal blood flow. Brit. Med. J. 280 (1980) 283–286
54. Eik-Nes, S.H., Marsal, K., Kristoffersen, K.: Methodology and basic problems related to blood flow studies in the human fetus. Ultrasound Med. Biol. 10 (1984) 329–334
55. Erskine, R.L.A., Ritchie, J.W.K.: Quantitative measurement of fetal blood flow using Doppler ultrasound. Brit. J. Obstet. Gynecol. 92 (1985) 600–604
56. Gembruch, U., Krapp, M., Baumann, P.: Changes of venous blood flow velocity waveforms in fetuses with supraventricular tachycardia. Ultrasound Obstet. Gynecol. 5 (1995) 394–399
57. Giles, W.B., Trudinger, B.J., Blaird, P.: Fetal umbilical artery flow velocity waveforms and placental resistance: Pathologic correlation. Brit. J. Obstet. Gynaecol. 92 (1985) 31–38
58. Gill, R.W., Trudinger, B.J., Gerrit, W.J., Kossow, G., Warren, P.S.: Fetal umbilical venous flow measured in utero by pulsed Doppler and B-mode ultrasound. Amer. J. Obstet. Gynecol. 139 (1981) 720–725
59. Gill, R.W., Kossoff, G., Warren, P.S., Garrett, W.J.: Umbilical venous flow in normal and complicated pregnancy. Ultrasound Med. Biol. 10 (1984) 349–363
60. Giussani, D.A., Spencer, J.A.D., Moore, P.J., Bennet, L., Hanson, M.A.: Afferent and efferent components of the cardiovascular reflex responses to acute hypoxia in term fetal sheep. J. Physiol. 461 (1993) 431–449
61. Goffinet, F., Paris-Llado, J., Nisand, I., Bréart, G.: A randomised controlled trial of Doppler ultrasound velocimetry of the umbilical artery in low risk pregnancies. Brit. J. Obstet. Gynaecol. 104 (1997) 419–424
62. Goffinet, F., Paris-Llado, J., Nisand, I., Bréart, G.: Umbilical artery Doppler velocimetry in unselected and low risk pregnancies: a review of randomised controlled trials. Brit. J. Obstet. Gynaecol. 104 (1997) 425–430
63. Goldin, E., Harel, S., Tomer, A., Yavin, E.: Thromboxan and prostacyclin levels in fetal rabbit brain and placenta after intrauterine partial ischemic episodes. J. Neurochem. 54 (1990) 587–591
64. Grab, D., Paulus, W.E., Erdmann, M. et al.: Intraobserver-Reproduzierbarkeit von dopplersonographischen Messungen im fetalen Ductus arterious. Z. Geburtsh. Neonatol. 203 (1999) 15–17
65. Gramellini, D., Folli, M.C., Raboni, S., Vadora, E., Merialdi, M.: Cerebral-umbilical Doppler ratio as predictor of adverse outcome. Obstet. Gynecol. 79 (1992) 416–420
66. Griffin, D., Bilardo, K., Masini, L. et al.: Doppler blood flow waveforms in the descending thoracic aorta of the human fetus. Brit. J. Obstet. Gynaecol. 91 (1984) 997–1006
67. Gudmundson, S., Huhta, J.C., Weiner, S., Wood, D.C., Tulzer, G., Cohen, A.: Cerebral Doppler velocimetry and fetal hydrocephalus. J. Matern. Fetal Invest. 1 (1991) 79–82
68. Gudmundson, S., Neerhof, M., Weiner, S., Tulzer, G., Wood, D., Hutha, J.C.: Fetal hydronephrosis and renal artery blood velocity. Ultrasound Obstet. Gynecol. 1 (1991) 413–416
69. Gudmundson, S., Hutha. J.C., Wood, D.C., Tulzer, G., Cohen, A.W., Weiner, S.: Doppler ultrasonography in the fetus with nonimmune hydrops. Amer. J. Obstet. Gynecol. 164 (1991) 33–37
70. Gudmundson, S., Tulzer, G., Hutha, J.C., Marsal, K.: Venous Doppler in the fetus with absent end-diastolic flow in the umbilical artery. Ultrasound Obstet. Gynecol. 7 (1996) 262–267
71. Hata, T., Mari, G., Reiter, A.A.: Doppler velocity waveforms of blood flow in the fetal renal artery in a case of Meckel syndrome. Amer. J. Roentgenol. 156 (1991) 408
72. Hecher, K., Campbell, S., Snijders, R., Nicolaides, K.: Reference ranges for fetal venous and atrioventricular blood flow parameters. Ultrasound Obstet. Gynecol. 4 (1994) 381–390
73. Hecher, K., Campbell, S., Doyle, P., Harrington, K., Nicolaides, K.: Assessment of fetal compromise by Doppler ultrasound investigation of the fetal circulation. Arterial, intracardiac, and venous blood flow velocity studies. Circulation 91 (1995) 129–138
74. Hecher, K., Snijders, R., Campbell, S., Nicolaides, K.: Fetal venous, arterial, and intracardiac blood flows in red blood cell isoimmunization. Obstet. Gynecol. 85 (1995) 122–128
75. Hecher, K., Snijders, R., Campbell, S., Nicolaides, K.: Fetal venous, intracardiac, and arterial blood flow measurements in intrauterine growth retardation; Relationship with fetal blood gases. Amer. J. Obstet. Gynecol. 173 (1995) 10–15
76. Hecher, K., Ville, Y., Snijders, R., Nicolaides, K.: Doppler studies of the fetal circulation in twin-twin transfusion syndrome. Ultrasound Obstet. Gynecol. 5 (1995) 318–324
77. Hendricks, S.K., Sorensen, T.K., Wang, K.Y., Bushnell, J.M., Seguin, E.M., Zingheim, R.W.: Doppler umbilical artery waveform indices – Normal values from fourteen to forty-two weeks. Amer. J. Obstet. Gynecol. 161 (1989) 761–765
78. Heymann, M.A., Lewis, A.B., Rudolph, A.M.: Pulmonary vascular responses during advancing gestation in fetal lambs in utero. Chest 71 (1977) 270–271
79. Hilder, L., Costeloe, K., Thilaganathan, B.: Prolonged pregnancy: evaluation gestation-specific risks of fetal and infant mortality. Brit. J. Obstet. Gynecol. 105 (1998) 169–173
80. Huisman, T.W.A., Stewart, P.A., Wladimiroff, J.W.: Flow velocity waveforms in the fetal inferior vena cava during the second half of normal pregnancy. Ultrasound Med. Biol. 17 (1991) 379–382
81. Huisman, T.W.A., Gittenberger-De Groot, A.C., Wladimiroff, J.W.: Recognition of a fetal subdiaphragmatic venous vestibulum essential for fetal venous Doppler assessment. Pediatr. Res. 32 (1992) 338–341

82. Huisman, T.W.A., Brezinka, C., Stewart, P.A., Wladimiroff, J.W.: Ductus venosus flow velocity waveforms in relation to fetal behavioural status. Brit. J. Obstet. Gynaecol. 101 (1994) 220–224

83. Indik, J., Chen, V., Reed, K.L.: Association of umbilical venous with inferior vena cava blood flow velocities. Obstet. Gynecol. 77 (1991) 551–557

84. Iwamoto, H., Kaufman, T., Keil, L., Rudolph, A.: Responses to acute hypoxemia in fetal sheep at 0.6–0.7 gestation. Amer. J. Physiol. 256 (1989) H613–H620

85. Jörn, H., Funk, A., Fendel, H.: Doppler-Ultraschalldiagnostik bei Terminüberschreitung. Geburtsh. u. Frauenheilk. 53 (1993) 603–608

86. Jouppila, P., Kirkinen, P.: Increased vascular resistance in the descending aorta of the human fetus in hypoxia. Brit. J. Obstet. Gynaecol. 91 (1984) 853–856

87. Jouppila, P., Kirkinen, P.: Blood velocity waveforms of the fetal aorta in normal and hypertensive pregnancies. Obstet. Gynecol. 67 (1986) 856–860

88. Kaminopetros, P., Dykes, E.H., Nicolaides, K.H.: Fetal renal artery blood velocimetry in multicystic kidney disease. Ultrasound Obstet. Gynecol. 1 (1991) 410–412

89. Kanzaki, T., Murakami, M., Kobayashi, H., Chiba, Y.: Characteristic abnormal blood flow patterns of the inferior vena cava in fetal arrhythmias. J. Matern. Fetal Invest. 1 (1991) 35–39

90. Karsdorp, V.H.M., van Vugt, J.M.G., Kostense, P.J., Arduini, D., Montenegro, N., Todros, T.: Clinical significance of absent or reversed end diastolic velocity waveforms in umbilical artery. Lancet 344 (1994) 1664–1668

91. Kenny, J.F., Plappert, T., Doubilet, P. et al.: Changes in intracardiac blood flow velocities and right and left ventricular stroke volumes with gestational age in the normal human fetus: A prospective Doppler echocardiographic study. Circulation 74 (1986) 1208–1216

92. Kirkinen, P., Jouppila, P.: Umbilical vein blood flow in rhesus-isoimmunization. Brit. J. Obstet. Gynaecol. 90 (1983) 640–643

93. Kirshon, B., Mari, G., Moise, K.J., Wasserstrum, N.: The effects of indomethacin on the fetal ductus arteriosus during treatment of symptomatic polyhydramnios. J. Reprod. Med. 35 (1990) 529–532

94. Kirshon, B., Moise, K.J., Mari, G., Willis, R.: Long term indomethacin decreases fetal urine output and results in oligohydramnios. Amer. J. Perinatol. 8 (1991) 86–88

95. Kiserud, T., Eik-Nes, S.H., Blaas, H.G., Hellevik, L.R.: Ultrasonographic velocimetry of the fetal ductus venosus. Lancet 338 (1991) 1412–1414

96. Kiserud, T., Eik-Nes, S.H., Hellevik, L.R., Blaas, H.G.: Ductus venosus – A longitudinal Doppler velocimetric study of the human fetus. J. Matern. Fetal Invest. 2 (1992) 5–11

97. Kiserud, T., Eik-Nes, S.H., Hellevik, L.R., Blaas, H.G.: Ductus venosus blood velocity changes in fetal cardiac diseases. J. Matern. Fetal Invest. 3 (1993) 15–20

98. Kiserud, T., Eik-Nes, S.H., Blaas, H.G., Hellevik, L.R., Simensen, B.: Ductus venosus blood velocity and the umbilical circulation in the seriously growth-retarded fetus. Ultrasound Obstet. Gynecol. 4 (1994) 109–114

99. Kofinas, A.D., Penry, M., Hatjis, C.G.: Umbilical vessel flow velocity waveforms in cord entanglement in a monoamniotic multiple gestation. J. Reprod. Med. 36 (1991) 314–316

100. Kurmanavicius, J., Florio, I., Wisser, J. et al.: Reference resistance indices of the umbilical, fetal middle cerebral and uterine arteries at 24–42 weeks of gestation. Ultrasound Obstet. Gynecol. 10 (1997) 112–120

101. Laudy, J.A.M., De Ridder M.A.J., Wladimiroff, J.W.: Doppler velocimetry in branch pulmonary arteries of normal human fetuses during the second half of gestation. Pediatr. Res. 41 (1997) 897–901

102. Laurin, J., Lingman, G., Marsal, K., Persson, P.H.: Fetal blood flow in pregnancy complicated by intrauterine growth retardation. Obstet. Gynecol. 69 (1987) 895–902

103. Larson, J.D., Rayburn, W.F., Crosby, S., Thurnau, G.R.: Multiple nuchal cord entanglements and intrapartum complications. Amer. J. Obstet. Gynecol. 173 (1995) 1228–1231

104. Lewinsky, R., Farine, D., Ritchie, J.W.: Transvaginal Doppler assessment of the fetal cerebral circulation. Obstet. Gynecol. 78 (1991) 637–640

105. Lingman, G., Marsal, K.: Fetal central blood circulation in the third trimester of normal pregnancy – a longitudinal study. II. Aortic blood velocity waveform. Early Hum. Develop. 13 (1986) 151–159

106. Low, J.A.: The current status of maternal and fetal blood flow velocimetry. Amer. J. Obstet. Gynecol. 164 (1991) 1049–1063

107. Macara, L., Kingdom, J.C.P., Kaufmann, P.: Structural analysis of placenta terminal villi from growth-restricted pregnancies with abnormal umbilical artery Doppler waveforms. Placenta 17 (1996) 37–48

108. Mackenzie, F.M., Kingston, G.O., Oppenheimer, L.: The early prenatal diagnosis of bilateral renal agenesis using transvaginal sonography and color Doppler ultrasonography. J. Ultrasound Med. 13 (1994) 49–53

109. Mai, R., Kristen, P., Rempen, A.: Der enddiastolische Blutfluß der A. renalis in der normalen Schwangerschaft. Ultraschall Klin. Prax. 8 (1994) 232–234

110. Malcus, P., van Beek, E., Marsal, K.: Umbilical artery velocimetry and non-stress test in monitoring high risk pregnancies. A comparative longitudinal study. Ultrasound Obstet. Gynecol. 1 (1991) 95–101

111. Mari, G., Moise, K.J., Deter, R.L., Kirshon, B., Carpenter, R.J., Hutha, J.C.: Doppler assessment of the pulsatility index in the cerebral circulation of the human fetus. Amer. J. Obstet. Gynecol. 160 (1989) 698–703

112. Mari, G., Moise, K.J., Deter, R.L., Kirshon, B., Carpenter, R.J.: Doppler Assessment of renal blood flow velocity waveform during indomethacin therapy for preterm labor and polyhydramnios. Obstet. Gynecol. 75 (1990) 199–201

113. Mari, G.: Arterial blood flow velocity waveforms of the pelvis and lower extremities in normal and growth-retarded fetuses. Amer. J. Obstet. Gynecol. 165 (1991) 143–151

114. Mari, G., Wasserstrum, N.: Flow velocity waveforms of the fetal circulation preceding fetal death in a case of lupus anticoagulant. Amer. J. Obstet. Gynecol. 164 (1991) 776–778

115. Mari, G., Kirshon, B., Abuhamad, A.: Fetal renal artery flow velocity waveforms in normal pregnancies and pregnancies complicated by polyhydramnios and oligohydramnios. Obstet. Gynecol. 81 (1993) 560–564

116. Mari, G., Abuhamad, A.Z., Keller, M., Verpairojkit, B., Ment, L., Copel, J.A.: Is the fetal brain-sparing effect a risk factor for the development of intraventricular hemorrhage in the preterm infant? Ultrasound Obstet. Gynecol. 8 (1996) 329–332

117. Mari, G.: Noninvasive diagnosis by Doppler ultrasonography of fetal anemia due to maternal red-cell alloimmunization. New Engl. J. Med. 342 (2000) 9–14

118. Marsal, K., Laurin, J., Lindblad, A., Lingman, G.: Blood flow in the fetal descending aorta. Sem. Perinat. 11 (1987) 322–334

119. Maulik, D., Yarlagadda, P., Downing, G.: Doppler velocimetry in obstetrics. Obstet. Gynecol. Clin. North Amer. 17 (1990) 163–186

120. Mielke, G., Steil, E., Kendziorra, H., Goelz, R.: Ductus arteriosus-dependent pulmonary circulation secondary to cardiac malformations in fetal life. Ultrasound Obstet. Gynecol. 9 (1997) 25–29

121. Mielke, G., Benda, N.: Blood flow velocity waveforms of the fetal pulmonary artery and the ductus arteriosus: reference ranges from 13 weeks to term. Ultrasound Obstet. Gynecol. 15 (2000) 213–218

122. Meyer, W.W., Lind, J.: Iliac arteries in children with a single umbilical artery. Structure, calcifications and early atherosclerotic lesions. Arch. Dis. Child 49 (1974) 671–679

123. Moise, K.J., Huhta, J.C., Sharif, D.S. et al.: Indomethacin in the treatment of premature labor. Effects on the fetal ductus arteriosus. New Engl. J. Med. 319 (1988) 327–331

124. Moise, K.J.; Effect of advancing gestational age on the frequency of the fetal ductus constriction in association with maternal indomethacin use. Amer. J. Obstet. Gynecol. 168 (1993) 1350–1353

125. Nadasy, G.L., Monos, E., Mohacsi, E., Csepli, J., Kovach, A.G.: Effect of increased luminal blood flow on the development of the human arterial wall. Comparison of mechanical properties of double and single arteries in vitro. Blood Vessels 18 (1981) 139–143

126. Nakai, Y., Miyazaki, Y., Matsuoka, Y.: Pulsatile umbilical venous flow and its clinical significance. Brit. J. Obstet. Gynaecol. 99 (1992) 977–980

127. Neilson, J.P., Alfirevic, Z.: Doppler ultrasound in high risk pregnancies (Cochrane Review). In: The Cochrane Library, Issue 1, 2000. Oxford: Update Software

128. Nicolaides, K.H., Campbell, S., Bradley, R.J., Bilardo, C.M., Soothill, P.W., Gibb, D.: Maternal oxygen therapy for intrauterine growth retardation. Lancet 28 (1987) 942–945

129. Noordam, M.J., Hoekstra, F.M.E., Hop, W.C.J., Wladimiroff, J.W.: Doppler colour flow imaging of fetal intracerebral arteries relative to fetal behavioural states in normal pregnancy. Early Hum. Dev. 39 (1994) 49–56

130. Oepkes, D., Vanderbussche, F.P., van Bel, F., Kanhai, H.H.H.: Fetal ductus venosus blood flow velocities before and after transfusion in red-cell alloimmunized pregnancies. Obstet. Gynecol. 82 (1993) 237–241

131. Oepkes, D., Brand, R., Vandenbussche, F.P., Meerman, R.H., Kanhai, H.H.H.: The use of ultrasonography and Doppler in the prediction of fetal haemolytic anaemia: a multivariate analysis. Brit. J. Obstet. Gynaecol. 101 (1994) 680–684

132. Parilla, B.V., Tamura, R.K., MacGregor, S.N., Geibel, L.J., Sabbagha, R.E.: The clinical significance of a singel umbilical artery as an isolated finding on prenatal ultrasound. Obstet. Gynecol. 85 (1995) 570–572

133. Persutte, W.H., Hobbins, J.: Single umbilical artery: a clinical enigma in modern prenatal diagnosis. Ultrasound Obstet. Gynecol. 6 (1995) 216–229

134. Pilu, G., Falco, P., Guazzarini, M., Sandri, F., Bovicelli, L.: Sonographic demonstration of nuchal cord and abnormal umbilical artery waveform heralding fetal distress. Ultrasound Obstet. Gynecol. 12 (1998) 125–127

135. Rasanen, J., Jouppila, P.: Fetal cardiac function and ductus arteriosus during indomethacin and sulindac therapy for threatened preterm labor: A randomized study. Amer. J. Obstet. Gynecol. 173 (1995) 20–25

136. Rasanen, J., Hutha, J.C., Weiner, S., Wood, D.C., Ludomirski, A.: Fetal branch pulmonary arterial vascular impedance during the second half of pregnancy. Amer. J. Obstet. Gynecol. 174 (1996) 1441–1449

137. Rasanen, J., Wood, D.C., Weiner, S., Ludormirski, A., Huhta, J.C.: Role of the pulmonary circulation in the distribution of human fetal cardiac output during the second half of pregnancy. Circulation 94 (1996) 1068–1073

138. Reed, K.L., Appleton, C.P., Anderson, C.F., Shenker, L., Sahn, D.L.: Doppler studies of vena cava flows in human fetuses. Circulation 81 (1990) 498–505

139. Reed, K.L., Chaffin, D.G., Anderson, C.F.: Umbilical venous Doppler velocity pulsations and inferior vena cava pressure elevations in fetal lamb. Obstet. Gynecol. 87 (1996) 617–620

140. Reed, K.L., Chaffin, D.G., Anderson, C.F., Newman, A.T.: Umbilical venous velocity pulsations are related to atrial contraction pressure waveforms in fetal lambs. Obstet. Gynecol. 89 (1997) 953–956

141. Respondek, M., Weil, S.R., Huhta, J.C.: Fetal echocardiography during indomethacin treatment. Ultrasound Obstet. Gynecol. 5 (1995) 86–89

142. Reuss, M.L., Rudolph, A.M., Dae, M.W.: Phasic blood flow patterns in the superior and inferior venae cavae and umbilical vein of fetal sheep. Amer. J. Obstet. Gynecol. 145 (1983) 70–78

143. Ribbert, L.S.M., van Lingen, R.A., Visser, G.H.A.: Continous maternal hyperoxygenation in the treatment of early fetal growth retardation. Ultrasound Obstet Gynecol 1 (1991) 331–335

144. Richardson, B.S., Rurak, D., Patrick, J.E., Homan, J., Carmichael, L.: Cerebral oxidative metabolism during sustained hypoxaemia in fetal sheep. J. Dev. Physiol. 11 (1989) 37–43

145. Righmire, D.A., Campbell, S.: Fetal and maternal Doppler blood flow parameters in postterm pregnancies. Obstet. Gynecol. 69 (1987) 891–894

146. Rizzo, G., Arduini, D., Romanini, C.: Umbilical vein pulsations: A physiologic finding in early gestation. Amer. J. Obstet. Gynecol. 167 (1992) 675–677

147. Rizzo, G., Arduini, D., Caforio, L., Romanini, C.: Effects of sampling sites on inferior vena cava flow velocity waveforms. J. Matern. Fetal Invest. 2 (1992) 153–156

148. Rizzo, G., Arduini, D., Romanini, C.: Inferior vena cava flow velocity waveforms in appropriate- and small-for-gestational-age fetuses. Amer. J. Obstet. Gynecol. 166 (1992) 1271–1280

149. Rizzo, G., Capponi, A., Arduini, D., Romanini, C.: Ductus venosus velocity waveforms in appropriate and small for gestational age fetuses. Early Hum. Develop. 39 (1994) 15–26

150. Rizzo, G., Capponi, A., Arduini, D., Romanini, C.: The value of fetal arterial, cardiac and venous flows in predicting pH and blood gases measured in umbilical blood at cordocentesis in growth retarded fetuses. Brit. J. Obstet. Gynaecol. 102 (1995) 963–969

151. Rizzo, G., Capponi, A., Talone, P.E., Arduini, D., Romanini, C.: Doppler indices from inferior vena cava and ductus venosus in predicting pH and oxygen tension in umbilical blood at cordocentesis in growth-retarded fetuses. Ultrasound Obstet. Gynecol. 7 (1996) 401–410

152. Rizzo, G., Capponi, A., Chaoui, R., Taddei, F., Arduini, D., Romanini, C.: Blood flow velocity waveforms from peripheral pulmonary arteries in normally grown and growth-retarded fetuses. Ultrasound Obstet. Gynecol. 8 (1996) 87–92

153. Robillard, J.E., Weitzman, R.E., Burmeister, L., Smith, F.G.: Developmental aspects of the renal response to hypoxemia in the lamb fetus. Circ. Res. 48 (1981) 128–138

154. Robinson, J.N., Abuhamad, A.Z.: Umbilical artery Doppler velocimetry waveform abnormality in fetal gastroschisis. Ultrasound Obstet. Gynecol. 10 (1997) 356–358

155. Rowlands, D.J., Vyas, S.K.: Longitudinal study of fetal middle cerebral artery flow velocity waveforms preceding fetal death. Brit. J. Obstet. Gynaecol. 102 (1995) 888–890

156. Rudolph, A.M., Heymann, M.A.: Circulatory changes during growth in the fetal lamb. Circ. Res. 26 (1970) 289–299

157. Rudolph, A.M.: Hepatic and ductus venosus blood flows during fetal life. Hepatology 3 (1983) 254–258

158. Scherjon, S.A., Smolders-DeHaas, H., Kok, J.H., Zondervan, H.A.: The „brain-sparing" effect: Antenatal cerebral Doppler findings in relation to neurologic outcome in very preterm infants. Amer. J. Obstet. Gynecol. 169 (1993) 169–175

159. Schröder, H., Gilbert, R.D., Power, G.G.: Urinary and hemodynamic responses to blood volume changes in fetal sheep. J. Dev. Physiol. 6 (1984) 131–141

160. Schulman, H., Fleischer, A., Stern, W., Farmakides, G., Jagani, N., Blattner, P.: Umbilical velocity wave ratios in human pregnancy. Amer. J. Obstet. Gynecol. 148 (1984) 985–989

161. Schulman, H., Winter, D., Farmakides, G.: Pregnancy surveillance with Doppler velocimetry of uterine and of uterine and umbilical arteries. Brit. J. Obstet. Gynecol. 160 (1990) 192–196

162. Sepulveda, W., Flack, N.J., Bower, S., Fisk, N.M.: The value of color doppler ultrasound in the prenatal diagnosis of hypoplastic umbilical artery. Ultrasound Obstet. Gynecol. 4 (1994) 143–146

163. Sepulveda, W., Bower, S., Flack, N.J., Fisk, N.M.: Discordant iliac and femoral artery flow velocity waveforms in fetuses with single umbilical artery. Amer. J. Obstet. Gynecol. 171 (1994) 521–525

164. Sepulveda, W., Platt, C.C., Fisk, N.M.: Prenatal diagnosis of cerebral arteriovenous malformations using color Doppler ultrasonography: Case report and review of the literature. Ultrasound Obstet. Gynecol. 6 (1995) 282–286

165. Sepulveda, W., Nicolaides, P., Bower, S., Ridout, D.A., Fisk, N.M.: Common iliac artery flow velocity waveforms in fetuses with a single umbilical artery: a longitudinal study. Brit. J. Obstet. Gynaecol. 103 (1996) 660–663

166. Sepulveda, W., Shennan, A.H., Peek, M.J.: Reverse end-diastolic flow in the middle cerebral artery: An agonal pattern in the human fetus. Amer. J. Obstet. Gynecol. 174 (1996) 1645–1647

167. Sheldon, R.E., Peters, L.L., Jones, M.D., Makowski, E.L., Meschia, G.: Redistribution of cardiac output and oxygen delivery in the hypoxemic fetal lamb. Amer. J. Obstet. Gynecol. 135 (1979) 1071–1078

168. Soothill, P.W., Nicolaides, K.H., Bilardo, C.M., Campbell, S.: Relation of fetal hypoxia in growth retardation to mean blood velocity in the fetal aorta. Lancet II (1986) 1118–1120

169. Soothill, P.W., Campbell, S.: Prediction of morbidity in small and normally grown fetuses by fetal heart rate variability, biophysical profil score and umbilical artery Doppler studies. Brit. J. Obstet. Gynaecol. 100 (1993) 742–745

170. Soregaroli, M., Rizzo, G., Danti, L., Arduini, D., Romanini, C.: Effects of maternal hyperoxygenation on ductus venosus flow velocity waveforms in normal third-trimester fetuses. Ultrasound Obstet. Gynecol. 3 (1993) 115–119

171. Strigini, F.A.L., de Luca, G., Lencion, G., Scida, P., Giusti, G., Genazzani, A.R.: Middle cerebral artery velocimetry: Different clinical relevance depending on umbilical velocimetry. Obstet. Gynecol. 90 (1997) 953–957

172. Teitel, D.F., Iwamoto, H.S., Rudolph, A.M.: Effects of birth-related events on central blood flow patterns. Pediatr. Res. 22 (1987) 557–566

173. Tonge, H.M., Struijk, P.C., Wladimiroff, J.W.: Blood flow measurements in the fetal descending aorta: technique and clinics. Clin. Cardiol. 7 (1984) 323–327

174. Tonge, H.M., Wladimiroff, J.W., Noordam, M.J., van Kooten, C.: Blood flow velocity waveforms in the descending fetal aorta: Comparison between normal and growth-retarded pregnancies. Obstet. Gynecol. 67 (1986) 851–855

175. Trudinger, B.J., Cook, C.M., Jones, L., Giles, W.B.: A comparison of fetal heart rate monitoring and umbilical artery waveforms in the recognition of fetal compromise. Brit. J. Obstet. Gynaecol. 93 (1986) 171–175

176. Trudinger, B.J., Cook, C.M., Giles, W.B., Connelly, A., Thompson, R.S.: Umbilical artery flow velocity waveforms in high risk pregnancy. Randomised controlled trial. Lancet I (1987) 188–190

177. Uerpairojkit, B., Chan, L., Reece, A.E., Martinez, E., Mari, G.: Cerebellar Doppler velocimetry in the appropriate- and small-for-gestational-age fetus. Obstet. Gynecol. 87 (1996) 989–993

178. Ulm, B., Ulm, M., Deutinger, J., Bernaschek, G.: Umbilical artery Doppler velocimetry in fetuses with a single umbilical artery. Obstet. Gynecol. 90 (1997) 205–209

179. Ulrich, S., Weiss, E., Kalder, M., Hitschold, T., Berle, P.: Doppler sonographic flow measurements of the middle cerebral artery in end-diastolic zero-flow in the umbilical arteries in relation to fetal outcome. Z. Geburtsh. Neonatol. 200 (1996) 21–24

180. Van den Wijngaard, J.A., Groenenberg, I.A., Wladimiroff, J.W., Hop, W.C.: Cerebral Doppler ultrasound of the human fetus. Brit. J. Obstet. Gynecol. 96 (1989) 845–849

181. Veille, J.C., Kanaan, C.: Duplex Doppler ultrasonographic evaluation of the fetal renal artery in normal and abnormal fetuses. Amer. J. Obstet. Gynecol. 161 (1989) 1502–1507

182. Veille, J.C., Penry, M., Mueller-Heubach, E.: Fetal renal pulsed Doppler waveform in prolonged pregnancies. Amer. J. Obstet. Gynecol. 169 (1993) 882–884

183. Vermillion, S.T., Scardo, J.A., Lashus, A.G., Wiles, H.B.: The effect of indomethacin tocolysis on fetal ductus arteriosus constriction with advancing gestational age. Amer. J. Obstet. Gynecol. 177 (1997) 256–261

184. Vetter, K., Favre, T., Suter, R., Huch, R., Huch, A.: Dopplersonographisch ermittelte spezifisch hämodynamische Veränderungen im Kreislauf von Feten in den letzten 4 Wochen vor Geburt. Z. Geburtsh. u. Perinat. 193 (1989) 215–218

185. Voigt, H.J., Deeg, K.H., Rupprecht, T.: Zerebrale Dopplersonographie beim fetalen Hydrozephalus. Z. Geburtsh. Neonat. 199 (1995) 23–29

186. Vyas, S., Nicolaides, K.H., Campbell, S.: Renal artery flow-velocity waveforms in normal and hypoxemic fetuses. Amer. J. Obstet. Gynecol. 161 (1989) 168–172

187. Vyas, S., Nicolaides, K.H., Bower, S., Campbell, S.: Middle cerebral artery flow velocity waveforms in fetal hypoxemia. Brit. J. Obstet. Gynecol. 97 (1990) 797–803

188. Vyas, S., Campbell, S., Bower, S., Nicolaides, K.H.: Maternal abdominal pressure alters fetal cerebral blood flow. Brit. J. Obstet. Gynaecol. 97 (1990) 740–742

189. Vyas, S., Nicolaides, K.H., Campbell, S.: Doppler examination of the middle cerebral artery in anemic fetuses. Amer. J. Obstet. Gynecol. 162 (1990) 1066–1068

190. Wang, K.G., Chen, C.P., Yang, J.M., Su, T.H.: Impact of reverse end-diastolic flow velocity in umbilical artery on pregnancy outcome after 28th gestational week. Acta Obstet. Gynecol. Scand. 77(5) (1998) 527–531

191. Weiss, E., Ulrich, S., Berle, P.: Blood flow velocity waveforms of the middle cerebral artery and abnormal neurological evaluations in live-born fetuses with absent or reverse end-diastolic flow velocities of the umbilical arteries. Eur. J. Obstet. Gynecol. Reprod. Biol. 45 (1992) 93–100

192. Wisser, J., Kurmanovicius, J., Müller, C., Huch, A., Huch, R.: Pulsatility index in the fetal anterior tibial artery during the second half of normal pregnancy. Ultrasound Obstet. Gynecol. 11 (1998) 199–203

193. Wladimiroff, J.W., Tonge, H.M., Stewart, P.A.: Doppler ultrasound assessment of cerebral blood flow in the human fetus. Brit. J. Obstet. Gynecol. 93 (1986) 471–475

194. Wladimiroff, J.W., van de Wijngaard, J.A., Degani, S., Noordam, M.J., Eyck, J., Tonge, H.M.: Cerebral and umbilical arterial blood flow velocity wave form in normal and growth retarded pregnancies. Obstet. Gynaecol. 69 (1987) 705–709

195. Wlodek, M.E., Brace, R.A., Cock, M.L., Hooper, S.B., Harding, R.: Endocrine responses of fetal sheep to prolonged hypoxemia with and without acidemia: Relation to urine production. Amer. J. Physiol. 268 (1995) F868–F875

196. Woo, J.S., Liang, S.T., Lo, R.L., Chan, F.Y.: Middle cerebral artery Doppler flow velocity waveforms. Obstet. Gynecol. 70 (1987) 613–616

197. Zikulnig, L., Hecher, K., Bregenzer, T., Bäz, E., Hackelöer, B.J.: Prognostic factors in severe twin-twin transfusion syndrome treated by endoscopic laser surgery. Ultrasound Obstet. Gynecol. 14 (1999) 380–387

198. Zimmermann, R., Eichhorn, K.H., Huch, A., Huch, R.: Zusammenhang zwischen verminderter Fruchtwassermenge und Dopplerspektren fetaler Gefäße am Termin. Geburtsh. u. Frauenheilk. 53 (1993) 479–482

44 Perinatal Abnormalities and Fetal Outcome in Cases with Severely Abnormal Doppler-Flow Findings in the Umbilical Artery and Fetal Aorta

High-Risk Pregnancies

Surveillance methods. Chronic placental insufficiency is considered the prototype of a disease causing fetal compromise and is often detected early by the combined use of antepartum surveillance methods, resulting in the saving of infant lives and the reduction of permanent disabilities (39). Growing experience with the use of these surveillance methods, along with recent discoveries in fetal pathophysiology and the pathologic anatomy of the placenta (33), show that this condition has an individual dynamic that must be recognized and understood in order to achieve successful obstetric management. Key factors in this regard are the degree of the placental changes, the age of the pregnancy, fetal organ maturity, and the ability of the fetus to mobilize compensatory reserves (15). Thus, besides the classic definition of a fetus with restricted intrauterine growth and a birth weight below the 5th or 10th percentile, there are many pregnancies with an intermediate- to short-term imbalance between the placental supply and fetal demand in which significant fetal compromise can develop in situations that require increased fetoplacental performance.

With this in mind, we should evaluate available surveillance methods from the standpoint of how well they can detect a more chronic, subtle form of fetal hypoxia (e.g., fetal biometry), impending hypoxia (e.g., movements, amniotic fluid volume, fetal Doppler flow), or acute fetal hypoxia (e.g., FHR monitoring) (8). There is a tradition of combining different examination methods to evaluate the degree of fetal compromise (42, 59). Developments such as Doppler ultrasound (20) and electronic FHR monitoring (60) have gained an established place in modern obstetrics and are very widely used.

Doppler ultrasound. Doppler ultrasound can be used in selecting high-risk obstetric cases and providing them with intensive surveillance. There is general agreement that perinatal management can be optimized by Doppler ultrasound surveillance, especially in high-risk pregnancies. A definite causal relationship exists between abnormal flow patterns and adverse fetal outcome (11, 64, 65, 68). Chronically increased resistance in the placental circulation leads to chronic fetal hypoxia resulting in growth retardation and altered fetal hemodynamics (77, 79). When an abnormal flow pattern is detected in a high-risk pregnancy, it can be used to identify hypoxemic fetal distress caused by a significant impairment of gas exchange in the placenta (57, 77). Thus, the detection of abnormal flow provides a means for the early diagnosis of a restricted fetal oxygen supply (31, 78).

Absent End-Diastolic Flow and Reverse Flow

Absent End-Diastolic Flow in the Umbilical Artery and/or Fetal Aorta

High-risk population. Cases in which Doppler ultrasound shows absent end-diastolic flow (AEDF) in the umbilical artery or fetal aorta are placed in the high-risk category. They are seen with an incidence of 2–8%. Various authors have described the presence of AEDF and have related it to intrauterine hypoxia (24, 50, 56, 68). A redistribution of fe-

tal blood flow is commonly observed in fetuses with AEDF. This centralization of blood flow, with an associated decrease in peripheral vascular perfusion accompanied by cerebrovascular autoregulation, is called the brain-sparing effect (2, 71, 75, 80). Studies have documented its association with higher rates of cesarean section, prematurity, neonatal ICU transfers, and increased morbidity and mortality rates (62, 68). By contrast, relatively little is known about long-term developmental problems in affected infants. Several authors have described increased neonatal morbidity with permanent neuromotor deficits (16, 17, 70).

Reverse Flow in the Umbilical Artery and/or Fetal Aorta

Extreme compromise. There is good reason to believe that the functional disturbance of the fetoplacental unit is a continuous, progressive process and that when compensatory reserves have been exhausted, this progression is reflected in increasingly abnormal Doppler indices. In this sense the severity of Doppler flow abnormalities correlates with the degree of fetal compromise. Accordingly, when end-diastolic reverse flow (RF) is detected in the umbilical artery and/or the fetal aorta, it is reasonable to expect that serious perinatal problems will arise (11, 13, 33, 62). Reverse flow is associated with a 50–100% perinatal mortality (5, 11, 62, 63) and therefore reflects a hazardous situation for the fetus. Most fetuses with RF will die within a few days of testing (13, 82). Suspicion of fetal distress (e.g., an abnormal FHR trace) is a frequent indication for cesarean delivery (11, 13, 63). The morbidity of these high-risk infants is particularly high.

Obstetric management. The relationship between fetal outcome and the occurrence of RF and its causes is still poorly understood due to the low prevalence of this finding (approximately 0.3–1%). Reports to date are unclear as to the pathophysiologic mechanisms of RF and its optimum obstetric management. How best to proceed in cases where RF is noted at an early gestational age remains an open question. Although the population with RF is very small, these fetuses warrant very close attention due to their high morbidity and mortality rate.

Pathoanatomic Changes and Technical Issues

Pathoanatomic Changes in Reverse Flow

Comparison of placentas. Fifteen cases with RF and 15 cases with a normal Doppler spectrum at comparable gestational ages were studied retrospectively to determine a possible causal relationship between abnormalities of the placental vessels and the occurrence of RF in the fetal vessels (20). Placental specimens were cut into sections 2–3 μm thick and stained with Masson-Goldner stain. A computer-assisted image analysis system was configured for placental morphometry. The object of the image analysis was the periphery of one placentone. Fifty approximately round villi were analyzed in each specimen.

Birth weight and placental weight. The mean gestational age at birth was 30 weeks, 4 days in the group with RF and 30 weeks, 6 days in the control group with normal flow. The statistical difference in birth weights between the two groups was highly significant: 985 g ± 115 g in the RF group versus 1780 g ± 141 g in the control group (*P* < 0.0001). Placental weight was 216 g ± 18 g in the RF group versus 385 g ± 32 g in the group with normal flow (*P* < 0.01). The ratio of placental weight to birth weight showed no significant difference between the two groups.

Metabolic membranes. The frequency of terminal villi with metabolic membranes was only 18.7% in RF group but was 44.6% in the control group (*P* < 0.01). The average number of metabolic membranes per villus was much lower in the RF cases than in the cases with normal flow (0.32 ± 0.07 versus 0.61 ± 0.10). The total number of metabolic membranes averaged only 3.54 in the RF cases, compared with 7.40 in the cases with normal flow (*P* = 0.02). The relationship of the metabolic membranes to the overall villus circumference also showed a statistically significant difference between the RF group (2.14 ± 0.64) and the group with normal flow (7.56 ± 3.59) (*P* < 0.05). Although the average number of vessels was smaller in the RF cases than in the controls (4.12 ± 0.33 versus 5.61 ± 0.42; *P* < 0.01), the differences between the two groups with regard to average vascular surface area or total vascular area in the terminal villi was not significant.

Technical Issues in the Diagnosis of AEDF and Reverse Flow

Figures 44.1–44.3 show a normal Doppler spectrum compared with spectra that illustrate AEDF and RF in the umbilical artery.

Meticulous technique. The detection of AEDF and RF in the fetal vessels requires a meticulous examination technique, as technical variables can very easily produce false-positive findings and prompt obstetric decisions with potentially far-reaching consequences. Whenever possible, the diagnosis should be confirmed by a second independent examiner.

Technical parameters. Key technical parameters that affect the test result are the insonation angle, which should be less than 60° (greater angles register less diastolic flow), and the high-pass–filter setting, which should not exceed 50–100 Hz. Setting the high-pass filter too high can cause the end-diastolic flow to be truncated, creating the appearance of AEDF (Fig. 44.4).

Gestational age. Another factor to be considered is gestational age. Decreased diastolic flow or even AEDF may well be a physiologic finding when noted very early in the pregnancy. Fetal breathing movements can cause a transient decrease in diastolic flow or can mimic reverse flow (Fig. 44.5). The end-diastolic flow may also show fluctuations that are described as "partial AEDF" or "partial RF."

Clinical Results of AEDF and RF in the Umbilical Artery and/or Fetal Aorta

Long-term neuromotor development. We conducted a 10-year follow-up of 120 fetuses and children with AEDF in the umbilical artery or fetal aorta and an additional 30 cases with RF in the umbilical artery or aorta. Besides prenatal abnormalities, we studied the perinatal outcomes and long-term neuromotor development of children who had these very abnormal Doppler findings during the last trimester of pregnancy. The results of our long-term follow-ups are particularly helpful in sorting out antepartum injury patterns from the perinatal problems that arose. Neuromotor development was evaluated with the Munich Functional Development Test (26, 37). Additional data were elicited from the parents and gleaned from the children's medical records.

Of the children in this high-risk population who survived, 30 cases with AEDF were tested postnatally for neuromotor development. Perinatal abnormalities and neuromotor developmental deficits in these children were compared with a matched-pair group of comparable gestational age with no abnormal Doppler findings (n = 30 children). Developmental status in each child was assessed in the categories of gross and fine motor skills, perception, independence, speech, speech comprehension, and social age.

Absent End-Diastolic Flow

The mean gestational age at delivery was 32 weeks and 5 days in this group of n = 120 children, and the mean birth weight was 1385 g. The rate of severely dystrophic infants (< 5th percentile) was 69%. Perinatal mortality was 18%. Ninety-seven percent of the liveborn infants with umbilical artery AEDF required transfer to neonatal ICU (Table 44.1).

Centralization of fetal circulation. It is noteworthy that 80% of the children with AEDF had an abnormal S/D ratio in the middle cerebral artery (indicating oxygen sparing), as compared with only 7% in the control group.

Neuromotor development. To evaluate the long-term morbidity associated with a severely abnormal antepartum Doppler test, the neuromotor development of these children was studied prospectively in two groups of comparable gestational age at delivery. Group I, consisting of 30 children with normal Doppler findings in the fetal vessels, was compared with group II, consisting of 30 children with AEDF in the umbilical artery and/or fetal aorta. Table 44.2 reviews the perinatal findings in both groups. The children were between 9 and 36 months of age at the time of neuromotor testing. For each functional category, the developmental age was determined and the deviation from the corrected age was calculated in months. The average neuromotor development of all the children with AEDF lagged behind the average development of equal-age children with no placental dysfunction: 32% of the children with AEDF showed impairment of neuromotor development, compared with just 17% of the children with normal Doppler findings (Fig. 44.6). The neuromotor deficits predominantly involved gross motor skills, perception, and speech.

When the two groups were compared for postpartum weight, longitudinal growth, and head circumference, a significant difference was found between the first examination of the newborn after birth and an examination at the age of 21 to 24 months.

Reverse Flow

Fetuses with AEDF in the umbilical artery or aorta constitute a high-risk population with serious perinatal abnormalities and a markedly

Table 44.1 Perinatal findings in children with absent end-diastolic flow (AEDF) in the umbilical artery or fetal aorta (n = 120)

Pregnancy-induced hypertension	62%
Oligohydramnios	60%
Abnormal FHR trace (Fischer score < 5)	70%
Gestational age at delivery (weeks + days)	32 + 5
Preterm delivery < 37 weeks' gestation	85%
Preterm delivery < 33 weeks' gestation	49%
Primary cesarean section	84%
Birthweight (average)	1385 g
5' Apgar score < 7	11%
pH (average)	7.24
Dystrophy < 5th percentile	69%
Perinatal mortality	18%
Congenital anomalies	22%

Table 44.**2** Comparison of perinatal findings in children with normal Doppler findings (group I: n = 30 children) and with AEDF in the fetal vessels (group II: n = 30 children) of comparable gestational age at delivery

Perinatal findings	Normal (group I)	Abnormal (group II)
Oligohydramnios	14%	23%
Abnormal FHR trace (Fischer score < 5)	14%	29%
Gestational age at delivery (weeks + days)	34+0	33+3
Preterm delivery < 37 weeks' gestation	82%	100%
Preterm delivery < 33 weeks' gestation	31%	53%
Primary cesarean section	44%	84%
Birthweight (average)	2570 g	1460 g
1' Apgar score < 7	27%	47%
pH (average)	7.26	7.29
Dystrophy < 10th percentile	23%	53%
Congenital anomalies	9%	24%
Transfer to neonatal ICU	57%	93%

increased risk of neuromotor handicap. In some cases with prolonged AEDF (e.g., patients with severe preeclampsia), we could also detect reverse flow (RF) in the fetal vessels for a period of several days. Other cases were referred to us in which RF was present in the umbilical artery or fetal aorta at the time of the examination. To compare the perinatal findings associated with AEDF and RF, we formed two groups of 30 cases each with comparable gestational ages at delivery. Besides prenatal surveillance methods, neonatal neurosonographic and echocardiographic tests were included in the evaluations.

Comparison of perinatal findings. RF in the fetal vessels was diagnosed in 30 cases at an average gestational age of 30 weeks, 1 day. The risk factors of pregnancy-induced hypertension (PIH), placental insufficiency, oligohydramnios, and nicotine abuse were significantly more prevalent in cases with RF than in cases with AEDF. The mean gestational age at delivery was 30 weeks, 6 days in both groups. For comparable modes of delivery, a higher incidence of acidosis (pH ≤ 7.2) was found in the RF group (31.3%) than in the AEDF group (8.8%). Severe intrauterine growth retardation (< 5th percentile) was present in 86% of the children with RF (odds ratio 9.7) versus 63% of the AEDF cases. Intrauterine fetal death (IUFD) occurred in 43% of the fetuses with RF (odds ratio 22.7). Pathologic examination revealed chronic placental insufficiency in 67% of these fetuses and a congenital anomaly in 25%. The incidence of IUFD in the group with AEDF was only 3.3%. Thus the perinatal mortality associated with RF, at 29%, is substantially higher than the 7% rate associated with AEDF.

Neonatal morbidity. Neonatal morbidity was 81% in the group with RF, compared with 63% in the group with AEDF. Forty-four percent of the RF cases had a cerebral abnormality at postnatal ultrasound (e.g., cysts, ventricular dilatation, or cerebral hemorrhage) versus 31% of the children with AEDF. The incidence of cerebral hemorrhage in the surviving newborns with antenatal RF was 25%, versus 17% in the AEDF group. Four of 10 children with cerebral hemorrhage died during the neonatal period. In children of comparable gestational age who had no seriously abnormal Doppler findings cerebral hemorrhage was not observed.

Clinical Implications

The introduction of Doppler flowmetry of the fetoplacental unit has made an important contribution to the assessment of intrauterine fetal well-being.

Early detection compared with FHR monitoring. Particularly in the immature fetus, suspicious FHR findings can be qualified by Doppler ultrasound, influencing clinical management to the benefit of the child (22, 62, 63). In our experience, the average interval between the appearance of a significant Doppler abnormality and the appearance of

abnormal FHR changes is approximately 12 days (62). Other authors report intervals of 4 to 21 days (8, 13, 31). In many cases an abnormal FHR recording is noted at the same time that abnormal flow is detected (62). Among our own patients, the FHR trace was already abnormal (Fischer score = 4) in 50% of cases with RF at the time of the initial Doppler examination, compared with only 17% of cases with AEDF. Several authors have stressed the advantage of the Doppler examination over FHR monitoring in the early detection of fetal compromise (2, 8, 61). It may be that the altered fetal hemodynamics in the umbilical artery induces an autoregulation of the cerebral artery which alters the central regulation of the fetal heart rate. The initial response is a biphasic change in the middle cerebral artery blood flow, followed by a loss of vasodilatation in the artery and a decrease in left ventricular output, with a resulting change in FHR variability (4).

Significance of AEDF. The occurrence of AEDF is an ominous clinical sign (7, 8, 50, 54, 63, 76, 78). This is demonstrated by a review of the literature on the abnormalities that are found when these infants are delivered (Table 44.**3**). The perinatal mortality and morbidity are markedly increased. In our own studies, we found subsequent neuromotor abnormalities in 33% of AEDF children that were tested using the Munich Functional Development Test (16) (Fig. 44.**6**).

Brain-sparing effect. Neuromotor development is also significantly affected by cerebral Doppler findings, particularly the brain-sparing effect. This refers to the appearance of end-diastolic velocities and a reduction of the S/D ratio and pulsatility index in the cerebral vessels (2, 58, 75). The brain-sparing effect involves a centralization of the fetal circulation with increased blood flow to the brain. In the literature, the brain-sparing effect is construed as a mechanism to protect the fetal brain from hypoxia (58). If this mechanism fails, the fetus with AEDF may exhibit terminal signs before 30 weeks' gestation (71).

Loss of end-diastolic flow. In our studies of AEDF and RF in the umbilical artery and fetal aorta, we noted a loss of end-diastolic flow in the cerebral vessels only in fetuses who had subsequent abnormalities. It is reasonable to assume that the brain-sparing effect ultimately failed in these fetuses. Their condition was so poor that centralization of the fetal circulation was no longer possible. An apparent normalization of abnormal cerebral Doppler findings is also described in the literature (12, 19, 75, 77).

Intrauterine growth retardation. When we compared immediate postnatal data such as Apgar score, pH, and blood gases in our study, we were surprised to find only very minor differences between children with normal and abnormal neuromotor scores. We may conclude that perinatal asphyxia led to an increase in perinatal morbidity but did not cause permanent developmental deficits. Intrauterine growth retardation has been identified as a predisposing factor for learning deficits between 9 and 11 years of age, unrelated to factors of perinatal morbidity (41). The problem of later neuromotor retardation, then, does not appear to arise during birth. It appears that the developmental disorder arises antenatally through the adverse effect of a deficient intrauterine blood supply on fetal brain development. The greater influence of the antenatal period is also emphasized in the literature (53, 66).

Dystrophy. Other adverse prognostic factors for postnatal development in our study were preterm delivery, a birth weight below the 3rd percentile, a head circumference below the 3rd percentile, and a low placental weight in relation to birth weight. Dystrophy and immaturity are also cited in the literature as causes of perinatal problems in fetuses with AEDF (1, 40, 56, 82, 83). Thirty-eight percent of abnormal infants and 24% of normal infants remained severely dystrophic in their size and weight until follow-up. Other authors have also described

Table 44.**3** Review of the literature on abnormalities associated with AEDF

Authors	Year	Cases	Gestational age at delivery	Cesarean rate (%)	IUGR (%)	Birth-weight (%)	Malformations
Reed (51)	1987	14	33	80	79	1227 g	29
Rochelson (55)	1987	15	34	80	60	1851 g	27
Ombelet (47)	1988	21	31	100	95	924 g	–
Johnstone (30)	1988	24	32	83	92	1282 g	–
Kirkinen (36)	1988	84	33+5	72	–	–	9
Arabin (3)	1988	30	33	100	100	–	–
Rochelson (56)	1989	10	34	80	60	1581 g	–
Jouppila (32)	1989	84	33+5	72	–	1820 g	9
Gudmundsson (23)	1990	14	37	100	86	2086 g	–
Pillai und James (49)	1990	4	32+1	100	100	1285 g	–
Wenstrom (81)	1991	22	29	–	45	1077 g	45
Trudinger (69)	1991	96	31+1	91	81	1198 g	9
Poulain (50)	1992	62	–	86	39	–	16
Pattinson (48)	1994	21	31+4	–	17	1014 g	–
Ashmead (6)	1993	5	33	–	–	1710 g	–
Valcamonico (72)	1994	26	31+4	–	100	1172 g	8
Rizzo (54)	1994	192	30+6	61	–	1124 g	13
Ulrich (70)	1994	68	31+	–	56	1225 g	–
Weiner (77)	1994	10	32+3	90	–	1258 g	–
Karsdorp (33)	1994	178	31+4	96	–	1209 g	–
Zelop (83)	1996	32	31+1	94	–	1139 g	–
Average values from all studies		52	32	72.1	87.5	1343 g	18.3
Our results	1998	120	32+5	84	69	1385 g	22

length and weight discrepancies that persisted with aging (41, 52, 73). Vohr and Oh (73) consider head circumference at one year of age to be a crucial prognostic factor for development.

Cerebral hemorrhage. Neurologic abnormalities at birth can affect the further development of the child (34). Cerebral hemorrhage occurred in 10% of the children with AEDF. Other authors (71, 78) have reported rates of 15%. The high rate of cerebral hemorrhage can be ascribed partly to increased cerebral perfusion from the brain-sparing effect (13). Cerebral hemorrhage in our study was more common in children with neuromotor deficits (25%) than in children with normal neuromotor function (4.5%) and is therefore considered to have causal significance in the deficits. Only Scherjon et al. (58) described fewer cerebral hemorrhages in children who had subsequent abnormalities. Ulrich et al. (70) found a significantly higher incidence of severe cerebral hemorrhage and significant neurologic developmental problems in a population with AEDF than in a matched group of preterm infants with normal Doppler findings. Thirty-one percent of the AEDF infants demonstrated neurologic and psychomotor deficits. This figure is comparable to the 33% incidence of developmental delays found in our population.

Developmental areas affected. The most pronounced deficits were noted in gross and fine motor skills and perception. Other authors have also found a preponderance of gross and fine motor deficits (10, 46, 74) and motor and perception deficits (44) in preterm infants. Independence was least impaired.

Reappearance of positive end-diastolic flow. Brar and Platt (11) reported that positive end-diastolic flow reappeared in approximately 15% of fetuses that previously showed AEDF in the umbilical artery. An improved fetal outcome was noted in these cases. This may result from a change in the status of placental blood flow. Bell et al. (9) found in their study that 11 of 40 (27.5%) fetuses with AEDF in the umbilical artery exhibited positive end-diastolic flow during the course of the pregnancy. The interval from AEDF registration to delivery, gestational age at delivery, and birth weight were greater in these fetuses while neonatal mortality was reduced. It was postulated that the outcome of

fetuses with AEDF may improve following the reappearance of a positive end-diastolic velocity. According to Weiss and Berle (80), a short interval from initial diagnosis to delivery is associated with a higher rate of fetal acidosis and a greater number of emergency cesarean sections. The prognosis of the fetuses could be improved through conservative management. An improvement in umbilical artery flow was recorded in IUGR fetuses following maternal oxygen therapy (4, 35). The reappearance of end-diastolic frequencies was also reported.

Karsdorp et al. (33) found rheologic improvement in the maternal circulation following antihypertensive medication and volume augmentation. Positive end-diastolic flow reappeared in all seven patients with AEDF in the umbilical artery, whereas AEDF persisted in the seven women who did not receive hemodilution. The difference in fetal outcomes was significant. Five of seven fetuses that showed a reappearance of positive end-diastolic flow following AEDF survived, versus only one of seven fetuses that continued to have AEDF. It is possible that blood flow through the placenta could have been improved in these fetuses.

Placental changes. An increased S/D ratio in the umbilical artery may be associated with a loss of small resistance vessels and tertiary villi in the placenta (34, 57, 68) or may lead to occlusion of the large vessels in the mainstem villi. Similar results were reported by McCowan et al. (45). Although a relatively small number of vessels were found in the terminal villi in cases with RF or AEDF, there was no statistically significant difference in the number of vessels in the terminal villi between small and normal-size placentas. Two other studies did not confirm this theory on the obliteration of small resistance vessels in the placenta, instead providing further evidence in support of the "vasoconstriction" or "hypovascularization" theory (34, 57). Decreased placental weight, a smaller area of placental attachment, and broader terminal villi with reduced epithelial plate formation and thicker diffusion paths have been discovered in cases with RF or AEDF (25). This means that the exchange capacity of the placenta is impaired in RF/AEDF cases. This can account for the adverse fetal outcome. Our pathomorphologic results and the associated serial Doppler ultrasound findings support the vasoconstriction theory.

Pathophysiology of RF. Although a high fetal mortality has been observed in cases with RF, the pathophysiology leading to the end-diastolic flow reversal is still unclear. Due to the low incidence of this phenomenon, very little epidemiologic data have been published to date. Nearly all authors have dealt with fewer than 30 cases in their studies. As a result, the data on AEDF and RF have usually been analyzed together. An exception is the study by Karsdorp et al. (33), who analyzed and compiled data from nine perinatal centers.

IUGR and PIH. Many factors that can affect both fetal and maternal hemodynamics will alter the flow pattern in the umbilical artery or fetal aorta (11). Pregnancies with intrauterine growth retardation (IUGR) (odds ratio 3.1), with pregnancy-induced hypertension (PIH), or with IUGR and PIH (odds ratio 7.4) have a significantly higher association with RF and/or AEDF (7, 18, 33, 63, 83). In the present study, a high risk for developing RF was found in cases with IUGR (odds ratio 22.6). Cases with severe IUGR were found to have either a small placenta or massive intervillous fibrin deposition within the placenta. This can account for the development of abnormal flow patterns. Patients in our study who had PIH had an increased risk for the occurrence of RF (odds ratio 3.8). A number of authors have speculated on a close association between severely abnormal Doppler flow patterns and PIH (18, 83). An increased production of prostacyclin and/or endothelium-derived relaxing factors has been found in patients with PIH. Reportedly, this can decrease placental blood flow by the reduction of active renin and angiotensin II in the peripheral circulation or by increased activity of the renin-angiotensin system in the uteroplacental circulation. The

Table 44.**4**   Review of the literature on mortality rates associated with reverse flow

Authors	Year	Cases	Delivery (weeks)	Total mortality (%)	IUFT (%)	Perinatal-mortality (%)	Post-partum mortality (%)
Brar (11)	1988	12	30+1	50	33	50	18
Illyes (29)	1988	5	32+2	100	100	100	–
Schmidt (62)	1991	4	30+4	100	75	50	25
Fouron (21)	1993	5	28+3	60	60	–	–
Valcamonico (72)	1994	5	30+1	–	20	40	20
Karsdorp (33) (multicenter study)	1994	67	29+0	75	24	–	51
Zelop (83)	1996	24	29+1	–	17	33	–
Average values from all studies		17	30	77	47	55	29
Our results	1998	30	30+6	53	40	27	22

result is local hypoxemia in the placenta. The formation of oxygen-free radicals is also induced. These compounds are known to act as mediators for local vasoconstriction of the placental vessels in PIH. Apparently this could explain the increased placental vascular resistance that is found in patients with PIH.

Nicotine abuse. RF was also found more frequently in women who smoke more than 10 cigarettes per day (odds ratio 9.4). These results contradict reports in the literature. Karsdorp et al. (33) found no relationship between the risk of RF and maternal nicotine abuse. Also, nicotine reportedly has no effect on hemodynamics prior to the occurrence of vascular lesions with morphologic changes (25). But nicotine can induce vasoconstriction in the placental vessels, thereby reducing uteroplacental blood flow. These changes are well documented by the available literature on placental studies (34, 57).

Intrauterine fetal death. An increased incidence of intrauterine fetal death (IUFD) has been described in fetuses with RF (7, 11, 63, 76). The average incidence reported by seven authors was 47%, meaning that IUFD occurred in almost half of fetuses with RF (Table 44.**4**). The interval between initial detection and fetal death ranged from one to several days. In our own study, intrauterine death occurred in 40% of the fetuses with RF. The average interval between RF registration and IUFD was only 2.5 days. Overall, 92% of IUFDs occurred within one week after diagnosis.

Todros et al. (67) found in their study that the detection of AEDF or RF had a very high predictive value for an adverse fetal outcome. They state that when absent or reverse end-diastolic flow is found, it is time to deliver the fetus.

Obstetric management. Doppler ultrasound, then, is an important method in prenatal diagnosis for the evaluation of high-risk pregnancies. Since severely abnormal Doppler spectra are often present in the initial flow examination, Doppler should be performed in high-risk pregnancies at the earliest possible time. It is possible, though somewhat unlikely, that some fetuses with AEDF or RF will show improvement of end-diastolic flow after appropriate therapy. This means that when optimum, intensive prenatal care is provided in cases with severely abnormal Doppler waveforms, it may not be necessary to deliver the baby right away, and there may be time to induce lung maturation with glucocorticoids in an immature fetus. In many cases, however, it will be necessary to perform an immediate cesarean section. The decision regarding the timing of the delivery and perinatal management should be tailored to the individual situation. The parents should be given detailed information on the prognosis, and the decision should be made in close consultation with neonatologists at a perinatal center.

Summary

Significant additional prognostic factor. The presence of absent or reverse end-diastolic flow in the fetal vessels appears to be a significant additional prognostic factor for high-risk pregnancies. These findings are associated with a marked increase of mortality and serious morbidity in the neonatal period (Table 44.**5**). They also signify a substantially higher risk of later neuromotor deficits compared with children of comparable gestational age who have normal Doppler findings.

Intracerebral hemorrhage. Long-term sequelae can also result from hypoxia-induced intracerebral hemorrhage, which is often based on increased cerebral blood flow due to the brain-sparing effect. Fetuses that are delivered in a compromised state (abnormal umbilical cord pH, abnormal Apgar score) have a significantly higher risk of hemorrhage than fetuses that receive optimum perinatal management. This includes prompt referral to a perinatal center and close consultation with a neonatologist.

Reduced placental perfusion. In the past, absent and reverse end-diastolic velocities have often been placed in a single diagnostic category because of the small case numbers. This practice should be discontinued. If these flow patterns are based on a decrease in placental blood flow, both phenomena should be viewed as the end points on a continuum of placental perfusion, with AEDF generally having more "innocent" clinical implications than RF. We must vigorously explore the underlying mechanisms of reduced placental perfusion, and we must better understand the dynamics of this process in order to avoid potential antepartum insults to maturing organs which set the stage for long-term morbidity. These efforts will continue to rely chiefly on proficient Doppler scanning of the fetomaternal vessels. It will also be necessary to employ other biophysical tests within the context of a biophysical profile (ABCD profile) (27, 28) in order to meet this important clinical challenge.

Table 44.**5**   Comparison of perinatal findings associated with RF and AEDF

	RF (8 authors)		AEDF (21 authors)		RF/AEDF (16 authors)	
Cases (n)	152		1062		560	
	Average	Median	Average	Median	Average	Median
Cases	19	9	51	30	35	32
Gestational age at delivery	30.1	30.1	31.9	31.6	31.2	31.2
Total mortality (%)	73.0	67.5	32.2	34	43.9	40
Perinatal mortality (%)	50.0	45	28.7	22	35.4	38
Neonatal mortality (%)	27.1	22	19.4	20	20.0	10
IUFD (%)	46.0	36.5	16.7	11	25.1	16
Malformations (%)	21.8	23	18.2	15	21	21
IUGR (%)	100	100	88.3	91	90	94
Birthweight (g)	997	983	1337	1225	1114	1037
Cesarean section (%)	93	96	72.7	80	74.4	75
1' Apgar = 7 (%)	84.3	78	63.8	66	68.5	72
pH ≤ 7.2 (%)	41.5	41.5	19.0	19	26.0	26

Absent end-diastolic flow and reverse flow

Fig. 44.**1**   Normal Doppler findings in the umbilical artery.

Fig. 44.**2**   Absent end-diastolic flow in the umbilical artery.

Fig. 44.**3**   Typical appearance of reverse flow in the umbilical artery.

Fig. 44.**4**   This "AEDF" is an artifact caused by setting the wall filter too high.

Fig. 44.**5**   Transient AEDF and RF caused by fetal breathing movements.

Fig. 44.**6**   Frequency of impaired neuromotor development in children with normal Doppler findings (n = 30) and with AEDF in fetal vessels (n = 30).

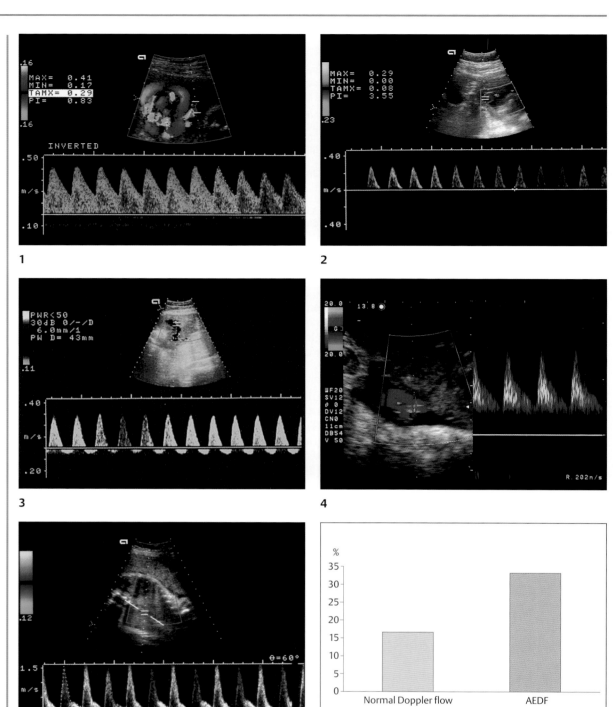

References

1. Adiotomre, P.N., Johnstone, F.D., Laing, I.A.: Effect of absent end diastolic flow velocity in the fetal umbilical artery on subsequent outcome. Arch. Dis. Child Fetal Neonatal. Ed. 76 (1997) 35–38
2. Arabin, B., Saling, E.: Die „Sparschaltung" des fetalen Kreislaufs dargestellt anhand von eigenen quantitativen Doppler-Blutflußparametern. Z. Geburtsh. Perinatol. 191 (1987) 213–218
3. Arabin, B., Siebert, M., Jimenez, E., Saling, E.: Obstetrical characteristics of a loss of end-diastolic velocities in the fetal aorta and/or umbilical artery using Doppler ultrasound. Gynecol. Obstet. Invest. 25 (1988) 173–180
4. Arduini, D., Rizzo, G.: Prediction of fetal outcome in small for gestational age fetuses: Comparision of Doppler measurements obtained from different fetal vessels. J. Perinat. Med. 20 (1992) 29–38
5. Ariyuki, Y., Hata, T., Kitao, M.: Reverse end-diastolic umbilical artery velocity in a case of intrauterine fetal death at 14 weeks' gestation. Amer. J. Obstet. Gynecol. 159 (1993) 1621–1622
6. Ashmead, G.G., Lazebnik, N., Ashmead, J.W., Stepanchak, W., Mann, L.I.: Normal blood gases in fetuses with absence of end-diastolic umbilical artery velocity. Amer. J. Perinatol. 10 (1993) 67–70
7. Battaglia, C., Artini, P.G., Galli, P.A., D'Ambrogio, G., Droghini, F., Genazzani, A.R.: Absent or reversed end diastolic flow in umbilical artery and severe intrauterine growth retardation. Acta Obstet. Gynecol. Scand. 72 (1993) 167–171
8. Bekedam, D.J., Visser, G.H.A., van der Zee, A.G.J., Snijders R.J.M., Poelmann-Weesjes, G.: Abnormal velocity waveforms of the umbilical artery in growth-retarded fetuses: Relationship to antepartum late heart rate decelerations and outcome. Early Hum. Dev. 24 (1990) 79–89
9. Bell, J.G., Ludomirsky, A., Bottalico, J., Weiner, S.: The effect of improvement of umbilical artery absent end-diastolic velocity on perinatal outcome. Amer. J. Obstet. Gynecol. 167 (1992) 1015–1020
10. Bjerre, F., Hansen, E.: Psychomotoric development and school adjustment of 7-year-old children with low birthweight. Acta Paediatr. Scand. 65 (1976) 88–96
11. Brar, H.S., Platt, L.D.: Reverse end-diastolic flow velocity on umbilical artery velocimetry in high-risk pregnancies: An ominous finding with adverse pregnancy outcome. Amer. J. Obstet. Gynecol. 159 (1988) 559–561
12. Chandran, R., Serra-Serra, V., Sellers, S.M., Redman, C.W.G.: Fetal middle cerebral artery flow velocity waveforms – a terminal pattern. Brit. J. Obstet. Gynaecol. 98 (1991) 937–938
13. Chaoui, R., Hoffmann, H., Zienert, A., Bollmann, R., Halle, H., Grauel, E.L.: Klinische Bedeutung und fetal outcome beim enddiastolischen Flowverlust in der A. umbilicalis und/oder fetale Aorta: Analyse von 51 Fällen. Geburtsh. u. Frauenheilkd. 51 (1991) 532–539
14. Comas, C., Carrera, M., Devesa, R. et al.: Early detection of reversed diastolic umbilical flow: should we offer karyotyping? Ultrasound Obstet. Gynecol. 10 (1997) 400–402
15. Edelstone, D.I.: Fetal compensatory response to reduced oxygen delivery. Sem. in Perinatol. 8 (1984) 184–191
16. Ertan, A.K., Jost, W., Hendrik, J., Lauer, S., Uhrmacher, S., Schmidt, W.: Perinatal events and neuromotoric development of children with zero flow in the fetal vessels during the last trimester. In: Cosmi, E.V., Di Renzo, G.C.: 2nd World Congress of Perinatal Medicine, Monduzzi Editore 1993; pp. 1049–1052
17. Ertan, A.K., Jost, W., Mink, D., Schmidt, W.: Neuromotoric development of children after AED-Flow during pregnancy. In: Kurjak, A., Latin, V., Rippmann, E. (eds.): Advances on the pathophysiology of pregnancy. CIC Edizioni internazionali 1995 pp. 55–62
18. Ertan, A.K., He, J.P., Tossounidis, I., Schmidt, W.: Einfluß der EPH-Gestose auf perinatale Faktoren bei Fällen mit „Reverse Flow" bzw. „enddiastolischem Block" in den fetalen Gefäßen. In: Künzel, W. (Hrsg.): Arch. Gynecol. Obstet. 258 (1996) 113
19. Erz, W., Gonser, M.: Dopplersonographie der fetalen Arteria cerebri media: Präfinale Normalisierung des zerebralen Blutflusses? Geburtsh. u. Frauenheilkd. 55 (1995) 407–410
20. Fitzgerald, D.E., Drumm, J.E.: Non-invasive measurement of human fetal circulation using ultrasound: a new method. Brit. Med. J. 2 (1977) 1450–1451
21. Fouron, J.C., Teyssier, G., Shalaby, L., Lessard, M., Van-Doesburg, N.H.: Fetal central blood flow alterations in human fetuses with umbilical artery reverse diastolic flow. Amer. J. Perinatol. 10 (1993) 197–207
22. Göschen, K.: Überwachung der Schwangerschaft aus forensischer Sicht. Gynäkologe 27 (1994) 197–207
23. Gudmundsson, S., Lindblad, A., Marsal, K.: Cord blood gases and absence of end-diastolic blood velocities in the umbilical artery. Early Hum. Dev. 24 (1990) 231–237
24. Gudmundsson, S., Tulzer, G., Huhta, J.C., Marsal, K.: Venous Doppler in the fetus with absent end-diastolic flow in the umbilical artery. Ultrasound Obstet. Gynecol. 7 (1996) 262–267
25. He, J.P., Ertan, A.K., Reitnauer, K., Mink, D., Schmidt, W.: Pathomorphologische Veränderungen der Endzotten: Vergleich bei Fällen mit „Reverse Flow"/enddiastolischem Block bzw. mit normalen Doppler-Flow-Befunden in den fetalen Gefäßen. Abstractband, Mittelrheinische Gesellschaft für Geburtshilfe und Gyn. (1997)
26. Hellbrügge, T., Lajosi, F., Menara, D., Schamberger, R., Rautenstrauch,T.: Münchner Funktionelle Entwicklungsdiagnostik. Erstes Lebensjahr. Lübeck: Hansisches Verlagskontor 1978
27. Hendrik, H.-J., Tossounidis, I., Boos, R., Schmidt, W.: Neuentwicklung eines fetalen biophysikalischen Profils unter Verwendung verschiedener sonographischer Parameter, Doppler-Flow und der Kinetocardiotokographie. Ultraschalldiagnostik, Dreiländertreffen, Bildgebung/Imaging 61 S. 2 (1994) 92
28. Hendrik, H.-J., Ertan, A.K., Schmidt, W.: Die Überwachung der Risikoschwangerschaft mit einem neuen biophysikalischen Profil (ABCD-Profil). Z. Geburtsh. Neonat. Zur Publikation eingereicht
29. Illyes, M., Gati, I.: Reverse Flow in the human fetal descending aorta as a sign of severe fetal asphyxia precending intrauterine deaths. J. clin. Ultrasound 16 (1988) 403–407
30. Johnstone, F.D., Haddad, N.G., Hoskins, P., McDicken, W., Chambers, S., Muir, B.: Umbilical artery Doppler flow velocity waveform: the outcome of pregnancies with absent end-diastolic flow. Eur. J. Obstet. Gynecol. Reprod. Biol. 28 (1988) 171–178
31. Jouppila, P., Kirkinen, P.: Increased vascular resistance in the descending aorta of the human fetus in hypoxia. Brit. J. Obstet. Gynaecol. 91 (1984) 853–856
32. Jouppila, P., Kirkinen, P.: Noninvasive assessment of fetal aortic blood flow in normal and abnormal pregnancies. Clin. Obstet. Gynecol. 32 (1989) 703–709
33. Karsdorp, V.H., van Vugt, J.M., van Geijn, H.P. et al.: Clinical significance of absent or reversed end diastolic velocity waveforms in umbilical artery. Lancet 344 (1994) 1664–1668
34. Karsdorp, V.H., Dirks, B.K., van der Linden, J.C., van Vugt, J.M., Baak, J.P., van Geijn, H.P.: Placenta morphology and absent or reversed end diastolic flow velocities in the umbilical artery: a clinical and morphometrical study. Placenta 17 (1996) 393–399
35. Kingdom, J.C., Kaufman, P.: Oxygen and placental villous development: origins of fetal hypoxia. Placenta 18 (1997) 613–621
36. Kirkinen, P., Muller, R., Baumann, H. et al.: Cerebral blood flow velocity waveforms in hydrocephalic fetuses. J. Clin. Ultrasound 16 (1988) 493–498
37. Köhler, G., Egelkraut, H.: Münchner Funktionelle Entwicklungsdiagnostik für das zweite und dritte Lebensjahr. Eigenverlag der Aktion Sonnenschein 1984
38. Krebs, C., Macara, L.M., Leiser, R., Bowman, A.W.F., Greer, I.A., Kingdom, J.C.P.: Intrauterine growth restriction and absent diastolic flow velocity in umbilical artery is associated with maldevelopment of the terminal placental villous tree. Amer. J. Obstet. Gynecol. 175 (1996) 1534–1542
39. Kubli, F., Schmidt, W.: Zustandsdiagnostik des Feten. In: Bachmann K.D., Ewerbeck, H., Kleihauer, E., Rossi, E., Stalder, G. (Hrsg.): Pädiatrie in Klinik und Praxis. Bd. 1. Stuttgart: Thieme 1987 S. 79–94
40. Kurkinen-Raty, M., Kivela, A., Jouppila, P.: The clinical significance of an absent end-diastolic velocity in the umbilical artery detected before the 34th week of pregnancy. Acta Obstet. Gynecol. Scand. 76 (1997) 398–404
41. Low, J.A., Handley-Derry, M.H., Burke, S.O. et al.: Association of intrauterine fetal growth retardation and learning deficits at age of 9 to 11 years. Amer. J. Obstet. Gynecol. 167 (1992) 1499–1505
42. Manning, F.A., Morrison, I., Lange, I.R.: Fetal biophysical profile scoring. A prospective study in 1184 high-risk patients. Amer. J. Obstet. Gynecol. 140 (1981) 289–293
43. Marlow, N., Hunt, L.P., Chiswick, M.L.: Clinical factors associated with adverse outcome for babies weighing 2000 g or less at birth. Arch. Dis. Child 63 (1988) 1131–1136
44. Matilainen, R., Heinonen, K., Siren-Tiusanen, H., Jokela, V., Launiala, K.: Neurodevelopmental screening of in utero growth-retarded prematurely born children before school age. Eur. J. Pediatr. 146 (1987) 453–457
45. McCowan, L.M., Mullre, B.M., Ritchie, K.: Umbilical artery flow velocity waveforms and the placental vascular bed. Amer. J. Obstet. Gynecol. 157 (1987) 900–902
46. Nickel, R.E., Bennett, F.G., Lawson, F.N.: School performance of children with birthweights of 1000 g or less. Amer. J. Dis. Child. 136 (1982) 105–110
47. Ombelet, W., Nuradi, S., Vandenberghe, K., Spitz, B.: Absent or reversed end diastolic flow in the umbilical arteries: a warning sign of serious fetal compromise. Clin. Exp. Hypertens. B7 (1988) 303–316
48. Pattinson, R.C., Norman, K., Odendaal, H.J.: The role of Doppler velocimetry in the management of high risk pregnancies. Brit. J. Obstet. Gynaecol. 101 (1994) 114–120
49. Pillai, M., James, D.: Continuation of normal neurobehavioural development in fetuses with absent umbilical arterial end diastolic velocities. Brit. J. Obstet. Gynaecol. 98 (1990) 277–281
50. Poulain, P., Palaric, J.C., Milon, J. et al.: Absent end diastolic flow of umbilical artery Doppler: pregnancy outcome in 62 cases. Eur. J. Obstet. Gynecol. Reprod. Biol. 53 (1992) 115–119
51. Reed, K.L., Anderson, C.F., Shenker, L.: Changes in intracardiac Doppler blood flow velocities in fetuses with absent umbilical artery diastolic flow. Amer. J. Obstet. Gynecol. 157 (1987) 774–779
52. Richter, T., Lietz, R., Beyreiss, K.: Gewichts- und Längenentwicklung ehemals hypotroph geborener Kinder in Abhängigkeit vom Schweregrad der intrauterinen Retardierung. Kinderärztl. Praxis 59 (1991) 341–345
53. Riegel, K.: Die Entwicklung des Kindes nach Schwangerschafts- und Geburtsrisiken. Diagnostik 14 (1981) 493–500
54. Rizzo, G., Pietropolli, A., Capponi, A., Arduini, D., Romanini, C.: Chromosomal abnormalities in fetuses with absent end-diastolic velocity in umbilical artery: analysis of risk factors for an abnormal karyotype. Amer. J. Obstet. Gynecol. 171 (1994) 827–831
55. Rochelson, B., Schulman, H., Farmakides, G. et al.: The significance of absent end-diastolic velocity in umbilical artery velocity waveforms. Amer. J. Obstet. Gynecol. 156 (1987) 1213–1218
56. Rochelson, B.: The clinical significance of absent end-diastolic velocity in the umbilical artery waveforms. Clin. Obstet. Gynecol. 32 (1989) 692–702
57. Salafia, C.M., Pezzullo, J.C., Minior, V.K., Divon, M.Y.: Placental pathology of absent and reversed end-diastolic flow in growth-restricted fetuses. Obstet. Gynecol. 90 (1997) 830–836
58. Scherjon, S.A., Smolders-De Haas, H., Kok, J.H., Zondervan, H.A.: The „brain-sparing" effect: Antenatal cerebral Doppler findings in relation to neurologic outcome in very preterm infants. Amer. J. Obstet. Gynecol. 169 (1993) 169–175
59. Schmidt, W., Kubli, F., Garoff, L., Hendrik, H.J., Leucht, W., Runnebaum, B.: Diagnose der intrauterinen Wachstumsretardierung – Vergleich von Klinik, Gesamtöstrogenbestimmung aus dem 24 h Urin und Ultraschallbiometrie (Distanzmessungen, biparietaler Kopfdurchmesser, thorako-abdominaler Querdurchmesser) unter Berücksichtigung des antepartalen und subpartalen CTGs. Geburtsh. u. Frauenheilk. 42 (1982) 709–716
60. Schmidt, W., Gnirs, J.: Fetale Bewegungsaktivität und akustische Stimulation. Gynäkologe 23 (1990) 289–297

61. Schmidt, W., Graf von Ballestrem, C.L., Ertan, A.K., Rühle, W., Gnirs, J., Boos, R.: Pathologische Doppler-Flow-Befunde und kardiotokographische Ergebnisse. Geburtsh. u. Frauenheilkd. 51 (1991) 523–531

62. Schmidt, W., Rühle, W., Ertan, A.K., Boos, R., Gnirs, J.: Doppler-Sonographie – Perinatologische Daten bei Fällen mit enddiastolischem Block bzw. Reverse Flow. Geburtsh. u. Frauenheilkd. 51 (1991) 288–292

63. Schmidt, W., Ertan, A.K., Rühle, W., von Ballestrem, C.L., Gnirs, J., Boos, R.: Dopplersonographie: „Enddiastolischer Block bzw. Reverse Flow" – Perinatologische Daten und geburtshilfliches Management. Jahrbuch der Gynäkologie und Geburtshilfe, Zülpich: Biermann; 1991 S. 99–106

64. Schmidt, W., Ertan, A.K.: Dopplersonographie in der Geburtsmedizin. Geburtshilfliches Management bei hochpathologischen Doppler-Flow-Befunden. In: Hillemans, H.G. (Hrsg.): Geburtshilfe – Geburtsmedizin. Eine umfassende Bilanz zukunftsweisender Enwicklungen am Ende des 20. Jahrhunderts. Berlin: Springer 1995; S. 317–325

65. Schulman, H., Fleischer, A., Stern, W., Farmakides, G., Jagani, N., Blattner, P.: Umbilical velocity wave ratios in human pregnancy. Amer. J. Obstet. Gynecol. 148 (1984) 985–990

66. Taylor, D.J., Howie, P.W.: Fetal growth achievement and neurodevelopmental disability. Brit. J. Obstet. Gynaecol. 96 (1989) 789–794

67. Todros, T., Ronco, G., Fianchino, O. et al.: Accuracy of the umbilical arteries Doppler flow velocity waveforms in detecting adverse perinatal outcomes in a high-risk population. Acta Obstet. Gynecol. Scand. 75 (1996) 113–119

68. Trudinger, B.J., Cook, C.M., Giles, W.B., Connelly, A., Thompson, R.S.: Umbilical artery flow velocity waveforms in high-risk pregnancy. Randomised controlled trial. Lancet. i (1987) 188–190

69. Trudinger, B.J., Cook, C.M., Giles, W.B. et al.: Fetal umbilical artery velocity waveforms and subsequent neonatal outcome. Brit. J. Obstet. Gynaecol. 98 (1991) 378–384

70. Ulrich, S., Ernst, J.P., Kalder, M., Weiss, E., Berle, P.: Neurologische Spätmorbidität von Frühgeburten mit intrauterin diagnostiziertem Null- oder Negativflow der Nabelarterien. Z. Geburtsh. Perinatol. 198 (1994) 100–103

71. Ulrich, S., Weiss, E., Kalder, M., Hitschold, T., Berle, P.: Doppler sonographic flow measurements of the middle cerebral artery in end-diastolic zero flow in the umbilical arteries in relation to fetal outcome. Z. Geburtsh. Neonatol. 200 (1996) 21–24

72. Valcamonico, A., Danti, L., Frusca, T. et al.: Absent end-diastolic velocity in umbilical artery: risk of neonatal morbidity and brain damage. Amer. J. Obstet. Gynecol. 170 (1994) 796–801

73. Vohr, B., Oh, W.: Growth and development in preterm infants small for gestational age. J. Pediatr. 103 (1983) 941–944

74. Vohr, B., Garcia-Coll, C.: Neurodevelopmental and school performance of very low-birthweight infants: a seven year longitudinal study. Pediatrics 76 (1985) 345–350

75. Vyas, S., Nicolaides, K.H., Bower, S., Campbell, S.: Middle cerebral artery flow velocity waveforms in fetal hypoxaemia. Brit. J. Obstet. Gynecol. 97 (1990) 797–803

76. Wang, K.G., Chen, C.P., Yang, J.M., Su, T.H.: Impact of reverse end-diastolic flow velocity in umbilical artery on pregnancy outcome after the 28th gestational week. Acta Obstet. Gynecol. Scand. 77 (1998) 527–531

77. Weiner, Z., Farmakides, G., Schulman, H., Penny, B.: Central and peripheral hemodynamic changes in fetuses with absent enddiastolic velocity in umbilical artery: correlation with computerized fetal heart rate pattern. Amer. J. Obstet. Gynecol. 170 (1994) 509–515

78. Weiss, E., Ulrich, S., Berle, P.: Condition at birth of infants with previously absent or reverse umbilical artery end-diastolic flow velocities. Arch. Gynecol. Obstet. 252 (1982) 37–43

79. Weiss, E., Hitschold, T., Müntefering, H., Berle, P.: Dopplersonographie der Art. umbilicalis: Differenzierte Diagnostik bei der intrauterinen Mangelentwicklung. Geburtsh. u. Frauenheilkd. 49 (1989) 466–471

80. Weiss, E., Berle, P.: Clinical management of fetuses with diastolic zero or Reverse Flow of the umbilical arteries: Duration of clinical surveillance and fetal outcome. Z. Geburtsh. Perinat. 195 (1991) 37–42

81. Wenstrom, K.D., Weiner, C.P., Williamson, R.A.: Diverse maternal and fetal pathology associated with absent diastolic flow in the umbilical artery of high-risk fetuses. Obstet. Gynecol. 77 (1991) 374–378

82. Woo, J.S.K., Liang, S.T., Lo, R.L.S.: Significance of an absent or reversed end diastolic flow in doppler umbilical artery waveforms. J. Ultrasound Med. 6 (1987) 291–297

83. Zelop, C.M., Richardson, D.K., Heffner, L.J.: Outcomes of severely abnormal umbilical artery doppler velocimetry in structurally normal singleton fetuses. Obstet. Gynecol. 87 (1996) 434–438

3-D Ultrasound

45 3-D Ultrasound in Prenatal Diagnosis

Capabilities of 3-D Ultrasound

With the development of high-performance transvaginal and abdominal transducers, the image quality in conventional two-dimensional (2-D) ultrasound has been dramatically improved in recent years. One drawback of 2-D ultrasound, however, is that images can be acquired in only two of the three cardinal planes. These are the sagittal and coronal (frontal) planes in transvaginal scanning and the sagittal and transverse planes in abdominal scanning. The transverse planes are not accessible to transvaginal scanning, and the coronal planes cannot be scanned transabdominally.

Another difficulty with 2-D ultrasound is that the examiner must be able to mentally assemble a two-dimensional set of cross-sectional images into a three-dimensional image. While an experienced sonographer will do this automatically, a less experienced examiner often finds it difficult to envision a three-dimensional image in this way, especially if the anatomic orientation is uncertain. Similar difficulties arise in trying to demonstrate a finding to the parents using a 2-D image. While this can be done in principle if the technology is adequately explained, the parents cannot be expected to form an accurate three-dimensional picture in their minds.

Storing volume data. Modern three-dimensional (3-D) ultrasound provides a routine method not only for storing single image planes as in 2-D ultrasound but also for storing complete sets of volume data in a computer memory. Once stored, these data sets can be accessed to reconstruct any desired image plane within the acquired volume. They can also be manipulated interactively, in virtual real time, to render three-dimensional surface images and transparent views.

Time requirement. For years, the major problem with 3-D ultrasound was the relatively large amount of time required for the computation of three-dimensional surface-rendered or transparent images. While a single image could be rendered in just 20–30 seconds, it took 20–30 minutes to render entire sequences consisting of up to 60 separate images. To keep the examination time within reasonable limits, most operators used only seven individual frames when computing an animated sequence.

With the latest generation of 3-D and 4-D scanners, which have powerful built-in computers, it is possible not only to view directly the surface of a stored object but also display extended image sequences of more than 60 frames within approximately 20 seconds.

Technique of Transvaginal and Abdominal 3-D Ultrasound

Generally a 3-D examination consists of four main steps: data acquisition, 3-D visualization, volume/image processing, and the storing of volumes, rendered images or sequences (Table 45.**1**).

Table 45.**1** Steps involved in transvaginal and transabdominal 3-D ultrasound

Data acquisition
- ➤ Orientation in the 2-D image
- ➤ Definition of the region of interest (ROI)
- ➤ Volume acquisition

3-D visualization
- ➤ Multiplanar display
- ➤ Surface-rendered image (surface mode, light mode)
- ➤ Transparent image (maximum mode, X-ray mode)
- ➤ Vascular image (combination of surface or transparent rendering and color Doppler)
- ➤ Animated image (rendering of image sequences)

Volume/image processing
- ➤ Electronic scalpel
- ➤ Filtering
- ➤ Contrast and brightness control
- ➤ Color image

Storage of volumes or rendered images/image sequences

■ Data Acquisition (Volume Acquisition)

All three-dimensional ultrasound technology is based on the acquisition of multiple adjacent, two-dimensional scans which are stored at correlative sites in an electronic memory, where they are assembled to produce a volume data set.

Two main technologies are currently available for the acquisition of ultrasound volumes. Their differences are reviewed in Table 45.**2**.

Table 45.**2** Differences between internal and external 3-D imaging systems

Internal (integrated) system	External system
3-D system built into the ultrasound system	A sensor is mounted on the transducer
Specialized 3-D transducers, which can be used only with a 3-D ultrasound scanner	Any transducer can be used, regardless of the manufacturer
Automated volume acquisition with a 3-D transducer	Freehand volume acquisition by the operator
High precision of volume acquisition, since all of the individual 2-D scan planes are acquired at equidistant intervals	Less precise due to the variable distance between the individual 2-D scan planes
Very fast volume acquisition	Speed of volume acquisition depends on manual transducer manipulation
No need for interpolation between the individual scan planes	Interpolation software is required
Independent of a magnetic field	The magnetic field may introduce geometric errors
Direct interactive control in the rendering of 3-D images	3-D image rendering is time-consuming due to the necessary conversion steps
Orthogonal display, surface-rendered and transparent views	(Orthogonal display), surface-rendered and transparent views
Excellent image quality	Acceptable image quality
Allows 4-D ("live 3-D") imaging	Does not allow 4-D imaging

Data Acquisition with an Internal or Integrated System

With an internal system (GE-Kretztechnik, Austria), the whole 3-D unit is built into the ultrasound imager, and a dedicated 3-D transducer is matched to the system (7, 9–19, 30, 32–36) (Fig. 45.**1**). Volume acquisition is activated by the touch of a button, at which point the transducer element within the probe casing is automatically swept through a fan-shaped pattern at a specified angle (Fig. 45.**2**). The sweep angle is adjustable from 10° to 90° with an endovaginal transducer and from 15° to 75° with an abdominal transducer. All of the image planes captured during volume acquisition are equidistant from one another. After signal processing and quantitation, the acquired planes are digitally stored at correlative sites in an electronic volume memory.

Display. All of the acquisition planes can be retrieved from the volume memory and displayed (multiplanar sectional image analysis), or three-dimensional surface images and transparent views can be rendered from the volume data. The three-dimensional images can be displayed on the monitor as separate images or rotated to create an animated display (8, 17).

Advantages. The advantages of this system are the very short acquisition time for abdominal and transvaginal volumes and the high precision of volume acquisition, in which successively acquired two-dimensional scan planes are stored at precisely equal intervals.

Currently this type of system provides the most accurate surface-rendered images for routine examinations. The electronic 3-D probes can display both gray-scale data and color Doppler information in three dimensions (17).

Disadvantage. The disadvantage of an internal system is that the 3-D probes are designed exclusively for a particular system; they cannot be used with other machines (17).

Technique. The examination with a dedicated 3-D probe starts with a two-dimensional B-mode scan to establish orientation. When an optimum image has been obtained, the desired object is framed with a superimposed volume box to define the region of interest (ROI). The desired sweep speed—fast, medium, or slow—is then selected. The acquisition times range from 0.3 to 4 seconds depending on the probe, volume size, and sweep speed. The best image quality is obtained with a slow sweep speed, as this acquires the highest number of image planes within a designated volume. But this also increases the risk of fetal movement during sweep acquisition, resulting in motion artifacts. A fast or medium sweep speed is satisfactory for routine examinations.

Data Acquisition with an External System

A specialized transducer is not used in external acquisition systems. Scans are obtained with a conventional 2-D probe, whose position and movement in space are tracked by an add-on system (e.g., TomTec system, Echotech, InViVo system). Manual parallel or sweeping movements of the transducer may be linked to an external mechanism or may be executed freehand using a tracking system. In the latter case an electromagnetic position sensor is mounted on the hand-held probe (6, 22–25, 31). This device can sense the exact position and movements of the probe by detecting changes in a magnetic field (Fig. 45.**3**).

Display. In an external system, a volume set is produced from the individual acquired images by storing and spatially encoding each of the two-dimensional scan planes in an external 3-D memory. In practical terms, this is done by transmitting the acquired image data via the video signal of the ultrasound unit to an external computer (workstation) that is equipped with a frame grabber. After the individual images have been digitized by the frame grabber, they are stored in the computer memory according to their known locations and are assembled into a volume (17).

Advantage. The advantage of an external system is that it can be used with any standard ultrasound transducer (17).

Disadvantage. The disadvantage of an external system is that the scanning process is more complicated than with an integrated system and the distances between the individual two-dimensional scan planes can vary due to the free-hand acquisition. Some of the planes may even overlap. Although the external systems as a whole have improved markedly in their quality, they still cannot compete with the precision of an internal system with automated volume acquisition in routine situations. Also, the external systems cannot yet generate real-time 3-D sequences.

3-D Visualization

Three different modes of 3-D visualization are available, depending on the system used:
- Multiplanar (orthogonal) display
- Surface rendering
- Transparent display (Table 45.**1**)

Multiplanar (Orthogonal) Display

Orthogonal planes. In the multiplanar display, all three mutually perpendicular scan planes (the "orthogonal" planes) are displayed simultaneously on the monitor immediately after volume acquisition. All conventional scan planes can be viewed, as well as planes that are unattainable with traditional 2-D abdominal or transvaginal ultrasound. These are the coronal planes in abdominal ultrasound and the transverse planes in vaginal ultrasound. When one plane is rotated or shifted, corresponding changes are displayed at once in the two other planes.

Textbook position, tomographic survey. Before the orthogonal planes are displayed, it is advantageous to rotate the object of interest within the volume using the appropriate rotation controls so that it is displayed in an upright or "textbook" position (16, 17) (Figs. 45.**4**, 45.**5**). The rotation control can now be used to manipulate a selected plane in all three directions with millimeter precision, permitting an accurate tomographic survey of a particular region (Figs. 45.**4**, 45.**5**).

Abnormalities. In the fetal profile, which can be accurately defined in the 2-D B-mode image only 69.9% of the time (16), an abnormal profile can be recognized with confidence only if it is certain that the scan is not an oblique cut (Fig. 45.**6**). This is a particular problem in 2-D examinations where there is insufficient amniotic fluid to clearly define the fetal profile (Fig. 45.**7**). Besides evaluating the fetal profile, the examiner can also selectively scrutinize all other anatomic regions such as the diaphragm (Fig. 45.**8**) and biometry planes in the orthogonal display (12–15, 26). With paired structures such as the orbits, biometric data can be optimally compared between the right and left sides in an accurate plane of section (Fig. 45.**6**), making it easier to recognize abnormalities such as orbital hypoplasia (16). Other abnormalities such as spinal defects (21) can also be accurately defined in the multiplanar display and clearly and completely evaluated.

Volume determinations. Finally, a simultaneous display of the three perpendicular planes permits a more accurate volume determination than can be achieved with two-dimensional ultrasound (5, 30).

Three-Dimensional Image Reconstruction (3-D Rendering)

Basically two different 3-D display modes are available:

- Surface rendering
- Transparent mode

The goal of these display modes is to provide the examiner with a three-dimensional spatial view of the object being examined. Different computation algorithms are used, depending on the type of information desired.

Surface Rendering

Both the surface and light modes are available for surface rendering (Table 45.**3**, Fig. 45.**9**).

Interactive display. The interactive display like that used in current integrated systems (Combison 530D, Voluson 530 MT, Voluson 730, GE-Kretztechnik, Austria) offers the examiner several advantages in surface rendering. First, the selected region of interest can be viewed directly in the current mode as a three-dimensional image. Also, the operator can instantly switch between two different computation algorithms to find the mode that best demonstrates the finding. There is also the option of fading between two modes, which in some cases provides a smoother, more visually appealing image.

Requirement. A basic requirement for all three-dimensional surface rendering is the presence of an adequate fluid pocket in front of the structure being imaged (Figs. 45.**6**, 45.**45**). Overlying structures such as a fetal arm or the umbilical cord and adjacent structures like the placenta tend to obscure the structure of interest, such as the fetal face (Fig. 45.**45**). This is comparable to a photograph in which the subject's face is partially blocked by a raised hand. Consequently, the obscuring object must be electronically deleted before surface rendering is performed (see Volume Analysis and Image Processing).

Clinical application. In clinical use, the transvaginal 3-D probe can provide a surface-rendered image of the embryo or the fetus (4, 19) (Figs. 45.**10**–45.**12**). The transabdominal probe can provide a good fetal surface image starting at about 20 weeks' gestation, and in some cases an acceptable image can be obtained even earlier (Fig. 45.**13**).

Besides demonstrating normal anatomy (1–3, 6, 13–15, 17, 22, 26–29, 32–34) (Figs. 45.**13**–45.**23**), the photo-realistic view of the fetus offers interesting opportunities for the detection of subtle abnormalities (9, 10–18, 21, 29, 35) (Figs. 45.**24**–45.**37**). The interactive display is particularly useful for the detection or exclusion of specific abnormalities, making it possible to identify fetal surface abnormalities and define the extent of a defect in all dimensions.

Abnormalities of the face and head. This particularly applies to the fetal head (10, 12, 15, 16, 18, 21, 28, 29), where a variety of changes such as an abnormal profile (flat profile, frontal bossing, depressed nasal bridge, retrognathia), cyclopia, facial dysmorphism, cleft lip and palate, auricular dysplasia, and low-set ears can be defined (Figs. 45.**24**–45.**29**). Specific abnormalities elsewhere in the fetal body surface can also be identified (12, 15, 18).

Clefts and organ surfaces. Dorsal and ventral clefts can be vividly defined in their full extent and differentiated by their surface structure (Figs. 45.**30**–45.**32**). The surfaces of fetal abdominal organs can also be defined in some cases. This requires the presence of intra-abdominal ascites or a conspicuous fluid-filled structure such as megalocystis. To visualize these external or internal organ surfaces, part of the body must be "sliced off" with an electronic scalpel. This can be done in a lateral or coronal longitudinal scan (Figs. 45.**33**, 45.**34**) or in a transverse scan.

Genital anomalies. Even subtle abnormalities in the fetal genital region can be appreciated in the surface-rendered image (Fig. 45.**35**).

Limb anomalies. Surface rendering has also created new capabilities in the diagnosis of limb anomalies (11, 12, 15, 35). Since the examination is not performed on a live, moving fetus but on a digitally stored limb that can be freely rotated in space, it is easy to recognize abnormal body proportions in skeletal dysplasias (11, 35) and angular deformities such as clubbing of the hand or foot (12, 15) (Fig. 45.**36**). These findings can be appreciated even more clearly in an animated rotating display.

The same applies to detailed examinations of the hand and foot. These structures, too, are often difficult to evaluate with conventional 2-D ultrasound because of arm and leg movements. But the 3-D surface analysis of the stored hand or foot can clearly reveal details such as the presence of an extra digit (15) (Fig. 45.**37**) or the absence of a finger (15) (Fig. 45.**36**).

Surface mode and color Doppler. Blood flow within the vessels, including the umbilical cord vessels, can be visualized in three dimensions by combining the surface mode with color Doppler or power Doppler (Fig. 45.**38**).

Transparent Mode

Maximum mode, x-ray mode. The transparent mode is another form of three-dimensional rendering. Unlike surface rendering, however, it displays the interior of a defined volume, similar to a glass figure. The transparent mode basically employs two computation algorithms, which may be used separately or blended (faded) together: the maximum mode and the x-ray mode (Table 45.**4**).

Skeletal imaging. The transparent mode chiefly displays hyperechoic structures while greatly attenuating less echogenic structures. This can provide a survey view of the fetal skeleton. Extraneous echoes are not a problem in the transparent mode, as they are automatically eliminated from the image.

Besides showing normal ossification (14, 17, 27) (Figs. 45.**39**, 45.**41**), this technique can reveal ossification defects (16) (Figs. 45.**40**, 45.**42**) and abnormal curvature of the fetal spine (12, 15) (Fig. 45.**42**).

Glass body rendering. The combination of the transparent mode and Power Doppler (Angio-mode) offers the possibility of presenting the fetal vascular system three-dimensionally as if viewed in a glass model (Fig. 45.**43**).

Image Animation

Animated rotating display. In both the surface and transparent modes or in an isolated vascular display, whole series of images can be reconstructed within a few seconds. This makes it possible to view the ob-

Table 45.**3**   Surface and light modes in surface rendering

Surface mode
In the surface mode, the volume elements (voxels) encountered first are displayed. As the name implies, this mode is used to render the fetal body surface (17) (Fig. 45.**9**).

Light mode
The light mode is a variant of the surface mode in which the subject appears to be illuminated by a virtual light source. The surface can be lighted from various angles. This mode can provide a softer image, but it can also create certain shadowing effects that enhance the impression of three-dimensional depth (17) (Fig. 45.**9**).

Table 45.**4**   Maximum and x-ray modes for transparent volume display

Maximum mode
In the maximum mode, the maximum value detected along each virtual ray through the volume is displayed. This predominantly displays hyperechoic structures like the fetal bones (17).

X-ray mode
This mode displays the mean gray-scale values that are encountered along the virtual rays through the volume. The resulting image resembles an x-ray film (17).

ject of interest from multiple angles in the form of an animated, rotating display (15, 17).

The operator selects the starting point and end point of the animated sequence and inputs the desired angle increment between the separate frames (Fig. 45.**44**). After the cine mode is activated, the desired images are computed. It takes about 10 seconds to render a series of 30 images with a modern, integrated 3-D system. With the latest technology, the first and last images in the sequence are displayed directly on the monitor, making it easier to select an optimum angle for animating the object about the x or y axis (Fig. 45.**45**).

Once the series of images has been computed, the rendered object can be viewed as an animated rotating display. Whether the rotation is done automatically or by manual incrementation, the examiner can view the object from numerous angles and can gain an even better three-dimensional impression of its features.

▣ *Volume Analysis and Image Processing*

Cartesian storage, electronic scalpel. Especially in surface rendering, structures located in front of the area of interest must be electronically "removed" to obtain unobstructed surface images of acceptable quality. Larger intervening structures can be deleted from the image by a process called Cartesian storage (14, 15, 17) or by using an electronic scalpel.

In Cartesian storage, unwanted structures are removed by eliminating all volume data outside a box that has been defined by the operator in Cartesian coordinates (Figs. 45.**46**, 45.**47**).

With the electronic scalpel (20, 23), the operator "cuts away" interposed structures by using an adjustable box or by outlining them with a cursor (Fig. 45.**48**). This process can be repeated several times until all the unwanted areas have been deleted.

Speckle. Small extraneous signals called "speckle" (e.g., caused by particles floating in the amniotic fluid) can be eliminated with a low-pass filter (Fig. 45.**49**). The necessary degree of filtering depends on the amplitude of the unwanted echoes and is adjusted with the threshold control. An optimum filter setting is just sufficient to remove the extraneous echoes (17).

Contrast and brightness. Contrast and brightness adjustments of the rendered surface image can be made and checked interactively—i.e., every manual adjustment of the contrast or brightness control is seen immediately on the monitor. This makes it easy to achieve optimum brightness and contrast in the surface-rendered image (Fig. 45.**50**).

▣ *4-D Imaging*

4-D imaging combines 3-D ultrasound and time. With acquisition rate of 6–25 volumes per second, it provides a "live" three-dimensional display of the fetus (real-time 3-D). All of the acquired volumes are captured sequentially in the electronic memory, making it possible to document entire sequences of fetal movements, which can be stored with digital image quality. The individual volumes can then be sequentially retrieved from the memory, similar to the cine loop used in two-

dimensional ultrasound. In this way the examiner can quickly locate the volume that gives the best three-dimensional view of a particular movement phase or anatomical area. Remarkable "snapshots" of fetal movements (facial expression or body movements) can be obtained with this technique (Fig. 45.**51**).

STIC technique (spatial–temporal image correlation). This technique allows 4-D fetal echocardiography in B-mode without the need of any external triggering devices. After performing a slow motion volume scan of the fetal heart the data of this scan are rearranged and stick together by correlation of their temporal and spatial domain. The result is a 4-D real time data set presenting one heart cycle in motion. After the storage of the data set the heart can be assessed off-line in an endless volume cine loop. The triplanar demonstration of the beating heart enables a comprehensive assessment of the fetal heart morphology including the great vessels. Due to the fact that the volume can be rotated and resliced in all three dimensions even complex anomalies of the fetal heart can be demonstrated precisely. The combination of STIC and Color Doppler allows an exact control of the cardiac blood flow while the heart in motion (Fig. 45.**52**).

▣ *Digital Storage of Volumes, Computed Images or Image Sequences*

Long-term storage. Three-dimensional ultrasound gives us the capability to store not just two-dimensional images but complete volumes. Today, various media are available for the long-term storage of these volumes, such as removable hard disks and magnetic optic disks.

When findings of interest are stored digitally on nondegrading media, the examiner can retrieve the volumes at any time and navigate through them in the absence of the patient (14). This is of particular value in the diagnosis of fetal anomalies, as it enables the examiner to scrutinize equivocal findings in an unhurried fashion without upsetting the patient by lingering at a particular site with the probe, which is frequently done in conventional 2-D examinations.

Problems with 3-D Ultrasound

Various kinds of problem may arise when 3-D ultrasound is used for prenatal diagnosis.

Fetal position and amniotic fluid volume. In 28% of cases, a high-quality surface image cannot be obtained with 3-D ultrasound because of an unfavorable fetal position or a deficient amniotic fluid volume (16). For example, if the face of the fetus is touching the placenta, a good surface-rendered image can be obtained only if the placenta is selectively "cut" from the head with the electronic scalpel. In cases of pronounced oligohydramnios or anhydramnios, surface rendering cannot be performed, and the examiner must be content with a multiplanar display.

Quality of 3-D images. The quality of three-dimensional surface images depends critically on the quality of the two-dimensional B-mode image and on gestational age. If the two-dimensional B-mode scan yields a poor fetal image because of maternal obesity, it is unreasonable to expect that the three-dimensional surface images will turn out better.

The fetus displays more prominent facial features with advancing gestational age, and surface-rendered images of those features become more impressive.

Motion artifacts. If the fetus moves during volume acquisition, various motion artifacts can occur depending on the type of movement, and in some cases this can mimic fetal defects (Fig. 45.**53**). The risk of motion artifacts can be significantly reduced by using a faster sweep speed, but this also causes some deterioration of image quality because fewer scan planes are acquired.

The electronic scalpel can also cause iatrogenic defects if the cut extends past the unwanted structures and unintentionally removes normal fetal structures as well (Fig. 45.**54**).

Cardiac diagnosis. Until recently, fetal cardiac prognosis was another problem area in 3-D ultrasound because the data acquisition time was still too long, even with rapid scanning. If the cardiac cycle is shorter than the time needed to digitally store the fetal heart, cardiac activity during data storage leads to wave-like motion artifacts (24). As a result, an accurate three-dimensional portrait of the fetal heart can be only achieved with new technologies (STIC) avoiding these motion-artifacts.

The advantages and problems of 3-D imaging are reviewed in Table 45.**5** and Fig. 45.**6**.

Table 45.**5** Advantages of 3-D ultrasound over conventional 2-D ultrasound (after 14)

Ability to store and retrieve a complete volume

> The examiner can navigate through the stored volume on line in all three planes with tomographic precision.
> Bedside scan time is reduced, as the stored volumes can be reviewed in the patient's absence.
> Digital volume storage on a hard disk without data loss; this allows for multiple analysis (including biometry) and retrospective analysis of the stored volume even weeks, months, or years after the examination.
> The volume can be shipped by removable hard disk for independent review by a second examiner.
> Stored volumes can be copied numerous times and used for training purposes (e.g., group practice in locating biometry planes or recognizing fetal anomalies).

Multiplanar display

> Visualization of the third plane, which is unattainable with conventional ultrasound.
> Ability to check the precise location of an imaged anatomic plane (facial profile, biometry planes).
> Accurate volumetry.

Surface rendering

Examiner
> Vivid depiction of fetal structures
> Detailed evaluation of surface structures (e.g., facial structures)
> Confident detection or exclusion of surface defects
> Visualization of complex malformations or of anomalies associated with angular deformity
> Object can be rotated and evaluated from various angles

Parents
> Entirely new experience from the photorealistic depiction of fetal structures
> Enhanced parental bonding to the fetus
> Better appreciation of the severity of a fetal anomaly
> Reassurance from the exclusion of a fetal anomaly

Transparent mode

> Fetal skeletal view provides a prenatal "infant radiograph"

4-D ultrasound

> Real-time 3-D display of fetal movements

Table 45.**6** Problems with 3-D ultrasound (after 14)

> The examiner must get used to the size of the probe
> Fetal or probe movements during data acquisition lead to motion artifacts
> Orientation problems may arise in the stored volume
> Surface rendering cannot be done in pronounced oligohydramnios
> Overlying or adjacent structures interfere with surface rendering and must first be removed by Cartesian storage or with an electronic scalpel
> Setting the threshold too high or faulty manipulation of the electronic scalpel leads to iatrogenic structural defects.
> The storage of 3-D volumes requires a high storage capacity (one vaginal 3-D volume = 5 to 18 MB, one abdominal volume = 3 to 10 MB).

Critical Appraisal and Outlook

Promising technology. Without question, 3-D ultrasound has profited greatly from the explosive advances that have occurred in computer technology. With the various display options that are now available with 3-D ultrasound, there is no doubt that this technology holds great promise for the future—especially in prenatal diagnosis, where it is often essential to detect subtle abnormalities. The precise tomographic examination of suspicious findings and the ability to scrutinize structures in surface-rendered and transparent views will particularly help examiners experienced with 2-D anomaly scans to obtain a clearer look at defects and evaluate them more precisely. This is especially true in the diagnosis of complex malformations and of anomalies that are associated with angular deformity.

Detection of fetal anomalies. In a comparative study of 458 fetuses (242 normal fetuses and 216 with anomalies) between 16 and 38 weeks' gestation, Merz et al. (14) found that 3-D ultrasound had advantages over conventional 2-D ultrasound in 64.2% of the cases. The orthogonal display alone yielded advantages in 46.2% of cases owing to the more accurate tomographic depiction of the desired plane and the easier recognition of an off-axis plane. When the orthogonal display was combined with surface-rendered or transparent views, advantages were noted in 71.5% of the cases. This higher percentage resulted from the additional information supplied by the vivid surface image and from the ability to evaluate the subject from multiple angles, determine the precise extent of a defect, image bony structures (in the transparent mode), and obtain a clearer overview of complex anomalies.

Chromosomal abnormalities. 3-D ultrasound may well bring interesting new aspects to the diagnosis of fetuses with chromosome disorders or syndromes, in which it is important to be able to detect subtle abnormalities.

Exclusion of fetal anomalies. The same applies to the targeted exclusion of fetal anomalies. Particularly in cases with an increased recurrence risk, the parents can see for themselves that the 3-D image demonstrates a normal fetus.

4-D technology. 4-D imaging provides a real-time 3-D view of the fetus, as if it were enclosed in a "glass abdomen." In the future, this will make it easier to confirm normal fetal movement patterns and to detect abnormal patterns.

It is reasonable to predict that 3-D and 4-D ultrasound will continue to profit from further advances in the computer sector as even faster and more powerful computer processors are developed. It is likely that even three-dimensional fetal cardiac diagnosis will become a routine procedure.

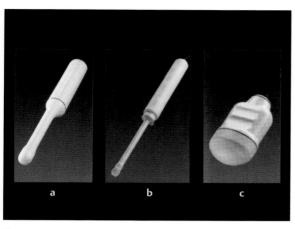

1

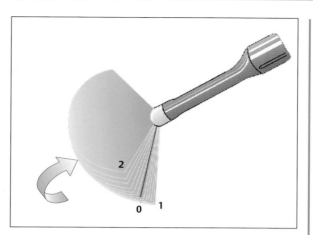

2

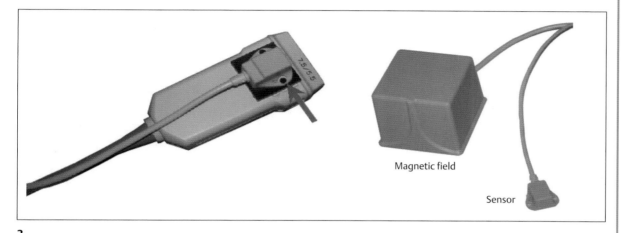

3

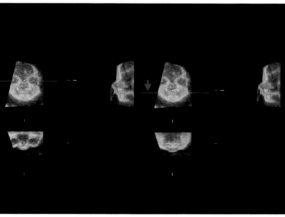

4

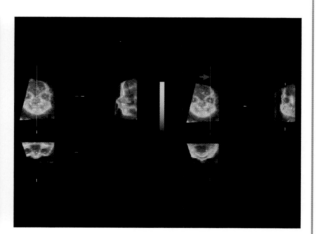

5

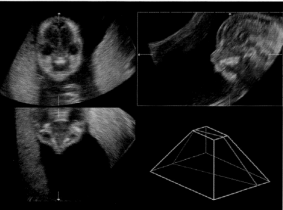

6

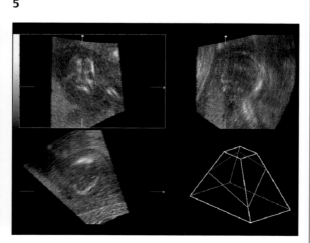

7

Data acquisition

Fig. 45.**1**   3D transducers.
a Vaginal transducer.
b Rectal transducer.
c Abdominal transducer (GE/Kretz-technik, Austria).

Fig. 45.**2**   Scanning principle with a transvaginal (shown) or transabdominal 3D transducer. With a forward scan direction, the 2D scan plane (point 0) is automatically deflected to point 1 and swept continuously from there to point 2.

Fig. 45.**3**   External system (TomTec). A position sensor is mounted on the probe. The position and movements of the probe are detected with a magnetic field.

Multiplanar display

Fig. 45.**4**   Face of a normal fetus (24 weeks) in the orthogonal display. The stored volume has been rotated so that the examiner can view the object of interest in a "textbook position".
Left half of figure: coronal scan (upper left), midsagittal scan (upper right), and transverse scan (lower left) at eye level through both orbits.
Right half of figure: the transverse scan plane has been moved downward in the lower image to the level of the maxilla, defining the tooth buds.

Fig. 45.**5**   Same fetus as in Fig. 45.**4**. The midsagittal plane in the left half of the figure is shifted to obtain a longitudinal scan through the left orbit (upper right).

Fig. 45.**6**   Accurate profile view of a fetus in the multiplanar display, showing pronounced retrognathia (20 weeks).

Fig. 45.**7**   Abnormally flat profile of a fetus with pronounced oligohydramnios (multiplanar display) at 17 weeks. Karyotype: trisomy 21.

Fig. 45.**8** Left diaphragmatic hernia in the multiplanar display, 34 weeks. The defect is clearly visualized in the longitudinal coronal plane (arrows).

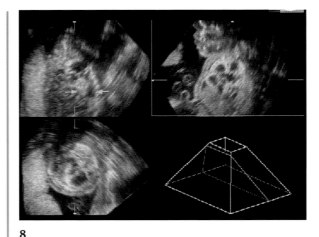

8

Surface rendering

Fig. 45.**9** Surface rendering of a fetal face using different algorithms.

Fig. 45.**10** Embryo with yolk sac at 7 weeks. Surface-rendered image.

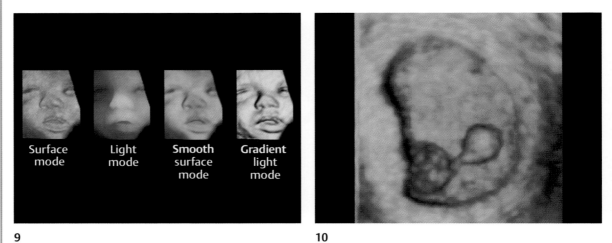

Surface mode   Light mode   Smooth surface mode   Gradient light mode

9   **10**

Fig. 45.**11** Embryo with yolk sac at 8 weeks, 5 days. Surface-rendered image. The face and limb buds of the embryo can already be discerned.

Fig. 45.**12** Lateral view of an embryo at 10 weeks.

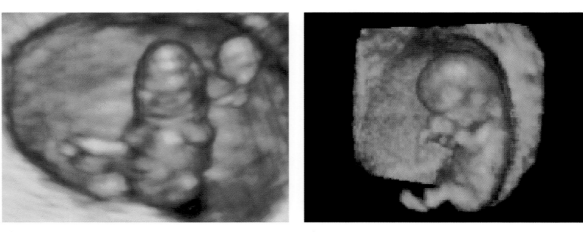

11   **12**

Fig. 45.**13** Fetus sucking its thumb. Surface-rendered image, 19 weeks.

Fig. 45.**14** Frontal view of a fetal face in the surface mode, 32 weeks.

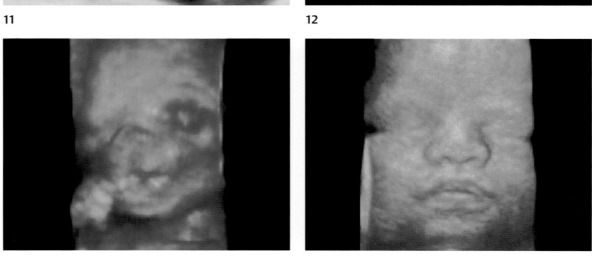

13   **14**

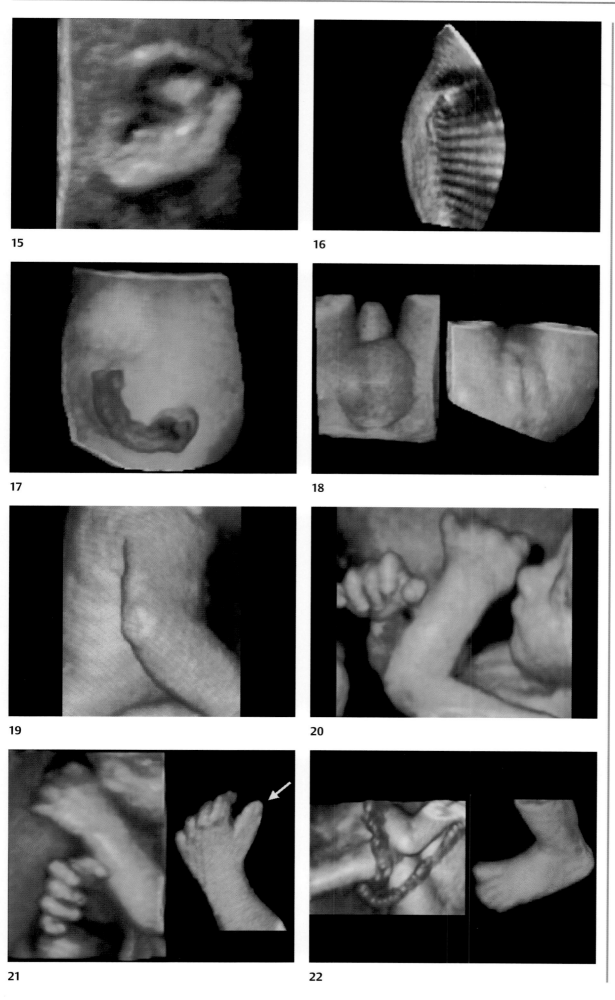

15

16

17

18

19

20

21

22

Fig. 45.**15**   Lateral view of a normal fetal ear, 24 weeks.

Fig. 45.**16**   Normal lateral view of the back, 24 weeks. A tangential electronic "cut" through the body can provide a surface-rendered view of the ribs.

Fig. 45.**17**   Coronal view of the fetal abdomen at 28 weeks, showing the umbilical cord insertion.

Fig. 45.**18**   *Left:* male genitalia, 32 weeks. *Right:* female genitalia, 31 weeks.

Fig. 45.**19**   Normal right upper arm, 27 weeks.

Fig. 45.**20**   Fetus with both upper limbs, 33 weeks.

Fig. 45.**21**   *Left:* view of the hands and fingers, 33 weeks. *Right:* view of the thumb with nail, 34 weeks.

Fig. 45.**22**   *Left:* loop of umbilical cord wrapped around the left leg, 33 weeks. *Right:* foot, 27 weeks.

Fig. 45.**23** Loop of umbilical cord, 32 weeks.

Fig. 45.**24** Comparison of abnormal fetal surface profiles.
a Flat profile in trisomy 18 (28 weeks).
b Flat profile in trisomy 21 (33 weeks).
c Retrognathia in osteogenesis imperfecta (29 weeks).
d Frontal bossing in thanatophoric dysplasia (24 weeks).

Fig. 45.**25** Cyclopia, 23 weeks.

Fig. 45.**26** Edematous facial swelling in nonimmune fetal hydrops, 31 weeks.

Fig. 45.**27** Dysmorphic face with open mouth. Karyotype: trisomy 21 (26 weeks).

Fig. 45.**28** Facial clefts.
a Right-sided cleft lip (33 weeks).
b Median cleft lip and palate (32 weeks).
c Bilateral cleft lip and palate (21 weeks).

Fig. 45.**29** Low-set ear with an abnormal shape ("question mark") in trisomy 18 (31 weeks).

Fig. 45.**30** *Left:* rachischisis involving the lower half of the spinal column, 14 weeks. *Right:* small lumbar myelomeningocele with a thin skin covering, 21 weeks.

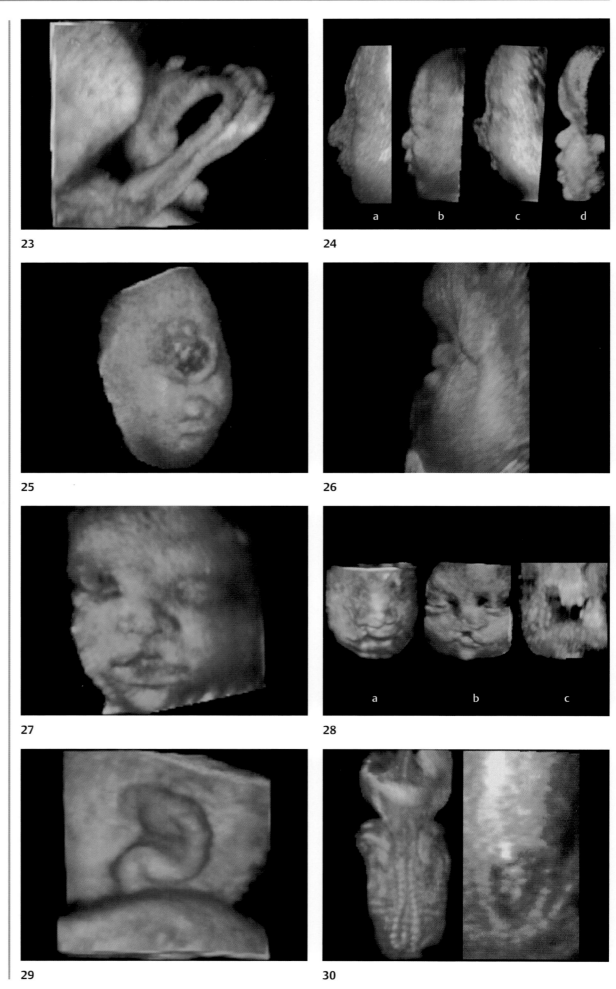

23

24

25

26

27

28

29

30

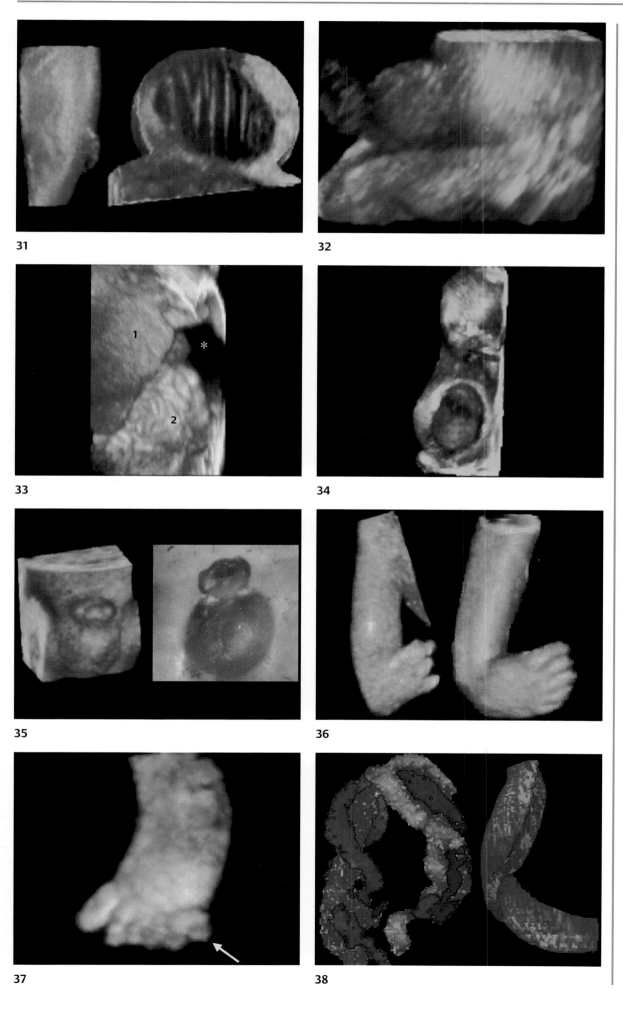

31

32

33

34

35

36

37

38

Fig. 45.**31** *Left:* small, flat lumbar myelomeningocele, 22 weeks. *Right:* large lumbar myelomeningocele, viewed from above. Cutaway surface image of the myelomeningocele shows nerve fibers running across the sac, 31 weeks.

Fig. 45.**32** Small omphalocele, 23 weeks.

Fig. 45.**33** Fetus with ascites (∗). The abdominal wall has been "removed" with the electronic scalpel, displaying a surface image of the abdominal organs.
1 = Liver, 2 = small bowel.

Fig. 45.**34** Coronal view of prune belly syndrome, 12 weeks. The megalocystis has been "sliced open" with the electronic scalpel.

Fig. 45.**35** *Left:* surface image of the clitoris and scrotum in hermaphroditism, 31 weeks. *Right:* postpartum appearance.

Fig. 45.**36** *Left:* malformation of the right arm with superior deviation of the hand, which has only four fingers, 27 weeks. *Right:* pes equinovarus on the right side with angular deviation of the foot, 22 weeks.

Fig. 45.**37** Postaxial hexadactyly with a sixth toe (arrow), 23 weeks.

Fig. 45.**38** Combining the surface mode with color Doppler gives a three-dimensional color image of the blood flow in the umbilical cord. *Left:* normal umbilical cord with 2 arteries and 1 vein. *Right:* single umbilical artery.

Transparent mode

Fig. 45.39 Maximum mode demonstrates the normal superior sutures in a 20-week fetus.

Fig. 45.40 Maximum mode at 20 weeks shows an ossification defect in the calvaria: an abnormally wide frontal suture in achondroplasia (arrows).

Fig. 45.41 *Left:* normal fetal skeleton in maximum mode, 20 weeks. *Right:* normal fetal skeleton in x-ray mode, 22 weeks.

Fig. 45.42 *Left:* thoracic scoliosis, maximum mode, 23 weeks. *Right:* marked ossification defect of the ribs (arrows) in osteochondrodysplasia, 22 weeks.

Animated display

Fig. 45.43 Glass body rendering. The combination of transparent mode and Power Doppler reveals the vascular system of the fetus.

Fig. 45.44 An animated display is created by defining the starting and end points of surface rendering and the angle increment between the frames. With a sweep angle of 180° and a 5° increment, 37 surface images are rendered.

Fig. 45.45 With the latest 3D technology, the initial frame (left) and end frame (right) of the desired animated sequence are immediately displayed along with the central frame (center).

Volume analysis and image processing

Fig. 45.46 Multiplanar display of a fetus with adjacent placenta (2) and intervening extremity (3). Amniotic fluid (1). 23 weeks. Original data set. The diagram at lower right shows the whole volume in the form of a truncated pyramid.

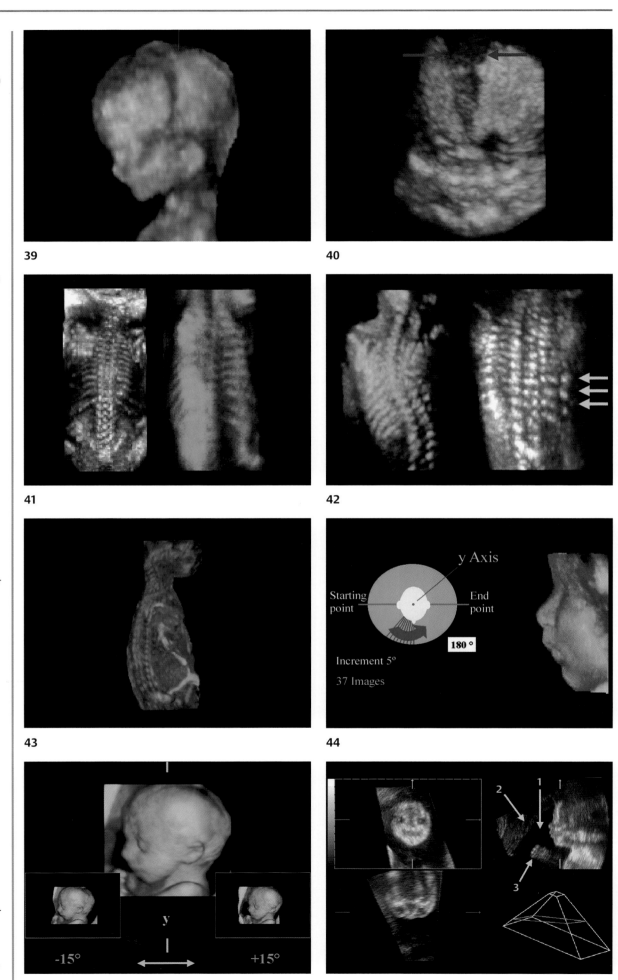

39

40

41

42

43

44

45

46

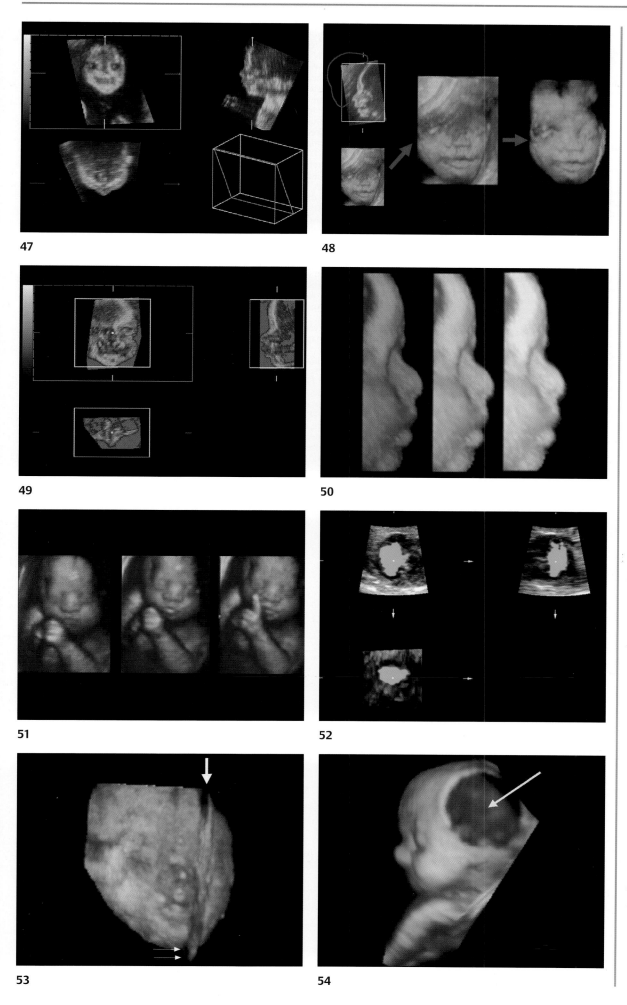

47

48

49

50

51

52

53

54

Fig. 45.**47**   Same case as in Fig. 45.**46**. Through Cartesian storage, the whole volume has been reduced to a box (lower right) to exclude the placenta from surface rendering.

Fig. 45.**48**   Upper *Left:* 2D lateral view of the fetal face abutting the placenta. Lower *Left:* interposed placenta prevents clear surface rendering of the face. Center: same surface image before use of the electronic scalpel. *Right:* facial image after use of the electronic scalpel.

Fig. 45.**49**   Removing fine extraneous echoes with the threshold control. All extraneous echoes within the pink area are eliminated with the low-pass filter.

Fig. 45.**50**   Fetal profile. The interactive brightness control is adjusted to give an optimum view of the facial surface (center image).

Fig. 45.**51**   4D imaging gives a "live" view of the moving fetus in real time. The operator can scroll through the digitally recorded volume sequences, picking out frames of special interest.

Fig. 45.**52**   AV-canal in a fetus with trisomy 21, 31 weeks. The STIC technique in combination with Color Doppler shows the blood flow in all three orthogonal planes at the same time.

Artifacts

Fig. 45.**53**   Fetal head in surface mode. The step-like artifact (arrow) was caused by fetal movement during volume acquisition.

Fig. 45.**54**   Fetal head in surface mode, with an artifact. A faulty cut with the electronic scalpel produced an apparent defect in the calvaria (arrow).

References

1. Baba, K., Okai, T.: Clinical applications of three-dimensional ultrasound in obstetrics. In: Baba, K., Jurkovic, D.: Three-dimensional Ultrasound in Obstetrics and Gynecology. London: Parthenon 1997; pp. 29–36
2. Benoit, B.: Three-dimensional surface mode for demonstration of normal fetal anatomy in the second and third trimesters. In: Merz, E. (ed.): 3-D ultrasound in obstetrics and gynecology. Philadelphia: Lippincott, Williams and Williams 1998; pp. 95–100
3. Blaas, H.G., Eik-Nes, S.H., Kiserud, T., Berg, S., Angelsen, B., Olstad, B.: Three-dimensional imaging of the brain-cavities in human embryos. Ultrasound Obstet. Gynecol. 5 (1995) 228–232
4. Bonilla-Musoles, F.: Three-dimensional visualization of the human embryo: a potential revolution in prenatal diagnosis. Ultrasound Obstet. Gynecol. 7 (1996) 393–397
5. Chang, F.M.: Three-dimensional ultrasound-assessed organ volumetry: clinical application in fetal medicine. In: Merz, E. (ed.): 3-D ultrasound in obstetrics and gynecology. Philadelphia: Lippincott, Williams and Wilkins 1998; pp. 101–104
6. Kelly, I.G., Gardener, J.E., Brett, A.D., Richards, R., Lees, W.R.: Three-dimensional ultrasound of the fetus. Radiology 192 (1994) 253–259
7. Kirbach, D., Whittingham, T.A.: 3D ultrasound – the Kretztechnik Voluson approachR. Eur. J. Ultrasound 1 (1994) 85–89
8. Kratochwil, A.: Importance and possibilities of multiplanar examination in three-dimensional sonography. In: Merz, E. (ed.): 3-D ultrasound in obstetrics and gynecology. Philadelphia: Lippincott, Williams and Wilkins 1998; pp. 105–108
9. Lee, A., Deutinger, J., Bernaschek, G.: Voluvision: Three-dimensional ultrasonography of fetal malformations. Amer. J. Obstet. Gynecol. 170 (1994) 1312–1314
10. Lee, A., Deutinger, J., Bernaschek, G.: Three dimensional ultrasound: abnormalities of the fetal face in surface and volume rendering mode. Brit. J. Obstet. Gynaecol. 102 (1995) 302–306
11. Lee, A., Kratochwil, A., Deutinger, J., Bernaschek, G.: Three dimensional ultrasound in diagnosing phocomelia. Ultrasound Obstet. Gynecol. 5 (1995) 238–240
12. Merz, E., Bahlmann, F., Weber, G.: Volume (3D)-scanning in the evaluation of fetal malformations – A new dimension in prenatal diagnosis. Ultrasound Obstet. Gynecol. 5 (1995) 222–227
13. Merz, E.: Einsatz der 3D-Ultraschalltechnik in der pränatalen Diagnostik. Ultraschall in Med. 16 (1995) 154–161
14. Merz, E., Bahlmann, F., Weber, G., Macchiella, D.: Three-dimensional ultrasonography in prenatal diagnosis. J. Perinatal Med. 23 (1995) 213–222
15. Merz, E.: Three-dimensional ultrasound in the evaluation of fetal anatomy and fetal malformations. In: Chervenak, F.A., Kurjak, A. (eds.): Current perspectives on the fetus as a patient. London: Parthenon 1996; pp. 75–87
16. Merz, E., Weber, G., Bahlmann, F., Miric-Tesanic, D.: Application of transvaginal and abdominal three-dimensional ultrasound for the detection or exclusion of malformations of the fetal face. Ultrasound Obstet. Gynecol. 9 (1997) 237–243
17. Merz, E.: Aktuelle technische Möglichkeiten der 3D-Sonographie in der Gynäkologie und Geburtshilfe. Ultraschall in Med. 18 (1997) 190–195
18. Merz, E.: Three-dimensional ultrasound in the evaluation of fetal malformations. for the detection or exclusion of malformations of the fetal face. In: Baba, K., Jurkovic, D.: Three-dimensional Ultrasound in Obstetrics and Gynecology. New York: Parthenon 1997; 29–36
19. Merz, E., Bahlmann, F., Welter, C., Miric-Tesanic, D.: Transvaginale 3D-Sonographie in der Frühgravidität. Gynäkologe 32 (1999) 213–219
20. Merz, E., Miric-Tesanic, D., Welter, C.: Value of the electronic scalpel (cut mode) in the evaluation of the fetal face. Ultrasound Obstet. Gynecol. 16 (2000) 364–368
21. Mueller, G.M., Weiner, C.P., Yankowitz, J.: Three-dimensional ultrasound in the evaluation of fetal head and spine anomalies. Obstet. Gynecol. 88 (1996) 372–378
22. Nelson, T.R., Pretorius, D.H.: Three-dimensional ultrasound of fetal surface features. Ultrasound Obstet. Gynecol. 2 (1992) 166–174
23. Nelson, T.R., Davidson, T.E., Pretorius, D.H.: Interactive electronical scalpel for extraction of organs from 3DUS data. Radiology 197(P) (1995) 191
24. Nelson, T.R., Pretorius, D.H., Sklansky, M., Hagen-Ansert, S.: Three-dimensional echocardiographic evaluation of fetal heart anatomy and function: acquisition, analysis and display. J. Ultrasound Med. 15 (1996) 1–9
25. Nelson, T.R., Pretorius, D.H.: Interactive acquisition, analysis and visualization of sonographic volume data. Int. J. Imag. Systems Technol. 8 (1997) 26–37
26. Ploeckinger-Ulm, B., Ulm, M.R., Lee, A., Kratochwil, A., Bernaschek, G.: Antenatal depiction of fetal digits with three-dimensional ultrasonography. Amer. J. Obstet. Gynecol. 175 (1996) 571–574
27. Pretorius, D.H., Nelson, T.R.: Prenatal visualization of superior sutures and fontanelles with 3-dimensional ultrasonography. J. Ultrasound Med. 13 (1994) 871–876
28. Pretorius, D.H., House, M., Nelson, T.R.: Fetal face visualization using three-dimensional ultrasonography. J. Ultrasound Med. 14 (1995) 349–356
29. Pretorius, D.H., House, M., Nelson, T.R., Hollenbach, K.A.: Evaluation of normal and abnormal lips in fetuses: Comparison between three- and two-dimensional sonography. AJR 165 (1995) 1233–1237
30. Riccabona, M., Nelson, T.R., Pretorius, D.H., Davidson, T.E.: Distance and volume measurement using threedimensional ultrasound. J. Ultrasound Med. 14 (1995) 881–886
31. Sakas, G., Schreyer, L., Grimm, M.: Pre-processing, segmenting and volume rendering 3D ultrasonic data. In: IEEE Computer Graphics and Applications, Vol. 15, 4 (1995) 47–54
32. Steiner, H., Staudach, A., Spitzer, D., Graf, A.H., Wienerroither, H.: Bietet die 3D-Sonographie neue Perspektiven in der Gynäkologie und Geburtshilfe? Geburtsh. u. Frauenheilk. 53 (1993) 779–782
33. Steiner, H., Staudach, A., Spitzer, D., Schaffer, H.: Three-dimensional ultrasound in obstetrics and gynaecology; technique, possibilities and limitations. Hum. Reprod. 9 (1994) 1773–1778
34. Steiner, H., Merz, E., Staudach, A.: Three-dimensional fetal facing. Human Reproduction (1995) (Video)
35. Steiner, H., Spitzer, D., Weiss-Wichert, P.H., Graf, A.H., Staudach, A.: Three-dimensional ultrasound in prenatal diagnosis of skeletal dysplasia. Prenat. Diagn. 15 (1995) 373–377
36. Steiner, H.: Potential der dreidimensionalen (3D-)Sonographie in der Fehlbildungsdiagnostik. Gynäkologe 28 (1995) 315–320

Invasive Diagnosis and Treatment in Pregnancy

46 Invasive Prenatal Diagnosis

WITHDRAWN

Procedures. Various invasive procedures are available for use in modern prenatal diagnosis, depending on the age of the pregnancy and the nature of the inquiry. They include conventional amniocentesis, early amniocentesis, chorionic villus sampling, cordocentesis, percutaneous procedures in the fetus, fetoscopy, and amnioinfusion (Fig. 46.1). All of these prenatal procedures are performed under continuous ultrasound guidance. They may employ needles of varying length and thickness (amniocentesis, abdominal chorionic villus sampling, cordocentesis, fetal aspiration or biopsy, amnioinfusion) (Table 46.1), a special catheter (transvaginal chorionic villus sampling), or an endoscope (fetoscopy). In the needle procedures, the needle may be inserted freehand with one hand holding the transducer and the other directing the needle, or it may be introduced through a needle guide that attaches to the transducer and defines the direction of the insertion.

It does not matter whether the needle is inserted freehand or with the help of a needle guide. In any case, the selection of the procedure depends chiefly on the experience of the individual examiner. The advantage of freehand insertion over the use of a needle guide is that the needle is easier to maneuver and there are fewer problems with asepsis. The disadvantage is that is requires greater manual dexterity.

Ultrasound examination. The ultrasound examinations that are performed before, during, and after an invasive procedure have various goals, which are summarized in Table 46.2.

Counseling. Every invasive procedure should be preceded by a detailed counseling session in which the procedure is explained to the patient along with the risks to the mother and fetus. Every invasive procedure requires written informed consent. With her signature, the patient attests that she consents to the procedure and has been adequately informed about the procedure and its risks.

Rh sensitization. An invasive procedure in every Rh-negative patient is followed by anti-D prophylaxis to prevent isoimmunization. The stan-

dard dose (without prior testing for infiltration of HbF cells) is 300 µg anti-D (= 1500 I.U.) administered by intramuscular injection within 72 hours after the procedure.

If antibodies have already been detected in the Rh-negative patient before the invasive procedure, anti-D prophylaxis is omitted.

Amniocentesis

Transabdominal amniocentesis to obtain an amniotic fluid sample is the most commonly performed invasive procedure for prenatal diagnosis. This is because it is a relatively simple technique with a low risk and a high diagnostic yield.

Indications

Amniocentesis has a broad range of indications (Table 46.3). It is performed in the second trimester to determine fetal karyotype in cases of advanced maternal age, to detect anterior or posterior fetal clefts (AFP, acetylcholinesterase (AChE)), and to detect intrauterine infections and known familial metabolic disorders. Other applications, which are becoming less frequent, are the investigation of Rh incompatibility (amniotic fluid bilirubin content) in the second and third trimesters and the assessment of fetal lung maturity (L/S ratio) in the third trimester.

Technique

Timing. Conventional genetic amniocentesis is usually performed between 15 and 18 weeks of gestation under ultrasound guidance. At this time a needle can be inserted into the uterus without too much risk of puncturing the bladder or bowel. Also, a sufficient amniotic fluid volume is present, ensuring that the sample will contain a sufficiently large number of cells. If the amniotic cell culture fails to grow, there is still enough time for a repeat amniocentesis

Gestational age. It is important to confirm the gestational age sonographically. Quantitative amniotic fluid parameters such as α-fetoprotein (AFP) can be corrected interpreted only if it can be related to the true gestational age in weeks.

If the calculated gestational age does not agree with the sonographically determined gestational age, only the latter (based on the

Table 46.1 Comparison of different units of measurement (gauge [54], inches, and millimeters) for needle thickness

Gauge	Inches	Millimeter
24	0.022	0.56
23	0.025	0.64
22	0.028	0.71
21	0.032	0.81
20	0.035	0.89
19	0.042	1.07
18	0.049	1.24
17	0.058	1.47
16	0.065	1.65

Table 46.2 Objectives of the ultrasound examination in relation to invasive procedures

> Confirm gestational age
> Exclude an abnormal pregnancy
> Detect gross fetal anomalies
> Detect amniotic fluid abnormalities
> Locate the placenta
> Locate the placental umbilical cord insertion
> Monitor the needle insertion
> Check the fetus and uterine puncture site after the procedure

Table 46.3 Indications for amniocentesis

> Chromosome analysis
  • Advanced maternal age (≥ 35 years)
  • Balanced chromosome rearrangement in the parents
  • History of a child with a chromosomal abnormality
  • Abnormal ultrasound finding
  • Psychological indication
> Detection of infection
> Metabolic disorders
> AFP/AChE determination in amniotic fluid (anterior and posterior clefts)
> Bilirubin determination in amniotic fluid (Rh incompatibility)
> L/S ratio to assess fetal lung maturity

crown–rump length) should be used to avoid a false-positive laboratory result. Ultrasound confirmation of gestational age is particularly important in cases where a borderline elevation of amniotic fluid AFP is found. If the previously elevated AFP is found to be within normal limits after the pregnancy has been redated, the patient can be spared a second amniocentesis.

Nonviable pregnancy. If the preliminary ultrasound scan indicates a nonviable pregnancy (e.g., blighted ovum, hydatidiform mole, intrauterine fetal death) or a gross fetal anomaly (e.g. anencephaly), there is no need to proceed with amniocentesis.

Unfavorable conditions. A reduced amniotic fluid volume (oligohydramnios) usually makes it more difficult to puncture the amniotic cavity. This also occurs with an unfavorable placental location (anterior placenta). If a complete anterior placenta is found, the patient may be advised of the slightly increased procedure risk (bleeding from the puncture site, amniotic fluid contamination by maternal cells), and the amniocentesis may be postponed by 1–2 weeks. Since some degree of placental migration usually occurs with further uterine enlargement, a 1- or 2-week postponement will often clear a path to the amniotic cavity, making it unnecessary to traverse the placenta. If the placenta cannot be avoided, care should be taken to insert the needle away from the placental insertion of the umbilical cord to avoid injury to that area.

Continuous ultrasound guidance. In contrast to the older technique of blind puncture following initial ultrasound localization of the fetus (49), amniocentesis today is always performed under continuous ultrasound guidance (46, 57, 76, 89, 108) (Figs. 46.**2**, 46.**3**). In this way the needle can be inserted a safe distance from the fetus. If the needle must pass close to the fetus because of amniotic fluid conditions, the fetus can be observed throughout the procedure to avoid injury. If the fetus changes its position suddenly, the operator should either wait until it has moved away from the needle insertion site or change to a different site.

Technique. The transducer is coupled to the abdominal wall with sterile ultrasound gel or a clear antiseptic solution. The advantage of the latter is that it provides good image quality for the procedure and also disinfects the abdominal skin and transducer.

Amniocentesis is performed with a 22- to 20-gauge disposable spinal needle with stylet. The ultrasound visibility of the needle while in utero depends on the insertion angle and needle type. The steeper the insertion angle, the more difficult it is to see the needle. After the stylet has been removed, usually only the needle tip or part of the needle shaft can be seen, but this is adequate for directing the procedure. With special cannulas that have a roughened surface, more of the needle can be seen (45). Local anesthesia is usually unnecessary but may be used in anxious or pain-sensitive patients.

For midtrimester amniocentesis, a fluid sample of approximately 15–18 mL (not to exceed 20 mL) is withdrawn.

Table 46.**4** Comparison of standard and early amniocentesis (AC) with chorionic villus sampling (CVS) (after 17)

	Standard AC	Early AC	CVS
Timing (weeks' gestation)	15–18	12–14	10–12
Needle route	TA	TA	TA/TC
➢ Success rate (first insertion)	> 99%	96–98%	TA 90–97% / TC 69–90%
➢ Bloody amniotic fluid	1–2%	1–5%	–
➢ Fetomaternal transfusion	2–7%	?	TA 18–68% / TC 5–23%
Fetal complications			
➢ Abortion ≤ 2 weeks	0.3–0.5%	0.3–0.9%	1.7–2.2%
➢ Abortion ≤ 28 weeks	0.6–1.0%	0.7–3.9%	2.3–4.9%
➢ Stillbirth (> 28 weeks/ neonatal death)	0.4%	0.4–0.8%	0.2–1.0%
➢ Pregnancy loss	2.5–4.3%	6.2–6.6%	5.6–10.1%
Cytogenetics			
➢ Chromosomal abnormality	1.0–4.0%	1.9–5.4%	2.4–6.1%
➢ Failed culture	0.1–0.7%	0–2.3%	0.4–2.4%
➢ Maternal cell contamination	0.2–0.3%	0.2–1.6%	0.2–1.0%
➢ Pseudomosaic	1.3–9.8%	4.3–9.9%	1.8–2.3%
➢ Mosaic	0.1–0.3%	0.1–0.7%	0.8–1.5%
➢ Discrepancy with fetal karyotype	0.2–0.5%	0.1–0.7%	1.2–2.1%
➢ Processing time (working days)	(5) 7–13	8–14	1–4 (DP) 6–14 (culture)
Second procedure required	1–2%	2–3%	2.5–6 (10)%

TA = transabdominal   TC = transcervical   DP = direct preparation

◼ *Risks of Amniocentesis*

Maternal risk. The maternal risk is small. Possible complications are amnionitis, which has an incidence of only one in 8000 (66), and peritonitis, which can result from accidental puncture of the bowel. One maternal death due to amniotic fluid embolism was reported in the early days of amniocentesis when larger needles were used (4), but this risk is negligible today owing to the use of 20- to 22-gauge needles.

If anti-D prophylaxis is omitted after amniocentesis in an Rh-negative patient with an Rh-positive fetus, there is a risk that sensitization may occur. This is particularly true in transplacental amniocentesis (Fig. 46.**2**) where there is an entry of fetal cells into the maternal circulation.

Fetal risk. The fetal risk is considerably higher than the maternal risk. The spontaneous abortion rate after 15 weeks' gestation is approximately 0.5–1% (121) (Table 46.**4**). Rupture of the fetal membranes occurs in 0.5–2% of cases (39, 121). Usually this is a short-term amniotic fluid leakage that will stop with a few hours or days of bed rest. Very rarely, however, the amniotic fluid leakage may persist for several weeks. Whenever a membrane rupture occurs, the inflammatory parameters (blood count; C-reactive protein, CRP) should be checked at frequent intervals.

Separation of the amniotic membrane (Fig. 46.**4**) and bleeding from the placenta following a transplacental puncture (Fig. 46.**5**) are complications that are usually of short duration.

If the amniocentesis is unsuccessful, it may be reattempted at a different site. More than two tries should not be made in one sitting, however, as this would increase the abortion risk.

Postprocedure ultrasound. An ultrasound examination should be performed after every amniocentesis to confirm the viability of the fetus and exclude possible complications such as a placental hematoma or separation of the amnion.

Fig. 46.**1** Timing of various invasive procedures in prenatal diagnosis.

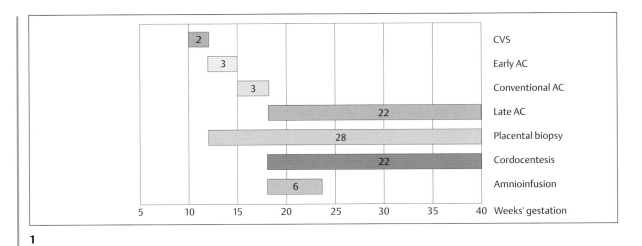

1

Amniocentesis

Fig. 46.**2** *Left:* early amniocentesis with a posterior placenta at 14 weeks, 4 days. *Right:* transplacental amniocentesis with a complete anterior placenta at 16 weeks, 2 days.

Fig. 46.**3** Late amniocentesis with a posterior placenta at 21 weeks, 2 days.

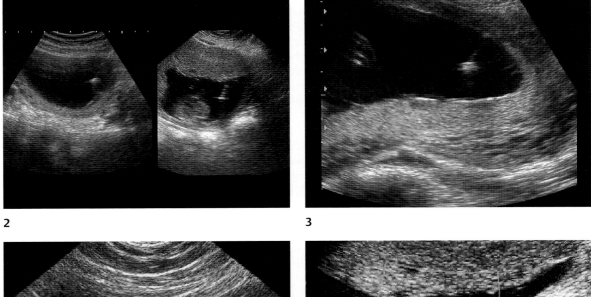

2

3

Fig. 46.**4** Separation of the amnion following amniocentesis (arrow).

Fig. 46.**5** Bleeding from the needle track after transplacental amniocentesis. Color Doppler image of the hemorrhage.

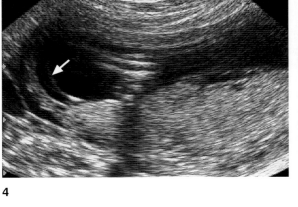

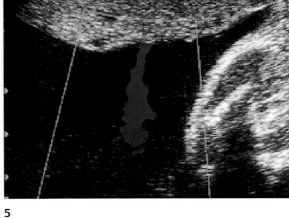

4

5

Fig. 46.**6** Amniocentesis in twins at 15 weeks, 2 days. The two amniotic cavities are punctured separately and in succession.

Chorionic villus sampling

Fig. 46.**7** Transvaginal and transabdominal routes for chorionic villus sampling: 1 = transvaginal sampling with a posterior placenta, 2 = transabdominal sampling with an anterior placenta, 3 = transabdominal sampling with a posterior placenta.

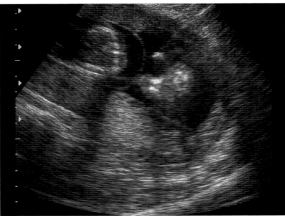

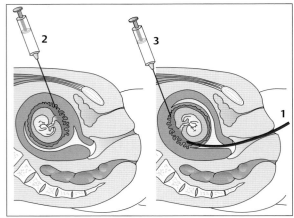

6

7

Amniocentesis in Multiple Pregnancy

Dye instillation. The current practice in diamniotic twin pregnancies is to instill a dye into the amniotic cavity after puncturing the first cavity and drawing a fluid sample (Fig. 46.**6**). Then if the fluid drawn from the second amniotic cavity (second needle insertion) is clear, this confirms that the second sac, and not the first, has been punctured. Methylene blue was initially used for this purpose. But after several groups of authors between 1998 and 1992 reported severe side effects such as hemolytic anemia (94) and an increased incidence of jejunal atresia (17–19%) (27, 67, 87, 95, 97), methylene blue was no longer used in prenatal diagnosis. The dye of choice today is indigo carmine, which is available in ampules; 1–2 mL is instilled into the amniotic fluid.

With the high resolution of modern ultrasound imagers, often the two amniotic cavities can be clearly distinguished from each other, making dye use unnecessary.

Using one insertion site. It is possible to pass a needle into both gestational sacs from a single insertion site (56). After fluid has been drawn from the first sac, the amniotic membrane is pierced and fluid is sampled from the second sac. The drawback of this technique is that there is a risk of cell cross-contamination, making cytogenetic interpretation more difficult.

Early Amniocentesis

Higher complication rate. Unlike conventional amniocentesis, early amniocentesis is performed between 12 weeks and 14 weeks, 6 days or in some cases as early as 11 completed weeks' gestation (24, 100, 135). The advantage of early amniocentesis is that it provides a cytogenetic finding as early as 13–15 weeks. The disadvantage of early amniocentesis is that the amniotic fluid volume is still relatively small, and therefore less fluid is sampled (10–14 mL, depending on gestational age). This increases the risk of a failed culture (24), and the complication rate is higher than in conventional amniocentesis (24, 100) (Table 46.**4**). Some authors combine early amniocentesis with a filtration technique (120) to increase the yield of cells.

In a Canadian multicenter study published in 1998, early amniocentesis was found to be associated with higher total fetal loss and a higher incidence of club foot deformities (32, 100) (Table 46.**5**). Therefore, early amniocentesis before 14 weeks of gestation is no longer recommended.

Cytogenetics

In both conventional and early amniocentesis, the cytogenetic result is usually available in 8–12 working days. A faster option is the "pipette method" (15), which yields a result in 48–72 hours.

Table 46.5 Comparison of early amniocentesis and conventional amniocentesis (after 100)

	Early amniocentesis	Conventional amniocentesis
Gestational age	11 weeks to 12 weeks + 6 days	15 weeks to 16 weeks + 6 days
Cases examined	n = 1916	n = 1775
Volume of amniotic fluid sample	11 mL	20 mL
Total fetal loss (spontaneous and induced abortions)	7.6%	5.9%
Clubfoot	1.3%	0.1%
Rupture of membranes	3.5%	1.7%

Chorionic Villus Sampling

Earlier prenatal diagnosis. Chorionic villus sampling (CVS) is a technique in which villi are sampled from the chorion frondosum (Figs. 46.**7**–46.**10**). The advantage of CVS over conventional amniocentesis is that it can be done much earlier in the pregnancy (between 10 and 12 weeks' gestation) (Fig. 46.**1**), making it possible to advance the prenatal diagnosis by 4–6 weeks. If pregnancy termination is necessary, it is easier for the parents to cope with at this early stage than later in the pregnancy.

The chorionic villus sample (Fig. 46.**9**) is composed of epithelial cells from the outer and inner trophoblastic layers (syncytiotrophoblast and cytotrophoblast) and of fibroblasts from the mesenchymal villous core. The cells of the outer and inner trophoblastic layers are analyzed by direct preparation, while the fibroblasts are analyzed by long-term culture.

Indications

The indications for CVS in the first trimester are similar to those for amniocentesis with regard to karyotyping. In addition, many monogenic disorders can be diagnosed when specifically looked for (Table 46.**6**). In contrast to amniocentesis, an AFP/AChE test for spina bifida diagnosis cannot be performed in CVS because the material is sampled outside the amniotic cavity. This is a minor drawback, however, since spina bifida can be detected or excluded with a targeted ultrasound scan.

Technique

Two main approaches are used for chorionic villus sampling: transcervical (8, 33, 60, 128) and transabdominal (9, 115, 116) (Figs. 46.**7**–46.**9**). The preferred route depends on the location of the targeted chorion, the position of the uterus (anteflexed or retroflexed), and the experience of the operator.

Transabdominal route. Transabdominal sampling (Figs. 46.**7**, 46.**8**) is appropriate for cases in which the chorion frondosum is easily accessible by an abdominal route. This particularly applies to anterior and lat-

Table 46.6 Indications for chorionic villus sampling

Chromosome analysis
➢ Advanced maternal age (≥ 35 years)
➢ Balanced chromosome rearrangement in the parents
➢ History of a child with a chromosomal abnormality
➢ Abnormal ultrasound finding (nuchal translucency)
➢ Psychological indication

Monogenic disorders (some examples are listed below)
➢ AGS
➢ Fragile X syndrome
➢ Galactosemia
➢ Hemophilia A and B
➢ Hemoglobinopathy
➢ Niemann–Pick disease
➢ Tay–Sachs disease
➢ Cystic fibrosis
➢ Duchenne type muscular dystrophy
➢ Pelizaeus–Merzbacher syndrome
➢ Phenylketonuria (PKU)
➢ Thalassemia
➢ Zellweger syndrome

eral placentas, although a posterior placenta is also accessible when the uterus is anteflexed (Fig. 46.**8**). A disposable spinal needle (18–20 gauge) with or without a stylet is used. After the abdominal skin is sterilely prepped with a clear antiseptic spray and local anesthesia is administered, the needle is advanced into the chorion frondosum under continuous ultrasound guidance. With slight in-and-out movements of the needle and negative pressure on the plunger, approximately 10–15 mg of villous tissue is aspirated into the disposable syringe, which contains about 4 mL of medium.

Transcervical route. Transcervical CVS (Figs. 46.**7**, 46.**9**) is preferred when it is difficult or impossible to reach the target with a transabdominal needle. This is the case with a low posterior placental location.

A flexible polyethylene catheter with stylet (outer diameter 1.5–1.7 mm) is usually employed for transcervical sampling. The catheter can be bent to match the degree of uterine flexion (Fig. 46.**9**). In some models a bismuth strip is embedded in the catheter wall for better ultrasound visualization (50). Other instruments formerly used for transcervical chorionic villus sampling, such as special endoscopes with biopsy forceps (38, 41) or rigid biopsy forceps alone (28, 60), are too traumatizing and have been abandoned in favor of catheters.

After the vagina has been flushed with saline, the anterior lip of the cervix is grasped with a single-tooth tenaculum, and the catheter is advanced into the chorion frondosum under constant ultrasound guidance (with a moderately distended urinary bladder). When the catheter tip has reached its target, the stylet is removed and chorionic villi are aspirated by manual suction into a disposable syringe containing some medium.

If insufficient chorionic villus material is obtained, the sampling should be repeated. No more than two attempts should be made in any one patient, however, as this would triple or quadruple the spontaneous abortion rate (96, 136).

▆ *Risks and Problems of Chorionic Villus Sampling*

The risks of CVS have been evaluated in several collaborative studies (12, 75, 103), which are reviewed in Crombach et al. (17).

Maternal risks. The principal maternal risks are bleeding and lower abdominal pain. Uterine bleeding is 2 to 6 times more common after transcervical CVS than after transabdominal sampling (6–9% vs. 1.5–5%) (17).

Fetal risks. Comparing the spontaneous abortion rates after first-trimester transabdominal and transcervical CVS in prospective randomized studies, it appears that transabdominal CVS has a slightly lower risk than transcervical CVS (2.6–4.1% vs. 2.7–7.7% (17).

Abortion risk. In clinically controlled single- and multicenter studies, the abortion risk after CVS and early amniocentesis is generally 1–2% higher than after standard amniocentesis (17). But if we also take into account the spontaneous miscarriage rate, which is significantly higher at 10–12 weeks than at 16 weeks, it is reasonable to assume that chorionic villus sampling and amniocentesis have comparable risks when performed by an experienced examiner.

Limb anomalies. Firth et al. (35) caused a sensation in 1991 when they reported an etiologic link between chorionic villus sampling and fetal limb anomalies. In a series of 539 chorionic villus aspirations that had been performed at 8 and 9 weeks' gestation (55–66 days menstrual age), 5 of the babies were subsequently found to have serious limb abnormalities. Local circulatory impairment and thromboembolic

processes have been discussed as possible causes of these anomalies (52, 111). Several studies have been published in recent years on the risk of limb anomalies following CVS (11, 36, 42, 62, 107). On the whole, however, investigators have been unable to establish a definite link between chorionic sampling after 9 weeks' gestation and an increased risk of limb anomalies. But when the frequency and severity of limb defects occurring after early CVS (≤ 9 weeks' gestation) are compared with those after CVS performed between 10 and 12 weeks' gestation, early CVS is associated with a much higher incidence of limb anomalies (0.3%) than later CVS (0.06%) (17). Because of this, it is currently recommended that CVS not be performed earlier than 10 weeks of gestation (36, 62).

▆ *Cytogenetics*

Today a cytogenetic diagnosis is available in 1–3 days when the direct preparation method is used and in 6–12 working days when a long-term culture is grown. A result is not obtained in only 0.3% of all cases (72). False-positive results (trisomies, mosaicism) are found in approximately 1–2% of all cases (61). Mosaicism can be observed in direct preparations of syncytiotrophoblastic and cytotrophoblastic cells and also in fibroblast cultures from the mesenchymal villous core. Most of these cases involve a confined placental mosaicism (CPM) (72, 75, 117). False-negative results are extremely rare, occurring in one in 1000 to one in 10,000 cases, and occur almost exclusively in direct preparations (61, 93).

If the findings are equivocal, either amniocentesis or cordocentesis (at 18 weeks or later) can be performed for further clarification.

Placental Biopsy in the Second and Third Trimesters

As in the first trimester, cytogenetic and molecular genetic results can be obtained quickly and dependably by sampling placental tissue in the second and third trimesters (3, 51, 55).

Indications. Placental biopsy is appropriate in cases where cordocentesis is difficult, not possible, or too risky. It may be done before 17 weeks' gestation, in cases of pronounced oligohydramnios or anhydramnios, or in fetuses with a single umbilical artery.

Technique. The technique of late placental biopsy is basically the same as that of transabdominal chorionic villus sampling in the first trimester (Fig. 46.**10**).

Risk and cytogenetics. Placental biopsy in the second and third trimesters is no riskier than amniocentesis and has the advantage of giving a faster preliminary result. As in first-trimester chorionic villus sampling, the result of a direct preparation should not be interpreted alone but should be combined with the long-term culture result.

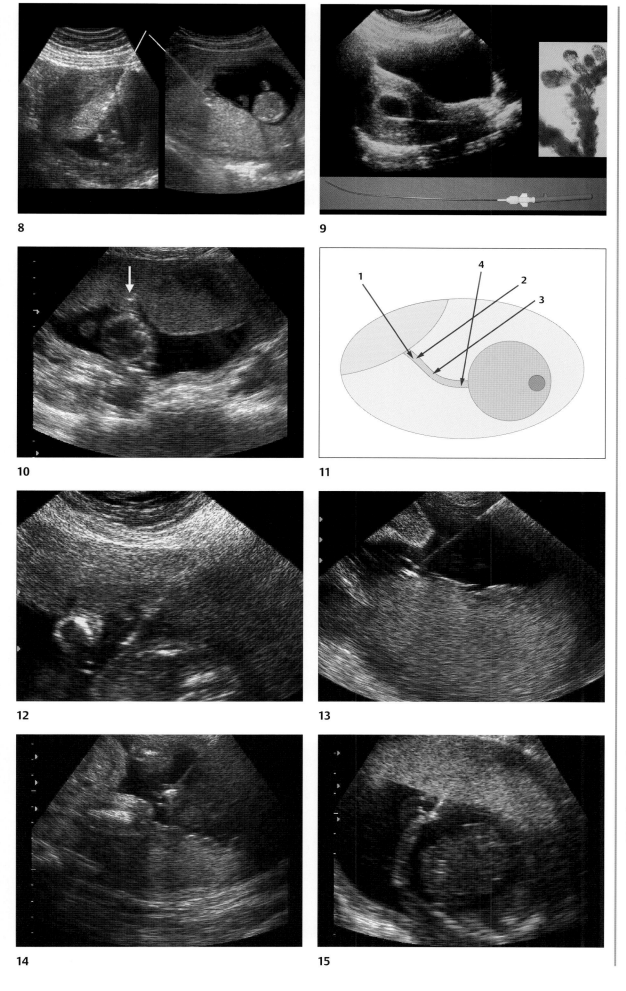

8

9

10

11

12

13

14

15

Fig. 46.**8** *Left:* transabdominal chorionic villus sampling with an anterior placenta, transverse scan. *Right:* transabdominal chorionic villus sampling with a posterior placenta, longitudinal scan.

Fig. 46.**9** *Left:* transvaginal chorionic villus sampling with a posterior placenta, using a polyethylene catheter (below). *Right:* close-up view of a chorionic villus.

Placental biopsy

Fig. 46.**10** Placental biopsy with a complete anterior placenta, done for the purpose of excluding trisomy 21 (17 weeks, 6 days). Needle tip (arrow).

Cordocentesis

Fig. 46.**11** Approaches to the umbilical cord for cordocentesis (after 69). 1 = transplacental route through an anterior placenta, 2 = transamniotic route to the placental umbilical cord insertion, 3 = transamniotic route to a free loop of umbilical cord, 4 = transamniotic route to the fetal umbilical cord insertion.

Fig. 46.**12** Transplacental cordocentesis with an anterior placenta. The umbilical vein is punctured at the placental insertion (23 weeks).

Fig. 46.**13** Cordocentesis with a posterior placenta. The umbilical vein is punctured at the placental insertion of the cord.

Fig. 46.**14** Cordocentesis with puncture of the umbilical vein in a free loop of umbilical cord.

Fig. 46.**15** Transplacental cordocentesis. The umbilical vein is punctured near the fetal cord insertion in fetal hydrops (19 weeks, 3 days).

Cordocentesis

Transabdominal puncture of the fetal umbilical cord under ultrasound guidance (cordocentesis) provides direct diagnostic and/or therapeutic access to the fetal circulation without posing a high maternal or fetal risk.

Development of the procedure. Valenti (125) reported on initial attempts to sample fetal blood from the umbilical cord in 1973. At that time, however, endoscopy was the only method available for accessing the cord. In subsequent years fetoscopy was used to direct the puncture of placental vessels (47) and umbilical vessels (104). This technique carried a relatively high abortion risk of 5–6%, however (53). In 1983, Daffos et al. (19) introduced transabdominal needle aspiration of the umbilical cord under ultrasound guidance, which significantly reduced the risk of fetal loss.

Direct access to the fetal circulation has yielded important insights into physiologic and pathologic changes in the blood of the growing fetus (22, 37).

▬ *Technique*

Timing. Depending on the indication, cordocentesis can be performed from about 18 completed weeks' gestation until the end of the pregnancy. When imaging and placental conditions are optimal, it can be done as early as 15 completed weeks (1).

Prerequisites. Cordocentesis is usually performed on an ambulatory basis. It requires a high-resolution ultrasound scanner (5-MHz transducer), an experienced cordocentesis team, and a laboratory specializing in fetal blood analysis. Especially in midtrimester cordocentesis, when the total fetoplacental volume is still low and only about 2–3 mL of fetal blood can be obtained, the laboratory must meet stringent criteria regarding the number of analyses performed and the time needed to report the results.

Procedure. Cordocentesis is performed in the supine patient under local anesthesia. The benefit of local anesthesia is that the direction of needle insertion can be adjusted if necessary without causing pain.

Fig. 46.**16**   The fetal source of a blood sample is confirmed by determining the red blood cell mean corpuscular volume (MCV). At 143.4 fL, the fetal MCV is well above that of the mother (MCV 86 fL), 19 weeks.

Fig. 46.**17**   Indications for diagnostic cordocentesis (authors' data; n = 356).

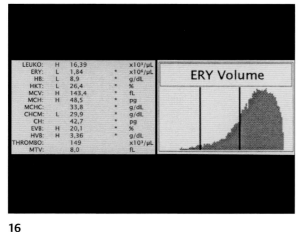

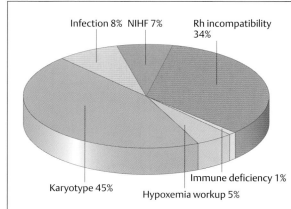

16

17

Fig. 46.**18**   Jet phenomenon (arrow) after puncture of the umbilical vein at the placental cord insertion. Posterior placenta.

Fig. 46.**19**   Complications of cordocentesis. *Left:* transient local narrowing of the vessel lumen at the umbilical vein puncture site (arrows). Single umbilical artery at 31 weeks, 6 days. *Right:* umbilical cord hematoma after prior cordocentesis (arrow), 17 weeks, 1 day.

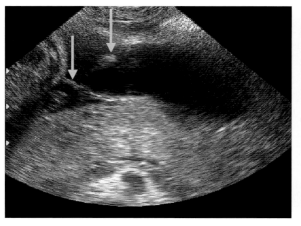

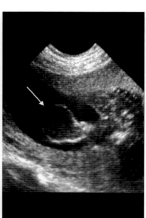

18

19

Umbilical vein. After the abdominal skin has been aseptically prepared and the umbilical cord identified with ultrasound, the needle is inserted into the abdomen freehand or using a needle guide under ultrasound guidance. It is advanced to the umbilical cord and into the umbilical vein. The most favorable puncture site is the placental insertion of the umbilical cord, as the cord is the least mobile at that location (Figs. 45.**11**–45.**13**). A free loop of umbilical cord or the fetal insertion of the cord can also be used (Figs. 46.**14**, 46.**15**). Intra-abdominal puncture of the umbilical vein is yet another option (2). It is most difficult to puncture a free loop of umbilical cord, which is easily pushed aside rather than pierced by the advancing needle tip. Fetal movements are usually accompanied by displacement of the umbilical cord, making it necessary to redirect the needle. At some centers, intramuscular or intravenous sedation of the fetus with pancuronium (0.3 mg/kg estimated body weight) is used to prevent fetal movements, especially during therapeutic procedures (129, 132).

Umbilical artery. Besides the large-caliber vein, it is also possible to sample blood from one of the two smaller-caliber umbilical arteries. This procedure carries a risk of vasospasm, however, with subsequent fetal bradycardia and/or profuse afterbleeding, and therefore puncture of the umbilical vein is always preferred.

Placental location. A needle 10–15 mm long (20–22 gauge) with stylet is used. With an anterior placenta, the needle may be advanced directly through the placenta into the umbilical cord insertion (Figs. 46.**11**, 46.**12**) or it may be passed through the amnion and into the umbilical cord insertion from the side (Fig. 46.**11**). With a lateral or posterior placenta, the needle is passed through the amnion to the placental insertion of the cord, and the cord is punctured about 0.5–1 cm from its insertion site (Figs. 46.**11**, 46.**13**). A stable needle is important, especially with a posterior placenta, so that the needle will not bend on the relatively long path to the umbilical cord insertion. Blood is drawn from the umbilical vein with a 1-mL tuberculin syringe.

Fetal blood. The easiest way to confirm that the blood is of fetal origin is by determining the red cell mean corpuscular volume (MCV) with a cell counter. The MCV of fetal blood in the second trimester should exceed 100 fL, while the MCV of maternal blood is less than 95 fL.

After cordocentesis and other invasive procedures, anti-D prophylaxis is mandatory in Rh-negative women. The only exceptions are patients in whom Rh antibodies are already present.

Indications

There are various indications for the diagnostic use of cordocentesis (69) (Table 46.**7**, Fig. 46.**17**).

Rapid Karyotyping

Cordocentesis is most commonly used for rapid determination of the fetal chromosome complement (1, 113). This is done in cases with equivocal chromosomal findings (mosaic-cell lines) from amniotic cell culture or chorionic villus sampling. A reliable chromosome analysis can be obtained in 48–72 hours by leukocyte culture of the sampled fetal blood. In this way abnormal findings can be confirmed within a short time or specifically excluded. This advantage of rapid karyotyping can also be utilized when ultrasound reveals an abnormality that has an association with chromosome disorders, such as growth retardation, nuchal cystic hygroma, omphalocele, duodenal atresia, vacuolated placental structure (triploidy), single umbilical artery, or in cases of late chromosome analysis (22–23 weeks' gestation) to investigate, say, an abnormal triple test.

Diagnosis of Infection

Various fetal infections can be diagnosed in the fetal blood: rubella (20, 31, 40, 74), cytomegalovirus (64), toxoplasmosis (22, 26), varicella (118), and infection with parvovirus B19 (79).

IgM antibodies. The prenatal diagnosis of infection is based on the detection of pathogen-specific IgM antibodies in the fetal blood. Because IgM antibodies cannot pass through the intact placental barrier, their detection is considered proof of a fetal infection. It should be noted, however, that IgM formation does not occur until the second trimester and that a measurable concentration is not present before 20 weeks' gestation (123). For this reason, cordocentesis to detect a fetal infection is not performed until 22 weeks' gestation at most prenatal centers. In all cases, contamination of the fetal blood by maternal blood should be avoided.

Rubella and cytomegalovirus. A positive IgM antibody test for rubella and cytomegalovirus in the fetal blood justifies pregnancy termination, as these fetal infections are associated with serious abnormalities in the newborn. Conversely, a negative fetal blood test means that a fetal infection is unlikely but does not rule it out with complete confidence.

Toxoplasmosis. Whether cordocentesis should be performed when a first toxoplasmosis infection is contracted during pregnancy is a question that requires critical discussion. On the one hand, an IgM determination in the fetal blood has a sensitivity of only 44% (26). Moreover, unlike rubella and cytomegalovirus infections, an effective treatment is available for toxoplasmosis. For forensic reasons alone, then, a pregnant woman who contracts an initial infection should be treated with spiramycin (< 16 weeks' gestation) or with sulfadiazine and pyrimethamine (> 16 weeks' gestation), regardless of whether or not cordocentesis is performed. It should also be considered that it can

Table 46.**7** Diagnostic applications of cordocentesis

> Rapid karyotyping
> Diagnosis of infection
> Diagnosis of blood diseases
> Diagnosis of fetal anemia
> Determination of fetal blood group
> Diagnosis of fetal hypalbuminemia
> Assessment of fetal condition in cases of growth retardation and/or abnormal Doppler flow

take up to 6 weeks to isolate the causative organism from the fetal blood and amniotic fluid. Hence there is no guarantee that the organism can be positively identified before viability is reached (at 24 weeks' gestation).

Parvovirus B19. With a parvovirus B19 infection, a hemoglobin determination in the cord blood provides rapid information on whether hemolysis has already occurred (79). If fetal anemia is confirmed, an intrauterine blood transfusion should be performed (see Chapter 47, Fetal Therapy).

Diagnosis of Blood Diseases

Various blood diseases can be diagnosed by analysis of the fetal blood: hemoglobinopathies, coagulopathies, immune deficiencies (severe combined immunodeficiency, SCID), and thrombocytopenias.

Hemoglobinopathies. The prenatal diagnosis of hemoglobinopathies is based on the detection of the different globulin chains. Fetuses with β-thalassemia major have a severe paucity of β chains due to impaired synthesis of the globulin β-peptide chain, resulting in an extremely low β/γ ratio with values less than 0.02 (82). In sickle-cell anemia, γ, α and βS chains are detected but no βA chains (82).

Coagulopathies. The most important fetal coagulopathies are the X-linked recessive disorders hemophilia A (factor VIII deficiency) and hemophilia B (factor IX deficiency) and the autosomal-dominant von Willebrand–Jürgens syndrome (decrease in factor VIII or IX).

Although the factor VIII and IX levels in the second trimester are lower than in the newborn, the factor deficiency in a particular coagulopathy can be positively detected or excluded antenatally (23, 71).

Immune deficiencies. Severe immune deficiencies, while rare, have profound consequences for the affected families, especially if one child has already died from an immune defect. Because most immune deficiencies are not detected by enzyme studies of amniotic or chorionic cells and gene-specific DNA probes are available for only a few immunodeficiency disorders (X-linked agammaglobulinemia, Wiskott–Aldrich syndrome, septic granulomatosis), today most immune deficiencies can be diagnosed only by fetal leukocyte studies. With simultaneous dual fluorescence flow cytometry, the diagnosis can be made the same day from minimal amounts of lysed fetal whole blood without having to know the exact type of immune deficiency present in the family (109).

Thrombocytopenias. Determination of the platelet count in congenital thrombocytopenias (amegakaryocytic thrombocytopenia, thrombocytopenia–radial aplasia syndrome, Wiskott–Aldrich syndrome, alloimmune thrombocytopenia, immune thrombocytopenia purpura) provides important information on the intrauterine risk to the fetus. This particularly applies to alloimmune thrombocytopenia (59), in which the PLA1-negative mother forms antibodies against the PLA1-positive fetus (analogous to Rh immunization). Fetal thrombocytopenia is detected by cordocentesis performed between 20 and 22 weeks' gestation. If thrombocytopenia is diagnosed, intrauterine therapy with platelet concentrate should be carried out to prevent fetal cerebral hemorrhage (see Chapter 47, Fetal Therapy).

Knowledge of the platelet count is also critical in selecting the mode of delivery. If the fetal platelet count is low, there is an increased risk of intracerebral hemorrhage during a spontaneous delivery. While it is possible to determine the platelet count intrapartum by microblood sampling from the fetal scalp, this can only be done relatively late in the delivery. Cordocentesis, on the other hand, can be performed before the onset of labor. If the platelet count in the fetus is below 50,000, a cesarean delivery is advised (73, 110).

Diagnosis of Fetal Anemia

Transfusion planning. In disorders that can lead to severe fetal anemia as a result of hemolysis (Rh or Kell erythroblastosis, parvovirus B19 infection), the fetal blood count (hematocrit, hemoglobin, reticulocytes) (131), erythropoietin determination (122), direct Coombs test, and fetal blood group supply important information on the condition of the fetus and the degree of fetal risk. Unlike the Liley procedure (65), an amniotic fluid bilirubin assay that only indirectly reflects the degree of fetal anemia and poorly evaluates fetal risk, especially in the second trimester (81), cordocentesis can directly determine the degree of anemia and provide a specific basis for planning an intrauterine transfusion.

Timing. The timing of the first cordocentesis depends on various factors such as a positive obstetric history, elevated antibody titers in the maternal serum (> 1 : 8), and antibody type and is therefore determined on an individual basis. If fetal ultrasound shows that ascites is already present, it may be assumed that the fetus has severe anemia (Hct < 15%, Hb < 4 g/dL) (14, 80).

Determination of Fetal Blood Group

The fetal blood group, including subgroups, can be successfully determined by 22 weeks' gestation. Since every irregular antibody in the maternal blood is not necessary due to fetal sensitization, the risk to the fetus can be clearly assessed only if the fetal blood group is accurately known. If the fetus belongs to the same blood group as the mother and if anemia is not present, there is no need for further invasive procedures.

Diagnosis of Fetal Hypoalbuminemia

In cases of nonimmune fetal hydrops (NIHF), it is helpful to determine albumin in addition to the hemoglobin and hematocrit, as this condition is often associated with marked hypoalbuminemia and leads to water retention in the fetus by altering the oncotic pressure.

Assessment of Fetal Condition in Cases of Growth Retardation and/or Abnormal Doppler Flow

Parameters. Direct access to the fetal circulation in the late second trimester and third trimester is opening new avenues in modern obstetric medicine. Especially in cases of significant fetal growth retardation, cordocentesis has gained increasing importance in the determination of fetal blood gases (16, 84, 90, 118), acid-base status (84, 118), lactate (16, 84, 118), reticulocytes (83, 85), amino acids (6, 13, 29), and triglycerides (30).

Correlations. Several groups of authors conducted comparative studies of Doppler and cordocentesis findings (7, 34, 90, 91, 130) as well as studies comparing fetal heart rate (FHR) patterns and cordocentesis findings (127). These authors found various correlations with pH values, blood gases, and lactate.

Detection of asphyxia. But because neither the FHR patterns (127) nor Doppler findings (90) provide clear-cut evidence of fetal compromise in all cases, cordocentesis can be a useful adjunct to the noninvasive tests, especially in cases of severe growth retardation. In cases with abnormal Doppler flow (absent end-diastolic flow in the umbilical artery and/or aorta, brain-sparing effect in the middle cerebral artery) with a normal-appearing FHR trace, chronic asphyxia can be specifically confirmed or excluded by cordocentesis (91).

Risks of Cordocentesis

The overall complication rate of cordocentesis is slightly higher than that of amniocentesis. Besides the risk of membrane rupture, chorioamnionitis, or abortion, there are additional risks relating to possible bleeding from the umbilical cord (Fig. 46.**18**), transient luminal narrowing (Fig. 46.**19**), umbilical cord hematoma (Fig. 46.**19**) or thrombosis, fetal bradycardia, fetomaternal transfusion, or intrauterine fetal death.

A risk of 0.5% has been reported for chorioamnionitis (132), 0.4% for rupture of the membranes (132), 6.6% for fetal bradycardia (132), and 0.8% for abortion (21). The risk of intrauterine fetal death in diagnostic cordocentesis is between 0.8% (132) and 1.1% (133).

Postprocedure bleeding. Transient bleeding from the umbilical cord puncture site, called the "jet phenomenon," is a relatively common, innocuous finding after cordocentesis (Fig. 46.**18**). Daffos et al. (21) found that the bleeding lasted 5–60 seconds in 32% of the cases, 1–2 min in 6%, and more than 2 min in 2%.

To minimize puncture risks, Whittle (134) recommends that cordocentesis be performed only at prenatal centers where at least 30 of these procedures are performed annually.

Contraindications. A maternal HIV or hepatitis B infection is a contraindication to cordocentesis, as the procedure could transmit the infection to the fetus.

Postprocedure ultrasound. Cordocentesis, like amniocentesis, should be followed by an ultrasound examination to confirm fetal viability.

Percutaneous Procedures in the Fetus

A percutaneous needle may be passed into a fetal organ to obtain material for diagnostic analysis. This applies mainly to the examination of fluid collections such as hydrothorax or chylothorax, an enlarging cystic structure in the renal area, an ovarian cyst, or ascites. In some cases the diagnostic procedure also has a therapeutic component.

If sufficient lymphocytes are found in the sampled fluid, the fetal karyotype can also be determined.

Fetal Hydrothorax or Chylothorax

Fetal thoracentesis for a pleural effusion (Fig. 46.**20**) is more therapeutic than diagnostic because hydrothorax and chylothorax cannot be reliably distinguished antenatally by the color of the aspirate (both are straw-colored) or by biochemical testing. Once the newborn infant begins to feed, chylothorax is distinguishable by the detection of chylomicrons in the aspirate. The aspirate in chylothorax also contains abundant lymphocytes.

Obstructive Uropathy, Renal Dysplasia

With a significant or progressive urinary tract obstruction or in cystic renal disease, the fetal urinary bladder, renal pelvis (Fig. 46.**21**), or a renal cyst can be percutaneously aspirated to obtain a urine sample. This procedure decompresses the affected organ, making it easier to evaluate sonographically. Also, biochemical analysis of the sampled urine makes it possible to evaluate fetal renal function.

Fetal urine values. The functional status of the fetal kidney(s) is evaluated by the analysis of electrolytes, osmolality, creatinine, urea, phos-

phate, microglobulins (α_1- and β_2-microglobulin), and total protein (70, 77, 86, 87, 124). It should be noted that some of these values change with increasing renal maturity, and an accurate assessment can be made only by taking into account the normal values for the corresponding gestational age in weeks. For example, sodium and phosphate values decline with advancing gestation, while creatinine rises and calcium and urea remain constant (88). Dysplastic renal changes are associated with elevated sodium and calcium levels and low urea and creatinine levels (86).

Cutoff levels. A poor prognosis is indicated when values exceed certain cutoff levels: sodium > 100 mg/dL, chloride > 90 mg/dL, osmolality > 200 mosmol/L, calcium > 8 mg/dL, β_2-microglobulin > 6 mg/dL, and total protein > 40 mg/dL (70). A knowledge of fetal urine values is particularly important in cases where the placement of a fetal shunt is being considered.

Ovarian Cyst

When an enlarging, indeterminate mass is detected in the fetal lower abdomen, it is appropriate to consider intrauterine aspiration (Fig. 46.**22**), which has both a diagnostic and therapeutic rationale. The detection of high estradiol levels in the aspirate confirms the diagnosis of an ovarian cyst (68).

Ascites

The percutaneous aspiration of fetal ascites is useful in differentiating simple ascites (Fig. 46.**23**), like that found in nonimmune hydrops, from ascites due to meconium peritonitis (Fig. 46.**24**). While simple ascites presents as a clear yellowish fluid, ascites due to meconium peritonitis has a brownish color.

Liver Biopsy

Fetal liver biopsies were performed in the past to detect certain metabolic disorders (48, 78, 98, 114). Today fetal liver biopsy is considered obsolete, since most disorders can be confirmed or excluded by the molecular genetic analysis of a chorionic villus sample or amniotic fluid cells.

Fetoscopy

Fetoscopy is a method for the direct visualization of the fetus. The term "fetoscopy" was coined by Scrimgeour (112). It was practiced chiefly in the 1970s and 1980s (5, 58, 92, 101, 105, 106) to detect fetal abnormalities and to obtain fetal blood or skin samples. With the dramatic improvement in ultrasound image quality, fetoscopy has become less important and today is used only for special investigations. Fetoscopy is performed mainly during the period from 18 to 24 weeks of gestation.

Indications. Today the only major role of diagnostic fetoscopy is in the diagnosis of hereditary skin diseases (e.g., epidermolysis bullosa or harlequin-type congenital ichthyosis) (102). In recent years, fetoscopy has attracted renewed interest in the selective laser coagulation of placental vessels in fetofetal transfusion syndrome (25, 43, 44, 126) (see Chapter 47, Fetal Therapy).

Technique. Following sedation and local anesthesia, a trocar is passed through the abdomen into the amniotic cavity under ultrasound guidance (Fig. 46.**25**). Then the fetoscope is introduced through the sheath into the amniotic cavity and directed to the targeted site under contin-

Percutaneous procedures in the fetus

Fig. 46.**20**   Right-sided hydrothorax following thoracentesis, 34 weeks. A straw-colored aspirate is obtained (below).

Fig. 46.**21**   Aspiration of the right renal pelvis in bilateral hydronephrosis for biochemical analysis of the fetal urine, 23 weeks.

Fig. 46.**22**   Large ovarian cyst on the right side (diameter 6 cm). The aspiration needle is introduced along the superimposed dotted line.

Fig. 46.**23**   Percutaneous aspiration of ascites in nonimmune fetal hydrops, 20 weeks.

Fig. 46.**24**   Percutaneous aspiration in suspected meconium peritonitis after bowel perforation (29 weeks, 6 days). The aspirate is dark brown (right), distinguishing it from the pale yellow color of simple ascites.

Fetoscopy

Fig. 46.**25**   Fetoscope with sheath and light source.

Amnioinfusion

Fig. 46.**26**   Amnioinfusion in original Potter syndrome with anhydramnios. The needle is introduced adjacent to the occiput (arrows). The fluid jet entering the amniotic cavity can be clearly visualized with color Doppler.

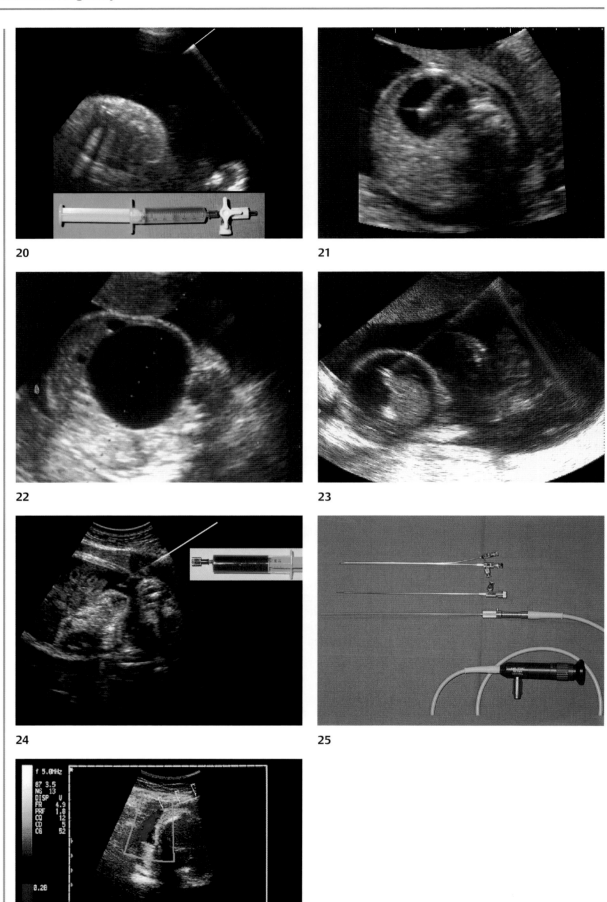

20

21

22

23

24

25

26

uous ultrasound control. This is necessary, since the fetoscope has only a limited field of view and orientation with the fetoscope alone is difficult.

After the fetal skin region of interest has been located and identified endoscopically, the biopsy forceps is introduced and the sample is taken under vision. Another option is to exchange the biopsy forceps for the endoscope and then perform the biopsy under ultrasound guidance (102). After the biopsy is completed, the cutaneous wound is inspected with the endoscope. With generalized skin disorders, fetoscopy can be omitted and the skin sample taken with a biopsy forceps under ultrasound guidance.

Risks. The reported abortion rate is < 5% and was 2% in the largest published series (106). Transvaginal amniotic fluid leakage occurs in 4–5% of patients, and premature labor occurs in approximately 10% (106). Prophylactic antibiotics are administered as a precaution against amnionitis.

Amnioinfusion

Pronounced oligohydramnios can seriously restrict imaging conditions and hamper fetal diagnosis. Infusing fluid into the amniotic cavity (e.g., physiologic saline solution) can greatly help the situation, especially when it is necessary to detect or exclude an original Potter syndrome (Fig. 46.**26**) (10, 63, 99, 119). When the amnioinfusion is completed, the surface of the fetus can be seen more clearly and it is also easier to observe physiologic functions such as stomach and bladder filling (see Chapter 47, Fetal Therapy).

References

1. Bald, R., Chatterjee, M.S., Gembruch, U., Schuh, S., Hansmann, M.: Antepartum fetal blood sampling with cordocentesis. Comparison with chorionic villus sampling and amniocentesis in diagnosing karyotype anomalies. J. Reprod. Med. 36 (1991) 655–658
2. Bang, J., Bock, T.E., Trolle, D.: Ultrasound guided fetal intravenous transfusion for severe rhesus haemolytic disease. Brit. Med. J. Clin. Res. Ed. 284 (1982) 373–374
3. Basaran, S., Miny, P., Pawlowitzki, I.H., Horst, J., Holzgreve, W.: Rapid karyotyping for prenatal diagnosis in the second and third trimester of pregnancy. Prenat. Diagn. 8 (1988) 315–320
4. Bell, J.A., Pearn, J.H., Wilson, B.H., Ansford, A.J.: Prenatal cytogenetic diagnosis: a current audit. A review of 2000 cases of prenatal cytogenetic diagnoses after amniocentesis, and comparisons with early experience. Med. J. Aust. 146 (1987) 12–15
5. Benzie, R.J., Doran, T.A.: The „fetoscope" – a new clinical tool for prenatal genetic diagnosis. Amer. J. Obstet. Gynecol. 121 (1975) 460–464
6. Bernardini, I., Evans, M.I., Nicolaides, K.H., Economides, D.L., Gahl, W.A.: The fetal concentrating index as a gestational age-independent measure of placental dysfunction in intrauterine growth retardation. Amer. J. Obstet. Gynecol. 164 (1991) 1481–1490
7. Bilardo, C.M., Nicolaides, K.H., Campbell, S.: Doppler measurements of fetal and uteroplacental circulations: Relationship with umbilical venous blood gases measured at cordocentesis. Amer. J. Obstet. Gynecol. 162 (1990) 115–120
8. Brambati, B., Oldrini, A., Aladerun, S.A.: Methods of chorionic villi sampling in first trimester fetal diagnosis. In: Albertinei, A., Rosignani, P.G. (eds.): Progress in perinatal medicine. Amsterdam: Excerpta Medica 1983; p. 275
9. Brambati, B., Lanzani, A., Tului, L.: Transaabdominal and transcervical chorionic villus sampling: efficiency and risk evaluation of 2,411 cases. Amer. J. Med. Genet. 35 (1990) 160–164
10. Burges, A., Strauss, A., Heer, I., Hasbargen, U., Hepp, H.: Amnioninfusion in der pränatalen Diagnostik und Therapie. Gynäkologe 32 (1999) 832–839
11. Burton, B.K., Schulz, C.J., Burd, L.I.: Limb anomalies associated with chorionic villus sampling. Obstet. Gynecol. 79 (1992) 726–730
12. Canadian collaborative CVS-amniocentesis clinical trial group. Multicentre randomised clinical trial of chorion villus sampling and amniocentesis. First report. Lancet I (1989) 1–6
13. Cetin, I., Corbetta, C., Sereni, L.P. et al.: Umbilical amino acid concentrations in normal and growth-retarded fetuses sampled in utero by cordocentesis. Amer. J. Obstet. Gynecol. 162 (1990) 253–261
14. Chitkara, U., Wilkins, I., Lynch, L., Mehalek, K., Berkowitz, R.H.: The role of sonography in assessing severity of fetal anaemia in Rh and Kell-isoimmunised pregnancies. Obstet. Gynecol. 71 (1988) 393–398
15. Clausen, U., Ulmer, R., Beinder, E., Voigt, H.J.: Schnelle Karyotypisierung im II. und III. Trimester: Ergebnisse und Erfahrungen. Geburtsh. u. Frauenheilk. 55 (1995) 41–48
16. Cox, W.L., Daffos, F., Forestier, F. et al.: Physiology and management of intrauterine growth retardation: A biologic approach with fetal blood sampling. Amer. J. Obstet. Gynecol. 159 (1988) 36–41
17. Crombach, G., von Eckardstein, S., Reihs, T., Röhrborn, G.: Stellenwert der invasiven Pränataldiagnostik im ersten Trimenon im Vergleich zur Standardamniozentese. Gynäkologe 28 (1995) 302–314
18. Cuthbertson, G., Weiner, C.P., Giller, R.H., Grose, C.: Prenatal diagnosis of second-trimester congenital varicella syndrome by virus-specific immunoglobulin M. J. Pediatr. 111 (1987) 592–595
19. Daffos, E., Capella-Pavlovsky, M., Forestier, F.: A new procedure for pure fetal blood sampling in utero. Prenat. Diagn. 3 (1983) 271–274
20. Daffos, E., Forestier, F., Grangeot-Keros, L. et al.: Prenatal diagnosis of congenital rubella. Lancet II (1984) 1–3
21. Daffos, E., Capella-Pavlovsky, M., Forestier, F.: Fetal blood sampling during pregnancy with use of a needle guided by ultrasound: A study of 606 consecutive cases. Amer. J. Obstet. Gynecol. 153 (1985) 655–660
22. Daffos, F., Forestier, F., Capella-Pavlovsky, M. et al.: Prenatal management of 746 pregnancies at risk for congenital toxoplasmosis. New Eng. J. Med. 318 (1988) 271–275
23. Daffos, F., Forestier, F., Kaplan, C., Cox, W.: Prenatal diagnosis and management of bleeding disorders with fetal blood samplings. J. Obstet. Gynecol. 158 (1988) 939–946
24. Daniel, A., Ng, A., Kuah, K.B., Reiha, S., Malafiej, P.: A study of early amniocentesis for prenatal cytogenetic diagnosis. Prenat. Diagn. 18 (1998) 21–28
25. De Lia, J.E., Kuhlmann, R.S., Harstad, T.W., Cruikshank, D.P.: Fetoscopic laser ablation of placental vessels in severe previable twin-twin transfusion syndrome. Amer. J. Obstet. Gynecol. 172 (1995) 1202–1211
26. Desmonts, G., Daffos, F., Forestier, F., Capella-Pavlovsky, M., Thulliez, P., Chartier, M.: Prenatal diagnosis of congenital toxoplasmosis. Lancet I (1985) 500–504
27. Dolk, H.: Methylene blue and atresia or stenosis of ileum and jejunum. Lancet 338 (1991) 1021–1022
28. Dumez, Y., Goosens, M., Boue, J. et al.: Chorion villi sampling using rigid forceps under ultrasound control. In: Fraccaro, M., Simoni, G., Brambati, B. (eds.): First trimester fetal diagnosis. Berlin: Springer 1985; p. 38
29. Economides, D.L., Nicolaides, K.H., Gahl, W.A., Bernardini, I., Evans, M.I.: Plasma amino acids in appropriate- and small-for-gestational-age fetuses. Amer. J. Obstet. Gynecol. 161 (1989) 1219–1227
30. Economides, D.L., Nicolaides, K.H., Campbell, S.: Metabolic and endocrine findings in appropriate and small for gestational age fetus. J. Perinat. Med. 19 (1991) 97–105
31. Enders, G., Jonatha, W.: Prenatal diagnosis of intrauterine rubella. Infection 15 (1987) 162–164
32. Farrell, S.A., Summers, A.M., Dallaire, L., Singer, J., Johnson, J.A., Wilson, R.D.: Club foot, an adverse outcome of early amniocentesis: disruption or deformation? CEMAT. Canadian Early and Mid-Trimester Amniocentesis Trial. J. Med. Genet. 36 (1999) 843–846
33. Ferguson II, J.E., Vick, D.J., Hogge, J.S., Hogge, W.A.: Transcervical chorionic villus sampling and amniocentesis: a comparison of reliablility, culture findings, and fetal outcome. Amer. J. Obstet. Gynecol. 163 (1990) 926–931

34. Ferrazzi, E., Pardi, G., Bauscaglia, M. et al.: The correlation of biochemical monitoring versus umbilical flow velocity measurements of the human fetus. Amer. J. Obstet. Gynecol. 159 (1988) 1081–1087
35. Firth, H.V., Boyd, P.A., Chamberlain, P., MacKenzie, I.Z., Lindenbaum, R.H., Hudson, S.M.: Severe limb abnormalities after chorionic villus sampling at 56–66 day's gestation. Lancet 337 (1991) 762–763
36. Firth, H.V., Boyd, P.A., Chamberlain, P., MacKenzie, I.Z., Morris-Kay, G.M., Hudson, S.M.: Analysis of limb reduction defects in babies exposed to chorionic villus sampling. Lancet 343 (1994) 1069–1071
37. Forestier, F., Daffos, F., Rainaut, M., Bruneau, M., Trivin, F.: Blood chemistry of normal human fetuses at midtrimester of pregnancy. Pediatr. Res. 21 (1987) 579–583
38. Ghirardini, G., Camurri, L., Gualerzi, C. et al.: Chorionic villi sampling by means of a new endoscopic device. In: Fraccara, M., Simoni, G., Brambati, B. (eds.): First trimester fetal diagnosis. Berlin: Springer 1985; p. 54
39. Giorlandino, C., Mobili, L., Bilancioni, E. et al.: Transplacental amniocentesis: is it really a higher-risk procedure? Prenat. Diagn. 14 (1994) 803–806
40. Grangeot-Keros, L., Pillot, J., Daffos, F., Forestier, F.: Prenatal and postnatal production of IgM and IgA antibodies to rubella virus studied by antibody capture immunoassay. J. Infect. Dis. 158 (1988) 138–143
41. Gustavii, B.: First trimester chromosomal analysis of chorionic villi obtained by direct vision technique. Lancet I (1983) 507–508
42. Halliday, J., Lumley, J., Sheffield, L.J., Lancaster, P.A.L.: Limb deficiencies, chorion villus sampling, and advanced maternal age. Amer. J. Med. Genet. 47 (1993) 1096–1098
43. Hecher, K., Zikulnig, L., Hackelöer, B.J.: Perspektiven der operativen Endoskopie in der Fetalmedizin. Gynäkologe 32 (1999) 855–865
44. Hecher, K., Plath, H., Bregenzer, T., Hansmann, M., Hackelöer, B.J.: Endoscopic laser surgery versus serial amniocenteses in the treatment of severe twin-twin transfusion syndrome. Amer. J. Obstet. Gynecol. 180 (1999) 717–724
45. Heckemann, R., Seidel, K.J.: The sonographic appearance and contrast enhancement of puncture needles. J. clin. Ultrasound 11 (1983) 265–268
46. Henkel, B.: Amniozentese unter permanenter sonographischer Sicht. Geburtsh. u. Frauenheilk. 44 (1984) 685–688
47. Hobbins, J.C., Mahoney, M.J.: In utero diagnosis of hemoglobinopathies. Technic for obtaining fetal blood. New Engl. J. Med. 290 (1974) 1065–1068
48. Holzgreve, W., Golbus, M.S.: Prenatal diagnosis of ornithine transcarbamylase deficiency utilizing fetal liver biopsy. Amer. J. Hum. Genet. 36 (1984) 320–328
49. Holzgreve, W., Hansmann, M.: Erfahrungen mit der „Free-Hand-Needle" Technik bei 3215 Amniocentesen im 2. Trimenon zur pränatalen Diagnostik. Gynäkologe 17 (1984) 77–82
50. Holzgreve, W., Miny, P.: Improved echogenicity of the catheter for chorionic villi sampling. In: Fraccara, M., Simoni, G., Brambati, B. (eds.): First trimester fetal diagnosis. Berlin: Springer 1985; p. 64
51. Holzgreve, W., Miny, P., Gerlach, B., Westendorp, A., Ahlert, D., Horst, J.: Benefits of placental biopsies for rapid karyotyping in the second and third trimester (late chorionic villus sampling) in high-risk pregnancies. Amer. J. Obstet. Gynecol. 162 (1990) 1188–1192
52. Hoyme, H.F., Jones, K.L., van Allen, M.I., Saunders, B.D., Benirschke, K.: Vascular pathogenesis of transverse limb reduction defects. J. Pediatr. 101 (1982) 839–843
53. International Fetoscopy Group: The status of fetoscopy and fetal tissue sampling. The results of the first meeting of the International Fetoscopy Group. Prenat. Diagn. 4 (1984) 79–81
54. Iserson, K.V.: The origins of the gauge system for medical equipment. J. Emerg. Med. 5 (1987) 45–48
55. Jahoda, M.G.J., Pijpers, L., Reuss, A., Sachs, E.S.: Transabdominale Chorionzentese für die schnelle pränatale Diagnostik im zweiten Trimenon: Erfahrungen bei 147 Schwangeren. Z. Geburtsh. Perinat. 192 (1988) 101–103
56. Jeanty, P., Shah, D., Roussis, P.: Single-needle insertion in twin amniocentesis. J. Ultrasound Med. 9 (1990) 511–517
57. Jonatha, W.D.: Amniozentese in der Frühschwangerschaft unter Sichtkontrolle mit Ultraschall. Elektromedica 3 (1974) 94
58. Jonatha, W.D.: Fetoskopien im Rahmen der pränatalen Diagnostik. In: Husslein, H. (Hrsg.): Gynäkologie und Geburtshilfe. Forschungen – Erkenntnisse. Wien: Egermann 1977; S. 657
59. Kaplan, C., Daffos, F., Forestier, F. et al.: Management of alloimmune thrombocytopenia: Antenatal diagnosis and in utero transfusion of maternal platelets. Blood 72 (1988) 340–343
60. Kazi, Z., Rozovskii, I.S., Bakharev, V.A.: Chorion biopsy in early prenatal diagnosis for inherited disorders. Prenat. Diagn. 2 (1982) 39
61. Kennerknecht, I., Baarbi, G., Wolf, M. et al.: Cytogenetic diagnoses after chorionic villus sampling are less reliable in very-high- or very-low-risk pregnancies. Prenat. Diagn. 13 (1993) 929–944
62. Kuliev, A.M., Modell, B., Jackson, L. et al.: Risk evaluation of CVS. Prenat. Diagn. 13 (1993) 197–209
63. Lameier, L., Katz, V.L.: Amnioninfusion: a review. Obstet. Gynecol. Surv. 48 (1993) 829–837
64. Lange, I., Rodeck, C.H., Morgan-Capner, P., Simmons, A., Kangro, H.O.: Prenatal serological diagnosis of intrauterine cytomegalovirus infection. Brit. med. J. 284 (1982) 1673–1674
65. Liley, A.W.: Liquor amnii analysis in the management of the pregnancy complicated by rhesus sensitisation. Amer. J. Obstet. Gynecol. 82 (1961) 1359–1370
66. MacLachlan, N.A.: Amniocentesis. In: Brock, D.J.H., Rodeck, C.H., Ferguson-Smith, M.A. (eds.): Prenatal diagnosis and screening. London: Livingstone 1992; pp. 13–24
67. McFadyen, I.: The dangers of intra-amniotic methylene blue. Brit. J. Obstet. Gynaecol. 99 (1992) 89–90
68. Meagher, S.E., Fisk, N.M., Boogert, A., Russell, P.: Fetal ovarian cysts: diagnostic and therapeutic role for intrauterine aspiration. Fetal Diagn. Ther. 8 (1993) 195–199
69. Merz, E.: Cordocentese – Indikationen und Konsequenzen. Gynäkologe 27 (1994) 174–180
70. Merz, E.: Intrauterine Therapie der obstruktiven Uropathie. Akt. Urol. 27 (1996) A15–A16
71. Mibashan, R.S., Rodeck, C.H.: Haemophilia and other genetic defects haemostasis. In: Rodeck, C.H., Nicolaides, K.H. (eds.): Prenatal Diagnosis. Proceedings of the Eleventh Study Group of the Royal College of Obstetricians and Gynaecologists. Chichester, England 1984; 179
72. Miny, P., Hammer, P., Schloo, R. et al.: Pränatale Diagnostik an Chorionzotten und Plazentapunktaten vom ersten bis zum dritten Schwangerschaftstrimenon: Diagnostische Zuverlässigkeit von Chromosomenuntersuchungen. Geburtsh. u. Frauenheilk. 51 (1991) 694–703
73. Moise, K.J.Jr., Carpenter, R.J.Jr., Cotton, D.B., Wasserstrum, N., Kirshon, B., Cano, L.: Percutaneous umbilical cord blood sampling in the evaluation of fetal platelet counts in pregnant patients with autoimmune thrombocytopenia purpura. Obstet. Gynecol. 72 (1988) 346–350
74. Morgan-Capner, P., Rodeck, C.H., Nicolaides, K., Cradock-Watson, J.E.: Prenatal detection of rubella-specific IgM in fetal sera. Prenat. Diagn. 5 (1985) 21–26
75. MRC Working Party on the evaluation of chorion villus sampling. Medical research council european trial of chorion villus sampling. Lancet 337 (1991) 1491–1499
76. Müller-Holve, W., Stöckenius, U., Popp, L.W., Fabinger, R., Martin, K.: Amniozentese unter permanenter Ultraschallsicht – Vorteile eines speziellen Verfahrens. Ultraschall 6 (1985) 200–207
77. Muller, F., Dommergues, M., Mandelbrot, L., Aubry, M.C., Nichoul-Fekete, C., Dumez, Y.: Fetal urine biochemistry predicts postnatal renal function in children with bilateral obstructive uropathies. Obstet. Gynecol. 82 (1993) 813–820
78. Murotsuki, J., Uehara, S., Okamura, K., Yajima, A., Oura, T., Miyabayashi, S.: Fetal liver biopsy for prenatal diagnosis of carbamyl phosphate synthetase deficiency. Amer. J. Perinatol. 11 (1994) 160–162
79. Naides, S.J., Weiner, C.P.: Antenatal diagnosis and palliative treatment of non-immune hydrops fetalis secondary to fetal parvovirus B 19 infection. Prenat. Diagn. 9 (1989) 105–114
80. Nicolaides, K.H., Rodeck, C.H., Millar, D.S., Mibashan, R.S.: Fetal haematology in rhesus isoimmunisation. Brit. Med. J. 220 (1985) 661–663
81. Nicolaides, K.H., Rodeck, C.H., Mibashan, R.S., Kemp, J.R.: Have Liley charts outlived their usefulness? Amer. J. Obstet. Gynecol. 155 (1986) 90–94
82. Nicolaides, K.H.: Cordocentesis. Clin. Obstet. Gynecol. 31 (1988) 123–135
83. Nicolaides, K.H., Thilaganathan, B.Sc., Rodeck, C.H., Mibashan, R.S.: Erythroblastosis and reticulocytosis in anaemic fetuses. Amer. J. Obstet. Gynecol. 159 (1988) 1063–1065
84. Nicolaides, K.H., Economides, D.L., Soothill, P.W.: Blood gases, pH, and lactate in appropriate- and small-for-gestational-age fetuses. Amer. J. Obstet. Gynecol. 161 (1989) 996–1001
85. Nicolaides, K.H., Thilaganathan, B.Sc., Mibashan, R.S.: Cordocentesis in the investigation of fetal erythropoiesis. Amer. J. Obstet. Gynecol. 161 (1989) 1197–1200
86. Nicolaides, K.H., Cheng, H.H., Snijders, R.S., Moniz, D.F.: Fetal urine biochemistry in the assessment of obstructive uropathy. Amer. J. Obstet. Gynecol. 166 (1992) 932–937
87. Nicolini, U., Monni, G.: Intestinal obstruction in babies exposed in utero to methylene blue. Lancet 336 (1990) 1258–1259
88. Nicolini, U., Fisk, N.M., Rodeck, C.H., Beacham, J.: Fetal urine biochemistry: an index of renal maturation and dysfunction. Brit. J. Obstet. Gynaecol. 99 (1992) 46–50
89. Nolan, G.H., Schmickel, R.D., Chantaratherakitti, P., Hamman, J., Louwsma, G.: The effect of ultrasonography on midtrimester genetic amniocentesis complications. Amer. J. Obstet. Gynecol. 140 (1981) 531–534
90. Okamura, K., Watanabe, T., Tanigawara, S. et al.: Biochemical evaluation of fetuses with hypoxia caused by severe preeclampsia using cordocentesis. J. Perinat. Med. 18 (1990) 441–447
91. Pardi, G., Cetin, I., Marconi, A.M. et al.: Diagnostic value of blood sampling in fetuses with growth retardation. New Engl. J. Med. 10 (1993) 692–696
92. Phillips, J.M.: Fetoscopy: an overview. J. Reprod. Med. 15 (1975) 69–72
93. Pittalis, M.C., Dalpra, L., Toricelli, F. et al.: The predictive value of cytogenetic diagnosis after CVS based on 4860 cases with both direct and culture methods. Prenat. Diagn. 14 (1994) 267–278
94. Poinsot, J., Buillois, B., Margis, D., Carlhant, D., Boog, G., Alix, D.: Neonatal hemolytic anemia after intraamniotic injection of methylene blue. Arch. Fr. Pédiatr. 45 (1988) 657–660
95. Pol, J.G., van der Wolf, H., Boer, K. et al.: Jejunal atresia related to the use of methylene blue in genetic amniocentesis in twins. Brit. J. Obstet. Gynaecol. 99 (1992) 141–143
96. Pränatale Diagnostik an Chorionzotten. Abschlußbericht über die Dokumentation der Untersuchungen innerhalb der Gemeinschaftsstudie in der Bundesrepublik Deutschland 1985–1991
97. Pruggmayer, M.R.K., Jahoda, M.G.J., Van der Pol, J.G. et al.: Genetic amniocentesis in twin pregnancies: results of a multicenter study of 529 cases. Ultrasound Obstet. Gynecol. 2 (1992) 6–10
98. Qu, Y., Abdenur, J.E., Eng, C.M., Desnick, R.J.: Molecular prenatal diagnosis of glycogen storage disease type Ia. Prenat. Diagn. 16 (1996) 333–336
99. Quetel, T.A., Mejides, A.A., Salman, F.A., Torres-Rodriguez, M.M.: Amnioinfusion: an aid in the ultrasonographic evaluation of severe oligohydramnios in pregnancy. Amer. J. Obstet. Gynecol. 167 (1992) 333–336
100. Randomised trial to assess safety and fetal outcome of early and midtrimester amniocentesis. The Canadian Early and Mid-trimester Amniocentesis Trial (CEMAT) Group. Lancet 351 (1998) 242–247
101. Rauskolb, R., Fuhrmann, W.: Die Fetoskopie. Z. Geburtsh. Perinat. 182 (1978) 243–262
102. Rauskolb, R.: Neues zur Fetoskopie als diagnostische Methode. Gynäkologe 17 (1984) 47–51
103. Rhoads, G.G., Jackson, L.G., Schlesselman, S.E. et al.: The safety and efficacy of chorionic villus sampling for early prenatal diagnosis of cytogenetic abnormalities. New Engl. J. Med. 320 (1989) 609–617
104. Rodeck, C.H., Campbell, S.: Sampling pure fetal blood by fetoscopy in second trimester of pregnancy. Brit. Med. J. II (1978) 728–730

105. Rodeck, C.H., Nicolaides, K.H.: Die Anwendung der Fetoskopie bei fetaler Therapie. Gynäkologe 17 (1984) 52–55
106. Rodeck, C.H., Nicolaides, K.H.: Fetoscopy. Brit. Med. Bull. 42 (1986) 296–300
107. Schloo, R., Miny, P. Holzgreve, W., Horst, J., Lenz, W.: Distal limb deficiency following chorionic villus sampling? Amer. J. Med. Genet. 42 (1992) 404–413
108. Schmidt, W., Gabelmann, J., Müller, U. et al.: Pränatale Diagnostik – Technik und Ergebnisse von 1000 Fruchtwasserpunktionen. Geburtsh. u. Frauenheilk. 40 (1980) 761–768
109. Schofer, O., Zepp, F., Merz, E. et al.: Simultane Doppelfluoreszenz-Flowzytometrie aus lysiertem Vollblut zur pränatalen Diagnostik eines kombinierten Immundefektes. Monatsschr. Kinderheilk. 137 (1989) 264–268
110. Scioscia, A.L., Grannum, P.A., Copel, J.A., Hobbins, J.C.: The use of percutaneous umbilical blood sampling in immune thrombocytopenic purpura. Amer. J. Obstet. Gynecol. 159 (1988) 1066–1068
111. Scott, R.: Limb abnormalities after chorionic villus sampling. Lancet 337 (1991) 1038–1039
112. Scrimgeour, J.B.: Fetoscopy. In: Motulsky, G.A., Lenz, W. (eds.): Birth defects. Amsterdam: Excerpta Medica 1974; 234
113. Shaw, D.M., Roussis, P., Ulm, J., Jeanty, Ph., Boehm, F.H.: Cordocentesis for rapid karyotyping. Amer. J. Obstet. Gynecol. 162 (1990) 1548–1553
114. Shulman, L.P., Elias, S.: Percutaneous umbilical blood sampling, fetal skin sampling, and fetal liver biopsy. Semin. Perinatol. 14 (1990) 456–464
115. Smidt-Jensen, S., Hahnemann, N.: Transabdominal fine needle biopsy from chorionic villi in the first trimester. Prenat. Diagn. 4 (1984) 163–169
116. Smidt-Jensen, S., Permin, M., Philip, J. et al.: Randomised comparison of amniocentesis and transabdominal and transcervical chorionic villus sampling. Lancet 340 (1992) 1237–1244
117. Smidt-Jensen, S., Lind., A.M., Permin, M., Zachary, J.M., Lundsteen, C., Philip, J.: Cytogenetic analysis of 2928 CVS samples and 1075 amnioceses from randomized studies. Prenat. Diagn. 13 (1993) 723–740
118. Soothill, P.W., Nicolaides, K.H., Rodeck, Ch.H., Campbell, S.: Effect of gestational age on fetal and intervillous blood gas and acid-base values in human pregnancy. Fetal Therapy 1 (1986) 32–35
119. Strang, T.H.: Amnioninfusion. J. Reprod. Med. 49 (1995) 108–114
120. Sundberg, K., Bang, J., Brocks, V., Jensen, F.R., Smidt-Jensen, S., Philip, J.: Early sonographically guided amnioceses with filtration technique. J. Ultrasound Med. 14 (1995) 585–590
121. Tabor, A., Madsen, M., Obel, E.B., Philip, J., Bang, J., Norgaard-Pedersen, B.: Randomised controlled trial of genetic amniocentesis in 4606 low-risk women. Lancet I (1986) 1287–1293
122. Thilaganathan, B., Salvesen, D.R., Abbas, A., Ireland, M., Nicolaides, K.H.: Fetal plasma erythropoietin concentration in red blood cell-isoimmunized pregnancies. Amer. J. Obstet. Gynecol. 167 (1992) 1292–1297
123. Toivanen, P., Rossi, T., Hirvonen, T.: Immunglobulins in human fetal sera at different stages of gestation. Experientia 25 (1969) 527–528
124. Tutschek, B., Rodeck, C.H.: Diagnostisch-therapeutisches Konzept bei Fehlbildungen der Nieren und der ableitenden Harnwege. Gynäkologe 28 (1995) 356–367
125. Valenti, C.: Antenatal detection of haemoglobinopathies. Amer. J. Obstet. Gynecol. 115 (1973) 851–853
126. Ville, Y., Hecher, K., Gagnon, A., Sebire, N., Hyett, J., Nicolaides, K.: Endoscopic laser coagulation in the mangement of severe twin-to-twin transfusion syndrome. Brit. J. Obstet. Gynaecol. 105 (1998) 446–453
127. Visser, G.H.A., Sadovsky, G., Nicolaides, K.H.: Antepartum heart rate patterns in small-for-gestational-age third-trimester fetuses: Correlations with blood gas values obtained at cordocentesis. Amer. J. Obstet. Gynecol. 162 (1990) 698–703
128. Ward, R.H.T., Modell, B., Petrou, M., Karagozlu, F., Douratsos, E.: Method of sampling chorionic villi in first trimester of pregnancy under guidance of realtime ultrasound. Brit. Med. J. Clin. Res. Ed. 286 (1983) 1542–1544
129. Weiner, C.P.: The role of cordocentesis in fetal diagnosis. Clin. Obstet. Gynecol. 31 (1988) 285–292
130. Weiner, C.P.: The relationship between the umbilical artery systolic/diastolic ratio and umbilical blood gas measurements in specimens obtained by cordocentesis. Amer. J. Obstet. Gynecol. 162 (1990) 1198–1202
131. Weiner, C.P., Williamson, R.A., Wenstrom, K.D., Sipes, S.L., Grant, S.S., Widness, J.A.: Management of fetal hemolytic disease by cordocentesis. I. Prediction of fetal anemia. Amer. J. Obstet. Gynecol. 165 (1991) 546–553
132. Weiner, C.P., Wenstrom, K.D., Sipes, S.L., Williamson, R.A.: Risk factors for cordocentesis and fetal intravascular transfusion. Amer. J. Obstet. Gynecol. 165 (1991) 1020–1025
133. Weiner, C.P., Williamson, R.A., Wenstrom, K.D. et al.: Management of fetal hemolytic disease by cordocentesis. II. Outcome of treatment. Amer. J. Obstet. Gynecol. 165 (1991) 1302–1307
134. Whittle, M.J.: Cordocentesis. Brit. J. Obstet. Gynaecol. 96 (1989) 262–264
135. Wilson, R.D., Johnson, J., Windrim, R. et al. The early amniocentesis study: A randomized clinical trial of early amniocentesis and midtimester amniocentesis. Fetal Diagn. Ther. 12 (1997) 97–101
136. Young, S.R., Shipley, C.F., Wade, R.V. et al.: Single-center comparison of results of 1000 prenatal diagnoses with chorionic villus sampling and 1000 diagnoses with amniocentesis. Amer. J. Obstet. Gynecol. 165 (1991) 255–263

47 Fetal Therapy and Treatment of Abnormal Amniotic Fluid Volume

Fetal Therapy

Fetal therapy is still a relatively young but constantly advancing field within prenatal medicine. There is still some controversy surrounding the use of prenatal therapy, however, depending on the condition and the treatments that are available for it.

Development. Fetal therapy was inaugurated in 1963 by Sir William Liley (75), who successfully treated fetal anemia in Rh incompatibility by passing a needle into the fetal abdomen under radiographic guidance and infusing a donor blood concentrate (0 Rh negative) into the abdomen.

Role of ultrasonography. Two factors played a key role in the further evolution of fetal therapy: (1) the development of high-resolution ultrasound, which permitted accurate needle guidance to the umbilical cord, and (2) the important discoveries about certain fetal diseases that were made in animal studies during the past 20 years.

The ultrasound examination has an indispensable role in fetal therapy, not only in investigating the fetal disorder but also in monitoring the treatment and assessing fetal response.

Prerequisites and Forms of Therapy

The term "fetal therapy" has acquired a very broad meaning. On the one hand, there are intrauterine forms of therapy that are well established, such as the treatment of supraventricular tachycardia or fetal anemia. But there are also therapies that are of uncertain efficacy (e.g., shunting) and others that are still in the experimental stage (e.g., various types of open fetal surgery) and cannot yet be considered standard procedures. Finally, there are therapeutic procedures that so far have been tested only in animal models (Table 47.1).

Weighing risks and benefits. The general goal of fetal therapy is to intervene as early as possible in fetal disease to prevent irreversible organ damage or intrauterine fetal death.

Because the fetus is always accessed through the mother, it is necessary to consider both the fetal and the maternal risks in every therapeutic intervention. Thus, fetal therapy always involves a potential conflict of interests between the fetus and mother (66). The procedure should significantly improve the prognosis for the fetus without adversely affecting maternal health. The physician must carefully weigh the risks of any proposed therapeutic procedure against the anticipated benefit.

To accurately evaluate the risks of fetal therapy and its prospect for success, it is essential to arrange close interdisciplinary teamwork among prenatal specialists, neonatologists, pediatric cardiologists, pediatric surgeons, pediatric neurologists, and neurosurgeons.

Indications. In deciding whether fetal treatment is appropriate, it is important to consider not only the severity of the disorder but also the current gestational age. For example, if a given disorder does not develop until an advanced gestational age (> 32 weeks), it must be considered whether premature delivery and neonatal treatment might be a better option than fetal therapy.

Because most fetal therapies require a specialized knowledge of indications and techniques, it is advisable to perform fetal therapeutic procedures only at a level III prenatal center where adequate experience and interdisciplinary teamwork are ensured. Optimum timing of the planned intervention is an important concern. Fetal therapy that is instituted too late is associated with a high risk to the fetus. Conversely, an active treatment that is undertaken precipitously is not only unnecessary but can jeopardize fetal and maternal health.

Parental counseling. Every fetal treatment should be preceded by thorough counseling of the parents. The role of the counseling physician is not to advocate an experimental treatment, nor is it to give the parents a value-neutral account of the options and leave the decision entirely up to them. If the only alternative to inaction is an unproven treatment, parental counseling should be comprehensive and interdisciplinary.

It should be made clear in parental counseling that a successful outcome cannot be guaranteed in all fetal diseases and disorders that are treatable in principle.

Prerequisites. The International Fetal Medicine and Surgery Society (IFMSS) consensus has established the following points as prerequisites for undertaking surgical procedures on the fetus, umbilical cord, or placenta (52, 60):

- The disease can be accurately diagnosed and its severity assessed, and associated anomalies are excluded.
- The natural history of the disease is known, and the prognosis can be assessed.
- Currently there is no known effective postnatal treatment for the disease, or such treatment would come too late.
- The feasibility of the intervention has been established in an animal model, and the reversibility of adverse effects of the disease has been proven.
- The procedures are performed at specialized multidisciplinary fetal treatment centers according to rigorous protocols and only with the full informed consent of the parents.

Ethical considerations on fetal therapy were published by the American Academy of Pediatrics in 1999 (26).

Every invasive antenatal procedure requires the written consent of the patient herself.

Two types of fetal therapy. Fetal therapy is classified into two main categories: indirect and direct.

Indirect fetal therapy. Indirect fetal therapy is a medical form of treatment in which the medication is administered to the fetus via the maternal circulation and the placenta (Table 47.2). In some cases the medication may also be administered by instilling it into the amniotic fluid.

Table 47.1 Classification of current fetal therapeutic procedures

> Procedures of definite efficacy
> Procedures of uncertain efficacy
> Procedures of an experimental nature
> Procedures tested only in animal models

Direct fetal therapy. Direct fetal therapy is an invasive procedure in which the fetus is treated directly. Access to the fetus can be gained in several ways:

- With a sonographically guided needle (usually directed into the umbilical vein)
- With a fetoscope (e.g., for laser treatment)
- By hysterotomy (open fetal surgery) or endoscopic surgery (Table 47.2)

Indirect Fetal Therapy

Induction of Fetal Lung Maturation

Glucocorticoid therapy. Glucocorticoids were first used to stimulate fetal lung maturation by Liggins and Howie (74) in 1972. The currently recommended dose is 2 · 8 mg betamethasone or 2 · 12 mg dexamethasone 24 hours apart (64, 72, 91). Both agents pass through the placenta with little difficulty (125). Hydrocortisone and prednisolone, on the other hand, are largely deactivated in the placenta. Caution should be used with the continuous intravenous administration of beta sympathicomimetics for tocolysis, as this can lead to maternal pulmonary edema.

Table 47.2 Indirect and direct fetal therapy

Form of therapy	Measures
Indirect fetal therapy	
Induction of fetal lung maturation	Glucocorticoid therapy (betamethasone, dexamethasone)
AGS	Dexamethasone therapy
Multiple carboxylase deficiency	Biotin replacement therapy
Hyperthyroidism	Propylthiouracil therapy
Hypothyroidism	L-thyroxine therapy (instilled into the amniotic fluid)
Cardiac arrhythmias	Digoxin, flecainide, etc.
First toxoplasmosis infection in pregnancy	Antimalarial pyrimethamine (Daraprim) and long-term sulfonamide sulfamethoxydiazine (Durenat)
Direct fetal therapy	
➢ Treatment via the umbilical cord	
Anemia	Transfusion of packed red blood cells
Alloimmune thrombocytopenia	Transfusion of platelet concentrate
NIHF	Protein replacement
➢ Percutaneous procedures in the fetus	
Anemia	Intra-abdominal transfusion
Anemia before 18 weeks' gestation	Intracardiac transfusion
Pleural effusion	Thoracocentesis
Ascites	Aspiration of ascites
Urinary tract obstruction	Aspiration of renal pelvis or bladder
Ovarian cyst	Cyst aspiration
➢ Shunt insertion	
Hydronephrosis	Renal or bladder shunt
Pleural effusion	Thoracic shunt
Large lung cyst	Pulmonary shunt
Hydrocephalus	Cerebral ventricular shunt
➢ Intrauterine laser therapy	
Fetofetal transfusion syndrome	Coagulation of communicating placental vessels
Acardius acephalus	Coagulation of second umbilical cord
Sacrococcygeal teratoma	Coagulation of the tumor-feeding vessels
➢ Open/endoscopic fetal surgery	
Congenital diaphragmatic hernia	Repair of defect
Myelomeningocele	Repair of defect
Cystic adenomatoid malformation	Removal of abnormal area
Sacrococcygeal teratoma	Removal of abnormal area

Fetal Metabolic Disorders

Adrenogenital Syndrome (AGS)

In AGS, a 21-hydroxylase defect is present in 80% of cases (100). The defective gene is located on chromosome 6 near the HLA-B and D locus. The metabolic disorder has an autosomal-recessive mode of inheritance. The syndrome is characterized by adrenocortical hyperplasia with increased androgen synthesis. The resulting high androgen levels lead in female fetuses to masculinization of the external genitalia ranging from clitoral hyperplasia to intersex genitals.

Detection. AGS is detected by the molecular genetic examination (83) of chorionic villi.

Treatment. Masculinization can be prevented by the early administration of dexamethasone. The associated suppression of the fetal adrenal cortex prevents the formation of elevated androgen levels (32, 38, 83).

Because sex identification by chorionic villus sampling cannot be done until about 10 weeks' gestation but the anatomic differentiation of the external genitalia begins as early as 7 weeks, treatment of the female embryo at 10 weeks to prevent masculinization comes too late. Therefore, dexamethasone therapy should be started at 6 weeks' gestation even before the sex of the embryo is known (83). The recommended dose is 3 · 0.5 mg/day (38).

If karyotyping at 10 weeks' gestation by CVS shows that the embryo is male, the cortisone therapy can be discontinued in a tapered dose. If a female is identified, the therapy is continued until the end of the pregnancy. Maternal serum cortisol and estradiol levels are determined (about every 4 weeks) to monitor therapeutic response. Also, the fetal adrenal glands and genitals are monitored sonographically as gestational age advances.

Multiple Carboxylase Deficiency

Carboxylase deficiency (= holocarboxylase synthetase defect) is an autosomal-recessive metabolic disorder marked by decreased activity of four biotin-sensitive carboxylases (propionyl CoA-, 3-methylcrotonyl CoA-, pyruvate- and acetyl-CoA-carboxylase). The decreased carboxylase activity leads to severe metabolic acidosis and exanthema formation during the first days of life (94).

Detection. Multiple carboxylase deficiency is diagnosed in amniotic cell culture (95, 114).

Treatment. Biotin replacement is started in the second half of pregnancy. Treatment consists of the maternal oral administration of 10 mg/day biotin (114).

Hyperthyroidism

The reported incidence of neonatal hyperthyroidism is between one in 4000 and one in 40,000 (35). Intrauterine hyperthyroidism occurs in mothers with autoimmune thyroiditis (Graves or Hashimoto thyroiditis). Although the mothers are under treatment for hyperthyroidism and may even have a euthyroid metabolic status (15), high titers of thyroid-stimulating immunoglobulins (TSIs) are found. These IgG antibodies are able to cross the placental barrier and stimulate the fetal thyroid. This can result in intrauterine growth retardation, premature delivery, fetal death, or stillbirth (68).

Fetal hyperthyroidism should be suspected whenever ultrasound reveals an enlarged fetal thyroid accompanied by tachycardia higher than 160 bpm (56, 124). Additional suggestive signs are growth retardation and nonimmune fetal hydrops (NIHF) (56, 124). Prolonged tachycardia in the fetus can lead to fetal heart failure.

Investigation. Fetal hyperthyroidism is investigated by cordocentesis (116, 130) with the determination of T4, thyroid-stimulating immunoglobulin (TSI), and thyroid-stimulating hormone (TSH). Typically this reveals elevated T4 and TSI levels accompanied by low TSH values (56).

Treatment. Intrauterine treatment consists of the maternal oral administration of propylthiouracil (101, 130). The recommended dose is 3 · 50–100 mg/day (116).

Further surveillance consists of regular ultrasound or FHR examinations of the fetus. Maternal serum thyroid values are determined concurrently.

Successful treatment is marked a regression of fetal tachycardia, goiter, heart failure, and NIHF.

Hypothyroidism

Fetal hypothyroidism occurs in between one in 4000 and one in 5000 births (115) and can have various causes (36, 63, 84): thyroid aplasia, hypoplasia or dysplasia in the fetus, an immune disorder, deficient maternal iodine intake (endemic iodine-deficient regions), hormonal synthesis disorders, and the ingestion of goitrogenic substances.

Newborns with hypothyroidism exhibit typical features: respiratory distress, cyanosis, jaundice, poor feeding, hoarse cry, umbilical hernia, and muscular hypotonia. It is suspected that fetal hypothyroidism adversely affects subsequent neurophysiologic development (46).

Investigation. Ultrasound demonstrates an intrauterine fetal goiter. There may be coexisting polyhydramnios due to goiter-induced esophageal obstruction and impaired swallowing.

Fetal hypothyroidism can be diagnosed by cordocentesis with the determination of T4 and TSH in the fetal blood (T4 ↓, TSH ↑) or by amniocentesis with the determination of amniotic fluid TSH (43, 98, 113). The amniotic fluid assay appears to be less reliable, however (108).

Hypothyroidism in newborns is detected by the hypothyroid screen, a TSH filter-paper radioimmunoassay of heel blood on the fifth day after birth.

Treatment. The weekly intra-amniotic administration of 200–500 mg of L-thyroxine is a promising treatment for a sonographically detected goiter and abnormal TSH values in the cord blood or amniotic fluid (1). Positive response is marked by a normalization of T4 and TSH values in the fetal serum, a reduction of TSH levels in the amniotic fluid, and regression of the fetal goiter (43).

Fetal Tachyarrhythmias

The principal forms of tachyarrhythmia are sinus tachycardia, paroxysmal supraventricular tachycardia, and atrial flutter. They can be differentiated by M-mode examination and Doppler echocardiography (see Chapter 25 and reviews of the literature 922, 23, 41, 42, 69, 79, 118]).

Sinus tachycardia. Sinus tachycardia usually has an exogenous cause (tocolysis, infection, hyperthyroidism).

Paroxysmal supraventricular tachycardia. This tachyarrhythmia is characterized by a heart rate of 210–300 bpm based on a reentry mechanism in the presence of accessory conduction pathways (see Chapter 25).

Atrial flutter. Atrial flutter is based on a reentry pathway in the atrium accompanied by a 2 : 1 to 4 : 1 AV block. This disorder is much less common than the other two forms of tachycardia.

Consequences. Supraventricular tachycardia of long duration causes severe shortening of the diastolic filling phase. With rising pressure in

the right atrium and a rise in systemic venous pressure, a nonimmune fetal hydrops develops with fetal heart failure and eventual intrauterine death.

The goal of treatment in tachyarrhythmias is to induce cardioversion to a persistent sinus rhythm, preferably before fetal hydrops has occurred. Once the fetus has become hydropic, it is more difficult for medications to reach the fetus via the maternal circulation.

Treatment. Fetal tachyarrhythmias are among the conditions that are usually responsive to intrauterine therapy. But the selection of an appropriate therapy requires a familiarity with the pharmacology, pharmacokinetics, and side effects of the proposed drug. Also, the therapy should always be preceded by an assessment of maternal electrolytes, renal excretory products, and liver values, and an ECG should be done to exclude maternal heart disease.

Various medications are available for the treatment of fetal tachyarrhythmias (43, 69, 71). Digoxin is generally considered the drug of first choice (Tables 47.**3** and 47.**4**), and digoxin therapy alone will successfully induce cardioversion in approximately 50% of fetuses (43) (Fig. 47.**1**).

In fetuses with hydrops and in nonhydropic cases where fetal tachyarrhythmia does not respond to treatment for 3–4 days, 300–400 mg/day flecainide can additionally be administered in 3 or 4 divided doses (43). The advantage of flecainide is that it will still reach the fetus in cases of fetal and placental hydrops (6).

Direct fetal treatment with amiodarone administered through the umbilical vein (40) should be considered a last recourse due to its side effects and extremely long half life (43).

Besides the antiarrhythmic drugs listed in Table 47.**3**, various other drugs have been described in the literature including verapamil, quinidine, disopyramide, procainamide, and propafenone (69, 70, 71). These agents are rarely used in fetal therapy, however, because of their side effects.

Acute First Toxoplasmosis Infection in Pregnancy

Toxoplasmosis is a danger to the unborn only when a first infection is contracted during pregnancy, because the organisms can cross the placental barrier only during the parasitemic phase. A toxoplasmosis infection that is acquired before pregnancy confers lifelong immunity (see Chapter 33, Infectious Diseases).

Treatment. Whenever a toxoplasmosis infection is detected serologically in pregnancy, treatment is necessary in addition to serum titer follow-ups and a detailed ultrasound evaluation. The treatment of choice depends on gestational age. Treatment with spiramycin is indicated up to 16 weeks' gestation. After 16 weeks, the antimalarial pyrimethamine (Daraprim) is given in conjunction with the long-term sulfonamide sulfamethoxydiazine (Durenat) (Table 47.**5**).

Pyrimethamine should not be used before 16 weeks' gestation due to its possible teratogenic effect. Because pyrimethamine occasionally causes bone-marrow side effects, platelet counts should be obtained weekly, starting before treatment is initiated. When present, these effects can be halted with 15 mg of calcium folinate without compromising the effect of the pyrimethamine (34).

With accurate diagnosis and prompt treatment, the fetal infection rate in maternal toxoplasmosis and the risk of congenital toxoplasmosis can be reduced by 60–100% (34).

Table 47.**3** Antiarrhythmic therapy for supraventricular tachycardia (adapted from 43)

Medication	Action	Metabolism, HL, plasma levels	Indications	Dosage	Fetomaternal ratio	Maternal side effects	Fetal side effects
Digoxin (Lanicor)	Inhibits the Na/K-ATPase pump	Renal excretion; HL 34–36 h; plasma level: 2.0–2.5 ng/mL	SVT	Loading dose for 2–3 days: 1–1.5 mg/24 h i.v. in 3 divided doses. Maintenance: 3 x 0.15–0.2 mg/24 h p.o. (dose reduction in renal failure based on creatinine clearance)	0.8–1.0; decreased in hydrops	Vomiting, dizziness, anorexia, nausea, diarrhea, fatigue, color visual disturbance, disorientation, sleeplessness, sinus bradycardia, AV block, ES, VT, increased glycoside toxicity in hypokalemia, hypomagnesemia and hypercalcemia. *Contraindication:* WPW syndrome, VT and 2nd or 3rd degree AV block	Low uptake in hydropic fetuses; WPW syndrome cannot be diagnosed in the fetus; no digitalis-induced fetal VT reported to date
β-Methyl-digoxin (Lanitop)	Inhibits the Na/K-ATPase pump	Demethylated in the liver to digoxin (first pass effect); otherwise like digoxin	SVT	Loading dose for 2–3 days: 1 mg/24 h i.v. in 3 divided doses. Maintenance: 500–600 μg/24 h p.o. in 3 divided doses (dose reduction in renal failure based on creatinine clearance)	0.8–1.0; decreased in hydrops	Same as digoxin	Same as digoxin
Flecainide (Tambocor)	Sodium channel blockade and conduction delay with normal repolarization	70% hepatic breakdown, 30% renal excretion; HL: 14–20 h; plasma level: 200–1000 ng/mL	SVT VT	3 or 4 x 100 mg p.o.	0.7–0.8	Proarrhythmia, dizziness, nausea, diplopia, headache	Negative inotropism (proarrhythmia)
Sotalol (Sotalex)	Prolongs repolarization by potassium channel blockade and β-adrenoreceptor blockade	Renal excretion; HL: 15–17 h; plasma level: 1.5–2.5 μg/mL	SVT VT	2 x 80–160 mg/24 h p.o. (dose reduction in renal failure based on creatinine clearance)	0.8–1.0	Proarrhythmia: VT; negative inotropism: bradycardia; AV block	Negative inotropism (proarrhythmia)
Amiodarone (Cordarex)	Prolongs repolarization by potassium channel blockade	Metabolized by liver to active desethylamiodarone; renal excretion of metabolites; HL: 14–100 d; plasma level: 1–2 μg/mL amiodarone; desethylamiodarone 0.5–2 times higher	SVT VT	Loading dose for 5–7 days: 1200 mg/24 h i.v., cont. infusion or 5–6 x 200 mg/24 h p.o. Maintenance: 3–4 x 200 mg/24 h p.o. Direct: 2.5–5 mg/kg estimated fetal weight (minus hydrops) into the umbilical vein for 10 min	0.1–0.25; decreased in hydrops	Proarrhythmia: VT; thyroid dysfunction, corneal deposits, photosensitization, hepatic dysfunction (with long-term use, also pulmonary fibrosis, neuropathy, and myopathy); contraception for at least 12 months after therapy	Thyroid dysfunction: transient hypothyroidism (may require monitoring of fetal thyroid values); corneal deposits, mild negative inotropism (proarrhythmia)
Propranolol (Dociton)	β-adrenoreceptor blockade	Rapid breakdown in the liver (first pass effect); HL: 3–5 h; plasma level: 50–1000 ng/mL	SVT VT	2 or 3 x 40–80 mg/24 h p.o.	0.1–0.3	Bronchospasm (not in asthmatics with increased bronchoreactivity); bradycardia, AV block; increased hypoglycemia in diabetics; cold hands and extremities (not in Raynaud disease)	Negative inotropism: bradycardia; AV block; neonate: hypoglycemia, bradycardia, and respiratory depression, possible low birthweight
Verapamil (Isoptin)	Calcium channel blockade	Broken down to mildly active and inactive metabolites in the liver; conjugated metabolites excreted via bile and urine, renal excretion ca. 4% unchanged; HL: 3–7 h; plasma level: 50–100 ng/mL	SVT VT	3 or 4 x 60–120 mg/24 h p.o.	0.3–0.4	AV block, hypotension, constipation, atonic bleeding (avoid concurrent use with magnesium sulfate or beta blockers)	Negative inotropism (contraindicated in hydrops and cardiomegaly), bradycardia, AV block (no direct fetal administration due to risk of cardiogenic shock)

HL = half life,   ES = extrasystole,   SVT = supraventricular tachycardia,   VT = ventricular tachycardia

Table 47.**4**   Guidelines for the intrauterine treatment of supraventricular tachycardia (SVT), supraventricular tachycardia with 1:1 AV conduction and atrial flutter (after 43)

Tachyarrhythmia	First choice	Second choice	Third choice
Paroxysmal supraventricular tachycardia (short-term)	Observation (at least twice weekly)	–	–
Paroxysmal supraventricular tachycardia (persistent, especially before 30 weeks' gestation)	Digoxin	Digoxin + flecainide	Digoxin + sotalol
SVT without hydrops	Digoxin	Digoxin + flecainide	Digoxin + sotalol Alternative: digoxin + amiodarone (direct and transplacental)
SVT with hydrops and without AV valve regurgitation	Digoxin + flecainide	Digoxin	
SVT with hydrops and/or with AV valve regurgitation and scant movements	Digoxin + flecainide	Digoxin + amiodarone (direct and transplacental)	

Table 47.**5**   Treatment of an initial toxoplasmosis infection during pregnancy (adapted from 34)

< 16 weeks Spiramycin (Rovamycine 500)	2–3 g/day for 4 weeks (= 2 or 3 tablets/b.i.d.)
Pyrimethamine (Daraprim) + Sulfamethoxydiazine (Durenat)	Pyrimethamine: Day 1: 50 mg (2 25-mg tablets) Days 2–30: 25 mg/day (1 25-mg tablet) Sulfamethoxydiazine: Day 1: 1.0 g/day (2 0.5-g tablets) Days 2–30: 0.5 g/day (1 0.5-g tablet)

▬ *Direct Fetal Therapy*

Five main types of invasive procedure are available for direct fetal therapy (Table 47.**2**):

- Treatment by cordocentesis
- Percutaneous procedures in the fetus
- Shunt procedures
- Intrauterine laser treatment
- Open and endoscopic fetal surgery

Treatment by Cordocentesis

The use of cordocentesis has created new and effective options in fetal therapy. This particularly applies to intrauterine transfusions for the treatment of fetal anemia. There are various other treatments that offer varying success rates, including platelet replacement for severe fetal thrombocytopenia (67, 93) and protein replacement for NIHF. Another option is direct intravascular therapy for severe fetal tachycardia or tachyarrhythmia (40) that has not responded to indirect treatment by maternal digitalization.

Treatment of Fetal Anemia

Today, fetal anemia is treated almost exclusively by intravascular transfusion via cordocentesis (46, 128). It does not matter whether the fetus has Rh or Kell erythroblastosis, nonimmune hydrops, or a severe parvovirus B19 infection (90).

Intra-abdominal and intravascular transfusion. Studies comparing intra-abdominal and intravascular transfusions have shown that the intravascular route yields a significantly better perinatal result than intra-abdominal transfusion (48). Particularly in cases where fetal hydrops has developed, intravascular transfusion is definitely superior to intra-abdominal transfusion.

Indication. A transfusion is indicated when the fetal hematocrit has fallen below 30% or the fetal hemoglobin is less than 8 g%. In extreme cases this may be seen as early as 18 weeks' gestation.

Technique. The fetus is transfused with washed, filtered, and irradiated Rh-negative type O erythrocytes (packed red blood cells) that are free of HIV and cytomegalovirus. This product minimizes the risk of viral contamination and a graft-versus-host reaction (Fig. 47.**2**). The transfusion is done as a "top-up" procedure–i.e., blood is not exchanged and the packed red cells are simply transfused into the umbilical vein (Fig. 47.**3**). This technique minimizes the risk of needle dislodgement due to fetal movements with possible complications such as umbilical cord hematoma, bleeding, or vasospasm.

The transfusion volume (TV) depends on the initial hematocrit (1st Hct), the donor hematocrit, and the fetoplacental blood volume (105):

$$TV = (desired\ Hct - 1st\ Hct)/donor\ Hct \cdot fetoplacental\ blood\ volume$$

From 20 to 50 mL is transfused per session, depending on fetal age and fetal hematocrit. The needle tip position and fetal heart rate are continually monitored during the transfusion. The transfusion rate is approximately 5 mL/min. The goal is to achieve a fetal hematocrit (desired Hct) of approximately 40%.

Transfusion interval. The need for a repeat transfusion depends on how low the fetal hematocrit is. Initially the transfusion interval may be from one day to two weeks, depending on severity. Later the interval may be increased to about three weeks, depending on the response (Fig. 47.**4**).

Treatment of Alloimmune Thrombocytopenia

Alloimmune thrombocytopenia occurs in one in 1000 to one in 5000 live births (89). In this condition, maternal antibodies against platelet-specific alloantigens lead to the destruction of fetal platelets. Because platelet antigens are already expressed by 16 weeks' gestation (45) and the placental transfer of IgG antibodies may occur as early as 14 weeks, it is possible for fetal thrombocytopenia to develop in early pregnancy (89).

The antibody most commonly found in Caucasian women is anti-HPA1a (78–89%) followed by anti-HPA5b (6–15%); the other antibodies are much less common (87, 126). It should be noted that the detection of platelet-specific antibodies does not necessarily mean that fetal or neonatal thrombocytopenia will develop (89). When autoimmune thrombocytopenic purpura is diagnosed in the mother, fetal thrombocytopenia will develop in 37–70% of cases (7, 97). The main risk to the fetus is that the low platelet count will lead to severe cerebral hemorrhage with neurologic sequelae or fetal death. Approximately 50% of cerebral hemorrhages occur in utero, usually between 30 and 35 weeks' gestation (87).

Detection. Fetal thrombocytopenia is detected by an initial cordocentesis performed between 20 and 22 weeks (89). Since normal platelet counts in the fetus are very similar to those in adults and do not vary appreciably with gestational age (65), normal adult values can be used as a reference for platelet evaluation. A platelet count below 150,000/μL means that fetal thrombocytopenia is present, and a count less than 50,000/μL indicates severe thrombocytopenia (85). The fetal blood group is also determined at initial cordocentesis.

Indication and technique. Intrauterine treatment is considered necessary when the fetal platelet count falls below 50,000/µL (88). An irradiated, cytomegalovirus-free concentrate of 2.5–4 million platelets/µL is injected with a 22-gauge needle into the umbilical vein at the placental insertion of the cord. Since the fetal platelet counts will fall again within a short time, weekly transfusions are required. The fetal platelet counts after each transfusion should be in the range of 300,000 to 500,000/µL (89).

The principal risks of this therapy are severe umbilical cord bleeding at the puncture site and hematoma formation in the umbilical cord with obstruction of the umbilical vessels. These risks can be minimized by immobilizing the fetus with curare derivatives (27).

Maternal treatment with immunoglobulins is considered less effective than the transfusion of platelet concentrate into the umbilical vein (44).

Treatment of Nonimmune Fetal Hydrops

In nonimmune fetal hydrops (NIHF), which can have a variety of underlying causes, the therapeutic approach depends critically on the diagnostic findings (cordocentesis, TORCH) (see Chapter 18, Nonimmune Fetal Hydrops).

Blood transfusion. When fetal anemia has been detected by cordocentesis, the intrauterine transfusion of O–Rh-negative donor blood is the treatment of choice.

Human albumin therapy. If cord blood analysis indicates a low albumin level, human albumin can be administered by cordocentesis for the correction of hypoproteinemia (Fig. 47.**5**). The treatment is of doubtful efficacy, however, because the serum albumin levels will quickly fall again and multiple cord punctures are necessary.

Medical therapy. If ultrasound shows evidence of fetal heart failure, maternal digitalization should be performed. If serologic testing reveals a fetal infection, therapy should be provided that is specific for the infecting organism (see Chapter 33, Infectious Diseases).

Needle aspiration of body cavities. The needle aspiration of fetal body cavities (hydrothorax, ascites) is more diagnostic than therapeutic because the fluid tends to reaccumulate within a short time. An exception is the therapeutic aspiration of fetal pleural effusions just prior to delivery.

Percutaneous Procedures in the Fetus

Intra-abdominal Transfusion for Rh Incompatibility

Practiced mainly in the 1960s and 1970s, puncture of the fetal abdomen for intra-abdominal blood transfusion in an anemic fetus has largely been abandoned because the survival rate was only 24–56% (14). The outlook is especially poor in cases of fetal hydrops, which hampers the absorption of red blood cells from the abdomen (127). Instead of an intra-abdominal transfusion, the current practice is to direct a needle into the umbilical vein under ultrasound guidance and transfuse the blood directly into the vessel. The advantage of intravenous over intra-abdominal transfusion is that the donor blood enters the circulation directly, providing the fastest possible correction of anemia. This method is effective even in fetal hydrops, where it is much less likely that an intra-abdominal transfusion would be successful.

Intracardiac Transfusion for Early Anemia

In cases of severe Rh incompatibility with onset of fetal anemia before 18 weeks' gestation, it is difficult to transfuse blood via the umbilical cord. If this is not possible, a last recourse is to introduce a needle into the fetal heart and transfuse blood directly into one of the ventricles (Fig. 47.**6**).

Chylothorax

The detection of pleural effusion in the fetus always warrants further investigation. The presence of an early, pronounced, persistent intrathoracic fluid collection can lead to pulmonary hypoplasia (21). One way to prevent this is to aspirate the effusion(s) with a percutaneous needle. A single, early aspiration is unlikely to be successful, however, as the fluid will quickly reaccumulate, and therefore serial aspirations are required. As an alternative, Rodeck et al. (106) recommend the intrauterine placement of a thoracoamniotic shunt.

Follow-up may be adequate for a moderate or nonprogressive pleural effusion. To prevent acute respiratory distress in the newborn, however, both pleural effusions in the fetus should be selectively aspirated just prior to delivery (by cesarean section) (99).

Technique. Following local anesthesia, a needle is introduced into the more favorably situated fetal pleural space, and most of the fluid is aspirated. Then, by external manipulation and repositioning the mother, the fetus is moved to a position in which the opposite pleural space can also be punctured and drained (Fig. 47.**7**). With the fluid thus removed, the neonatal lungs can adequately expand without the need for emergency postpartum thoracentesis.

Severe Fetal Ascites

Percutaneous aspiration of the fetal abdomen in ascites is done more for diagnostic than therapeutic intent. But when the ascites is severe, prenatal decompression of the fetal abdomen may be appropriate just before delivery to lower the risk of respiratory problems in the newborn.

Fetal Urinary Tract Obstruction

Moderate, unilateral hydronephrosis that is not compressing the fetal thoracic organs generally does not require intrauterine intervention if the amniotic fluid volume is normal. But if the hydronephrosis is progressive and of early onset (renal pelvis > 3 cm in diameter) or if there is significant bilateral urinary tract obstruction, severe damage may occur to the renal parenchyma, resulting in serious compromise of renal function.

Urine analysis. In principle, the obstructed renal pelvis or greatly distended urinary bladder can be decompressed by percutaneous drainage (Fig. 47.**8**). But because the fluid quickly reaccumulates, the percutaneous aspiration of fetal urine is done more to assist the diagnostic evaluation of renal function than as a therapeutic procedure. If urine analysis (Na, Cl, microglobulins, osmolality) indicates severe renal function impairment, there is little rationale for further treatment. Several urinary parameters are available for the assessment of fetal renal function. Levels that are above designated threshold values indicate a poor prognosis: sodium > 100 mg/dL, chloride > 90 mg/dL, osmolality > 200 mosmol/L, calcium > 8 mg/dL, β2-microglobulin > 6 mg/dL, and total protein > 40 mg/dL. It should be noted that the urine values change with advancing gestational age.

If urine analysis shows that one kidney is still functional, a shunt procedure may be considered.

Indirect fetal therapy

Fig. 47.1 Treatment of fetal cardiac arrhythmias.
a Supraventricular tachycardia (214 bpm), 32 weeks.
b Cardioversion on third day after starting digitalis. Heart rate 125 bpm.

Direct fetal therapy

Fig. 47.2 *Left:* intrauterine blood transfusion under ultrasound guidance. *Right:* transfusion of packed red blood cells (0 Rh negative).

Fig. 47.3 Intrauterine blood transfusion with a needle passed into the umbilical vein at the placental cord insertion (large arrow = needle tip). When the needle is correctly placed in the umbilical vein, ultrasound during the transfusion will show small turbulent zones moving toward the fetus (short arrows).

Fig. 47.4 Transfusion of a hydropic fetus with an initial Hb of 3.7 g%. After a total of four transfusions, the Hb rises to 14.8 g%.

Fig. 47.5 Unsuccessful albumin replacement in nonimmune fetal hydrops. The replacement produces only a brief rise in albumin, which soon returns to the original level.

Fig. 47.6 Intracardiac transfusion in an hydropic fetus at 17 weeks, 1 day. The needle tip appears as a bright echo within the cardiac ventricle (arrow).

Fig. 47.7 Percutaneous drainage of fetal hydrothorax at 36 weeks.
Left: after successful aspiration of the left side, the needle is passed into the right pleural space (arrow = needle tip). Vertex presentation with the spine to the left. *Right:* following the aspiration, only a small fluid crescent is visible in the right pleural space. Both lungs are well expanded.

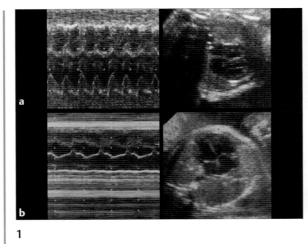

1

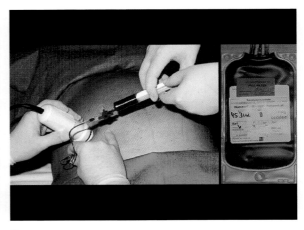

2

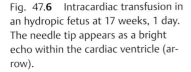

3

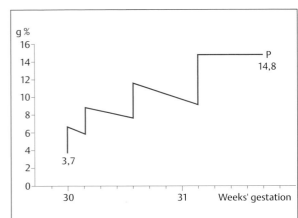

4

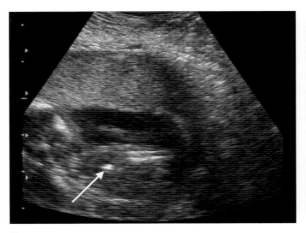

5

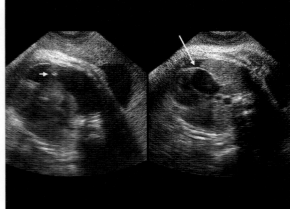

6

7

Ovarian Cyst

Fetal ovarian cysts usually do not require prenatal treatment when they are small. But a rapidly enlarging cyst will cause the displacement of other abdominal organs, and percutaneous drainage of the cyst can be of therapeutic benefit in these cases (Fig. 47.**9**).

Shunt Procedures

Today it is believed that an intrauterine shunt procedure is appropriate only in selected cases. Basically, the placement of a shunt may be considered in a fetal organ that has become cystically expanded by an extensive fluid collection. Shunts are an option for urinary tract obstruction, severe hydrothorax, a large pulmonary cyst, and hydrocephalus. The goal of shunting is to decompress the obstructed cavity system, thereby preventing damage to the surrounding parenchyma.

Disadvantages of shunting are that coexisting oligohydramnios makes intrauterine shunt placement more difficult and that shunt dislodgement or obstruction occurs in 29% of cases (10). Other possible complications are the development of oligohydramnios accompanied by maternal ascites (107) or migration of the shunt into the uterine wall or maternal abdomen (8).

Shunting for Urinary Tract Obstruction

Controversial therapy. The intrauterine treatment of obstructive uropathy has sparked considerable debate among prenatal diagnosticians, pediatricians, and urologists in recent years. Intrauterine vesicoamniotic shunting was first described in the early 1980s by Harrison et al. (50) as a treatment for fetal urinary tract obstruction and oligohydramnios. In subsequent years various other groups of authors all over the world attempted this invasive procedure (9, 10). A lack of selection criteria and various complications (shunt dislodgement or obstruction) cast doubt on the benefits of antenatal shunting, especially among pediatricians and urologists. Although the improved resolution of modern ultrasound equipment and specific biochemical tests on fetal uterine aspirated from the obstructed bladder or kidney provided significantly better criteria for the evaluation of fetal renal function, invasive prenatal urologic procedures have been increasingly abandoned in recent years due to the risk of complications and the questionable fetal benefit.

Prerequisites. Today it appears that intrauterine shunting for obstructive uropathy is appropriate only if several basic criteria are satisfied (80):
- Urinary tract obstruction has been diagnosed with ultrasound.
- Ultrasound has excluded associated anomalies.
- abnormal karyotype has been excluded.
- Fetal urinalysis has excluded irreversible renal damage.
- The procedure is performed at a center where interdisciplinary follow-up is available.
- The infant is delivered at a perinatal center.

Goal. The goal of intrauterine shunting is to prevent permanent renal damage and pulmonary hypoplasia by decompressing the obstructed urinary tract. Harrison et al. (51) demonstrated that this was possible in 1982.

Bilateral hydronephrosis. In cases where there is early onset of bilateral hydronephrosis with megalocystis and oligohydramnios, the placement of a vesicoamniotic shunt (pigtail catheter) in the distended urinary bladder can provide complete urinary tract decompression (Fig. 47.**10**). If giant unilateral hydronephrosis has developed, displacing the abdominal organs and compressing the fetal lung, the greatly distended renal pelvis can be decompressed by the direct insertion of a pigtail catheter (Figs. 47.**11**, 47.**12**).

Shunting for unilateral hydronephrosis, unlike that for bilateral hydronephrosis, is a controversial issue. The placement of a shunt after 34 weeks' gestation is not appropriate due to the risk of a fetal complication. At that stage it is better to deliver the infant early and provide appropriate neonatal treatment.

Shunting for Isolated Chylothorax

If an isolated pleural effusion forms and subsequently enlarges, fetal pulmonary hypoplasia and significant cardiac displacement can be prevented by establishing continuous shunt drainage from the pleural space into the amniotic fluid (8, 92, 104, 106, 109, 110). Similar to the procedure for a bilateral urinary tract obstruction, the shunt consists of a double pigtail catheter (Rocket, London) (outer diameter 21 mm, inner diameter 0.15 mm) placed into the midthoracic pleural space using local anesthesia and aseptic technique (109). It is unnecessary to induce fetal paralysis for this procedure (12). Sebire and Nicolaides (109) reported a survival rate of 100% (31/31) in thoracoamniotic shunting for pleural effusions in nonhydropic fetuses and 50% (27/54) in hydropic fetuses. With thoracentesis, on the other hand, they achieved a survival rate of only 50% (4/8) in nonhydropic fetuses and 33% (3/9) in hydropic fetuses.

Shunting for Cystic Adenomatoid Malformation

Analogous to a pleural effusion, a shunt can be placed in a large pulmonary cyst to prevent compression of the surrounding lung tissue (13).

Shunting for Hydrocephalus

Introduced during the 1980s, intrauterine shunting for hydrocephalus (Denver shunt with a one-way valve) (25) was later abandoned when it was discovered that a large percentage of fetuses with hydrocephalus had associated anomalies and undetected cerebral malformations and that ultimately less than 5% of hydrocephalus cases are suitable for an intrauterine shunt procedure. From 1982 to 1985, a total of 37 shunt procedures were listed in the International Fetal Surgery Registry (78). The treatment-associated mortality rate for these procedures was 10.25%.

Intrauterine Laser Treatment

Laser Treatment in Fetofetal Transfusion Syndrome

When used in fetofetal transfusion syndrome of early onset, intrauterine laser treatment (28, 61, 122, 123) permits the selective coagulation of superficial vascular anastomoses on the placenta, thereby correcting the unbalanced blood flow between the donor and recipient fetuses.

Technique. Using local anesthesia and aseptic technique, a trocar is inserted transabdominally into the amniotic cavity of the recipient (polyhydramnios), and the amniotic membrane separating the two sacs is located with a fetoscope. A 0.4-mm fiber is introduced, and all anastomoses are individually identified and coagulated with the laser (Nd:YAG) (Fig. 47.**13**). This can effectively halt the unilateral perfusion across the anastomoses. After the anastomoses have been coagulated, the polyhydramnios is drained until a normal amniotic fluid volume is restored.

Comparison with serial amniocentesis. In a comparative study of laser treatment and serial decompression amniocentesis, Hecher et al. (61) showed that the laser treatment can not only successfully treat polyhydramnios but can significantly increase the likelihood of at least one surviving twin. Polyhydramnios recurred in only one of 73 cases

Fig. 47.**8** Percutaneous drainage of bilateral hydronephrosis, 33 weeks.
1 = Dilated right renal pelvis,
2 = dilated left renal pelvis,
3 = urinary bladder. Arrow = needle.

Fig. 47.**9** Therapeutic drainage of a giant ovarian cyst that has caused significant internal organ displacement, 35 weeks.

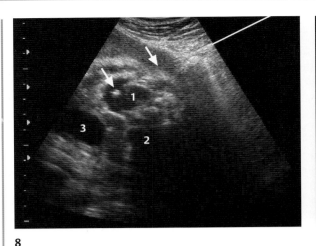

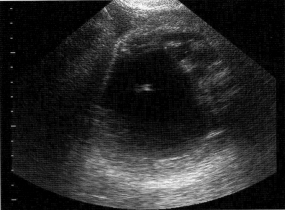

8

9

Fig. 47.**10** Placement of a vesicoamniotic shunt for bilateral hydronephrosis and megalocystis. *Left:* puncture of the fetal bladder for insertion of the shunt (lower inset). *Right:* shunt in place, providing effective drainage of urine into the amniotic cavity.

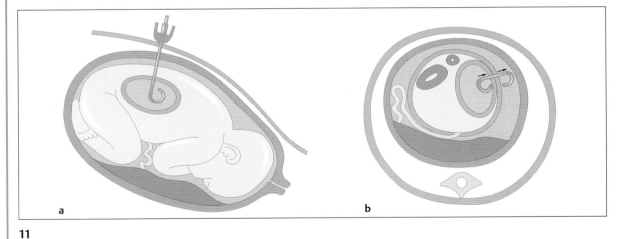

10

Fig. 47.**11** Bilateral hydronephrosis treated with a shunt inserted into the dilated renal pelvis.

a Longitudinal section during shunt placement.

b Cross section with the shunt in place. Urine flows through the shunt (arrows) directly into the amniotic fluid.

a

b

11

Fig. 47.**12** *Left:* normal shunt position, 9 weeks after placement. The right renal pelvis shows only mild residual dilatation. *Right:* postpartum appearance with the shunt still in place.

Fig. 47.**13** Laser therapy in fetofetal transfusion syndrome. Inset: after the vascular anastomoses are identified, they are coagulated with the laser near the membrane separating the two amniotic sacs.

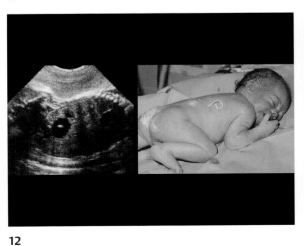

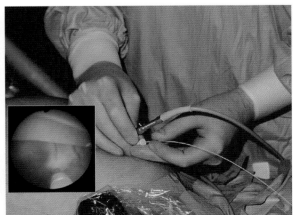

12

13

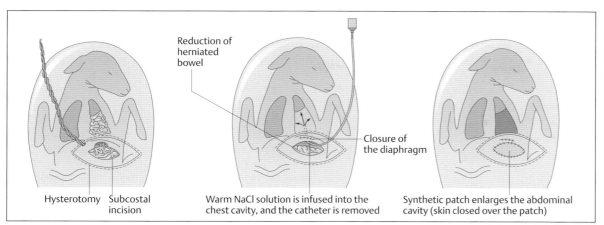

14

Fig. 47.**14** Open intrauterine repair of a congenital diaphragmatic hernia (in a lamb model) (after 49).

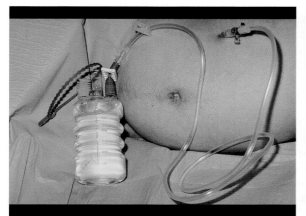

15

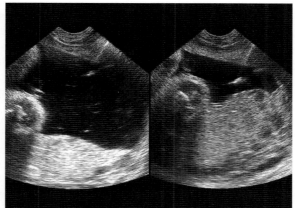

16

Treatment of abnormal amniotic fluid volume

Fig. 47.**15** Decompression amniocentesis for massive polyhydramnios. Patient is in left lateral decubitus.

Fig. 47.**16** Decompression amniocentesis for severe polyhydramnios, 36 weeks. *Left:* before decompression. *Right:* after drainage of 3000 cc amniotic fluid.

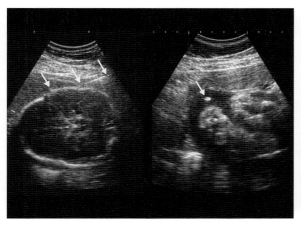

17

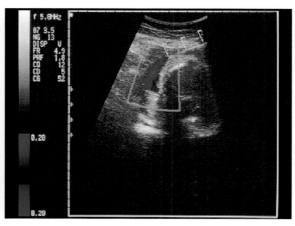

18

Fig. 47.**17** Amnioinfusion for anhydramnios at 31 weeks.
Left: the needle is inserted tangentially, bypassing the right side of the fetal cranium (arrows). *Right:* appearance after instillation of 400 mL NaCl. The needle tip (arrow) is now clearly surrounded on all sides by amniotic fluid.

Fig. 47.**18** Amnioinfusion. The instillation jet (blue) is visualized with color Doppler. Arrows = needle.

treated by endoscopic laser coagulation. The rate of pregnancies with at least one surviving twin in the laser group, at 79%, was significantly higher than in the group treated by serial amniocentesis (60%). Regarding the timing of the delivery, laser treatment added an average of three weeks to the length of the pregnancy compared with serial amniocentesis. The percentage of cases with the intrauterine death of both twins was only 3% in the laser group versus 19% in the amniocentesis group. In both groups, ultrasound revealed brain abnormalities in some of the newborns: 6% in the laser-treated group and 18% in the group treated by serial amniocentesis (61).

Laser Treatment in Acardius Acranius

Acardius acranius is a condition that poses a high risk to the healthy twin. Because of the greatly increased circulatory load imposed on the healthy "pump twin," the latter suffers early cardiac failure with an approximately 50% rate of intrauterine death (86, 119). One treatment option is to occlude the umbilical cord vessels in the acardiac twin. This can be done with N-butyl-2-cyanoacrylate glue (Histoacryl), endoscopic ligation, or by endoscopic laser coagulation (58, 121). The laser occlusion should be done as early as possible (by about 16 weeks' gestation) (59) because as the pregnancy advances and the umbilical cord becomes edematous, it is no longer possible to coagulate the cord vessels even with a high-energy beam. One alternative in these cases is to coagulate the communicating vessels directly on the placental surface (58).

Laser Treatment of Sacrococcygeal Teratoma

Most fetuses with a sacrococcygeal teratoma are hemodynamically stable, and intervention is unnecessary until after the baby is delivered. But with extensive intrauterine tumor growth and large AV shunts in the tumor, there will likely be a massive increase in fetal cardiac output leading to heart failure and intrauterine fetal death. The goals of endoscopic fetal surgery are to diminish blood flow to the tumor and thus reduce the AV anastomoses, arrest further tumor growth, prevent intratumoral hemorrhage, and improve fetal cardiac function (60). In some cases this can be accomplished by laser coagulation of the tumor vessels (57). At present, however, laser treatment cannot eliminate the need for definitive postpartum resection of the tumor.

Open and Endoscopic Fetal Operations

Open fetal surgery is still limited to animal models in many areas. For certain conditions, however, successful results have already been reported in human fetuses. At present, this type of fetal therapy is considered only for cases that would otherwise have a poor prognosis.

The main problem with open fetal surgery is that techniques that are successful in animal models cannot be directly applied to humans. For example, fetal surgery can be performed in sheep with relatively few problems because the risk of premature labor is much lower than in primates. In humans, however, uterine contractions are a serious and frequent sequela to open fetal surgery. Besides high-dose tocolysis with risk of pulmonary edema and a prolonged hospital stay, the only appropriate mode of delivery is by cesarean section.

The procedures that have been performed in human fetuses with varying degrees of success include the open repair of diaphragmatic hernia and spina bifida and the open resection of cystic adenomatoid malformation and sacrococcygeal teratoma.

Diaphragmatic Hernia

As early as 1981, Harrison et al. (49) of San Francisco showed that the intrauterine surgical repair of diaphragmatic hernia in the fetal lamb (Fig. 47.**14**) could result in normal lung development, substantially improving the otherwise poor chance of survival.

Nonherniated liver. Based on the clinical experience that Harrison et al. (54) acquired in humans as part of a prospective study, we now know that the survival rate of fetuses with a diaphragmatic hernia and no intrathoracic herniation of liver tissue is not improved by open fetal surgery compared with delaying the surgery until after the baby is delivered (3/4 versus 6/7).

Herniated left lobe. Cases in which the left lobe of the liver has herniated into the chest cavity (approximately 50% of cases) pose a major challenge to open fetal surgery. Returning the liver to the abdominal cavity in these cases causes a kinking of the umbilical vein, leading to obstruction of venous flow and subsequent death (53). After it was shown in animal models that transient occlusion of the trachea with an external clip or internal balloon leads to enlargement of the lungs and induces a gradual reduction of the abdominal organs that have herniated into the chest (30, 111, 120), new treatment strategies have been devised based on the use of endoscopic techniques. Fetoscopic transient occlusion of the fetal trachea with a clip, performed in a total of 16 human fetuses, yielded a significantly better survival rate (75%) than in babies that were managed postnatally by extracorporeal membrane oxygenation (38%) (55).

Spina Bifida

Experiments in fetal sheep in 1995 showed that the early closure of spina bifida can prevent serious neurologic sequelae (81). Since then, the first successful results have been reported in human fetuses. Adzick et al. (5) described the successful open repair of spina bifida in a 23-week-old fetus. A shunt was additionally placed to prevent hydrocephalus. Bruner et al. (16) reported on the intrauterine endoscopic repair of spinal defects in four fetuses with a myelomeningocele.

Cystic Adenomatoid Malformation

After it was shown in animal models that lung tissue could be successfully resected in the fetus (2), open lobectomies were subsequently performed in human fetuses (3). In 1998, Adzick et al. (4) reported on the open surgical treatment of 13 hydropic fetuses. In eight of these fetuses, lobectomy was followed by a rapid clearing of hydrops and significant compensatory intrauterine lung growth. All eight of the fetuses survived.

Sacrococcygeal Teratoma

Open fetal surgery was performed in five hydropic fetuses with giant sacrococcygeal teratomas at the Fetal Treatment Center in San Francisco. All of the fetuses were born prematurely. Two of the babies died from causes relating to prematurity. Of the remaining three, who initially did well, one died during the resection of residual tumor and another died on the day before the scheduled release date from complications relating to a central venous catheter. The remaining child developed normally (96). A new therapeutic approach is based on minimally invasive coagulation of the tumor vessels (96).

Other Animal Models

Cleft lip and palate. The treatment of cleft lip and palate in the fetal stage has been tested in various animal models (mouse [47], rabbit [76], lamb [20]). These experiments have shown that the correction of this defect in the fetal stage leads to an essentially complete recovery–i.e., the defect can be repaired without scarring. This may relate to various antenatal factors such as abundant epidermal growth factor, high fibronectin levels, an immature reticuloendothelial system, a mild inflammatory response, and the presence of amniotic fluid.

Skeletal malformations. Research in a primate model has shown that intrauterine bone grafting can be performed in fetal monkeys, inasmuch as the fetal immune system is still immature and will tolerate bone allografts (82).

Future of Fetal Surgery

Despite the enthusiasm for open fetal surgery and its advances, it should be kept in mind that so far these procedures have been performed only at a few centers and that despite some success in humans, they are still of an experimental nature due to their uncertain outcome. It may be that endoscopic techniques will be the key to controlling the problem of postoperative uterine contractions as well as finding new approaches that entail less risk to the pregnant woman.

Treatment of Abnormal Amniotic Fluid Volume

Both an increase and decrease in amniotic fluid volume are associated with increased rates of perinatal morbidity and mortality for the child. If the cause of the condition cannot be corrected, the only other option is to provide symptomatic treatment aimed at establishing a normal amniotic fluid volume and thus reducing the overall risk to the fetus. In polyhydramnios, this means treating the condition medically or by amniotic drainage. In oligohydramnios, symptomatic treatment consists of amnioinfusion.

Medical Treatment of Polyhydramnios

Indomethacin. If the development of polyhydramnios is based on increased fetal urine production, it can be treated with indomethacin, a prostaglandin synthetase inhibitor (19, 77). The amniotic fluid volume can be reduced within a few days by the maternal oral administration of $4 \cdot 25$ mg/day.

If the polyhydramnios has a cause other than excessive urine production, such as a gastrointestinal obstruction, indomethacin therapy is less effective. A better option in these cases is serial amniocentesis. Indomethacin therapy is contraindicated in fetofetal transfusion syndrome, as it would further compromise the already oliguric donor (17).

Possible maternal side effects of indomethacin therapy are gastrointestinal disturbances, impaired renal function, and pulmonary edema. In the fetus, the main risk is premature closure of the ductus arteriosus (62). Consequently, the patency of the ductus arteriosus should be checked regularly with Doppler ultrasound.

Decompression Amniocentesis in Polyhydramnios

Serial Amniocentesis in a Singleton Pregnancy

Severe polyhydramnios is associated with maternal and fetal complications (31). A significant increase in amniotic fluid volume leads not only to serious maternal complaints (feeling of pressure, urinary stasis, respiratory problems) but can also trigger early labor with risk of premature membrane rupture and an increased risk of preterm delivery.

Technique. To relieve maternal complaints and lengthen the gestation of the still-immature fetus, an excessive amniotic fluid volume can be corrected by serial amniocentesis (Figs. 47.**15**, 47.**16**). This consists of draining between 2 and 4 L of amniotic fluid at intervals of 1–2 weeks, depending on the gestational age and amniotic fluid volume, with the goal of restoring and maintaining an approximately normal fluid volume. The drainage is performed with the patient in a lateral decubitus position to prevent a vena cava syndrome. After sterile preparation of the abdomen, a 19-gauge needle is inserted into the amniotic cavity under ultrasound guidance, and the amniotic fluid is sterilely aspirated into 500-mL negative-pressure bottles. Following the procedure, the decompression of the uterine cavity will usually incite brief uterine contractions, which can be stopped with 6–12 hours of intravenous tocolysis. If the pressure is relieved too rapidly and a very large fluid volume is withdrawn, placental abruption is likely to occur.

An ultrasound examination should be performed immediately after the procedure. FHR monitoring is also recommended after the ultrasound.

Serial Amniocentesis in Fetofetal Transfusion Syndrome

Symptomatic treatment. Untreated, a severe fetofetal transfusion syndrome in the second trimester will cause a large amniotic fluid pocket to form around the recipient twin with severe oligohydramnios around the donor (the "stuck twin"). The polyhydramnios at just 20–24 weeks' gestation will cause significant maternal complaints ranging to respiratory distress. An alternative to laser treatment in these cases is serial amniocentesis (24, 33, 60, 103, 117). Unlike laser coagulation, this is only a symptomatic treatment. It involves the sterile drainage of amnio-tic fluid at intervals of about one week, each time withdrawing enough fluid to restore a normal amniotic fluid volume (see above).

Fetal outcome. In a comparative study of laser treatment and serial amniocentesis, Hecher et al. (61) found that the average delivery time in the amniocentesis group was 30.7 weeks' gestation. The rate of pregnancies with at least one surviving child was 60%, and there was a 19% rate of intrauterine death of both twins. Neonatal ultrasound revealed brain abnormalities in 18% of the infants. Denbow et al. (29) found signs of antenatally acquired cerebral lesions in 35% of the infants surviving after amniotic drainage and signs of perinatally acquired lesions in 23%.

Amniotic septostomy. Berry et al. (11) recommend that in fetofetal transfusion syndrome with polyhydramnios and a stuck twin, incision of the amniotic septum (amniotic septostomy) should be done in addition to amniocentesis in order to permanently equalize the pressures between the two amniotic cavities. Reportedly, this technique also results in a higher survival rate.

Amnioinfusion

In cases with pronounced oligohydramnios and no evidence of membrane rupture, the infusion of fluid into the amniotic cavity has both a diagnostic and therapeutic benefit (18, 37, 39, 73, 102, 112) (Fig. 47.**17**).

Improved diagnosis. From a diagnostic standpoint, the added intrauterine fluid significantly improves ultrasound visualization of the fetus, allowing better scrutiny of the fetal body surface and better assessment of swallowing and excretory functions (gastric and bladder filling). Amnioinfusion also facilitates fluid sampling for fetal karyotyping, although the karyotype cannot always be determined from the aspirated fluid.

Therapeutic goals. From a therapeutic standpoint, it is hoped that amnioinfusion for oligohydramnios (barring fetal nonviability due to anomalies) can prevent fetal pulmonary hypoplasia, prevent joint contractures, prevent umbilical cord compression with associated FHR changes, and prolong the duration of the pregnancy.

Technique. Usually a 0.9% NaCl solution is infused into the amniotic cavity. Other options are Ringer solution or 5% glucose. First the maternal abdomen and transducer are sterilely prepared. Local anesthesia is not strictly necessary but is helpful in case the needle position has to be adjusted during the procedure. Then a 19-gauge needle is introduced into the amniotic cavity under ultrasound guidance. This can be done relatively easily if a residual amniotic fluid pocket is still present. But if oligohydramnios is severe, the insertion will be much more difficult. To avoid fetal injury or inadvertent umbilical cord puncture in these cases, the needle should not be introduced from the front of the fetus or in an area of looped cord, but should be carefully directed past the fetal occiput into the amniotic cavity. The needle is advanced in a tangential direction between the amnion and the fetal scalp. If the needle is correctly positioned within the cavity, the initial infusion will produce a good fluid stream that is clearly visible with color Doppler ultrasound (Fig. 47.**18**). A weak stream indicates faulty placement of the needle tip. The fluid volume necessary for amnioinfusion ranges from 300 to 600 mL, depending on the severity of the oligohydramnios and the gestational age. Potential complications of amnioinfusion are fetal injury, misdirected infusion, bleeding, infection, uterine contractions, FHR alterations, and rupture of the membranes.

Serial amnioinfusions. Serial infusions may be necessary depending on how quickly the amniotic fluid volume declines following the procedure. The additional infusions are performed at intervals of 1–2 weeks, depending on the situation.

References

1. Abuhamad, A.Z., Fisher, D.A., Warsof, S.L. et al.: Antenatal diagnosis and treatment of fetal goitrous hypothyroidism: case report and review of the literature. Ultrasound Obstet. Gynecol. 6 (1995) 368–371
2. Adzick, N.S., Hu, L.M., Davies, P., Flake, A.W., Reid, L.M., Harrison, M.: Compensatory lung growth after pneumonectomy in the fetus. Surg. Forum 37 (1986) 648
3. Adzick, N.S.: Fetal cystic adenomatoid malformation of the lung: diagnosis, perinatal management, and outcome. Semin. Thorac. Cardiovasc. Surg. 6 (1994) 247–252
4. Adzick, N.S., Harrison, M.R., Crombleholme, T.M., Flake, A.W., Howell, L.J.: Fetal lung lesions: management and outcome. Amer. J. Obstet. Gynecol. 179 (1998) 884–889
5. Adzick, N.S., Sutton, L.N., Crombleholme, T.M., Flake, A.W.: Successful fetal surgery for spina bifida. Lancet 352 (1998) 1675–1676
6. Allan, L.D., Chita, S.K., Sharland, G.K., Maxwell, D., Priestley, K.: Flecainide in the treatment of fetal tachycardias. Brit. Heart J. 65 (1991) 46–48
7. Beck, R.: Perinatal and neonatal aspects of maternal idiopathic thrombocytopenia purpura. Amer. J. Perinatol. 1 (1984) 251–258
8. Becker, R., Arabin, B., Novak, A., Entezami, M., Weitzel, H.K.: Successful treatment of primary fetal hydrothorax by long-time drainage from week 23. Fetal Diagn. Ther. 8 (1993) 331–337
9. Berkowitz, R.L., Glickman, M.G., Smith, G.J. et al.: Fetal urinary tract obstruction: what is the role of surgical intervention in utero? Amer. J. Obstet. Gynecol. 144 (1982) 367–375
10. Bernaschek, G., Deutinger, J., Hansmann, M., Bald, R., Holzgreve, W., Bollmann, R.: Feto-amniotic shunting – report of the experience of four European centres. Prenat. Diagn. 14 (1994) 821–833
11. Berry, D., Montgomery, L., Johnson, A., Saade, G., Moise, K.: Amniotic septostomy for the treatment of the stuck twin sequence. Amer. J. Obstet. Gynecol. 176 (1997) A44
12. Blott, M., Nicolaides, K.H., Greenough, A.: Pleuroamniotic shunting for decompression of fetal pleural effusions. Obstet. Gynecol. 71 (1988) 798–800
13. Blott, M., Nicolaides, K.H., Greenough, A.: Postnatal respiratory function after chronic drainage of fetal pulmonary cyst. Amer. J. Obstet. Gynecol. 159 (1988) 858–859
14. Bock, J.T.: Intrauterine transfusions in severe rhesus hemolytic disease. Acta Obstet. Gynecol. Scand. Suppl. 53 (1976) 29–36
15. Bruinse, H.W., Vermeulen-Meiners, C., Wit, J.M.: Fetal treatment for thyreotoxicosis in non-thyreotoxic pregnant women. Fetal Ther. 3 (1988) 152–157
16. Bruner, J.P., Richards, W.O., Tulipan, N.B., Arney, T.L.: Endoscopic coverage of fetal myelomeningocele in utero. Amer. J. Obstet. Gynecol. 180 (1999) 153–158
17. Buderus, S., Thomas, B., Fahnenstich, H., Kowalewski, S.: Renal failure in two preterm infants: toxic effect of prenatal maternal indomethacin treatment? Brit. J. Obstet. Gynaecol. 100 (1993) 97–98
18. Burges, A., Strauss, A., Heer, I., Hasbargen, U., Hepp, H.: Amnioninfusion in der pränatalen Diagnostik und Therapie. Gynäkologe 32 (1999) 832–839
19. Cabrol, D., Landesmann, R., Müller, J., Uzan, M., Sureau, C., Saxena, B.B.: Treatment of polyhydramnios with prostaglandin synthetase inhibitor (indomethacin). Amer. J. Obstet. Gynecol. 157 (1987) 422–426
20. Canady, J.W., Thompson, S.A., Colburn, A.: Craniofacial growth after iatrogenic cleft palate repair in a fetal ovine model. Cleft Palate Craniofac. J. 34 (1997) 69–72
21. Castillo, R.A., Devoe, L.D., Falls, G., Holzmann, G.B., Hadi, H.A., Fadel, H.E.: Pleural effusions and pulmonary hypoplasia. Amer. J. Obstet. Gynecol. 1547 (1987) 1252–1255
22. Chan, F.Y., Woo, S.K., Ghosh, A., Tang, M., Lam, C.: Prenatal diagnosis of congenital fetal arrhythmias by simultaneous pulsed Doppler velocimetry of the fetal abdominal aorta and inferior vena cava. Obstet. Gynecol. 76 (1990) 200–204
23. Chaoui, R., Bollmann, R., Hoffmann, H., Göldner, B.: Fetale Echokardiographie: Teil III. Die fetalen Arrhythmien. Zentralbl. Gynäkol. 113 (1991) 1335–1350
24. Cincotta, R., Oldharn, J., Sampson, A.: Antepartum and postpartum complications of twin-twin transfusion. Aust. NZ. J. Obstet. Gynaecol. 36 (1996) 303–308
25. Clewell, W.H., Johnson, M.L., Meier, P.R. et al.: A surgical approach to the treatment of fetal hydrocephalus. N. Engl. J. Med. 306 (1982) 1320–1325
26. Committee on bioethics, American academy of pediatrics: Fetal therapy – ethical considerations. Pediatrics (1999) 1061–1063
27. De Crespigny, L.C., Robinson, H.P., Ross, A., Quinn, M.: Curarisation of fetus for intrauterine procedures. Lancet 1 (1985) 1164
28. De Lia, J.E., Kuhlmann, R.S., Harstad, T.W., Cruikshank, D.P.: Fetoscopic laser ablation of placental vessels in severe previable twin-twin transfusion syndrome. Amer. J. Obstet. Gynecol. 172 (1995) 1202–1211
29. Denbow, M.L., Battin, M.R., Cowan, F., Azzopardi, D., Edwards, A.D., Fisk, N.M.: Neonatal cranial ultrasound findings in preterm twins complicated by severe fetofetal transfusion syndrome. Amer. J. Obstet. Gynecol. 178 (1998) 479–483
30. Deprest, J.A., Evrard, V.A., Van Ballaer, P.P. et al.: Tracheoscopic endoluminal plugging using an inflatable device in the fetal lamb model. Eur. J. Obstet. Gynecol. Reprod. Biol. 81 (1998) 165–169
31. Desmedt, E.J., Henry, D.A., Beischer, N.A.: Polyhydramnios and associated maternal and fetal complications in singleton pregnancies. Brit. J. Obstet. Gynecol. 97 (1990) 1115–1122
32. Dorr, H.G., Sippell, W.G., Willig, R.P.: Pränatale Diagnostik und Therapie des Adrenogenitalen Syndroms (AGS) mit 21-Hydroxylase-Defekt. Geburtsh. u. Frauenheilkd. 52 (1992) 586–588
33. Elliott, J.P., Urig, M.A., Clewell, W.H.: Aggressive therapeutic amniocentesis tor treatment of twin-twin transfusion syndrome. Obstet. Gynecol. 77 (1991) 537–540
34. Enders, G.: Infektionen und Impfungen in der Schwangerschaft. München: Urban & Schwarzenberg 1988; S. 143–161
35. Fisher, D.A.: Neonatal thyroid disease of women with autoimmune thyroid disease. Thyroid Today 9 (1986) 1–7
36. Fisher, D.A., Polk, D.H.: Development of the thyroid. Baillieres Clin. Endocrinol. MeTab. 3 (1989) 627–657
37. Fisk, N.M., Ronderos-Dumit, D., Soliani, A., Nicolini, U., Vaughan, J., Rodeck, C.H.: Diagnostic and therapeutic transabdominal amnioinfusion in oligohydramnios. Obstet. Gynecol. 78 (1991) 270–278

38. Forest, M.G., David, M., Morel, Y.: Prenatal diagnosis and treatment of 21-hydroxylase deficiency. J. Steroid. Biochem. Mol. Biol. 45 (1993) 75–82

39. Gembruch, U., Hansmann, M.: Artificial instillation of amniotic fluid as a new technique for the diagnostic evaluation of cases of oligohydramnios. Prenat. Diagn. 8 (1988) 33–45

40. Gembruch, U., Manz, M., Bald, R. et al.: Repeated intravascular treatment with amiodarone in a fetus with refractory supraventricular tachycardia and hydrops fetalis. Amer. Heart J. 118 (1989) 1335–1338

41. Gembruch, U., Bald, R., Hansmann, M.: Die farbkodierte M-mode-Doppler-Echokardiographie bei der Diagnostik fetaler Arrhythmien. Geburtsh. u. Frauenheilkd. 50 (1990) 286–290

42. Gembruch. U., Somville, T.: Intrauterine Diagnostik und Therapie fetaler Arrhythmien. Gynäkologe 28 (1995) 329–345

43. Gembruch, U., Geipel, A.: Die indirekte und direkte medikamentöse Therapie des Feten. Gynäkologe 32 (1999) 840–854

44. Giers, G., Hoch, J., Bauer, H. et al.: Therapy with intravenous immunoglobulin G (ivIgG) during pregnancy for fetal alloimmune (HPA-1a (Zwa)) thrombocytopenic purpura. Prenat. Diagn. 16 (1996) 495–502

45. Gruel, Y., Boizard, B., Daffos, F., Forestier, F., Caen, J., Wautier, J.L.: Determination of platelet antigens and glycoproteins in the human fetus. Blood 68 (1986) 488–492

46. Haddow, J.E., Palomaki, G.E., Allan, W.C. et al.: Maternal thyroid deficiency during pregnancy and subsequent neuropsychological development of the child. N. Engl. J. Med. 341(1999) 549–555

47. Hallock, G.G.: In utero cleft lip repair in A/J mice. Plast. Reconstr. Surg. 75 (1985) 785–790

48. Harman, C.R., Bowman, J.M., Manning, F.A., Menticoglou, S.M.: Intrauterine transfusion – intraperitoneal versus intravascular approach: a case-control comparison. Amer. J. Obstet. Gynecol. 162 (1990) 1053–1059

49. Harrison, M.R., Ross, N.A., de Lorimier, A.A.: Correction of congenital diaphragmatic hernia in utero. III. Development of a successful surgical technique using abdominoplasty to avoid compromise of umbilical blood flow. J. Pediatr. Surg. 16 (1981) 934–942

50. Harrison, M.R., Golbus, M.S., Filly, R.A. et al.: Fetal surgery for congenital hydronephrosis. N. Engl. J. Med. 306 (1982) 591–593

51. Harrison, M.R., Nakayama, D.K., Noall, R., de Lorimier, A.A.: Correction of congenital hydronephrosis in utero. Decompression reverses the effects of obstruction on the fetal lung and urinary tract. J. Pediatr. Surg. 17 (1982) 965–974

52. Harrison, M.R.: Professional considerations in fetal treatment. In: Harrison, M.R., Golbus, M.S., Filly, R.A (eds.): The unborn patient. Philadelphia: Saunders 1991; pp. 8–13

53. Harrison, M.R., Adzick, N.S., Flake, A.W., Jennings, R.W.: The CDH two-step: a dance of necessity. J. Pediatr. Surg. 28 (1993) 813–816

54. Harrison, M.R., Adzick, N.S., Bullard, K.M. et al.: Correction of congenital diaphragmatic hernia in utero VII: a prospective trial. J. Pediatr. Surg. 32 (1997) 1637–1642

55. Harrison, M.R., Mychaliska, G.B., Albanese, C.T. et al.: Correction of congenital diaphragmatic hernia in utero IX: fetuses with poor prognosis (liver herniation and low lung-to-head ratio) can be saved by fetoscopic temporary tracheal occlusion. J. Pediatr. Surg. 33 (1998) 1017–1022

56. Hatijs, C.G.: Diagnosis and successful treatment of fetal goitrous hyperthyroidism caused by maternal Graves disease. Obstet. Gynecol. 81 (1993) 837–839

57. Hecher, K., Hackelöer, B.J.: Intrauterine endoscopic laser surgery for fetal sacrococcygeal teratoma. Lancet 347 (1996) 470

58. Hecher, K., Reinold, U., Gbur, K., Hackelöer, B.J.: Unterbrechung des umbilikalen Blutflusses bei einem akardischen Zwilling durch endoskopische Laserkoagulation. Geburtsh. u. Frauenheilk. 5 (1996) 97–100

59. Hecher, K., Hackelöer, B.-J., Ville, Y.: Umbilical cord coagulation by operative microendoscopy at 16 weeks' gestation in an acardiac twin. Ultrasound Obstet. Gynecol. 10 (1997) 130–132

60. Hecher, K., Zikulnig, L., Hackelöer, B.J.: Perspektiven der operativen Endoskopie in der Fetalmedizin. Gynäkologe 32 (1999) 855–865

61. Hecher, K., Plath, H., Bregenzer, T., Hansmann, M., Hackelöer, B.J.: Endoscopic laser surgery versus serial amniocenteses in the treatment of severe twin-twin transfusion syndrome. Amer. J. Obstet. Gynecol. 180 (1999) 717–724

62. Hendricks, S.D., Smith, J.R., Moore, D.E., Brown, Z.A.: Oligohydramnios associated with prostaglandin synthetase inhibitors in preterm labour. Brit. J. Obstet. Gynaecol. 97 (1990) 312–316

63. Hetzel, B.S.: Progress in the prevention and control of iodine-deficiency disorders. Lancet 2 (1987) 266

64. Hildebrand, K., Hösli, I., Holzgreve, W.: Pränatale Lungenreifung mit Corticosteroiden – ein Überblick. Z. Geburtsh. Neonatol. 200 (1996) 207–212

65. Hohlfeld, P., Forestier, F., Kaplan, C., Tissot, J.D., Daffos, F.: Fetal thrombocytopenia: a retrospective survey of 5194 fetal blood samplings. Blood 84 (1994) 1851–1856

66. Johnsen, D.E.: The creation of fetal rights: conflicts with womens constitutional rights to liberty, privacy, and equal protection. Yale Law Journal 95 (1986) 599–625

67. Kaplan, C., Daffos, F., Forestier, F. et al.: Management of alloimmune thrombocytopenia: Antenatal diagnosis and in utero transfusion of maternal platelets. Blood 72 (1988) 340–343

68. Kaplan, M.M., Meier, D.A.: Thyroid diseases in pregnancy. In: Gleicher, N. (ed.): Principles and practice of medical therapy in pregnancy, 3rd ed. Stamford, Conneticut: Appleton & Lange 1998; pp. 432–448

69. Kleinman, C.S., Copel, J.A., Weinstein, E.M., Santulli, T.V., Hobbins, J.: In utero diagnosis and treatment of fetal supraventricular tachycardia. Semin. Perinatol. 9 (1985) 113–129

70. Kleinman, C.S., Copel, J.A.: Electrophysiological principles and fetal antiarrhythmic therapy. Ultrasound Obstet. Gynecol. 1 (1991) 286–297

71. Kleinman, C.S., Nehgme, R., Copel, J.A.: Fetal cardiac arrhythmias: diagnosis and therapy. In: Creasy, R.K., Resnik, R. (eds.): Maternal-fetal medicine. 4th ed. Philadelphia: Saunders 1999; 301–318

72. Külz, Th.: Medikamentöse Therapie des Feten. Gynäkologe 31 (1998) 970–979

73. Lameier, L., Katz, V.L.: Amnioninfusion: a review. Obstet. Gynecol. Surv. 48 (1993) 829–837

74. Liggins, G.C., Howie, R.N.: A controlled trial of antepartum glucocorticoid treatment for prevention of the respiratory distress syndrome in premature infants. Pediatrics 50 (1972) 515–525

75. Liley, A.W.: Intrauterine transfusion of the fetus in hemolytic disease. Brit. Med. J. 2 (1963) 1107–1109

76. Longaker, M.T., Dodson, T.B., Kaban, L.B.: A rabbit model for fetal cleft lip repair. J. Oral Maxillofac. Surg. 48 (1990) 714–719

77. Mamopoulos, M., Assimakopoulos, E., Reece, E.A., Andreou, A., Zheng, X.Z., Mantalenakis, S.: Maternal indomethacin therapy in the treatment of polyhydramnios. Amer. J. Obstet. Gynecol. 162 (1990) 1225–1229

78. Manning, F.A., Harrison, M.R., Rodeck, C.: Catheter shunts for fetal hydronephrosis and hydrocephalus. Report of the International Fetal Surgery Registry. N. Engl. J. Med. 315 (1986) 336–340

79. McCurdy, C.M., Reed, K.L.: Fetal arrhythmias. In: Copel, J.A., Reed, K.L. (eds.): Doppler ultrasound in obstetrics and gynecology. New York: Raven Press 1995; pp. 252–270

80. Merz, E.: Intrauterine Therapie der obstruktiven Uropathie. Akt. Urologie 27 (1996) A15–A16

81. Meuli, M., Meuli-Simmen, C., Hutchins, G.M. et al.: In utero surgery rescues neurological function at birth in sheep with spina bifida. Nature Med. 1 (1995) 342–347

82. Michejda, M., Bacher, J., Kuwabara, R., Hodgen, G.D.: In utero allogenic bone transplantation in primates. Transplantation 32 (1982) 96–100

83. Miller, W.L.: Genetics, diagnosis, and management of 21-hydroxylase deficiency. J. Clin. Endocrinol. MeTab. 78 (1994) 241–246

84. Miyai, K., Connely, J.F., Foley, T.P. Jr. et al. An analysis of the variation of incidence of congenital dysgenetic hypothyroidism in various countries. Endocrinol. Jpn. 31 (1984) 77–81

85. Moise, K.J. Jr., Carpenter, R.J. Jr., Cotton, D.B., Wasserstrum, N., Kirshon, B., Cano, L.: Percutaneous umbilical cord blood sampling in the evaluation of fetal platelet counts in pregnant patients with autoimmune thrombocytopenia purpura. Obstet. Gynecol. 72 (1988) 346–350

86. Moore, T.R., Gale, S., Benirschke, K.: Perinatal outcome of forty-nine pregnancies complicated by acardiac twinning. Amer. J. Obstet. Gynecol. 163 (1990) 907–912

87. Mueller-Eckhardt, C., Kiefel, V., Grubert, A. et al.: 348 cases of suspected neonatal alloimmune neonatal thrombocytopenia. Lancet 1 (1989) 363–366

88. Murphy, M.F., Waters, A.H., Doughty, H.A. et al.: Antenatal management of fetomaternal alloimmune thrombocytopenia – report of 15 affected pregnancies. Transfusion Med. 4 (1994) 281–292

89. Murphy, M.F.: Management of fetal and neonatal alloimmune thrombocytopenia. In: Kurjak, A. (ed.): Textbook of Perinatal Medicine. London: Parthenon 1998; pp. 1081–1087

90. Naides, S.J., Weiner, C.P.: Antenatal diagnosis and palliative treatment of non-immune hydrops fetalis secondary to fetal parvovirus B 19 infection. Prenat. Diagn. 9 (1989) 105–114

91. National Institutes of Health Consensus Development Conference Statement. Effects of corticosteroids for fetal maturation on perinatal outcomes. Amer. J. Obstet. Gynecol. 173 (1995) 246

92. Nicolaides, K.H., Azar, G.B.: Thoraco-amniotic shunting. Fetal Diagn. Ther. 5 (1990) 153–164

93. Nicolini, U., Rodeck, C.H., Kochenour, N.K. et al.: In-utero platelet transfusion for alloimune thrombocytopenia. Lancet 2 (1988) 506

94. Nyhan, W.L., Sakati, N.A.: Multiple carboxylase deficiency: holocarboxylase synthetase. In: Diagnostic recognition of genetic disease. Philadelphia: Lea & Febiger 1987; pp. 50–57

95. Packman, S., Golbus, M.S., Cowan, M.J. et al.: Prenatal treatment of biotin-responsive multiple carboxylase deficiency. Lancet 2 (1982) 1435–1438

96. Paek, B., Strauss, A., Hasbargen, U., Hepp, H., Harrison, M.R.: Invasive fetale Therapie. Gynäkologe 32 (1999) 866–878

97. Patriarco, M., Yeh, S.: Immunological thrombocytopenia in pregnancy. Obstet. Gynecol. Surv. 41 (1986) 661–671

98. Perelman, A.H., Johnson, R.L., Clemons, R.D., Finberg, H.G., Clewell, W.H., Trujillo, L.: Intrauterine diagnosis and treatment of fetal goitrous hypothyroidism. J. Clin. Endocrinol. MeTab. 71 (1990) 618–621

99. Petres, R.E., Redwine, J.P., Cruikshank, J.P.: Congenital bilateral chylothorax. J. Amer. med. Ass. 248 (1982) 1360–1361

100. Pollack, M.S., Maurer, D., Levine, L.S. et al.: Prenatal diagnosis of congenital adrenal hyperplasia (21-hydroxylase deficiency) by HLA typing. Lancet 1 (1979) 1107–1108

101. Porreco, R.P., Bloch, C.A.: Fetal blood sampling in the management of intrauterine thyrotoxicosis. Obstet. Gynecol. 76 (1990) 509–512

102. Quetel, T.A., Mejides, A.A., Salman, F.A., Torres-Rodriguez, M.M.: Amnioinfusion: an aid in the ultrasonographic evaluation of severe oligohydramnios in pregnancy. Amer. J. Obstet. Gynecol. 167 (1992) 333–336

103. Reisner, D.P., Mahony, B.S., Petty, C.N. et al.: Stuck twin syndrome: outcome in thirty-seven consecutive cases. Amer. J. Obstet. Gynecol. 169 (1993) 991–995

104. Roberts, A.B., Clarkson, P.M., Pattison, N.S., Jamieson, M.G., Mok, P.M.: Fetal hydrothorax in the second trimester of pregnancy: successful intra-uterine treatment at 24 weeks gestation. Fetal Ther. 1 (1986) 203–209

105. Rodeck, C.H., Nicolaides, K.H.: Die Anwendung der Fetoskopie bei fetaler Therapie. Gynäkologe 17 (1984) 52–55

106. Rodeck, C.H., Fisk, N.M., Fraser, D.I., Nicolini, U.: Long-term in utero drainage of fetal hydrothorax. N. Engl. J. Med. 319 (1988) 1135–1138

107. Ronderos-Dumit, D., Nicolini, U., Vaughan, J., Fisk, N.M., Chamberlain, P.F., Rodeck, C.H.: Uterine-peritoneal amniotic fluid leakage: an unusual complication of intrauterine shunting. Obstet. Gynecol. 78 (1991) 913–915

108. Sack, J., Fisher, D.A., Hobel, C.J., Lam, R.: Thyroxine in human amniotic fluid. J. Pediatr. 87 (1975) 364–368
109. Sebire, N.J., Nicolaides, K.H.: Thoracoamniotic shunting for fetal pleural effusions. In: Chervenak, F.A., Kurjak, A. (eds.): The fetus as a patient. New York: Parthenon 1996; pp. 317–326
110. Seeds, J.W., Bowes, W.A.Jr.: Results of treatment of severe fetal hydrothorax with bilateral pleuroamniotic catheters. Obstet. Gynecol. 68 (1986) 577–579
111. Skarsgard, E.D., Meuli, M., van der Wall, K.J., Bealer, J.F., Adzick, N.S., Harrison, M.R.: Fetal endoscopic tracheal occlusion („Fetendo-Plug") for congenital diaphragmatic hernia. J. Pediatr. Surg. 31 (1996) 1335–1338
112. Strang, T.H.: Amnioinfusion. J. Reprod. Med. 49 (1995) 108–114
113. Thorpe-Beeston, J.G., Nicolaides, K.H., McGregor, A.M.: Fetal thyroid function. Thyroid 2 (1992) 207–217
114. Thuy, L.P., Belmont, J., Nyhan, W.L.: Prenatal diagnosis and treatment of holocarboxylase synthetase deficiency. Prenat. Diagn. 19 (1999) 108–112
115. Trainer, T.D., Howard, P.L.: Thyroid function tests in thyroid and nonthyroid disease. Crit. Rev. Clin. Lab. Sci. 19 (1983) 135–171
116. Treadwell, M.C., Sherer, D.M., Sacks, A.J., Ghezzi, F., Romero, R.: Successful treatment of recurrent non-immune hydrops secondary to fetal hyperthyroidism. Obstet. Gynecol. 87 (1996) 838–840
117. Trespidi, L., Boschetto, C., Caravelli, E., Villa, L., Kustermann, A., Nicolini, U.: Serial amniocenteses in the management of twin-twin transfusion syndrome: when is it valuable? Fetal Diagn. Ther. 12 (1997) 15–20
118. Ulmer, H.E., Mandelbaum, A., Schmidt, W.: Pränatale Behandlung fetaler Herzerkrankungen. Gynäkologe 21 (1988) 138–147
119. Van Allen, M.I., Smith, D.W., Shepard, T.H.: Twin reversed arterial perfusion (TRAP) sequence: A study of 14 twin pregnancies with acardius. Sem. Perinat. 7 (1983) 285–293
120. van der Wall, K.J., Bruch, S.W., Meuli, M. et al.: Fetal endoscopic („Fetendo") tracheal clip. J. Pediatr. Surg. 31 (1996) 1101–1104
121. Ville, Y., Hyett, J., Vandenbusche, F.P.A., Nicolaides, K.H.: Endoscopic laser coagulation of umbilical cord vessels in twin reversed arterial perfusion sequence. Ultrasound Obstet. Gynecol. 4 (1994) 396–398
122. Ville, Y., Hyett, J., Hecher, K., Nicolaides, K.: Preliminary experience with endoscopic laser surgery for severe twin-twin transfusion syndrome. New Engl. J. Med. 332 (1995) 224–227
123. Ville, Y., Hecher, K., Gagnon, A., Sebire, N., Hyett, J., Nicolaides, K.: Endoscopic laser coagulation in the management of severe twin-to-twin transfusion syndrome. Brit. J. Obstet. Gynaecol. 105 (1998) 446–453
124. Wallace, C., Couch, R., Ginsberg, J.: Fetal thyrotoxicosis: a case report and recommendations for prediction, diagnosis and treatment. Thyroid 5 (1995) 125–128
125. Ward, R.M.: Pharmacologic enhancement of fetal lung maturation. Clin. Perinatol. 21 (1994) 523–542
126. Waters, A., Murphy, M., Hambley, H. et al.: Management of alloimmune thrombocytopenia in the fetus and neonate. In: Nance, S.T. (ed.): Clinical and Basic Science Aspects of immunohaematology. Arlington: American Association of Blood Banks 1991; pp. 155–177
127. Watts, D.H., Luthy, D.A., Benedetti, T.J., Cyr, D.R., Easterling, T.R., Hickok, D.: Intraperitoneal fetal transfusion under direct ultrasound guidance. Obstet. Gynecol. 71 (1988) 84–88
128. Weiner, C.P., Wenstrom, K.D., Sipes, S.L., Williamson, R.A.: Risk factors for cordocentesis and fetal intravascular transfusion. Amer. J. Obstet. Gynecol. 165 (1991) 1020–1025
129. Weiner, C.P., Williamson, R.A., Wenstrom, K.D. et al.: Management of fetal hemolytic disease by cordocentesis. II. Outcome of treatment. Amer. J. Obstet. Gynecol. 165 (1991) 1302–1307
130. Wenstrom, K., Weiner, C.P., Williamson, R.A., Grant, S.S.: Prenatal diagnosis of fetal hyperthyroidism using funipuncture. Obstet. Gynecol. 76 (1990) 513–517

Safety and Genetic and Ethical Aspects of Prenatal Ultrasound Diagnosis

48 Safety Aspects of Diagnostic Ultrasound in Pregnancy

Historical Development

Intensity. The risks of ultrasound use in medicine have been discussed for more than 50 years. At the first symposium on medical ultrasound held 50 years ago, it was already clear that, in contrast to ionizing radiation, the dose (total energy absorbed during the exposure time) was not the key factor. Instead, the intensity of the ultrasound field (Table 48.**1**) was identified as the critical parameter in terms of producing biological effects (8).

Heating and cavitation. When pulsed diagnostic ultrasound was introduced in the early 1960s, it became necessary to distinguish between average intensity and pulse intensity. It was assumed that the average intensity determined heat generation while the pulse intensity determined harmful mechanical effects, especially those due to cavitation. This concept had major weaknesses, however, because when a narrow ultrasound field is emitted, the degree of tissue heating is determined more by the power of the ultrasound than by its intensity (Fig. 48.**1**), while cavitation is determined by the peak negative pressure of the sound. Also, both effects are dependent on the sound frequency and on tissue properties. As a result, biological safety during the 1980s was evaluated in terms of heating and cavitation, which were identified as the two major, primary biophysical effects of diagnostic ultrasound (14, 15). These phenomena correlate much better with desired or undesired

bioeffects, but their disadvantage is that they depend on several parameters of the ultrasound field, and a complex methodology is needed to analyze these effects in exposed tissue.

Computer models were therefore developed to determine tissue heating. These models are designed to estimate the degree of heating based on known parameters of the ultrasound field and the manner in which the ultrasound is used (2). Because a comparable mathematical model cannot yet be devised for ultrasound-induced cavitation due to the lack of a theoretical foundation, the amplitude of the negative pressure in the tissue has been taken as the critical quantity for purposes of safety evaluation.

Threshold values. The bioeffects of ultrasound are dependent on threshold values. Adverse thermal effects can be excluded at temperatures up to 38.5° C. Temperatures above 41° C inhibit cell division and produce teratogenic effects in experimental animals, depending on the timing of the exposure (1, 14). Cavitation is not observed in diagnostic ultrasound procedures whose sound fields do not exceed negative pressure amplitudes of 5.5 MPa. The threshold for cavitation in vivo is assumed to be 10 MPa. In tissues that contain gases, such as the lung and bowel after birth and tissues that have been treated with gas-containing ultrasound contrast agents, the cavitation threshold is considerably lower. Thus, the goal of all safety efforts in diagnostic ultrasound should be to avoid exceeding the biologically relevant threshold values.

Risk Assessment for Various Ultrasound Procedures

Given the variety of methods employed in diagnostic ultrasound, it is no longer possible to make a blanket risk assessment for ultrasonography. Different ultrasound procedures must be individually analyzed according to the level of exposure and clinical use.

A-Mode, B-Mode and M-Mode Ultrasound

Tissue heating. The power settings and intensities (spatial peak temporal average intensity, I_{spta}) used in A-mode, B-mode and M-mode ultrasound (and in 3-D ultrasound as an extension of B-mode) are so low that exposed tissues are not heated to an appreciable degree. This also applies to endoscopic and transvaginal examinations, which are not associated with thermal effects.

Negative pressure amplitudes. The negative pressure amplitudes in these modes do not exceed 5.5 MPa (7) and are not sufficient to induce cavitation. However, exposure of the aerated lung in laboratory animals has led to subpleural capillary erythrocyte extravasation in cases where the peak negative pressure exceeded 1 MPa. The underlying mechanism is unclear, but apparently the effect is not thermally induced and requires aerated alveoli—hence there is no danger to the fetal lung (11). So far these extravasations have been described only in animal models, and the lesions were more severe in small laboratory mammals than in large mammals. In humans, they presumably do not occur in clinical examinations because the human pleura is thicker and appears to be more resistant to mechanical stresses.

Table 48.**1** Physical terms used in describing ultrasound fields (after 10)

1. Power

$$\text{Power} = \frac{\text{energy}}{\text{time}} \qquad \text{Unit of measure} = \frac{\text{joule}}{\text{second}}$$

Energy is the ability to do work. It has the same unit of measure as work, namely the joule. In diagnostic ultrasound equipment, power (or output) is usually rated in mW = 10^{-3} W.

2. Intensity

$$\text{Intensity} = \frac{\text{energy}}{\text{time} \cdot \text{area}} = \frac{\text{power}}{\text{area}} \qquad \text{Unit of measure:} \frac{\text{joule}}{\text{second} \cdot \text{m}^2}$$

In diagnostic ultrasound equipment, intensity is usually rated in mW/cm² (1 mW/cm² = 0.1 W/cm²). The maximum intensity of solar radiation on earth is 100 mW/cm².
The intensity in a pulsed ultrasound field is not temporally or spatially constant. Therefore, it is usually stated as the temporal and/or spatial peak intensity or as average values. The following intensity ratings are most commonly used (where S = space, T = time, P = peak, and A = averaged):

I(SATA) Spatial average temporal average intensity
I(SPTA) Spatial peak temporal average intensity
I(SPTP) Spatial peak temporal peak intensity

3. Acoustic pressure

Ultrasound propagates through tissue as a longitudinal wave. This creates an alternating pressure that is superimposed upon the resting pressure of the tissue.

$$\text{Pressure} = \frac{\text{force}}{\text{area}} \qquad \text{Unit of measure: pascal} = \frac{\text{newton}}{\text{m}^2}$$

In the compression phase of the wave, the pressure rises above the resting pressure. In the suction phase, the pressure falls below the resting pressure. Acoustic pressure is rated in megapascal (1 MPa = 10⁶ newtons/m² = 9.87 atm).

Doppler Techniques

Electronic FHR Monitoring

The power outputs, intensities, and pressure amplitudes used in electronic FHR monitoring are so low that they do not raise safety concerns, even when monitoring is continued for an extended period of time (6).

Pulsed Doppler (Color Doppler, Power Doppler, Duplex)

Intensities. The exposure levels in Doppler procedures are higher than in B-mode and M-mode examinations. The intensities that are emitted in these three procedures overlap considerably, with duplex producing the highest intensities. Some machines emit intensities that are equal to those of therapeutic ultrasound or even higher (7), although the ultrasound field is considerably narrower and the power output lower. At these intensities, it is conceivable that stationary scanning for pulsed Doppler flowmetry may raise the temperature of the insonated tissue (6, 14). Flowmetry is more problematic than color Doppler and power Doppler imaging, because these modes employ a moving Doppler beam that distributes the heating effect over a larger tissue volume. A useful rule of thumb is that color Doppler produces approximately 10 times the intensity (spatial peak temporal average intensity, I_{spta}) of simple B-mode ultrasound, while pulsed Doppler flowmetry produces approximately 100 times the B-mode intensity.

Heating relevant to safety. At present, we cannot answer the key question of what conditions in diagnostic ultrasound will definitely cause tissue heating that is relevant to patient safety. In animal studies, different independent groups of investigators using pulsed Doppler have measured temperature increases of more than 5° C in various nonperfused soft tissues. Exposure times of 60–90 seconds were sufficient to produce this effect. In all of these studies, the greatest tissue heating occurred during the first 30 seconds. It was also discovered that the power setting of the ultrasound emitter was a much more important determinant of tissue heating than the average intensity (Fig. 48.**1**) (3, 14).

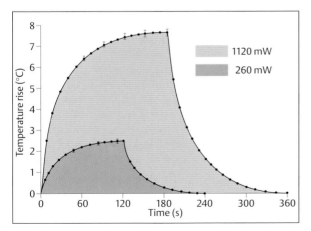

Fig. 48.**1**　Temperature rise plotted over time at the center of isolated fetal guinea pig brain exposed to ultrasound. The ultrasound exposure corresponds roughly to that of duplex scanning (field parameters: 3.2 MHz, pulse duration 6.25 µs, PRF 4 kHz). Upper curve: total power output 1120 mW, SPTA intensity 2.5 Wcm^{-2}. Lower curve: total power output 26 mW, SPTA intensity 2.9 Wcm^{-2} (after [3]).

Bone mineralization. When fetal brain was insonated through the skull, the temperature in the tissue directly bordering the proximal temporal bone was heated by secondary warming from the insonated bone more strongly than tissue that was more centrally located. For equal power settings, this heating near bone increased with progressive mineralization of the fetal bone (3). Acoustically, the embryo behaves like a soft-tissue structure and absorbs very little sound energy. Once the bone starts to mineralize in the 12th week of gestation, absorption rises steadily. As a result, there is less thermal risk to the embryo than to the fetus.

The Doppler techniques are comparable to B-mode and M-mode from the standpoint of possible mechanical injuries.

Ultrasound Contrast Agents

Cavitation. Contrast agents that contain gas are sometimes used in diagnostic ultrasound to increase acoustic backscattering from the blood. These agents lower the cavitation threshold of aqueous solutions in vitro and can induce the formation of chemical radicals like those that occur with ionizing radiation. It is unclear at present whether this implies risks for clinical use. Blood in vivo is considerably more resistant to cavitation than solutions in vitro. It is uncertain whether the administration of contrast agents enables cavitation to occur in vivo.

The contrast agents in current use have bubble sizes less than 10 µm, which should not interfere with capillary perfusion. To date, the clinical use of these agents has shown no evidence of any other risks, including problems of immune tolerance (9). But since new contrast agents are constantly being developed and their possible clinical applications are expanding, it is not yet possible to make a definitive assessment of risk. An individual risk/benefit analysis should be made whenever ultrasound contrast agents are used.

Safety Indices

Since biosafety is dependent on numerous boundary conditions of the ultrasound field and the exposed tissue, there have been attempts to make this problem simpler and more transparent for users. Safety indices have been defined for this purpose, although their practical implementation is not yet complete.

Two independent indices. Heating and cavitation are the two key physical mechanisms for the production of bioeffects by ultrasound. Accordingly, two independent indices have been devised for monitoring these effects (2). Both indices are calculated on the basis of very simple models of the tissue and its acoustic properties. Here we shall review only the basic concept of these indices. A detailed description and evaluation can be found in the literature (5). The display of these indices for the user is regulated by the Online Display Standard (ODS), which became a criterion for the approval of diagnostic ultrasound equipment in the United States on January 1, 1996. Most European manufacturers have also equipped newer devices with ODS.

Thermal Index (TI)

Tissue heating. The thermal index (TI) is designed to warn the user of possible heating of the exposed tissue during the examination when certain equipment settings are used. It is defined as the ratio of the actual acoustic output to the output that would be necessary to heat a given tissue by 1° C under unfavorable conditions. It is assumed that the exposure time is long enough to establish a thermal equilibrium. The TI was deliberately defined as a dimensionless quantity. A TI of 0.8 means that a tissue volume may be heated by a maximum of 0.8° C under the given insonation conditions.

Variants. Three variants of the TI have been defined:
- The thermal index for soft tissues (TIS)
- The thermal index for bone (TIB), which is used when strongly absorbing bone is located near the beam focus
- The thermal index for cranium (TIC), which is used when bone is located near the transducer, especially in transcranial examinations

In obstetric examinations, it is normally best to use the TIS. During the second half of pregnancy, however, the TIB should be used as a safety indicator for the exposure of fetal bone.

Calculating a thermal index. A simple formula is used to calculate each thermal index. The formula for TIS is as follows:

$$TIS = W \cdot f \cdot k$$

In this equation W is the acoustic output measured in water, f is frequency, and k is a factor that covers all the parameters of the model being used. Attenuation is assumed to be only 0.3 dB/cm MHz, so that tissue heating tends to be overestimated. The two other indices (TIB and TIC) are independent of frequency, and only different k values are used.

■ *Mechanical Index (MI)*

Cavitation. This index tries to estimate the likelihood that cavitation will occur in the exposed tissue. The local negative pressure peak p in the tissue is calculated from pressures measured in water. Again, soft-tissue attenuation is assumed to be only 0.3 dB/cm MHz. The p value is entered in the formula as a positive value in MPa, the frequency f in MHz:

$$MI = \frac{p}{\sqrt{f}}$$

The MI is also a dimensionless quantity. It tells the user about the amplitude of the pulse at any given time. Higher pulse amplitudes lead to proportionately higher MI values. This index is based on the assumption that there is a threshold for the negative acoustic pressure beyond which cavitation, and thus harmful bioeffects, can be produced. At present, however, we do not know the MI threshold beyond which cavitation is likely to occur in living mammalian tissue. In the United States, a maximum MI of 1.9 is permitted in ultrasound examinations. At a frequency of 5 MHz, this corresponds to a negative pressure amplitude of 4.2 MPa. Ultrasound devices marketed in Europe reach a maximum of 5.5 MPa (7).

■ *Display of the Indices*

Online Display Standard (ODS). Most modern ultrasound devices display the safety indices in conformance with ODS requirements (2). The ODS stipulates that only one index be displayed on the monitor screen. The decision of which index to display depends on the operating mode of the equipment and its clinical application. The index that is best for a particular type of examination should be selected. For example, only the MI is displayed for B-mode imaging.

Selection of appropriate TI. The TI takes precedence in pulsed Doppler and M-mode examinations. The specific application determines which TI is displayed. The TIC is used strictly in transcranial examinations. The TIS or TIB is displayed in all other examinations, depending on which is more appropriate for the given study. Of course, the TIB will always indicate higher values than the TIS because bone is a stronger sound absorber than soft tissue. In some examinations such as scans of the eye or breast, TIS is the default because soft tissues are being exa-

Table 48.**2**   Guidelines for diagnostic ultrasound use in pregnancy

General
➢ The power output of the device should be as low as possible, and a high gain setting should be used.
➢ The examiner must know whether the device continues to emit while in the freeze-frame mode. If necessary, the transducer should be lifted from the skin.
➢ Ultrasound examinations should be medically indicated. There is no objection to the routine screening of every pregnancy with B-mode ultrasound.
➢ The lung should not be exposed unnecessarily in postnatal cardiologic examinations.

Pulsed Doppler examinations
➢ Doppler flowmetry should be activated only after the vessel has been located with color Doppler and the sample volume has been defined. The depth of the sampling site should be kept small, as some machines have TGC to compensate for attenuation.
➢ If a safety index is not available, the sampling time should be kept short and should not exceed 30 s if at all possible. The operator should wait at least 30 s before acquiring a second sample at the same site.
➢ More deeply situated bone should be minimally exposed in fetal and neonatal pulsed Doppler examinations.
➢ Thermal effects should be considered more likely to occur in febrile patients, and the sampling times should be shortened accordingly.
➢ The routine screening of every pregnancy with pulsed Doppler to determine fetal and placental blood flow cannot be recommended at present due to the potential risks. This examination should be reserved for selected patients.
➢ The use of ultrasound contrast agents requires a special indication and a preliminary, individual risk/benefit analysis.

mined, but the TIB is more suitable because bone may be incidentally exposed. Thus, the examiner should be able to modify the default display that is selected by the machine.

Threshold of 1.0. As a general rule, the ODS requires that an index be displayed in a particular machine or mode only if can reach a value ≥ 1.0. Under these conditions, values of 0.4 or more are displayed. This applies equally to the TI and MI.

■ *Interpreting the Indices*

The displayed safety indices can provide the user with valuable, hitherto unavailable information on how changing the settings on the control panel affects the pulse amplitude (and thus the MI) and the time-averaged intensity or total power output, and thus the heating capacity of the ultrasound field. But as with any new method of risk assessment, a certain caution should be exercised when interpreting the index values. At present, both the TI and MI can be interpreted only as general indicators of possible risks. They are based on computations and not on valid measurements of the true heating or cavitation potential that exists in tissues while an examination is in progress (5).

Initial experimental tests of the TI have shown that the value estimated from the index generally conveys a good approximation of reality, but that the calculated TI can significantly over- or underestimate the heating that actually occurs in specific clinical situations (12). The MI has not yet been tested for its practical value as a safety indicator.

Conclusions and Recommendations

A number of epidemiologic studies have been done on possible adverse intrauterine effects from ultrasound exposure, but the majority have dealt with B-mode examinations. So far, none of these studies have demonstrated adverse postnatal effects (4). Nevertheless, to be completely safe and to avoid exceeding the thresholds for thermal and cavitational effects, the guidelines listed in Table 48.2 should be followed in prenatal ultrasound examinations (10, 13). Diagnostic ultrasound is safe and effective when these guidelines are observed. Another important prerequisite, of course, is adequate user training.

References

1. AIUM (American Institute of Ultrasound in Medicine): Bioeffects & Safety of Diagnostic Ultrasound. AIUM, Laurel MD 1993
2. AIUM/NEMA (American Institute of Ultrasound in Medicine/National Electrical Manufactures Association): Standard for real time display of thermal and mechanical acoustic output indices on diagnostic ultrasound equipment. AIUM, Rockville MD 1992
3. Bosward, K.L., Barnett, S.B., Wood, A.K.W., Edwards, M.I., Kossoff, G.: Heating of guinea-pig fetal brain during exposure to pulsed ultrasound. Ultrasound Med. Biol. 19 (1993) 415–424
4. EFSUMB (European Federation of Societies for Ultrasound in Medicine and Biology): tutorial: epidemiology of diagnostic ultrasound exposure during human pregnancy. Eur J Ultrasound 1996; 4: 69–73
5. tutorial: thermal and mechanical indices. Eur J Ultrasound 1996; 4: 145–50
6. EFSUMB (European Federation of Societies for Ultrasound in Medicine and Biology): Clinical Safety Statement 1998. Europ. J. Ultrasound 8 (1998) 67–68
7. Henderson, I., Willson, K., Iago, I.R., Whittingham, T.A.: A survey of the acoustic outputs of diagnostic ultrasound equipment in current clinical use. Ultrasound Med. Biol. 21 (1995) 699–705
8. Matthes, K., Rech, W.: Der Ultraschall in der Medizin. Kongressbericht der Erlanger Ultraschall-Tagung 1949. Zürich: S. Hirzel 1949
9. Nanda, N.C.: Echocontrast enhancers: How safe are they? Advances in Echo-Contrast 2 (1992) 19–24
10. Rott, H.-D.: Ultraschalldiagnostik: Neuere Bewertung der biologischen Sicherheit. Dtsch. Ärztebl. 93 (1996) A-1533–1537
11. Rott, H.-D.: Lungenhämorrhagien durch diagnostischen Ultraschall. Ultraschall in Med. 18 (1997) 226–228
12. Shaw, A., Pay, N.M., Preston, R.C.: Assessment of the likely thermal index values for pulsed Doppler ultrasound equipment. – Stages II and III: experimental assessment of scanner/-transducer combinations. National Physical Laboratory (NPL): NPL Report CMAM 12, Teddington U.K. 1998
13. SSK (Strahlenschutzkomission): Empfehlungen zur Patientensicherheit bei Anwendung der Ultraschalldiagnostik in der Medizin. Empfehlungen der Strahlenschutzkommission. Berichte der Strahlenschutzkommission des Bundesministers für Umwelt, Naturschutz und Reaktorsicherheit. Heft 14. Stuttgart: Gustav Fischer 1998
14. WFUMB (World Federation for Ultrasound in Medicine and Biology): Symposium on Safety and Standardisation in Medical Ultrasound: Issues and Recommendations Regarding Thermal Mechanisms for Biological Effects of Ultrasound (eds.: Barnett, S.B., Kossoff, G.) Ultrasound Med. Biol. 18/9 (Special Issue) 1992
15. WFUMB (World Federation for Ultrasound in Medicine and Biology): Symposium on Safety of Ultrasound in Medicine: Emphasis on Non-thermal Mechanisms (eds.: Barnett, S.B., Kossoff, G.) Ultrasound Med. Biol. 24 (1998) 1–55

49 Genetic Counseling for a Fetal Anomaly

Aims of Genetic Counseling

Finding abnormalities in a fetal ultrasound scan gives rise to various differential diagnostic considerations. These include the reasons for conducting the prenatal examination, such as advanced maternal age, the previous birth of a child with a neural tube defect, or definite maternal carriership for sex-linked hereditary hydrocephalus due to aqueductal stenosis. At the same time, the nature of the detected anomaly will prompt a search for coexisting abnormalities that may signal the presence of a syndromic condition. The severity of the observed anomaly and/or its treatability are criteria that determine how the examiner will proceed from there.

Counseling during a pregnancy. In some cases at this point a genetic counselor is called in to provide additional diagnostic help. The laboratory tests available to him or her—cytogenetics and molecular genetics—are informative and helpful in many cases. The genetic counselor can also assist in gathering family data not previously interpreted as risk factors and identifying the symptoms that may be expected to accompany the disorder. He or she can also provide referrals to therapeutic specialists and support groups.

Counseling after a pregnancy. Ordinarily, the function of the genetic counselor is to provide counseling after the termination of a pregnancy with a malformed fetus or after the delivery of an affected child, informing the parents about the etiology of the disorder and any risks of recurrence in a future pregnancy. Genetic counseling is offered in a variety of family situations (Fig. 49.**1**). The prevalence figures shown for the various situations are based on more than 19,000 comprehensive counseling cases over a 26-year period. The situation of an affected fetus, as addressed here, accounts for approximately 15–20% of counseling cases.

Guiding principles. The following two principles should be kept in mind when genetic counseling is offered for a congenital anomaly:
- Not all congenital conditions are hereditary.
- Not all hereditary conditions are detectable at birth.

General basic risk. The general basic risk should always be considered in genetic counseling. It describes the occurrence of disorders that cannot be predicted or prevented. This type of disorder cannot be inferred from the most thorough and meticulous family history, nor can it be detected with the formidable tools of modern prenatal diagnosis. The basic risk defined by these criteria is on the order of 5% and is higher in cases of parental consanguinity.

Our scope is too limited to allow a comprehensive discussion of the many different anomalies and malformations that are detectable with ultrasound. We can only cite examples drawn from the various etiologic groups, some of which are supplemented by table listings.

▬ Key Questions

Several key questions must be addressed in genetic counseling (Table 49.**1**).

What Information is Available on the Child?

It should always be determined whether the disorder is an isolated anomaly or part of a syndrome of multiple disorders that have a common cause. Additionally, there are patterns of disturbances in which various organ systems are affected by changes whose pathogenesis cannot be readily understood. Cases in which the diagnosis rests entirely on ultrasound findings are naturally more difficult to interpret than cases for which postmortem findings are already available. Occasionally, radiographs of the fetus or chromosomal findings can supply critical information.

What Was the Course of the Pregnancy?

The prior obstetric history is an important factor in evaluating etiologic factors. It includes prior miscarriages, unsuccessful attempts to con-

Table 49.**1** Procedures in genetic counseling for a fetal anomaly

Prerequisites
- ➤ Accurate documentation of the nature and severity of existing abnormalities (e.g., photographs, radiographs)
- ➤ Postmortem findings
- ➤ Chromosome analysis

Points addressed by the counselor
- ➤ Prior obstetric history
- ➤ Delivery
- ➤ Exposure to drugs and other exogenous factors
- ➤ Vaccinations
- ➤ Infectious diseases
- ➤ Personal history of the parents
- ➤ Age
- ➤ Family history
- ➤ Consanguinity

Additional diagnostic tests (as needed)
- ➤ Parental chromosome analysis
- ➤ Molecular genetics
- ➤ Biochemical analyses
- ➤ Comparison of typical family appearance

Diagnostic classification
- ➤ Isolated anomaly or syndromic occurrence
- ➤ Asymmetrical/symmetrical involvement
- ➤ Syndrome/association/sequence
- ➤ Physical abnormalities with/without mental retardation
- ➤ Chromosomal or monogenic pathogenesis
- ➤ Sporadic occurrence or precedent(s) in the family tree
- ➤ Evidence of an exogenous cause or disruption

Assessing the risk of recurrence
- ➤ Mendelian principles
- ➤ Empirical risk figures with multifactorial inheritance
- ➤ Definite carriership in parents
- ➤ Effective measures for treatment or early detection
- ➤ Capabilities of prenatal diagnosis
- ➤ Explanation of general basic risk

Table 49.2 Medications that should be avoided during pregnancy (selection)

Hazardous	Use with great caution
➤ Retinoids	➤ Lithium
➤ Coumarin derivatives	➤ Tetracycline
➤ Vitamin A	➤ Anticonvulsants combined with barbiturates
➤ Cytostatic drugs	➤ Oral antidiabetics

Table 49.3 Fetal anomalies linked to rubella infection during pregnancy. Type of anomaly related to the timing of maternal infection

Timing of infection	Type of anomaly
Week 6 of gestation	Ocular lens changes, cataract
Week 9 of gestation	Inner ear abnormalities
Week 5–10 of gestation	Cardiac anomalies
Week 6–9 of gestation	Dental anomalies

ceive, pharmacologic induction of ovulation, and the long-term use of oral contraceptives. Medication use (Table 49.2), recreational drug and alcohol use, workplace exposures, trips abroad, vaccinations, infectious diseases, surgical operations, and radiation exposure should be closely scrutinized in each case and analyzed in their temporal relationship to the stage of pregnancy. It should be considered, for example, that the severity of rubella embryopathy varies with the timing of the infection (Table 49.3). Another consideration is the relationship between the "timetable" of limb development and the timing of thalidomide exposure (Fig. 49.2).

What Does the Personal History of the Parents Show?

Maternal diseases such as diabetes mellitus, epilepsy, renal diseases, hypertension, or Crohn's disease are significant risk factors for pregnancy and the occurrence of anomalies, although the etiologic relationships can be difficult to define. For example, inferior regression and macrosomia in the fetus are known to occur in association with poorly controlled maternal diabetes. Epilepsy in the father increases the basic risk to the child, as does maternal epilepsy, although the underlying pathogenic mechanism is poorly understood. The question "is it the disease itself and/or its necessary treatment, or it is both factors combined?" is an important issue and has not yet been resolved.

Folic acid prophylaxis. The importance of paternal alcohol abuse as a causal factor in congenital anomalies has been overestimated in the past and is still overstated today. So far there is no convincing proof that the risk of anomalies is increased. The prophylactic use of folic acid during the first 3 months of pregnancy should be considered in cases of maternal Crohn's disease or epilepsy. If Crohn's disease has been treated by resection of the terminal ileum, vitamin absorption will be decreased. We conclude from our own observations that the risk of spina bifida aperta may be increased, and we have made it a policy to recommend folic acid prophylaxis in maternal Crohn's disease, preferably starting the therapy even before the patient becomes pregnant.

What Does the Family History Show?

Drawing up a comprehensive family tree is a basic tool for the genetic counselor. The record should include previous abnormal pregnancies that the counseled couple has had, along with any affected parents and siblings. Attention should be given to anomalies or malformations of a similar nature and to current diseases, bearing in mind that varying expression of monogenic traits or syndromes in different affected individuals can make classification and interpretation much more difficult. Some disorders are associated with microsymptoms that are easily overlooked if their existence is unknown and they are not specifically sought, such as a notch in the vermilion border or a bifid uvula signifying a genetic predisposition for cleft lip and palate.

Parental consanguinity or parents who originate from enclaves or from isolated ethnic, religious, or linguistic groups are significant findings. The age of the parents when the child was conceived can also furnish important clues. Affected persons in the same family who were not diagnosed antenatally due to a lack of diagnostic facilities or who manifest a different symptom pattern based on age-related factors can seriously distort the estimation of recurrence risk. Childhood photographs of the parents can be of substantial value in differentiating a typical family appearance from syndromic features.

▦ *Estimating Risks of Recurrence*

Working from the above information, the genetic counselor proceeds with the actual disease analysis and the estimation of possible recurrence risks.

Figure 49.3 illustrates the various possible causes to be considered when a fetal anomaly is detected. In a fairly large number of case, a cause can be established at once because a chromosome analysis is already available or the pediatric pathologist has made a definitive diagnosis. In many cases, though, these "hard data" are unavailable, and it is the task of the genetic counselor to attempt an etiologic classification from which any risks of recurrence can be derived.

Counseling in Various Disorders

▦ *Sporadic (Random) Disorders*

Examples of disorders that are classified as "random" because of an unknown cause are unilateral hand, finger and arm anomalies such as ectrodactyly, atypical cleft hand, acheiria with finger buds, and peromelia. These anomalies are always unilateral and represent isolated occurrences in the family. Today some of these cases are attributed to embolic vascular occlusions that may have occurred during the embryonic period. It is very likely that this category also includes Poland syndrome, a unilateral symbrachydactyly with atrophy of the forearm muscles, absence of the sternal head of the pectoralis muscle, and occasional smallness of the ipsilateral breast in women or axillary migration of the nipple.

This group also includes the unilateral aplasia of individual muscles, usually the pectoralis, or the asymmetrical absence of a long tubular bone such as the fibula or femur.

None of the above anomalies is considered to have an increased risk of recurrence, either in siblings or in the offspring of affected persons.

▦ *Anomalies with a Definite Exogenous Cause*

Two classic examples in this category are thalidomide embryopathy and rubella embryopathy, which unfortunately still occurs today. Chondrodysplasia punctata can result from the use of anticoagulant medication. Abnormal growth of the long tubular bones and dental enamel defects due to maternal tetracycline use after 11 weeks' gestation and the otherwise rare condition of an Ebstein anomaly in the right heart following lithium therapy are known examples of exogenously induced congenital abnormalities (Table 49.2). Alcoholic embryopathy is another familiar and relatively common example. There is no risk of recurrence if exposure is avoided in future pregnancies.

Chromosome Disorders

A usually variegated pattern of dysmorphic features and anomalies involving various organ systems, especially when associated with intrauterine growth restriction, should raise suspicion of a chromosomal abnormality. If a corresponding cytogenetic analysis has not been performed on the child, parental karyotyping is necessary to exclude carriership. The anomalies that are seen in the classic trisomies (13, 18, 21) are so well known that simple physical examination can provide a high index of suspicion. Advanced maternal age at conception is a suggestive factor. When a free trisomy is present, the risk of recurrence is usually small.

Balanced chromosomal abnormality. Before a definite prognosis is offered for future pregnancies, it should be confirmed that one of the parents does not have a balanced chromosome rearrangement, such as a 13/14 translocation. Increased miscarriage rates or prolonged inability to conceive provide historical clues (Figs. 49.**4**, 49.**5**).

Differential diagnosis. The differential diagnosis should include the presence of severe genetic syndromes, some of which have a monogenic inheritance with a high risk of recurrence. When complex-appearing malformation syndromes are detected by ultrasound, amniocentesis with fetal karyotyping should definitely be performed as this study can greatly advance the differential diagnosis.

Monogenic Hereditary Disorders

This category includes anomalies or malformation syndromes that are caused by *one* gene and thus can be considered hereditary diseases in the strict sense. They are very rare. Mendelian principles of inheritance should be applied in assessing the risk of these disorders.

Autosomal and X-linked inheritance. While traits and diseases that have an autosomal-dominant or autosomal-recessive inheritance can be found in both sexes (the genes are located on the autosomes), conditions that have an X-linked mode of inheritance occur as diseases predominantly in males, while females tend to be carriers with no disease manifestations. Today these carriers can be identified in many cases by using special analytical methods, including biochemical stress tests, indirect molecular genetic family studies, and occasionally by direct detection (e.g., of a deletion in the corresponding gene).

X-linked dominant inheritance. In the very rare X-linked dominant traits, both sexes are affected but the traits are consistently more pronounced in males than females. Some of these disorders are fatal in the male (e.g., Bloch-Sulzberger incontinentia pigmenti).

Autosomal-dominant inheritance. In very general terms, it is reasonable to say that gross physical dysmorphias tend to have an autosomal-dominant mode of inheritance whereas metabolic disorders, which usually produce no physical abnormalities at birth, tend to have an autosomal-recessive inheritance. Symmetrical anomalies, especially those involving the extremities, should also raise suspicion of an autosomal-dominant disorder. This type of disorder is either transmitted by an affected parent or occurs as a (dominant) new mutation. The degrees of trait expression in dominant disorders are particularly variable, often making it difficult to recognize the familial nature of the disease. Examples of anomalies with an autosomal-dominant inheritance are shown in Table 49.**4**.

Dominant new mutations, which are more common with advanced paternal age, are particularly easy to recognize when the traits are conspicuous, and an initial occurrence in the family can often be confirmed by looking at photographs.

Autosomal-recessive inheritance. Table 49.**5** lists examples of hereditary anomalies that have an autosomal-recessive mode of inheritance.

X-linked recessive inheritance. In the group of sex-linked hereditary anomalies, hydrocephalus based on aqueductal stenosis in boys merits special attention due to the severity of the disease and its high risk of recurrence. This condition is frequently associated with thumb anomalies such as a triphalangeal thumb, a finger-shaped thumb, and contractures in the metacarpophalangeal joint of the thumb. The absence of these anomalies is not uncommon, but their presence suggests the correct diagnosis. Given the many other, largely exogenous causes of aqueductal stenosis leading to hydrocephalus, it is important to recognize this somewhat rare hereditary form, which has a 50% risk of re-

Table 49.4   Examples of fetal anomalies with an autosomal-dominant inheritance (1–8, 10)

Name	Ultrasound features	Additional features
Holt–Oram syndrome	Radial aplasia, clubbed hand, cardiac anomaly (?)	Triphalangeal thumb, usually ASD and VSD
Cleft hand/cleft foot	Both hands and feet affected, third ray missing	Often syndactyly D I and D II or D IV and D V
Franceschetti syndrome	Auricular deformities, large mouth, small chin, narrow zygomatic arches	Lid coloboma, prominent nose
Apert syndrome	Spoon hands and feet, turricephaly, frontal bossing	Syndactyly of the toes, deep-set eyes
Chondrodystrophy	Intrauterine growth retardation, large head, high forehead, short extremities	Trident hand, lumbar hyperlordosis
Marfan syndrome	Long fingers and toes, thin extremities	Scoliosis, funnel chest, aortic insufficiency, mitral valve prolapse

Table 49.5   Examples of fetal anomalies with an autosomal-recessive inheritance (3, 4, 5, 10)

Name	Ultrasound features	Additional features
Achondrogenesis	Hydropic appearance, growth retardation, short limbs	Short neck, very short life expectancy
Fryns syndrome	Diaphragmatic defect, holoprosencephaly	Cardiac anomalies, hypoplastic fingernails, small fingertips, lens opacity
Ellis–van Creveld syndrome	Hexadactyly, distal limb shortening, occasional cleft lip and palate	Cardiac anomalies (ASD), oral frenula, small nails
Pena–Shokeir syndrome	Intrauterine growth retardation, joint contractures, clubfoot, pulmonary hypoplasia	Depressed nasal tip, low-set ears
Osteogenesis imperfecta	Multiple fractures in utero	Blue sclerae

Table 49.6   Examples of fetal anomalies with an X-linked recessive inheritance (only males affected) (3, 8, 9)

Name	Ultrasound features	Additional features
Aqueductal stenosis	Internal hydrocephalus of first through third ventricles	Thumb anomalies
Lenz microphthalmos	Bilateral microphthalmos	Prominent ears, hanging shoulders
Bloch–Sulzberger incontinentia pigmenti	Ocular anomalies such as microphthalmos, may be unilateral	Streak-like vesicles predominantly on the arms, head, and trunk

currence in the brothers of affected individuals. Molecular genetic tests are available. Other disorders are shown in Table 49.**6**.

Classification aids. Certain facts can be helpful in the classification of monogenic disorders, such as advanced paternal age at conception (> 40 years), which may suggest the presence of a dominant new mutation. Parental consanguinity can be useful in recognizing an autosomal-recessive disorder. The occurrence of other affected males in the maternal family may signal an X-linked recessive mode of inheritance.

Recurrence risk. In counseling for monogenic disorders, the following information is helpful in predicting the recurrence risk in a future pregnancy:

Dominant trait. If the child has inherited a disorder as a dominant trait that has already occurred in the family (i.e., one of the parents is affected), the recurrence risk for future offspring is 50%, regardless of gender (Fig. 49.**6**).

Dominant new mutation. If there is no prior familial occurrence and the paternal age is advanced, a dominant new mutation should be suspected. The likelihood of recurrence in another child is small (exception: mosaicism).

Autosomal-recessive inheritance. If there is a definite genetic syndrome with an autosomal-recessive mode of inheritance (e.g., parents are blood relatives or come from an isolated group), the recurrence risk is 25%, regardless of the gender of the offspring (Fig. 49.**7**).

Sex-linked recessive inheritance. If a sex-linked recessive disease has been observed in a family, the recurrence risk is 25% in future offspring and 50% in males (Fig. 49.**8**).

Prenatal testing. Prenatal testing is currently available for a number of monogenic disorders in established index cases. It is based on various diagnostic measures such as biochemical testing or indirect or direct molecular genetic testing, and gross anomalies are accessible to ultrasound analysis.

■ *Anomalies with Multifactorial Inheritance*

"Multifactorial inheritance" refers to an increased familial occurrence of certain diseases and anomalies that are not classifiable in terms of Mendelian inheritance. For many years, efforts were made to establish a dominant inheritance for most of these cases by reference to phenomena such as decreased penetrance and variable expressivity. But in the early 1960s, the concept was altered to emphasize the interaction between hereditary disposition and environmental factors (Fig. 49.**9**).

Environmental factors. Different environmental factors are active in different disorders. The importance of a folic acid deficiency in the pathogenesis of neural tube defects has been well established, while a vitamin deficiency (especially of B vitamins) has been implicated in the pathogenesis of cleft lip and palate. Overweight, certain medications (e.g., corticosteroids), and serious diseases have long been known to precipitate diabetes mellitus. Lack of sleep, fever, alcohol abuse, and flickering illumination are known for their significance in triggering epileptic seizures.

The two most important congenital anomalies with multifactorial inheritance in genetic counseling are neural tube defects and cleft lip and palate, both of which are clearly detectable with ultrasound. Neural tube defects occur in one in 1000 newborns, cleft lip and palate in one in 600–700 newborns. Other examples are club foot, pyloric stenosis, scoliosis, congenital heart defects, and congenital hip dislocation.

Recurrence risks. Recurrence risks for multifactorial disorders and diseases can be calculated as empirical risk figures by applying statistical methods in a large family tree. Sex predilections are known to exist for some diseases, such as hip dysplasia and scoliosis in females and pyloric stenosis in males.

It is important to determine whether the abnormal trait is an isolated occurrence in the affected child or is found in conjunction with other abnormalities or malformations, suggesting a syndromic pattern. These cases require a different risk calculation, and additional options are often available for antenatal detection (Table 49.**7**).

Table 49.**7** Syndromes in which the cardinal feature is cleft lip and palate or a neural tube defect (selection) (1, 2, 3, 8, 10)

Syndromes with cleft lip and palate	Syndromes with a neural tube defect
➤ Trisomy 13	➤ Trisomy 18
➤ Ellis–van Creveld syndrome	➤ Arnold–Chiari syndrome
➤ Chondrodysplasia punctata	➤ Dandy–Walker syndrome
➤ Trisomy 18 (rare)	➤ Meckel–Gruber syndrome

■ *Specific Genetic Syndromes, Associations, and Sequences*

Syndromes. There are a number of syndromes with characteristic features that cannot be ascribed to any other modes of inheritance or specific causal factors. It is noteworthy that affected individuals are more similar to one another than to their biological siblings. They also deviate markedly from their typical family phenotype. Usually these syndromes are named for their initial describer and occasionally for the first person affected. There are some syndromes for which causal factors have not yet been identified. Prenatal detection is difficult because even a quality ultrasound examination cannot detect most typical syndrome-associated dysmorphias.

Ultrasound is usually helpful in syndromes characterized by severe anomalies. Not infrequently, these are sporadic cases that have little risk of recurrence, but most parents still experience significant and understandable concern (Table 49.**8**).

Table 49.**8** Genetic syndromes with different recurrence risks and a characteristic pattern of symptoms (selection) (3, 8, 10)

Name	Ultrasound features	Additional features
Ivemark syndrome	Complex cardiac anomaly, asplenia, situs inversus	Trilobed lung, occasional polysplenia
Rubinstein–Taybi syndrome	Microcephaly, abnormal profile (?)	Broad thumbs and big toes
Weaver syndrome	Intrauterine macrosomia (without maternal diabetes mellitus)	Broad forehead, hypertelorism, long philtrum
Silver–Russell syndrome	Intrauterine growth retardation, relatively large head	Triangular face, limb asymmetries

Associations. "Association" refers to patterns of disturbances that are distinguished by a number of malformations for which a pathogenetic connection cannot be identified. Because the same pattern is observed again and again, these disorders are often designated by acronyms derived from the first letters of the various features. Figures on recurrence risks vary greatly and are based partly on empirical data (Table 49.**9**).

Sequence. For pathogenetic reasons, some characteristic congenital disorders are called a "sequence" because the pattern of abnormalities results from a succession of conditions. Observations in the literature indicate a slightly increased recurrence risk. Close relatives should be scrutinized for microsymptoms to ensure that a familial disposition with an increased recurrence risk is not overlooked (Table 49.**10**).

▬ *Imprinting*

Disorders caused by imprinting are not detectable with ultrasound. They are mentioned here for completeness and because of their special causal mechanism.

The best known examples are Prader–Willi syndrome and Angelman syndrome. They are caused by uniparental disomy, in which the child inherits two paternal copies (Prader–Willi) or two maternal copies (Angelman) of a very small segment of chromosome 15. There is a deletion of the corresponding chromosome segment in the father or mother. When crossover occurs, the chromosome that is present reconstructs the DNA segment on the partner chromosome as a duplicate of itself. The affected child is homozygous for the genes located on this chromosome segment that are responsible for the disorders.

Conclusions

Risk figures. Figure 49.**10**, which is based on Fig. 49.**3**, shows the risk figures that should be presented in genetic counseling when the congenital anomaly has been assigned to one of the causes indicated. They can be very diverse. Unfortunately, there are still counseling cases in which an exact cause cannot be identified, and so a definite recurrence risk cannot be stated. Because the genetic counselor always presents the couple with the highest risk figure, which they must use in deciding whether to conceive, the result is a very unsatisfactory situation for the counselor and clients alike.

Counseling situation. The variety of possible causes of congenital anomalies have been presented in this chapter. It is obvious that the more accurately the pattern of abnormalities has been determined or documented by a postmortem examination, the easier it will be to counsel the parents of an affected child and present them with a clear picture.

If a primary diagnosis cannot be established, an effort should be made to focus as much as possible on information pertaining to the family history and prior obstetric history during the counseling session. Principal features should be distinguished from accompanying features, and isolated disorders from complex disorders, so that the counselor and couple can work together to weigh and prioritize the risk factors for a future pregnancy (Table 49.**1**).

It is clear that the discussion of the various causal possibilities can be very stressful and challenging for laypersons. The clients must not be spared this process, however, if they are to understand how the risk estimates were arrived at and why, in some cases, it is impossible to offer a clear assessment of the recurrence risk.

Special ultrasound examinations. In all cases, however, the parents in the new pregnancy will have fears and apprehensions and will seek reassurance. These are the cases in which the genetic counselor will recommend an additional ultrasound study, preferably a special scan at 20 weeks' gestation, to look for and exclude abnormalities. Despite the limits of what it can achieve, this scan will in many cases provide the worried parents with needed reassurance for the rest of the pregnancy.

Table 49.**9** Associations: a selection of fetal anomalies with undetermined pathogenesis (3, 10)

Name	Acronym	Features
VATER/VACTERL	V	Vertebral and vascular anomalies
	A	Anal and auricular deformities
	C	Cardiac anomalies
	T	Tracheoesophageal fistula
	E	Esophageal atresia
	R	Radial aplasia, renal and rib anomalies
	L	Limb anomalies
CHARGE	C	Coloboma (unilateral or bilateral)
	H	Heart defects
	A	Atresia of the choanae
	R	Retarded growth and psychomotoric development
	G	Genital hypoplasia
	E	Ear deformities and deafness
CHILD (X-linked dominant)	C	Congenital
	H	Hemidysplasia
	I	Ichthyosiform nevus
	L	Limb
	D	Defect

Table 49.**10** Sequences: fetal anomalies in which the symptom patterns are interpreted as a succession of disturbances (2, 3, 10)

Name	Ultrasound features	Additional features
Potter I syndrome	Renal agenesis, oligohydramnios, clubfeet	Abnormal face with a flattened nose and canthobuccal fold
Prune belly syndrome	Greatly dilated bladder, megaureters, hydronephrosis	Urethral valve or stenosis, flaccid abdominal wall
Pierre Robin syndrome	Small chin, glossoptosis	Cleft palate, postnatal respiratory problems

References

1. Gorlin, R.J., Cohen, M.M.jr., Levin, L.S.: Syndromes of the head and neck. 3rd. ed. Oxford: University Press 1990
2. Goodman, R.M., Gorlin, R.J.: Atlas of the face in genetic disorders. St. Louis: Mosby 1977
3. Leiber, B.: Die klinischen Syndrome. 8. Aufl. München: Urban & Schwarzenberg 1996
4. McKusick, V.A.: Mendelian inheritance in man. 11th ed. Baltimore & London: Hopkins University Press 1994
5. Spranger, J.W., Langer, L.O., Wiedemann, H.R.: Bone dysplasias. An Atlas of Constitutional Disorders of Skeletal Development. Stuttgart: Gustav Fischer 1974
6. Temtamy, S., McKusick, V.A.: The genetics of hand malformations. Birth Defects, Orig. Art. Ser., Vol. XIV Nr. 3. The National Foundation – March of Dimes. New York: Alan R. Liss. Inc. 1978
7. Theile, U.: Checkliste Genetische Beratung. Stuttgart: Thieme 1992
8. Warkany, J.: Congenital malformations. Chicago: Year Books Medical Publishers 1975
9. Warkany, J., Lemire, R.J., Cohen M.M.jr.: Mental Retardation and Congenital Malformations of the Central Nervous System. Chicago: Year Book Medical Publishers 1981
10. Wiedemann, H.R., Kunze, J.: Atlas der klinischen Syndrome. 4. Aufl. Stuttgart: Schattauer 1995

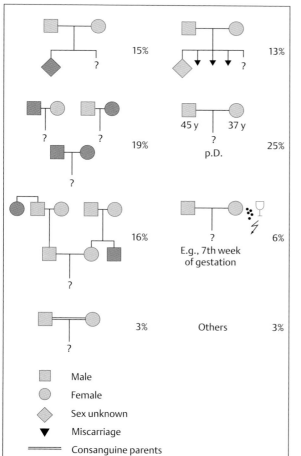

1

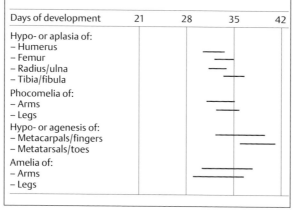

2

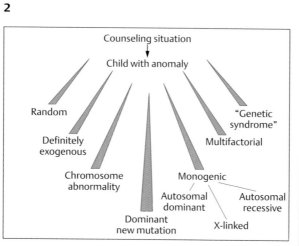

3

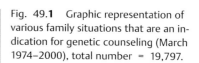

Fig. 49.**1** Graphic representation of various family situations that are an indication for genetic counseling (March 1974–2000), total number = 19,797.

Fig. 49.**2** Critical periods for the development of limb anomalies following thalidomide exposure during pregnancy (after Pliess 1962).

Fig. 49.**3** Various causes of a fetal anomaly from a genetic standpoint.

Fig. 49.**4**   Karyogram of an unbalanced 13/14 translocation. Karyotype 46,XX,-14,+t(13q;14q).

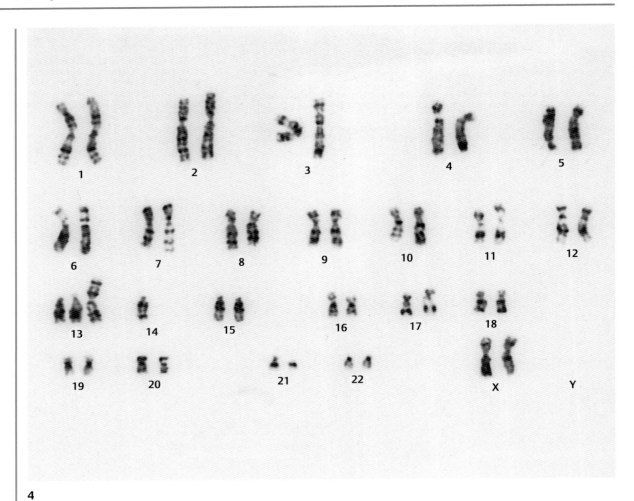

4

Fig. 49.**5**   Karyogram of a balanced 13/14 translocation. Karyotype 45,XX,-13,-14,+t(13q;14q).

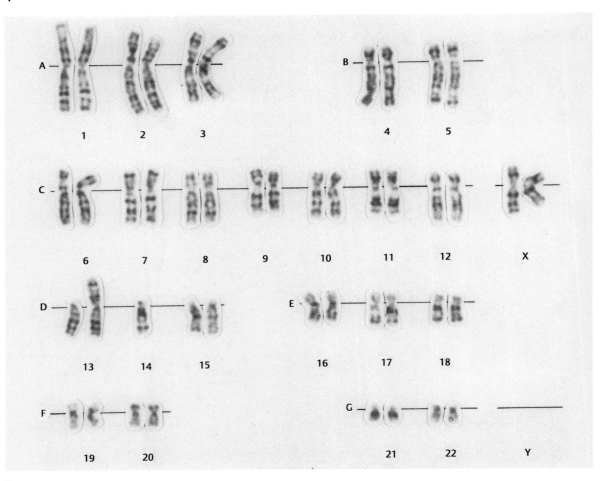

5

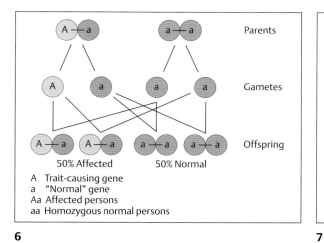

A Trait-causing gene
a "Normal" gene
Aa Affected persons
aa Homozygous normal persons

6

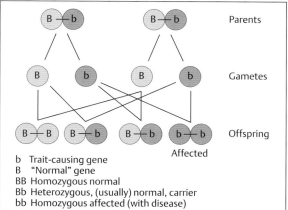

b Trait-causing gene
B "Normal" gene
BB Homozygous normal
Bb Heterozygous, (usually) normal, carrier
bb Homozygous affected (with disease)

7

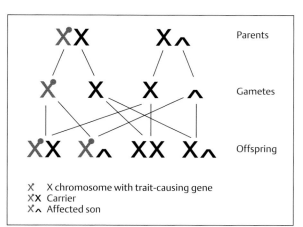

X̍ X chromosome with trait-causing gene
X̍X Carrier
X̍ʌ Affected son

8

Heredity

Environment

Blood groups,
monogenic
disorders

Accident (?)
Infection (?)

Traits and diseases in which a hereditary
disposition and a certain environmental influence
must coincide

9

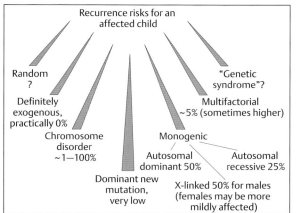

Recurrence risks for an
affected child

Random
?

"Genetic
syndrome"?

Definitely
exogenous,
practically 0%

Multifactorial
~5% (sometimes higher)

Chromosome
disorder
~1–100%

Monogenic

Autosomal
dominant 50%

Autosomal
recessive 25%

Dominant new
mutation,
very low

X-linked 50% for males
(females may be more
mildly affected)

10

Modes of inheritance

Fig. 49.**6** Autosomal-dominant inheritance.

Fig. 49.**7** Autosomal-recessive inheritance.

Fig. 49.**8** X-linked recessive inheritance.

Fig. 49.**9** Multifactorial inheritance. Interaction of hereditary disposition and environmental factors.

Fig. 49.**10** Risk figures for the various causes of fetal anomalies in genetic counseling, corresponding to Fig. 49.**3**.

50 Ethical Considerations in Obstetric Ultrasound

Value System

Very generally, ethics refers to the rational foundation for rules of conduct. Establishing rules for medical conduct, as in evidence-based medicine, would conform to this definition of ethics in the broadest sense, although the ethical issues of this aspect basically involve deciding between right and wrong medical actions from a technical standpoint. For most physicians, this kind of decision is so prominent that it eclipses ethical considerations in the narrower sense—i.e., issues that address good and bad or go beyond technical aspects to question what is good or bad for the well-being of man. The usual scientific criteria that are applied in medicine are not adequate for this purpose, because they are devoid of values which go beyond the technical but are crucial for making ethical decisions in the strict sense.

Values can be neither proved nor justified using categories of the natural sciences. For ethical justifications in the strict sense, one is forced to leave the solid ground of the physical and enter the uncertain realm of the metaphysical, where the physician, often trained only in the natural sciences, must forego the accustomed security of provable facts and theorems. As a result, physicians are reluctant to base vitally important decisions on philosophical maxims or even on religious beliefs, which some hold and others do not. They still seek to base their actions on the natural sciences, even in areas where scientific criteria can at best provide only an apparent ethical rationale.

This attitude overlooks the fact that in western culture, which fostered the development of the natural sciences in the first place, a system of values prevails to which every contemporary person owes his or her physical and social existence. One aspect of this basically truth-oriented value system is that the natural sciences mandate a strict prohibition of all subjectivity and of any value-related incursions on the research process. The practical implementation of scientific knowledge cannot (and must not) occur without reference to values, however.

The Western value system traces its roots to the Judeo-Christian belief that God created man—and every human being—in his own likeness. Later the Enlightenment and especially the French Revolution secularized the implications of this belief. They formulated the concept of human rights, upon which the constitutions of present-day western nations and communities are based. They became—at least as ideals—the foundation for the peaceful coexistence of human beings.

A central aspect of this belief system is the concept of human dignity, which states only that human beings have a special place in the universe without defining specifically what that place may be. Every person has an equal share in this privileged place, giving rise to the concepts of equal rights and the right to life. The absolute prohibition against killing is society's response to this notion, as is the relative claim of all persons to the resources of this earth and to human services, to which society responds with the principle of solidarity, or mutual responsibility. Human dignity also implies the right to self-determination.

Thus, the right to life in the defensive sense (prohibition against killing) and in the sense of having a claim to resources (solidarity) and autonomy cannot be justified from a physical standpoint. At the same time, they require no metaphysical justification if they are accepted as the basis for societal living simply because people from western cultures find themselves to be a product of these rights and interpret them as an historical given rather than a man-made system that is at

their disposal. Those who recognize and acknowledge their existence as the product of a concrete historical process may do without a rigorous metaphysical foundation for their ethics.

Principles

We may now list several basic principles for ethical issues relating to obstetric ultrasound, especially in the area of prenatal diagnosis:

1. The right to life of every human being in the defensive sense. Aside from war, self-protection, and the death penalty, this right is absolute and is not subject to circumstances, situations, or conditions.
2. The right to life of every human being in the sense of a claim to resources. This right affirms the principle of solidarity, which is subject to limitations based on circumstances, situations, and conditions.
3. The right to life of every human being to self-determination, which is not absolute but is also subject to limitations.

In the area of obstetric ultrasound, these rights compete and conflict with one another because on the one hand, the mother and child are independent beings and are incommensurable bearers of these rights. But at the same time, the pregnant woman and her unborn child are interconnected in such a way that what benefits one may harm the other.

Ethical Issues Relating to Autonomy

Autonomy of the Patient

The ultrasound examination is comparable to simple external observation in the sense that it causes no physical changes and certainly no permanent ones. It assumes the status of an "intervention" from the patient's viewpoint only when the transducer is introduced into a natural body orifice such as the vagina. But regardless of this, the very fact that every ultrasound examination is done to collect information on a physical condition is sufficient to require the consent of the patient. Generally this is easily secured, provided the examination is indicated and is done solely for the health of the pregnant woman. Generally this indication exists if the examination is expected to produce a result that has therapeutic implications (even the absence of a condition that may require treatment has a therapeutic implication—i.e., that no treatment is required).

Nevertheless, an ultrasound examination, even when indicated (perhaps urgently) for the benefit of the patient, may be refused by her. She need give no reason for this refusal. Of course, the physician is obliged in such cases to inform the patient of the possible consequences of her refusal (and not merely to avoid liability claims). It is also incumbent upon the physician to allay the fears that laypersons may have regarding the harmful effects of ultrasound. In other cases, the pregnant woman may refuse ultrasound because she does not wish to know the sex of her child. In this regard, she has the right not only to be unaware of her child's gender but also to request that no such determination be made. Her "right not to know" can be affirmed by assuring her that, even though the examination itself is necessary, any inadvertent gender identification will be kept confidential.

Some pregnant women who reject pregnancy termination as an option will exercise their general right not to know by refusing to be confronted with findings that would raise pregnancy termination as a possible issue to be considered. In theory, the physician could promise such women to withhold this type of finding from them. From a practical standpoint, however, we would advise strongly against this. The reality with which the mother may be confronted after the delivery might be such that she may regard its nondisclosure as not being covered by her initial refusal of information. It is better for the physician to handle this type of case either by withholding prenatal ultrasound altogether or by securing the pregnant woman's consent to have all findings, except for gender, reported to her.

While the focus of our discussions so far have been on the welfare of the pregnant woman, questions of autonomy become more difficult to answer when dealing with the welfare of the unborn child. Does the pregnant woman have an obligation to act or tolerate actions for the benefit of her child? At first sight, one might regards this question as self-evident and answer in the affirmative, reasoning that the pregnant woman, like a mother, has a definite obligation to her child. And this is obviously the case—but only for an internal frame of reference—i.e., the woman's own conscience. The question of whether any external authority can demand that the pregnant woman act or tolerate actions on behalf of her child requires further scrutiny.

Let us consider the extreme case of whether the pregnant woman must tolerate a treatment that threatens her life for the benefit of her child, and thus whether an obligation that may be ethically binding upon her internally can also be imposed on her from the outside. Some physicians believe that this is the case. They include those who claim that, in some situations, a pregnant woman must tolerate a cesarean section for a fetal indication. Ultimately this would mean that it may become necessary to force the patient to undergo a cesarean section for the sake of the child—a proposition that is in gross violation of her autonomy. With this in mind, it appears justified to enforce the obligation to act or tolerate actions only in the "internal" frame of reference, meaning the patient's own conscience, while granting no one the right to impose an external will, even if it would be life-saving for the child.

Only action by the pregnant woman (or someone appointed by her) aimed at causing the death of the child is ethically proscribed. Similarly, while there are laws that prohibit "abortion," there are no laws against the negligent killing of the unborn or against causing deliberate (or negligent) bodily injury to a fetus.

In the future, these considerations will go beyond the diagnostic importance of obstetric ultrasound and will assume growing significance as more prenatal treatments become available. Because no such treatment is conceivable that does not act on the child by going "through the mother" in some way, inevitably invading the physical integrity of the pregnant woman, her consent will always be necessary. She will owe her child this consent in varying degrees according to the internal dictates of her conscience. This tolerance cannot ethically be imposed from the outside, not even indirectly. Therefore the mother is not held responsible for the consequences of not treating the child, and she must not be sanctioned for such an omission. Beyond the prohibition against killing, she is subject to no externally imposed ethical obligations to act or to tolerate actions. It may seem contradictory, then, that the pregnant woman is prohibited from killing her child by external constraints, yet she has the external right to refuse to act or tolerate actions, even if this results in the death of her child. This contradiction does exist if we judge actions and omissions only by their consequences. It disappears, however, when we truly respect the autonomy of the human being: the negative behavioral norm (here, the prohibition against killing) limits the freedom of conduct only for a very specific act. On the other hand, a positive behavioral norm (the obligation to take action or tolerate a procedure) precludes all other possible actions and brooks no other ethically responsible arrangement. To this extent it revokes autonomy, whereas a negative behavioral norm (a

prohibition) merely restraints autonomy by setting a defined limit. For the "inner frame of reference" or conscience, the woman's state of mind continues to have ethical meaning. This may even include her intention to kill her child by taking no action or withholding consent. From the outside, respect for the pregnant woman's autonomy and ultimately respect for her as a moral individual who can choose between good and bad will prevent any unwarranted interference and moral constraints.

This concept will continue to be valid even when future methods of prenatal treatment offer greater success and are less risky and invasive for the pregnant woman. The incursion into her physical integrity requires and will continue to require her consent, and the refusal of that consent will not be subject to ethical scrutiny from the outside. It must simply be respected by virtue of the patient's autonomy, regardless of the emergency situation that may threaten her child. This same reasoning should apply to legal judgments as well.

Autonomy of the Unborn Child

At first it seems ridiculous to grant autonomy to a being that does not have the slightest opportunity to make its own decisions. But autonomy is an essential and inherent human trait, regardless of whether or not it is exercised. If necessary, it must be asserted by others in a representative capacity. Where health issues are concerned, the mother, father, physician, or the state may feel called to this responsibility. Ultimately, however, this representative authority must be subordinate to the maternal right of self-determination over her own body, if only because anything done to the child has to "go through" the mother. In the final analysis, then, only the mother can represent her child where prenatal treatment is concerned. This means that an inherent conflict exists between the interests of the mother and those of the child. Thus, the possibility of exercising in a representative capacity the autonomy of a person unable to form or express his own will is limited to consenting to measures that are of benefit to that person. Consent to measures that benefit someone else, such as live organ donation or a diagnostic procedure for someone else's benefit, and consent for killing the child could be given only by the child and could therefore not be substituted.

The statements made above are by no means undisputed in ethical discussions. But if we accept the principle of human autonomy, the above statements follow with reasonable certainty. To refute them, it would be necessary to refute autonomy.

▪ *Ethical Issues Regarding the Right to Life in the Defensive Sense*

Aside from the justifiable exceptions noted above, the right to life is absolute, and the prohibition against killing is considered to be independent of all circumstances and always valid. In an historical context, this does not mean that anyone can justify such an exception and lay claim to it. Tradition acknowledges only the three above-named exceptions to the prohibition against killing, and even these are not uncontested. Moreover, in the Judeo-Christian tradition and in the tradition of the Enlightenment derived from it, there are no justifiable reasons for making exceptions to the prohibition against killing. It follows, then, that anyone wishing to make such an exception must seek justification for it outside the tradition of the Enlightenment, thereby abandoning the common foundation for the norms of peaceful human coexistence in the western tradition. Such a person is entirely on his own.

Because this can have harsh, emotionally intolerable implications for the killing of the unborn, solutions are sought which do not conflict with the prohibition against killing.

One such attempt is to consider the prohibition against killing to be inapplicable to the unborn, especially in early pregnancy, on the grounds that the "object" of the killing is not yet a human being and the prohibition against killing is not relevant until the conceptus has attained human status. This cutoff point cannot be defined scientifically, however, because such a determination involves value judgments. At best, science can tell us the point or developmental stage before which a human being definitely does not exist because a human organism is not yet present. In normal sexual reproduction, the completion of fertilization (union of the pronuclei) adequately defines this point in time. It must be conceded that, from a biological perspective, human life did exist in the gametes before that point. But the real issue is not human life but the life of a human being—a distinction that is easily overlooked with indiscriminate language use. A human organism is not present before fertilization is completed, and a living human being does not yet exist.

In principle, this (negative) statement also applies to the inception of human life in monozygotic multiples and, at least conceivably, to a cloned human being. The conditions of a cloned organism's asexual reproduction make it clear, however, that the reverse conclusion that "a human being starts with the completion of fertilization" cannot be conclusive and that an additional criterion is required. In a pragmatic sense, we can accept the end of fertilization in sexual reproduction as the beginning of human life, just to be certain that we do no injustice. But this is not a rigorous biological argument, merely a biologically oriented attribution. A rigorous biological rationale cannot be offered because, as we noted earlier, it entails a value judgment that is not grounded in the natural sciences. While it is generally accepted in the community of western values that a human being is a human being from his or her inception, this assertion cannot simply be projected on the biological level. So then, the consensus that human life begins when fertilization ends is not a biological claim but an ethical decision which conforms to the high value ascribed to man and seeks to remain on the "safe side." This decision is supported by the fact that as development continues after fertilization, there is no other single event that could better characterize the point where human life begins.

Against this background, there is simply no way that one can ethically justify the direct and deliberate killing of an unborn child. One cannot even point to circumstances where one life must be weighed against another—the life of the pregnant woman against that of her child—because the life of every human being is of equal value. In cases where pregnancies are terminated for a "medical indication," differentiated ethical considerations must be applied.

A medical indication in a narrow sense exists when the pregnancy poses an immediate danger to the life or health of the mother, and the danger can be eliminated by terminating the pregnancy. This reasoning disregards the child and deals strictly with the pregnancy itself. If a child were not at issue, it would be an easy matter to justify the termination. In reality, of course, we cannot simply disregard the child. If killing the child is the means for ending the pregnancy, it cannot be justified. But if killing the child is a necessary or likely outcome of terminating the pregnancy—i.e., it is not the deliberate goal of the attending physician but is seen as an unintended, possibly unavoidable consequence of the procedure, then there is room for making a different ethical interpretation. One may consider it splitting hairs to question whether the child is killed deliberately or as an unintended side effect. But from an ethical standpoint, the essential difference becomes clear when we ask about the success of the procedure. If the physician considers the procedure a failure if the child survives, then he must have intended it to die, which cannot be justified. But if he views the child's survival in a positive light, then he did not intend to kill the child but only end the pregnancy. Taking fetal death as a necessary, unintended, but ultimately acceptable consequence of the procedure when the mother's life is threatened or her health is seriously jeopardized may seem ethically justified in a liberal interpretation. If we apply stricter criteria, then we might accept a variable degree of risk to the life of the child by making an effort to ensure that the child actually has a chance

to survive (postponing the procedure, using a less traumatizing technique). These considerations are based on the assumption that the prohibition against killing protects the child from deliberate killing, but that the concern for his life may well be subject to a choice between conflicting rights.

But the ethics break down if we broaden the medical indication, as the law does, and include "fetal indication" under the heading of medical indications. If the life and health of the pregnant woman are not immediately threatened by the pregnancy itself but only by the child that will issue from it, then killing the child becomes an ethically unacceptable means of treatment. If, contrary to intentions, the child were to survive the procedure, the physician would have to judge the procedure a failure because the child is not dead. In this instance what is justified legally cannot be justified ethically without resorting to interpretations that contradict the traditional prohibition against killing.

Accordingly, pregnancy termination for a "fetal indication" cannot be ethically justified. But can it at least be tolerated? Let us take the case of an existing pregnancy in which the fetus is discovered (e.g., by ultrasound) to have such a serious defect that the pregnant woman may not reasonably be expected to carry the child to term (raising another question of what is "reasonable" and who defines it). In this instance it becomes humanly difficult to put our high ethical principles into practice. There is a tendency in such cases to accept and tolerate a pregnancy termination aimed at the death of the child due to the overwhelming nature of the situation from the standpoint of the responsible parties. This acknowledgment of human limitations has been applied by the Catholic Church, which condemns medically indicated abortions regardless of the circumstances or intentions, yet is more lenient toward them in pastoral practice. The Church concedes that the affected parties are in a "status perplexus"—a confusing and overwhelming situation that does not justify killing the unborn but does mitigate its culpability, perhaps to a level of practical tolerance. In a similar way, pregnancy termination may be tolerated in difficult and unforeseen cases following prenatal diagnosis.

From this perspective, however, it would be ethically untenable to conceive a child with a known risk while holding out the option of an "indicated termination" based on the results of prenatal diagnosis. In such a case, the parents would conceive a child while reserving the right to kill it if it does not conform to certain health criteria. This "conditional conception" is ethically untenable because the right to life that a child possesses by its very existence is made dependent upon conditions that it must fulfill.

It may be countered that the parents have a right to a healthy child, but there is no inherent right to health or even to have a child. As far as health is concerned, the most that one can claim is access to the means for preserving or restoring health. But this right is not absolute and does not outweigh the defensive right to life of the child. As far as the right to a child is concerned, at most there is a right not to be hindered by a third party from conceiving and bearing a child; but under no circumstances can one argue that the "right to a child" justifies killing a (different) child in order to exercise that right. It follows that parents should give up their wish to conceive if they are unwilling to assume the (potentially high) risk of having a handicapped child. Advising them to have a "trial conception" would be ethically wrong.

But when a physician is called upon to administer prenatal tests in such a "conditional" program, he cannot ethically refuse. He may not ask whether or not his patient has deliberately (in an ethically unjustified manner) orchestrated a condition of medical need. Whether willing or not, he is obliged to provide his services to the conditionally conceiving parents. In any case, he may not refuse them on the grounds that he disapproves of their conditional gestation. At most he may threaten such refusal in a future instance, although this threat cannot be carried out in a future pregnancy any more than it can in the present one. The principle of not questioning his patients' motives makes the physician an instrument for the unethical conduct of others.

Selective Fetocide in Multiple Pregnancy

Higher-order multiple pregnancies are considered a medical indication for pregnancy termination because they directly endanger the life and health of the mother. If other means are available to reduce or eliminate the danger, they are of course preferable to ending the pregnancy. One such means is a procedure intended to reduce the number of fetuses in a multiple gestation. The term "selective fetocide" is somewhat misleading in that the selection is basically limited to the most favorably located fetus(es), and this would have to be considered a rather nonselective process. But the critical consideration is that the procedure is designed to kill, and the affected fetus has no chance of survival. Such a procedure cannot be ethically justified, therefore, although it may be tolerated by noting that ultimately the killing is not deliberate and, at least in theory, would be avoided if at all possible. Another mitigating factor is that eliminating one or more fetuses avoids the necessity of aborting the entire pregnancy. Even so, there is no ethically satisfactory solution in this kind of situation.

Physicians other than the gynecologist attending the multiple pregnancy should make every effort to spare their patients and colleagues from having to deal with these dilemmas. In the treatment of infertility, the risk of a high-order multiple pregnancy must be scrupulously avoided. In practice this means foregoing an immediate chance for a pregnancy if hormonal stimulation has induced the maturation of too many oocytes. A physician who allows the pregnancy to occur at the cost of a high-order multiple gestation makes his colleagues, who must then help the mother out of danger, the instrument of his irresponsible conduct.

Prenatal Diagnosis

General reservations against any prenatal diagnosis (PND) misconstrue its purpose and reduce it to the role of eliminating children that are unwanted for health reasons. PND derives its justification from the fact that it allows the pregnancy to be monitored (e.g., to detect multiple gestation) in preparation for the birth. It is also used to monitor fetal development and is justified by the therapeutic implications that these findings may have. PND would be morally objectionable only if it were used for the selective killing of fetuses, but this has no practical significance because this purpose of PND is inseparable from its other functions. Other ethical issues relating to PND were addressed above under Autonomy.

Prenatal Therapy and Medical Experimentation

Ethical considerations on prenatal therapy were also discussed under Autonomy. With regard to the child, the difficulty is that it is unable to give its consent, which therefore must be given by a representative. Only the mother can act in this capacity, because a decision made by anyone else, be it the father or a court-appointed guardian, would be limited by the autonomy of the pregnant woman. Thus, no prenatal therapy can be provided without her consent, and conversely no one can prevent her from accepting prenatal treatment for her child. Possible inability of the pregnant woman to form or express her will in these matters is certainly a very rare situation and would further complicate the ethical picture, but the general mechanisms for this contingency are in place. In cases where the pregnant woman is brain-dead, the risk/benefit appraisal on behalf of the unborn child should be done with particular care. It should be determined whether or not the risks appear to be acceptable from the standpoint of the child and whether the means necessary for preserving the life of the unborn child are commensurate with the outcome that can reasonably be achieved. The claim of the unborn child to such means, which include ultrasound monitoring, is only a relative claim, and therefore the reasonable withholding of such means is not considered "killing by neglect." The attending physician is the only party competent to make this decision. Whether appointing a guardian for the unborn child would be of legal help is a controversial issue.

Prenatal therapy that is still in the experimental stage also requires a risk/benefit appraisal for both the mother and the child. It also requires approval by a competent ethical commission. This applies only to planned therapeutic trials, however, in which a protocol is followed that also takes into account the expected scientific gain. Experimental therapies that are tried in individual cases without systematic controls are not subject to this oversight, but they do require rigorous self-review by the responsible physician. In both types of experiment, measures are prohibited that are not of direct fetal benefit, such as biopsies or other ancillary procedures that are done only for purposes of scientific investigation. Two exceptions to this principle are recognized:

- Cases in which the risk and discomfort of the procedure are negligible.
- Cases in which the experimental treatment has a very high chance of a successful outcome for the child, and only those willing to assume the risks and discomfort necessary for a successful scientific outcome are enrolled.

Anyone who may consent to this risk assumption in a representative capacity should receive careful and detailed counseling.

These discussions make it clear that a general withholding of experimental therapies from those unable to give their consent is too undiscriminating and wastes opportunities for those involved. On the other hand, the participation of those unable to give consent (the unborn) in experiments that do not directly benefit them but serve the interests of other parties is ethically objectionable at a fundamental level. It is also true, however, that institutionally sanctioned exceptions may be allowed (consent from a guardian, approval by an ethical commission) in cases where the risks and discomfort are minimal.

Appendix

51 Biometry Curves and Tables

Synopsis

Table 53.**1** Synopsis of biometric data (mean values for completed weeks of gestation, weeks = weeks postmenstrual age), length and circumference measurements in mm, weight in g

Weeks	CCD[1]	CRL[1]	BPD[1,2]	OFD[2]	HC[2]	ATD[2]	ASD[2]	AC[2]	Fe[2]	Ti[2]	Fi[2]	Hu[2]	Ra[2]	Ul[2]	Foot[3]	Wt[4] m.	Wt[4] f.	L[4] m.	L[4] f.	Weeks
5	5	1																		5
6	13	4																		6
7	21	8	3																	7
8	29	14	7																	8
9	36	22	10																	9
10	44	32	14																	10
11	51	43	17																	11
12	57	55	20																	12
13	63	66	26	32	96	22	21	67	11	9	8	10	6	8	12					13
14			29	35	106	25	24	78	15	12	11	13	10	11	16					14
15			32	39	118	29	28	89	18	15	14	17	13	15	19					15
16			35	43	130	32	31	100	21	18	17	20	16	18	22					16
17			39	47	143	36	35	111	24	21	20	23	18	21	25					17
18			42	52	155	39	38	122	27	24	23	26	21	23	28					18
19			46	56	168	43	42	132	30	26	25	28	23	26	31					19
20			49	60	181	46	45	143	33	29	28	31	25	28	33					20
21			52	65	193	50	48	154	36	31	30	33	28	31	36					21
22			56	69	206	53	52	165	39	34	33	36	30	33	39					22
23			59	73	218	56	55	175	41	36	35	38	32	35	41	600	580	31	31	23
24			62	77	230	60	59	186	44	38	37	40	33	37	44	690	670	32	32	24
25			65	81	241	63	62	196	46	41	39	42	35	39	46	800	760	34	33	25
26			68	84	253	66	65	207	49	43	41	45	37	41	49	940	880	35	35	26
27			71	88	263	70	68	217	51	45	43	47	39	43	52	1080	1000	36	36	27
28			74	91	273	73	72	227	53	47	45	48	40	45	54	1220	1120	38	37	28
29			77	94	283	76	75	237	56	49	47	50	42	47	56	1350	1250	39	39	29
30			80	97	292	79	78	247	58	51	49	52	43	49	59	1520	1420	41	40	30
31			82	100	301	82	81	257	60	52	51	54	44	50	61	1690	1590	42	42	31
32			85	102	309	85	84	266	62	54	52	55	46	52	64	1890	1790	43	43	32
33			87	105	316	88	87	276	64	56	54	57	47	53	66	2130	2030	45	44	33
34			89	107	323	91	90	285	66	57	56	59	48	55	69	2390	2270	47	46	34
35			91	109	329	94	93	294	68	59	57	60	49	56	71	2640	2550	48	48	35
36			92	110	335	97	96	303	70	60	58	61	50	57	73	2860	2760	49	49	36
37			94	112	339	100	98	311	71	62	60	63	51	58	76	3090	2970	50	50	37
38			95	113	343	102	101	319	73	63	61	64	52	59	78	3300	3160	51	50	38
39			96	114	346	105	103	327	74	64	62	65	53	60	81	3470	3320	52	51	39
40			97	114	349	107	106	334	76	65	63	66	53	61	83	3600	3450	52	52	40

[1] After Bahlmann, F., Merz, E., Weber, G., Wellek, S., Engelhardt, O.: Transvaginal ultrasound biometry in early pregnancy: a growth model. Ultraschall in Med. 18 (1997) 196–204
[2] After Merz., E., Wellek, S.: Normal fetal growth profile: a uniform model for calculating normal growth curves for current head and abdomen parameters and long limb bones. Ultraschall in Med. 17 (1996) 153–162
[3] After Merz., E., Oberstein, A., Wellek, S.: Age-related reference ranges for fetal foot length. Ultraschall in Med. 21 (2000) 79–85
[4] After Volgt, M., Schneider, K.T.M., Jährig, K.: Analysis of babies born in the Federal Republic of Germany in 1992. Part 1: new percentiles for body measurements in newborns. Geburtsh. u. Frauenheilk. 56 (1996) 550–558

CCD = chorionic cavity diameter
CRL = crown–rump length
BPD = biparietal diameter
OFD = occipitofrontal diameter
HC = head circumference
ATD = abdominal transverse diameter
ASD = abdominal sagittal diameter
AC = abdominal circumference
Fe = femur
Ti = tibia
Fi = fibula
Hu = humerus
Ra = radius
Ul = ulna
Wt = weight
L = length
m = male
f = female

Biometry and Gestational Age Estimation in the First Trimester

Table 53.**2** Normal range for chorionic cavity diameter (CCD) as a function of gestational age (in completed weeks + days), data in mm, lower limit 5th percentile, upper limit 95th percentile

Weeks +days	Days	CCD (mm) 5%	50%	95%	Weeks +days	Days	CCD (mm) 5%	50%	95%	Weeks +days	Days	CCD (mm) 5%	50%	95%	Weeks +days	Days	CCD (mm) 5%	50%	95%	Weeks +days	Days	CCD (mm) 5%	50%	95%
4+0	28	–	–	–	6+0	42	6.5	13.0	19.6	8+0	56	21.8	28.6	35.4	10+0	70	36.5	43.6	50.6	12+0	84	49.8	57.1	64.4
4+1	29	–	–	–	6+1	43	7.6	14.1	20.7	8+1	57	22.9	29.7	36.5	10+1	71	37.5	44.6	51.6	12+1	85	50.7	58.0	65.3
4+2	30	–	0.1	6.2	6+2	44	8.7	15.3	21.8	8+2	58	24.0	30.8	37.6	10+2	72	38.5	45.6	52.7	12+2	86	51.5	58.8	66.2
4+3	31	–	0.9	7.2	6+3	45	9.8	16.4	23.0	8+3	59	25.1	31.9	38.8	10+3	73	39.5	46.6	53.7	12+3	87	52.3	59.7	67.0
4+4	32	–	1.9	8.3	6+4	46	10.9	17.5	24.1	8+4	60	26.1	33.0	39.9	10+4	74	40.5	47.6	54.7	12+4	88	53.1	60.5	67.9
4+5	33	–	3.0	9.4	6+5	47	12.0	18.6	25.3	8+5	61	27.2	34.1	41.0	10+5	75	41.5	48.6	55.7	12+5	89	53.9	61.3	68.7
4+6	34	–	4.1	10.5	6+6	48	13.1	19.8	26.4	8+6	62	28.2	35.1	42.0	10+6	76	42.4	49.6	56.7	12+6	90	54.7	62.1	69.5
5+0	35	–	5.2	11.6	7+0	49	14.2	20.9	27.5	9+0	63	29.3	36.2	43.1	11+0	77	42.4	50.6	57.7	13+0	91	55.4	62.8	70.3
5+1	36	–	6.3	12.7	7+1	50	15.3	22.0	28.7	9+1	64	30.3	37.3	44.2	11+1	78	44.3	51.5	58.7	13+1	92	56.1	63.6	71.0
5+2	37	1.0	7.4	13.9	7+2	51	16.4	23.1	29.8	9+2	65	31.4	38.3	45.3	11+2	79	45.3	52.5	59.7	13+2	93	56.8	64.2	71.7
5+3	38	2.1	8.5	15.0	7+3	52	17.5	24.1	30.9	9+3	66	32.4	39.4	46.4	11+3	80	46.2	53.4	60.7	13+3	94	57.4	64.8	72.3
5+4	39	3.2	9.7	16.1	7+4	53	18.6	25.3	32.1	9+4	67	33.4	40.4	47.4	11+4	81	47.1	54.4	61.6	13+4	95	57.8	65.3	72.8
5+5	40	4.3	10.8	17.3	7+5	54	19.7	26.4	33.2	9+5	68	34.5	41.5	48.5	11+5	82	48.0	55.3	62.5					
5+6	41	5.4	11.9	18.4	7+6	55	20.7	27.5	34.3	9+6	69	35.5	42.5	49.6	11+6	83	48.9	56.2	63.5					

After Bahlmann, F., Merz, E., Weber, G., Wellek, S., Engelhardt, O.: Transvaginal ultrasound biometry in early pregnancy: a growth model. Ultraschall in Med. 18 (1997) 196–204

Table 53.**3** Normal range for amniotic cavity diameter (ACD) as a function of gestational age (in completed weeks + days), data in mm, lower limit 5th percentile, upper limit 95th percentile

Weeks +days	Days	ACD (mm) 5%	50%	95%	Weeks +days	Days	ACD (mm) 5%	50%	95%	Weeks +days	Days	ACD (mm) 5%	50%	95%	Weeks +days	Days	ACD (mm) 5%	50%	95%
6+0	42	–	2.4	9.0	8+0	56	10.0	17.4	24.8	10+0	70	25.8	34.0	42.2	12+0	84	42.3	51.3	60.3
6+1	43	–	3.4	10.1	8+1	57	11.0	18.5	26.0	10+1	71	26.9	35.2	43.5	12+1	85	43.4	52.5	61.6
6+2	44	–	4.4	11.1	8+2	58	12.1	19.7	27.2	10+2	72	28.1	36.4	44.8	12+2	86	44.6	53.7	62.8
6+3	45	–	5.4	12.2	8+3	59	13.2	20.8	28.5	10+3	73	29.3	37.7	46.0	12+3	87	45.8	55.0	64.1
6+4	46	–	6.4	13.3	8+4	60	14.4	22.0	29.7	10+4	74	30.4	38.9	47.3	12+4	88	47.0	56.2	65.4
6+5	47	0.5	7.5	14.4	8+5	61	15.5	23.2	30.9	10+5	75	31.6	40.1	48.6	12+5	89	48.1	57.4	66.7
6+6	48	1.6	8.5	15.5	8+6	62	16.6	24.4	32.1	10+6	76	32.8	41.4	49.6	12+6	90	49.3	58.6	68.0
7+0	49	2.6	9.6	16.7	9+0	63	17.7	25.6	33.4	11+0	77	34.0	42.6	51.2	13+0	91	50.4	59.8	69.2
7+1	50	3.7	10.7	17.8	9+1	64	18.9	26.7	34.6	11+1	78	35.2	43.8	52.5	13+1	92	51.6	61.0	70.5
7+2	51	4.6	11.8	18.9	9+2	65	20.0	27.9	35.9	11+2	79	36.3	45.1	53.8	13+2	93	52.7	62.2	71.7
7+3	52	5.7	12.9	20.1	9+3	66	21.1	29.1	37.1	11+3	80	37.5	46.3	55.1	13+3	94	53.8	63.3	72.9
7+4	53	6.7	14.0	21.3	9+4	67	22.3	30.3	38.4	11+4	81	38.7	47.5	56.4	13+4	95	54.7	64.4	74.0
7+5	54	7.8	15.1	22.4	9+5	68	23.4	31.6	39.7	11+5	82	39.9	48.8	57.7					
7+6	55	8.9	16.3	23.6	9+6	69	24.6	32.8	40.9	11+6	83	41.1	50.0	59.0					

After Bahlmann, F., Merz, E., Weber, G., Wellek, S., Engelhardt, O.: Transvaginal ultrasound biometry in early pregnancy: a growth model. Ultraschall in Med. 18 (1997) 196–204

Table 53.**4** Normal range for the yolk sac (YS) as a function of gestational age (in completed weeks + days), data in mm, lower limit 5th percentile, upper limit 95th percentile

Weeks +days	Days	YS (mm) 5%	50%	95%	Weeks +days	Days	YS (mm) 5%	50%	95%	Weeks +days	Days	YS (mm) 5%	50%	95%	Weeks +days	Days	YS (mm) 5%	50%	95%	Weeks +days	Days	YS (mm) 5%	50%	95%
4+0	28	–	–	–	6+0	42	–	3.3	4.5	8+0	56	3.9	5.0	6.1	10+0	70	4.6	5.7	6.8	12+0	84	4.7	5.8	6.8
4+1	29	–	–	–	6+1	43	–	3.5	4.6	8+1	57	4.0	5.1	6.2	10+1	71	4.7	5.7	6.8	12+1	85	4.7	5.8	6.8
4+2	30	0.6	1.8	3.0	6+2	44	3.0	3.6	4.8	8+2	58	4.1	5.2	6.3	10+2	72	4.7	5.8	6.8	12+2	86	4.7	5.7	6.8
4+3	31	0.7	1.9	3.1	6+3	45	3.1	3.8	4.9	8+3	59	4.1	5.2	6.4	10+3	73	4.7	5.8	6.9	12+3	87	4.7	5.7	6.8
4+4	32	0.8	1.9	3.1	6+4	46	3.1	3.9	5.0	8+4	60	4.2	5.3	6.4	10+4	74	4.7	5.8	6.9	12+4	88	4.6	5.6	6.7
4+5	33	0.9	2.0	3.2	6+5	47	3.2	4.0	5.2	8+5	61	4.3	5.4	6.5	10+5	75	4.7	5.8	6.9	12+5	89	4.6	5.6	6.7
4+6	34	1.0	2.2	3.3	6+6	48	3.3	4.2	5.3	8+6	62	4.3	5.4	6.5	10+6	76	4.7	5.8	6.9	12+6	90	4.6	5.6	6.7
5+0	35	1.1	2.3	3.5	7+0	49	3.5	4.3	5.4	9+0	63	4.4	5.5	6.6	11+0	77	4.8	5.8	6.9	13+0	91	4.5	5.5	6.6
5+1	36	1.2	2.4	3.6	7+1	50	3.6	4.4	5.5	9+1	64	4.4	5.5	6.6	11+1	78	4.8	5.8	6.9	13+1	92	4.5	5.5	6.6
5+2	37	1.4	2.6	3.7	7+2	51	3.7	4.5	5.7	9+2	65	4.5	5.6	6.7	11+2	79	4.8	5.8	6.9	13+2	93	4.5	5.5	6.6
5+3	38	1.5	2.7	3.9	7+3	52	3.9	4.6	5.8	9+3	66	4.5	5.6	6.7	11+3	80	4.8	5.8	6.9	13+3	94	4.4	5.4	6.5
5+4	39	1.7	2.9	4.0	7+4	53	4.0	4.7	5.9	9+4	67	4.5	5.6	6.7	11+4	81	4.8	5.8	6.9	13+4	95	4.4	5.4	6.5
5+5	40	1.8	3.0	4.2	7+5	54	4.2	4.8	6.0	9+5	68	4.6	5.7	6.8	11+5	82	4.8	5.9	6.9					
5+6	41	2.0	3.2	4.3	7+6	55	4.3	4.9	6.1	9+6	69	4.6	5.7	6.8	11+6	83	4.8	5.9	6.9					

After Bahlmann, F., Merz, E., Weber, G., Wellek, S., Engelhardt, O.: Transvaginal ultrasound biometry in early pregnancy: a growth model. Ultraschall in Med. 18 (1997) 196–204

Table 53.**5** Normal range for crown–rump length (CRL) as a function of gestational age (in completed weeks + days), data in mm, lower limit 5th percentile, upper limit 95th percentile

Weeks +days	Days	CRL (mm) 5%	50%	95%	Weeks +days	Days	CRL (mm) 5%	50%	95%	Weeks +days	Days	CRL (mm) 5%	50%	95%	Weeks +days	Days	CRL (mm) 5%	50%	95%	Weeks +days	Days	CRL (mm) 5%	50%	95%
5+0	35	–	1.2	4.3	7+0	49	3.8	7.9	11.9	9+0	63	17.4	22.4	27.4	11+0	77	37.1	43.1	49.1	13+0	91	58.6	65.5	72.5
5+1	36	–	1.4	4.6	7+1	50	4.5	8.7	12.8	9+1	64	18.6	23.7	28.8	11+1	78	38.6	44.7	50.8	13+1	92	59.9	66.9	73.9
5+2	37	–	1.7	4.9	7+2	51	5.3	9.5	13.7	9+2	65	19.9	25.0	30.2	11+2	79	40.2	46.3	52.5	13+2	93	61.1	68.1	75.2
5+3	38	–	2.0	5.3	7+3	52	6.1	10.4	14.6	9+3	66	21.2	26.4	31.6	11+3	80	41.8	48.0	54.2	13+3	94	62.1	69.2	76.4
5+4	39	–	2.3	5.7	7+4	53	6.9	11.3	15.6	9+4	67	22.5	27.8	33.1	11+4	81	43.4	49.6	55.6	13+4	95	62.8	70.2	77.2
5+5	40	–	2.7	6.1	7+5	54	7.8	12.2	16.6	9+5	68	23.8	29.2	34.6	11+5	82	45.0	51.3	57.6					
5+6	41	–	3.1	6.6	7+6	55	8.7	13.2	17.7	9+6	69	25.2	30.7	36.1	11+6	83	46.5	52.9	59.3					
6+0	42	–	3.5	7.1	8+0	56	9.7	14.2	18.8	10+0	70	26.6	32.1	37.6	12+0	84	48.1	54.6	61.1					
6+1	43	0.4	4.0	7.7	8+1	57	10.7	15.3	19.9	10+1	71	28.1	33.6	39.2	12+1	85	49.7	56.2	62.8					
6+2	44	0.8	4.6	8.3	8+2	58	11.7	16.4	21.1	10+2	72	29.5	35.2	40.8	12+2	86	51.2	57.9	64.5					
6+3	45	1.3	5.1	8.9	8+3	59	12.8	17.5	22.3	10+3	73	31.0	36.7	42.4	12+3	87	52.8	59.5	66.1					
6+4	46	1.9	5.8	9.6	8+4	60	13.9	18.7	23.5	10+4	74	32.5	38.3	44.1	12+4	88	54.3	61.0	67.8					
6+5	47	2.5	6.4	10.4	8+5	61	15.0	19.9	24.8	10+5	75	34.0	39.9	45.7	12+5	89	55.8	62.6	69.4					
6+6	48	3.1	7.1	11.1	8+6	62	16.2	21.1	26.1	10+6	76	35.5	41.5	47.4	12+6	90	57.2	64.1	71.0					

After Bahlmann, F., Merz, E., Weber, G., Wellek, S., Engelhardt, O.: Transvaginal ultrasound biometry in early pregnancy: a growth model. Ultraschall in Med. 18 (1997) 196–204

Table 53.**6** Normal range for biparietal diameter (BPD) as a function of gestational age (in completed weeks + days), data in mm, lower limit 5th percentile, upper limit 95th percentile

Weeks +days	Days	BPD (mm) 5%	50%	95%	Weeks +days	Days	BPD (mm) 5%	50%	95%	Weeks +days	Days	BPD (mm) 5%	50%	95%	Weeks +days	Days	BPD (mm) 5%	50%	95%
6+0	42	–	–	–	8+0	56	4.6	6.8	9.6	10+0	70	11.3	13.6	15.9	12+0	84	17.9	20.3	22.7
6+1	43	–	–	–	8+1	57	5.1	7.3	9.6	10+1	71	11.7	14.0	16.4	12+1	85	18.4	20.8	23.2
6+2	44	–	–	–	8+2	58	5.6	7.8	10.1	10+2	72	12.2	14.5	16.8	12+2	86	18.9	21.3	23.7
6+3	45	–	1.3	3.4	8+3	59	6.0	8.3	10.6	10+3	73	12.7	15.0	17.3	12+3	87	19.4	21.8	24.2
6+4	46	–	1.8	4.0	8+4	60	6.5	8.8	11.0	10+4	74	13.1	15.5	17.8	12+4	88	19.9	22.3	24.7
6+5	47	0.1	2.3	4.5	8+5	61	7.0	9.3	11.5	10+5	75	13.6	15.9	18.3	12+5	89	20.4	22.8	25.2
6+6	48	0.6	2.8	5.0	8+6	62	7.5	9.7	12.0	10+6	76	14.1	16.4	18.8	12+6	90	20.9	23.3	25.7
7+0	49	1.1	3.3	5.5	9+0	63	7.9	10.2	12.5	11+0	77	14.6	16.6	19.2	13+0	91	21.5	23.9	26.3
7+1	50	1.6	3.8	6.1	9+1	64	8.4	10.7	13.0	11+1	78	15.0	17.4	19.7	13+1	92	22.0	24.4	26.8
7+2	51	2.6	4.3	6.6	9+2	65	8.9	11.2	13.5	11+2	79	15.5	19.9	20.2	13+2	93	22.6	25.0	27.4
7+3	52	2.6	4.8	7.1	9+3	66	9.4	11.7	14.0	11+3	80	16.0	18.3	20.7	13+3	94	23.2	25.6	28.0
7+4	53	3.1	5.3	7.6	9+4	67	9.8	12.1	14.4	11+4	81	16.5	18.8	21.2	13+4	95	23.9	26.3	28.7
7+5	54	3.6	5.8	8.1	9+5	68	10.3	12.6	14.9	11+5	82	17.0	19.3	21.7					
7+6	55	4.1	6.3	8.6	9+6	69	10.8	13.1	15.4	11+6	83	17.4	19.8	22.2					

After Bahlmann, F., Merz, E., Weber, G., Wellek, S., Engelhardt, O.: Transvaginal ultrasound biometry in early pregnancy: a growth model. Ultraschall in Med. 18 (1997) 196–204

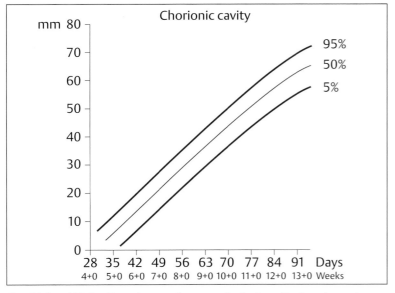

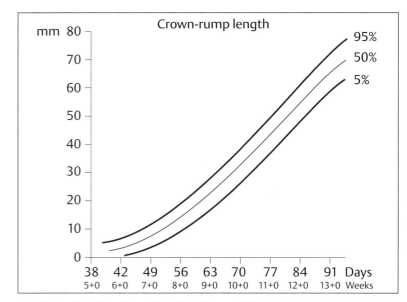

Figs. 53.**1** and 53.**2** Normal ranges for mean chorionic cavity diameter and crown–rump length as a function of gestational age (in completed weeks + days), data in mm, lower limit 5th percentile, upper limit 95th percentile

After Bahlmann, F., Merz, E., Weber, G., Wellek, S., Engelhardt, O.: Transvaginal ultrasound biometry in early pregnancy—a growth model. Ultraschall in Med. 18 (1997) 196–204

Table 53.**7** Estimation of gestational age based on the crown–rump length (CRL) and biparietal diameter (BPD) in the first trimester (gestational age in completed weeks + days), lower limit 5th percentile, upper limit 95th percentile

	CRL Weeks + days p.m.				CRL Weeks + days p.m.				BPD Weeks + days p.m.		
mm	5%	50%	95%	mm	5%	50%	95%	mm	5%	50%	95%
1	–	–	–	31	8+6	9+5	10+3	1	–	–	–
2	5+2	6+0	6+4	32	9+0	9+6	10+4	2	–	–	–
3	5+4	6+1	6+5	33	9+1	9+6	10+5	3	6+1	6+6	7+3
4	5+5	6+2	7+0	34	9+1	10+0	10+6	4	6+3	7+1	7+6
5	5+6	6+3	7+1	35	9+2	10+1	11+0	5	6+5	7+3	8+1
6	6+0	6+4	7+2	36	9+3	10+2	11+0	6	7+0	7+5	8+4
7	6+1	6+5	7+3	37	9+4	10+2	11+1	7	7+2	8+0	8+6
8	6+2	6+6	7+4	38	9+4	10+3	11+2	8	7+4	8+2	9+1
9	6+3	7+0	7+5	39	9+5	10+4	11+3	9	7+6	8+4	9+3
10	6+4	7+1	7+6	40	9+6	10+5	11+4	10	8+1	8+6	9+5
11	6+4	7+2	8+0	41	10+0	10+5	11+4	11	8+2	9+1	10+1
12	6+5	7+3	8+1	42	10+0	10+6	11+5	12	8+4	9+3	10+3
13	6+6	7+4	8+2	43	10+1	11+0	11+6	13	8+6	9+5	10+5
14	7+0	7+5	8+3	44	10+2	11+1	12+0	14	9+1	10+0	11+0
15	7+1	7+6	8+4	45	10+2	11+1	12+0	15	9+3	10+2	11+2
16	7+2	8+0	8+5	46	10+3	11+2	12+1	16	9+4	10+4	11+5
17	7+3	8+0	8+6	47	10+4	11+3	12+2	17	9+6	10+6	12+0
18	7+3	8+1	9+0	48	10+5	11+4	12+3	18	10+1	11+1	12+2
19	7+4	8+2	9+0	49	10+5	11+4	12+3	19	10+3	11+3	12+4
20	7+5	8+3	9+1	50	10+6	11+5	12+4	20	10+5	11+5	13+0
21	7+6	8+4	9+2	51	11+0	11+6	12+5	21	11+0	12+1	13+2
22	7+6	8+5	9+3	52	11+0	11+6	12+6	22	11+2	12+3	13+5
23	8+0	8+5	9+4	53	11+1	12+0	12+6	23	–	–	–
24	8+1	8+6	9+5	54	11+2	12+1	13+0	24	–	–	–
25	8+2	9+0	9+6	55	11+2	12+2	13+1	25	–	–	–
26	8+3	9+1	9+6	56	11+3	12+2	13+2	26	–	–	–
27	8+3	9+2	10+0	57	11+4	12+3	13+3	27	–	–	–
28	8+4	9+2	10+1	58	11+5	12+4	13+3	28	–	–	–
29	8+5	9+3	10+2	59	11+5	12+5	13+4	29	–	–	–
30	8+6	9+4	10+3	60	11+6	12+5	13+5	30	–	–	–

After Rempen, A. (1997); in: Rempen, A., Chaoui, R., Kozlowski, P., Häusler, M., Terinde, R., Wisser, J.: Standards for ultrasound examination in early pregnancy. Ultraschall in Med. 22 (2001) M1–M5

Biometry and Gestational Age Estimation in the Second and Third Trimesters

▬ Superior and Abdominal Parameters and Long Extremity Bones

Table 53.**8**   Normal data for superior parameters (biparietal diameter, occipitofrontal diameter, head circumference) and abdominal parameters (abdominal transverse and sagittal diameters, abdominal circumference) as a function of gestational age (in completed weeks), data in mm, lower limit 5th percentile, upper limit 95th percentile. * Outer-to-outer measurement

Weeks	BPD 5%	BPD 50%	BPD 95%	OFD 5%	OFD 50%	OFD 95%	HC 5%	HC 50%	HC 95%	ATD 5%	ATD 50%	ATD 95%	ASD 5%	ASD 50%	ASD 95%	AU 5%	AU 50%	AU 95%	Weeks
12.5	21	25	29	26	30	34	80	92	104	17	20	24	15	19	23	50	62	74	12.5
13.0	23	26	30	28	32	36	84	96	108	18	22	26	17	21	25	55	67	80	13.0
13.5	24	28	31	29	34	38	89	101	113	20	24	28	18	23	27	60	73	85	13.5
14.0	25	29	33	31	35	40	94	106	119	21	25	29	20	24	28	65	78	91	14.0
14.5	27	31	35	33	37	41	100	112	124	23	27	31	22	26	30	71	83	96	14.5
15.0	28	32	36	35	39	43	105	118	130	25	29	33	23	28	32	76	89	102	15.0
15.5	30	34	38	37	41	46	111	124	137	26	31	35	25	29	34	81	94	108	15.5
16.0	31	35	39	39	43	48	117	130	143	28	32	37	27	31	36	86	100	114	16.0
16.5	33	37	41	41	45	50	123	136	149	30	34	38	28	33	37	91	105	119	16.5
17.0	35	39	43	43	47	52	130	143	156	31	36	40	30	35	39	96	111	125	17.0
17.5	36	40	45	45	50	54	136	149	162	33	38	42	32	36	41	102	116	131	17.5
18.0	38	42	46	47	52	56	142	155	168	35	39	44	33	38	43	107	122	136	18.0
18.5	40	44	48	49	54	59	148	162	175	36	41	46	35	40	45	112	127	142	18.5
19.0	41	46	50	51	56	61	155	168	181	38	43	48	37	42	47	117	132	148	19.0
19.5	43	47	52	54	58	63	161	174	188	39	44	49	38	43	48	122	138	153	19.5
20.0	45	49	53	56	60	65	167	181	194	41	46	51	40	45	50	127	143	159	20.0
20.5	46	51	55	58	63	67	173	187	201	43	48	53	42	47	52	133	149	165	20.5
21.0	48	52	57	60	65	69	180	193	207	44	50	55	43	48	54	138	154	170	21.0
21.5	49	54	59	62	67	72	186	200	214	46	51	57	45	50	55	143	159	176	21.5
22.0	51	56	60	64	69	74	192	206	220	48	53	58	46	52	57	148	165	181	22.0
22.5	53	57	62	66	71	76	198	212	226	49	55	60	48	54	59	153	170	187	22.5
23.0	54	59	64	68	73	78	204	218	232	51	56	62	50	55	61	158	175	193	23.0
23.5	56	61	65	70	75	80	210	224	238	52	58	64	51	57	63	163	181	198	23.5
24.0	57	62	67	72	77	82	216	230	244	54	60	65	53	59	64	168	186	204	24.0
24.5	59	64	69	74	79	84	221	236	250	56	61	67	54	60	66	173	191	209	24.5
25.0	61	65	70	75	81	86	227	241	256	57	63	69	56	62	68	178	196	215	25.0
25.5	62	67	72	77	82	88	232	247	262	59	65	71	57	63	69	183	202	220	25.5
26.0	64	68	73	79	84	90	238	253	267	60	66	72	59	65	71	188	207	226	26.0
26.5	65	70	75	81	86	91	243	258	273	62	68	74	61	67	73	193	212	231	26.5
27.0	66	71	77	82	88	93	248	263	278	63	70	76	62	68	75	198	217	236	27.0
27.5	68	73	78	84	90	95	253	268	284	65	71	78	64	70	76	202	222	242	27.5
28.0	69	74	79	86	91	97	258	273	289	67	73	79	65	72	78	207	227	247	28.0
28.5	71	76	81	87	93	98	263	278	294	68	75	81	67	73	80	212	232	252	28.5
29.0	72	77	82	89	94	100	268	283	299	70	76	83	68	75	81	217	237	257	29.0
29.5	73	78	84	90	96	101	272	288	303	71	78	84	70	76	83	221	242	263	29.5
30.0	74	80	85	92	97	103	277	292	308	73	79	86	71	78	85	226	247	268	30.0
30.5	76	81	86	93	99	104	281	297	313	74	81	88	73	79	86	231	252	273	30.5
31.0	77	82	88	94	100	106	285	301	317	76	82	89	74	81	88	235	257	278	31.0
31.5	78	83	89	96	101	107	289	305	321	77	84	91	76	82	89	240	262	283	31.5
32.0	79	85	90	97	102	108	293	309	325	78	85	92	77	84	91	244	266	288	32.0
32.5	80	86	91	98	104	110	297	313	329	80	87	94	78	85	93	249	271	293	32.5
33.0	81	87	92	99	105	111	300	316	333	81	88	96	80	87	94	253	276	298	33.0
33.5	82	88	93	100	106	112	303	320	336	83	90	97	81	88	96	258	280	303	33.5
34.0	83	89	95	101	107	113	307	323	340	84	91	99	83	90	97	262	285	308	34.0
34.5	84	90	96	102	108	114	310	326	343	85	93	100	84	91	99	266	289	313	34.5
35.0	85	91	97	103	109	115	313	329	346	87	94	102	85	93	100	270	294	317	35.0
35.5	86	92	97	103	110	116	315	332	349	88	96	103	87	94	102	275	298	322	35.5
36.0	87	92	98	104	110	116	318	335	352	89	97	105	88	96	103	279	303	327	36.0
36.5	87	93	99	105	111	117	320	337	354	91	98	106	89	97	105	283	307	331	36.5
37.0	88	94	100	105	112	118	322	339	356	92	100	108	90	98	106	287	311	336	37.0
37.5	89	95	101	106	112	119	324	341	359	93	101	109	92	100	107	290	315	340	37.5
38.0	89	95	101	106	113	119	326	343	361	94	102	110	93	101	109	294	319	344	38.0
38.5	90	96	102	107	113	120	327	345	362	95	104	112	94	102	110	298	323	348	38.5
39.0	90	96	103	107	114	120	329	346	364	97	105	113	95	103	111	301	327	352	39.0
39.5	91	97	103	108	114	120	330	348	365	98	106	114	96	105	113	305	331	356	39.5
40.0	91	97	103	108	114	121	331	349	366	99	107	116	97	106	114	308	334	360	40.0
40.5	91	97	104	108	114	121	332	349	367	100	108	117	98	107	115	311	338	364	40.5
41.0	91	98	104	108	115	121	332	350	368	101	109	118	99	108	116	314	341	367	41.0
41.5	92	98	104	108	115	121	332	350	369	102	110	119	100	109	117	317	343	370	41.5

After Merz., E., Wellek, S.: Normal fetal growth profile: a uniform model for calculating normal growth curves for current head and abdomen parameters and long limb bones. Ultraschall in Med. 17 (1996) 153–162

Table 53.**9**   Normal data for the long extremity bones (femur, tibia, fibula, humerus, radius, ulna) as a function of gestational age (in completed weeks), data in mm, lower limit 5th percentile, upper limit 95th percentile

Weeks	Fe 5%	Fe 50%	Fe 95%	Ti 5%	Ti 50%	Ti 95%	Fi 5%	Fi 50%	Fi 95%	Hu 5%	Hu 50%	Hu 95%	Ra 5%	Ra 50%	Ra 95%	Ul 5%	Ul 50%	Ul 95%	Weeks
12.5	6	9	12	4	7	10	3	6	9	5	8	11	1	4	7	3	5	8	12.5
13.0	8	11	14	6	9	12	5	8	11	7	10	13	3	6	9	5	8	11	13.0
13.5	10	13	16	7	10	13	6	9	12	9	12	15	5	8	11	7	10	13	13.5
14.0	11	15	18	9	12	15	8	11	14	10	13	17	6	10	13	8	11	14	14.0
14.5	13	16	20	11	14	17	9	13	16	12	15	18	8	11	14	10	13	16	14.5
15.0	15	18	21	12	15	18	11	14	17	14	17	20	10	13	16	12	15	18	15.0
15.5	16	20	23	14	17	20	12	16	19	15	18	22	11	14	17	13	16	19	15.5
16.0	18	21	25	15	18	21	14	17	20	17	20	23	12	16	19	15	18	21	16.0
16.5	19	23	26	16	20	23	15	18	22	18	21	25	14	17	20	16	19	22	16.5
17.0	21	24	28	18	21	24	17	20	23	20	23	26	15	18	22	17	21	24	17.0
17.5	22	26	29	19	22	26	18	21	24	21	24	28	16	20	23	19	22	25	17.5
18.0	24	27	31	21	24	27	19	23	26	22	26	29	17	21	24	20	23	27	18.0
18.5	25	29	32	22	25	29	21	24	27	24	27	30	19	22	25	21	25	28	18.5
19.0	27	30	34	23	26	30	22	25	29	25	28	32	20	23	26	23	26	29	19.0
19.5	28	32	35	24	28	31	23	26	30	26	30	33	21	24	28	24	27	31	19.5
20.0	29	33	37	26	29	32	24	28	31	27	31	34	22	25	29	25	28	32	20.0
20.5	31	35	38	27	30	34	25	29	32	29	32	36	23	26	30	26	30	33	20.5
21.0	32	36	40	28	31	35	27	30	34	30	33	37	24	28	31	27	31	34	21.0
21.5	33	37	41	29	33	36	28	31	35	31	35	38	25	29	32	29	32	35	21.5
22.0	35	39	42	30	34	37	29	33	36	32	36	39	26	30	33	30	33	37	22.0
22.5	36	40	44	31	35	39	30	34	37	33	37	40	27	31	34	31	34	38	22.5
23.0	37	41	45	33	36	40	31	35	38	34	38	42	28	32	35	32	35	39	23.0
23.5	39	43	46	34	37	41	32	36	40	36	39	43	29	32	36	33	36	40	23.5
24.0	40	44	48	35	38	42	33	37	41	37	40	44	30	33	37	34	37	41	24.0
24.5	41	45	49	36	40	43	34	38	42	38	41	45	31	34	38	35	38	42	24.5
25.0	42	46	50	37	41	44	35	39	43	39	42	46	32	35	39	36	39	43	25.0
25.5	43	48	52	38	42	45	36	40	44	40	43	47	32	36	40	37	40	44	25.5
26.0	45	49	53	39	43	47	38	41	45	41	45	48	33	37	41	38	41	45	26.0
26.5	46	50	54	40	44	48	38	42	46	42	46	49	34	38	41	39	42	46	26.5
27.0	47	51	55	41	45	49	39	43	47	43	47	50	35	39	42	40	43	47	27.0
27.5	48	52	57	42	46	50	40	44	48	44	47	51	36	39	43	41	44	48	27.5
28.0	49	53	58	43	47	51	41	45	49	45	48	52	36	40	44	41	45	49	28.0
28.5	50	55	59	44	48	52	42	46	50	45	49	53	37	41	45	42	46	50	28.5
29.0	51	56	60	45	49	53	43	47	51	46	50	54	38	42	45	43	47	51	29.0
29.5	52	57	61	46	50	54	44	48	52	47	51	55	39	42	46	44	48	52	29.5
30.0	53	58	62	46	51	55	45	49	53	48	52	56	39	43	47	45	49	52	30.0
30.5	54	59	63	47	51	56	46	50	54	49	53	57	40	44	48	46	49	53	30.5
31.0	55	60	64	48	52	56	47	51	55	50	54	58	41	44	48	46	50	54	31.0
31.5	56	61	66	49	53	57	47	52	56	51	55	59	41	45	49	47	51	55	31.5
32.0	57	62	67	50	54	58	48	52	57	51	55	60	42	46	50	48	52	56	32.0
32.5	58	63	68	51	55	59	49	53	57	52	56	60	43	46	50	49	53	56	32.5
33.0	59	64	69	51	56	60	50	54	58	53	57	61	43	47	51	49	53	57	33.0
33.5	60	65	70	52	56	61	51	55	59	54	58	62	44	48	52	50	54	58	33.5
34.0	61	66	71	53	57	62	51	56	60	54	59	63	44	48	52	51	55	59	34.0
34.5	62	67	72	54	58	62	52	56	61	55	59	63	45	49	53	51	55	59	34.5
35.0	63	68	73	54	59	63	53	57	61	56	60	64	45	49	53	52	56	60	35.0
35.5	64	69	74	55	59	64	53	58	62	56	61	65	46	50	54	52	57	61	35.5
36.0	65	70	74	56	60	65	54	58	63	57	61	66	46	50	54	53	57	61	36.0
36.5	66	70	75	56	61	65	54	59	63	58	62	66	47	51	55	54	58	62	36.5
37.0	66	71	76	57	62	66	55	60	64	58	63	67	47	51	55	54	58	63	37.0
37.5	67	72	77	58	62	67	56	60	65	59	63	68	48	52	56	55	59	63	37.5
38.0	68	73	78	58	63	67	56	61	65	59	64	68	48	52	56	55	59	64	38.0
38.5	69	74	79	59	63	68	57	61	66	60	64	69	48	52	57	56	60	64	38.5
39.0	69	74	79	59	64	69	57	62	66	60	65	69	49	53	57	56	60	65	39.0
39.5	70	75	80	60	64	69	58	62	67	61	65	70	49	53	57	57	61	65	39.5
40.0	71	76	81	60	65	70	58	63	67	61	66	70	49	53	58	57	61	66	40.0
40.5	71	76	81	61	65	70	58	63	68	61	66	71	49	54	58	57	62	66	40.5
41.0	72	77	82	61	66	71	59	63	68	62	66	71	50	54	58	58	62	66	41.0
41.5	72	77	83	61	66	71	59	64	68	62	67	71	50	54	58	58	62	67	41.5

After Merz., E., Wellek, S.: Normal fetal growth profile: a uniform model for calculating normal growth curves for current head and abdomen parameters and long limb bones. Ultraschall in Med. 17 (1996) 153–162

Table 53.**10**   Normal data for the ratio of abdominal circumference (AC) to head circumference (HC) as a function of gestational age (in completed weeks), data in mm, lower limit 5th percentile, upper limit 95th percentile

Weeks	AC/HC 5%	AC/HC 50%	AC/HC 95%	Weeks	AC/HC 5%	AC/HC 50%	AC/HC 95%
12.0	0.64	**0.71**	0.79	25.5	0.75	**0.82**	0.89
12.5	0.66	**0.73**	0.80	26.0	0.76	**0.83**	0.90
13.0	0.66	**0.73**	0.81	26.5	0.76	**0.83**	0.90
13.5	0.67	**0.74**	0.81	27.0	0.76	**0.83**	0.90
14.0	0.67	**0.74**	0.82	27.5	0.77	**0.84**	0.90
14.5	0.68	**0.75**	0.82	28.0	0.77	**0.84**	0.91
15.0	0.68	**0.75**	0.82	28.5	0.77	**0.84**	0.91
15.5	0.69	**0.76**	0.83	29.0	0.78	**0.85**	0.91
16.0	0.69	**0.76**	0.83	29.5	0.78	**0.85**	0.92
16.5	0.69	**0.76**	0.84	30.0	0.78	**0.85**	0.92
17.0	0.70	**0.77**	0.84	30.5	0.79	**0.86**	0.92
17.5	0.70	**0.77**	0.84	31.0	0.79	**0.86**	0.93
18.0	0.70	**0.78**	0.85	31.5	0.79	**0.86**	0.93
18.5	0.71	**0.78**	0.85	32.0	0.80	**0.87**	0.94
19.0	0.71	**0.78**	0.85	32.5	0.80	**0.87**	0.94
19.5	0.71	**0.79**	0.86	33.0	0.81	**0.87**	0.94
20.0	0.72	**0.79**	0.86	33.5	0.81	**0.88**	0.95
20.5	0.72	**0.79**	0.86	34.0	0.81	**0.88**	0.95
21.0	0.72	**0.79**	0.86	34.5	0.82	**0.89**	0.95
21.5	0.73	**0.80**	0.87	35.0	0.82	**0.89**	0.96
22.0	0.73	**0.80**	0.87	35.5	0.83	**0.89**	0.96
22.5	0.73	**0.80**	0.87	36.0	0.83	**0.90**	0.97
23.0	0.74	**0.81**	0.88	36.5	0.84	**0.90**	0.97
23.5	0.74	**0.81**	0.88	37.0	0.84	**0.91**	0.98
24.0	0.74	**0.81**	0.88	37.5	0.85	**0.91**	0.98
24.5	0.75	**0.82**	0.89	38.0	0.85	**0.92**	0.99
25.0	0.75	**0.82**	0.89	38.5	0.86	**0.93**	0.99
				39.0	0.87	**0.93**	1.00
				39.5	0.87	**0.94**	1.01
				40.0	0.88	**0.95**	1.02
				40.5	0.89	**0.96**	1.03
				41.0	0.90	**0.97**	1.04

Adapted from Merz, E.: Thesis: Sonographic monitoring of fetal bone development in the second and third trimesters. A study on the growth of the long tubular bones compared with head and trunk growth and on the possible applications of fetal bone length in obstetric ultrasound. Mainz (1988).

Table 53.**11** Calculation of the head circumference (HC) from the biparietal diameter (BPD) and occipitofrontal diameter (OFD) using the formula $HC = 2.325 \sqrt{BPD^2 + OFD^2}$ (after Hansmann, M.; in: Huch, A., Huch, R., Duc, G., Rooth, G.: Klinisches Management des Frühgeborenen [Clinical Management of the Preterm Infant). Thieme Stuttgart 1982, p. 31)

OFD (mm)	BPD (mm) 10	11	12	13	14	15	16	17	18	19	20	21	22	23	24	25	26	27	28	29	30	OFD (mm)
20	52	53	54	55	57	58	60	61	63	64	66	67	69	71	73	74	76	78	80	82	84	20
21	54	55	56	57	59	60	61	63	64	66	67	69	71	72	74	76	78	80	81	83	85	21
22	56	57	58	59	61	62	63	65	66	68	69	71	72	74	76	77	79	81	83	85	86	22
23	58	59	60	61	63	64	65	66	68	69	71	72	74	76	77	79	81	82	84	86	88	23
24	60	61	62	63	65	66	67	68	70	71	73	74	76	77	79	81	82	84	86	88	89	24
25	63	64	64	66	67	68	69	70	72	73	74	76	77	79	81	82	84	86	87	89	91	25
26	65	66	67	68	69	70	71	72	74	75	76	78	79	81	82	84	85	87	89	91	92	26
27	67	68	69	70	71	72	73	74	75	77	78	80	81	82	84	86	87	89	90	92	94	27
28	69	70	71	72	73	74	75	76	77	79	80	81	83	84	86	87	89	90	92	94	95	28
29	71	72	73	74	75	76	77	78	79	81	82	83	85	86	88	89	91	92	94	95	97	29
30	74	74	75	76	77	78	79	80	81	83	84	85	86	88	89	91	92	94	95	97	99	30
31	76	76	77	78	79	80	81	82	83	85	86	87	88	90	91	93	94	96	97	99	100	31
32	78	79	79	80	81	82	83	84	85	87	88	89	90	92	93	94	96	97	99	100	102	32
33	80	81	82	82	83	84	85	86	87	89	90	91	92	94	95	96	98	99	101	102	104	33
34	82	83	84	85	85	86	87	88	89	91	92	93	94	95	97	98	100	101	102	104	105	34
35	85	85	86	87	88	89	89	90	92	93	94	95	96	97	99	100	101	103	104	106	107	35
36	87	88	88	89	90	91	92	93	94	95	96	97	98	99	101	102	103	105	106	107	109	36
37	89	90	90	91	92	93	94	95	96	97	98	99	100	101	103	104	105	106	108	109	111	37
38	91	92	93	93	94	95	96	97	98	99	100	101	102	103	104	106	107	108	110	111	113	38
39	94	94	95	96	96	97	98	99	100	101	102	103	104	105	106	108	109	110	112	113	114	39
40	96	96	97	98	99	99	100	101	102	103	104	105	106	107	108	110	111	112	114	115	116	40
41	98	99	99	100	101	102	102	103	104	105	106	107	108	109	110	112	113	114	115	117	118	41
42	100	101	102	102	103	104	104	105	106	107	108	109	110	111	112	114	115	116	117	119	120	42
43	103	103	104	104	105	106	107	108	108	109	110	111	112	113	114	116	117	118	119	121	122	43
44	105	105	106	107	107	108	109	110	111	111	112	113	114	115	117	118	119	120	121	123	124	44
45	107	108	108	109	110	110	111	112	113	114	114	115	116	117	119	120	121	122	123	124	126	45
46	109	110	111	111	112	112	113	114	115	116	117	118	119	120	121	122	123	124	125	126	128	46
47	112	112	113	113	114	115	115	116	117	118	119	120	121	122	123	124	125	126	127	128	130	47
48	114	114	115	116	116	117	118	118	119	120	121	122	123	124	125	126	127	128	129	130	132	48
49	116	117	117	118	118	119	120	121	121	122	123	124	125	126	127	128	129	130	131	132	134	49
50	119	119	120	120	121	121	122	123	124	124	125	126	127	128	129	130	131	132	133	134	136	50
51	121	121	122	122	123	124	124	125	126	127	127	128	129	130	131	132	133	134	135	136	138	51
52	123	124	124	125	125	126	126	127	128	129	130	130	131	132	133	134	135	136	137	138	140	52
53	125	126	126	127	127	128	129	129	130	131	132	133	133	134	135	136	137	138	139	140	142	53
54	128	128	129	129	130	130	131	132	132	133	134	135	136	136	137	138	139	140	141	143	144	54
55	130	130	131	131	132	133	133	134	135	135	136	137	138	139	140	140	141	142	143	145	146	55
56	132	133	133	134	134	135	135	136	137	137	138	139	140	141	142	143	144	145	146	147	148	56
57	135	135	135	136	136	137	138	138	139	140	140	141	142	143	144	145	146	147	148	149	150	57
58	137	137	138	138	139	139	140	141	141	142	143	143	144	145	146	147	148	149	150	151	152	58
59	139	140	140	140	141	142	142	143	143	144	145	146	146	147	148	149	150	151	152	153	154	59
60	141	142	142	143	143	144	144	145	146	146	147	148	149	149	150	151	152	153	154	155	156	60

Table 53.**11** (continued)   Calculation of the head circumference (HC) from the BPD and OFD (data in mm)

OFD (mm)	BPD (mm) 30	31	32	33	34	35	36	37	38	39	40	41	42	43	44	45	46	47	48	49	50	OFD (mm)
40	116	118	119	121	122	124	125	127	128	130	132	133	135	137	138	140	142	143	145	147	149	40
41	118	120	121	122	124	125	127	128	130	132	133	135	136	138	140	142	143	145	147	149	150	41
42	120	121	123	124	126	127	129	130	132	133	135	136	138	140	141	143	145	147	148	150	152	42
43	122	123	125	126	127	129	130	132	133	135	137	138	140	141	143	145	146	148	150	152	153	43
44	124	125	126	128	129	131	132	134	135	137	138	140	141	143	145	146	148	150	151	153	155	44
45	126	127	128	130	131	133	134	135	137	138	140	142	143	145	146	148	150	151	153	155	156	45
46	128	129	130	132	133	134	136	137	139	140	142	143	145	146	148	150	151	153	155	156	158	46
47	130	131	132	134	135	136	138	139	141	142	143	145	147	148	150	151	153	155	156	158	160	47
48	132	133	134	135	137	138	140	141	142	144	145	147	148	150	151	153	155	156	158	159	161	48
49	134	135	136	137	139	140	141	143	144	146	147	149	150	152	153	155	156	158	159	161	163	49
50	136	137	138	139	141	142	143	145	146	147	149	150	152	153	155	156	158	160	161	163	164	50
51	138	139	140	141	143	144	145	146	148	149	151	152	154	155	157	158	160	161	163	164	166	51
52	140	141	142	143	144	146	147	148	150	151	153	154	155	157	158	160	161	163	165	166	168	52
53	142	143	144	145	146	148	149	150	152	153	154	156	157	159	160	162	163	165	166	168	169	53
54	144	145	146	147	148	150	151	152	154	155	156	158	159	160	162	163	165	166	168	170	171	54
55	146	147	148	149	150	152	153	154	155	157	158	159	161	162	164	165	167	168	170	171	173	55
56	148	149	150	151	152	154	155	156	157	159	160	161	163	164	166	167	168	170	171	173	175	56
57	150	151	152	153	154	156	157	158	159	161	162	163	165	166	167	169	170	172	173	175	176	57
58	152	153	154	155	156	158	159	160	161	163	164	165	166	168	169	171	172	174	175	177	178	58
59	154	155	156	157	158	159	161	162	163	164	166	167	168	170	171	173	174	175	177	178	180	59
60	156	157	158	159	160	161	163	164	165	166	168	169	170	172	173	174	176	177	179	180	182	60
61	158	159	160	161	162	164	165	166	167	168	170	171	172	174	175	176	178	179	180	182	183	61
62	160	161	162	163	164	166	167	168	169	170	172	173	174	175	177	178	179	181	182	184	185	62
63	162	163	164	165	166	168	169	170	171	172	174	175	176	177	179	180	181	183	184	186	187	63
64	164	165	166	167	168	170	171	172	173	174	175	177	178	179	181	182	183	185	186	187	189	64
65	166	167	168	169	171	172	173	174	175	176	177	179	180	181	182	184	185	186	188	189	191	65
66	169	170	171	172	173	174	175	176	177	178	179	181	182	183	184	186	187	188	190	191	193	66
67	171	172	173	174	175	176	177	178	179	180	181	183	184	185	186	188	189	190	192	193	194	67
68	173	174	175	176	177	178	179	180	181	182	183	185	186	187	188	190	191	192	194	195	196	68
69	175	176	177	178	179	180	181	182	183	184	185	187	188	189	190	192	193	194	195	197	198	69
70	177	178	179	180	181	182	183	184	185	186	187	189	190	191	192	193	195	196	197	199	200	70
71	179	180	181	182	183	184	185	186	187	188	189	191	192	193	194	195	197	198	199	201	202	71
72	181	182	183	184	185	186	187	188	189	190	191	193	194	195	196	197	199	200	201	202	204	72
73	183	184	185	186	187	188	189	190	191	192	194	195	196	197	198	199	201	202	203	204	206	73
74	186	187	187	188	189	190	191	192	193	194	196	197	198	199	200	201	203	204	205	206	208	74
75	188	189	190	191	191	192	193	194	195	197	198	199	200	201	202	203	205	206	207	208	210	75
76	190	191	192	193	194	195	196	197	198	199	200	201	202	203	204	205	207	208	209	210	212	76
77	192	193	194	195	196	197	198	199	200	201	202	203	204	205	206	207	209	210	211	212	213	77
78	194	195	196	197	198	199	200	201	202	203	204	205	206	207	208	209	211	212	213	214	215	78
79	196	197	198	199	200	201	202	203	204	205	206	207	208	209	210	211	213	214	215	216	217	79
80	199	199	200	201	202	203	204	205	206	207	208	209	210	211	212	213	215	216	217	218	219	80

Table 53.**11** (continued)   Calculation of the head circumference (HC) from the BPD and OFD (data in mm)

OFD (mm)	BPD (mm) 50	51	52	53	54	55	56	57	58	59	60	61	62	63	64	65	66	67	68	69	70	OFD (mm)
60	182	183	185	186	188	189	191	192	194	196	197	199	201	202	204	206	207	209	211	213	214	60
61	183	185	186	188	189	191	193	194	196	197	199	201	202	204	206	207	209	211	212	214	216	61
62	185	187	188	190	191	193	194	196	197	199	201	202	204	206	207	209	211	212	214	216	217	62
63	187	188	190	191	193	194	196	198	199	201	202	204	206	207	209	210	212	214	216	217	219	63
64	189	190	192	193	195	196	198	199	201	202	204	206	207	209	210	212	214	215	217	219	221	64
65	191	192	194	195	196	198	199	201	203	204	206	207	209	210	212	214	215	217	219	220	222	65
66	193	194	195	197	198	200	201	203	204	206	207	209	211	212	214	215	217	219	220	222	224	66
67	194	196	197	199	200	202	203	205	206	208	209	211	212	214	215	217	219	220	222	224	225	67
68	196	198	199	200	202	203	205	206	208	209	211	212	214	216	217	219	220	222	224	225	227	68
69	198	199	201	202	204	205	207	208	210	211	213	214	216	217	219	220	222	224	225	227	229	69
70	200	201	203	204	206	207	208	210	211	213	214	216	217	219	221	222	224	225	227	229	230	70
71	202	203	205	206	207	209	210	212	213	215	216	218	219	221	222	224	225	227	229	230	232	71
72	204	205	206	208	209	211	212	214	215	216	218	219	221	222	224	226	227	229	230	232	233	72
73	206	207	208	210	211	213	214	215	217	218	220	221	223	224	226	227	229	230	232	234	235	73
74	208	209	210	212	213	214	216	217	219	220	221	223	224	226	227	229	231	232	234	235	237	74
75	210	211	212	214	215	216	218	219	220	222	223	225	226	228	229	231	232	234	235	237	239	75
76	212	213	214	215	217	218	219	221	222	224	225	227	228	230	231	233	234	236	237	239	240	76
77	213	215	216	217	219	220	221	223	224	226	227	228	230	231	233	234	236	237	239	240	242	77
78	215	217	218	219	221	222	223	225	226	227	229	230	232	233	235	236	238	239	241	242	244	78
79	217	219	220	221	222	224	225	226	228	229	231	232	233	235	236	238	239	241	242	244	245	79
80	219	221	222	223	224	226	227	228	230	231	233	234	235	237	238	240	241	243	244	246	247	80
81	221	223	224	225	226	228	229	230	232	233	234	236	237	239	240	241	243	244	246	247	249	81
82	223	225	226	227	228	230	231	232	234	235	236	238	239	240	242	243	245	246	248	249	251	82
83	225	226	228	229	230	231	233	234	235	237	238	239	241	242	244	245	247	248	249	251	252	83
84	227	228	230	231	232	233	235	236	237	239	240	241	243	244	246	247	248	250	251	253	254	84
85	229	230	232	233	234	235	237	238	239	241	242	243	245	246	247	249	250	252	253	255	256	85
86	231	232	234	235	236	237	239	240	241	242	244	245	246	248	249	251	252	253	255	256	258	86
87	233	234	236	237	238	239	241	242	243	244	246	247	248	250	251	252	254	255	257	258	260	87
88	235	236	238	239	240	241	243	244	245	246	248	249	250	252	253	254	256	257	259	260	261	88
89	237	238	240	241	242	243	244	246	247	248	250	251	252	254	255	256	258	259	260	262	263	89
90	239	241	242	243	244	245	246	248	249	250	251	253	254	255	257	258	259	261	262	264	265	90
91	241	243	244	245	246	247	248	250	251	252	253	255	256	257	259	260	261	263	264	266	267	91
92	243	245	246	247	248	249	250	252	253	254	255	257	258	259	261	262	263	265	266	267	269	92
93	245	247	248	249	250	251	252	254	255	256	257	259	260	261	262	264	265	266	268	269	271	93
94	248	249	250	251	252	253	254	256	257	258	259	261	262	263	264	266	267	268	270	271	272	94
95	250	251	252	253	254	255	256	258	259	260	261	262	264	265	266	268	269	270	272	273	274	95
96	252	253	254	255	256	257	258	260	261	262	263	264	266	267	268	270	271	272	274	275	276	96
97	254	255	256	257	258	259	260	262	263	264	265	266	268	269	270	271	273	274	275	277	278	97
98	256	257	258	259	260	261	262	264	265	266	267	268	270	271	272	273	275	276	277	279	280	98
99	258	259	260	261	262	263	264	266	267	268	269	270	272	273	274	275	277	278	279	281	282	99
100	260	261	262	263	264	265	266	268	269	270	271	272	274	275	276	277	279	280	281	282	284	100

Table 53.**11** (continued)   Calculation of the head circumference (HC) from the BPD and OFD (data in mm)

OFD (mm)	70	71	72	73	74	75	76	77	78	79	80	81	82	83	84	85	86	87	88	89	90	OFD (mm)
80	247	249	250	252	253	255	257	258	260	261	263	265	266	268	270	271	273	275	277	278	280	80
81	249	250	252	254	255	257	258	260	261	263	265	266	268	270	271	273	275	276	278	280	282	81
82	251	252	254	255	257	258	260	262	263	265	266	268	270	271	273	275	276	278	280	281	283	82
83	252	254	255	257	259	260	262	263	265	266	268	270	271	273	275	276	278	280	281	283	285	83
84	254	256	257	259	260	262	263	265	267	268	270	271	273	275	276	278	280	281	283	285	286	84
85	256	257	259	261	262	264	265	267	268	270	271	273	275	276	278	279	281	283	284	286	288	85
86	258	259	261	262	264	265	267	268	270	272	273	275	276	278	280	281	283	284	286	288	289	86
87	260	261	263	264	266	267	269	270	272	273	275	276	278	280	281	283	284	286	288	289	291	87
88	261	263	264	266	267	269	270	272	273	275	277	278	280	281	283	284	286	288	289	291	293	88
89	263	265	266	268	269	271	272	274	275	277	278	280	281	283	285	286	288	289	291	293	294	89
90	265	267	268	269	271	272	274	275	277	278	280	282	283	285	286	288	289	291	293	294	296	90
91	267	268	270	271	273	274	276	277	279	280	282	283	285	286	288	290	291	293	294	296	298	91
92	269	270	272	273	275	276	277	279	280	282	283	285	287	288	290	291	293	294	296	298	299	92
93	271	272	273	275	276	278	279	281	282	284	285	287	288	290	291	293	295	296	298	299	301	93
94	272	274	275	277	278	280	281	283	284	285	287	288	290	292	293	295	296	298	299	301	303	94
95	274	276	277	279	280	281	283	284	286	287	289	290	292	293	295	296	298	300	301	303	304	95
96	276	278	279	280	282	283	285	286	288	289	291	292	294	295	297	298	300	301	303	304	306	96
97	278	279	281	282	284	285	287	288	289	291	292	294	295	297	298	300	301	303	305	306	308	97
98	280	281	283	284	286	287	288	290	291	293	294	296	297	299	300	302	303	305	306	308	309	98
99	282	283	285	286	287	289	290	292	293	294	296	297	299	300	302	303	305	306	308	310	311	99
100	284	285	286	288	289	291	292	293	295	296	298	299	301	302	304	305	307	308	310	311	313	100
101	286	287	288	290	291	292	294	295	297	298	300	301	302	304	305	307	308	310	311	313	315	101
102	288	289	290	292	293	294	296	297	299	300	301	303	304	306	307	309	310	312	313	315	316	102
103	290	291	292	294	295	296	298	299	300	302	303	305	306	308	309	310	312	313	315	316	318	103
104	291	293	294	295	297	298	299	301	302	304	305	306	308	309	311	312	314	315	317	318	320	104
105	293	295	296	297	299	300	301	303	304	306	307	308	310	311	313	314	316	317	319	320	322	105
106	295	297	298	299	301	302	303	305	306	307	309	310	312	313	314	316	317	319	320	322	323	106
107	297	299	300	301	302	304	305	306	308	309	311	312	313	315	316	318	319	321	322	324	325	107
108	299	301	302	303	304	306	307	308	310	311	312	314	315	317	318	320	321	322	324	325	327	108
109	301	302	304	305	306	308	309	310	312	313	314	316	317	319	320	321	323	324	326	327	329	109
110	303	304	306	307	308	310	311	312	314	315	316	318	319	320	322	323	325	326	328	329	330	110
111	305	306	308	309	310	311	313	314	315	317	318	319	321	322	324	325	326	328	329	331	332	111
112	307	308	310	311	312	313	315	316	317	319	320	321	323	324	326	327	328	330	331	333	334	112
113	309	310	312	313	314	315	317	318	319	321	322	323	325	326	327	329	330	332	333	334	336	113
114	311	312	313	315	316	317	319	320	321	322	324	325	326	328	329	331	332	333	335	336	338	114
115	313	314	315	317	318	319	320	322	323	324	326	327	328	330	331	332	334	335	337	338	340	115
116	315	316	317	319	320	321	322	324	325	326	328	329	330	332	333	334	336	337	339	340	341	116
117	317	318	319	321	322	323	324	326	327	328	330	331	332	334	335	336	338	339	340	342	343	117
118	319	320	321	323	324	325	326	328	329	330	331	333	334	335	337	338	339	341	342	344	345	118
119	321	322	323	325	326	327	328	330	331	332	333	335	336	337	339	340	341	343	344	345	347	119
120	323	324	325	327	328	329	330	331	333	334	335	337	338	339	341	342	343	345	346	347	349	120

Table 53.11 (continued)   Calculation of the head circumference (HC) from the BPD and OFD (data in mm)

OFD (mm)	BPD (mm) 90	91	92	93	94	95	96	97	98	99	100	101	102	103	104	105	106	107	108	109	110	OFD (mm)
100	313	314	316	318	319	321	322	324	326	327	329	330	332	334	335	337	339	341	342	344	346	100
101	315	316	318	319	321	322	324	326	327	329	330	332	334	335	337	339	340	342	344	345	347	101
102	316	318	319	321	322	324	326	327	329	330	332	334	335	337	339	340	342	344	345	347	349	102
103	318	320	321	323	324	326	327	329	331	332	334	335	337	339	340	342	344	345	347	349	350	103
104	320	321	323	324	326	327	329	331	332	334	335	337	339	340	342	344	345	347	349	350	352	104
105	322	323	325	326	328	329	331	332	334	336	337	339	340	342	344	345	347	349	350	352	354	105
106	323	325	326	328	329	331	332	334	336	337	339	340	342	344	345	347	349	350	352	353	355	106
107	325	327	328	330	331	333	334	336	337	339	341	342	344	345	347	349	350	352	353	355	357	107
108	327	328	330	331	333	334	336	338	339	341	342	344	345	347	349	350	352	353	355	357	358	108
109	329	330	332	333	335	336	338	339	341	342	344	345	347	349	350	352	353	355	357	358	360	109
110	330	332	333	335	336	338	339	341	343	344	346	347	349	350	352	354	355	357	358	360	362	110
111	332	334	335	337	338	340	341	343	344	346	347	349	350	352	354	355	357	358	360	362	363	111
112	334	336	337	338	340	341	343	344	346	348	349	351	352	354	355	357	359	360	362	363	365	112
113	336	337	339	340	342	343	345	346	348	349	351	352	354	355	357	359	360	362	363	365	367	113
114	338	339	341	342	344	345	347	348	350	351	353	354	356	357	359	360	362	364	365	367	368	114
115	340	341	342	344	345	347	348	350	351	353	354	356	357	359	360	362	364	365	367	368	370	115
116	341	343	344	346	347	349	350	352	353	355	356	358	359	361	362	364	365	367	368	370	372	116
117	343	345	346	347	349	350	352	353	355	356	358	359	361	362	364	366	367	369	370	372	373	117
118	345	346	348	349	351	352	354	355	357	358	360	361	363	364	366	367	369	370	372	373	375	118
119	347	348	350	351	353	354	355	357	358	360	361	363	364	366	367	369	371	372	374	375	377	119
120	349	350	352	353	354	356	357	359	360	362	363	365	366	368	369	371	372	374	375	377	378	120
121	351	352	353	355	356	358	359	361	362	363	365	366	368	369	371	372	374	376	377	379	380	121
122	352	354	355	357	358	360	361	362	364	365	367	368	370	371	373	374	376	377	379	380	382	122
123	354	356	357	359	360	361	363	364	366	367	369	370	372	373	374	376	378	379	381	382	384	123
124	356	358	359	360	362	363	365	366	367	369	370	372	373	375	376	378	379	381	382	384	385	124
125	358	359	361	362	364	365	366	368	369	371	372	374	375	377	378	380	381	383	384	386	387	125
126	360	361	363	364	365	367	368	370	371	373	374	375	377	378	380	381	383	384	386	387	389	126
127	362	363	365	366	367	369	370	372	373	374	376	377	379	380	382	383	385	386	388	389	391	127
128	364	365	366	368	369	371	372	373	375	376	378	379	381	382	383	385	386	388	389	391	392	128
129	366	367	368	370	371	372	374	375	377	378	379	381	382	384	385	387	388	390	391	393	394	129
130	368	369	370	372	373	374	376	377	379	380	381	383	384	386	387	389	390	391	393	394	396	130
131	370	371	372	374	375	376	378	379	380	382	383	385	386	387	389	390	392	393	395	396	398	131
132	371	373	374	375	377	378	379	381	382	384	385	386	388	389	391	392	394	395	397	398	399	132
133	373	375	376	377	379	380	381	383	384	385	387	388	390	391	393	394	395	397	398	400	401	133
134	375	377	378	379	381	382	383	385	386	387	389	390	392	393	394	396	397	399	400	402	403	134
135	377	379	380	381	382	384	385	386	388	389	391	392	393	395	396	398	399	401	402	403	405	135
136	379	380	382	383	384	386	387	388	390	391	392	394	395	397	398	399	401	402	404	405	407	136
137	381	382	384	385	386	388	389	390	392	393	394	396	397	399	400	401	403	404	406	407	408	137
138	383	384	386	387	388	390	391	392	394	395	396	398	399	400	402	403	405	406	407	409	410	138
139	385	386	388	389	390	391	393	394	395	397	398	399	401	402	404	405	406	408	409	411	412	139
140	387	388	389	391	392	393	395	396	397	399	400	401	403	404	405	407	408	410	411	413	414	140

Table 53.**11** (continued)   Calculation of the head circumference (HC) from the BPD and OFD (data in mm)

OFD (mm)	BPD (mm) 110	111	112	113	114	115	116	117	118	119	120	121	122	123	124	125	126	127	128	129	130	OFD (mm)
120	378	380	382	383	385	386	388	390	391	393	395	396	398	400	401	403	405	406	408	410	411	120
121	380	382	383	385	387	388	390	391	393	395	396	398	400	401	403	404	406	408	410	411	413	121
122	382	383	385	387	388	390	391	393	395	396	398	400	401	403	404	406	408	409	411	413	415	122
123	384	385	387	388	390	391	393	395	396	398	400	401	403	404	406	408	409	411	413	414	416	123
124	385	387	388	390	392	393	395	396	398	400	401	403	404	406	408	409	411	413	414	416	418	124
125	387	389	390	392	393	395	396	398	400	401	403	404	406	408	409	411	413	414	416	418	419	125
126	389	390	392	394	395	397	398	400	401	403	405	406	408	409	411	413	414	416	418	419	421	126
127	391	392	394	395	397	398	400	401	403	405	406	408	409	411	413	414	416	418	419	421	423	127
128	392	394	395	397	399	400	402	403	405	406	408	410	411	413	414	416	418	419	421	423	424	128
129	394	396	397	399	400	402	403	405	406	408	410	411	413	414	416	418	419	421	423	424	426	129
130	396	397	399	400	402	404	405	407	408	410	411	413	415	416	418	419	421	423	424	426	427	130
131	398	399	401	402	404	405	407	408	410	411	413	415	416	418	419	421	423	424	426	427	429	131
132	399	401	402	404	406	407	409	410	412	413	415	416	418	419	421	423	424	426	427	429	431	132
133	401	403	404	406	407	409	410	412	413	415	416	418	420	421	423	424	426	428	429	431	432	133
134	403	405	406	408	409	411	412	414	415	417	418	420	421	423	424	426	428	429	431	432	434	134
135	405	406	408	409	411	412	414	415	417	418	420	421	423	425	426	428	429	431	433	434	436	135
136	407	408	410	411	413	414	416	417	419	420	422	423	425	426	428	429	431	433	434	436	437	136
137	408	410	411	413	414	416	417	419	420	422	423	425	427	428	430	431	433	434	436	438	439	137
138	410	412	413	415	416	418	419	421	422	424	425	427	428	430	431	433	434	436	438	439	441	138
139	412	414	415	416	418	419	421	422	424	425	427	428	430	432	433	435	436	438	439	441	442	139
140	414	415	417	418	420	421	423	424	426	427	429	430	432	433	435	436	438	439	441	443	444	140
141	416	417	419	420	422	423	425	426	427	429	430	432	434	435	437	438	440	441	443	444	446	141
142	418	419	420	422	423	425	426	428	429	431	432	434	435	437	438	440	441	443	444	446	448	142
143	419	421	422	424	425	427	428	430	431	433	434	436	437	439	440	442	443	445	446	448	449	143
144	421	423	424	426	427	428	430	431	433	434	436	437	439	440	442	443	445	446	448	449	451	144
145	423	425	426	427	429	430	432	433	435	436	438	439	441	442	444	445	447	448	450	451	453	145
146	425	426	428	429	431	432	434	435	436	438	439	441	442	444	445	447	448	450	451	453	455	146
147	427	428	430	431	433	434	435	437	438	440	441	443	444	446	447	449	450	452	453	455	456	147
148	429	430	432	433	434	436	437	439	440	442	443	444	446	447	449	450	452	453	455	456	458	148
149	431	432	433	435	436	438	439	440	442	443	445	446	448	449	451	452	454	455	457	458	460	149
150	432	434	435	437	438	439	441	442	444	445	447	448	450	451	452	454	455	457	458	460	461	150
151	434	436	437	438	440	441	443	444	446	447	448	450	451	453	454	456	457	459	460	462	463	151
152	436	438	439	440	442	443	445	446	447	449	450	452	453	455	456	458	459	461	462	464	465	152
153	438	439	441	442	444	445	446	448	449	451	452	454	455	456	458	459	461	462	464	465	467	153
154	440	441	443	444	445	447	448	450	451	452	454	455	457	458	460	461	463	464	466	467	469	154
155	442	443	445	446	447	449	450	452	453	454	456	457	459	460	462	463	464	466	467	469	470	155
156	444	445	446	448	449	451	452	453	455	456	458	459	460	462	463	465	466	468	469	471	472	156
157	446	447	448	450	451	452	454	455	457	458	459	461	462	464	465	467	468	470	471	472	474	157
158	448	449	450	452	453	454	456	457	458	460	461	463	464	466	467	468	470	471	473	474	476	158
159	450	451	452	454	455	456	458	459	460	462	463	465	466	467	469	470	472	473	475	476	478	159
160	451	453	454	455	457	458	459	461	462	464	465	466	468	469	471	472	474	475	476	478	479	160

Table 53.**12**   Calculation of the abdominal circumference based on the mean abdominal diameter AM = (ATD + ASD)/2 using the formula AC = AM x π (mm)

AM (mm)	AC (mm)	AM (mm)	AC (mm)	AM (mm)	AC (mm)	AM (mm)	AC (mm)	AM (mm)	AC (mm)	AM (mm)	AC (mm)	AM (mm)	AC (mm)
11	35	31	97	51	160	71	223	91	286	111	349	131	412
12	38	32	101	52	163	72	226	92	289	112	352	132	415
13	41	33	104	53	167	73	229	93	292	113	355	133	418
14	44	34	107	54	170	74	232	94	295	114	358	134	421
15	47	35	110	55	173	75	236	95	298	115	361	135	424
16	50	36	113	56	176	76	239	96	302	116	364	136	427
17	53	37	116	57	179	77	242	97	305	117	368	137	430
18	57	38	119	58	182	78	245	98	308	118	371	138	434
19	60	39	123	59	185	79	248	99	311	119	374	139	437
20	63	40	126	60	188	80	251	100	314	120	377	140	440
21	66	41	129	61	192	81	254	101	317	121	380	141	443
22	69	42	132	62	195	82	258	102	320	122	383	142	446
23	72	43	135	63	198	83	261	103	324	123	386	143	449
24	75	44	138	64	201	84	264	104	327	124	390	144	452
25	79	45	141	65	204	85	267	105	330	125	393	145	456
26	82	46	145	66	207	86	270	106	333	126	396	146	459
27	85	47	148	67	210	87	273	107	336	127	399	147	462
28	88	48	151	68	214	88	276	108	339	128	402	148	465
29	91	49	154	69	217	89	280	109	342	129	405		
30	94	50	157	70	220	90	283	110	346	130	408		

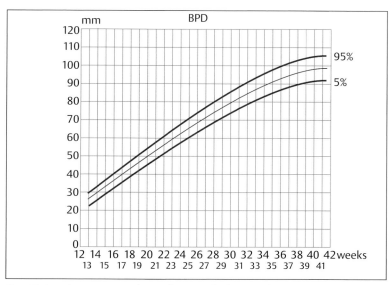

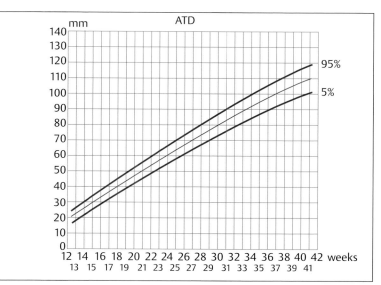

Figs. 53.3 and 53.4 Normal growth curves for biparietal diameter and abdominal transverse diameter (weeks = completed weeks gestation), lower limit 5th percentile, upper limit 95th percentile

After Merz., E., Wellek, S.: The normal fetal growth profile—a unified model to calculate normal growth curves for standard head and abdominal parameters and the long extremity bones. Ultraschall in Med. 17 (1996) 153–162

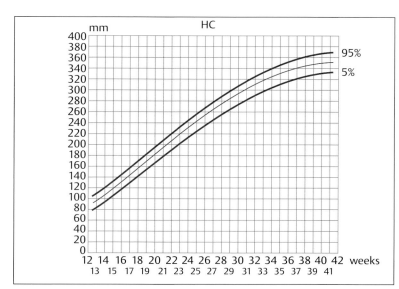

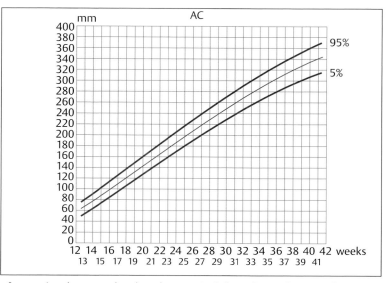

Figs. 53.5 and 53.6 Normal growth curves for head circumference and abdominal circumference (weeks = completed weeks gestation), lower limit 5th percentile, upper limit 95th percentile

After Merz., E., Wellek, S.: The normal fetal growth profile—a unified model to calculate normal growth curves for standard head and abdominal parameters and the long extremity bones. Ultraschall in Med. 17 (1996) 153–162

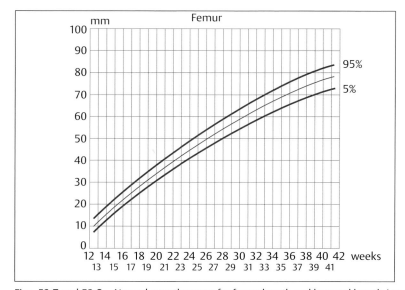

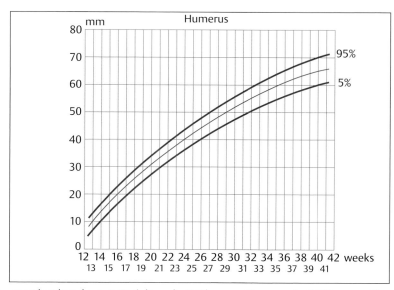

Figs. 53.7 and 53.8 Normal growth curves for femur length and humeral length (weeks = completed weeks gestation), lower limit 5th percentile, upper limit 95th percentile

After Merz., E., Wellek, S.: Normal fetal growth profile: a uniform model for calculating normal growth curves for current head and abdomen parameters and long limb bones. Ultraschall in Med. 17 (1996) 153–162

Organ Biometry in the Head and Neck

Table 53.**13** Normal data for the anterior and posterior cerebral lateral ventricles (LV), the cerebral hemisphere, and the ventricular–hemispheric ratio as a function of gestational age (in completed weeks), data in mm, lower limit 5th percentile, upper limit 95th percentile

| | LV anterior | | | LV posterior | | | Hemisphere | | | V/H ratio | | | |
Weeks	5%	50%	95%	5%	50%	95%	5%	50%	95%	5%	50%	95%	Weeks
14	5.2	6.7	8.1	5.1	6.7	8.4	13	15	16	0.39	0.47	0.56	14
15	5.3	6.8	8.3	5.1	6.8	8.5	15	16	18	0.36	0.43	0.51	15
16	5.4	6.9	8.4	5.2	6.9	8.6	16	18	19	0.33	0.40	0.48	16
17	5.6	7.0	8.5	5.3	7.0	8.7	17	19	21	0.31	0.37	0.44	17
18	5.7	7.2	8.6	5.4	7.1	8.8	19	21	23	0.29	0.35	0.41	18
19	5.8	7.3	8.8	5.5	7.2	8.8	20	22	24	0.27	0.32	0.39	19
20	5.9	7.4	8.9	5.6	7.2	8.9	22	24	26	0.26	0.31	0.37	20
21	6.1	7.5	9.0	5.6	7.3	9.0	23	25	28	0.24	0.29	0.35	21
22	6.2	7.7	9.2	5.7	7.4	9.1	25	27	30	0.23	0.28	0.33	22
23	6.3	7.8	9.3	5.8	7.5	9.2	26	29	31	0.22	0.27	0.32	23
24	6.4	7.9	9.4	5.9	7.6	9.3	28	30	33	0.21	0.26	0.31	24
25	6.6	8.1	9.5	6.0	7.7	9.3	29	32	35	0.21	0.25	0.30	25
26	6.7	8.2	9.7	6.1	7.7	9.4	31	34	37	0.20	0.24	0.29	26
27	6.8	8.3	9.8	6.1	7.8	9.5	32	35	38	0.19	0.23	0.28	27
28	7.0	8.4	9.9	6.2	7.9	9.6	34	37	40	0.19	0.23	0.27	28
29	7.1	8.5	10.1	6.3	8.0	9.7	35	38	41	0.19	0.22	0.27	29
30	7.2	8.7	10.2	6.4	8.1	9.8	36	40	43	0.18	0.22	0.26	30
31	7.3	8.8	10.3	6.5	8.2	9.9	38	41	44	0.18	0.21	0.26	31
32	7.5	9.0	10.4	6.6	8.3	9.9	39	42	46	0.18	0.21	0.26	32
33	7.6	9.1	10.6	6.7	8.3	10.0	40	43	47	0.18	0.21	0.25	33
34	7.7	9.2	10.7	6.7	8.4	10.1	41	44	48	0.17	0.21	0.25	34
35	7.9	6.7	10.8	6.8	8.5	10.2	42	45	49	0.17	0.21	0.25	35
36	8.0	6.8	10.9	6.9	8.6	10.3	42	46	50	0.17	0.21	0.25	36
37	8.1	6.9	11.1	7.0	8.7	10.4	43	47	51	0.17	0.21	0.25	37
38	8.2	7.0	11.2	7.1	8.8	10.4	43	47	51	0.17	0.21	0.25	38
39	8.3	7.2	11.3	7.2	8.8	10.5	44	48	52	0.17	0.21	0.25	39

Adapted from Sniders, R.J.M., Nicolaides, K.H.: Fetal biometry at 14–40 weeks' gestation. Ultrasound Obstet. Gynec. 4 (1994) 34–48

Table 53.**14** Normal data for the transverse cerebellar diameter and cisterna magna as a function of gestational age (in completed weeks), data in mm, lower limit 5th percentile, upper limit 95th percentile

| | Transverse cerebellar diameter | | | Cisterna magna | | | |
Weeks	5%	50%	95%	5%	50%	95%	Weeks
14	12	14	15	1.9	3.5	5.3	14
15	13	15	17	2.1	3.8	5.7	15
16	14	16	18	2.4	4.1	6.0	16
17	15	17	19	2.6	4.3	6.3	17
18	16	18	21	2.8	4.6	6.6	18
19	17	20	22	3.1	4.9	6.9	19
20	19	21	24	3.3	5.1	7.2	20
21	20	22	25	3.5	5.4	7.5	21
22	21	24	27	3.7	5.6	7.7	22
23	22	25	28	3.9	5.8	8.0	23
24	24	26	30	4.1	6.0	8.2	24
25	25	28	31	4.3	6.2	8.5	25
26	26	29	33	4.4	6.4	8.7	26
27	27	31	34	4.6	6.6	8.9	27
28	29	32	36	4.7	6.8	9.1	28
29	30	33	37	4.9	6.9	9.3	29
30	31	35	39	5.0	7.0	9.4	30
31	32	36	40	5.1	7.2	9.6	31
32	34	37	42	5.2	7.3	9.7	32
33	35	39	43	5.3	7.4	9.8	33
34	36	40	44	5.3	7.5	9.9	34
35	37	41	46	5.4	7.5	10.0	35
36	38	42	47	5.4	7.6	10.0	36
37	39	43	48	5.4	7.6	10.1	37
38	40	44	49	5.5	7.6	10.1	38
39	41	45	51	5.5	7.6	10.1	39

Adapted from Sniders, R.J.M., Nicolaides, K.H.: Fetal biometry at 14 to 40 weeks' gestation. Ultrasound Obstet. Gynec. 4 (1994) 34–48

Table 53.**15** Normal data for the cavum septi pellucidi as a function of gestational age (in completed weeks), data in mm, lower limit –2 SD, upper limit +2 SD

| Cavum septi pellucidi | | | |
Weeks	Mean –2 SD	Mean	Mean +2 SD
19-20	2.08	3.40	4.72
21-22	2.60	4.06	5.52
23-24	3.02	4.74	6.46
25-26	3.96	5.56	7.16
27-28	4.12	6.42	8.72
29–30	4.37	6.11	8.05
31–32	4.43	6.51	8.59
33-34	4.04	6.48	8.92
35-36	4.37	6.45	8.53
37-38	3.81	6.37	8.93
39-40	4.64	6.30	7.96
41-42	3.62	5.48	7.34

After Jou, H.-J. et al.: Ultrasound measurement of the fetal cavum septi pellucidi. Ultrasound Obstet. Gynec. 12 (1998) 419–421

Table 53.**16** Normal data for the fetal nasal width as a function of gestational age (in completed weeks), data in mm, lower limit 10th percentile, upper limit 90th percentile

| Nasal width | | | |
Weeks	10%	50%	90%
14-15	5.5	7.6	10.2
16-17	6.5	7.9	10.5
18-19	8.5	10.0	11.0
20-21	10.2	12.0	13.0
22	13.0	14.0	15.0
23	13.0	14.0	15.0
24	13.0	15.0	16.0
25	14.2	16.3	17.0
26	14.1	16.3	18.4
27	13.4	17.2	19.0
28	15.1	17.6	20.2
29-30	16.5	18.1	20.6
31-32	16.6	19.6	21.4
33-34	17.4	20.5	23.1
35-37	17.6	20.5	23.3
38-40	17.4	18.9	23.4

After Goldstein, I., Tamir, A., Itskovitz-Eldor, J., Zimmer, E.Z.: Growth of the fetal nose width and nostril distance in normal pregnancies. Ultrasound Obstet. Gynec. 9 (1997) 35–38

Table 53.**17**   Normal data for the transverse diameter of both thyroid lobes (including the trachea), the transverse diameter of the right and left lobes, and the AP diameter of the right and left lobes as a function of gestational age (in completed weeks), data in mm

| Weeks | Thyroid diameter in mm (mean ± 1 SD) | | | | |
	Right + left lobes, transverse	Right lobe, transverse	Left lobe, transverse	Right lobe, a.p.	Left lobe, a.p.
20 – 23	11.29 ± 1.90	4.64 ± 0.77	4.57 ± 0.77	4.99 ± 0.87	4.97 ± 0.80
24 – 27	14.34 ± 2.05	5.82 ± 0.62	5.71 ± 0.58	6.12 ± 0.86	6.07 ± 0.86
28 – 31	16.24 ± 2.06	6.42 ± 0.51	6.40 ± 0.56	6.81 ± 0.80	6.86 ± 0.86
32 – 35	18.02 ± 2.08	7.17 ± 0.83	7.11 ± 0.81	7.42 ± 0.99	7.59 ± 0.96
36 – 40	21.27 ± 2.62	8.49 ± 0.96	8.46 ± 1.04	8.49 ± 0.84	8.59 ± 0.87

Based on data from Meinel, K., Döring, K.: Growth of the fetal thyroid gland in the second half of pregnancy: ultrasound biometric studies. Ultraschall in Med. 18 (1997) 258–261

Organ Biometry in the Thorax

Table 53.**18** Normal data for the bony transverse (BTTD) and sagittal thoracic diameter (BTSD), bony thoracic circumference (BTC), and oblique lung diameter (LD) (in continuity with the long cardiac axis) as a function of gestational age (in completed weeks), data in mm, normal data for the ratio of lung diameter and bony chest circumference, lower limit 5th percentile, upper limit 95th percentile

Weeks	BTTD			BTSD			BTC			LD			LD/BTC			Weeks
	5%	50%	95%	5%	50%	95%	5%	50%	95%	5%	50%	95%	5%	50%	95%	
12.0	15	20	26	13	18	23	44	60	77	4	6	9	0.096	0.115	0.134	12.0
12.5	16	21	27	14	19	25	46	63	80	4	7	10	0.096	0.115	0.134	12.5
13.0	16	22	28	15	20	26	49	66	83	5	8	10	0.096	0.115	0.134	13.0
13.5	17	23	29	16	22	27	53	70	87	5	8	11	0.096	0.115	0.134	13.5
14.0	18	24	30	17	23	28	56	74	91	6	9	11	0.096	0.115	0.134	14.0
14.5	20	25	31	19	24	30	60	77	95	6	9	12	0.096	0.115	0.134	14.5
15.0	21	26	32	20	25	31	64	81	99	7	10	13	0.096	0.115	0.134	15.0
15.5	22	28	33	21	27	33	68	85	103	7	10	13	0.096	0.115	0.134	15.5
16.0	23	29	35	22	28	34	72	89	107	8	11	14	0.096	0.115	0.134	16.0
16.5	24	30	36	24	29	35	76	93	111	8	11	14	0.096	0.115	0.134	16.5
17.0	25	31	37	25	31	37	80	98	116	8	11	14	0.096	0.115	0.133	17.0
17.5	27	33	39	26	32	38	83	102	120	9	12	15	0.096	0.115	0.133	17.5
18.0	28	34	40	28	34	39	87	106	124	9	12	15	0.096	0.115	0.133	18.0
18.5	29	35	41	29	35	41	92	110	128	9	13	16	0.096	0.114	0.133	18.5
19.0	30	37	43	30	36	42	96	114	133	10	13	16	0.095	0.114	0.133	19.0
19.5	32	38	44	31	38	44	100	118	137	10	13	17	0.095	0.114	0.133	19.5
20.0	33	39	45	33	39	45	103	122	141	11	14	17	0.095	0.113	0.132	20.0
20.5	34	40	47	34	40	46	107	127	146	11	14	18	0.094	0.113	0.132	20.5
21.0	35	42	48	35	41	48	111	131	150	11	15	18	0.094	0.113	0.131	21.0
21.5	37	43	49	37	43	49	115	135	154	12	15	18	0.093	0.112	0.131	21.5
22.0	38	44	51	38	44	50	119	139	158	12	15	19	0.093	0.112	0.130	22.0
22.5	39	46	52	39	45	52	123	143	162	12	16	19	0.092	0.111	0.130	22.5
23.0	40	47	53	40	47	53	127	147	167	13	16	20	0.092	0.110	0.129	23.0
23.5	41	48	55	42	48	54	131	151	171	13	17	20	0.091	0.110	0.129	23.5
24.0	43	49	56	43	49	56	135	155	175	13	17	20	0.091	0.109	0.128	24.0
24.5	44	51	57	44	51	57	139	159	179	14	17	21	0.090	0.109	0.128	24.5
25.0	45	52	59	45	52	58	142	163	183	14	18	21	0.090	0.108	0.127	25.0
25.5	46	53	60	46	53	60	146	167	187	14	18	22	0.089	0.108	0.127	25.5
26.0	47	54	61	48	54	61	150	170	191	15	18	22	0.089	0.108	0.126	26.0
26.5	48	55	62	49	55	62	153	174	195	15	19	22	0.088	0.107	0.126	26.5
27.0	50	57	63	50	57	63	157	178	199	15	19	23	0.088	0.107	0.126	27.0
27.5	51	58	65	51	58	65	160	181	203	16	19	23	0.088	0.107	0.126	27.5
28.0	52	59	66	52	59	66	164	185	206	16	20	24	0.088	0.107	0.125	28.0
28.5	53	60	67	53	60	67	167	189	210	16	20	24	0.088	0.106	0.125	28.5
29.0	54	61	68	54	61	68	171	192	214	16	20	24	0.088	0.106	0.125	29.0
29.5	55	62	69	55	62	69	174	196	217	17	21	25	0.088	0.106	0.125	29.5
30.0	56	63	70	56	64	71	177	199	221	17	21	25	0.087	0.106	0.125	30.0
30.5	57	64	71	57	65	72	180	202	224	17	21	25	0.087	0.106	0.125	30.5
31.0	58	65	72	59	66	73	183	206	228	18	22	26	0.087	0.106	0.125	31.0
31.5	59	66	73	60	67	74	187	209	231	18	22	26	0.087	0.106	0.125	31.5
32.0	60	67	74	61	68	75	189	212	234	18	22	27	0.087	0.106	0.125	32.0
32.5	61	68	75	61	69	76	192	215	237	18	23	27	0.087	0.106	0.125	32.5
33.0	61	69	76	62	70	77	195	218	240	19	23	27	0.087	0.106	0.125	33.0
33.5	62	70	77	63	71	78	198	221	243	19	23	28	0.087	0.106	0.125	33.5
34.0	63	70	78	64	72	79	201	223	246	19	24	28	0.087	0.106	0.125	34.0
34.5	64	71	79	65	73	80	203	226	249	20	24	28	0.087	0.106	0.125	34.5
35.0	64	72	80	66	74	81	205	229	252	20	24	29	0.087	0.106	0.125	35.0
35.5	65	73	81	67	74	82	208	231	254	20	25	29	0.087	0.106	0.125	35.5
36.0	66	73	81	68	75	83	210	234	257	20	25	29	0.087	0.106	0.125	36.0
36.5	66	74	82	68	76	84	212	236	259	21	25	30	0.087	0.106	0.125	36.5
37.0	67	75	83	69	77	85	214	238	262	21	25	30	0.087	0.106	0.125	37.0
37.5	67	75	83	70	78	85	216	240	264	21	26	30	0.087	0.106	0.125	37.5
38.0	68	76	84	70	78	86	218	242	266	21	26	31	0.087	0.106	0.125	38.0
38.5	68	76	84	71	79	87	220	244	268	22	26	31	0.087	0.106	0.125	38.5
39.0	69	77	85	72	80	88	221	245	270	22	27	31	0.087	0.106	0.125	39.0
39.5	69	77	85	72	80	88	223	247	271	22	27	32	0.087	0.106	0.125	39.5
40.0	69	78	86	73	81	89	224	248	273	22	27	32	0.087	0.106	0.125	40.0
40.5	70	78	86	73	81	89	225	250	274	23	27	32	0.087	0.106	0.125	40.5
41.0	70	78	86	74	82	90	226	251	275	23	28	33	0.087	0.106	0.125	41.0

After Merz, E., Miric-Tesanic, D., Bahlmann, F., Weber, G., Hallermann, C.: Prenatal sonographic chest and lung measurements for predicting severe pulmonary hypoplasia. Prenatal Diagnosis 19 (1999) 614–619

Table 53.**19**   Normal data for fetal heart length and heart width, the ratio of fetal heart width/thoracic width, and the ratio of fetal heart area/thoracic area as a function of gestational age

Weeks	Fetal heart length 5%	50%	95%	Fetal heart width 5%	50%	95%	Fetal heart width/ thoracic width 5%	50%	95%	Fetal heart area/ thoracic area 5%	50%	95%	Weeks
20	16.14	**23.02**	29.90	11.73	**17.53**	23.33	0.36	**0.44**	0.53	0.19	**0.25**	0.31	20
22	19.18	**26.06**	32.94	14.35	**20.15**	25.95	0.36	**0.45**	0.54	0.19	**0.25**	0.31	22
24	22.22	**29.10**	35.98	16.97	**22.77**	28.57	0.37	**0.46**	0.55	0.20	**0.26**	0.32	24
26	25.26	**32.14**	39.02	19.59	**25.39**	31.19	0.38	**0.47**	0.55	0.20	**0.26**	0.32	26
28	28.30	**35.18**	42.06	22.21	**28.01**	33.81	0.38	**0.47**	0.56	0.21	**0.27**	0.33	28
30	31.34	**38.22**	45.10	24.83	**30.63**	36.43	0.39	**0.48**	0.57	0.22	**0.28**	0.34	30
32	34.38	**41.26**	48.14	27.45	**33.25**	39.05	0.40	**0.49**	0.57	0.22	**0.28**	0.34	32
34	37.42	**44.30**	51.18	30.07	**35.87**	41.67	0.41	**0.49**	0.58	0.23	**0.29**	0.35	34
36	40.46	**47.34**	54.22	32.69	**38.49**	44.29	0.41	**0.50**	0.59	0.23	**0.29**	0.35	36
38	43.50	**50.38**	57.26	35.31	**41.11**	46.91	0.42	**0.51**	0.60	0.24	**0.30**	0.36	38
40	46.98	**53.42**	60.30	37.93	**43.73**	49.53	0.43	**0.52**	0.60	0.25	**0.31**	0.37	40

Adapted from Chaoui, R., Heling, K.S., Bollmann, R.: Sonographic measurements of the fetal heart in the plane of the four-chamber view. Geburtsh. u. Frauenheilk. 54 (1994) 145–151

Table 53.**20**   Left and right transverse cardiac ventricular diameters and right–left ratio in the end-diastolic (ED) and end-systolic (ES) phases of the cardiac cycle as a function of gestational age (in completed weeks), mean values ± 1 SD

		Transverse cardiac ventricular diameters (mm)						
Weeks	n	Left ED	ES	Right ED	ES	Right–left ratio ED	ES
---	---	---	---	---	---	---	---
28	17	11.3 ± 1.7	7.9 ± 1.6	11.2 ± 2.0	8.0 ± 1.6	0.99 ± 0.05	0.99 ± 0.07
29	18	11.6 ± 1.6	8.3 ± 1.2	11.7 ± 1.5	8.3 ± 1.3	0.99 ± 0.03	1.00 ± 0.03
30	18	12.4 ± 1.4	8.9 ± 1.1	12.4 ± 1.5	9.0 ± 1.1	1.01 ± 0.04	1.02 ± 0.03
31	16	12.7 ± 1.6	9.3 ± 1.3	12.6 ± 1.5	9.3 ± 1.1	0.99 ± 0.03	1.00 ± 0.04
32	19	13.0 ± 1.6	9.6 ± 1.4	13.1 ± 1.6	9.7 ± 1.4	1.01 ± 0.04	1.00 ± 0.05
33	18	13.5 ± 2.2	9.9 ± 2.0	13.5 ± 2.2	9.8 ± 2.0	1.00 ± 0.03	0.99 ± 0.33
34	18	13.6 ± 1.3	10.1 ± 1.4	13.6 ± 1.5	9.9 ± 1.4	1.01 ± 0.04	0.98 ± 0.04
35	18	14.8 ± 2.0	11.0 ± 2.0	14.8 ± 2.0	11.0 ± 2.0	1.00 ± 0.03	1.00 ± 0.05
36	17	15.9 ± 1.5	11.8 ± 1.7	15.9 ± 1.6	11.7 ± 1.6	1.01 ± 0.04	1.00 ± 0.04
37	17	16.2 ± 1.6	12.2 ± 1.6	16.2 ± 1.5	12.3 ± 1.6	1.00 ± 0.04	0.98 ± 0.04
38	18	16.3 ± 1.7	12.3 ± 1.6	16.1 ± 1.5	12.5 ± 1.8	0.99 ± 0.03	1.01 ± 0.04
39	18	16.7 ± 1.5	12.5 ± 1.4	16.6 ± 1.3	12.7 ± 1.4	1.00 ± 0.03	0.99 ± 0.03
40	15	18.2 ± 1.2	14.4 ± 1.4	18.1 ± 1.2	14.2 ± 1.3	0.99 ± 0.03	0.99 ± 0.03

After Wladimiroff, J.W. et al.: Normal cardiac ventricular geometry and function during the last trimester of pregnancy and early neonatal period. Brit J. Gynaecol. 89 (1982) 839–844

Table 53.**21**   Normal data for the diameters of the aorta and pulmonary trunk (inner-to-inner measurement) as a function of gestational age (in completed weeks), data in mm, lower limit 5th percentile, upper limit 95th percentile

Weeks	Aortic diameter (mm) 5%	50%	95%	Pulmonary trunk diameter (mm) 5%	50%	95%	Weeks
14	1.2	**1.50**	1.8	1.5	**1.91**	2.2	14
15	1.6	**1.96**	2.4	1.8	**2.20**	2.8	15
16	1.8	**1.98**	2.2	2.0	**2.15**	2.5	16
17	2.1	**2.32**	2.6	2.1	**2.32**	2.6	17
18	2.4	**2.56**	2.8	2.7	**2.83**	2.9	18
19	2.5	**2.66**	2.9	2.8	**3.06**	3.4	19
20	2.4	**2.74**	3.0	2.7	**3.21**	3.8	20
21	2.6	**2.97**	3.3	3.3	**3.42**	3.7	21
22	2.8	**3.38**	3.8	3.5	**3.95**	4.5	22
23	3.3	**3.45**	3.7	3.0	**3.91**	4.4	23
24	3.4	**3.98**	4.6	4.0	**4.38**	4.8	24
25	3.7	**3.96**	4.3	4.0	**4.48**	5.1	25
26	4.2	**4.43**	4.7	4.8	**4.90**	5.2	26

Adapted from data supplied by Achrion, R. et al.: In utero ultrasonographic measurements of fetal aortic and pulmonary artery diameters during the first half of gestation. Ultrasound Obstet. Gynecol. 11 (1998) 180–184

Table 53.**22**   Normal data for the diameters of the aorta and pulmonary trunk (inner-to-inner measurement) as a function of gestational age, data in mm, lower limit 5th percentile, upper limit 95th percentile

Weeks	Aortic diameter (mm) 5%	50%	95%	Pulmonary trunk diameter (mm) 5%	50%	95%	Weeks
20	2.14	**3.45**	4.76	2.64	**4.10**	5.56	20
22	2.55	**3.86**	5.17	3.23	**4.69**	6.15	22
24	2.96	**4.27**	5.58	3.82	**5.28**	6.82	24
26	3.37	**4.68**	5.99	4.41	**5.87**	7.33	26
28	3.78	**5.09**	6.40	5.00	**6.46**	7.92	28
30	4.19	**5.50**	6.81	5.59	**7.05**	8.51	30
32	4.60	**5.91**	7.22	6.18	**7.64**	9.10	32
34	5.01	**6.32**	7.63	6.77	**8.23**	9.69	34
36	5.42	**6.73**	8.04	7.36	**8.82**	10.28	36
38	5.83	**7.14**	8.45	7.95	**9.41**	10.87	38
40	6.24	**7.55**	8.86	8.54	**10.00**	11.46	40

Adapted from Chaoui, R., Heling, K.S., Bollmann, R.: Sonographic measurements of the fetal heart in the plane of the four-chamber view. Geburtsh. u. Frauenheilk. 54 (1994) 145–151

Organ Biometry in the Abdomen

Table 53.23 Normal data for hepatic length (mm) as a function of gestational age (in completed weeks), mean values ± 2 SD

Weeks	Hepatic length (mm) Mean −2 SD	Mean	Mean +2 SD	Weeks	Hepatic length (mm) Mean −2 SD	Mean	Mean +2 SD
20	20.9	27.3	33.7	31	33.9	39.6	45.3
21	26.5	28.0	29.5	32	35.2	42.7	50.2
22	23.9	30.6	37.3	33	37.2	43.8	50.4
23	26.4	30.9	35.4	34	37.7	44.8	51.9
24	26.2	32.9	39.6	35	38.7	47.8	56.9
25	28.3	33.6	38.9	36	40.6	49.0	57.4
26	29.4	35.7	42.0	37	45.2	52.0	58.8
27	33.3	36.6	39.9	38	48.7	52.9	57.1
28	34.4	38.4	42.4	39	48.7	55.4	62.1
29	34.1	39.1	44.1	40	–	59.0	–
30	33.7	38.7	43.7	41	46.9	49.3	51.7

Based on data from Vintzileos, A.M. et al.: Fetal liver ultrasound measurements during normal pregnancy. Obstet. Gynecol 66 (1985) 477–480

Table 53.24 Normal data for longitudinal and transverse gallbladder diameters as a function of gestational age (in completed weeks), data in mm, lower limit 10th percentile, upper limit 90th percentile

Weeks	Gallbladder diameter Longitudinal diameter (mm) 10%	50%	90%	Transverse diameter (mm) 10%	50%	90%	Weeks
15-19	5	10	15	2	3	3.5	15-19
20-22	10	15	20	3	4	6	20-22
23-24	10	19	22	4	6	7	23-24
25-26	14.5	21	28	4	6	8	25-26
27-30	17	21	30	5	7	9	27-30
31-34	19	26	32	5	7	10	31-34
35-40	21	27	33	4	6.5	9	35-40

Adapted from data supplied by Goldstein, I. et al.: Growth of the fetal gallbladder in normal pregnancies. Ultrasound Obstet. Gynecol. 4 (1994) 289–293

Table 53.25 Normal data for the spleen as a function of gestational age (in completed weeks), data in mm, lower limit 5th percentile, upper limit 95th percentile

Weeks	Spleen Length 5%	50%	95%	Sagittal 5%	50%	95%	Transverse 5%	50%	95%	Weeks
18	7	14	21	3	8	11	4	9	13	18
19	12	16	23	4	8	12	4	9	14	19
20	11	18	26	5	8	12	5	10	15	20
21	12	20	27	5	9	13	6	11	16	21
22	15	22	29	6	10	13	7	12	16	22
23	16	23	31	7	10	14	8	12	17	23
24	19	25	32	7	11	15	8	13	18	24
25	19	26	33	7	11	15	9	14	19	25
26	20	27	34	8	12	15	10	15	19	26
27	22	29	37	9	13	17	10	15	20	27
28	24	31	38	10	13	17	11	16	21	28
29	25	33	40	10	14	18	12	17	21	29
30	27	34	41	11	15	19	13	17	22	30
31	30	36	43	12	15	19	13	18	23	31
32	31	38	45	12	16	20	14	19	24	32
33	33	40	47	13	16	20	15	20	24	33
34	35	43	50	13	17	21	16	20	25	34
35	38	45	52	14	18	22	16	21	26	35
36	41	48	55	15	19	22	17	22	27	36
37	44	51	58	15	19	23	18	23	27	37
38	47	54	62	16	20	23	18	23	28	38
39	51	58	65	17	20	24	19	24	29	39
40	55	62	70	17	21	25	20	25	29	40

After Schmidt, W., Yarkoni, S., Jeanty, P., Grannum, P., Hobbins, J.C.: Sonographic measurements of the fetal spleen: clinical implications. J. Ultrasound Med. 4 (1985) 667–672

Table 53.26 Normal data for the transverse colon diameter (mm) as a function of gestational age (in completed weeks), data in mm (outer-to-outer measurement), lower limit 10th percentile, upper limit 90th percentile

Weeks	Transverse colon diameter (mm) 10%	50%	90%	Weeks	Transverse colon diameter (mm) 10%	50%	90%
26	1	5	9	36	9	12	16
27	2	5	9	37	10	13	17
28	3	6	10	38	11	14	18
29	4	7	11	39	12	15	19
30	4	8	11	40	13	16	20
31	5	8	12	41	14	17	21
32	6	9	13	42	15	19	22
33	6	10	13				
34	7	11	14				
35	8	11	15				

Based on data from Goldstein, I. et al.: Ultrasound assessment of fetal intestinal development in the evaluation of gestational age. Obstet. Gynecol. 70 (1987) 682–686

Organ Biometry in the Urogenital System

Table 53.**27** Normal data for longitudinal and sagittal (anteroposterior) renal diameters (in mm, predicted values) as a function of gestational age (in completed weeks), lower limit = mean − 2 SD, upper limit = mean +2 SD

Weeks	Longitudinal renal diameter (mm)			Sagittal renal diameter (mm)			Weeks
	Mean −2 SD	**Mean**	Mean +2 SD	Mean −2 SD	**Mean**	Mean +2 SD	
22	–	–	–	8.9	**11.3**	13.7	22
23	–	–	–	9.3	**11.7**	14.1	23
24	22.0	**24.5**	27.0	9.7	**12.1**	14.5	24
25	22.6	**25.1**	27.7	10.2	**12.6**	15.0	25
26	23.3	**25.8**	28.3	10.7	**13.1**	15.5	26
27	24.0	**26.5**	29.0	11.3	**13.7**	16.1	27
28	24.7	**27.2**	29.8	11.9	**14.3**	16.7	28
29	25.5	**28.0**	30.5	12.5	**15.0**	17.4	29
30	26.3	**28.8**	31.3	13.2	**15.6**	18.0	30
31	27.1	**29.6**	32.1	14.0	**16.4**	18.8	31
32	27.9	**30.4**	32.9	14.8	**17.2**	19.6	32
33	28.8	**31.3**	33.8	15.6	**18.0**	20.4	33
34	29.6	**32.2**	34.7	16.5	**18.9**	21.3	34
35	30.5	**33.1**	35.6	17.5	**19.9**	22.3	35
36	31.5	**34.0**	36.5	18.5	**20.9**	23.3	36
37	32.4	**35.0**	35.0	19.5	**21.9**	24.4	37
38	33.4	**36.0**	38.5	20.7	**23.1**	25.5	38
39	34.5	**37.0**	39.5	21.8	**24.3**	26.7	39
40	35.5	**38.0**	40.5	23.1	**25.5**	27.9	40
41	36.6	**39.1**	41.6	–	–	–	41
42	37.7	**40.2**	42.7	–	–	–	42

Based on data from Bertagnoli, L. et al.: Quantitative characterization of the growth of the fetal kidney. J. Clin. Ultrasound 11 (1983) 349–356

■ *Organ Biometry in the Skeleton*

Table 53.**28**   Normal data for the orbital diameter (OD), inner interorbital distance (IID) and outer interorbital distance (OID) as a function of gestational age (in completed weeks), data in mm, lower limit 5th percentile, upper limit 95th percentile

Weeks	OD 5%	OD 50%	OD 95%	IID 5%	IID 50%	IID 95%	OID 5%	OID 50%	OID 95%	Weeks
12.0	1.3	3.1	5.0	3.5	5.8	8.2	5.8	10.7	15.5	12.0
12.5	2.1	3.9	5.8	4.2	6.6	8.9	8.7	13.5	18.3	12.5
13.0	2.7	4.5	6.4	4.8	7.1	9.5	10.6	15.4	20.3	13.0
13.5	3.2	5.1	6.9	5.3	7.6	10.0	12.3	17.1	21.9	13.5
14.0	3.7	5.6	7.4	5.7	8.1	10.4	13.8	18.6	23.5	14.0
14.5	4.2	6.0	7.9	6.1	8.5	10.8	15.2	20.1	24.9	14.5
15.0	4.7	6.5	8.3	6.5	8.9	11.2	16.6	21.4	26.2	15.0
15.5	5.1	6.9	8.7	6.9	9.3	11.6	17.8	22.7	27.5	15.5
16.0	5.5	7.3	9.2	7.3	9.6	12.0	19.0	23.9	28.7	16.0
16.5	5.9	7.7	9.6	7.6	10.0	12.3	20.2	25.0	29.9	16.5
17.0	6.3	8.1	9.9	8.0	10.3	12.7	21.3	26.2	31.0	17.0
17.5	6.7	8.5	10.3	8.3	10.7	13.0	22.4	27.2	32.1	17.5
18.0	7.0	8.9	10.7	8.6	11.0	13.3	23.5	28.3	33.1	18.0
18.5	7.4	9.2	11.0	9.0	11.3	13.7	24.5	29.3	34.1	18.5
19.0	7.7	9.5	11.4	9.3	11.6	14.0	25.5	30.3	35.1	19.0
19.5	8.1	9.9	11.7	9.6	11.9	14.3	26.5	31.3	36.1	19.5
20.0	8.4	10.2	12.0	9.9	12.2	14.6	27.4	32.2	37.1	20.0
20.5	8.7	10.5	12.3	10.2	12.5	14.9	28.3	33.2	38.0	20.5
21.0	9.0	10.8	12.6	10.5	12.8	15.2	29.2	34.1	38.9	21.0
21.5	9.3	11.1	12.9	10.8	13.1	15.5	30.1	34.9	39.8	21.5
22.0	9.6	11.4	13.2	11.1	13.4	15.8	31.0	35.8	40.6	22.0
22.5	9.9	11.7	13.5	11.3	13.7	16.0	31.8	36.7	41.5	22.5
23.0	10.2	12.0	13.8	11.6	14.0	16.3	32.7	37.5	42.3	23.0
23.5	10.4	12.2	14.1	11.9	14.2	16.6	33.5	38.3	43.1	23.5
24.0	10.7	12.5	14.3	12.2	14.5	16.9	34.2	39.1	43.9	24.0
24.5	10.9	12.8	14.6	12.4	14.8	17.1	35.0	39.8	44.7	24.5
25.0	11.2	13.0	14.8	12.7	15.0	17.4	35.8	40.6	45.4	25.0
25.5	11.4	13.3	15.1	13.0	15.3	17.6	36.5	41.3	46.2	25.5
26.0	11.7	13.5	15.3	13.2	15.6	17.9	37.2	42.1	46.9	26.0
26.5	11.9	13.7	15.5	13.5	15.8	18.2	37.9	42.8	47.6	26.5
27.0	12.1	13.9	15.8	13.7	16.1	18.4	38.6	43.5	48.3	27.0
27.5	12.3	14.2	16.0	14.0	16.3	18.7	39.3	44.1	49.0	27.5
28.0	12.6	14.4	16.2	14.2	16.6	18.9	40.0	44.8	49.6	28.0
28.5	12.8	14.6	16.4	14.5	16.8	19.1	40.6	45.5	50.3	28.5
29.0	13.0	14.8	16.6	14.7	17.0	19.4	41.3	46.1	50.9	29.0
29.5	13.2	15.0	16.8	14.9	17.3	19.6	41.9	46.7	51.5	29.5
30.0	13.3	15.2	17.0	15.2	17.5	19.9	42.5	47.3	52.1	30.0
30.5	13.5	15.3	17.2	15.4	17.7	20.1	43.1	47.9	52.7	30.5
31.0	13.7	15.5	17.3	15.6	18.0	20.3	43.7	48.5	53.3	31.0
31.5	13.9	15.7	17.5	15.9	18.2	20.5	44.3	49.1	53.9	31.5
32.0	14.0	15.9	17.7	16.1	18.4	20.8	44.8	49.6	54.4	32.0
32.5	14.2	16.0	17.8	16.3	18.7	21.0	45.3	50.2	55.0	32.5
33.0	14.3	16.2	18.0	16.5	18.9	21.2	45.9	50.7	55.5	33.0
33.5	14.5	16.3	18.1	16.7	19.1	21.4	46.4	51.2	56.0	33.5
34.0	14.6	16.4	18.3	17.0	19.3	21.7	46.9	51.7	56.5	34.0
34.5	14.8	16.6	18.4	17.2	19.5	21.9	47.4	52.2	57.0	34.5
35.0	14.9	16.7	18.5	17.4	19.7	22.1	47.8	52.6	57.5	35.0
35.5	15.0	16.8	18.6	17.6	19.9	22.3	48.3	53.1	57.9	35.5
36.0	15.1	16.9	18.8	17.8	20.1	22.5	48.7	53.5	58.4	36.0
36.5	15.2	17.0	18.9	18.0	20.3	22.7	49.1	54.0	58.8	36.5
37.0	15.3	17.1	19.0	18.2	20.5	22.9	49.5	54.4	59.2	37.0
37.5	15.4	17.2	19.1	18.4	20.7	23.1	49.9	54.8	59.6	37.5
38.0	15.5	17.3	19.2	18.6	20.9	23.3	50.3	55.1	59.9	38.0
38.5	15.6	17.4	19.2	18.8	21.1	23.5	50.7	55.5	60.3	38.5
39.0	15.7	17.5	19.3	19.0	21.3	23.7	51.0	55.8	60.6	39.0
39.5	15.7	17.5	19.4	19.2	21.5	23.8	51.3	56.1	60.9	39.5
40.0	15.8	17.6	19.4	19.3	21.7	24.0	51.6	56.4	61.2	40.0
40.5	15.8	17.6	19.5	19.5	21.9	24.2	51.8	56.7	61.5	40.5
41.0	15.9	17.7	19.5	19.7	22.0	24.4	52.1	56.9	61.7	41.0

After Merz, E., Wellek, S., Püttmann, S., Bahlmann, F., Weber, G.: Orbital diameter, inner and outer interorbital distances. A growth model for fetal orbital dimensions. Ultraschall in Med. 16 (1995) 12–17

Table 53.**29** Normal data for clavicle length as a function of gestational age (in completed weeks), data in mm, lower limit 5th percentile, upper limit 95th percentile

Weeks	Clavicle length (mm)		
	5%	50%	95%
15	11	16	21
16	12	17	22
17	13	18	23
18	14	19	24
19	15	20	25
20	16	21	26
21	17	22	27
22	18	23	28
23	19	24	29
24	20	25	30
25	21	26	31
26	22	27	32
27	23	28	33
28	24	29	34
29	25	30	35
30	26	31	36
31	27	32	37
32	28	33	38
33	29	34	39
34	30	35	40
35	31	36	41
36	32	37	42
37	33	38	43
38	34	39	44
39	35	40	45
40	36	41	46

Based on data from Yarkoni, S. et al.: Clavicle measurement: a new biometric parameter for fetal evaluation. J. Ultrasound Med. 4 (1985) 467–470

Table 53.**30** Normal data for rib length (mm) as a function of gestational age (in completed weeks), mean values and ± 2 SD from the mean

Weeks	Rib length (mm)		
	Mean −2 SD	Mean	Mean +2 SD
14	12.6	22.6	32.6
15	14.6	24.6	34.6
16	16.6	26.6	36.6
17	18.7	28.7	38.7
18	20.7	30.7	40.7
19	22.7	32.7	42.7
20	24.8	34.8	44.8
21	26.8	36.8	46.8
22	28.8	38.8	48.8
23	30.9	40.9	50.9
24	32.9	42.9	52.9
25	34.9	44.9	54.9
26	36.9	46.9	56.9
27	39.0	49.0	59.0
28	41.0	51.0	61.0
29	43.0	53.0	63.0
30	45.1	55.1	65.1
31	47.1	57.1	67.1
32	49.1	59.1	69.1
33	51.2	61.2	71.2
34	53.2	63.2	73.2
35	55.2	65.2	75.2
36	57.2	67.2	77.3
37	59.3	69.3	79.3
38	61.3	71.3	81.3
39	63.3	73.3	83.3
40	65.4	75.4	85.4

Based on data from Abuhamad, A.Z. et al.: Prenatal ultrasonographic fetal rib length measurement: correlation with gestational age. Ultrasound Obstet. Gynecol. 7 (1996) 193–196

Table 53.**31** Normal data for the total height of six vertebral bodies (five lumbar vertebrae + last thoracic vertebra) as a function of gestational age (in completed weeks), data in mm, mean values (x) with minimum and maximum

Weeks	Six vertebral bodies (five lumbar + last thoracic [mm])		
	Min.	Mean	Max.
13	11	13.0	14
14	13	14.5	16
15	14	16.8	22
16	16	19.7	25
17	18	21.8	25
18	19	22.6	29
19	22	25.6	31
20	23	27.7	33
21	22	28.5	33
22	27	31.2	35
23	29	33.3	38
24	30	35.5	41
25	35	37.8	44
26	35	49.7	45
27	37	41.4	48
28	40	44.0	49
29	41	45.0	52
30	42	47.4	54
31	43	48.1	54
32	45	50.0	56
33	46	51.6	56
34	48	53.2	57
35	49	54.5	61
36	52	56.5	61
37	52	57.8	63
38	52	58.4	63
39	54	60.1	65
40	57	61.8	66

Adapted from Issel, E.P.: Measurement of the height of six vertebral bodies as a new parameter in fetal biometry. Ultraschall Klin. Prax. 4 (1989) 21–15

Table 53.**32** Normal data for fetal foot length as a function of gestational age (in completed weeks), data in mm, normal data for the femur/foot ratio, lower limit 5th percentile, upper limit 95th percentile

Weeks	Foot length			Femur–foot ratio			Weeks
	5%	50%	95%	5%	50%	95%	
12.5	6	10	14	0.85	1.01	1.18	12.5
13.0	8	12	16	0.85	1.01	1.18	13.0
13.5	10	14	18	0.85	1.01	1.17	13.5
14.0	11	16	20	0.86	1.01	1.17	14.0
14.5	13	17	21	0.86	1.01	1.17	14.5
15.0	15	19	23	0.86	1.01	1.17	15.0
15.5	16	20	25	0.86	1.01	1.17	15.5
16.0	18	22	26	0.86	1.01	1.17	16.0
16.5	19	23	28	0.86	1.01	1.17	16.5
17.0	20	25	29	0.86	1.01	1.16	17.0
17.5	22	26	31	0.86	1.01	1.16	17.5
18.0	23	28	32	0.86	1.01	1.16	18.0
18.5	25	29	34	0.86	1.01	1.16	18.5
19.0	26	31	35	0.86	1.01	1.16	19.0
19.5	27	32	37	0.86	1.01	1.16	19.5
20.0	29	33	38	0.86	1.01	1.15	20.0
20.5	30	35	39	0.86	1.01	1.15	20.5
21.0	31	36	41	0.86	1.01	1.15	21.0
21.5	33	37	42	0.86	1.01	1.15	21.5
22.0	34	39	44	0.86	1.00	1.15	22.0
22.5	35	40	45	0.86	1.00	1.14	22.5
23.0	36	41	46	0.86	1.00	1.14	23.0
23.5	38	43	48	0.86	1.00	1.14	23.5
24.0	39	44	49	0.86	1.00	1.14	24.0
24.5	40	45	50	0.86	1.00	1.13	24.5
25.0	41	46	52	0.86	1.00	1.13	25.0
25.5	43	48	53	0.86	1.00	1.13	25.5
26.0	44	49	54	0.86	0.99	1.13	26.0
26.5	45	50	56	0.86	0.99	1.12	26.5
27.0	46	52	57	0.86	0.99	1.12	27.0
27.5	47	53	58	0.86	0.99	1.12	27.5
28.0	49	54	59	0.86	0.99	1.12	28.0
28.5	50	55	61	0.86	0.99	1.11	28.5
29.0	51	56	62	0.86	0.99	1.11	29.0
29.5	52	58	63	0.86	0.98	1.11	29.5
30.0	53	59	64	0.86	0.98	1.11	30.0
30.5	54	60	66	0.86	0.98	1.10	30.5
31.0	56	61	67	0.86	0.98	1.10	31.0
31.5	57	63	68	0.85	0.97	1.10	31.5
32.0	58	64	70	0.85	0.97	1.09	32.0
32.5	59	65	71	0.85	0.97	1.09	32.5
33.0	60	66	72	0.85	0.97	1.08	33.0
33.5	61	67	73	0.85	0.96	1.08	33.5
34.0	63	69	75	0.85	0.96	1.08	34.0
34.5	64	70	76	0.84	0.96	1.07	34.5
35.0	65	71	77	0.84	0.95	1.07	35.0
35.5	66	72	78	0.84	0.95	1.06	35.5
36.0	67	73	80	0.84	0.95	1.06	36.0
36.5	68	75	81	0.83	0.94	1.05	36.5
37.0	70	76	82	0.83	0.94	1.05	37.0
37.5	71	77	83	0.83	0.93	1.04	37.5
38.0	72	78	84	0.82	0.93	1.04	38.0
38.5	73	79	86	0.82	0.92	1.03	38.5
39.0	74	81	87	0.81	0.92	1.02	39.0
39.5	75	82	88	0.81	0.91	1.01	39.5
40.0	77	83	90	0.80	0.90	1.00	40.0
40.5	78	84	91	0.79	0.89	0.99	40.5
41.0	79	86	92	0.78	0.88	0.98	41.0

After Merz, E., Oberstein, A., Wellek, S.: Age-related reference ranges for fetal foot length. Ultraschall in Med. 21 (2000) 79–85

Umbilical Cord and Amniotic Fluid

Table 53.**33** Normal data for the umbilical cord diameter (outer-to-outer measurement) and the diameters of the umbilical artery and umbilical vein (inner-to-inner measurement) as a function of gestational age (in completed weeks), data in mm, lower limit 5th percentile, upper limit 95th percentile

Weeks	Umbilical cord			Umbilical artery			Umbilical vein			Weeks
	5%	50%	95%	5%	50%	95%	5%	50%	95%	
8	1.52	2.5	3.48							8
10	2.32	3.3	4.28							10
12	2.44	4.4	6.36							12
14	4.14	6.1	8.06	0.42	1.2	1.98	0.82	2.0	3.18	14
16	4.14	6.1	8.06	0.32	1.1	1.88	1.22	2.4	3.58	16
18	7.36	10.1	12.84	1.12	1.9	2.68	2.42	3.6	4.78	18
20	8.76	11.9	15.04	1.22	2.0	2.78	2.73	4.1	5.47	20
22	10.55	12.9	15.25	1.42	2.4	3.38	3.33	4.7	6.07	22
24	12.33	13.9	15.47	1.42	2.6	3.78	4.22	5.4	6.58	24
26	12.26	15.2	18.14	1.23	2.8	4.37	4.04	6.0	7.96	26
28	12.37	15.9	19.43	2.12	3.1	4.08	4.84	6.6	8.36	28
30	13.95	16.3	18.65	1.83	3.4	4.97	5.73	7.3	8.87	30
32	14.27	17.6	20.93	2.23	3.6	4.97	5.94	7.7	9.46	32
34	15.44	17.4	19.36	2.12	3.3	4.48	5.83	7.4	8.97	34
36	15.24	17.4	19.56	2.33	3.7	5.07	6.03	7.6	9.17	36
38	16.24	18.0	19.76	3.42	4.2	4.98	6.63	8.2	9.77	38
40	14.65	17.0	19.35	2.14	3.9	5.66	6.43	7.8	9.17	40

After Weismann, A., Jakobi, P., Bronsthein, M., Goldstein, L.: Sonographic measurement of the umbilical cord and vessels during normal pregnancies. J. Ultrasound Med. 13 (1994) 11–14

Table 53.**34** Normal data for the amniotic fluid index as a function of gestational age (in completed weeks), data in mm, lower limit 5th percentile, upper limit 95th percentile

Weeks	Amniotic fluid index		
	5%	50%	95%
16	79	121	185
17	83	127	194
18	87	133	202
19	90	137	207
20	93	141	212
21	95	143	214
22	97	145	216
23	98	146	218
24	98	147	219
25	97	147	221
26	97	147	223
27	95	146	226
28	94	146	228
29	92	145	231
30	90	145	234
31	88	144	238
32	86	144	242
33	83	143	245
34	81	142	248
35	79	140	249
36	77	138	249
37	75	135	244
38	73	132	239
39	72	127	226
40	71	123	214
41	70	116	194
42	69	110	175

After Moore, T.R. and Cayle, J.E.: The amniotic fluid index in normal human pregnancy. Am. J. Obstet. Gynecol. 162 (1990) 1168–1173

Gestational Age Estimation in the Second and Third Trimesters

Table 53.35 Estimation of gestational age based on the biparietal diameter (BPD, outer-to-outer measurement), gestational age in completed weeks + days (5%, 50%, 95%)

BPD (mm)	5%	50%	95%	BPD (mm)	5%	50%	95%
22	11 + 5	12 + 4	13 + 4	57	20 + 5	22 + 5	24 + 5
23	12 + 0	12 + 6	13 + 6	58	21 + 0	23 + 0	25 + 1
24	12 + 1	13 + 1	14 + 1	59	21 + 2	23 + 2	25 + 4
25	12 + 3	13 + 3	14 + 3	60	21 + 4	23 + 5	25 + 6
26	12 + 5	13 + 4	14 + 5	61	21 + 6	24 + 0	26 + 2
27	12 + 6	13 + 6	15 + 0	62	22 + 1	24 + 2	26 + 5
28	13 + 1	14 + 1	15 + 2	63	22 + 4	24 + 5	27 + 0
29	13 + 3	14 + 3	15 + 4	64	22 + 6	25 + 0	27 + 3
30	13 + 4	14 + 5	15 + 6	65	23 + 1	25 + 2	27 + 6
31	13 + 6	15 + 0	16 + 1	66	23 + 3	25 + 5	28 + 2
32	14 + 1	15 + 2	16 + 3	67	23 + 5	26 + 0	28 + 4
33	14 + 3	15 + 4	16 + 5	68	24 + 0	26 + 3	29 + 0
34	14 + 4	15 + 5	17 + 0	69	24 + 2	26 + 5	29 + 3
35	14 + 6	16 + 0	17 + 2	70	24 + 4	27 + 1	29 + 6
36	15 + 1	16 + 2	17 + 5	71	25 + 0	27 + 3	30 + 2
37	15 + 3	16 + 4	18 + 0	72	25 + 2	27 + 6	30 + 4
38	15 + 4	16 + 6	18 + 2	73	25 + 4	28 + 1	31 + 0
39	15 + 6	11 + 1	18 + 4	74	25 + 6	28 + 4	31 + 3
40	16 + 1	17 + 3	19 + 0	75	26 + 2	28 + 6	31 + 6
41	16 + 3	17 + 5	19 + 2	76	26 + 4	29 + 2	32 + 2
42	16 + 4	18 + 0	19 + 4	77	26 + 6	29 + 5	32 + 5
43	16 + 6	18 + 2	19 + 6	78	27 + 1	30 + 0	33 + 1
44	17 + 1	18 + 4	20 + 2	79	27 + 4	30 + 3	33 + 4
45	17 + 3	19 + 0	20 + 4	80	27 + 6	30 + 5	34 + 0
46	17 + 5	19 + 2	20 + 6	81	28 + 1	31 + 1	34 + 3
47	18 + 0	19 + 4	21 + 2	82	28 + 3	31 + 4	34 + 6
48	18 + 2	19 + 6	21 + 4	83	28 + 6	31 + 6	35 + 2
49	18 + 4	20 + 1	22 + 0	84	29 + 1	32 + 2	35 + 6
50	18 + 5	20 + 3	22 + 2	85	29 + 4	32 + 5	36 + 2
51	19 + 0	20 + 5	22 + 4	86	29 + 6	33 + 1	36 + 5
52	19 + 2	21 + 1	23 + 0	87	30 + 1	33 + 3	37 + 1
53	19 + 4	21 + 3	23 + 2	88	30 + 4	33 + 6	37 + 4
54	19 + 6	21 + 5	23 + 5	89	30 + 6	34 + 2	38 + 1
55	20 + 1	22 + 0	24 + 0	90	31 + 1	34 + 5	38 + 4
56	20 + 2	22 + 3	24 + 3	91	31 + 4	35 + 1	39 + 0

Adapted from data supplied by Altman, D.G. and Chitty, L.S.: New charts for ultrasound dating of pregnancy. Ultrasound Obstet. Gynecol. 10 (1997) 174–191

Table 53.36 Estimation of gestational age based on the head circumference (HC), gestational age in completed weeks + days (5%, 50%, 95%)

HC (mm)	5%	50%	95%	HC (mm)	5%	50%	95%
80	11 + 3	12 + 4	13 + 5	200	21 + 0	22 + 2	23 + 5
85	11 + 6	12 + 6	14 + 1	205	21 + 3	22 + 5	24 + 2
90	12 + 2	13 + 2	14 + 4	210	21 + 5	23 + 1	24 + 5
95	12 + 4	13 + 5	15 + 0	215	22 + 1	23 + 4	25 + 1
100	13 + 0	14 + 1	15 + 3	220	22 + 4	24 + 0	25 + 5
105	13 + 3	14 + 4	15 + 5	225	22 + 6	24 + 3	26 + 1
110	13 + 6	15 + 0	16 + 1	230	23 + 2	24 + 6	26 + 5
115	14 + 2	15 + 3	16 + 4	235	23 + 5	25 + 3	27 + 1
120	14 + 5	15 + 6	17 + 0	240	24 + 1	25 + 6	27 + 5
125	15 + 1	16 + 2	17 + 3	245	24 + 3	26 + 2	28 + 2
130	15 + 4	16 + 4	17 + 6	250	24 + 6	26 + 5	28 + 6
135	15 + 6	17 + 0	18 + 2	255	25 + 2	27 + 2	29 + 3
140	16 + 2	17 + 3	18 + 5	260	25 + 5	27 + 5	30 + 0
145	16 + 5	17 + 6	19 + 1	265	26 + 1	28 + 2	30 + 4
150	17 + 1	18 + 2	19 + 3	270	26 + 4	28 + 6	31 + 2
155	17 + 4	18 + 5	19 + 6	275	27 + 0	29 + 3	32 + 0
160	17 + 6	19 + 1	20 + 2	280	27 + 3	30 + 0	32 + 4
165	18 + 2	19 + 3	20 + 5	285	27 + 6	30 + 4	33 + 3
170	18 + 5	19 + 6	21 + 1	290	28 + 3	31 + 1	34 + 1
175	19 + 1	20 + 2	21 + 4	295	28 + 6	31 + 5	35 + 0
180	19 + 3	20 + 5	22 + 0	300	29 + 3	32 + 3	35 + 6
185	19 + 6	21 + 1	22 + 3	305	30 + 0	33 + 1	36 + 5
190	20 + 2	21 + 4	22 + 6	310	30 + 3	33 + 6	37 + 4
195	20 + 4	22 + 0	23 + 2	315	31 + 0	34 + 4	38 + 4
				320	31 + 5	35 + 3	39 + 4

Adapted from data supplied by Altman, D.G. and Chitty, L.S.: New charts for ultrasound dating of pregnancy. Ultrasound Obstet. Gynecol. 10 (1997) 174–191

Table 53.38 Estimation of gestational age based on length of the femoral shaft, gestational age in completed weeks + days (5%, 50%, 95%)

Femur (mm)	5%	50%	95%	Femur (mm)	5%	50%	95%
10	12 + 1	13 + 0	13 + 6	40	21 + 1	22 + 6	24 + 6
11	12 + 3	13 + 2	14 + 1	41	21 + 3	23 + 2	25 + 2
12	12 + 5	13 + 4	14 + 4	42	21 + 6	23 + 5	25 + 5
13	13 + 0	13 + 6	14 + 6	43	22 + 1	24 + 1	26 + 1
14	13 + 1	14 + 1	15 + 1	44	22 + 4	24 + 3	26 + 4
15	13 + 3	14 + 3	15 + 3	45	22 + 6	24 + 6	27 + 1
16	13 + 5	14 + 5	15 + 6	46	23 + 2	25 + 2	27 + 4
17	14 + 0	15 + 0	16 + 1	47	23 + 4	25 + 5	28 + 0
18	14 + 2	15 + 2	16 + 3	48	24 + 0	26 + 1	28 + 3
19	14 + 4	15 + 5	16 + 6	49	24 + 3	26 + 4	29 + 0
20	14 + 6	16 + 0	17 + 1	50	24 + 5	27 + 0	29 + 3
21	15 + 1	16 + 2	17 + 3	51	25 + 1	27 + 3	30 + 0
22	15 + 3	16 + 4	17 + 6	52	25 + 4	27 + 6	30 + 3
23	15 + 5	16 + 6	18 + 1	53	26 + 0	28 + 2	31 + 0
24	16 + 0	17 + 2	18 + 4	54	26 + 2	28 + 5	31 + 3
25	16 + 2	17 + 4	18 + 6	55	26 + 5	29 + 2	32 + 0
26	16 + 4	17 + 6	19 + 2	56	27 + 1	29 + 5	32 + 3
27	16 + 6	18 + 2	19 + 5	57	27 + 4	30 + 1	33 + 0
28	17 + 1	18 + 4	20 + 0	58	28 + 0	30 + 4	33 + 4
29	17 + 4	18 + 6	20 + 3	59	28 + 3	31 + 1	34 + 1
30	17 + 6	19 + 2	20 + 5	60	28 + 6	31 + 4	34 + 4
31	18 + 1	19 + 4	21 + 1	61	29 + 2	32 + 1	35 + 1
32	18 + 3	20 + 0	21 + 4	62	29 + 5	32 + 4	35 + 5
33	18 + 5	20 + 2	22 + 0	63	30 + 1	33 + 1	36 + 2
34	19 + 1	20 + 5	22 + 2	64	30 + 4	33 + 4	36 + 6
35	19 + 3	21 + 0	22 + 5	65	31 + 0	34 + 1	37 + 3
36	19 + 5	21 + 3	23 + 1	66	31 + 3	34 + 4	38 + 0
37	20 + 1	21 + 5	23 + 4	67	32 + 0	35 + 1	38 + 5
38	20 + 3	22 + 1	24 + 0				
39	20 + 5	22 + 4	24 + 3				

Adapted from data supplied by Altman, D.G. and Chitty, L.S.: New charts for ultrasound dating of pregnancy. Ultrasound Obstet. Gynecol. 10 (1997) 174–191

Table 53.37 Estimation of gestational age based on the transverse cerebellar diameter (TCD), gestational age in completed weeks + days (5%, 50%, 95%)

TCD (mm)	5%	50%	95%	TCD (mm)	5%	50%	95%
13	13 + 1	14 + 3	16 + 0	25	22 + 2	24 + 2	26 + 3
14	14 + 0	15 + 2	16 + 6	26	23 + 0	25 + 0	27 + 3
15	14 + 6	16 + 2	17 + 5	27	23 + 4	25 + 6	28 + 2
16	15 + 4	17 + 0	18 + 4	28	24 + 1	26 + 4	29 + 2
17	16 + 3	17 + 6	19 + 3	29	24 + 5	27 + 2	30 + 2
18	17 + 2	18 + 5	20 + 2	30	25 + 1	28 + 0	31 + 2
19	18 + 0	19 + 4	21 + 1	31	25 + 5	28 + 6	32 + 2
20	18 + 6	20 + 3	22 + 0	32	26 + 1	29 + 4	33 + 3
21	19 + 4	21 + 1	22 + 6	33	26 + 4	30 + 2	34 + 4
22	20 + 2	22 + 0	23 + 5	34	26 + 6	31 + 0	35 + 5
23	21 + 0	22 + 5	24 + 4	35	27 + 2	31 + 5	36 + 6
24	21 + 5	23 + 4	25 + 4	36	27 + 4	32 + 3	38 + 1

Adapted from data supplied by Altman, D.G. and Chitty, L.S.: New charts for ultrasound dating of pregnancy. Ultrasound Obstet. Gynecol. 10 (1997) 174–191

Weight Estimation

Table 53.**39** Estimation of fetal weight based on the biparietal diameter (BPD) and abdominal circumference (AC) using the formula W = −3200.40479 + 167.07186 × AC (cm) + 15.90391 × BPD^2 (cm); weight indicated in grams

AC (cm)	7.0	7.1	7.2	7.3	7.4	7.5	7.6	7.7	7.8	7.9	8.0	8.1	8.2	8.3	8.4	8.5	8.6	8.7	8.8	8.9	9.0	OFD (cm)
21.0	877	900	923	946	969	993	1017	1041	1066	1091	1116	1142	1167	1194	1220	1247	1274	1302	1330	1358	1386	21.0
21.1	893	916	938	961	985	1008	1032	1057	1081	1106	1132	1157	1183	1209	1236	1263	1290	1318	1345	1374	1402	21.1
21.2	909	931	954	977	1000	1024	1048	1072	1097	1122	1147	1173	1199	1225	1252	1279	1306	1333	1361	1389	1418	21.2
21.3	925	947	970	993	1016	1040	1064	1088	1113	1138	1163	1189	1215	1241	1267	1294	1321	1349	1377	1405	1433	21.3
21.4	940	963	985	1008	1032	1056	1080	1104	1129	1153	1179	1204	1230	1257	1283	1310	1337	1365	1393	1421	1449	21.4
21.5	956	978	1001	1024	1048	1071	1095	1120	1144	1169	1194	1220	1246	1272	1299	1326	1353	1380	1408	1436	1465	21.5
21.6	972	994	1017	1040	1063	1087	1111	1135	1160	1185	1210	1236	1262	1288	1315	1341	1369	1396	1424	1452	1481	21.6
21.7	987	1010	1033	1056	1079	1103	1127	1151	1176	1201	1226	1252	1277	1304	1330	1357	1384	1412	1440	1468	1496	21.7
21.8	1003	1025	1048	1071	1095	1118	1142	1167	1191	1216	1242	1267	1293	1319	1346	1373	1400	1428	1455	1484	1512	21.8
21.9	1019	1041	1064	1087	1110	1134	1158	1182	1207	1232	1257	1283	1309	1335	1362	1389	1416	1443	1471	1499	1528	21.9
22.0	1034	1057	1080	1103	1126	1150	1174	1198	1223	1248	1273	1299	1325	1351	1377	1404	1431	1459	1487	1515	1543	22.0
22.1	1050	1073	1095	1118	1142	1165	1189	1214	1238	1263	1289	1314	1340	1367	1393	1420	1447	1475	1502	1531	1559	22.1
22.2	1066	1088	1111	1134	1157	1181	1205	1230	1254	1279	1304	1330	1356	1382	1409	1436	1463	1490	1518	1546	1575	22.2
22.3	1082	1104	1127	1150	1173	1197	1221	1245	1270	1295	1320	1346	1372	1398	1424	1451	1479	1506	1534	1562	1591	22.3
22.4	1097	1120	1142	1166	1189	1213	1237	1261	1286	1311	1336	1361	1387	1414	1440	1467	1494	1522	1550	1578	1606	22.4
22.5	1113	1135	1158	1181	1205	1228	1252	1277	1301	1326	1352	1377	1403	1429	1456	1483	1510	1537	1565	1593	1622	22.5
22.6	1129	1151	1174	1197	1220	1244	1268	1292	1317	1342	1367	1393	1419	1445	1472	1498	1526	1553	1581	1609	1638	22.6
22.7	1144	1167	1190	1213	1236	1260	1284	1308	1333	1358	1383	1409	1435	1461	1487	1514	1541	1569	1597	1625	1653	22.7
22.8	1160	1183	1205	1228	1252	1275	1299	1324	1348	1373	1399	1424	1450	1476	1503	1530	1557	1585	1612	1641	1669	22.8
22.9	1176	1198	1221	1244	1267	1291	1315	1339	1364	1389	1414	1440	1466	1492	1519	1546	1573	1600	1628	1656	1685	22.9
23.0	1192	1214	1237	1260	1283	1307	1331	1355	1380	1405	1430	1456	1482	1508	1534	1561	1589	1616	1644	1672	1700	23.0
23.1	1207	1230	1252	1275	1299	1323	1347	1371	1396	1421	1446	1471	1497	1524	1550	1577	1604	1632	1660	1688	1716	23.1
23.2	1223	1245	1268	1291	1315	1338	1362	1387	1411	1436	1462	1487	1513	1539	1566	1593	1620	1647	1675	1703	1732	23.2
23.3	1239	1261	1284	1307	1330	1354	1378	1402	1427	1452	1477	1503	1529	1555	1582	1608	1636	1663	1691	1719	1748	23.3
23.4	1254	1277	1300	1323	1346	1370	1394	1418	1443	1468	1493	1519	1544	1571	1597	1624	1651	1679	1707	1735	1763	23.4
23.5	1270	1293	1315	1338	1362	1385	1409	1434	1458	1483	1509	1534	1560	1586	1613	1640	1667	1695	1722	1751	1779	23.5
23.6	1286	1308	1331	1354	1377	1401	1425	1449	1474	1499	1524	1550	1576	1602	1629	1656	1683	1710	1738	1766	1795	23.6
23.7	1301	1324	1347	1370	1393	1417	1441	1465	1490	1515	1540	1566	1592	1618	1644	1671	1698	1726	1754	1782	1810	23.7
23.8	1317	1340	1362	1385	1409	1433	1457	1481	1505	1530	1556	1581	1607	1634	1660	1687	1714	1742	1770	1798	1826	23.8
23.9	1333	1355	1378	1401	1425	1448	1472	1497	1521	1546	1571	1597	1623	1649	1676	1703	1730	1757	1785	1813	1842	23.9
24.0	1349	1371	1394	1417	1440	1464	1488	1512	1537	1562	1587	1613	1639	1665	1691	1718	1746	1773	1801	1829	1858	24.0
24.1	1364	1387	1409	1433	1456	1480	1504	1528	1553	1578	1603	1628	1654	1681	1707	1734	1761	1789	1817	1845	1873	24.1
24.2	1380	1402	1425	1448	1472	1495	1519	1544	1568	1593	1619	1644	1670	1696	1723	1750	1777	1805	1832	1860	1889	24.2
24.3	1396	1418	1441	1464	1487	1511	1535	1559	1584	1609	1634	1660	1686	1712	1739	1765	1793	1820	1848	1876	1905	24.3
24.4	1411	1434	1457	1480	1503	1527	1551	1575	1600	1625	1650	1676	1702	1728	1754	1781	1808	1836	1864	1892	1920	24.4
24.5	1427	1450	1472	1495	1519	1542	1566	1591	1615	1640	1666	1691	1717	1743	1770	1797	1824	1852	1879	1908	1936	24.5
24.6	1443	1465	1488	1511	1534	1558	1582	1607	1631	1656	1681	1707	1733	1759	1786	1813	1840	1867	1895	1923	1952	24.6
24.7	1459	1481	1504	1527	1550	1574	1598	1622	1647	1672	1697	1723	1749	1775	1801	1828	1856	1883	1911	1939	1967	24.7
24.8	1474	1497	1519	1542	1566	1590	1614	1638	1663	1688	1713	1738	1764	1791	1817	1844	1871	1899	1927	1955	1983	24.8
24.9	1490	1512	1535	1558	1582	1605	1629	1654	1678	1703	1729	1754	1780	1806	1833	1860	1887	1914	1942	1970	1999	24.9
25.0	1506	1528	1551	1574	1597	1621	1645	1669	1694	1719	1744	1770	1796	1822	1849	1875	1903	1930	1958	1986	2015	25.0
25.1	1152	1544	1567	1590	1613	1637	1661	1685	1710	1735	1760	1786	1811	1838	1864	1891	1918	1946	1974	2002	2030	25.1
25.2	1537	1560	1582	1605	1629	1652	1676	1701	1725	1750	1776	1801	1827	1853	1880	1907	1934	1962	1989	2018	2046	25.2
25.3	1553	1575	1598	1621	1644	1668	1692	1716	1741	1766	1791	1817	1843	1869	1896	1923	1950	1977	2005	2033	2062	25.3
25.4	1569	1591	1614	1637	1660	1684	1708	1732	1757	1782	1807	1833	1859	1885	1911	1938	1965	1993	2021	2049	2077	25.4
25.5	1584	1607	1629	1652	1676	1700	1724	1748	1773	1797	1823	1848	1874	1901	1927	1954	1981	2009	2037	2065	2093	25.5
25.6	1600	1622	1645	1668	1692	1715	1739	1764	1788	1813	1838	1864	1890	1916	1943	1970	1997	2024	2052	2080	2109	25.6
25.7	1616	1638	1661	1684	1707	1731	1755	1779	1804	1829	1854	1880	1906	1932	1959	1985	2013	2040	2068	2096	2125	25.7
25.8	1631	1654	1677	1700	1723	1747	1771	1795	1820	1845	1870	1896	1921	1948	1974	2001	2028	2056	2084	2112	2140	25.8
25.9	1647	1669	1692	1715	1739	1762	1786	1811	1835	1860	1886	1911	1937	1963	1990	2017	2044	2072	2099	2128	2156	25.9
26.0	1663	1685	1708	1731	1754	1778	1802	1826	1851	1876	1901	1927	1953	1979	2006	2033	2060	2087	2115	2143	2172	26.0
26.1	1678	1701	1724	1747	1770	1794	1818	1842	1867	1892	1917	1943	1969	1995	2021	2048	2075	2103	2131	2159	2187	26.1
26.2	1694	1717	1739	1762	1786	1809	1833	1858	1882	1907	1933	1958	1984	2010	2037	2064	2091	2119	2146	2175	2203	26.2
26.3	1710	1732	1755	1778	1801	1825	1849	1874	1898	1923	1948	1974	2000	2026	2053	2080	2107	2134	2162	2190	2219	26.3
26.4	1726	1748	1771	1794	1817	1841	1865	1889	1914	1939	1964	1990	2016	2042	2068	2095	2123	2150	2178	2206	2235	26.4
26.5	1741	1764	1786	1810	1833	1857	1881	1905	1930	1955	1980	2005	2031	2058	2084	2111	2138	2166	2194	2222	2250	26.5
26.6	1757	1779	1802	1825	1849	1872	1896	1921	1945	1970	1996	2021	2047	2073	2100	2127	2154	2181	2209	2237	2266	26.6
26.7	1773	1795	1818	1841	1864	1888	1912	1936	1961	1986	2011	2037	2063	2089	2116	2142	2170	2197	2225	2253	2282	26.7
26.8	1788	1811	1834	1857	1880	1904	1928	1952	1977	2002	2027	2053	2078	2105	2131	2158	2185	2213	2241	2269	2297	26.8
26.9	1804	1827	1849	1872	1896	1919	1943	1968	1992	2017	2043	2068	2094	2120	2147	2174	2201	2229	2256	2285	2313	26.9

→

Table 53.**39** (continued)   Estimation of fetal weight based on the biparietal diameter (BPD) and abdominal circumference (AC)

AC (cm)	7.0	7.1	7.2	7.3	7.4	7.5	7.6	7.7	7.8	7.9	8.0	8.1	8.2	8.3	8.4	8.5	8.6	8.7	8.8	8.9	9.0	OFD (cm)
27.0	1820	1842	1865	1888	1911	1935	1959	1983	2008	2033	2058	2084	2110	2136	2163	2190	2217	2244	2272	2300	2329	27.0
27.1	1836	1858	1881	1904	1927	1951	1975	1999	2024	2049	2074	2100	2126	2152	2178	2205	2232	2260	2288	2316	2344	27.1
27.2	1851	1874	1896	1919	1943	1967	1991	2015	2040	2065	2090	2115	2141	2168	2194	2221	2248	2276	2304	2332	2360	27.2
27.3	1867	1889	1912	1935	1959	1982	2006	2031	2055	2080	2106	2131	2157	2183	2210	2237	2264	2291	2319	2347	2376	27.3
27.4	1883	1905	1928	1951	1974	1998	2022	2046	2071	2096	2121	2147	2173	2199	2226	2252	2280	2307	2335	2363	2392	27.4
27.5	1898	1921	1944	1967	1990	2014	2038	2062	2087	2112	2137	2163	2188	2215	2241	2268	2295	2323	2351	2379	2407	27.5
27.6	1914	1936	1959	1982	2006	2029	2053	2078	2102	2127	2153	2178	2204	2230	2257	2284	2311	2339	2366	2395	2423	27.6
27.7	1930	1952	1975	1998	2021	2045	2069	2093	2118	2143	2168	2194	2220	2246	2273	2300	2327	2354	2382	2410	2439	27.7
27.8	1945	1968	1991	2014	2037	2061	2085	2109	2134	2159	2184	2210	2236	2262	2288	2315	2342	2370	2398	2426	2454	27.8
27.9	1961	1984	2006	2029	2053	2076	2101	2125	2149	2174	2200	2225	2251	2278	2304	2331	2358	2386	2413	2442	2470	27.9
28.0	1977	1999	2022	2045	2069	2092	2116	2141	2165	2190	2215	2241	2267	2293	2320	2347	2374	2401	2429	2457	2486	28.0
28.1	1993	2015	2038	2061	2084	2108	2132	2156	2181	2206	2231	2257	2283	2309	2335	2362	2390	2417	2445	2473	2502	28.1
28.2	2008	2031	2053	2077	2100	2124	2148	2172	2197	2222	2247	2272	2298	2325	2351	2378	2405	2433	2461	2489	2517	28.2
28.3	2024	2046	2069	2092	2116	2139	2163	2188	2212	2237	2263	2288	2314	2340	2367	2394	2421	2448	2476	2504	2533	28.3
28.4	2040	2062	2085	2108	2131	2155	2179	2203	2228	2253	2278	2304	2330	2356	2383	2409	2437	2464	2492	2520	2549	28.4
28.5	2055	2078	2101	2124	2147	2171	2195	2219	2244	2269	2294	2320	2346	2372	2398	2425	2452	2480	2508	2536	2564	28.5
28.6	2071	2094	2116	2139	2163	2186	2210	2235	2259	2284	2310	2335	2361	2387	2414	2441	2468	2496	2523	2552	2580	28.6
28.7	2087	2109	2132	2155	2178	2202	2226	2251	2275	2300	2325	2351	2377	2403	2430	2457	2484	2511	2539	2567	2596	28.7
28.8	2103	2125	2148	2171	2194	2218	2242	2266	2291	2316	2341	2367	2393	2419	2445	2472	2500	2527	2555	2583	2611	28.8
28.9	2118	2141	2163	2186	2210	2234	2258	2282	2307	2332	2357	2382	2408	2435	2461	2488	2515	2543	2571	2599	2627	28.9
29.0	2134	2156	2179	2202	2226	2249	2273	2298	2322	2347	2373	2398	2424	2450	2477	2504	2531	2558	2586	2614	2643	29.0
29.1	2150	2172	2195	2218	2241	2265	2289	2313	2338	2363	2388	2414	2440	2466	2493	2519	2547	2574	2602	2630	2659	29.1
29.2	2165	2188	2211	2234	2257	2281	2305	2329	2354	2379	2404	2430	2455	2482	2508	2535	2562	2590	2618	2646	2674	29.2
29.3	2181	2204	2226	2249	2273	2296	2320	2345	2369	2394	2420	2445	2471	2497	2524	2551	2578	2606	2633	2662	2690	29.3
29.4	2197	2219	2242	2265	2288	2312	2336	2360	2385	2410	2435	2461	2487	2513	2540	2567	2594	2621	2649	2677	2706	29.4
29.5	2213	2235	2258	2281	2304	2328	2352	2376	2401	2426	2451	2477	2503	2529	2555	2582	2609	2637	2665	2693	2721	29.5
29.6	2228	2251	2273	2296	2320	2344	2368	2392	2417	2441	2467	2492	2518	2545	2571	2598	2625	2653	2681	2709	2737	29.6
29.7	2244	2266	2289	2312	2336	2359	2383	2408	2432	2457	2482	2508	2534	2560	2587	2614	2641	2668	2696	2724	2753	29.7
29.8	2260	2282	2305	2328	2351	2375	2399	2423	2448	2473	2498	2524	2550	2576	2603	2629	2657	2684	2712	2740	2769	29.8
29.9	2275	2298	2321	2344	2367	2391	2415	2439	2464	2489	2514	2539	2565	2592	2618	2645	2672	2700	2728	2756	2784	29.9
30.0	2291	2313	2336	2359	2383	2406	2430	2455	2479	2504	2530	2555	2581	2607	2634	2661	2688	2716	2743	2771	2800	30.0
30.1	2307	2329	2352	2375	2398	2422	2446	2470	2495	2520	2545	2571	2597	2623	2650	2677	2704	2731	2759	2787	2816	30.1
30.2	2322	2345	2368	2391	2414	2438	2462	2486	2511	2536	2561	2587	2613	2639	2665	2692	2719	2747	2775	2803	2831	30.2
30.3	2338	2361	2383	2406	2430	2453	2477	2502	2526	2551	2577	2602	2628	2654	2681	2708	2735	2763	2790	2819	2847	30.3
30.4	2354	2376	2399	2422	2445	2469	2493	2518	2542	2567	2592	2618	2644	2670	2697	2724	2751	2778	2806	2834	2863	30.4
30.5	2370	2392	2415	2438	2461	2485	2509	2533	2558	2583	2608	2634	2660	2686	2712	2739	2767	2794	2822	2850	2879	30.5
30.6	2385	2408	2430	2454	2477	2501	2525	2549	2574	2599	2624	2649	2675	2702	2728	2755	2782	2810	2838	2866	2894	30.6
30.7	2401	2423	2446	2469	2493	2516	2540	2565	2589	2614	2640	2665	2691	2717	2744	2771	2798	2825	2853	2881	2910	30.7
30.8	2417	2439	2462	2485	2508	2532	2556	2580	2605	2630	2655	2681	2707	2733	2760	2786	2814	2841	2869	2897	2926	30.8
30.9	2432	2455	2478	2501	2524	2548	2572	2596	2621	2646	2671	2697	2722	2749	2775	2802	2829	2857	2885	2913	2941	30.9
31.0	2448	2471	2493	2516	2540	2563	2587	2612	2636	2661	2687	2712	2738	2764	2791	2818	2845	2873	2900	2929	2957	31.0
31.1	2464	2486	2509	2532	2555	2579	2603	2627	2652	2677	2702	2728	2754	2780	2807	2834	2861	2888	2916	2944	2973	31.1
31.2	2480	2502	2525	2548	2571	2595	2619	2643	2668	2693	2718	2744	2770	2796	2822	2849	2876	2904	2932	2960	2988	31.2
31.3	2495	2518	2540	2563	2587	2611	2635	2659	2684	2709	2734	2759	2785	2812	2838	2865	2892	2920	2948	2976	3004	31.3
31.4	2511	2533	2556	2579	2603	2626	2650	2675	2699	2724	2750	2775	2801	2827	2854	2881	2908	2935	2963	2991	3020	31.4
31.5	2527	2549	2572	2595	2618	2642	2666	2690	2715	2740	2765	2791	2817	2843	2870	2896	2924	2951	2979	3007	3036	31.5
31.6	2542	2565	2588	2611	2634	2658	2682	2706	2731	2756	2781	2807	2832	2859	2885	2912	2939	2967	2995	3023	3051	31.6
31.7	2558	2580	2603	2626	2650	2673	2697	2722	2746	2771	2797	2822	2848	2874	2901	2928	2955	2983	3010	3039	3067	31.7
31.8	2574	2596	2619	2642	2665	2689	2713	2737	2762	2787	2812	2838	2864	2890	2917	2944	2971	2998	3026	3054	3083	31.8
31.9	2589	2612	2635	2658	2681	2705	2729	2753	2778	2803	2828	2854	2880	2906	2932	2959	2986	3014	3042	3070	3098	31.9
32.0	2605	2628	2650	2673	2697	2720	2745	2769	2793	2818	2844	2869	2895	2922	2948	2975	3002	3030	3057	3086	3114	32.0
32.1	2621	2643	2666	2689	2713	2736	2760	2785	2809	2834	2859	2885	2911	2937	2964	2991	3018	3045	3073	3101	3130	32.1
32.2	2637	2659	2682	2705	2728	2752	2776	2800	2825	2850	2875	2901	2927	2953	2979	3006	3034	3061	3089	3117	3146	32.2
32.3	2652	2675	2697	2721	2744	2768	2792	2816	2841	2866	2891	2916	2942	2969	2995	3022	3049	3077	3105	3133	3161	32.3
32.4	2668	2690	2713	2736	2760	2783	2807	2832	2856	2881	2907	2932	2958	2984	3011	3038	3065	3092	3120	3148	3177	32.4
32.5	2684	2706	2729	2752	2775	2799	2823	2847	2872	2897	2922	2948	2974	3000	3027	3053	3081	3108	3136	3164	3193	32.5
32.6	2699	2722	2745	2768	2791	2815	2839	2863	2888	2913	2938	2964	2990	3016	3042	3069	3096	3124	3152	3180	3208	32.6
32.7	2715	2738	2760	2783	2807	2830	2854	2879	2903	2928	2954	2979	3005	3031	3058	3085	3112	3140	3167	3196	3224	32.7
32.8	2731	2753	2776	2799	2822	2846	2870	2894	2919	2944	2969	2995	3021	3047	3074	3101	3128	3155	3183	3211	3240	32.8
32.9	2747	2769	2792	2815	2838	2862	2886	2910	2935	2960	2985	3011	3037	3063	3089	3116	3144	3171	3199	3227	3255	32.9
33.0	2762	2785	2807	2830	2854	2878	2902	2926	2951	2976	3001	3026	3052	3079	3105	3132	3159	3187	3215	3243	3271	33.0
33.1	2778	2800	2823	2846	2870	2893	2917	2942	2966	2991	3017	3042	3068	3094	3121	3148	3175	3202	3230	3258	3287	33.1
33.2	2794	2816	2839	2862	2885	2909	2933	2957	2982	3007	3032	3058	3084	3110	3137	3163	3191	3218	3246	3274	3303	33.2
33.3	2809	2832	2855	2878	2901	2925	2949	2973	2998	3023	3048	3074	3099	3126	3152	3179	3206	3234	3262	3290	3318	33.3
33.4	2825	2848	2870	2893	2917	2940	2964	2989	3013	3038	3064	3089	3115	3141	3168	3195	3222	3250	3277	3306	3334	33.4
33.5	2841	2863	2886	2909	2932	2956	2980	3004	3029	3054	3079	3105	3131	3157	3184	3211	3238	3265	3293	3321	3350	33.5
33.6	2857	2879	2902	2925	2948	2972	2996	3020	3045	3070	3095	3121	3147	3173	3199	3226	3253	3281	3309	3337	3365	33.6
33.7	2872	2895	2917	2940	2964	2988	3012	3036	3061	3085	3111	3136	3162	3189	3215	3242	3269	3297	3325	3353	3381	33.7
33.8	2888	2910	2933	2956	2980	3003	3027	3052	3076	3101	3126	3152	3178	3204	3231	3258	3285	3312	3340	3368	3397	33.8
33.9	2904	2926	2949	2972	2995	3019	3043	3067	3092	3117	3142	3168	3194	3220	3247	3273	3301	3328	3356	3384	3413	33.9

→

Table 53.**39** (continued)   Estimation of fetal weight based on the biparietal diameter (BPD) and abdominal circumference (AC)

AC (cm)	BPD (cm) 7.0	7.1	7.2	7.3	7.4	7.5	7.6	7.7	7.8	7.9	8.0	8.1	8.2	8.3	8.4	8.5	8.6	8.7	8.8	8.9	9.0	OFD (cm)
34.0	2919	2942	2964	2988	3011	3035	3059	3083	3108	3133	3158	3183	3209	3236	3262	3289	3316	3344	3372	3400	3428	34.0
34.1	2935	2957	2980	3003	3027	3050	3074	3099	3123	3148	3174	3199	3225	3251	3278	3305	3332	3360	3387	3415	3444	34.1
34.2	2951	2973	2996	3019	3042	3066	3090	3114	3139	3164	3189	3215	3241	3267	3294	3321	3348	3375	3403	3431	3460	34.2
34.3	2966	2989	3012	3035	3058	3082	3106	3130	3155	3180	3205	3231	3257	3283	3309	3336	3363	3391	3419	3447	3475	34.3
34.4	2982	3005	3027	3050	3074	3097	3121	3146	3170	3195	3221	3246	3272	3298	3325	3352	3379	3407	3434	3463	3491	34.4
34.5	2998	3020	3043	3066	3089	3113	3137	3162	3186	3211	3236	3262	3288	3314	3341	3368	3395	3422	3450	3478	3507	34.5
34.6	3014	3036	3059	3082	3105	3129	3153	3177	3202	3227	3252	3278	3304	3330	3356	3383	3411	3438	3466	3494	3522	34.6
34.7	3029	3052	3074	3098	3121	3145	3169	3193	3218	3243	3268	3293	3319	3346	3372	3399	3426	3454	3482	3510	3538	34.7
34.8	3045	3067	3090	3113	3137	3160	3184	3209	3233	3258	3284	3309	3335	3361	3388	3415	3442	3469	3497	3525	3554	34.8
34.9	3061	3083	3106	3129	3152	3176	3200	3224	3249	3274	3299	3325	3351	3377	3404	3430	3458	3485	3513	3541	3570	34.9
35.0	3076	3099	3122	3145	3168	3192	3216	3240	3265	3290	3315	3341	3366	3393	3419	3446	3473	3501	3529	3557	3585	35.0
35.1	3092	3115	3137	3160	3184	3207	3231	3256	3280	3305	3331	3356	3382	3408	3435	3462	3489	3517	3544	3573	3601	35.1
35.2	3108	3130	3153	3176	3199	3223	3247	3271	3296	3321	3346	3372	3398	3424	3451	3478	3505	3532	3560	3588	3617	35.2
35.3	3124	3146	3169	3192	3215	3239	3263	3287	3312	3337	3362	3388	3414	3440	3466	3493	3520	3548	3576	3604	3632	35.3
35.4	3139	3162	3184	3207	3231	3255	3279	3303	3328	3353	3378	3403	3429	3456	3482	3509	3536	3564	3592	3620	3648	35.4
35.5	3155	3177	3200	3223	3247	3270	3294	3319	3343	3368	3393	3419	3445	3471	3498	3525	3552	3579	3607	3635	3664	35.5
35.6	3171	3193	3216	3239	3262	3286	3310	3334	3359	3384	3409	3435	3461	3487	3514	3540	3568	3595	3623	3651	3680	35.6
35.7	3186	3209	3232	3255	3278	3302	3326	3350	3375	3400	3425	3451	3476	3503	3529	3556	3583	3611	3639	3667	3695	35.7
35.8	3202	3224	3247	3270	3294	3317	3341	3366	3390	3415	3441	3466	3492	3518	3545	3572	3599	3627	3654	3683	3711	35.8
35.9	3218	3240	3263	3286	3309	3333	3357	3381	3406	3431	3456	3482	3508	3534	3561	3588	3615	3642	3670	3698	3727	35.9
36.0	3233	3256	3279	3302	3325	3349	3373	3397	3422	3447	3472	3498	3524	3550	3576	3603	3630	3658	3686	3714	3742	36.0
36.1	3249	3272	3294	3317	3341	3364	3388	3413	3437	3462	3488	3513	3539	3566	3592	3619	3646	3674	3701	3730	3758	36.1
36.2	3265	3287	3310	3333	3356	3380	3404	3429	3453	3478	3503	3529	3555	3581	3608	3635	3662	3689	3717	3745	3774	36.2
36.3	3281	3303	3326	3349	3372	3396	3420	3444	3469	3494	3519	3545	3571	3597	3623	3650	3678	3705	3733	3761	3790	36.3
36.4	3296	3319	3341	3365	3388	3412	3436	3460	3485	3510	3535	3560	3586	3613	3639	3666	3693	3721	3749	3777	3805	36.4
36.5	3312	3334	3357	3380	3404	3427	3451	3476	3500	3525	3551	3576	3602	3628	3655	3682	3709	3736	3764	3792	3821	36.5
36.6	3328	3350	3373	3396	3419	3443	3467	3491	3516	3541	3566	3592	3618	3644	3671	3697	3725	3752	3780	3808	3837	36.6
36.7	3343	3366	3389	3412	3435	3459	3483	3507	3532	3557	3582	3608	3634	3660	3686	3713	3740	3768	3796	3824	3852	36.7
36.8	3359	3382	3404	3427	3451	3474	3498	3523	3547	3572	3598	3623	3649	3675	3702	3729	3756	3784	3811	3840	3868	36.8
36.9	3375	3397	3420	3443	3466	3490	3514	3538	3563	3588	3613	3639	3665	3691	3718	3745	3772	3799	3827	3855	3884	36.9
37.0	3391	3413	3436	3459	3482	3506	3530	3554	3579	3604	3629	3655	3681	3707	3733	3760	3788	3815	3843	3871	3899	37.0

$\rightarrow$

Table 53.**39** (continued)   Estimation of fetal weight based on the biparietal diameter (BPD) and abdominal circumference (AC)

AC (cm)	BPD (cm) 9.0	9.1	9.2	9.3	9.4	9.5	9.6	9.7	9.8	9.9	10.0	10.1	10.2	10.3	10.4	10.5	10.6	10.7	10.8	10.9	11.0	OFD (cm)
21.0	1386	1415	1444	1474	1503	1533	1564	1595	1626	1657	1688	1720	1753	1785	1818	1852	1885	1919	1953	1988	2022	21.0
21.1	1402	1431	1460	1489	1519	1549	1580	1610	1641	1673	1704	1736	1768	1801	1834	1867	1901	1935	1969	2003	2038	21.1
21.2	1418	1447	1476	1505	1535	1565	1595	1626	1657	1688	1720	1752	1784	1817	1850	1883	1916	1950	1985	2019	2054	21.2
21.3	1433	1462	1491	1521	1550	1581	1611	1642	1673	1704	1736	1768	1800	1832	1865	1899	1932	1966	2000	2035	2070	21.3
21.4	1449	1478	1507	1536	1566	1596	1627	1657	1688	1720	1751	1783	1816	1848	1881	1914	1948	1982	2016	2050	2085	21.4
21.5	1465	1494	1523	1552	1582	1612	1642	1673	1704	1735	1767	1799	1831	1864	1897	1930	1964	1997	2032	2066	2101	21.5
21.6	1481	1509	1538	1568	1598	1628	1658	1689	1720	1751	1783	1815	1847	1880	1913	1946	1979	2013	2047	2082	2117	21.6
21.7	1496	1525	1554	1584	1613	1643	1674	1704	1735	1767	1798	1830	1863	1895	1928	1961	1995	2029	2063	2098	2132	21.7
21.8	1512	1541	1570	1599	1629	1659	1689	1720	1751	1783	1814	1846	1878	1911	1944	1977	2011	2045	2079	2113	2148	21.8
21.9	1528	1556	1586	1615	1645	1675	1705	1736	1767	1798	1830	1862	1894	1927	1960	1993	2026	2060	2095	2129	2164	21.9
22.0	1543	1572	1601	1631	1660	1691	1721	1752	1783	1814	1846	1878	1910	1942	1975	2009	2042	2076	2110	2145	2180	22.0
22.1	1559	1588	1617	1646	1676	1706	1737	1767	1798	1830	1861	1893	1926	1958	1991	2024	2058	2092	2126	2160	2195	22.1
22.2	1575	1604	1633	1662	1692	1722	1752	1783	1814	1845	1877	1909	1941	1974	2007	2040	2074	2107	2142	2176	2211	22.2
22.3	1591	1619	1648	1678	1708	1738	1768	1799	1830	1861	1893	1925	1957	1990	2022	2056	2089	2123	2157	2192	2227	22.3
22.4	1606	1635	1664	1694	1723	1753	1784	1814	1845	1877	1908	1940	1973	2005	2038	2071	2105	2139	2173	2208	2242	22.4
22.5	1622	1651	1680	1709	1739	1769	1799	1830	1861	1892	1924	1956	1988	2021	2054	2087	2121	2155	2189	2223	2258	22.5
22.6	1638	1666	1696	1725	1755	1785	1815	1846	1877	1908	1940	1972	2004	2037	2070	2103	2136	2170	2204	2239	2274	22.6
22.7	1653	1682	1711	1741	1770	1800	1831	1862	1893	1924	1956	1987	2020	2052	2085	2119	2152	2186	2220	2255	2289	22.7
22.8	1669	1698	1727	1756	1786	1816	1847	1877	1908	1940	1971	2003	2035	2068	2101	2134	2168	2202	2236	2270	2305	22.8
22.9	1685	1714	1743	1772	1802	1832	1862	1893	1924	1955	1987	2019	2051	2084	2117	2150	2184	2217	2252	2286	2321	22.9
23.0	1700	1729	1758	1788	1818	1848	1878	1909	1940	1971	2003	2035	2067	2099	2132	2166	2199	2233	2267	2302	2337	23.0
23.1	1716	1745	1774	1803	1833	1863	1894	1924	1955	1987	2018	2050	2083	2115	2148	2181	2215	2249	2283	2317	2352	23.1
23.2	1732	1761	1790	1819	1849	1879	1909	1940	1971	2002	2034	2066	2098	2131	2164	2197	2231	2265	2299	2333	2368	23.2
23.3	1748	1776	1805	1835	1865	1895	1925	1956	1987	2018	2050	2082	2114	2147	2180	2213	2246	2280	2314	2349	2384	23.3
23.4	1763	1792	1821	1851	1880	1910	1941	1971	2002	2034	2065	2097	2130	2162	2195	2228	2262	2296	2330	2365	2399	23.4
23.5	1779	1808	1837	1866	1896	1926	1956	1987	2018	2050	2081	2113	2145	2178	2211	2244	2278	2312	2346	2380	2415	23.5
23.6	1795	1823	1853	1882	1912	1942	1972	2003	2034	2065	2097	2129	2161	2194	2227	2260	2293	2327	2362	2396	2431	23.6
23.7	1810	1839	1868	1898	1927	1958	1988	2019	2050	2081	2113	2145	2177	2209	2242	2276	2309	2343	2377	2412	2447	23.7
23.8	1826	1855	1884	1913	1943	1973	2004	2034	2065	2097	2128	2160	2193	2225	2258	2291	2325	2359	2393	2427	2462	23.8
23.9	1842	1871	1900	1929	1959	1989	2019	2050	2081	2112	2144	2176	2208	2241	2274	2307	2341	2374	2409	2443	2478	23.9
24.0	1858	1886	1915	1945	1975	2005	2035	2066	2097	2128	2160	2192	2224	2257	2289	2323	2356	2390	2424	2459	2494	24.0
24.1	1873	1902	1931	1961	1990	2020	2051	2081	2112	2144	2175	2207	2240	2272	2305	2338	2372	2406	2440	2475	2509	24.1
24.2	1889	1918	1947	1976	2006	2036	2066	2097	2128	2159	2191	2223	2255	2288	2321	2354	2388	2422	2456	2490	2525	24.2
24.3	1905	1933	1963	1992	2022	2052	2082	2113	2144	2175	2207	2239	2271	2304	2337	2370	2403	2437	2471	2506	2541	24.3
24.4	1920	1949	1978	2008	2037	2067	2098	2129	2160	2191	2223	2255	2287	2319	2352	2386	2419	2453	2487	2522	2557	24.4
24.5	1936	1965	1994	2023	2053	2083	2114	2144	2175	2207	2238	2270	2302	2335	2368	2401	2435	2469	2503	2537	2572	24.5
24.6	1952	1981	2010	2039	2069	2099	2129	2160	2191	2222	2254	2286	2318	2351	2384	2417	2451	2484	2519	2553	2588	24.6
24.7	1967	1996	2025	2055	2085	2115	2145	2176	2207	2238	2270	2302	2334	2367	2399	2433	2466	2500	2534	2569	2604	24.7
24.8	1983	2012	2041	2071	2100	2130	2161	2191	2222	2254	2285	2317	2350	2382	2415	2448	2482	2516	2550	2585	2619	24.8
24.9	1999	2028	2057	2086	2116	2146	2176	2207	2238	2269	2301	2333	2365	2398	2431	2464	2498	2532	2566	2600	2635	24.9
25.0	2015	2043	2072	2102	2132	2162	2192	2223	2254	2285	2317	2349	2381	2414	2447	2480	2513	2547	2581	2616	2651	25.0
25.1	2030	2059	2088	2118	2147	2177	2208	2238	2270	2301	2332	2364	2397	2429	2462	2496	2529	2563	2597	2632	2666	25.1
25.2	2046	2075	2104	2133	2163	2193	2224	2254	2285	2317	2348	2380	2412	2445	2478	2511	2545	2579	2613	2647	2682	25.2
25.3	2062	2091	2120	2149	2179	2209	2239	2270	2301	2332	2364	2396	2428	2461	2494	2527	2560	2594	2629	2663	2698	25.3
25.4	2077	2106	2135	2165	2194	2225	2255	2286	2317	2348	2380	2412	2444	2476	2509	2543	2576	2610	2644	2679	2714	25.4
25.5	2093	2122	2151	2180	2210	2240	2271	2301	2332	2364	2395	2427	2460	2492	2525	2558	2592	2626	2660	2694	2729	25.5
25.6	2109	2138	2167	2196	2226	2256	2286	2317	2348	2379	2411	2443	2475	2508	2541	2574	2608	2641	2676	2710	2745	25.6
25.7	2125	2153	2182	2212	2242	2272	2302	2333	2364	2395	2427	2459	2491	2524	2557	2590	2623	2657	2691	2726	2761	25.7
25.8	2140	2169	2198	2228	2257	2287	2318	2348	2379	2411	2442	2474	2507	2539	2572	2605	2639	2673	2707	2742	2776	25.8
25.9	2156	2185	2214	2243	2273	2303	2333	2364	2395	2426	2458	2490	2522	2555	2588	2621	2655	2689	2723	2757	2792	25.9
26.0	2172	2200	2230	2259	2289	2319	2349	2380	2411	2442	2474	2506	2538	2571	2604	2637	2670	2704	2738	2773	2808	26.0
26.1	2187	2216	2245	2275	2304	2334	2365	2396	2427	2458	2490	2522	2554	2586	2619	2653	2686	2720	2754	2789	2824	26.1
26.2	2203	2232	2261	2290	2320	2350	2381	2411	2442	2474	2505	2537	2570	2602	2635	2668	2702	2736	2770	2804	2839	26.2
26.3	2219	2248	2277	2306	2336	2366	2396	2427	2458	2489	2521	2553	2585	2618	2651	2684	2718	2751	2786	2820	2855	26.3
26.4	2235	2263	2292	2322	2352	2382	2412	2443	2474	2505	2537	2569	2601	2634	2666	2700	2733	2767	2801	2836	2871	26.4
26.5	2250	2279	2308	2338	2367	2397	2428	2458	2489	2521	2552	2584	2617	2649	2682	2715	2749	2783	2817	2852	2886	26.5
26.6	2266	2295	2324	2353	2383	2413	2443	2474	2505	2536	2568	2600	2632	2665	2698	2731	2765	2799	2833	2867	2902	26.6
26.7	2282	2310	2340	2369	2399	2429	2459	2490	2521	2552	2584	2616	2648	2681	2714	2747	2780	2814	2848	2883	2918	26.7
26.8	2297	2326	2355	2385	2414	2444	2475	2506	2537	2568	2600	2631	2664	2696	2729	2763	2796	2830	2864	2899	2933	26.8
26.9	2313	2342	2371	2400	2430	2460	2491	2521	2552	2584	2615	2647	2679	2712	2745	2778	2812	2846	2880	2914	2949	26.9
27.0	2329	2358	2387	2416	2446	2476	2506	2537	2568	2599	2631	2663	2695	2728	2761	2794	2827	2861	2896	2930	2965	27.0
27.1	2344	2373	2402	2432	2462	2492	2522	2553	2584	2615	2647	2679	2711	2743	2776	2810	2843	2877	2911	2946	2981	27.1
27.2	2360	2389	2418	2447	2477	2507	2538	2568	2599	2631	2662	2694	2727	2759	2792	2825	2859	2893	2927	2961	2996	27.2
27.3	2376	2405	2434	2463	2493	2523	2553	2584	2615	2646	2678	2710	2742	2775	2808	2841	2875	2908	2943	2977	3012	27.3
27.4	2392	2420	2449	2479	2509	2539	2569	2600	2631	2662	2694	2726	2758	2791	2824	2857	2890	2924	2958	2993	3028	27.4
27.5	2407	2436	2465	2495	2524	2554	2585	2615	2646	2678	2709	2741	2774	2806	2839	2872	2906	2940	2974	3009	3043	27.5
27.6	2423	2452	2481	2510	2540	2570	2600	2631	2662	2694	2725	2757	2789	2822	2855	2888	2922	2956	2990	3024	3059	27.6
27.7	2439	2467	2497	2526	2556	2586	2616	2647	2678	2709	2741	2773	2805	2838	2871	2904	2937	2971	3006	3040	3075	27.7
27.8	2454	2483	2512	2542	2571	2602	2632	2663	2694	2725	2757	2789	2821	2853	2886	2920	2953	2987	3021	3056	3091	27.8
27.9	2470	2499	2528	2557	2587	2617	2648	2678	2709	2741	2772	2804	2837	2869	2902	2935	2969	3003	3037	3071	3106	27.9

→

Table 53.39 (continued) Estimation of fetal weight based on the biparietal diameter (BPD) and abdominal circumference (AC)

AC (cm)	9.0	9.1	9.2	9.3	9.4	9.5	9.6	9.7	9.8	9.9	10.0	10.1	10.2	10.3	10.4	10.5	10.6	10.7	10.8	10.9	11.0	OFD (cm)
28.0	2486	2515	2544	2573	2603	2633	2663	2694	2725	2756	2788	2820	2852	2885	2918	2951	2985	3018	3053	3087	3122	28.0
28.1	2502	2530	2559	2589	2619	2649	2679	2710	2741	2772	2804	2836	2868	2901	2933	2967	3000	3034	3068	3103	3138	28.1
28.2	2517	2546	2575	2605	2634	2664	2695	2725	2756	2788	2819	2851	2884	2916	2949	2982	3016	3050	3084	3119	3153	28.2
28.3	2533	2562	2591	2620	2650	2680	2710	2741	2772	2803	2835	2867	2899	2932	2965	2998	3032	3066	3100	3134	3169	28.3
28.4	2549	2577	2607	2636	2666	2696	2726	2757	2788	2819	2851	2883	2915	2948	2981	3014	3047	3081	3115	3150	3185	28.4
28.5	2564	2593	2622	2652	2681	2711	2742	2773	2804	2835	2867	2899	2931	2963	2996	3030	3063	3097	3131	3166	3201	28.5
28.6	2580	2609	2638	2667	2697	2727	2758	2788	2819	2851	2882	2914	2946	2979	3012	3045	3079	3113	3147	3181	3216	28.6
28.7	2596	2625	2654	2683	2713	2743	2773	2804	2835	2866	2898	2930	2962	2995	3028	3061	3095	3128	3163	3197	3232	28.7
28.8	2611	2640	2669	2699	2729	2759	2789	2820	2851	2882	2914	2946	2978	3011	3043	3077	3110	3144	3178	3213	3248	28.8
28.9	2627	2656	2685	2715	2744	2774	2805	2835	2866	2898	2929	2961	2994	3026	3059	3092	3126	3160	3194	3229	3263	28.9
29.0	2643	2672	2701	2730	2760	2790	2820	2851	2882	2913	2945	2977	3009	3042	3075	3108	3142	3176	3210	3244	3279	29.0
29.1	2659	2687	2716	2746	2776	2806	2836	2867	2898	2929	2961	2993	3025	3058	3091	3124	3157	3191	3225	3260	3295	29.1
29.2	2674	2703	2732	2762	2791	2821	2852	2882	2914	2945	2976	3008	3041	3073	3106	3139	3173	3207	3241	3276	3310	29.2
29.3	2690	2719	2748	2777	2807	2837	2868	2898	2929	2961	2992	3024	3056	3089	3122	3155	3189	3223	3257	3291	3326	29.3
29.4	2706	2735	2764	2793	2823	2853	2883	2914	2945	2976	3008	3040	3072	3105	3138	3171	3204	3238	3273	3307	3342	29.4
29.5	2721	2750	2779	2809	2838	2869	2899	2930	2961	2992	3024	3056	3088	3120	3153	3187	3220	3254	3288	3323	3358	29.5
29.6	2737	2766	2795	2824	2854	2884	2915	2945	2976	3008	3039	3071	3104	3136	3169	3202	3236	3270	3304	3338	3373	29.6
29.7	2753	2782	2811	2840	2870	2900	2930	2961	2992	3023	3055	3087	3119	3152	3185	3218	3252	3285	3320	3354	3389	29.7
29.8	2769	2797	2826	2856	2886	2916	2946	2977	3008	3039	3071	3103	3135	3168	3201	3234	3267	3301	3335	3370	3405	29.8
29.9	2784	2813	2842	2872	2901	2931	2962	2992	3023	3055	3086	3118	3151	3183	3216	3249	3283	3317	3351	3386	3420	29.9
30.0	2800	2829	2858	2887	2917	2947	2977	3008	3039	3070	3102	3134	3166	3199	3232	3265	3299	3333	3367	3401	3436	30.0
30.1	2816	2844	2874	2903	2933	2963	2993	3024	3055	3086	3118	3150	3182	3215	3248	3281	3314	3348	3382	3417	3452	30.1
30.2	2831	2860	2889	2919	2948	2978	3009	3040	3071	3102	3134	3166	3198	3230	3263	3297	3330	3364	3398	3433	3468	30.2
30.3	2847	2876	2905	2934	2964	2994	3025	3055	3086	3118	3149	3181	3214	3246	3279	3312	3346	3380	3414	3448	3483	30.3
30.4	2863	2892	2921	2950	2980	3010	3040	3071	3102	3133	3165	3197	3229	3262	3295	3328	3362	3395	3430	3464	3499	30.4
30.5	2879	2907	2936	2966	2996	3026	3056	3087	3118	3149	3181	3213	3245	3278	3310	3344	3377	3411	3445	3480	3515	30.5
30.6	2894	2923	2952	2982	3011	3041	3072	3102	3133	3165	3196	3228	3261	3293	3326	3359	3393	3427	3461	3496	3530	30.6
30.7	2910	2939	2968	2997	3027	3057	3087	3118	3149	3180	3212	3244	3276	3309	3342	3375	3409	3443	3477	3511	3546	30.7
30.8	2926	2954	2984	3013	3043	3073	3103	3134	3165	3196	3228	3260	3292	3325	3358	3391	3424	3458	3492	3527	3562	30.8
30.9	2941	2970	2999	3029	3058	3088	3119	3150	3181	3212	3244	3275	3308	3340	3373	3407	3440	3474	3508	3543	3577	30.9
31.0	2957	2986	3015	3044	3074	3104	3135	3165	3196	3228	3259	3291	3323	3356	3389	3422	3456	3490	3524	3558	3593	31.0
31.1	2973	3002	3031	3060	3090	3120	3150	3181	3212	3243	3275	3307	3339	3372	3405	3438	3471	3505	3540	3574	3609	31.1
31.2	2988	3017	3046	3076	3106	3136	3166	3197	3228	3259	3291	3323	3355	3387	3420	3454	3487	3521	3555	3590	3625	31.2
31.3	3004	3033	3062	3091	3121	3151	3182	3212	3243	3275	3306	3338	3371	3403	3436	3469	3503	3537	3571	3605	3640	31.3
31.4	3020	3049	3078	3107	3137	3167	3197	3228	3259	3290	3322	3354	3386	3419	3452	3485	3519	3552	3587	3621	3656	31.4
31.5	3036	3064	3093	3123	3153	3183	3213	3244	3275	3306	3338	3370	3402	3435	3468	3501	3534	3568	3602	3637	3672	31.5
31.6	3051	3080	3109	3139	3168	3198	3229	3259	3290	3322	3353	3385	3418	3450	3483	3516	3550	3584	3618	3653	3687	31.6
31.7	3067	3096	3125	3154	3184	3214	3244	3275	3306	3338	3369	3401	3433	3466	3499	3532	3566	3600	3634	3668	3703	31.7
31.8	3083	3111	3141	3170	3200	3230	3260	3291	3322	3353	3385	3417	3449	3482	3515	3548	3581	3615	3650	3684	3719	31.8
31.9	3098	3127	3156	3186	3215	3246	3276	3307	3338	3369	3401	3433	3465	3497	3530	3564	3597	3631	3665	3700	3735	31.9
32.0	3114	3143	3172	3201	3231	3261	3292	3322	3353	3385	3416	3448	3481	3513	3546	3579	3613	3647	3681	3715	3750	32.0
32.1	3130	3159	3188	3217	3247	3277	3307	3338	3369	3400	3432	3464	3496	3529	3562	3595	3629	3662	3697	3731	3766	32.1
32.2	3146	3174	3203	3233	3263	3293	3323	3354	3385	3416	3448	3480	3512	3545	3577	3611	3644	3678	3712	3747	3782	32.2
32.3	3161	3190	3219	3249	3278	3308	3339	3369	3400	3432	3463	3495	3528	3560	3593	3626	3660	3694	3728	3763	3797	32.3
32.4	3177	3206	3235	3264	3294	3324	3354	3385	3416	3447	3479	3511	3543	3576	3609	3642	3676	3710	3744	3778	3813	32.4
32.5	3193	3221	3251	3280	3310	3340	3370	3401	3432	3463	3495	3527	3559	3592	3625	3658	3691	3725	3759	3794	3829	32.5
32.6	3208	3237	3266	3296	3325	3355	3386	3417	3448	3479	3511	3542	3575	3607	3640	3674	3707	3741	3775	3810	3845	32.6
32.7	3224	3253	3282	3311	3341	3371	3402	3432	3463	3495	3526	3558	3590	3623	3656	3689	3723	3757	3791	3825	3860	32.7
32.8	3240	3269	3298	3327	3357	3387	3417	3448	3479	3510	3542	3574	3606	3639	3672	3705	3739	3772	3807	3841	3876	32.8
32.9	3255	3284	3313	3343	3373	3403	3433	3464	3495	3526	3558	3590	3622	3655	3687	3721	3754	3788	3822	3857	3892	32.9
33.0	3271	3300	3329	3358	3388	3418	3449	3479	3510	3542	3573	3605	3638	3670	3703	3736	3770	3804	3838	3873	3907	33.0
33.1	3287	3316	3345	3374	3404	3434	3464	3495	3526	3557	3589	3621	3653	3686	3719	3752	3786	3820	3854	3888	3923	33.1
33.2	3303	3331	3360	3390	3420	3450	3480	3511	3542	3573	3605	3637	3669	3702	3735	3768	3801	3835	3869	3904	3939	33.2
33.3	3318	3347	3376	3406	3435	3465	3496	3526	3557	3589	3620	3652	3685	3717	3750	3783	3817	3851	3885	3920	3954	33.3
33.4	3334	3363	3392	3421	3451	3481	3511	3542	3573	3605	3636	3668	3700	3733	3766	3799	3833	3867	3901	3935	3970	33.4
33.5	3350	3379	3408	3437	3467	3497	3527	3558	3589	3620	3652	3684	3716	3749	3782	3815	3848	3882	3917	3951	3986	33.5
33.6	3365	3394	3423	3453	3482	3513	3543	3574	3605	3636	3668	3700	3732	3764	3797	3831	3864	3898	3932	3967	4002	33.6
33.7	3381	3410	3439	3468	3498	3528	3559	3589	3620	3652	3683	3715	3748	3780	3813	3846	3880	3914	3948	3982	4017	33.7
33.8	3397	3426	3455	3484	3514	3544	3574	3605	3636	3667	3699	3731	3763	3796	3829	3862	3896	3929	3964	3998	4033	33.8
33.9	3413	3441	3470	3500	3530	3560	3590	3621	3652	3683	3715	3747	3779	3812	3844	3878	3911	3945	3979	4014	4049	33.9
34.0	3428	3457	3486	3516	3545	3575	3606	3636	3667	3699	3730	3762	3795	3827	3860	3893	3927	3961	3995	4030	4064	34.0
34.1	3444	3473	3502	3531	3561	3591	3621	3652	3683	3714	3746	3778	3810	3843	3876	3909	3943	3977	4011	4045	4080	34.1
34.2	3460	3488	3518	3547	3577	3607	3637	3668	3699	3730	3762	3794	3826	3859	3892	3925	3958	3992	4026	4061	4096	34.2
34.3	3475	3504	3533	3563	3592	3622	3653	3684	3715	3746	3778	3810	3842	3874	3907	3941	3974	4008	4042	4077	4112	34.3
34.4	3491	3520	3549	3578	3608	3638	3669	3699	3730	3762	3793	3825	3858	3890	3923	3956	3990	4024	4058	4092	4127	34.4
34.5	3507	3536	3565	3594	3624	3654	3684	3715	3746	3777	3809	3841	3873	3906	3939	3972	4006	4039	4074	4108	4143	34.5
34.6	3522	3551	3580	3610	3640	3670	3700	3731	3762	3793	3825	3857	3889	3922	3954	3988	4021	4055	4089	4124	4159	34.6
34.7	3538	3567	3596	3626	3655	3685	3716	3746	3777	3809	3840	3872	3905	3937	3970	4003	4037	4071	4105	4140	4174	34.7
34.8	3554	3583	3612	3641	3671	3701	3731	3762	3793	3824	3856	3888	3920	3953	3986	4019	4053	4087	4121	4155	4190	34.8
34.9	3570	3598	3628	3657	3687	3717	3747	3778	3809	3840	3872	3904	3936	3969	4002	4035	4068	4102	4136	4171	4206	34.9

→

Table 53.**39** (continued)   Estimation of fetal weight based on the biparietal diameter (BPD) and abdominal circumference (AC)

AC (cm)	BPD (cm) 9.0	9.1	9.2	9.3	9.4	9.5	9.6	9.7	9.8	9.9	10.0	10.1	10.2	10.3	10.4	10.5	10.6	10.7	10.8	10.9	11.0	OFD (cm)
35.0	3585	3614	3643	3673	3702	3732	3763	3794	3825	3856	3888	3919	3952	3984	4017	4051	4084	4118	4152	4187	4221	35.0
35.1	3601	3630	3659	3688	3718	3748	3779	3809	3840	3872	3903	3935	3967	4000	4033	4066	4100	4134	4168	4202	4237	35.1
35.2	3617	3646	3675	3704	3734	3764	3794	3825	3856	3887	3919	3951	3983	4016	4049	4082	4115	4149	4184	4218	4253	35.2
35.3	3632	3661	3690	3720	3750	3780	3810	3841	3872	3903	3935	3967	3999	4031	4064	4098	4131	4165	4199	4234	4269	35.3
35.4	3648	3677	3706	3735	3765	3795	3826	3856	3887	3919	3950	3982	4015	4047	4080	4113	4147	4181	4215	4249	4284	35.4
35.5	3664	3693	3722	3751	3781	3811	3841	3872	3903	3934	3966	3998	4030	4063	4096	4129	4163	4196	4231	4265	4300	35.5
35.6	3680	3708	3737	3767	3797	3827	3857	3888	3919	3950	3982	4014	4046	4079	4112	4145	4178	4212	4246	4281	4316	35.6
35.7	3695	3724	3753	3783	3812	3842	3873	3903	3934	3966	3997	4029	4062	4094	4127	4160	4194	4228	4262	4297	4331	35.7
35.8	3711	3740	3769	3798	3828	3858	3888	3919	3950	3982	4013	4045	4077	4110	4143	4176	4210	4244	4278	4312	4347	35.8
35.9	3727	3755	3785	3814	3844	3874	3904	3935	3966	3997	4029	4061	4093	4126	4159	4192	4225	4259	4294	4328	4363	35.9
36.0	3742	3771	3800	3830	3859	3890	3920	3951	3982	4013	4045	4077	4109	4141	4174	4208	4241	4275	4309	4344	4379	36.0
36.1	3758	3787	3816	3845	3875	3905	3936	3966	3997	4029	4060	4092	4125	4157	4190	4223	4257	4291	4325	4359	4394	36.1
36.2	3774	3803	3832	3861	3891	3921	3951	3982	4013	4044	4076	4108	4140	4173	4206	4239	4273	4306	4341	4375	4410	36.2
36.3	3790	3818	3847	3877	3907	3937	3967	3998	4029	4060	4092	4124	4156	4189	4221	4255	4288	4322	4356	4391	4426	36.3
36.4	3805	3834	3863	3893	3922	3952	3983	4013	4044	4076	4107	4139	4172	4204	4237	4270	4304	4338	4372	4407	4441	36.4
36.5	3821	3850	3879	3908	3938	3968	3998	4029	4060	4091	4123	4155	4187	4220	4253	4286	4320	4354	4388	4422	4457	36.5
36.6	3837	3865	3895	3924	3954	3984	4014	4045	4076	4107	4139	4171	4203	4236	4269	4302	4335	4369	4403	4438	4473	36.6
36.7	3852	3881	3910	3940	3969	3999	4030	4061	4092	4123	4155	4186	4219	4251	4284	4318	4351	4385	4419	4454	4489	36.7
36.8	3868	3897	3926	3955	3985	4015	4046	4076	4107	4139	4170	4202	4234	4267	4300	4333	4367	4401	4435	4469	4504	36.8
36.9	3884	3913	3942	3971	4001	4031	4061	4092	4123	4154	4186	4218	4250	4283	4316	4349	4383	4416	4451	4485	4520	36.9
37.0	3899	3928	3957	3987	4017	4047	4077	4108	4139	4170	4202	4234	4266	4298	4331	4365	4398	4432	4466	4501	4536	37.0

After Merz, E., Lieser, H., Schicketanz, K.H., Härle, J.: Intrauterine fetal weight assessment with ultrasound. A comparison of several weight assessment methods and development of a new formula for the determination of fetal weight. Ultraschall 9 (1988) 15–24

Table 53.**40** Fetal weight estimation based on abdominal circumference (AC), $W = 0.1 \times AC^3$

AC (cm)	W (g)	AC (cm)	W (g)
22.9	1201	28.6	2339
23.0	1217	28.7	2364
23.1	1233	28.8	2389
23.2	1249	28.9	2414
23.3	1265	29.0	2439
23.4	1281	29.1	2464
23.5	1298	29.2	2490
23.6	1314	29.3	2515
23.7	1331	29.4	2541
23.8	1348	29.5	2567
23.9	1365	29.6	2593
24.0	1382	29.7	2620
24.1	1400	29.8	2646
24.2	1417	29.9	2673
24.3	1435	30.0	2700
24.4	1453	30.1	2727
24.5	1471	30.2	2754
24.6	1489	30.3	2782
24.7	1507	30.4	2809
24.8	1525	30.5	2837
24.9	1544	30.6	2865
25.0	1563	30.7	2893
25.1	1581	30.8	2922
25.2	1600	30.9	2950
25.3	1619	31.0	2979
25.4	1639	31.1	3008
25.5	1658	31.2	3037
25.6	1678	31.3	3066
25.7	1697	31.4	3096
25.8	1717	31.5	3126
25.9	1737	31.6	3155
26.0	1758	31.7	3186
26.1	1778	31.8	3216
26.2	1798	31.9	3246
26.3	1819	32.0	3277
26.4	1840	32.1	3308
26.5	1861	32.2	3339
26.6	1882	32.3	3370
26.7	1903	32.4	3401
26.8	1925	32.5	3433
26.9	1947	32.6	3465
27.0	1968	32.7	3497
27.1	1990	32.8	3529
27.2	2012	32.9	3561
27.3	2035	33.0	3594
27.4	2057	33.1	3626
27.5	2080	33.2	3659
27.6	2102	33.3	3693
27.7	2125	33.4	3726
27.8	2148	33.5	3760
27.9	2172	33.6	3793
28.0	2195	33.7	3827
28.1	2219	33.8	3861
28.2	2243	33.9	3896
28.3	2267	34.0	3930
28.4	2291	34.1	3965
28.5	2315	34.2	4000

After Merz, E., Lieser, H., Schicketanz, K.H., Härle, J.: Intrauterine weight assessment with ultrasound. A comparison of several weight assessment methods and development of a new formula for the determination of fetal weight. Ultraschall 9 (1988) 15–24

Table 53.**41** Weight table for underweight fetuses (weight indicated in grams). log10G = −1.7492 + 0.166 x AC − 2.646 + (AC x BPD)/100 (in cm, kg)

BPD (cm)	\multicolumn{21}{c}{Abdominal circumference (cm)}																			
	16.0	16.5	17.0	17.5	18.0	18.5	19.0	19.5	20.0	20.5	21.0	21.5	22.0	22.5	23.0	23.5	24.0	24.5	25.0	25.5	26.0	26.5
4.5	349	363	377	393	408	425	442	459	478	497	517	538	559	581	605	629	654	680	708	736	765	796
4.6	359	373	388	404	420	436	454	472	490	510	530	551	573	596	620	644	670	696	724	753	783	814
4.7	369	384	399	415	431	448	466	484	503	523	544	565	588	611	635	660	686	713	741	770	801	832
4.8	380	395	410	426	443	460	478	497	517	537	558	580	602	626	650	676	702	730	758	788	819	851
4.9	391	406	422	438	455	473	491	510	530	551	572	594	617	641	666	692	719	747	776	806	837	870
5.0	402	418	434	451	468	486	505	524	544	565	587	610	633	657	683	709	736	765	794	824	856	889
5.1	414	430	446	463	481	499	518	538	559	580	602	625	649	674	699	726	754	783	812	843	876	909
5.2	426	442	459	476	494	513	532	552	573	595	618	641	665	690	717	744	772	801	831	863	895	929
5.3	438	455	472	489	508	527	547	567	589	611	634	657	682	708	734	762	790	820	851	883	916	950
5.4	451	468	485	503	522	541	561	582	604	627	650	674	699	725	752	780	809	839	870	903	936	971
5.5	464	481	499	517	536	556	577	598	620	643	667	691	717	743	771	799	828	859	891	924	958	993
5.6	477	495	513	532	551	571	592	614	636	660	684	709	735	762	789	818	848	879	911	945	979	1015
5.7	491	509	527	547	566	587	608	630	653	677	701	727	753	780	809	838	869	900	933	966	1001	1038
5.8	505	524	542	562	582	603	625	647	670	695	719	745	772	800	829	858	889	921	954	989	1024	1061
5.9	520	539	558	578	598	619	642	664	688	713	738	761	792	820	849	879	911	943	977	1011	1047	1085
6.0	535	554	573	594	615	636	659	682	706	731	757	784	811	840	870	900	932	965	999	1035	1071	1109
6.1	550	570	590	610	632	654	677	700	725	750	777	804	832	861	891	922	955	988	1023	1058	1095	1134
6.2	566	586	606	627	649	672	695	719	744	770	797	824	853	882	913	945	977	1011	1046	1083	1120	1159
6.3	583	603	624	645	667	690	714	738	764	790	817	845	874	904	935	967	1001	1035	1071	1107	1145	1185
6.4	600	620	641	663	686	709	733	758	784	811	838	867	896	927	958	991	1025	1059	1096	1133	1171	1211
6.5	617	638	659	682	705	728	753	778	805	832	860	889	919	950	982	1015	1049	1084	1121	1159	1198	1238
6.6	635	656	678	701	724	748	773	799	826	853	882	911	914	973	1006	1039	1074	1110	1147	1185	1225	1266
6.7	653	675	697	720	744	769	794	820	848	876	905	935	965	997	1030	1065	1100	1136	1174	1213	1253	1294
6.8	672	694	717	740	765	790	816	842	870	898	928	958	990	1022	1056	1090	1126	1163	1201	1241	1281	1323
6.9	691	714	737	761	786	811	838	865	893	922	952	983	1015	1048	1082	1117	1153	1190	1229	1269	1310	1353
7.0	711	734	758	782	807	833	860	888	916	946	976	1008	1040	1074	1108	1144	1181	1219	1258	1298	1340	1383
7.1	732	755	779	804	830	856	883	912	941	971	1002	1033	1066	1100	1135	1171	1209	1247	1287	1328	1370	1414
7.2	763	777	801	827	853	880	907	936	965	996	1027	1060	1093	1128	1163	1200	1238	1277	1317	1358	1401	1445
7.3	775	799	824	850	876	904	932	961	991	1022	1054	1087	1121	1156	1192	1229	1267	1307	1348	1390	1433	1478
7.4	797	822	847	874	901	928	957	987	1017	1049	1081	1114	1149	1184	1221	1259	1297	1338	1379	1421	1465	1511
7.5	820	845	871	898	925	954	983	1013	1044	1076	1109	1143	1178	1214	1251	1289	1328	1369	1411	1454	1499	1544
7.6	844	870	896	923	951	980	1009	1040	1072	1104	1137	1172	1207	1244	1281	1320	1360	1401	1444	1487	1533	1579
7.7	868	894	921	949	977	1007	1037	1068	1100	1133	1167	1202	1238	1275	1313	1352	1393	1434	1477	1522	1567	1614
7.8	894	920	947	975	1004	1034	1065	1096	1129	1162	1197	1232	1269	1306	1345	1385	1426	1468	1512	1557	1603	1650
7.9	919	946	974	1003	1032	1062	1094	1126	1159	1193	1228	1264	1301	1339	1378	1418	1460	1503	1547	1592	1639	1687
8.0	946	973	1002	1031	1061	1091	1123	1156	1189	1224	1259	1296	1333	1372	1412	1453	1495	1538	1583	1629	1676	1725
8.1	973	1001	1030	1060	1090	1121	1153	1187	1221	1256	1292	1329	1367	1406	1446	1488	1531	1575	1620	1666	1714	1763
8.2	1001	1030	1059	1089	1120	1152	1185	1218	1253	1288	1325	1363	1401	1441	1482	1524	1567	1612	1657	1704	1753	1803
8.3	1030	1059	1089	1120	1151	1183	1217	1251	1286	1322	1359	1397	1436	1477	1518	1561	1605	1650	1696	1744	1793	1843
8.4	1060	1090	1120	1151	1183	1216	1249	1284	1320	1356	1394	1433	1473	1513	1555	1599	1643	1689	1735	1784	1833	1884
8.5	1091	1121	1151	1183	1216	1249	1283	1318	1355	1392	1430	1469	1510	1551	1594	1637	1682	1728	1776	1825	1875	1926
8.6	1122	1153	1184	1216	1249	1283	1318	1354	1390	1428	1467	1507	1548	1589	1633	1677	1722	1769	1817	1866	1917	1969
8.7	1155	1186	1218	1250	1284	1318	1353	1390	1427	1465	1505	1545	1586	1629	1673	1717	1764	1811	1859	1909	1960	2013
8.8	1188	1220	1252	1285	1319	1354	1390	1427	1465	1504	1543	1584	1626	1669	1714	1759	1806	1854	1903	1953	2005	2058
8.9	1222	1254	1287	1321	1356	1391	1428	1465	1503	1543	1583	1625	1667	1711	1756	1802	1849	1897	1947	1998	2050	2104
9.0	1258	1290	1324	1358	1393	1429	1456	1504	1543	1583	1624	1666	1709	1753	1799	1845	1893	1942	1992	2044	2097	2151

After Shepard, M.J., Richards, V.A., Berkowitz, R.L., Warsof, S.L., Hobbins, J.C.: An evaluation of two equations for predicting fetal weight by ultrasound. J. Obstet. Gynec. 142 (1982) 47–54

Weight and Length of Newborn Infants

▬ *Singletons*

Table 53.**42a** Birthweight percentiles for **male newborns** versus duration of pregnancy (Federal Republic of Germany, 1992, singletons)

Pregnancy duration (weeks)	Birthweight percentiles (g)				
	5th	10th	50th	90th	95th
23	420	450	600	720	770
24	480	510	690	840	880
25	540	600	800	970	1030
26	610	680	940	1120	1180
27	690	770	1080	1280	1360
28	750	860	1220	1450	1520
29	830	960	1350	1630	1710
30	940	1070	1520	1830	1910
31	1070	1180	1690	2020	2110
32	1200	1340	1890	2260	2360
33	1360	1550	2130	2550	2690
34	1600	1790	2390	2850	3000
35	1870	2060	2640	3140	3320
36	2140	2330	2860	3390	3550
37	2400	2570	3090	3620	3770
38	2620	2780	3300	3840	4000
39	2790	2950	3470	4010	4180
40	2910	3070	3600	4170	4350
41	3010	3160	3700	4290	4470
42	3030	3200	3760	4350	4520

Table 53.**42b** Birthweight percentiles for female newborns versus duration of pregnancy (Federal Republic of Germany, 1992, singletons)

Pregnancy duration (weeks)	Birthweight percentiles (g)				
	5th	10th	50th	90th	95th
23	400	430	580	700	750
24	460	490	670	800	860
25	520	560	760	930	990
26	590	640	880	1060	1140
27	650	710	1000	1220	1300
28	710	800	1120	1390	1460
29	790	900	1250	1570	1650
30	900	990	1420	1770	1850
31	1010	1100	1590	1960	2050
32	1140	1260	1790	2180	2280
33	1300	1470	2030	2470	2610
34	1530	1710	2270	2770	2920
35	1790	1980	2550	3060	3230
36	2060	2230	2760	3290	3460
37	2290	2460	2970	3500	3660
38	2500	2660	3160	3690	3850
39	2670	2820	3320	3850	4020
40	2800	2940	3450	4000	4180
41	2890	3020	3540	4100	4300
42	2900	3050	3580	4180	4360

Adapted from Voigt, M., Schneider, K.T.M., Jährig, K.: Analysis of children born in 1992 in the Federal Republic of Germany. Part 1: new biometry percentiles for newborns. Geburtsh. u. Frauenheilk. 56 (1996) 550–558

Table 53.**43a** Length percentiles for **male newborns** versus duration of pregnancy (Federal Republic of Germany, 1992, singletons)

Pregnancy duration SSW	Length percentiles (cm)		
	5th	50th	90th
23	28	31	34
24	29	32	36
25	30	34	37
26	31	35	38
27	32	36	39
28	34	38	41
29	35	39	43
30	36	41	44
31	38	42	45
32	39	43	46
33	41	45	48
34	42	47	49
35	45	48	51
36	46	49	52
37	47	50	53
38	48	51	54
39	49	52	55
40	50	52	55
41	50	53	56
42	50	53	56

Table 53.**43b** Length percentiles for **female newborns** versus duration of pregnancy (Federal Republic of Germany, 1992, singletons)

Pregnancy duration SSW	Length percentiles (cm)		
	5th	50th	90th
23	28	31	34
24	28	32	35
25	30	33	37
26	30	35	37
27	32	36	39
28	34	37	40
29	34	39	42
30	36	40	43
31	38	42	45
32	39	43	46
33	40	44	48
34	42	46	49
35	44	48	50
36	45	49	51
37	47	50	52
38	48	50	53
39	48	51	54
40	49	52	54
41	50	52	55
42	50	52	55

Adapted from Voigt, M., Schneider, K.T.M., Jährig, K.: Analysis of children born in 1992 in the Federal Republic of Germany. Part 1: new biometry percentiles for newborns. Geburtsh. u. Frauenheilk. 56 (1996) 550–558

Twins

Table 53.**44**   Combined birthweight percentiles for newborn twins of both sexes, 28–42 weeks' gestation

Weeks	Combined percentiles				
	10th	25th	50th	75th	90th
28	–	–	**1162**	–	–
29	–	–	**1240**	–	–
30	1007	1151	**1341**	1599	1865
31	1053	1202	**1437**	1731	2018
32	1147	1317	**1565**	1880	2165
33	1236	1455	**1695**	2062	2310
34	1370	1588	**1847**	2226	2486
35	1505	1717	**2010**	2391	2653
36	1636	1890	**2170**	2546	2800
37	1786	2057	**2337**	2700	2970
38	1935	2210	**2460**	2848	3105
39	2098	2315	**2580**	2967	3235
40	2209	2440	**2705**	3085	3363
41	2338	2562	**2825**	3129	3398
42	2307	2544	**2801**	3104	3367

After Bazso, J., Dolhay, B., Pohanka, Ö.: Weight gain in twins between 28 and 42 weeks of gestation. Zbl. Gynäkol. 20 (1970) 628–633

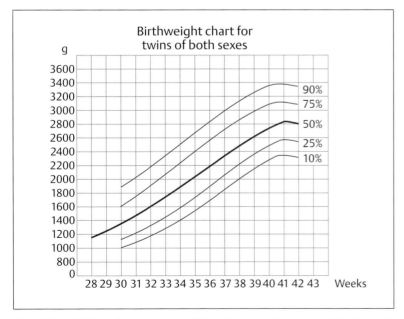

Figs. 53.**9**   Weight gain in twins from 28 to 42 weeks of gestation. After Bazso, J., Dolhay, B., Pohanka, Ö.: Zbl. Gynäkol. 20 (1970) 628–633.

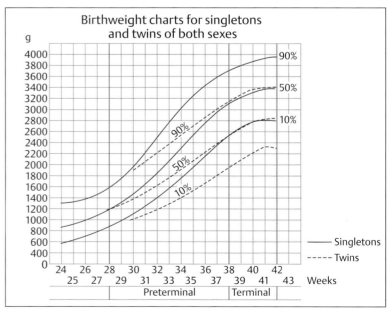

Figs. 53.**10**   Comparison of standard growth curves in singletons and twins from 28 to 42 weeks of gestation. After Bazso, J., Dolhay, B., Pohanka, Ö.: Zbl. Gynäkol. 20 (1970) 628–633.

Doppler Ultrasound during Pregnancy

Uterine Artery

Table 53.**45**   Pulsatility index (PI), resistance index (RI), and intensity-weighted mean flow velocity (Vmean [cm/s]) of the uterine artery

Weeks	PI Mean*	PI 90% interval	RI Mean*	RI 90% interval	Vmean Mean*	Vmean 90% interval
18	0.888	(0.509-1.407)	0.447	(0.222-0.659)	43.458	(20.659-71.901)
19	0.838	(0.460-1.356)	0.429	(0.204-0.641)	44.025	(21.202-72.500)
20	0.812	(0.436-1.328)	0.419	(0.194-0.630)	44.831	(21.982-73.337)
21	0.795	(0.420-1.309)	0.411	(0.186-0.622)	45.704	(22.830-74.240)
22	0.781	(0.407-1.293)	0.405	(0.180-0.615)	46.545	(23.647-75.113)
23	0.769	(0.397-1.280)	0.400	(0.175-0.610)	47.301	(24.377-75.899)
24	0.759	(0.388-1.268)	0.395	(0.171-0.605)	47.945	(24.997-76.575)
25	0.751	(0.381-1.258)	0.391	(0.167-0.601)	48.473	(25.500-77.133)
26	0.743	(0.374-1.248)	0.387	(0.163-0.597)	48.889	(25.891-77.580)
27	0.736	(0.369-1.239)	0.384	(0.160-0.593)	49.206	(26.183-77.928)
28	0.729	(0.363-1.230)	0.380	(0.157-0.590)	49.439	(26.391-78.192)
29	0.722	(0.358-1.222)	0.378	(0.154-0.587)	49.604	(26.532-78.388)
30	0.716	(0.354-1.214)	0.375	(0.152-0.584)	49.716	(26.619-78.532)
31	0.711	(0.349-1-207)	0.372	(0.150-0.581)	49.790	(26.668-78.637)
32	0.705	(0.345-1.999)	0.370	(0.147-0.578)	49.836	(26.689-78.714)
33	0.700	(0.341-1.192)	0.368	(0.145-0.576)	49.863	(26.692-78.772)
34	0.695	(0.337-1.185)	0.366	(0.144-0.574)	49.878	(26.682-78.818)
35	0.690	(0.333-1.178)	0.364	(0.142-0.571)	49.886	(26.664-78.856)
36	0.684	(0.330-1.171)	0.362	(0.140-0.569)	49.889	(26.643-78.891)
37	0.679	(0.326-1.164)	0.360	(0.139-0.567)	49.891	(26.620-78.923)
38	0.674	(0.322-1.157)	0.358	(0.137-0.566)	49.891	(26.595-78.955)
39	0.669	(0.318-1.150)	0.357	(0.136-0.564)	49.891	(26.571-78.986)
40	0.663	(0.313-1.143)	0.355	(0.135-0.562)	49.891	(26.546-79.017)
41	0.657	(0.308-1.134)	0.354	(0.134-0.561)	49.894	(26.521-79.048)
42	0.649	(0.302-1.125)	0.353	(0.133-0.559)	49.891	(26.496-79.079)

After Bahlmann, F., Neubert, S., Merz, E., Wellek, S.: The uteroplacental Doppler spectrum in a normal population: calculation of reference ranges for uterine artery resistance indices. (In preparation)

* Smoothed by nonlinear regression

Umbilical Artery

Table 53.**46**   Normal values for the uterine artery resistance index as a function of gestational age and placental location

	Resistance index					
	Uterine artery (placental side)			Uterine artery (nonplacental side)		
Weeks	5%	50%	95%	5%	50%	95%
24	0.33	**0.45**	0.61	0.35	**0.49**	0.69
26	0.33	**0.45**	0.61	0.34	**0.49**	0.69
28	0.33	**0.44**	0.60	0.34	**0.48**	0.68
30	0.32	**0.44**	0.60	0.34	**0.48**	0.67
32	0.32	**0.44**	0.59	0.33	**0.47**	0.67
34	0.32	**0.43**	0.59	0.33	**0.47**	0.66
36	0.32	**0.43**	0.58	0.33	**0.46**	0.65
38	0.32	**0.43**	0.57	0.32	**0.46**	0.65
40	0.32	**0.42**	0.57	0.32	**0.45**	0.64
42	0.31	**0.42**	0.56	0.32	**0.45**	0.63

In: Kurmanavicius, J., Florio, I., Wisser, J., Hebisch, G., Zimmermann, R., Müller, R., Huch, R., Huch, A.: Reference resistance indices of the umbilical, fetal middle cerebral and uterine arteries at 24–42 weeks of gestation. Ultrasound Obstet. Gynecol. 10 (1997) 112–120

Table 53.**47**   Pulsatility index (PI) and resistance index (RI) of the umbilical artery

Weeks	PI Mean*	PI 90% interval	RI Mean*	RI 90% interval
18	1.018	(1.361-1.652)	0.713	(0.591-0.825)
19	1.250	(0.972-1.539)	0.700	(0.577-0.812)
20	1.216	(0.940-1.505)	0.690	(0.567-0.802)
21	1.189	(0.913-1.476)	0.680	(0.557-0.793)
22	1.165	(0.890-1.450)	0.671	(0.548-0.784)
23	1.142	(0.869-1.427)	0.663	(0.539-0.776)
24	1.122	(0.849-1.405)	0.655	(0.530-0.768)
25	1.102	(0.831-1.385)	0.646	(0.522-0.760)
26	1.084	(0.813-1.365)	0.639	(0.514-0.752)
27	1.065	(0.797-1.346)	0.631	(0.506-0.745)
28	1.048	(0.780-1.327)	0.623	(0.498-0.737)
29	1.031	(0.764-1.308)	0.615	(0.490-0.730)
30	1.014	(0.748-1.290)	0.608	(0.082-0.723)
31	0.997	(0.732-1.272)	0.600	(0.474-0.715)
32	0.980	(0.716-1.254)	0.592	(0.465-0.707)
33	0.963	(0.700-1.236)	0.584	(0.457-0.700)
34	0.946	(0.684-1.218)	0.576	(0.449-0.692)
35	0.928	(0.668-1.199)	0.567	(0.440-0.684)
36	0.910	(0.651-1.180)	0.559	(0.431-0.675)
37	0.891	(0.634-1.160)	0.550	(0.422-0.667)
38	0.872	(0.615-1.139)	0.540	(0.412-0.657)
39	0.851	(0.595-1.117)	0.530	(0.402-0.648)
40	0.828	(0.573-1.093)	0.519	(0.390-0.637)
41	0.801	(0.547-1.065)	0.506	(0.377-0.624)
42	0.765	(0.513-1.028)	0.490	(0.360-0.608)

After Bahlmann, F., Reinhardt, I., Krummenauer, F., Neubert, S., Macchiella, D., Wellek, S.: Blood flow velocity waveforms of the umbilical artery in a normal population: reference values from 18 weeks to 42 weeks of gestation. (In preparation)

* Smoothed by nonlinear regression

Table 53.**48**   Peak systolic flow velocity (Vmax), intensity-weight mean flow velocity (Vmean), and end-diastolic flow velocity (Vmin) of the umbilical artery (in cm/s)

Weeks	Vmax Mean* 90% interval	Vmean Mean*	Vmean 90% interval	Vmin Mean* 90% interval
18	33.722 (20.328-55.388)	18.188	(8.738-32.244)	8.217 (3.195-15.819)
19	35.800 (21.880-58.315)	19.336	(9.441-34.053)	9.136 (3.789-17.231)
20	37.396 (22.952-60.760)	20.403	(10.064-35.781)	9.919 (4.247-18.506)
21	38.787 (23.818-63.000)	21.425	(10.641-37.465)	10.644 (4.646-19.724)
22	40.058 (24.564-65.120)	22.415	(11.187-39.116)	11.337 (5.014-20.909)
23	41.250 (25.231-67.161)	23.380	(11.707-40.742)	12.011 (5.363-22.075)
24	42.387 (25.843-69.147)	24.323	(12.206-42.347)	12.675 (5.702-23.232)
25	43.485 (26.416-71.094)	25.248	(12.686-43.933)	13.335 (6.036-24.383)
26	44.555 (26.961-73.013)	26.156	(13.150-45.502)	13.995 (6.371-25.536)
27	45.605 (27.487-74.912)	27.049	(13.598-47.056)	14.659 (6.710-26.692)
28	46.643 (28.000-76.799)	27.927	(14.032-48.596)	15.331 (7.057-27.857)
29	47.675 (28.507-78.680)	28.792	(14.452-50.122)	16.015 (7.416-29.033)
30	48.706 (29.014-80.561)	29.643	(14.858-51.634)	16.715 (7.790-30.225)
31	49.743 (29.525-82.446)	30.481	(15.252-53.134)	17.434 (8.184-31.437)
32	50.789 (30.047-84.341)	31.307	(15.632-54.620)	18.178 (8.603-32.673)
33	51.852 (30.585-86.253)	32.119	(16.000-56.094)	18.952 (9.051-33.939)
34	52.939 (31.146-88.189)	32.918	(16.354-57.554)	19.763 (9.537-35.242)
35	54.057 (31.739-90.156)	33.703	(16.695-59.000)	20.620 (10.069-36.592)
36	55.217 (32.375-92.165)	34.473	(17.021-60.432)	21.536 (10.660-38.000)
37	56.433 (33.066-94.230)	35.228	(17.331-61.848)	22.527 (11.325-39.483)
38	57.725 (33.834-96.371)	35.966	(17.625-63.247)	23.618 (12.092-41.067)
39	59.125 (34.709-98.620)	36.685	(17.899-64.627)	24.852 (13.000-42.793)
40	60.688 (35.747-101.032)	37.380	(18.149-65.984)	26.303 (14.126-44.736)
41	62.531 (37.064-103.723)	38.044	(18.369-67.309)	28.143 (15.640-47.068)
42	65.043 (39.052-107.085)	38.661	(18.541-68.587)	30.995 (18.167-50.413)

After Bahlmann, F., Reinhardt, I., Krummenauer, F., Neubert, S., Macchiella, D., Wellek, S.: Blood flow velocity waveforms of the umbilical artery in a normal population: reference values from 18 weeks to 42 weeks of gestation. (In preparation)

* Smoothed by nonlinear regression

Descending Aorta

Table 53.**49** Pulsatility index (PI) and resistance index (RI) of the descending aorta, measured at the level of the diaphragm

	PI		RI	
Weeks	Mean*	90% interval	Mean*	90% interval
18	1.788	(1.496-2.149)	0.799	(0.694-0.874)
19	1.788	(1.493-2.155)	0.798	(0.691-0.873)
20	1.790	(1.492-2.161)	0.796	(0.689-0.872)
21	1.793	(1.491-2.168)	0.795	(0.687-0.872)
22	1.796	(1.491-2.176)	0.794	(0.686-0.871)
23	1.801	(1.492-2.184)	0.794	(0.684-0.871)
24	1.806	(1.493-2.194)	0.793	(0.683-0.871)
25	1.812	(1.496-2.205)	0.792	(0.681-0.870)
26	1.819	(1.499-2.216)	0.791	(0.680-0.870)
27	1.826	(1.503-2.228)	0.791	(0.679-0.870)
28	1.835	(1.508-2.241)	0.790	(0.677-0.870)
29	1.826	(1.513-2.254)	0.790	(0.676-0.870)
30	1.819	(1.519-2.268)	0.789	(0.675-0.870)
31	1.812	(1.525-2.282)	0.789	(0.674-0.870)
32	1.806	(1.532-2.296)	0.788	(0.673-0.870)
33	1.801	(1.538-2.311)	0.788	(0.671-0.870)
34	1.796	(1.545-2.325)	0.787	(0.670-0.870)
35	1.793	(1.552-2.340)	0.787	(0.669-0.870)
36	1.790	(1.558-2.354)	0.786	(0.668-0.870)
37	1.923	(1.564-2.369)	0.786	(0.667-0.870)
38	1.932	(1.570-2.382)	0.785	(0.666-0.870)
39	1.941	(1.575-2.395)	0.785	(0.665-0.870)
40	1.948	(1.579-2.407)	0.785	(0.664-0.870)
41	1.954	(1.581-2.417)	0.784	(0.663-0.871)

After Bahlmann, F., Wellek, S., Reinhardt, I., Krummenauer, F., Merz, E., Welter, C: Reference values of fetal aortic flow velocity waveforms and associated intraobserver reliability in normal pregnancies. Ultrasound Obstet. Gynecol. 17 (2000) 42–49

* Smoothed by nonlinear regression

Middle Cerebral Artery

Table 53.**50** Peak systolic flow velocity (Vmax), intensity-weight mean flow velocity (Vmean), and end-diastolic flow velocity (Vmin) of the descending aorta, measured at the level of the diaphragm (in cm/s)

	Vmax		Vmean		Vmin	
Weeks	Mean*	90% interval	Mean*	90% interval	Mean*	90% interval
18	48.218	(24.540-77.073)	19.982	(5.692-36.843)	7.628	(2.684-14.103)
19	51.815	(27.536-81.403)	24.270	(9.823-41.317)	8.914	(3.821-15.585)
20	55.635	(30.755-85.954)	26.880	(12.275-44.112)	9.885	(4.643-16.752)
21	59.517	(34.037-90.568)	28.870	(14.109-46.289)	10.709	(5.317-17.771)
22	63.392	(37.311-95.175)	30.522	(15.603-48.126)	11.439	(5.898-18.697)
23	67.218	(40.536-99.733)	31.955	(16.879-49.744)	12.100	(6.410-19.554)
24	70.966	(43.685-104.214)	33.233	(18.000-51.208)	12.707	(6.868-20.357)
25	74.617	(45.223-108.596)	34.397	(19.007-52.558)	13.270	(7.282-21.115)
26	78.151	(49.668-112.863)	35.472	(19.924-53.818)	13.796	(7.657-21.836)
27	81.556	(52.473-117.000)	36.476	(20.770-55.008)	14.288	(8.000-22.524)
28	84.820	(55.136-120.996)	37.422	(21.559-56.139)	14.750	(8.313-23.182)
29	87.932	(57.647-124.840)	38.320	(22.300-57.223)	15.185	(8.599-23.812)
30	90.882	(59.997-128.522)	39.178	(23.001-58.267)	15.595	(8.859-24.418)
31	93.662	(62.176-132.034)	40.003	(23.668-59.277)	15.981	(9.096-25.000)
32	96.264	(64.177-135.368)	40.800	(24.308-60.260)	16.345	(9.311-25.560)
33	98.679	(64.992-138.515)	41.574	(24.925-61.219)	16.688	(9.504-26.098)
34	100.901	(67.612-141.468)	42.329	(25.522-62.160)	17.009	(9.676-26.614)
35	102.921	(69.032-144.220)	43.069	(26.105-63.085)	17.309	(9.827-27.111)
36	104.731	(70.241-146.763)	43.798	(26.677-64.000)	17.589	(9.957-27.586)
37	106.324	(71.234-149.088)	44.520	(27.242-64.908)	17.848	(10.067-28.040)
38	107.691	(72.000-151.187)	45.241	(27.805-65.815)	18.084	(10.154-28.473)
39	108.822	(72.531-153.050)	45.967	(28.374-66.726)	18.298	(10.218-28.882)
40	109.707	(72.814-154.666)	46.707	(28.957-67.651)	18.486	(10.257-29.265)
41	110.330	(72.837-156.022)	47.479	(29.571-68.609)	18.644	(10.266-29.619)

After Bahlmann, F., Wellek, S., Reinhardt, I., Krummenauer, F., Merz, E., Welter, C: Reference values of fetal aortic flow velocity waveforms and associated intraobserver reliability in normal pregnancies. Ultrasound Obstet. Gynecol. 17 (2000) 42–49

* Smoothed by nonlinear regression

Table 53.**51** Pulsatility index (PI) and resistance index (RI) of the middle cerebral artery

	PI		RI	
Weeks	Mean*	90% interval	Mean*	90% interval
18	1.848	(1.391-2.385)	0.782	(0.642-0.882)
19	1.848	(1.388-2.389)	0.782	(0.641-0.883)
20	1.848	(1.386-2.392)	0.782	(0.640-0.884)
21	1.848	(1.383-2.395)	0.782	(0.639-0.885)
22	1.848	(1.381-2.398)	0.782	(0.638-0.885)
23	1.848	(1.378-2.401)	0.782	(0.637-0.886)
24	1.848	(1.375-2.404)	0.782	(0.636-0.887)
25	1.848	(1.373-2.407)	0.782	(0.635-0.888)
26	1.848	(1.370-2.410)	0.782	(0.634-0.888)
27	1.848	(1.367-2.413)	0.782	(0.633-0.889)
28	1.848	(1.365-2.416)	0.782	(0.632-0.890)
29	1.848	(1.362-2.419)	0.782	(0.631-0.891)
30	1.847	(1.359-2.422)	0.782	(0.630-0.891)
31	1.845	(1.354-2.423)	0.782	(0.628-0.892)
32	1.840	(1.347-2.422)	0.781	(0.627-0.892)
33	1.829	(1.333-2.413)	0.780	(0.625-0.892)
34	1.805	(1.306-2.392)	0.777	(0.621-0.890)
35	1.762	(1.260-2.352)	0.771	(0.614-0.884)
36	1.696	(1.192-2.290)	0.758	(0.600-0.872)
37	1.612	(1.105-2.209)	0.737	(0.578-0.852)
38	1.524	(1.014-2.123)	0.708	(0.547-0.823)
39	1.453	(0.941-2.056)	0.676	(0.514-0.792)
40	1.414	(0.899-2.020)	0.651	(0.489-0.768)
41	1.403	(0.885-2.012)	0.640	(0.477-0.758)

After Bahlmann, F., Reinhardt, I., Krummenauer, F., Neubert, S., Macchiella, D., Wellek, S.: Blood flow velocity waveforms of the fetal middle cerebral artery in a normal population: reference values from 18 weeks to 42 weeks of gestation. Perinat. Med. 30 (2002), 490–501

* Smoothed by nonlinear regression

Table 53.**52** Peak systolic flow velocity (Vmax), intensity-weight mean flow velocity (Vmean), and end-diastolic flow velocity (Vmin) of the middle cerebral artery (in cm/s)

	Vmax		Vmean		Vmin	
Weeks	Mean*	90% interval	Mean*	90% interval	Mean*	90% interval
18	26.833	(13.377-44.205)	11.202	(4.292-18.642)	4.945	(1.940-9.445)
19	26.863	(13.248-44.440)	11.245	(4.048-18.994)	4.945	(1.801-9.652)
20	26.985	(13.211-44.767)	11.355	(3.871-19.413)	4.945	(1.663-9.860)
21	27.257	(13.324-45.244)	11.543	(3.771-19.910)	4.945	(1.524-10.067)
22	27.730	(13.638-45.922)	11.816	(3.757-20.493)	4.945	(1.386-10.275)
23	28.439	(14.188-46.837)	12.179	(3.833-21.165)	4.946	(1.248-10.484)
24	29.410	(15.000-48.012)	12.633	(4.000-21.928)	4.950	(1.114-10.695)
25	30.651	(16.082-49.458)	13.180	(4.259-22.784)	4.961	(0.986-10.914)
26	32.159	(17.432-51.172)	13.817	(4.609-23.731)	4.989	(0.875-11.149)
27	33.919	(19.033-53.137)	14.543	(5.048-24.766)	5.046	(0.794-11.414)
28	35.904	(20.859-55.327)	15.353	(5.571-25.885)	5.155	(0.764-11.730)
29	38.075	(22.871-57.703)	16.243	(6.174-27.084)	5.345	(0.816-12.127)
30	40.387	(25.024-60.220)	17.206	(6.850-28.357)	5.650	(0.982-12.640)
31	42.785	(27.263-62.822)	18.235	(7.591-29.695)	6.107	(1.301-13.305)
32	45.210	(29.529-65.453)	19.320	(8.389-31.090)	6.750	(1.805-14.155)
33	47.600	(31.761-68.048)	20.452	(9.234-32.531)	7.600	(2.516-15.212)
34	49.892	(33.894-70.545)	21.618	(10.113-34.006)	8.654	(3.432-16.475)
35	52.023	(35.866-72.881)	22.804	(11.011-35.501)	9.883	(4.523-17.911)
36	53.937	(37.621-75.000)	23.994	(11.914-37.000)	11.218	(5.719-19.453)
37	55.582	(39.108-76.851)	25.168	(12.801-38.484)	12.557	(6.920-21.000)
38	56.921	(40.288-78.395)	26.305	(13.650-39.929)	13.776	(8.000-22.426)
39	57.930	(41.138-79.609)	27.374	(14.433-41.308)	14.751	(8.836-23.608)
40	58.606	(41.655-80.489)	28.342	(15.113-42.585)	15.395	(9.342-24.460)
41	58.974	(41.864-81.062)	29.156	(15.640-43.708)	15.704	(9.512-24.976)

After Bahlmann, F., Reinhardt, I., Krummenauer, F., Neubert, S., Macchiella, D., Wellek, S.: Blood flow velocity waveforms of the fetal middle cerebral artery in a normal population: reference values from 18 weeks to 42 weeks of gestation. Perinat. Med. 30 (2002), 490–501

* Smoothed by nonlinear regression

Table 53.**53**   Normal values for the umbilicocerebral ratio and aortocerebral ratio as a function of gestational age

Weeks	Umbilicocerebral ratio (umbilical artery/ middle cerebral artery)			Aortocerebral ratio (descending aorta/ middle cerebral artery)		
	5%	50%	95%	5%	50%	95%
20	0.24	**0.67**	1.11	0.45	**0.94**	1.43
22	0.22	**0.66**	1.09	0.48	**0.96**	1.45
24	0.20	**0.64**	1.08	0.50	**0.99**	1.48
26	0.19	**0.62**	1.06	0.52	**1.01**	1.50
28	0.17	**0.61**	1.04	0.55	**1.03**	1.52
30	0.15	**0.59**	1.02	0.57	**1.06**	1.55
32	0.14	**0.57**	1.01	0.59	**1.08**	1.57
34	0.12	**0.56**	0.99	0.62	**1.10**	1.59
36	0.10	**0.54**	0.97	0.64	**1.13**	1.62
38	0.09	**0.52**	0.96	0.66	**1.15**	1.64
40	0.07	**0.50**	0.94	0.69	**1.18**	1.66
42	0.05	**0.49**	0.92	0.71	**1.20**	1.69

After Arduini, D., Rizzo, G.: Normal values of pulsatility index from fetal vessels: a cross-sectional study on 1556 healthy fetuses. J. Perinat. Med. 18 (1990) 165–172

Renal Artery

Table 53.**54**   Pulsatility index (PI) and resistance index (RI) of the renal artery

Weeks	PI			RI		
	5%	50%	95%	5%	50%	95%
		Percentiles			Percentiles	
20	1.61	2.52	3.43			
21	1.59	2.50	3.41			
22	1.57	2.48	3.39			
23	1.55	2.46	3.36			
24	1.54	2.44	3.34			
25	1.52	2.42	3.32			
26	1.50	2.40	3.29			
27	1.48	2.38	3.27			
28	1.46	2.35	3.25			
29	1.44	2.33	3.23			
30	1.42	2.31	3.20	0.79	0.89	0.99
31	1.40	2.29	3.18	0.79	0.88	0.98
32	1.38	2.27	3.16	0.78	0.88	0.97
33	1.36	2.25	3.14	0.77	0.87	0.97
34	1.34	2.23	3.12	0.77	0.86	0.96
35	1.32	2.21	3.10	0.76	0.86	0.95
36	1.30	2.19	3.08	0.75	0.85	0.95
37	1.28	2.17	3.06	0.75	0.84	0.94
38	1.25	2.15	3.04	0.74	0.84	0.93
39	1.23	2.13	3.02	0.73	0.83	0.93
40	1.21	2.11	3.00	0.73	0.82	0.92
41	1.19	2.08	2.96			

After Arduini, D., Rizzo, G.: Normal values of pulsatility index from fetal vessels: a cross-sectional study on 1556 healthy fetuses. J. Perinat. Med. 18 (1990) 165–172. And after Mai, R., Kristen, P., Rempen, A.: End-diastolic blood flow of the renal artery in normal pregnancy. Ultraschall Klin. Prax. 8 (1994) 232–234

Ductus venosus

Table 53.**55** Peak flow velocity during ventricular systole (S), peak end-diastolic flow velocity (SD), and peak diastolic flow velocity (D) of the ductus venosus (in cm/s)

Weeks	S Mean*	S 90% interval	SD Mean*	SD 90% interval	D Mean*	D 90% interval
14	48.000	(31.478-65.432)	35.479	(23.000-50.114)	41.742	(26.453-57.326)
15	49.458	(32.757-67.080)	37.832	(25.190-52.658)	42.737	(27.286-58.486)
16	51.504	(34.623-69.315)	39.169	(26.364-54.185)	44.526	(28.914-60.440)
17	53.730	(36.669-71.730)	40.154	(27.187-55.362)	46.700	(30.925-62.779)
18	55.904	(38.663-74.093)	40.955	(27.825-56.353)	48.928	(32.991-65.172)
19	57.894	(40.474-76.273)	41.640	(28.347-57.229)	50.994	(34.895-67.402)
20	59.636	(42.037-78.205)	42.245	(28.789-58.025)	52.780	(36.519-69.353)
21	61.108	(42.717-79.866)	42.792	(29.174-58.762)	54.242	(37.819-70.981)
22	62.313	(44.354-81.260)	43.295	(29.514-59.456)	55.385	(38.801-72.289)
23	63.272	(45.134-82.409)	43.763	(29.819-60.115)	56.243	(39.497-73.312)
24	64.016	(45.698-83.342)	44.204	(30.097-60.747)	56.862	(39.953-74.096)
25	64.577	(46.080-84.093)	44.622	(30.353-61.356)	57.291	(40.221-74.690)
26	64.990	(46.312-84.695)	45.022	(30.591-61.947)	57.578	(40.346-75.142)
27	65.284	(46.427-85.178)	45.408	(30.814-62.524)	57.762	(40.368-75.491)
28	65.488	(46.451-85.572)	45.782	(31.025-63.088)	57.875	(40.319-75.769)
29	65.624	(46.408-85.897)	46.146	(31.226-63.643)	57.941	(40.223-76.000)
30	65.712	(46.316-86.175)	46.503	(31.421-64.191)	57.978	(40.098-76.202)
31	65.766	(46.191-86.418)	46.855	(31.610-64.734)	57.997	(39.995-76.386)
32	65.798	(46.043-86.640)	47.204	(31.796-65.273)	58.006	(39.803-76.561)
33	65.816	(45.881-86.847)	47.551	(31.981-65.812)	58.011	(39.645-76.730)
34	65.825	(45.711-87.045)	47.900	(32.166-66.351)	58.012	(39.485-76.897)
35	65.829	(45.536-87.239)	48.251	(32.355-66.893)	58.013	(39.324-77.063)
36	65.831	(45.358-87.431)	48.609	(32.550-67.442)	58.013	(39.162-77.228)
37	65.832	(45.179-87.621)	48.976	(32.755-68.000)	58.013	(39.000-77.393)
38	65.832	(45.000-87.810)	49.359	(32.975-68.573)	58.013	(38.838-77.558)
39	65.832	(44.820-88.000)	49.764	(33.217-69.170)	58.013	(38.676-77.723)
40	65.832	(44.641-88.189)	50.206	(33.496-69.802)	58.013	(38.514-77.888)
41	65.832	(44.461-88.379)	50.711	(33.839-70.498)	58.013	(38.352-78.053)

After Bahlmann, F., Wellek, S., Reinhardt, I., Merz, E., Steiner, E., Welter, C: Reference values of ductus venosus flow velocity waveforms and various calculated waveform indices. Prenat. Diagn. 20 (2000) 623–634

* Smoothed by nonlinear regression

Table 53.**56** Peak flow velocity during atrial contraction (a) and intensity-weighted mean flow velocity (Vmean) of the ductus venosus (in cm/s)

Weeks	a Mean*	a 90% interval	Vmean Mean*	Vmean 90% interval
14	11.165	(1.872-21.571)	18.722	(30.025-41.737)
15	13.753	(4.189-24.462)	21.398	(32.826-44.669)
16	16.274	(6.438-27.286)	23.566	(35.120-47.093)
17	18.637	(8.530-29.953)	25.398	(37.078-49.181)
18	20.815	(10.437-32.434)	26.965	(38.771-51.004)
19	22.799	(12.150-34.721)	28.311	(40.241-52.604)
20	24.589	(13.669-36.815)	29.464	(41.521-54.014)
21	26.191	(15.000-38.720)	30.450	(42.632-55.255)
22	27.612	(16.151-40.445)	31.287	(43.595-56.348)
23	28.864	(17.131-42.000)	31.993	(44.426-57.309)
24	29.956	(17.952-43.395)	32.581	(45.140-58.153)
25	30.900	(18.625-44.643)	33.065	(45.749-58.893)
26	31.709	(19.163-45.756)	33.456	(46.266-59.539)
27	32.394	(19.578-46.745)	33.764	(46.700-60.103)
28	32.968	(19.880-47.622)	34.000	(47.061-60.595)
29	33.443	(20.084-48.400)	34.172	(47.359-61.023)
30	33.829	(20.199-49.089)	34.288	(47.600-61.394)
31	34.137	(20.236-49.701)	34.356	(47.794-61.718)
32	34.379	(20.207-50.247)	34.382	(47.946-62.000)
33	34.564	(20.121-50.735)	34.374	(48.062-62.247)
34	34.702	(19.988-51.176)	34.336	(48.150-62.465)
35	34.800	(19.815-51.578)	34.273	(48.213-62.658)
36	34.868	(19.612-51.949)	34.192	(48.257-62.832)
37	34.911	(19.384-52.296)	34.095	(48.286-62.991)
38	34.937	(19.139-52.626)	33.987	(48.304-63.139)
39	34.951	(18.882-52.943)	33.872	(48.314-63.279)
40	34.957	(18.617-53.253)	33.751	(48.318-63.414)
41	34.959	(18.348-53.558)	33.627	(48.320-63.545)

After Bahlmann, F., Wellek, S., Reinhardt, I., Merz, E., Steiner, E., Welter, C: Reference values of ductus venosus flow velocity waveforms and various calculated waveform indices. Prenat. Diagn. 20 (2000) 623–634

* Smoothed by nonlinear regression

Table 53.**57** Venous indices (S-a)/S, (S-a)/Vmean, and (S-a)/D, calculated from the peak flow velocities of the ductus venosus

Weeks	(S-a)/S Mean*	(S-a)/S 90% interval	(S-a)/Vmean Mean*	(S-a)/Vmean 90% interval	(S-a)/D Mean*	(S-a)/D 90% interval
14	0.766	(0.653-0.888)	1.208	(0.970-1.499)	0.889	(0.738-1.073)
15	0.723	(0.609-0.846)	1.123	(0.885-1.414)	0.843	(0.690-1.029)
16	0.688	(0.573-0.814)	1.054	(0.816-1.346)	0.802	(0.647-0.989)
17	0.659	(0.542-0.786)	0.997	(0.758-1.289)	0.764	(0.609-0.953)
18	0.634	(0.516-0.763)	0.947	(0.708-1.239)	0.731	(0.574-0.922)
19	0.612	(0.492-0.742)	0.904	(0.664-1.197)	0.701	(0.543-0.894)
20	0.592	(0.471-0.724)	0.866	(0.626-1.160)	0.676	(0.516-0.870)
21	0.575	(0.452-0.708)	0.834	(0.594-1.128)	0.653	(0.492-0.849)
22	0.559	(0.435-0.694)	0.806	(0.565-1.100)	0.633	(0.471-0.831)
23	0.546	(0.420-0.682)	0.782	(0.540-1.076)	0.617	(0.453-0.816)
24	0.534	(0.406-0.672)	0.761	(0.519-1.056)	0.602	(0.437-0.803)
25	0.523	(0.394-0.663)	0.743	(0.501-1.039)	0.590	(0.423-0.793)
26	0.514	(0.384-0.655)	0.728	(0.486-1.024)	0.580	(0.412-0.785)
27	0.506	(0.374-0.649)	0.715	(0.472-1.012)	0.572	(0.402-0.778)
28	0.499	(0.366-0.643)	0.704	(0.461-1.001)	0.565	(0.394-0.773)
29	0.493	(0.358-0.639)	0.696	(0.452-0.993)	0.559	(0.387-0.769)
30	0.488	(0.352-0.636)	0.688	(0.445-0.986)	0.555	(0.381-0.766)
31	0.484	(0.346-0.633)	0.683	(0.438-0.981)	0.551	(0.376-0.765)
32	0.480	(0.341-0.631)	0.678	(0.434-0.977)	0.549	(0.372-0.764)
33	0.477	(0.336-0.630)	0.674	(0.430-0.974)	0.547	(0.369-0.763)
34	0.475	(0.333-0.629)	0.672	(0.427-0.971)	0.546	(0.366-0.764)
35	0.473	(0.329-0.629)	0.670	(0.424-0.970)	0.545	(0.364-0.765)
36	0.472	(0.326-0.629)	0.668	(0.423-0.969)	0.544	(0.362-0.766)
37	0.471	(0.324-0.629)	0.668	(0.421-0.969)	0.544	(0.360-0.767)
38	0.470	(0.322-0.630)	0.667	(0.420-0.968)	0.543	(0.358-0.768)
39	0.469	(0.320-0.631)	0.667	(0.420-0.969)	0.543	(0.357-0.770)
40	0.469	(0.318-0.633)	0.667	(0.419-0.969)	0.543	(0.355-0.772)
41	0.469	(0.317-0.634)	0.667	(0.419-0.969)	0.543	(0.354-0.773)

After Bahlmann, F., Wellek, S., Reinhardt, I., Merz, E., Steiner, E., Welter, C: Reference values of ductus venosus flow velocity waveforms and various calculated waveform indices. Prenat. Diagn. 20 (2000) 623–634

* Smoothed by nonlinear regression

Table 53.**58** Venous indices S/D, a/S, and S/a calculated from the peak flow velocities of the ductus venosus

Weeks	S/D Mean*	S/D 90% interval	a/S Mean*	a/S 90% interval	S/a Mean*	S/a 90% interval
14	1.150	(1.066-1.276)	0.234	(0.112-0.347)	4.497	(3.583-5.780)
15	1.148	(1.064-1.276)	0.277	(0.153-0.391)	4.047	(3.153-5.304)
16	1.148	(1.063-1.275)	0.312	(0.186-0.427)	3.641	(2.767-4.871)
17	1.147	(1.062-1.275)	0.341	(0.214-0.458)	3.295	(2.440-4.497)
18	1.146	(1.061-1.275)	0.366	(0.237-0.484)	3.007	(2.171-4.182)
19	1.145	(1.060-1.275)	0.388	(0.258-0.508)	2.771	(1.955-3.919)
20	1.145	(1.059-1.274)	0.408	(0.276-0.529)	2.582	(1.785-3.703)
21	1.144	(1.058-1.274)	0.425	(0.292-0.548)	2.432	(1.654-3.526)
22	1.143	(1.057-1.274)	0.441	(0.306-0.565)	2.315	(1.557-3.381)
23	1.143	(1.056-1.274)	0.454	(0.318-0.580)	2.225	(1.486-3.264)
24	1.142	(1.055-1.274)	0.466	(0.328-0.594)	2.157	(1.437-3.169)
25	1.142	(1.054-1.274)	0.477	(0.337-0.606)	2.107	(1.406-3.092)
26	1.141	(1.053-1.274)	0.486	(0.345-0.616)	2.070	(1.389-3.028)
27	1.141	(1.052-1.274)	0.494	(0.351-0.626)	2.044	(1.382-2.974)
28	1.140	(1.051-1.274)	0.501	(0.357-0.634)	2.025	(1.383-2.929)
29	1.140	(1.051-1.274)	0.507	(0.361-0.642)	2.013	(1.390-2.889)
30	1.139	(1.050-1.274)	0.512	(0.364-0.648)	2.005	(1.401-2.854)
31	1.139	(1.049-1.274)	0.516	(0.367-0.654)	1.999	(1.415-2.821)
32	1.138	(1.048-1.274)	0.520	(0.369-0.659)	1.996	(1.431-2.791)
33	1.138	(1.047-1.274)	0.523	(0.370-0.664)	1.994	(1.449-2.762)
34	1.137	(1.046-1.274)	0.525	(0.371-0.667)	1.993	(1.467-2.734)
35	1.137	(1.046-1.274)	0.527	(0.371-0.671)	1.993	(1.486-2.706)
36	1.136	(1.045-1.274)	0.528	(0.371-0.673)	1.993	(1.505-2.678)
37	1.136	(1.044-1.274)	0.529	(0.371-0.676)	1.992	(1.524-2.651)
38	1.135	(1.043-1.274)	0.530	(0.370-0.678)	1.992	(1.543-2.624)
39	1.134	(1.040-1.274)	0.531	(0.369-0.680)	1.992	(1.563-2.597)
40	1.134	(1.041-1.274)	0.531	(0.367-0.682)	1.992	(1.582-2.570)
41	1.133	(1.040-1.274)	0.531	(0.366-0.683)	1.992	(1.601-2.542)

After Bahlmann, F., Wellek, S., Reinhardt, I., Merz, E., Steiner, E., Welter, C: Reference values of ductus venosus flow velocity waveforms and various calculated waveform indices. Prenat. Diagn. 20 (2000) 623–634

* Smoothed by nonlinear regression

Index

WITHDRAWN

Note: page numbers in *italics* refer to figures and tables. All anatomical terms and conditions refer to the fetus, unless indicated as maternal.

A

A-mode ultrasound 560
abdomen
  abdominal ultrasound 122, *123–125*
  biometry 144–145, *156–158, 596*
  embryology 122, *123*
  growth pattern 27, *31*
  masses
    cystic 129
    differential diagnosis *326*
  ultrasound anatomy 122, *123–125*
  wall defects 10
    ventral 301, *302,* 303–304, *305–306,* 307
abdominal circumference 13, 141
  crown–rump length relationship 27, *31*
  gestational age *582*
    estimation 161, *162*
  growth curves *591*
  head circumference ratio *584*
  mean abdominal diameter *590*
  weight estimation 163, *603–608, 609*
abdominal diameter
  gastroschisis 304, *306*
  mean *590*
  sagittal 141
    gestational age *582*
  transverse 13, 141
    gestational age *582*
    growth curves *591*
abdominal pain, maternal 438, 439, *441, 442*
abdominal pregnancy 41, *42,* 74, 77
abdominal transducer 3, *6*
abdominal ultrasound 3–4, *6–7*
  adnexal masses 77, *78*
  adrenal glands 126, *127*
  choriocarcinoma 68, *73*
  circulatory system 100, *101,* 102, *103–105*
  3-D ultrasound 516–519
  ectopic pregnancy 72, *73*–74, *75–77*
  examination 3
  fetal anomalies 77, *78, 79*
  fetal position 4
  first trimester abnormalities 67–68, *69–72,*
  73–74, 75–77, 78, 79
  genitalia 129, *130–131*
  head 82–83, *84–89*
  heart 106–121
  image orientation 3–4, *7*
  IUD in early pregnancy 68, *70–71*
  limbs 132–133, *134–136*
  molar pregnancy 68, *71*
  pelvimetry 55
  pelvis 126, *128*
  pregnancy detection 60–61, *63–64*
  puerperium 443, *444–445*
  scan planes 4, *7*
  spinal column 90, *91–92*

  thorax 97, *98–99*
  transducer 3, *6*
  transverse scans 4, *7*
  urinary tract 126, *127–128*
  uterine fibroids 77, *78, 79*
abdominometry 141, *148–149*
abortion
  abembryonic 33
  complete 33, *34–35,* 67, 69, 464
  incomplete 33, *35,* 464
  inevitable 33, *34,* 67, *69*
  missed 33, *35,* 36, 68, *70,* 464–465, *466*
    blood flow 459, *460,* 461
  prognostic factors 33
  risk 26
    cervical implantation 60
  spontaneous 32–33
    abdominal ultrasound 67–68, *69–70*
    amniocentesis risk 531
    chorionic villus sampling 534
    fetoscopy 541
    spiral artery abnormal transformation 462
  threatened 32–33, 67, *69*
  tubal 38, *40,* 74, *76*
acardia *429,* 430
acetylcholinesterase (AChE) 253
  epidermolysis bullosa hereditaria 360
achondrogenesis 337, 341, *345*
achondroplasia 337
  3-D ultrasound *526*
  heterozygous 344, *346–347*
  homozygous 344
acidemia, fetal 490, *492*
ACOG (American College of Obstetricians and
Gynecologists) 8
ADAM syndrome *see* amniotic band
sequence/syndrome
adnexal mass 74, *75–76*
  abdominal ultrasound 77, *78*
  benign 49, *52*
  detection in early pregnancy 77, *78*
  malignant 49, *52*
  see also ovarian *entries*
adrenal glands 126, *127*
  biometry 144, *157*
  congenital neuroblastoma *324,* 325–326
  intra-adrenal hemorrhage *324,* 326
  tumors *324,* 325–326
adrenogenital syndrome 545
  clitoral hypertrophy 330, *332*
age
  maternal 416
  see also gestational age
Aicardi syndrome 235
albumin replacement fetal therapy 549, *550*
alcohol abuse 206
  paternal 565
alcohol embryopathy 565

alkaline phosphatase activity 340
allylestrenol, oral maternal 176
alpha fetoprotein (AFP)
  amniotic fluid 10
  gestational age 530–531
  maternal serum 10
    uterine artery waveforms 475
alpha fetoprotein (AFP) assay
  anencephaly 212
  cephalocele 213
  epidermolysis bullosa hereditaria 360
  exencephaly 213
  gastroschisis 304
  iniencephaly 214
  maternal diabetes 178
  omphalocele 303
  spina bifida 253
amelia 349, *350*
American College of Obstetricians and Gynecologists (ACOG) 8
amino acids, intra-amniotic instillation 176
amiodarone fetal therapy 546, *547–548*
amniocentesis 13, 530–531, *532,* 533
  amniotic fluid volume 531
  continuous ultrasound guidance 531, *532*
  cytogenetics 533
  decompression *553,* 555
  duodenal atresia 298
  early 533
  high-risk pregnancy 14
  hypothyroidism 546
  indications 530
  nonviable pregnancy 531
  postprocedure ultrasound 531
  rhesus incompatibility 186
  risks 531, *532*
  serial *553,* 555
  spina bifida 253
  technique 530–531, *532*
  transplacental 531
  twin–twin transfusion syndrome 426–427
amnioinfusion 314, *316,* 540, 541, *553,* 555–556
  autosomal–recessive polycystic kidney disease
  315
  serial 556
amnion, unfused 364, *365, 400,* 401
amnionicity 416, *417*
  assessment in second/third trimester 423, *424*
amnioperitoneal sleeve 304, *306*
amniotic band sequence/syndrome 213, *215, 306,*
307, 401–402
  anencephaly differential diagnosis 212
  body stalk anomaly differential diagnosis 304,
  306
  club foot 353
  exencephaly differential diagnosis 213
  extremity anomalies 336
  pentalogy of Cantrell differential diagnosis 264

amniotic band sequence/syndrome 213, *215, 306,*
307, 401–402
  peromelia 351, *352*
amniotic bands, unfused *400,* 401, *402*
amniotic cavity 19, *24,* 60, *63*
  diameter 27, *29, 579*
  growth pattern 27, *30*
amniotic epithelium 26
amniotic fluid 409–411, *411–413*
  absorption 409
  biophysical profile *171*
  drainage 426–427
  functions 409
  index 410, *412, 601*
  missed abortion *35,* 36
  production 409
  quantification methods 409–410, *411–413*
  swallowing 169
  third screening 13
  volume 11
    abnormal 13, 207, 410–411, *412–413, 553,*
    555–556
      amniocentesis 531
      assessment 409–411, *411–413*
      3-D ultrasound 519
      determination 312
      fetal therapy for abnormal *553,* 555–556
      normal 409
      regulation 409, *411*
      spina bifida detection 253
  see also anhydramnios; oligohydramnios; polyhydramnios
amniotic membrane
  development 18, *22*
  nuchal translucency detection *77,* 78
  separation 531, *532*
amniotic septostomy 555
anal atresia *299,* 300, 321
anasarca 359
anemia
  cordocentesis diagnosis 538
  fetal 12
  fetal therapy 548
  intracardiac transfusion 549, *550*
  nonimmune hydrops 191
  rhesus incompatibility 501, *502,* 503
anencephaly 212, *214*
  chromosomal abnormalities 370
  detection 10, 11
    first trimester 45, *47*
  diagnosis 208
  exencephaly differential diagnosis 213
  fetal movement 12, 208
  microcephaly differential diagnosis 225
Angelman syndrome 568
angiography, color power 120, *121*
anhydramnios 208, *211,* 312, *313,* 410–411, *413*
  amnioinfusion *553,* 555–556
  causes 411
  multicystic dysplastic kidneys 318
  Potter sequence 314
  umbilical cord coiling 484
anti-D prophylaxis 184, 208
  amniocentesis 531
  cordocentesis 537
anticoagulant medication 565

anticonvulsants 212, 370
aorta 107
  ascending 100, *103*
  coarctation 278, 280, *282*
  color Doppler 112, *117*
  descending 102, *103–104, 109,* 111
    anemia 501, *502*
    arrhythmia evaluation 497, *500*
    blood flow classes 488
    blood flow quantitative analysis 484
    Doppler ultrasound 484, *486–487,* 488, 497,
    500, 614
      end-diastolic flow *487,* 488
      pulsatility index *487,* 488
      resistance index *487,* 488
  dextroposition 112
  diameter 144, *155, 595*
  embryo 462, *463*
  end-diastolic flow
    absent 507, 508–511, *512*
    reverse 508–511, *512*
  origin *108, 110,* 112
  overriding *273*
    tetralogy of Fallot *283,* 284
  reverse flow 507
  stenosis 278, *279,* 491, *494*
  vascular caliber 112
aortic arch 102, *103, 108, 110,* 112
  anomalies 278, 280, *282*
  course *117,* 118
  hypoplasia *273,* 278
aortic valve 113
aortocerebral ratio *615*
aqueductal stenosis 218, *228*
arachnoid cyst 220–221, *230*
  agenesis of corpus callosum differential diagnosis 221
araphia 253
arcadius acranius, laser treatment 554
Arnold–Chiari malformation 222–223, *231–232*
  type II 254, *260*
arrhinencephaly 235, *239*
arrhinia 235, *239*
arrhythmias *see* cardiac arrhythmias
arteriovenous shunts 190
arthrogryposis multiplex congenita 12, 208, 353,
354, 355
  camptodactyly 353, *354*
  club foot *338*
  forms 353
aryepiglottis 93
ascites, fetal 194–195, *195, 196, 197*
  3-D ultrasound *525*
  needle aspiration 549
  percutaneous aspiration 539, *540,* 549
  see also urinary ascites
asphyxia 171
  detection with cordocentesis 538
aspiration, amniotic fluid regulation 409
aspirin therapy in preeclampsia 474–475
asplenia syndrome *see* isomerism
assisted reproductive technologies 416
atrial extrasystole, blocked *291,* 292
atrial fibrillation 501, *502*
atrial flutter 293, *295,* 501, *502*
  fetal therapy 546

atrial natriuretic peptide (ANP) 189
atrial septal defect 280, *282–283*
atrial septum *109,* 111
atrioventricular block, second-/third-degree
292–293, *295*
atrioventricular canal 281, *283,* 284
  complete *283,* 284
  karyotyping 380
  STIC technique *527*
atrioventricular concordance 107
atrioventricular septal defect 281, *283,* 284
atrioventricular valve 114, *115*
auricle *see* ear
auricular root 83, *89*
  anomalies 238, *241*
autonomy 572–573
axillary vessels *104*

B

B-mode ultrasound
  aortic stenosis 278, *279*
  atrial septal defect 280, *282*
  atrioventricular septal defect 281, *283,* 284
  cardiac biometry 113
  coarctation of aorta 280
  descending aorta 484, *486–487,* 488
  DORV 285, *287*
  fetal breathing 97
  heart 106, *108–109*
  heterotaxia syndromes 286, *288,* 289, *291*
  hypoplastic left heart syndrome *276, 277, 279*
  IUGR 497
  neck structures 93–94
  placental insufficiency 497
  procedure 454
  pulmonary atresia *274,* 275
  pulmonary stenosis 277
  risk assessment 560
  tetralogy of Fallot *283,* 284
  total/partial anomalous pulmonary venous
  return 289–290, *291*
  transposition of the great arteries 285, 286,
  287
  tricuspid atresia 273, *274*
  tricuspid dysplasia 275
  truncus arteriosus 286
  ventricular septal defects 281, *282*
bag sign 200, *201*
Ballantyne syndrome 193
banana sign 12, *16*
  Arnold–Chiari malformation 222, *231*
  spina bifida 255
Bart hemoglobin 191
Beckwith–Wiedemann syndrome
  macroglossia 237
  omphalocele 303
behavior, fetal 168–172, *173*
  states 170–171, *173*
Belgian Multicenter Study 9
beta mimetics 475
betamethasone
  fetal behavior 171
  fetal lung maturation 545
biliary anomaly, intrahepatic 315

biliary dysgenesis 315
biometry
  abdomen 144–145, *156–158*
  abdominometry 141, *148–149*
  amniotic cavity diameter 27, *29, 579*
  basic 140–142, *147–150*
  bone 145–146, *158–159*
  documentation 140
  equipment settings 139
  extended 142–146, *151–159*
  first trimester 61–62, *66*
    gestational age *579–581*
  gestational age 139
    first trimester *579–581*
    second/third trimesters *582–601*
  growth charts 140
  growth disturbances 175, *179*
  head 142–143, *151–153*
  heart 113
  indications 139
  neck 142–143, *151–153*
    structures 94, *96*
  organ 142–146, *151–159*
  pelvis 144–145, *156–158*
  placenta 389, *391*
    abnormal 393, *396, 397, 398*
  points 139–140
  prerequisites 139–140
  reference plane 140, 141
    defining 139
  second/third trimesters 139–159
    gestational age *582–601*
  serial 13
  skeletal 141–142, *149–150*
  synopsis *578*
  thorax 143–144, *154–155*
  transvaginal 26–28, *29–31*
  umbilical cord 404, *407*
  see also biparietal diameter (BPD); cephalometry; crown–rump length; *specific organs*
biophysical profile 171
biotin fetal therapy 545
biparietal diameter (BPD) 9, 13, 27, *29, 31,*
140–141
  11th week of menstrual age 19, *24*
  crown–rump length relationship 27
  gestational age 28, *31, 580, 581, 582, 602*
    estimation 161, *162*
  growth curves 140–141, *148, 591*
  head circumference *585–590*
  outer-to-inner/outer-to-outer 139
  pelvimetry true conjugate 56
  weight estimation 163, *603–608*
birth
  circulatory system changes 100
  length 163, *166, 611*
birth weight 163, *166, 611*
  neonatal mortality 163
  twins *612*
blastopathies 204
blood flow, antegrade/retrograde 448
blood group determination 538
blood loss, fetal 191
blood transfusion
  intra-abdominal for rhesus incompatibility
  549

intracardiac for anemia 549, *550*
intrauterine
  intravascular 503, *550*
    ultrasound guidance *550*
  intravascular via cordocentesis 548
  nonimmune fetal hydrops 549
  planning 538
blood vessels, development 19, *25*
body contour, abnormal 208, *211*
body parameters, third ultrasound screening 13
body stalk anomaly 304, *306*
bone(s)
  biometry 145–146, *158–159*
  cartilaginous epiphyses 132, *133*
  disorders 142
  fractures in osteogenesis imperfecta 343, 344,
  346–347
  length and gestational age *583*
  long tubular 132, *133*
    measurement 141–142, *149–150*
  mineralization and pulsed Doppler *561*
  tissue 132
Bourneville–Pringle disease 190
  nonimmune hydrops 193
bowel
  biometry 144, *157*
  congenital closure of segment 297
  embryology 122
  hyperechoic structure *366*, 367
  loop
    extrusion 303–304, *305–306*
    floating 304, *305*
  ultrasound anatomy 122, *125*
brachial artery *104*
brachial palsy 163
brachiocephalic trunk 93, *96*
brachycephaly 225
bradyarrhythmias 292–293
  fetal anomalies *211*
  management *294*
  nonimmune hydrops 190
  severe 501, *502*
brain
  anatomy 82, 83, *84, 86, 87, 88*
  development 18, *21–22, 23*
  embryology 81
  malformations in Mohr syndrome 236
  mantle 83, *89*
brain death syndrome, intrauterine 171, *173*
brain-sparing effect
  cerebral vessels 490–491, *492*
  hypoxemia 490
  neuromotor development 509
branchiogenic cyst 248, *251*
breathing 83, *87, 94, 96, 97, 99*
  movements 168–169
    biophysical profile *171*
    end-diastolic flow 508
breech presentation 3–4, *7*
  fetal–pelvic index 55
  head shape 13, 82, *84*
  spina bifida detection 253
  third screening 13
bronchogenic cyst 262–263, *266*
  CCAM differential diagnosis 262
bubble sign *201*

C

calcaneus, rocker-bottom foot 353, *354*
calcification
  hepatic 307, *308*
  intra-abdominal 382, *384*
  intracranial
    cytomegalovirus 380
    neoplasms 223
  meconium peritonitis 301
  sacrococcygeal teratoma 333
calcium antagonists 476
calvaria
  hypomineralization *339*, 340
  ossification defect *526*
  osteogenesis imperfecta 343, 344, *347*
Campbell–Wilkin formula for weight estimation
164
camptodactyly 353, *354*
  Pena–Shokeir syndrome 355
camptomelic dysplasia *338*, 343
  hermaphroditism 329, *331*
carboxylase deficiency, multiple 545
cardiac apex 111
cardiac arrhythmias 118, *119*, 290, *291*, 292–293,
294–295
  classification 490
  descending aorta Doppler tracing 497, *500*
  diagnosis 490
  differential diagnosis 292
  Doppler ultrasound 501, *502*
  fetal therapy 550
  heart defects 208
  inferior vena cava Doppler tracing 497, *500*
  nonimmune hydrops 190, *197*
  see also specific arrhythmias
cardiac axis 111
cardiac compensation, TRAP sequence 430
cardiac output 143
cardiac preload 497, *499–500, 502*
cardiac preset 106
cardiac rhythm 111
cardiac volume overload 190
cardiomegaly 113
  Coxsackie infection 378
cardiomyopathy 118
  dilatative 278, *279*, 290
  hypertrophic 290
  nonimmune hydrops 190, *197*
cardiothoracic (CT) ratio 113, 144, *155*
cardiotocography 169
Carnegie classification 17
carotid artery
  common 93, 488
    Doppler ultrasound 490, *492*
  internal 462, 488
    brain-sparing effect 490
    Doppler ultrasound *489*, 490
inferior regression syndrome
  diabetes mellitus 178
  sirenomelia 351
cavitation 561, *562*
cavum septi pellucidi 82, 83, *85, 86, 89*
  biometry 142, *151, 152, 592*
cebocephaly 235, *239*

central nervous system (CNS)
anomalies 217–226, *227–233*
chromosomal abnormalities 370
cephalic presentation 3, *7*
cephalocele 213, *215–216*
cephalometry 46, 140–141, *147–148*
cephalopelvic disproportion 55
prediction 56
cephalothoracopagus *429, 431*
cerebellar artery, superior 490
cerebellar diameter, transverse 142, *151, 152*
gestational age estimation 161, *592, 602*
cerebellum
biometry 142, *151, 152*
bowing 12, *16*
ultrasound anatomy 82, 83, *86, 89*
cerebral arteries 462, *463*
anterior 490
brain-sparing effect 490–491, *492*
Doppler ultrasound *487*, 488, *489*, 490–491, *492*
end-diastolic flow *489*, 490
frequency spectrum recording 488, *489*
middle 488–489, *492*
anemia 501
arteriovenous malformations 491, *492*
brain-sparing effect 490, *492*
cerebroplacental ratio 490
Doppler ultrasound *614*
resistance indices predictive value 490–491
pulsatility index *489*, 490
resistance index *489*, 490
cerebral arteriovenous malformations 491, *492*
cerebral autoregulation loss 490, *492*
cerebral blood flow 102, *103*, 488
cerebral dysfunction, cavum septi pellucidi size 142
cerebral hemispheres
biometry 142, *151–152*
development 18, *24*
ultrasound anatomy 82, *84, 86, 88*
cerebral hemorrhage
absent end-diastolic flow 510
intrauterine 223, *232*
premature labor 491
cerebral ventricles 83, *88*
biometry 142, *151*
dilatation *366*, 367
lateral 82, 83, *83, 84, 89*
biometry 142, *151*
cerebral ventricular–hemispheric ratio 142, *151, 152*
hydrocephalus 217
cerebral ventriculomegaly 376
hydrocephalus 381, *384*
cerebro-oculofacioskeletal (COFS) syndrome 353
cerebromedullary cistern 83, *89*
cerebroplacental ratio 490
cervical carcinoma 49, *52*
cervical cerclage 50
cervical incompetence 14, 438, *439*
diagnosis 49–50, *52–53*
cervical os, internal 2
cervical pregnancy 38, 41, *42*, 74, *76*
cervical vessels 93
cervix

anatomy 49
length 438
opening 50, *53*
palpation 50
physiology 49
shortening 50
ultrasound 50, *52–53*
cesarean section
follow-up 443, *445*
intrauterine death of one twin 427
champagne-cork phenomenon 337, *338*, 342, *345*
chemotherapy monitoring 465
chickenpox *see* varicella syndrome
cholecystolithiasis 438, *441*
choledochal cysts *308*, 309
chondrodysplasia punctata
anticoagulant medication 565
Conradi–Hünermann type 348
embryopathica 348
nonfatal 340
rhizomelic type *338*, 340–341, *345*
X-linked dominant 360
chondroectodermal dysplasia *see* Ellis–van Creveld syndrome
choriocarcinoma 36, *37*, 68, *72, 73*
abdominal ultrasound 68, *73*
chorion, unfused 364, *365, 400*, 401
chorion frondosum *17*, 388, 458
chorionic villus sampling 533–534
chorion laeve 60
chorion villus sampling
chondrodysplasia punctata 341
rhesus incompatibility 186
chorionic cavity 60, *63–64*
diameter *579, 580*
chorionic sac *17, 20*
detection 26
growth rate 26, *30*
mean diameter 26, *29*
gestational age 28
missed abortion *35*, 36
chorionic villus sampling 13, *532*, 533–534, *535*
high-risk pregnancy 14
problems 534
risks 534
technique *532*, 533–534, *535*
chorionicity 416, *417*, 418
assessment in second/third trimester 423
chorioretinitis 380
choroid plexus 18, *22*
blood flow 462
cyst 221–222, *231*
chromosomal abnormalities 364, *365*
ultrasound anatomy 82, 83, *83, 84, 89*
chromosomal abnormalities 205
3-D ultrasound 520
empty gestational sac 33
genetic counseling 566, *570*
growth retardation 381
high-risk pregnancy 14
multiple pregnancies *421*, 423
nonimmune hydrops 190
nuchal translucency 10–11, *16*, 78, 363–364, *365*
trisomy 45, 78
phenotypic expression *368*, 371, *372*
proportional growth retardation 12, 176

renal anomalies *320*, 321
spina bifida 255
twins 427, 430
ultrasound suggestive signs 363–372
16–24 weeks 364, *365–366*, 367
abdominal wall 371
borderline dilatations *366*, 367
early 363–364, *365*
gastrointestinal tract 371
limbs *366, 368*, 369
pelvic bones *366, 368*, 369
placental 369
specific 370–371
umbilical cord *368*, 369
urogenital system 371
chromosome analysis, abortion products 32
chyloperitoneum 194
chylothorax 192, *196, 197*, 261–262, *265*
percutaneous drainage 549, *550*
percutaneous procedures 539, *540*
shunt procedures 551
cine loop 106
heart biometry 143, *154*
circle of Willis *487*, 488, *489*, 490
circulation/circulatory system 100, *101*, 102, *103–105*, 481–503
arterial system 481–496
changes at birth 100
embryology 100, *101*
hyperdynamic 501
physiology 481, *482*
shunts 481
streamlining of blood flow 481
ultrasound anatomy 100, 102, *103–105*
venous system 495, *496*, 497, *498–500*
cisterna magna 82, *86*
biometry 142, *151, 152, 592*
obliteration 222, *232*
clavicles 97, *98*
biometry 145, *158, 599*
ossification 347, *349*
cleft lip/palate 83, 236–237, *240–241*
chromosomal abnormalities 370
differential diagnosis *339*
intrauterine surgery 554
syndromes *567*
clefts, dorsal/ventral, 3-D ultrasound 518, *524–525*
cleidocranial dysplasia 145, *347*, 348–349
clinodactyly 353, *354*
clitoris 129, *131*
hypertrophy 330, *332*
cloaca
malformation 319
persistent 321
clotting factors 538
cloverleaf skull 224, *232*
differential diagnosis *339*
thanatophoric dysplasia 341, *346*
coagulation disorders 202
coagulation tests, maternal 427
coagulopathy
fetal 538
maternal 427
coarctation of aorta 278, 280, *282*
collodion baby 360

colon
  atresia 298, *299*, 300
  diameter *596*
  loops 144, *157*
color Doppler 280, *282*, 289, *291*, 449, *450*
  aliasing 116, *450*, 451
  aorta 112, *117*
  aortic stenosis 278, *279*
  atrioventricular septal defect *283*, 284
  blighted ovum 464
  chemotherapy monitoring 465
  circulatory system 100, 102, *103–105*
  coarctation of aorta 280
  color encoding 449, *450*
  DORV 285, *287*
  early pregnancy loss 464–465, *466*
  echocardiography 116, *117*, 118, *119*
  equipment settings 449
  great vessels 112, *117*
  hypoplastic left heart syndrome 277, *279*
  intervillous blood flow 459, *460*, 461
  M-mode 118, *119*
  molar pregnancy 36, *37*
  neck structures 94
  power 120, *121*
  pulmonary atresia *274*, 275
  pulmonary stenosis *276*, 277
  pulmonary trunk 112, *117*
  tetralogy of Fallot *283*, 284
  total/partial anomalous pulmonary venous
  return 290, *291*
  transposition of the great arteries 285, 286,
  287
  transvaginal ultrasound 458
  tricuspid atresia 273, *274*
  tricuspid dysplasia 275
  truncus arteriosus 286
  twin–twin transfusion syndrome 426, *428*
  umbilical artery *482*
  umbilical vein *482*
  ventricular septal defects 281, *282*
  yolk sac blood flow *460*, 461
complete congenital heart block 292–293, *295*
computed tomography (CT), pelvimetry 56
conception 60
conceptual age 17
condition, fetal 171
congenital cystic adenomatoid malformation
(CCAM) 192, 262, *265–266*
  chromosomal abnormalities 370
congenital high airway obstruction syndrome
(CHAOS) 192, 249
Conradi–Hünermann disease 340, 348
continuous-wave Doppler 449
contrast agents 561
cordocentesis *535*, 536–539
  blood disease diagnosis 538
  complications *536*, 539
  fetal therapy 548–549
  high-risk pregnancy 14
  hydrocephalus diagnosis 381
  hyperthyroidism 546
  hypothyroidism 546
  indications *536*, 537–538
  infection diagnosis 537–538
  karyotyping 537

placenta location 537
rhesus incompatibility 185–186
risks *536*, 539
technique *535*, 536–537
thrombocytopenia fetal therapy 548–549
umbilical artery 537
umbilical vein *535*, 537
umbilical waveforms 483
Cornelia de Lange syndrome 237
corpus callosum 83, *87*, *89*
  agenesis 221, *230*
    arachnoid cyst differential diagnosis 221
    chromosomal abnormalities 370
corpus luteum cyst *77*, 78
corpus luteum of pregnancy 61, *64*, *65*
cortex 82, *83*, *84*
corticosteroids
  fetal behavior 171
  toxoplasmosis 376
counseling
  aims 564–565
  chromosomal abnormalities 566, *570*
  fetal anomalies
    genetic 564–568, *569–571*
    prenatal diagnosis 208
  genetic syndromes/associations/sequences
  567–568
  imprinting 568
  invasive prenatal diagnosis 530
  key questions 564–565
  monogenic hereditary disorders 566–567, *571*
  recurrence risk estimation 565
  risk 568
  specific disorders 565–568
Coxsackie infection 378
  pericardial effusion 382, *384*
superior bones 81, *83*
  sutures *526*
superior roentgen signs 200, *201*
cranium concavities *16*
critical periods
  fetal anomalies 204
  limb defects 565, *569*
Crohn's disease, maternal 565
crown–rump length 9, 27, *29*, *30*
  abdomen circumference relationship 27, *31*
  biometry *580*
  biparietal diameter relationship 27
  femur length relationship 28, *31*
  first trimester 62, *66*
  gestational age 28, *31*, *580*, *581*
  growth curves 62, *66*
cyclopia 235
cystic adenomatoid malformation 551
  intrauterine surgery 554
cystic fibrosis 300
  hyperechoic bowel structure 367
cystic hygroma 246–247, *250*
  chromosome disorders 364, *365*, 381, *383*
  detection 45, *47*, 208
  nonimmune hydrops 190, 192
  unfused amnion and chorion 364
cystic masses, intrafetal 12, 208
cystoma, ovarian *77*, 78
cytogenetics
  amniocentesis 533

chorionic villus sampling 534
  placental biopsy 534
cytomegalovirus (CMV) 206, 380–381
  cordocentesis 537
  diagnosis 381
  growth retardation 381
  hepatomegaly 382
  hyperechoic bowel structure 367
  intraperitoneal calcifications 382
  microcephaly 380, 382
  nonimmune hydrops 191
cytotrophoblastic plugs 458

D

4-D imaging 519, 520, *527*
3-D ultrasound
  capabilities 516
  cardiac diagnosis 520
  Cartesian storage 519, *526–527*
  chromosomal abnormalities 520
  data acquisition 516–517, *521*
  digital storage 519
  electronic scalpel 519, *525*, *527*
  external system 517, *521*
  fetal anomalies 520
  glass body rendering 518, *526*
  image
    animation 518–519, *526*
    digital storage 519
    processing 519, *526–527*
    quality 519
  internal system 517, *521*
  motion artifacts 519–520, *527*
  multiplanar display 517, *521*
  prenatal diagnosis 516–520, *521–527*
  problems 519–520, *527*
  surface rendering 518, *521–525*
  techniques 516–519
  transparent mode 518, *526*
  visualization 517–519, *521–527*
  volume
    analysis 519, *526–527*
    data storing 516
    digital storage 519
  weight estimation 165
Dandy–Walker malformation 142, 222, *231*
  arachnoid cyst differential diagnosis 221
  posterior fossa cyst differential diagnosis *366*,
  367
death, intrauterine 200, *201*, 202, 424
  causes 200
  cerebral autoregulation loss 490
  complications 427
  end-diastolic flow, reverse/absent 511
  fetal Doppler use 481, *482*
  management 427
  multiple pregnancy 202
  one of twins 427, *428*
  ultrasound detection 200, *201*
death, maternal with ectopic pregnancy 73
decidua, trophoblast invasion 462
deglutition 94
DEGUM (German Society for Ultrasound in Medicine) 8

delivery
  arthrogryposis multiplex congenita 355
  gastroschisis 304
  intrauterine death of one twin 427
  omphalocele 303
  sacrococcygeal teratoma 334
dermoid cyst
  facial 236, *240*
  ovarian *77*, 78
dexamethasone
  adrenogenital syndrome 545
  fetal behavior 171
  fetal lung maturation 545
dextro-transposition of the great arteries (D-TGA) 285, *287–288*
dextrocardia 208
diabetes mellitus
  disproportional IUGR 176
  maternal 370
    macrosomia 177–178, *182*
  polyhydramnios *413*
  teratogenic effect 206
diaphragm 97, *99*
diaphragmatic hernia 208, 263–264, *267*
  bronchogenic cyst differential diagnosis 262–263, *266*
  chromosomal abnormalities 371
  intrauterine surgery *553*, 554
  polyhydramnios *413*
diastolic blood flow, ductus arteriosus 491
diastolic notch
  persistent 471, *472*, 477
  physiologic 471, *472*
diastrophic dysplasia *347*, 348
dicoumarin 348
diencephalon 81
digitalization, maternal 549
digoxin 293, *295*
  fetal therapy 546, *547–548*, 550
dihydralazine 476
diphenylhydantoin 336
disseminated intravascular coagulation (DIC) 427
dolichocephaly 13, 82, *84*, 225, *233*
  camptomelic syndrome 343
  head circumference 140, *147*
  IUGR erroneous diagnosis 177, *181*
Doppler effect 448
Doppler gain 451, *452*
Doppler shift 448
Doppler ultrasound
  aliasing 113, 116, *450*, 451
  arrhythmias 501, *502*
  arterial system 481–496
  cerebral arteries 487, 488, *489*, 490–491, *492*
    middle *614*
  color filter *453*, 454
  color gain 451, *452*
  common carotid artery 490, *492*
  concepts 448–449
  descending aorta 484, *486–487*, 488, *614*
  development 448
  ductus venosus 495, *496*, 497, *498–500*, 616
  equipment-related factors 449, *450*, 451, *452–453*, 454
  examination procedure 454

examination technique effects on spectrum *453*, 454–455
  fetal factors *453*, 454–455
  fetoplacental unit 509–511
  flow profile 451, *452*
  frequency spectrum *453*, 454
  high-risk pregnancy 507
  hydrops 501
  indications 497, *500*, 501, *502*, 503
  inferior vena cava 497, *500*
  insonation angle 451, *452–453*, 454
  instrument settings 454, 469
  internal carotid artery *489*, 490
  intracardiac waveforms 451, *453*
  intrauterine growth retardation 473, 477
  jugular vein 490, *492*
  maternal factors 454
  multiple pregnancies 501, *502*
  preeclampsia 473–474
  principles 448–457
  pulmonary arteries 491, *492*, 494
  pulmonary veins 491, *494*
  pulse repetition frequency 449, 451
  renal artery *615*
  resistance indices 448
  risk assessment 561
  sacrococcygeal teratoma 501
  sample volume 451, *452*, 469, 471
  techniques 449
  third screening 13
  transducer handling 469
  twin–twin transfusion syndrome 426
  umbilical arteries 481, *482*, 483–484, *613*
    velocimetry 483, *485*, *486*
  umbilical vein 495, *496*, 497, *498*, *500*
  uterine artery 469, *470*, 471, 476, 477, *613*
    screening 476
  uteroplacental circulation 469, *470*, 471
  variance encoding *450*, 451
  vein of Galen aneurysm 501
  venous system 495, *496*, 497, *498–500*
  wall filter setting *453*, 454
double bubble sign 298, *299*, 371
double-outlet right ventricle (DORV) 275, 284–285, *287*
  karyotyping 380
Down syndrome *see* trisomy 21
dropout effect 281
ductus arteriosus 100, *103*
  constriction 190
  Doppler flow measurement 114, *115*, 491, 493, *494*
  premature closure 190
  pulmonary atresia 275
  pulsatility index 491
  systolic blood flow 491
ductus venosus 100, *101*, *102*
  anemia 501, *502*
  Doppler flow measurement 114, *115*
  Doppler ultrasound 495, *496*, 497, *498–500*, 616
  frequency spectrum 495, *496*, 497, *498*
  shunt 481
duodenal atresia 297–298, *299*
  chromosomal abnormalities 371
dwarfism 177, *181*

achondrogenesis 341, *345*
  differential diagnosis *338*, 344, *346*
  growth disproportion 208
  mesomelic 343
  rhizomelic type chondrodysplasia punctata 340
  thanatophoric 208
  thanatophoric dysplasia 341, *345–346*
dysmelia 349
dysraphia 253
dystrophy 509–510

E

ear 82, 83, *86*, *88*
  anomalies 238, *241*
  auricular tag 238
  development 82
  length 143, *153*
  see also auricular root
Ebstein anomaly 275, *276*, 277, 382
  fetal hydrops 381, *383*
echocardiography, fetal 14, 270–271
  color Doppler 116, *117*, 118, *119*
  4-D 519, *527*
  M-mode scanning 118, *119*
  planes 107, *108*, *109*
  power color Doppler 120, *121*
  scan planes 106–107, *108–110*, 111–112
  transvaginal ultrasound 118, *119*, 120
  see also spectral Doppler echocardiography; tissue Doppler echocardiography
ectopia cordis 264, *267*
ectopic pregnancy 2, 36, 38, *39*
  abdominal 41, *42*, 74, 77
  abdominal ultrasound 72, 73–74, *75–77*
    role 74, 77
  causes 36
  cervical 38, 41, *42*, 74, 76
  conservative treatment 41, *42–43*
  detection *72*, 73, 75
    rate 36, 38
  diagnosis 36, 73
  diagnostic management 38, *40*
  frequency 73
  β-hCG test 73, *76*
  incidence 36
  indirect signs 38, *39*
  interstitial 38, *42*, 74
  location 73
  methotrexate transvaginal instillation 38, 41, *42–43*
  ovarian 41, *42*
  signs 73
  sites 36, *39*
  ultrasound detection 38
ectromelia 349, *350*, 351, *352*
Edwards syndrome *see* trisomy 18
electronic scalpel 519, *525*, *527*
Ellis–van Creveld syndrome *347*, 348
  short rib–polydactyly syndrome differential diagnosis 343
embryo/embryo development 61, *63–64*
  C-shaped 18, *20–21*
  Carnegie classification 17
  early circulation 462, *463*

first trimester 61, *64*
heart activity detection 61, *64*
maximum length 27, *29*
menstrual age
5th week 17, *20*
6th week 17–18, *20*
7th week 18, *20–21*
8th week 18, *21–22*
9th week 18, *22–23*
10th week 18–19, *23–24*
movement detection 61
vessel examination 462
embryology
circulatory system 100, *101*
esophagus 93
head 81–82, *83*
principles 60
spinal column 90, *91*
ultrasound 17–19, *20–25*
embryonic disk development 60
embryopathies 204, 206
radiation 206–207
embryotoxic insult 204
encephalocele 213, *215*
enchondral ossification 132
defect 341
end-diastolic flow
abnormal umbilical waveform 483, *485–486*
absent 483, *485*, 507, 508, *512*
diagnosis 508, *512*
neuromotor development 508–511, *512*
obstetric management 511
breathing movements 508
carotid arteries 488
cerebral arteries *489*, 490
descending aorta *487*, 488
gestational age 508
reappearance of positive 510
reverse 483, 507, 508, *512*
neuromotor development 508
obstetric management 511
pathoanatomic changes 507–508
umbilical artery *485*, 501
reference range *485*
endocardial fibroelastosis 118, 278, *279*
endometrium, implantation 458
endovaginal scanners 55
endovasculitis, hemorrhagic 193
enteropathic cytopathic human orphan (ECHO)
viruses 378
environmental factors
fetal anomalies 207
multifactorial inheritance 567, *571*
enzyme deficiencies 191
epidermolysis bullosa hereditaria 360, *361*
fetoscopy 539
epiglottis 93, *95*
epignathus 237, *241, 431*
epilepsy, maternal 565
erythema infectiosum 191, 376–377
see also parvovirus B19 infection
esophageal atresia 169, 248, *251–252*, 297, *299*
chromosomal abnormalities 371
esophagus 93
ethics 572–575
fetal therapy 575

medical experimentation 575
prenatal diagnosis 575
principles 572–575
right to life 573–574
value system 572
ethyl alcohol
limb malformations 336
see also alcohol abuse
EUROCAT (European Union Registry of Congenital Anomalies and Twins) 8, 204
eutrophic fetus 411
eventration 304, *306*, 307
exencephaly 212–213, *215*
anencephaly differential diagnosis 212
chromosomal abnormalities 370
microcephaly differential diagnosis 225
exogenous agents
extremity anomalies 336
proportional IUGR 176
expiration 94, *96*
extra-amniotic coelom 19, *24*
extrasystoles *291*, 292
extremities, anomalies 336–355
exogenous agents 336
genetic defects 336
limb defects 349, *350*, 351, *352*, 353, *354*, 355
osteochondrodysplasias *336*, 337, *338*,
339–344, *345–347*, 348–349
eyes
anatomy 83, *89*
anomalies 370
development 81
movements 83, 169

F

face embryology 81–82
facial anomalies 234–238, *239–241*, 370
3-D ultrasound 518, *524*
facial cleft anomalies 236–238, *240–241*, 370
facial profile
11th week of menstrual age 19, *24*
12th week 19, *25*
13th week 19, *25*
second/third trimesters 82–83, *86–87*
facial region tumors 235–236, *239–240*
epignathus 237, *241*
facial skeleton development 18, *24*
fallopian tube
intact 72, 74, *76*
rupture 38, *40*, 74, *76*
falx cerebri 18, *24*, 82
family history 565
fat, body 165
fatal multiple pterygium syndrome 246
favism 191
femoral artery *105*
vascular resistance 493, *496*
femoral circumflex artery *105*
femur 132, *133–134*
biometrics 141–142, *149, 150*
gestational age estimation *602*
fracture *338*
length 27–28, *31*
crown–rump length relationship 28, *31*

dwarfism *181*
gestational age estimation 161, *162*
growth curves *591*
ossification centers 132, *133, 134*
shortening 369
heterozygous achondroplasia 344, *346, 347*
femur–fibula–ulna syndrome 349, 351
femur–foot ratio 145, *158*, 337, *338*
fetal abnormalities, late-onset 13
fetal alcohol syndrome, cystic hygroma 246
fetal anomalies 2
3-D ultrasound 520
cardiac biometry 113
critical periods 204, 565, *569*
definition 204
detection 204–209, *207–208, 211*
before 24 weeks 9
first trimester 45–46, *47, 77, 78, 79*
rate 9
second screening 11
second trimester 46, *48*
third trimester 46, *48*
diabetes mellitus 178
diagnostic windows 207
early detection 10
multiple pregnancies 423
embryotoxic insult 204
environmental factors 207
equivocal findings 45–46, *47*
etiologic classification 205
exogenous cause 206
genetic causes 205–206, 565, *569*
genetic counseling 564–568, *569–571*
growth discordance 424
high-risk pregnancy 14
incidence 8, 207
incompatible with life 208
intrauterine treatment 208
likelihood of postnatal survival 208
limited postnatal survival 207–208
major 78, 204
minor 204
morphogenetic classification 205
multifactorial cause 206, 207
multifactorial inheritance 567
multiple 205
neonatal management 208
obstetric management 208
oligohydramnios 411
ontogenic classification 204
parvovirus B19 377
prenatal diagnosis counseling 208
prenatal screening 8–9
proportional IUGR 176
recurrence risk 208
estimation 565
structural defects 11
suggestive signs 208–209
teratogenic insult 204
three-level concept 8
transvaginal detection 45–46, *47–48*
treatable after birth 208
twins *427, 428–429*, 430, *431*, 432
ultrasound diagnosis 207–208
undetectable 208
see also specific organs and regions

fetal indication 574
fetal membranes
    retained 443
    rupture 531
fetal pole 17, *20*
fetal therapy
    direct 545, 548–549, *550*, 551, *552–553*,
        554–555
        cordocentesis 548–549
        laser treatment 551, *552*, 554
        percutaneous procedures 549, *550*, 551, *552*
        shunt procedures 551, *552*
    ethics 575
    indirect 544, 545–546, *547–548*
    prerequisites 544
    surgery *553*, 554–555, *555*
    see also amnioinfusion
fetal–pelvic index 55
fetocide, selective 575
fetofetal syndrome *see* twin–twin transfusion
syndrome
fetofetal vascular anastomoses *417*, 418
fetomaternal transfusion 191
fetopathies 204
fetoplacental unit, Doppler ultrasound 509–511
fetoscopy 539, *540*, 541
    high-risk pregnancy 14
fetus
    abnormal structures 12
    autonomy 573
    brain structures 2
    development
        11th week 19, *24*
        12th week 19, *25*
        13th week 19, *25*
        first trimester 61, *65*
    head 2
    malformations 204
    ossification 61, *65*
    position
        abdominal ultrasound 4
        third screening 13
    scan planes 4, 7
    skull 61, *65*
    spinal column 61, *65*
fetus papyraceus *201*, 202, 427, *428*
fibrin 473
fibula 132, *134*
fingers 133, *136*
    amputation in amniotic band syndrome 401
    thumb radial aplasia 351, *352*
    see also polydactyly
flecainide fetal therapy 546, *547–548*
folic acid
    neural tube defect prevention 256
    prophylaxis 565
    toxoplasmosis 376
folic acid antagonists 370
foot 132, *134–135*
    biometry 145–146, *158, 159, 600*
    club *338*, 353, *354*
        amniocentesis 533
        3-D ultrasound 518, *525*
        diastrophic dysplasia 348
        Pena–Shokeir syndrome *354*, 355
    deformities *368*, 369

spina bifida 255
growth curves 145, *158*
polydactyly *339*
position anomalies *368*, 369
rocker-bottom 353, *354*
sandal gap *368*
split 351, *352*
toe amputation in amniotic band syndrome
401
foramen ovale 111
    closure 100
Frank Starling law 501, *502*
frontal bossing, thanatophoric dysplasia 342, *345*

G

gain setting 139
gallbladder
    biometry 144, *157, 596*
    embryology 122
    ultrasound anatomy 122, *124*
gallstones *308*, 309
gametopathies 204
gastric filling 169
gastrointestinal tract
    anomalies 297–309
    atresias 297–298, *299*, 300
    disease 195
gastroschisis 303–304, *305–306*
    bladder exstrophy *313*
    body stalk anomaly differential diagnosis 304
    chromosomal abnormalities 371
genetic syndromes/associations/sequences 567–
568
genital tract 129
    anomalies 329–330, *331–332*
        3-D ultrasound 518, *525*
genitalia
    camptomelic syndrome 343
    embryology 129
    external 129
    ultrasound anatomy 129, *130–131*
German Society for Ultrasound in Medicine
(DEGUM) 8
gestation, multiple 2
gestational age
    abdominal circumference *582*
    abdominal sagittal diameter *582*
    amniocentesis 530–531
    assignment 28, *31*
        first trimester 61–62, *66*
        second/third trimesters 161, *162*
    biometrics 139, *579*
    biophysical profile 171
    biparietal diameter 28, *31, 580, 581, 582*
    chorionic cavity diameter 579, *580*
    chorionic sac mean diameter 28
    crown–rump length 27, 28, *31, 580, 581*
    dates
        confirmation 176
        error 175, 176, *179, 180*
        uncertain 177
    determination 9–10
    end-diastolic flow 508
    estimation curves 161, *162*

head circumference *582*
long bone length *583*
occipitofrontal diameter *582*
redating 175
second/third trimesters *602*
skeletal biometry 141
umbilical artery waveform patterns 481, *482*
ventricular–hemispheric ratio 142
yolk sac *579*
gestational edema, proteinuria and hypertension
(GEPH) 176
    intrauterine fetal death 200
gestational sac 60, *63–64*
    diameter 61–62, *66*
    empty 33, *35*
    growth curve 61, *66*
    identification 60
    measurement technique 61, *66*
    multiple pregnancy 418, *419*
    transvaginal scan *460*
    unequal size *421*, 423
    volume 62, *66*
glucocorticoid fetal therapy 545
glucose-6-phosphate dehydrogenase deficiency
191
    nonimmune hydrops 193
glucose tolerance test 178
goiter 247, *250–251*
golfball phenomenon *366*, 367
Goltz syndrome 145
gonads 129
Graves disease 545
great arteries, transposition of
    complete 285, *287–288*
    corrected 285–286, *288*
great vessels
    evaluation 112
    visualization *108, 110*, 112
Gregg syndrome 379–380
growth
    abnormal 11–12
    disproportional 208
    disturbances 175–178, *179–182*, 208
    phases 175
    third ultrasound screening 13
    see also intrauterine growth retardation
growth charts 140
growth curves 140
growth models 140
    long bones 142
Guérin–Stern syndrome 224

H

habituation, fetal 171
half twin peak *420*, 422
halo sign 200, *201*
hand 133, *136*
    deformities *368*, 369
    position anomalies *368*, 369
    split 351, *352*
    see also fingers; polydactyly
Hanhart syndrome 351
harlequin fetus 360, *361*
Hashimoto thyroiditis 545

head
  anomalies 212–241
    3-D ultrasound 518, *524*
  biometry 140–141, 142–143, *151–153, 592–593*
    spina bifida 255, *259, 260*
  camptomelic syndrome 343
  coronal scans 83, *88–89*
  development 18, *24*
  embryology 81–82, *83*
  growth
    discordant 424
    isolated retardation 177, *180, 181*
    low-profile pattern 175, 176, *179, 182*
  neural tube defects 212–214, *214–216*
  osteogenesis imperfecta 343
  sagittal scans 82–83, *86–88*
  second/third trimesters 81–83, *84–89*
  shape 82, *84*
    abnormal 12
  transverse scans 82, *84–86*
  ultrasound anatomy 82–83, *84–89*
  see also biparietal diameter (BPD); dolichocephaly; occipitofrontal diameter (OFD)
head circumference 13, 140, *147, 148*
  abdominal circumference ratio *584*
  biparietal diameter *585–590*
  dwarfism *181*
  gestational age *582*
    estimation 161, *162, 602*
  growth curves 140–141, *148, 591*
  occipitofrontal diameter *585–590*
head/trunk ratio 141, *149*
  IUGR 176
heart
  abdominal ultrasound 106–121
  abnormality differential diagnosis *339*
  activity detection 32
  anatomic forms of structures 107
  anomalies 107, 270–295
    chromosomal abnormalities 370, 380, *384*
    diagnosis 271, *272–273*
    epidemiology 270
    fetal hydrops 381, *383*
    with impaired intracardiac blood flow 278
    infections 382, *384*
    nuchal translucency 364
    position *272*
    prognosis 271, *272*
    rubella 380
    survival rates *272*
    symptoms 271, *272–273*
  atria 107, *110*, 111, 112
  B-mode ultrasound 106, *108–109*
  biometry 113, 143–144, *154–155, 595*
  blood flow 100, *101, 103*
  color Doppler 116, *117*, 118
  contractility 111
  cystic hygroma congenital defect 246
  3-D ultrasound 120, *121, 520*
  detection of embryonic 61, *64*
  development 18, 19, *20, 23, 25*
  dimensions 113
  examination technique 106
  five-chamber plane *110*, 112, *117*, 118
  four-chamber plane 106, 107, *108, 109*, 111, *117*,
  118, *119*

  abnormal 208, *211*
    biometry 143, *154*
  golfball phenomenon *366*, 367
  hemodynamics 491
  imagers 106
  indications for examination 106
  intracardiac waveforms 451, *453*, 462
  location in chest 111
  normal 116, *117*, 118
  output percentage distribution 481, *482*
  prenatal screening 12
  right heart dominance 481
  screening 106
  segmental approach 107, *109–110*, 111–112
  settings 106
  situs inversus 301
  size 111
  systematic analysis of structures 107, *109–110*,
  111–112
  tissue Doppler image *456*
  transducers 106
  tumors 190, 290, *291*
  ultrasound anatomy 97, *98*
  ventricles 107, *110*, 111
    diameters 143
  3-vessel view 118
  see also cardiac *entries;* echocardiography, fetal
heart block, complete congenital 292–293, *295*
heart disease in nonimmune hydrops 190
heart failure
  congestive 501
  diaphragmatic hernia 263
  fetal 12
  maternal digitalization 549
  nonimmune hydrops 189
  twin–twin transfusion syndrome *425*, 426
heart rate
  anemia 501, *502*
  biophysical profile *171*
  documentation 462, *463*
  Doppler spectrum effects *453, 454–455*
  embryonic 18, *23*, 61, *64*
  IUGR 497, *500*
  monitoring 483, *486*
  patterns 169–170, *173*
  placental insufficiency 497, *500*
  reference range 481, *485*
  silent pattern 171, *172, 173*
  sinusoidal pattern 171, *172*
HELLP syndrome 438, *441*
  acidemia *492*
Helsinki Study 9
hemangioma 213
  cervical 247–248, *251*
  hepatic 307, *308*
hematocele, retrouterine 74, *75, 76*
hematoma
  abdominal scar 51
  marginal-sinus 33, *34*
  peritubal 38, *40*, 74, *76*
  retroplacental 33, *34*
  serial scans 33
  subchorionic 33, *34*
hemodynamics, spectral Doppler echocardiography 113, *115*

hemoglobin, twin–twin transfusion syndrome 426
hemoglobinopathies 538
hemolytic disease, fetal hydrops 184–187
hemophilia 538
hepatic veins 100, *102*
hepatoblastoma 307
hepatomegaly 307, *308*
  differential diagnosis 382
hepatosplenomegaly 307
  Down syndrome detection 190
heptadactyly *338*, 353
hereditary disorders
  monogenic 205, 566–567
  sex-linked 129
Herlitz junctional epidermolysis bullosa 360, *361*
hermaphroditism 329, *331*
  3-D ultrasound 518, *525*
herpes zoster 378
heterotaxia syndromes 286, *288*, 289, *291*
  sinus bradycardia 292
hiccups, fetal 169
Hirschsprung disease 298, *299*, 300
hitchhiker thumbs *347*, 348
holoprosencephaly 219–220, *229*
  arachnoid cyst differential diagnosis 221
  arhinia 235, *239*
  chromosomal abnormalities 370
  cleft lip/palate *241*
  hypertelorism 234, *238*
  microcephaly 380
  proboscis 235
Holtermüller–Wiedemann syndrome 224
Holt–Oram syndrome 145
human albumin therapy *see* albumin replacement fetal therapy
β-human chorionic gonadotrophin (β-hCG) 11,
32, 68
  ectopic pregnancy 38
  molar pregnancy 36, *37*
  serum assay 60
    ectopic pregnancy 73, *76*
human chorionic gonadotrophin (hCG) 475
humans, radiosensitivity 206–207
humerus 132, *135*
  length growth curves *591*
  shortening 369
hydatiform mole *see* molar pregnancy
hydranencephaly 219, *228*
hydrocephalus 12, 13, 217–218, *227, 232*
  aqueductal stenosis 218, *228*
  arachnoid cyst differential diagnosis 221
  Arnold–Chiari malformation 222
  communicating 217, 218–219, *228*
  cytomegalovirus 380
  Dandy–Walker malformation 222, *231*
  differential diagnosis 381, *384*
  disproportional growth 208
  external 217
  eye movements 169
  internal 217
  intrauterine shunt procedures 551
  lymphocytic choriomeningitis 379
  macrocephaly 177, *182*
  misdiagnosis 217, *227*
  spina bifida 255, *260*
  ventricular–hemispheric ratio 142

hydronephrosis 13, 321
  bilateral 298, *299, 313*, 549, *552*
    shunt procedures 551, *552*
  chromosomal abnormalities 371
  percutaneous drainage 549, *552*
  unilateral 549, 551
hydrops
  cardiac arrhythmias 501, *502*
  congenital adrenal neuroblastoma 326
  diagnostic algorithm 381, *384*
  Doppler ultrasound 501
  immune 12, 381, *384*
    delivery 187
    diagnosis 185–186
    exchange transfusion 186–187
    hypoxia 184
    postpartum management 187
    rhesus incompatibility 184–187
    ultrasound features 184–185
  intracardiac transfusion *550*
  Klippel–Trenaunay–Weber syndrome 359
  maternal syndrome 193
  nonimmune 12, 188–195, *196–198*
    abdominal disease 192
    albumin replacement *550*
    anemias 191
    associated diseases 189–193
    blood transfusion *550*
    body cavity aspiration 194
    chromosomal abnormalities 190, 364
    cordocentesis 549
    cutaneous edema *195*, 359
    cytomegalovirus 380
    definition 188
    diagnosis 185, 193, *198*
    differential diagnosis 381–382, *383–384*
    fetal therapy 549
    fluid retention 188, *189*
    heart disease 190
    heart failure 189
    hypoalbuminemia 538
    incidence 188
    infections 191
    intrauterine blood transfusion 194
    maternal disorders 193
    myotonic dystrophy 193
    neoplasms 193
    parvovirus B19 375
    pathogenesis 188–189
    pharmacologic therapy 194
    placental conditions 193
    prognosis 193
    pulmonary diseases 192, *196, 197*
    skeletal dysplasias 192
    testicular hydrocele 329, *331*
    thoracic diseases 192, *196, 197*
    treatment 194
    ultrasound features 188
    umbilical cord changes 193
  parvovirus B19 375, 376–377, 381, *383*
  placental 13
  placental chorioangioma *400*, 401
  rhesus incompatibility 503
  sacrococcygeal teratoma 333, *335*
  transposition of the great arteries 286
  twin–twin transfusion syndrome *425*, 426

hydrothorax 192, *196, 197*, 261–262, *265*
  aspiration 194
  needle aspiration 549
  percutaneous drainage 539, *540*, 549, *550*
21-hydroxylase deficiency 330, 545
17-hydroxyprogesterone 330
hygroma, cervical 213
hypertelorism 234, *238*, 339
hypertension, pregnancy-induced 510–511
hyperthyroidism 247
  fetal therapy 545–546
hypoalbuminemia 538
hypochondrogenesis 341, *345*
hypofibrinogenemia 202
hypophosphatasia *338*, 339–340, *345*
hypoplastic left heart syndrome *276*, 277–278, *279*
  pulmonary vein Doppler flow 491, *494*
hypotelorism 234, *238*
hypothyroidism 247, *250–251*
  fetal therapy 546
hypoxemia
  brain-sparing effect 490, *492*
  peripheral vasoconstriction 493
hypoxia, vasopressin levels 493

I

ichthyosis congenita 360, *361*
  fetoscopy 539
ileal atresia 298, *299*
iliac artery
  common 484, *486*
  external 471, *472*
immune deficiencies 538
immunoglobulin M (IgM) antibodies 537
implantation 60, 458, *460*
  bleed 60, *64*
imprinting 568
in-vitro fertilization (IVF) 416
indigo carmine 533
indomethacin 476
  polyhydramnios treatment 555
  therapy response monitoring 491, 493
induction, preterm for rhesus incompatibility 186
infections 375
  congenital 191
  cordocentesis 537–538
  differential diagnosis 381–382, *383–384*
  malformations 206
  sequelae of intrauterine 375
  see also specific organisms and conditions
inferior vena cava 100, *102*
  Doppler flow measurement 114, *115*
  Doppler ultrasound 497, *500*
  streamlining of blood flow 481
inheritance 566–567, *571*
  multifactorial 567, 571
iniencephaly 213, *216*
inspiration 94, *96*
intercostal arteries 102, *104*
intercostal-to-phrenic inhibitory reflex 171
interorbital distance 598
  diameter 143, *152–153*

interstitial pregnancy 38, *42*, 74
intertracheal pressure changes 94
intervillous circulation
  commencement 458–459
  development 458–459, *460, 461*, 465
  maternal 469, *470*
intervillous space 459
intracranial blood vessels 462, *463*
intracranial tumors 223, *232*
intraplacental hematoma 397, *399*
intrauterine brain death syndrome 171, *173*
intrauterine contraceptive device (IUD), pregnancy with 36, *37*
  abdominal ultrasound 68, *70–71*
intrauterine growth retardation (IUGR) 163, 175–177, *179–182*
  brain-sparing effect 490, *492*
  causes 175, 176
  cordocentesis 538
  cytomegalovirus 380
  definition 175
  diagnosis 175, 176
  differential diagnosis 381
  differentiation 176–177
  disproportional 12, 175–176, *180, 182*
    chromosomal abnormalities 364, *365*
    Ellis–van Creveld syndrome *347*, 348
    heterozygous achondroplasia 344
  Doppler ultrasound 473, *477*, 497, *500*, 501
  early and chromosomal abnormalities 364, *365*
  end-diastolic flow, absent /reverse 510–511
  etiology 473, *477*
  eye movements 169
  fetal anomalies 208
  gestational age determination 10
  growth parameters 175
  hyperechoic bowel structure 367
  isolated retardation of growth
    head 177, *180, 181*
    limb 177, *181*
  Mohr syndrome 236
  neuromotor development 509
  oligohydramnios 411
  oxygen therapy 503
  pathogenesis 473, *477*
  placental chorioangioma *400*, 401
  placental insufficiency 497, *500*, 501
  placental maturity 389
  prognosis 175
  proportional 11, 175–176, *179, 182*
  quantification 176–177
  rubella 380
  single umbilical artery 404
  tests 176
  third ultrasound screening 13
  treatment 176
  types 175–176, *179–180, 182*
  urine production 145
  weight estimation 164
intrauterine hematoma *419*, 423
intrauterine pregnancy detection 73, *76*
intrauterine pressure 475
isomerism 284, 286, *288, 289, 291*

J

jaw development 81
jejunal atresia 298, *299*
jet phenomenon *536, 539*
Jeune syndrome 342
    hypophosphatasia differential diagnosis 340
joint contractures
    arthrogryposis multiplex congenita 353, *354*
    diastrophic dysplasia 348
    Pena–Shokeir syndrome 355
    varicella syndrome 375
jugular vein, Doppler velocimetry 490, *492*

K

Kartagener syndrome 301
karyograms *570*
karyotyping
    chromosome disorders 566, *570*
    cordocentesis 537
Kell antigen 184
kidneys
    anomalies 312–326
    biometry 144, *156, 157, 597*
    cystic diseases 315, *316*, 317–318
        Doppler ultrasound 493
    cysts 312, *313*
    development 19, *25*
    diseases 314–315, *316*, 317–318
        nonimmune hydrops 192, *196*
    dysplasia 319
        multicystic 371
    embryology 126, 312, *313*
    growth curves 144, *156*
    migration 126
    multicystic dysplastic *316*, 317–318
    multicystic obstructive 318, *320*
    nonvisualization in Potter syndrome 314
    polycystic in syndromes 318
    size 126
    tumors *324*, 325–326
    ultrasound anatomy 126, *127*
    see also renal *entries*
killing, prohibition against 573–574
Klippel-Feil syndrome 213
Klippel–Trenaunay–Weber syndrome 359, *361*
Kousseff syndrome 237
kyphoscoliosis 304
    diastrophic dysplasia 348

L

labia majora/minora 129, *131*
labor
    induction
        pregnancy dating 10
        preterm for rhesus incompatibility 186
    see also premature labor
lacrimal duct cysts 235, *239*
lambda sign 10, *16, 420, 422, 423*
laryngeal atresia 192, 249, *252*
laryngeal width *96*
larynx 93, *95*

biometry 94, *96*
laser therapy, intrauterine 551, *552*, 554
    arcadius acranius 555
    sacrococcygeal teratoma 554
    twin–twin transfusion syndrome 426–427,
    551, *552*
leg function, impaired in spina bifida 255–256
leiomyoma *see* uterine fibroids
lemon sign *16*, 208, *211*
    Arnold–Chiari malformation 222, *231, 232*
    spina bifida 255
leukemia risk with x-ray pelvimetry 55
levo-transposition of the great arteries (L-TGA)
285–286, *288*
limb buds 132
limbs
    amputation in amniotic band syndrome 401
    chromosomal abnormalities *366, 368*, 369
    defects 349, *350*, 351, *352*, 353, *354*, 355
        chorionic villus sampling 534
        critical periods 565, *569*
        3-D ultrasound 518, *525*
        isolated 349, *350*, 351, *352*, 353
    development 18, *22, 24*
    differentiation 18, *22*
    embryo 61, *64*
    embryology 132, *133*
    hypoplasias in varicella syndrome 375, 378,
    383
    isolated growth retardation 177, *181*
    lower 132, *133–135*
        vessels 102, *104–105*
    malformations
        differential diagnosis *339*
        exogenous agents 336
        Mohr syndrome 236
    ossification centers 61, *65*
    osteogenesis imperfecta 343
    positional abnormalities 353, *354*, 355
    restricted motion 353, *354*, 355
    shortening
        diastrophic dysplasia 348
        Ellis–van Creveld syndrome *347*, 348
        patterns 337, *338*
    ultrasound anatomy 132–133, *134–136*
    upper 132–133, *135–136*
        vessels 102, *104–105*
    see also joint contractures
lipoma, lumbosacral 255, *260*
lips
    integrity 83, *88*
    see also cleft lip/palate
lissencephaly 220, *229*
Listeria monocytogenes 206
liver
    adenoma 307
    autosomal–recessive polycystic kidney disease
    315
    biometry 144, *156, 596*
    biopsy 539
    calcifications 307, *308, 382, 384*
    cysts 307
    disease and nonimmune hydrops 192, 195
    embryology 122
    growth curves 144, *156*
    hemangioma 307, *308*

hemorrhage/hematoma 438, *441*
    intrauterine surgery 554
    mesenchymal hamartoma 307
    tumors 307, *308*
    ultrasound anatomy 122, *124*
lochia retention 443, *445*
lung 97, *99*
    development 261
    diameter *594*
        growth curves 143, *154*
    fluid 261
    maturation induction 545
    maturity 389
    oblique diameter 261
    see also pulmonary *entries*
lymphadenopathy, cervical 248
lymphocytic choriomeningitis 379, 381

M

M-mode ultrasound
    breathing movements 168
    color Doppler 118, *119*
    echocardiography 118, *119*
    embryonic heart activity 61
    eye movements 169
    fetal breathing 97, *99*
    heart biometry 143
    risk assessment 560
maceration, fetal 200, *201*
macrocephaly 177, *182*, 223–224, *232*
    differential diagnosis *339*
    heterozygous achondroplasia 344
    thanatophoric dysplasia 342, *345*
macroglossia 237, *241*
macrosomia 177–178, *181–182*
    causes 177, *178*
    detection 13
    diagnosis 177
    disproportional 177, *182*
    fetal anomalies 208
    maternal diabetes mellitus 177–178, *182*
    neonatal mortality/morbidity 163
    prognosis 177
    proportional 177, *181*
    weight estimation 165
Maffucci syndrome 359
magnesium 476
magnetic resonance imaging (MRI), pelvimetry 56
malnutrition, fetal 176
malrotation anomalies 286
mandible, development 18, *24*
marginal sinus hematoma 397, *398, 399*
maternal age 11, *16*
maternal death, ectopic pregnancy 73
maternal disorders 49–51, *52–54*
    diagnosis 438–439, *439–442*
    nonimmune hydrops 193
maternal plasma volume 409
maxilla 18, *24*
    defect 236, *241*
mechanical index 562
Meckel–Gruber syndrome 213, *215, 216*
    camptodactyly 353
    clinodactyly 353

Meckel–Gruber syndrome 213, *215, 216*
  holoprosencephaly 219
  renal artery resistance index 493
meconium, echogenic 300
meconium ileus 298, 300–301, *302*
meconium peritonitis 195, 298, 301, *302*
  ascites 539, *540*
medical experimentation 575
megacystis *320*, 518
megacystis–microcolon–hypoperistalsis syndrome 321
megaureter 319, *320*
Melnick–Needles syndrome 145
membranous ossification 132
meningocele 254
meningoencephalitis in toxoplasmosis 376
menstrual age 17
meromelia 349, *350*
Merz formula for weight estimation 164, 165
mesencephalon 81
mesomelia 337, *338*
  differential diagnosis *339*
mesonephros 312
metabolic disorders
  fetal therapy 545–546, *547–548*
  nonimmune hydrops 192, 193
metabolic membranes 508
metacarpals 133, *136*
metanephros 312
metencephalon 81
methotrexate, ectopic pregnancy management 38, 41, *42–43*
methyldopa 476
microcephaly 177, *180*, 224–225, *233*
  chondrodysplasia punctata 340
  chromosomal abnormalities 370
  cytomegalovirus 380, 382
  differential diagnosis *339*
  disproportional growth 208
  Meckel–Gruber syndrome *216*
  rubella 380, 382
  skeletal biometry 141
  transient growth 224
β_2-microglobulin 322, *323*
micrognathia 237–238, *241*
  chromosomal abnormalities 370
  differential diagnosis *339*
micromelia 337, *338*
  achondrogenesis 341, *345*
  differential diagnosis *339*
micropenis 329, *331*
microphthalmos 234–235, *239*
microphthalmos–microcephaly syndrome 234
micturition, fetal 129, *131*, 169
midbrain flexure 18
midline echo 82, *83–85*
mirror syndrome 193
miscarriage, recurrent 32
mitral valve 111
Mohr syndrome 236
molar pregnancy 36, *37*, 68, *71–72*
  abdominal ultrasound 68, *71*
  diagnosis 465
  incidence 68, *72*
  invasive 36, *37*, 68, *72*
  partial 68, *71*

monopodia 351, *352*
mortality, perinatal
  multiple pregnancies 416
  prolonged pregnancy 503
mouth
  movements 169
  opening 83, *86*
movement, fetal 168, *169, 173*
  biophysical profile *171*
  fetal anomalies 208
  prenatal screening 12
  see also breathing, movements
müllerian (paramesonephric) duct 129
multiple pregnancy 416–433
  amniocentesis *532, 533*
  amnionicity 416
    assessment in second/third trimester 423
  chorionicity 416, 418
    assessment in second/third trimester 423
  chromosomal abnormalities *421*, 423
  crown–rump length 27
  diagnosis 418, *419*
  Doppler ultrasound 501, *502*
  fetal anomalies 427, *428–429, 430, 431, 432*
  fetal weight estimation 165
  first trimester 418, *419–421, 422–423*
    abnormal *421*, 423
  frequency 416
  growth
    curves *421*, 423
    discordance *421*, 423, *424, 425*
  high-risk 416
  higher-order 418, *419*
  intrauterine fetal death 202
  management 432–433
  nuchal translucency 364, *421*, 423
  second/third trimester
    abnormal *421*, 424, *425, 426–427, 428–429, 430, 431, 432*
    normal *421*, 423
  selective fetocide 575
  sex determination 423
  see also twin pregnancy
multiple pterygium syndrome, fatal 246
multisystem failure 191
mummification 202
mutations, sporadic new 205
myelencephalon 81
myelocele 253, *258*
myelomeningocele 12, *16*, 253, 254, *259–260*
  Arnold–Chiari malformation 222
  3-D ultrasound *524–525*
  detection 208
  fetal movement 208
  iniencephaly differential diagnosis 213
  paralysis 255
myocardial contractility 378
myocardial insufficiency 497
myocardial motion imaging 455, *456*
myometrium 458
  infiltration in trophoblastic disease 465
myotonic dystrophy, nonimmune hydrops 193

N

nasal processes 81
neck
  anomalies 246–249, *250–252*
  biometry 142–143, *151–153, 592–593*
  cysts *48*
  diseases and nonimmune hydrops 192
  embryology 93
  functional impairment 248–249, *251–252*
  malignant tumors 248
  neoplasms 246–248, *250–251*
  pouch sign of upper 297
  ultrasound anatomy 93–94, *95–96*
negative pressure amplitudes 560
neonatal mortality, birth weight 163
neoplasms
  intracranial 223, *232*
  neck 246–248, *250–251*
  nonimmune hydrops 193
nephroma, congenital mesoblastic *324*, 325
nephrosis, congenital (Finnish type) 192, *196*
neural tube defects
  chromosomal abnormalities 370
  diabetes mellitus 178
  head 212–214, *214–216*
  syndromes *567*
neuroblastoma
  cervical 248
  nonimmune hydrops 193
neurocranium 81, *83*
neurology, fetal 171
neuromotor development, absent end-diastolic flow 508–511, *512*
neuron-specific enolase 326
nicotine abuse 511
nifedipine 476
nitric oxide (NO) donors 476
Noonan syndrome
  cystic hygroma 246
  pulmonary stenosis 277
nose 83, *89*
  anomalies 235, *239*, 370
  development 81
  width *592*
notochord 18
nuchal fold
  biometry 142–143, *152*
  thickened 225, *233*
nuchal ligament 246, *250*
nuchal translucency 10–11, *16*, 226
  chromosomal abnormalities 10–11, *16*, 78, 363–364, *365*
    trisomy 45, 78, 82
  detection in first trimester 45, *47, 77*, 78
  measurement 363, *365*
  multiple pregnancy 364, *421*, 423
  thickness 10–11, *16, 77*, 78
    transverse scan 82
    trisomy 21 *211*
  trisomies 363
  unfused amnion and chorion 364

O

obesity, maternal 454
obstetric management, fetal weight 163
occipitofrontal diameter (OFD) 140, *147, 148*
   gestational age *582*
   growth curves 140–141, *148*
   head circumference *585–590*
occipitofrontal midline echo 82, *85*
OEIS (omphalocele, exstrophy, imperforate anus, spinal defects) complex 303, *305*
oligohydramnios 11, *48,* 312, *313,* 410–411, *413*
   amniocentesis 531
   amnioinfusion 555–556
   causes 410–411
   club foot 353
   complications 411
   extremity anomalies 337
   fetal anomalies 207, 411
   fetal movement 208
   fetofetal transfusion syndrome 501
   heart rate pattern 483
   hyperechoic bowel structure 367
   multicystic dysplastic kidneys 318
   obstructive uropathy 319, 322
   Potter sequence 314
   pulmonary hypoplasia 261
   renal artery resistance 493
   sirenomelia 351
   twin–twin transfusion syndrome 426
   umbilical cord coiling 484
omphalocele 13, *267,* 301, *302,* 303, *305*
   body stalk anomaly differential diagnosis 304
   chromosomal abnormalities 371
   3-D ultrasound *525*
   detection 45, *47,* 208
   ruptured 304
omphaloenteric duct *see* vitelline duct
orbit 83, *89*
   anomalies 234–235, *238–239*
   diameter 143, *152–153, 598*
organogenesis 60
   completion 18–19, *23*
organotropism 204–205
ossification 61, *65*
   centers 90, *91, 92*
     femur 132, *134, 135*
     tibia 132, *134*
   3-D ultrasound 518, *526*
   enchondral 132
   membranous 132
   perichondral 132
   vertebrae 90
osteochondrodysplasias 337, *338,* 339–344, *345–347,* 348–349
   classification *336*
   3-D ultrasound *526*
   see also skeletal dysplasias
osteogenesis imperfecta 337, *338*
   hypophosphatasia differential diagnosis 340
   type II 343–344
ovarian cyst 129, 330, *331–332*
   percutaneous procedures 539, *540,* 551, *552*
   see also adnexal mass
ovarian pregnancy 41, *42*
ovarian torsion 330

ovarian tumors *77,* 78
ovum, blighted 33, *35,* 67–68, *70,* 464
   blood flow 459, *460,* 461
oxygen therapy, transmaternal 503, 510
oxytocin stress level 475

P

packed red blood cell transfusion 377
palate development 81
Pallister–Hall syndrome 329
pancreas
   annular 298
   biometry 144, *157*
   embryology 122
parental history 565
parenteral nutrition, fetal growth restoration 176
Parkes–Weber syndrome 359
paroxysmal supraventricular tachycardia 293, *295*
parvovirus B19 infection 191, 193, *195,* 376–377, *383*
   cordocentesis 538
   diagnosis 377
   fetal hydrops 375, 381, *383*
   hepatomegaly 382
   intraperitoneal calcifications 382
   management 377
   prognosis 377
Patau syndrome *see* trisomy 13
pelvic floor, maternal 443
pelvic inlet, transverse diameter 56
pelvimetry 55–56, *58*
pelvis
   abdominal ultrasound 126, *128*
   biometry 144–145, *156–158*
   broadening *366,* 369
   chromosomal abnormalities *366, 368,* 369
   ultrasound anatomy 126, *128*
Pena–Shokeir syndrome *241, 354,* 355
penis 129, *130*
pentalogy of Cantrell 264, *267*
   omphalocele 303
percutaneous procedures in fetus 539, *540,* 549, *550,* 551, *552*
   shunt procedures 551, *552*
pericardial effusion
   chromosomal abnormalities *366,* 367
   Coxsackie infection 378
   nonimmune hydrops *196*
pericardium 111
perichondral ossification 132
peripheral blood vessels 493, *496*
peritoneal cyst 129
periventricular lines 82, *84*
peromelia 336, 349, *350,* 351, *352*
peroneal artery *105*
pes equinovarus *see* foot, club
phalanges 133, *136*
pharyngeal diameter *96*
pharynx 93, *95*
   biometry 94, *96*
   embryology 93
phocomelia 349, *350,* 351
Pierre Robin syndrome
   micrognathia 237

microphthalmos 235
piriform recesses 93, *95*
placenta
   abnormalities 393, *395–396,* 397, *398–400,* 401–402
     structure 12
     thickness 13
   abruption 397, *400,* 401
   accreta 397, *398*
   area 397
   arteriovenous anastomoses 501
   biometry 389, *391*
     abnormal 393, *396,* 397, *398*
   biopsy 534, *535*
   bipartite 393, *395*
   bleeding following amniocentesis 531, *532*
   calcification 389
   chorioangioma 193, *400,* 401
   chromosomal abnormalities 369
   circulation 388
   circumvallate 393, *395*
   cotyledons 388
   decidual plate *390*
   definitive 458
   development 60, 388–389, *390*
   diameter 389
   dichorionic *420,* 422
   early 461
   end-diastolic flow, absent/reverse 510
   fetal anomalies 208, *211*
   fetal part 388
   fused 416
   grades 389, *391–392*
   hematomas 397, *398–399*
     abruption *400,* 401
   increta 397, *398*
   infarction *400,* 401
   intrauterine fetal death 200
   localization 50, *54,* 471, *472*
   location 13, 389, *390*
     abnormalities 393, *395–396*
     cordocentesis 537
   low-lying 393, *395*
   maternal part 388
   maturation 389, *391–392,* 393
   metastases 401
   monochorionic *420,* 422
   morphology 388, *390*
   nonimmune hydrops 193
   pathology 471
   perfusion 393, *394,* 397, *398*
   Po2 levels 459
   polyps 51, *54*
   precreta 397, *398*
   prenatal screening 12–13
   retained 443, *445*
   shape 393, *395*
   small 393, *396*
   structural changes 13
   structure 389, *391–392,* 393
   succenturiate 393, *395*
   teratoma 401
   terminal villi 508
   thick 393, *396*
   thickness 389, *391*
   thin 393, *398*

placenta
  third screening 13
  tripartite 393, *395*
  tumors *400*, 401
  vacuolated 369, 393, *396*
  vascular anastomoses 424, 426
  venous blood exit 469, *470*
placenta previa 13
  central 13
  complete 393, *396*
  low-lying 13
  marginal 13, 393, *395*
  partial 393, *396*
  placental localization 50, *54*
placental hydrops 393, *396*
placental insufficiency 13
  growth discordance 424, *425*
  high-risk pregnancy 507
  hyperechoic bowel structure 367
  IUGR 176, *180*, 497, *500*, 501
  oligohydramnios 411, *413*
placentation
  uterine blood flow changes 461–462, *463*
  uteroplacental circulation 469
placentocentesis, high-risk pregnancy 14
placentomegaly 393, *396*
placentones 389, 393, *394*
plantar artery, medial *105*
platelet count 538
pleural effusion
  hydrothorax 262
  nonimmune hydrops *195*, *196*
  percutaneous drainage 549, *550*
  pulmonary hypoplasia 261
  shunt procedures 551
  thoracentesis 539, *540*
pleuroperitoneal duct closure 263
polycystic kidney disease
  autosomal–dominant *316*, 317
  autosomal–recessive 315, *316*, 317
polydactyly *339*, 351, *352*, 353
  associations 369
  3-D ultrasound 518, *525*
  differential diagnosis *339*
  Ellis–van Creveld syndrome *347*, 348
  heptadactyly *338*, 353
  see also short rib–polydactyly syndrome
polyhydramnios 11, 410, *413*
  anal atresia 300
  arthrogryposis multiplex congenita 353, *354*, 355
  causes 410
  CCAM 262, *266*
  cervical teratoma 247
  chylothorax 262
  decompression amniocentesis *553*, 555
  duodenal atresia 298
  esophageal atresia 248, 297
  fetal anomalies 207, *211*
  fetofetal transfusion syndrome 501
  intrauterine laser treatment 551, 554
  Klippel–Trenaunay–Weber syndrome 359
  macrosomia in maternal diabetes 178
  medical treatment 555
  Pena–Shokeir syndrome 355
  placental chorioangioma *400*, 401
  sacrococcygeal teratoma 333

treatment 410
  twin–twin transfusion syndrome 426
polynomials, high-order 140
polysplenia syndrome *see* isomerism
porencephaly 220, *229*
  arachnoid cyst differential diagnosis 221
portal vein 100, *102*
posterior fossa cyst, chromosomal abnormalities
364, *365*, 367
Potter syndrome 11, 207, 208
  amnioinfusion *540*, 541
  anhydramnios 411, *413*
  classic 314–315, *316*
  oligohydramnios *413*
  type II *316*, 317–318
  type IIA 493
  type IV 318, *320*
power color Doppler 455, *456*
  amplitude analysis 455, *456*
  echocardiography 120, *121*
  ventricular septal defects 281
Prader–Willi syndrome 568
preeclampsia 473–475
  aspirin therapy 474–475
  nonimmune hydrops 193
pregnancy
  complications and nonimmune hydrops 193
  corpus luteum 61, *64*, *65*
  counseling 564
  dating accuracy 10
  detection by abdominal ultrasound 60–61,
  63–64
  early
    abnormalities 10, 32–43
    diagnostic approach 32
    hemodynamic evaluation 458–466
    normal 17–19, *20–25*
    ultrasound parameters 32
  early loss 464–465, *466*
  ectopic 36
  first trimester
    abnormalities 67–68, *69–72*, *73–74*, *75–77*,
    78, *79*
    biometry 61–62, *66*
    crown–rump length 62, *66*
    development 61, *64–65*
    developmental milestones *19*
    gestational age assignment 61–62, *66*
  high-risk
    Doppler ultrasound 507
    IUD in place 36
    surveillance 507
    targeted imaging 14
    vascular surveillance 481, *482*
  hypertensive disorders 476
  interstitial 38, *42*, 74
  intrauterine 73, *76*
  IUD in place 36, *37*, 68, *70–71*
  late and transvaginal ultrasound 2
  nonviable 531
  pain 438–439, *441*
  prolonged 503
  singleton 27, *29*, *31*
  subsequent to intrauterine death 202
  symphyseal distension 439, *442*
  termination

arthrogryposis multiplex congenita 355
  chondrodysplasia punctata 341
  conjoined twins 432
  ethics 573
  fetal indication 574
  omphalocele 303
  Pena–Shokeir syndrome 355
  short rib–polydactyly syndrome 343
  tubal 38, *40*
  ultrasound dating 161, *162*
  see also ectopic pregnancy; multiple pregnancy;
  twin pregnancy
pregnancy-associated plasma protein-A (PAPP-A)
11
pregnant woman, autonomy 572–573
premature labor
  cerebral hemorrhage 491
  intrauterine death of one twin 427
  placental chorioangioma *400*, 401
premature rupture of the membranes 411, *413*
prematurity 163
  duodenal atresia 298
  multiple pregnancies 416
prenatal care
  gestational age estimation 161
  rhesus incompatibility 186–187
  ultrasound screening 8–14, *16*
    examiner proficiency 8
    fetal anomalies 8–9
    first 9–11, *16*
    second 11–13
    third 13–14
    timing 8
prenatal diagnosis, ethics 575
prenatal diagnosis, invasive 530–541
  amniocentesis 530–531, *532*, 533
  amnioinfusion *540*, 541
  chorionic villus sampling *532*, 533–534, *535*
  cordocentesis *535*, 536–539
  counseling 530
  early 533
  fetoscopy 539, *540*, 541
  percutaneous 539, *540*
  placental biopsy 534, *535*
  procedures 530
preterm induction for rhesus incompatibility 186
proboscis 235, *239*
pronephros 312
propranolol *546*
propylthiouracil fetal therapy 546
prostacyclin 490
prostaglandin I$_2$ 473, 474
prostaglandin synthesis inhibitors 190, 193
protein, oral maternal 176
prune belly syndrome 129, 208, 319, *320*
  3-D ultrasound *525*
  prognosis 322
pseudoascites 122, *124*, 194
pseudogestational sac 73–74, *75*
pseudomicrocephaly 224
puerperium
  abdominal ultrasound 443, *444–445*
  complications 443, *445*
  x-ray pelvimetry 55
pulmonary arteries, Doppler flow measurement
114, *115*, 491, *492*, *494*

pulmonary atresia *274*, 275
  pulmonary stenosis differential diagnosis 277
pulmonary diseases, nonimmune hydrops 192, *196*, *197*
pulmonary Doppler ultrasound 94, *96*
pulmonary function test, fetal 94
pulmonary hypoplasia 113, 261, *264*
  CCAM 262
  diaphragmatic hernia 263
  lung measurement 143
  Pena–Shokeir syndrome *354*, 355
  short rib–polydactyly syndrome 343
  thoracometry 143
pulmonary sequestration 263, *266*
  CCAM differential diagnosis 262, *266*
pulmonary stenosis *276*, 277
  tetralogy of Fallot *283*, 284
pulmonary trunk 100, *103*, 107, *110*, 112
  color Doppler 112, *117*
  course *117*, 118
  diameter 144, *155*, 595
  origin *108*, *110*, 112, 118
  vascular caliber 112
pulmonary valve 113
pulmonary valvular stenosis 491
pulmonary veins 111
  Doppler flow measurement 114, *115*, 116, *117*, 491, *494*
pulmonary venous return, total/partial anomalous 289–290, *291*
pulsatility index 114, 448, 449
  cerebral arteries *489*, 490
  descending aorta *487*, 488
  ductus arteriosus 491
  intracranial vessels 462
  renal artery 493, *494*
  trophoblastic disease *465*
  umbilical artery *485*
  uterine waveform 471
pulse repetition frequency 449, 451
pulsed Doppler 449, *450*
  cerebral blood flow 488
  guidelines *562*
  intensity 561
  risk assessment 561
  uterine artery 462
pyelectasis 321
pyrimethamine 376
  fetal therapy 546, *548*

Q

quiescent phases 168

R

rachischisis 253, 255, *259*
  3-D ultrasound *524*
radial alveolar count (RAC) 261
radial artery *104*
radiation embryopathy 206–207
radiation injuries/exposure 207
radius 132–133, *135*
  aplasia 351, *352*

RADIUS study 9
rectal atresia 321
renal agenesis
  bilateral
    anhydramnios *313*
    see also Potter syndrome
  chromosomal abnormalities 371
  renal vessel imaging 493
  unilateral 314, 315
renal aplasia 314–315, *316*
renal artery, Doppler ultrasound 493, *494*, *615*
renal circumference 144
renal diameter 144
renal dysplasia, percutaneous procedures 539, *540*
renal pelvic dilatation, fetal 312, *313*, *320*, 321
  chromosomal abnormalities *366*, 367
renal pelvic dilatation, maternal 438–439, *441*
renal pelvis
  expansion 126, *127*
  obstruction 549, *552*
renal vessels 102, *104*
renal volume, weight estimation 164
resistance index 448–449
  cerebral arteries *489*, 490
  descending aorta *487*, 488
  prolonged pregnancy 503
  renal artery 493, *494*
  trophoblastic disease 465
  umbilical artery 481, *485*
  uterine Doppler ultrasound 471
  uterine waveform 471
respiratory excursions
  fetal *97*, *99*, *453*, 454
  maternal 454
respiratory tract
  embryology 93
  obstruction and nonimmune hydrops 192
retrochorionic hematoma *466*
retrognathia 237–238, *241*
  differential diagnosis 339
retroplacental hematoma 393, 397, *398–399*, *400*
rhabdomyoma 190
  cardiac 290, *291*
rhesus incompatibility 184, 501, *502*, 503
  compensatory mechanisms 184
  delivery 187
  diagnosis 185–186
  exchange transfusion 186–187
  immune fetal hydrops 184–187
  intra-abdominal transfusion 549
  postpartum management 187
  prenatal management 186–187
  prognosis 186
  recurrence risk 186
  transfusion intervals 187
rhesus prophylaxis 186, 208
  amniocentesis 531
  cordocentesis 537
rhizomelia 337, *338*
  differential diagnosis 339
rhombencephalon 18, *22*, *23*
ribs
  length 145, *159*, 599
  ossification defect *526*
  see also short rib–polydactyly syndrome

right to life 573–574
risk assessment 560–561
Roberts syndrome 213
  clitoral hypertrophy 330
  cystic hygroma 246
  tetraphocomelia 351
Routine Antenatal Diagnostic Imaging Ultrasound Study (RADIUS) 9
rubella 379–380
  cordocentesis 537
  embryopathy 382, *384*, 565
  growth retardation 381
  hepatomegaly 382
  intraperitoneal calcifications 382
  microcephaly 380, 382

S

S/D (systole/diastole) ratio 448
sacrococcygeal teratoma 255, *260*, *320*, 333–334, *335*
  Doppler ultrasound 501
  laser treatment 554
  and lipoma 255, *260*
  malignant transformation 334
  surgery 334, *335*, 554
safety indices 561–562
safety of diagnostic ultrasound 560–563
sandal gap 368
scale calibration 139
scanner, real-time 2
scapula 97, *98*
Schillinger formula for weight estimation 165
scoliosis *339*
  3-D ultrasound *526*
scrotum 129, *130*
  edema *196*
Seckel syndrome *180*
  auricular dysplasia 238
semilunar valve 114, *115*
septoaortic continuity 112
sex identification 129
Shepard formula for weight estimation 164
short rib–polydactyly syndrome 145, 192, 342, *346*
  forms 342
  heptadactyly *338*
  humerus *338*
  micropenis 329, *331*
shoulder dystocia 163
shunt procedures 551, *552*
sickle-cell anemia 538
sinus arrhythmias 292
sinus bradycardia 292
sinus tachycardia 293
  fetal therapy 546
sirenomelia 351, *352*
situs inversus 286, *288*, 289, *291*, 301, *302*
Sjögren–Larsson syndrome 360
Sjögren's syndrome 193
skeletal dysplasias 337, *338*, 339–344, *345–347*, 348–349
  classification *336*
  3-D ultrasound 518, *525*
  fatal 337, 339–341

skeletal dysplasias 337, *338*, 339–344, *345–347*, 348–349
  frequency 337, *338*
  intrauterine surgery 555
  nonfatal 344, *347*, 348–349
  nonimmune hydrops 192
  pulmonary hypoplasia 261
  rib length 145
  ultrasound differentiation 337
  vertebral bodies 145
skeleton, biometry *598–600*
skin
  amniotic fluid regulation 409
  anomalies 359–360, *361*
  bullous changes 360, *361*
  disorders 359–360, *361*
  edema 359, *361*
    fetal hydrops *195*, 359
  hereditary disease 539
  hyperechoic focal changes 360, *361*
  hyperkeratotic disorders 360, *361*
  tumors 359, *361*
skull
  cloverleaf 224, *232*, 339
    thanatophoric dysplasia 341, *346*
  deformable *339*
  embryology 81, *83*
  fetal 61, *65*
  frontal bossing in thanatophoric dysplasia 342, *345*
  shape abnormalities 223–225, *232–233*
    differential diagnosis *339*
  strawberry-shaped 225, *233*, 368
  see also superior bones
small bowel loops 144
small for gestational age (SGA) 163
  see also intrauterine growth retardation
Smith–Lemli–Opitz syndrome
  auricular dysplasia 238
  micrognathia 237
sodium, obstructive uropathy levels 322, *323*
Sotos syndrome 177
Spalding's sign 200, *201*
spectral Doppler echocardiography 113–114, *115*, 116
  aliasing 113, 116, *450*, 451
  aortic stenosis 278, *279*
  coarctation of aorta 280
  DORV 285
  hypoplastic left heart syndrome 277, *279*
  pulmonary atresia *274*, 275
  pulmonary stenosis 277
  tetralogy of Fallot 284
  transposition of the great arteries 285, 286, *287*
  tricuspid atresia 273, *274*
  tricuspid dysplasia 275
  truncus arteriosus 286
  ventricular septal defects 281, *282*
spina bifida 253–256, *257–260*
  aperta 253, *258*
  chromosomal abnormalities 370
  club foot association 353
  complete 253
  cystica 253, *259*
  diagnosis 255, *259*, *260*

head growth retardation 177
high 12
intrauterine surgery 554
lemon sign *211*
management 256
occulta 253, *257*
partial 253
prognosis 255–256
spinal column 90, *91–92*
  embryology 90, *91*
  fetal 61, *65*
  ultrasound anatomy 90, *91–92*
spinal cord, unequal growth with spinal column 90, *91*
spine, angulation 200, *201*
  spina bifida 255, *259*
spiral arteries 389, 393, *394*
  after placentation 461
  changes 458
  intrauterine growth retardation 473
  opening 458
  trophoblast invasion 462
  trophoblastic plugs 461
  waveform changes 462
spiramycin 376
  fetal therapy 546, *548*
spleen
  biometry 144, *156*, *157*, 596
  embryology 122
  growth curves 144, *156*
  ultrasound anatomy 122, *124*
splenomegaly 144, 307
  see also hepatosplenomegaly
startles 168, *169*
STIC (spatial–temporal image correlation) technique 519, 520, *527*
stomach
  biometry 144, *157*
  development 19, *25*
  growth curves 144
  situs inversus 301, *302*
  small 297
  ultrasound anatomy 122, *124*
stroke volume 143
stuck twin *425*, 426, 501
subamniotic hematoma 397, *399*
subchorionic cystic space 389, *392*
subchorionic hematoma 464, *466*
sucking movements 169
sulfadiazine 376
sulfamethoxydiazine fetal therapy 546, *548*
superior vena cava 112
  persistent left 112, 290, *291*
supraventricular extrasystoles *453*, 455, 501, *502*
supraventricular tachycardia 501, *502*
  fetal therapy 546, *548*, *550*
  paroxysmal 293, *295*
surgery, fetal *553*, 554–555
swallowing 94
  amniotic fluid regulation 409
  esophageal atresia 248
  movements 169
symmelia 351, *352*
symphyseal distension, maternal 439, *442*
sympodia 351
syndactyly *339*, 353, *354*

synophthalmia 235, *239*
syphilis 379
  hepatomegaly 382
  intraperitoneal calcifications 382
  nonimmune hydrops 191
systemic lupus erythematosus (SLE)
  complete congenital heart block 293
  nonimmune hydrops 193
systolic blood flow, ductus arteriosus 491

T

T sign *420*, 422
tachyarrhythmias 293, *295*
  fetal therapy 546, *547–548*
  management *294*
  nonimmune hydrops 190, 193, *197*
telencephalon 18, *22*, *23*
  development 18, *24*
  embryology 81
teratogenic insult 204
teratogens 206
  exencephaly 212
teratologic determination period 204
teratomas
  cardiac 290, *291*
  cephalocele differential diagnosis 213
  cervical 247, *251*
  classification 333
  congenital 237
  etiology 333
  intrathoracic 262
  malignant transformation 333
  nonhomogenous echo structure 333, *335*
  nonimmune hydrops 193
  pathogenesis 333
  placental 401
  umbilical cord 405
  see also sacrococcygeal teratoma
testes 129, *130*
testicular hydrocele 329, *331*
tetralogy of Fallot *283*, 284
  extreme 275
  rubella 382
tetrasomy 9, partial *240*
α-thalassemia 191
β-thalassemia 538
thalidomide 336
  embryopathy 349, 565
  exposure timing 565, *569*
thanatophoric dysplasia 224, 337, 341, *345–346*
  frontal bossing *338*
theca lutein cysts 68
thermal index 561–562
thoracentesis 539, *540*
thoracic anomalies 261–264, *265–267*
  hypoplasia 343
thoracic circumference, bony *594*
thoracic diameter
  sagittal 261, *594*
  transverse 261
    bony *594*
thoracic diseases, nonimmune hydrops 192, *196*, *197*
thoracoamniotic shunt 262, 551

thoracocentesis, before delivery 262
thoracometry 143, *154*
thoracopagus 45, *47, 429, 431*
thorax 97, *98–99*
  biometry 143–144, *154–155, 594–595*
  chromosomal abnormalities 370–371
  growth curves 143, *154*
  narrow *338, 344, 346*
    Ellis–van Creveld syndrome *347*, 348
    Pena–Shokeir syndrome *354, 355*
thrombocytopenias 538, 548–549
thromboxane A₂ 473, 474, 490
thumb, radial aplasia 351, *352*
thyroglossal duct cyst 248
thyroid gland biometry 143, *153, 593*
thyroiditis, autoimmune maternal 545
L-thyroxine fetal therapy 546
tibia 132, *134*
  fracture *338*
  ossification centers 132, *134*
tibial artery *105*
  vascular resistance 493, *496*
tidal volumes 94
tissue Doppler echocardiography 455, *456*
tissue heating 560, *561–562*
  pulsed Doppler 561
tocolytic therapy 190, 193
toes, amputation in amniotic band syndrome 401
tone, fetal *171*
tongue 83, *86*
tooth buds 82
TORCH infections 301, 375
  hepatic calcifications 307
  intrauterine fetal death 381
toxoplasmosis 376
  cordocentesis 537–538
  fetal therapy 546, *548*
  hepatomegaly 382
  intraperitoneal calcifications 382
  malformations 206
  nonimmune hydrops 191
  ventriculomegaly *384*
trachea 93, *95*
  biometry 94, *96*
  diameter *96*
  embryology 93
tracheal cartilages 93, *95*
transducers, heart imaging 106
transplacental therapy, intrauterine 376
transvaginal fetal echocardiography 462
transvaginal pelvimetry 55–56, *58*
transvaginal ultrasound 2–3, *5*
  applications 2
  color Doppler 458
  3-D ultrasound 45–46, 516–519
  early pregnancy abnormalities 32
  echocardiography 118, *119*, 120
  examination 3
  fetal anomalies 45–46, *47–48*
  first trimester 2
  image orientation 3, *5*
  maternal disorders 49–51, *52–54*
  pelvimetry 55–56, *58*
  scan planes *5*
  scanning sequence 3
  technique 17

transducer 3, *5*
  uteroplacental vessels 471
transverse lie
  dorsoinferior 4
  dorsosuperior 4, 7
TRAP sequence 192, *428*, 430
Treacher–Collins syndrome
  auricular dysplasia 238
  micrognathia 237
  microphthalmos 234
Treponema pallidum 206, 379
tricuspid valve 111
  atresia 273, *274*, 275
  dysplasia *274*, 275, *276*, 277
  incompetency 501
  insufficiency *273*
triple test 10
triploidy 12
  chromosomal abnormalities 371
  early growth retardation 364
  nuchal translucency 45
  placenta abnormality *211*
    vacuolation 369
  posterior fossa cyst *365*
  proportional IUGR 176
  spina bifida 370
  suggestive signs *372*
trisomy
  anembryonic abortion 33
  nuchal translucency 45, 78, 82, 363
trisomy 13
  cisterna magna widening 142
  corpus callosum agenesis 370
  early growth retardation 364
  holoprosencephaly 219, 370
  microcephaly 370
  microphthalmos *235, 239*
  nonimmune hydrops 190
  posterior fossa cyst 364
  proportional IUGR 176
  renal anomalies 318
  renal pelvic dilatation *313*
  spina bifida 370
  suggestive signs *372*
trisomy 18
  auricular dysplasia 238, *241*
  camptodactyly 353
  cisterna magna widening 142
  cleft lip/palate *240*
  clinodactyly *354*
  clitoral hypertrophy 330
  club foot association 353
  corpus callosum agenesis 370
  early growth retardation 364
  esophageal atresia 297
  holoprosencephaly 370
  micrognathia 237, *241*
  nonimmune hydrops 190
  nuchal translucency 363
  phenotypic expression *368*, 371, *372*
  posterior fossa cyst 364
  proportional IUGR 176, *182*
  renal anomalies 318
  rocker-bottom foot 353, *354*
  spina bifida 255, 370
  suggestive signs *372*

trisomy 21 *211*, 371
  fetal hydrops 364
  golfball phenomenon 367
  hand deformities *368*
  Hirschsprung disease 300
  hyperechoic bowel 300, *302*
  macroglossia 237, *241*
  nonimmune hydrops 190, *195*
  nuchal fold
    size 142
    thickening 225, *233*
  nuchal translucency 45, 363
  pelvis broadening *366*, 369
  pericardial effusion *366*, 367
  phenotypic expression 371, *372*
  proportional IUGR 176
  renal pelvic dilatation 367
  sandal gap *368*
  twin pregnancy 427, 430
  unfused amniotic bands *400*
trophoblast invasion, impaired 473, *477*
trophoblastic cells 458
trophoblastic diseases 465, *466*
trophoblastic layers 533
trophoblastic plugs 459, 461
truncus arteriosus 286, *288*
trunk
  camptomelic syndrome 343
  development 18–19, *24*
tubal pregnancy 38, *40*
  see also fallopian tube
Turner syndrome
  cystic hygroma 246, 364, *365*
  fetal hydrops 364
  hydrothorax *265*
  nonimmune hydrops 190
  nuchal translucency 363
  suggestive signs *372*
twin pregnancy
  amniocentesis *532*, 533
  amnionicity 416, *417*, 423, *424*
  autosite 432
  chorionicity 416, *417*, 418, 423, *424*
  conjoined 418, *429*, 430, *431*, 432
  detection 10, *16*
  dichorionic diamniotic 418, *420*, 422, 432
  dizygotic 416, *417*, 422–423, 427, *428*, 430
  dye instillation 533
  false-positive diagnosis 418, *419*, 422
  fetal anomalies 427, *428–429*, 430, *431*, 432
  fetofetal vascular anastomoses *417*, 418
  frequency 416
  genetic predisposition 416
  growth discordance 13, 423, 424, *425*
  intrauterine fetal death 202
    one twin *201*, 202, 427
  management 432–433
  maternal age 416
  monochorionic 418, *420–421*, 422, 423, 427
    diamniotic 432–433
  monochorionicity 426
  monozygotic 416, *417*, 418, 422–423, *428–429*, 430, *431*, 432
  nonimmune hydrops 192
  parasitic *428*, 430, 432, *432*

twin pregnancy
  rate 416
  zygosity *424*
twins
  birth weight *612*
  blighted 423
  conjoined 45, *47*
  dead second *201*
  stuck *425*, 426, 501
  vanishing 416
twin–twin transfusion syndrome 416, *417*, 418,
423, 424, *425*, 426–427
  abdominal ultrasound 190, 191, 192, *195*
  diagnosis 426, *428*
  donor twin 426
  fetal circulation 501, *502*
  fetoscopy 539
  growth discordance 424, 426
  intrauterine death of one twin *201*, 427
  laser treatment 551, *552*
  monochorionicity 426
  nuchal translucency 364
  recipient twin 426
  serial amniocentesis 555
  TRAP sequence *428*, 430
  treatment 426–427

U

ulna 132–133, *135*
ulnar artery *104*
umbilical arteries 100, 102, *105*, 404, *406*
  cerebroplacental ratio 490
  color Doppler *482*
  cordocentesis 537
  diameter *601*
  Doppler ultrasound 481, *482*, 483–484, *613*
  Doppler velocimetry 483, *485*, *486*
  embryo 462, *463*
  end-diastolic flow *485*, 501
    abnormal 483, *485–486*
    absent 507, 508–511, *512*
    reference range *485*
    reverse 507, 508–511, *512*
  single 304, 404–405, *407*, 484, *486*
    chromosomal abnormalities *368*, 369, 404
    compensatory dilatation 484
    diagnosis 208, *211*
  waveform patterns
    abnormalities 483, *485–486*
    gestational age 481, *482*
umbilical cord
  abnormalities 404–405, *407–408*
  absent 304, *306*
  anatomy 404, *406*
  biometry 404, *407*, 601
  chromosomal abnormalities *368*, 369
  coiling 405, *408*, 484
  compression 483, *486*
  cysts *368*, 369, 405, *408*
  hemangioma 405
  hematoma 405, *408*
  insertion 19, *25*, 122, *125*
    variations 405, *408*
  knotting 405, *408*

looping 202, 213, *215*
nonimmune hydrops 193
occlusion 554
packed red blood cell transfusion 377
physiology 404
prenatal screening 12
short 304
teratoma 405
tumors 405
twin–twin transfusion syndrome *425*, 426
umbilical artery Doppler spectrum 481, 483
vasa previa 405
umbilical hernia 301, *302*, 303, *305*
umbilical hernia, physiologic 10, 18–19, *22–23*, *24*
  detection 27, 61, *64*
  embryology 122, *123*
  omphalocele differential diagnosis *302*, 303
umbilical vein 100, *101*, *102*, 404, *406*
  color Doppler *482*
  cordocentesis *535*, 537
  diameter *601*
  Doppler ultrasound 495, *496*, 497, *498*, *500*
  persistent right 405, *407*
  thrombosis 405
umbilicocerebral ratio *615*
urachal cyst 319, 321
ureter
  dilated 321
  subpelvic obstruction 319
ureteral bud 312, *313*
ureterocele 319
urethra, obstruction 319
urethral valve *320*
urinalysis
  obstructive uropathy 322, *323*, 539
  renal dysplasia 539
urinary ascites 192, 194, *195*, *196*
urinary bladder, fetal
  biometry 144–145, *158*
  development 19, *24*, *25*
  dilated 321
  embryology 126, 319
  emptying 145
  exstrophy 312, *313*, 321
  nonvisualization in Potter syndrome 314
  ultrasound anatomy 126, *127–128*
  volume 145, *158*
urinary bladder dysfunction, maternal 443
urinary tract
  abdominal ultrasound 126, *127–128*
  anomalies 312–326
    obstructive 319, *320*, 321–322, *323–324*, 325
  outflow obstruction 319
urine
  fetal production 409
    twin–twin transfusion syndrome 426
  hourly production rate 145
  production 169
urogenital system
  biometrics *597*
  chromosomal abnormalities 371
uropathy, obstructive 319, *320*, 321–322, *323–
324*, 325
  management 322, *324*
  percutaneous drainage 549, *552*
  percutaneous procedures 539, *540*

prenatal management 322
shunt procedures 551, *552*
uterine artery, maternal
  Doppler ultrasound 469, *470*, 471, 476, *477*, *613*
    screening 476
  end-diastolic blood flow velocity 475, 477
  pulsed Doppler 462
  waveform
    maternal serum AFP levels 475
    medication effects 475–476
    uterine contractions 475, *477*
uterine fibroids, maternal 49, *52*
  detection in early pregnancy 77, 78, *79*
uteroplacental circulation 458, 459, *460*, 461,
469–477
  abnormal waveforms *471*
  development 469, *470*
  Doppler ultrasound 469, *470*, 471
  exchange processes 469, *470*
  transvaginal ultrasound 471
uterus, maternal
  angulation 443, *444*
  anomalies
    placenta location 393, *396*
    twin pregnancy mimicking 418, *419*
  bicornuate 38, *42*
  bleeding 2
  blood flow changes after placentation
  461–462, *463*
  contractions 475, *477*
    local 78, *79*
  Doppler ultrasound clinical significance 471,
  473–476, *477*
  involution 443, *444*
  leiomyoma 438, *440*
  length 443, *444*
  malignant tumors 49, *52*
  mass diagnosis 49, *52*
  postpartum 50–51, *54*
  retroflexed 2
  rupture 38, *42*
    risk with cervical implantation 60
  third screening 14
  wall vascularity 393, *394*

V

VACTERL syndrome 297, *299*, 300
  sirenomelia 351, *352*
vaginal bleeding, maternal 32, *33*
  placenta previa investigation 50
vaginal transducers 2, 3
valproic acid 212
value system 572
vanishing twin 416
varicella syndrome 375, 378, *383*
  diagnosis 378
  growth retardation 381
  hepatomegaly 382
  intraperitoneal calcifications 382
vasopressin 493
vein of Galen aneurysm 221, *230*, 456, *492*
  arachnoid cyst differential diagnosis 221
  Doppler ultrasound 501
vein of Galen malformation 491, *492*

velocity calibration 139
venous Doppler 501
ventricle
  diameter *595*
  output 481
  right
    right ventricular outflow tract (RVOT) obstruction 275
    ventricular hypertrophy *283,* 284
    ventricular output 481
  see also atrioventricular *entries;* cerebral ventricles; double-outlet right ventricle (DORV)
ventricular septal defects (VSD) 112, 280–281, *282*
  aortic arch anomalies 278
  DORV 285
  rubella 382
  tetralogy of Fallot *283,* 284
  tricuspid atresia 273, *274*
ventricular septum *109,* 111
ventriculoarterial concordance 107, 112
ventriculocoronary fistula 275
verapamil 546, *547*
vernix caseosa 409, *411*
vertebrae, ossification 90
vertebral arch 90, *92*
vertebral body 90, *92*
  biometry 145, *158, 159, 599*
  deficient ossification *339*
vesicoamniotic shunts 322, *324*
vesicocutaneous fistula 321
vesicourethral reflux 319
viral infections
  meconium ileus differential diagnosis 300
  proportional IUGR 176
visceroatrial situs 107
viscerocranium 81
vitelline duct 26
  blood flow *460,* 461
von Willebrand–Jürgens syndrome 538

W

Weaver syndrome 177
weight, fetal
  estimation 163–165, *166, 603–610*
    formulas 164
  low-weight infants 164, *610*
  normal-weight infants 164
  phases of gain 163
Wiedemann–Beckwith syndrome 177
Wilms tumor *324,* 325
wolffian (mesonephric) duct 129

Y

yawning, fetal 83, *86*
yolk sac 19, *24,* 26–27, *29*
  abnormal 33, *34*
  biometry *579*
  blood flow *460,* 461, *463*
  detection 26, 61, *64, 65*
  gestational age *579*
  growth pattern 26, *30*
  separation 18, *20–21*
  size/shape discrepancies 26–27

WITHDRAWN

WITHDRAWN

WITHDRAWN